Challenges and Opportunities for Effective Cancer Immunotherapies

Challenges and Opportunities for Effective Cancer Immunotherapies

Editors

Michael Kershaw
Clare Slaney

MDPI • Basel • Beijing • Wuhan • Barcelona • Belgrade • Manchester • Tokyo • Cluj • Tianjin

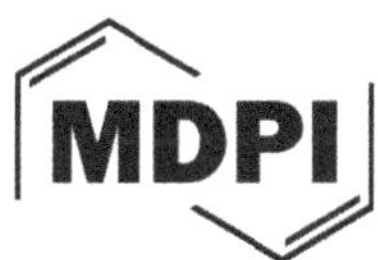

Editors
Michael Kershaw
Peter MacCallum Cancer
Centre
Australia

Clare Slaney
Peter MacCallum Cancer
Centre
Australia

Editorial Office
MDPI
St. Alban-Anlage 66
4052 Basel, Switzerland

This is a reprint of articles from the Special Issue published online in the open access journal *Cancers* (ISSN 2072-6694) (available at: https://www.mdpi.com/journal/cancers/special_issues/ Challenges_Opportunities_Immunotherapies).

For citation purposes, cite each article independently as indicated on the article page online and as indicated below:

LastName, A.A.; LastName, B.B.; LastName, C.C. Article Title. *Journal Name* **Year**, *Volume Number*, Page Range.

ISBN 978-3-0365-6960-4 (Hbk)
ISBN 978-3-0365-6961-1 (PDF)

Contents

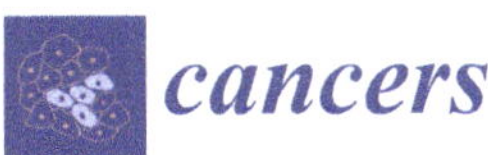 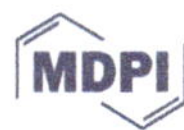

Editorial

Insights into Cancer Immunotherapies: Recent Breakthroughs, Opportunities, and Challenges

Evan G. Pappas [1,2], Michael H. Kershaw [1,2] and Clare Y. Slaney [1,2,*]

1   Cancer Immunology Program, Peter MacCallum Cancer Centre, Melbourne, VIC 3000, Australia
2   Sir Peter MacCallum Department of Oncology, University of Melbourne, Parkville, VIC 3010, Australia
*   Correspondence: clare.slaney@petermac.org

Citation: Pappas, E.G.; Kershaw, M.H.; Slaney, C.Y. Insights into Cancer Immunotherapies: Recent Breakthroughs, Opportunities, and Challenges. *Cancers* **2023**, *15*, 1322. https://doi.org/10.3390/cancers15041322

Received: 1 February 2023
Accepted: 14 February 2023
Published: 19 February 2023

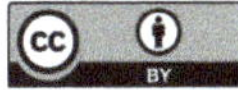

This Special Issue reminds us that, although incredible developments have occurred in the field of cancer immunotherapy, there is still plenty of room for improvement. Although many otherwise untreatable patients have benefited from novel therapies, we still do not completely understand why some patients respond while others do not. Here, experts in the field summarize recent breakthroughs, but they also examine the challenges and opportunities in improving current therapies. These discussions are increasingly important because cancer immunotherapy has become a focal point in the race toward a cure.

Many manuscripts from this Special Issue focus on improving and better understanding current immunotherapies. For example, Lau and colleagues lay the groundwork for enhancing the clinical efficacy of adoptive cell transfers [1], and others identify novel antigens [2]. An innovative approach by Jazowiecka-Rakus and collaborators boosted the effectiveness of oncolytic viruses [3], while Ponath et al. redeployed histone deacetylase inhibitors to improve natural killer cell immunotherapy [4]. Such advancements rely on understanding existing therapies to identify suitable opportunities. This is exemplified by the work of Wu et al., who revealed avenues for improving chimeric antigen receptor (CAR) T cells by elucidating how they differ from conventional T cells [5]. In addition to iterative improvements, Maruoka and colleagues also embraced new technologies by leveraging recently developed photoimmunotherapy [6]. Together, these studies pave the way for future clinical advancement.

Once a treatment completes clinical trials, it must continue to be scrutinized for efficacy and safety. Notably, Choi and colleagues studied an immune checkpoint inhibitor (ICI) that may be less effective than previously reported [7]. They demonstrated the importance of retrospectively studying real-life clinical experiences beyond trials. An opinion piece featured here also discusses current knowledge in the field of ICIs and how they can be leveraged to improve clinical outcomes for patients with HER2-positive breast cancer [8]. These articles promote the idea that the bench-to-bedside process is indeed circular and not linear.

In recent years, a wealth of knowledge has been generated and many of the included reviews focus on the key cellular players underpinning tumor immunology and the cytokines that control them. Examples include the importance of understanding metabolism in CAR T cells [9] and not minimizing the physical properties of the CARs and their direct impact on clinical outcomes [10]. Similarly, the use of CARs in a variety of other cell types beyond T cells is reviewed [11], reminding us that the pursuit of innovation is within reach. While cells play a central role in immunotherapies, we must not underestimate the complex contribution of the cytokines that influence them. For example, the interleukin 12 family of cytokines, and their roles in both improving and suppressing immune responses, are discussed in depth [12]. Similarly, a pleiotropic cytokine, tumor necrosis factor alpha, is also implicated in many processes that can promote or hinder effective anti-cancer responses [13]. Such reviews help demystify complicated cellular interactions, in turn informing better future therapies.

The potential of non-T cells in immunotherapy is increasingly appreciated, including natural killer cells [14] and dendritic cells [14]. The success of these strategies relies on the immune recognition of cancer cells. It is imperative that we better understand the mechanisms involved in the frequent failure to recognize tumor antigens [15] and the evasion of immune responses [16].

Emerging strategies to modulate the immune system are also dissected in this issue. For instance, the use of nonreplicating adenovirus for gene therapy is explored [17], while another manuscript addressed the opportunity of targeting dynamic kinases expressed on both immune and tumor cells [18]. New immunotherapies can be associated with toxicity and, thus, clinical tolerance was discussed in some reports included in this issue. For example, the use of pattern recognition receptors (PRR) to improve immune responses must be balanced against potential harm and side effects. Some intratumorally administered PRR agonists have recently been investigated, and they possess more favorable safety profiles [19]. Complications have also been reported with the use of other immunotherapies, such as anti-CD3-bispecific antibodies [20]. Reviewed by Middelburg et al., anti-CD3-bispecific antibody therapies, like CAR T cells, are therapeutically effective in hematological cancers, but they fail to treat solid tumors [21]. Hurdles include the immunosuppressive tumor microenvironment and the difficulty for T cells to infiltrate the tumors [22]. Another innovative strategy involves the use of nanoparticles and, more recently, combining them with immunotherapies [23].

Glioblastoma, an aggressive tumor of the brain, is characterized by poor clinical outcomes. Many animal studies failed to capture key human disease features, and the results were not successfully translated clinically. One article from this issue discusses the complexity of conducting and interpreting clinical trials featuring immunotherapies for glioblastomas [24], while another article focuses on key limitations in the animal models informing these trials [25].

Overall, the field of cancer immunotherapy represents an exciting breakthrough. Improved understanding has resulted in novel therapeutics, which have, in turn, been optimized. Despite such impressive advancements, many patients either lack access to or fail to benefit from treatment. Future work must improve accessibility, as well as stratify patients to better address their individual needs. This will allow a golden age of personalized immunotherapy in oncology.

Funding: National Health and Medical Research Council (NHMRC) of Australia, the National Breast Cancer Foundation (NBCF) of Australia, mRNA Victoria, and the Peter Mac Foundation.

Acknowledgments: We are grateful for the contributing authors and institutions for their work contributing to this Special Issue and the support for the *Cancers* editorial office.

Conflicts of Interest: The authors declare no conflict of interest.

References

1. Lau, P.K.H.; Cullinane, C.; Jackson, S.; Walker, R.; Smith, L.K.; Slater, A.; Kirby, L.; Patel, R.P.; von Scheidt, B.; Slaney, C.Y.; et al. Enhancing Adoptive Cell Transfer with Combination BRAF-MEK and CDK4/6 Inhibitors in Melanoma. *Cancers* **2021**, *13*, 6342. [CrossRef]
2. Duarte, J.D.G.; Woods, K.; Quigley, L.; Deceneux, C.; Tutuka, C.; Witkowski, T.; Ostrouska, S.; Hudson, C.; Tsao, S.; Pasam, A.; et al. Ropporin-1 and 1B Are Widely Expressed in Human Melanoma and Evoke Strong Humoral Immune Responses. *Cancers* **2021**, *13*, 1805. [CrossRef]
3. Jazowiecka-Rakus, J.; Hadrys, A.; Rahman, M.; McFadden, G.; Fidyk, W.; Chmielik, E.; Pazdzior, M.; Grajek, M.; Kozik, V.; Sochanik, A. Myxoma Virus Expressing LIGHT (TNFSF14) Pre-Loaded into Adipose-Derived Mesenchymal Stem Cells Is Effective Treatment for Murine Pancreatic Adenocarcinoma. *Cancers* **2021**, *13*, 1394. [CrossRef]
4. Ponath, V.; Frech, M.; Bittermann, M.; Al Khayer, R.; Neubauer, A.; Brendel, C.; Von Strandmann, E.P. The Oncoprotein SKI Acts as A Suppressor of NK Cell-Mediated Immunosurveillance in PDAC. *Cancers* **2020**, *12*, 2857. [CrossRef]
5. Wu, L.; Brzostek, J.; Sankaran, S.; Wei, Q.; Yap, J.; Tan, T.; Lai, J.; MacAry, P.; Gascoigne, N. Targeting CAR to the Peptide-MHC Complex Reveals Distinct Signaling Compared to That of TCR in a Jurkat T Cell Model. *Cancers* **2021**, *13*, 867. [CrossRef]

6. Maruoka, Y.; Furusawa, A.; Okada, R.; Inagaki, F.; Wakiyama, H.; Kato, T.; Nagaya, T.; Choyke, P.L.; Kobayashi, H. Interleukin-15 after Near-Infrared Photoimmunotherapy (NIR-PIT) Enhances T Cell Response against Syngeneic Mouse Tumors. *Cancers* **2020**, *12*, 2575. [CrossRef]

7. Choi, M.; Kim, Y.-M.; Lee, J.-W.; Lee, Y.; Suh, D.; Lee, S.; Lee, T.; Lee, M.; Park, D.; Kim, M.; et al. Real-World Experience of Pembrolizumab Monotherapy in Patients with Recurrent or Persistent Cervical Cancer: A Korean Multi-Center Retrospective Study (KGOG1041). *Cancers* **2020**, *12*, 3188. [CrossRef]

8. Solinas, C.; Fumagalli, D.; Dieci, M. Immune Checkpoint Blockade in HER2-Positive Breast Cancer: What Role in Early Disease Setting? *Cancers* **2021**, *13*, 1655. [CrossRef]

9. Rad SM, A.R.S.; Halpin, J.; Mollaei, M.; Bell, S.S.; Hirankarn, N.; McLellan, A.D. Metabolic and Mitochondrial Functioning in Chimeric Antigen Receptor (CAR)—T Cells. *Cancers* **2021**, *13*, 1229. [CrossRef]

10. Davey, A.S.; Call, M.E.; Call, M.J. The Influence of Chimeric Antigen Receptor Structural Domains on Clinical Outcomes and Associated Toxicities. *Cancers* **2020**, *13*, 38. [CrossRef]

11. Qin, V.M.; D'Souza, C.; Neeson, P.J.; Zhu, J.J. Chimeric Antigen Receptor beyond CAR-T Cells. *Cancers* **2021**, *13*, 404. [CrossRef]

12. Mirlekar, B.; Pylayeva-Gupta, Y. IL-12 Family Cytokines in Cancer and Immunotherapy. *Cancers* **2021**, *13*, 167. [CrossRef]

13. Mercogliano, M.; Bruni, S.; Mauro, F.; Elizalde, P.; Schillaci, R. Harnessing Tumor Necrosis Factor Alpha to Achieve Effective Cancer Immunotherapy. *Cancers* **2021**, *13*, 564. [CrossRef]

14. Toffoli, E.; Sheikhi, A.; Höppner, Y.; de Kok, P.; Yazdanpanah-Samani, M.; Spanholtz, J.; Verheul, H.; van der Vliet, H.; de Gruijl, T. Natural Killer Cells and Anti-Cancer Therapies: Reciprocal Effects on Immune Function and Therapeutic Response. *Cancers* **2021**, *13*, 711. [CrossRef]

15. Apavaloaei, A.; Hardy, M.-P.; Thibault, P.; Perreault, C. The Origin and Immune Recognition of Tumor-Specific Antigens. *Cancers* **2020**, *12*, 2607. [CrossRef]

16. Baugh, R.; Khalique, H.; Seymour, L.W. Convergent Evolution by Cancer and Viruses in Evading the NKG2D Immune Response. *Cancers* **2020**, *12*, 3827. [CrossRef]

17. Tessarollo, N.; Domingues, A.; Antunes, F.; Luz, J.; Rodrigues, O.; Cerqueira, O.; Strauss, B. Nonreplicating Adenoviral Vectors: Improving Tropism and Delivery of Cancer Gene Therapy. *Cancers* **2021**, *13*, 1863. [CrossRef]

18. Aehnlich, P.; Powell, R.; Peeters, M.; Rahbech, A.; Straten, P.T. TAM Receptor Inhibition–Implications for Cancer and the Immune System. *Cancers* **2021**, *13*, 1195. [CrossRef]

19. Burn, O.; Prasit, K.; Hermans, I. Modulating the Tumour Microenvironment by Intratumoural Injection of Pattern Recognition Receptor Agonists. *Cancers* **2020**, *12*, 3824. [CrossRef]

20. Middelburg, J.; Kemper, K.; Engelberts, P.; Labrijn, A.; Schuurman, J.; van Hall, T. Overcoming Challenges for CD3-Bispecific Antibody Therapy in Solid Tumors. *Cancers* **2021**, *13*, 287. [CrossRef]

21. Slaney, C.Y.; Wang, P.; Darcy, P.K.; Kershaw, M.H. CARs versus BiTEs: A Comparison between T Cell–Redirection Strategies for Cancer Treatment. *Cancer Discov.* **2018**, *8*, 924–934. [CrossRef]

22. Slaney, C.Y.; Kershaw, M.H.; Darcy, P.K. Trafficking of T Cells into Tumors. *Cancer Res.* **2014**, *74*, 7168–7174. [CrossRef]

23. Gong, P.; Wang, Y.; Zhang, P.; Yang, Z.; Deng, W.; Sun, Z.; Yang, M.; Li, X.; Ma, G.; Deng, G.; et al. Immunocyte Membrane-Coated Nanoparticles for Cancer Immunotherapy. *Cancers* **2020**, *13*, 77. [CrossRef]

24. Van Gool, S.; Makalowski, J.; Fiore, S.; Sprenger, T.; Prix, L.; Schirrmacher, V.; Stuecker, W. Randomized Controlled Immunotherapy Clinical Trials for GBM Challenged. *Cancers* **2020**, *13*, 32. [CrossRef]

25. Wouters, R.; Bevers, S.; Riva, M.; De Smet, F.; Coosemans, A. Immunocompetent Mouse Models in the Search for Effective Immunotherapy in Glioblastoma. *Cancers* **2020**, *13*, 19. [CrossRef]

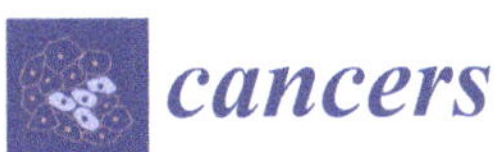

Article

Enhancing Adoptive Cell Transfer with Combination BRAF-MEK and CDK4/6 Inhibitors in Melanoma

Peter Kar Han Lau [1,2,3], Carleen Cullinane [1,3], Susan Jackson [1], Rachael Walker [1], Lorey K. Smith [1,3], Alison Slater [1], Laura Kirby [1], Riyaben P. Patel [1,3], Bianca von Scheidt [1], Clare Y. Slaney [1,3], Grant A. McArthur [1,2,3] and Karen E. Sheppard [1,3,4,*]

[1] Research Division, Peter MacCallum Cancer Centre, Melbourne, VIC 3000, Australia; peter.lau@petermac.org (P.K.H.L.); carleen.cullinane@petermac.org (C.C.); susan.jackson@petermac.org (S.J.); rachael.walker@petermac.org (R.W.); lorey.smith@petermac.org (L.K.S.); alison.slater@petermac.org (A.S.); laura.kirby@petermac.org (L.K.); Riyaben.patel@petermac.org (R.P.P.); bianca.vonscheidt@petermac.org (B.v.S.); clare.slaney@petermac.org (C.Y.S.); grant.mcarthur@petermac.org (G.A.M.)
[2] Department of Medical Oncology, Peter MacCallum Cancer Centre, Melbourne, VIC 3000, Australia
[3] Sir Peter MacCallum Department of Oncology, University of Melbourne, Parkville, VIC 3010, Australia
[4] Department of Biochemistry and Pharmacology, University of Melbourne, Melbourne, VIC 3010, Australia
*   Correspondence: karen.sheppard@petermac.org

Citation: Lau, P.K.H.; Cullinane, C.; Jackson, S.; Walker, R.; Smith, L.K.; Slater, A.; Kirby, L.; Patel, R.P.; von Scheidt, B.; Slaney, C.Y.; et al. Enhancing Adoptive Cell Transfer with Combination BRAF-MEK and CDK4/6 Inhibitors in Melanoma. *Cancers* **2021**, *13*, 6342. https://doi.org/10.3390/cancers13246342

Academic Editor: Adam C. Berger

Received: 4 November 2021
Accepted: 11 December 2021
Published: 17 December 2021

Publisher's Note: MDPI stays neutral with regard to jurisdictional claims in published maps and institutional affiliations.

Simple Summary: Adoptive cell transfer (ACT) is a potentially robust treatment option for patients with advanced melanoma that is resistant to immune checkpoint inhibitors. The addition of cyclin-dependent kinase 4/6 inhibitors to combination BRAF-MEK inhibitors can also greatly improve the duration of response against melanoma. The aim of our study was to investigate adoptive cell transfer with combination BRAF-MEK and CDK4/6 inhibitors. We show triplet targeted therapy is highly efficacious against BRAF^{V600} melanoma in YOVAL1.1 and the BRAFi resistant SM1WT1 model. Combination ACT with BRAF-MEK-CDK4/6i led to prolonged and deep anti-tumor responses in YOVAL1.1. This work provides additional evidence for BRAF-MEK-CDK4/6i in clinical trials and in combination with ACT.

Abstract: Despite the success of immune checkpoint inhibitors that target cytotoxic lymphocyte antigen-4 (CTLA-4) and programmed-cell-death-1 (PD-1) in the treatment of metastatic melanoma, there is still great need to develop robust options for patients who are refractory to first line immunotherapy. As such there has been a resurgence in interest of adoptive cell transfer (ACT) particularly derived from tumor infiltrating lymphocytes. Moreover, the addition of cyclin dependent kinase 4/6 inhibitors (CDK4/6i) have been shown to greatly extend duration of response in combination with BRAF-MEK inhibitors (BRAF-MEKi) in pre-clinical models of melanoma. We therefore investigated whether combinations of BRAF-MEK-CDK4/6i and ACT were efficacious in murine models of melanoma. Triplet targeted therapy of BRAF-MEK-CDK4/6i with OT-1 ACT led to sustained and robust anti-tumor responses in BRAFi sensitive YOVAL1.1. We also show that BRAF-MEKi but not CDK4/6i enhanced MHC Class I expression in melanoma cell lines in vitro. Paradoxically CDK4/6i in low concentrations of IFN-γ reduced expression of MHC Class I and PD-L1 in YOVAL1.1. Overall, this work provides additional pre-clinical evidence to pursue combination of BRAF-MEK-CDK4/6i and to combine this combination with ACT in the clinic.

Keywords: melanoma; adoptive cell transfer; targeted therapy; cell cycle; immuno-oncology

1. Introduction

While immune checkpoint inhibitors (ICI) targeting cytotoxic lymphocyte antigen-4 (CTLA-4) and anti-programmed death-1 (anti-PD1) have taken center stage in the treatment of advanced melanoma, there is a paucity of robust systemic treatment options in the refractory setting. Combination ipilimumab-nivolumab is generally favored as first line treatment for BRAF^{V600} metastatic melanoma given its five-year progression free survival (PFS) rate is double that of upfront BRAF-MEK inhibitors such as dabrafenib-trametinib (38% vs. 19%) [1,2]. As such, targeted therapy with BRAF-MEKi is increasingly used as second line therapy after immune checkpoint inhibitors but has relatively short duration of response of around 11–12 months [2]. Adoptive cell transfer (ACT) derived from tumor infiltrating lymphocytes (TIL) is a potentially robust option in the ICI refractory setting. Original studies by Rosenberg and colleagues, showed an objective response rate of approximately 50% with almost 30% of patients alive at the five-year timepoint in a pooled analysis of 3 trials [3,4]. Owing to the high labor requirements of extraction and production, TIL ACT has been limited to highly specialized academic centers. However, lifileucel is a commercial, centrally manufactured TIL ACT product that has shown promising activity in pre-treated ICI patients (n = 66) with an objective response of 36% [5]. Although median PFS was 4.1 months, the median duration of response was not reached after 18 months indicating the potential of long-term responses.

Combining BRAF-MEKi with ACT could therefore harness the advantages of targeted therapy with its high response rate (60–70%) and immunotherapy with its capacity for long term disease control. Findings from earlier pre-clinical studies support this approach. The addition of BRAFi (vemurafenib) to pmel-1 and OT-1 ACT treatments enhanced anti-tumor responses against the BRAFi resistant murine melanoma SM1 and SM1-ova tumors, respectively [6]. In a subsequent study, Hu-Lieskovan et al. [7], demonstrated synergy of combination BRAF-MEKi (dabrafenib and trametinib) with pmel-1 ACT against SM1 tumors. By itself, pmel-1 ACT had modest activity, but once combined with BRAF-MEKi, substantial tumor control was observed. Although anti-tumor responses to BRAF-MEKi are largely attributable to the sequential blockade of the mitogen activated protein kinase (MAPK) pathway, pre-clinical and patient studies show targeted therapy can exert a range of immunomodulatory effects on melanoma which are potentially synergistic with ACT [8]. BRAFi upregulates melanoma differentiation antigens such as gp100, MART-1 and tyrosinase in murine models [7], in vitro human cell lines [9,10], and in patient biopsy samples [11]. Additionally, expression of MHC I expression can be upregulated by melanoma in response to BRAFi treatment [10]. Hence targeted therapy may enhance the immunogenicity of melanoma and potentially augment the activity of ACT.

Cyclin dependent kinase 4/6 inhibitors (CDK4/6i) may also play a role in enhancing duration of response in combination with BRAF-MEKi via blockade of the cell cycle and exerting immunomodulatory effects on melanoma. The addition of CDK4/6i such as palbociclib [12] or ribociclib [13] to endocrine therapy almost doubles progression free survival compared to aromatase inhibitors alone in metastatic oestrogen receptor positive breast cancer. Approximately 90% of melanoma exhibit some cell cycle pathway dysregulation [14] which provides a strong rationale to combine CDK4/6i with BRAF-MEKi. Studies in our laboratory have shown encouraging in vivo anti-melanoma activity of palbociclib in combination with BRAF-MEKi [15,16]. Additional pre-clinical studies also demonstrate potential immuno-modulation by CDK4/6 inhibitors (CDK4/6i) in breast cancer and melanoma with upregulation of MHC Class I expression, T regulatory cell reduction, increased IFN-γ release in the tumor microenvironment and enhanced long-term anti-tumor immunity [17–21].

Building upon previous studies showing synergistic activity of BRAF-MEKi with ACT, we investigated whether the addition of CDK4/6i could further improve anti-tumor responses. We use two pre-clinical models, YOVAL1.1 which expresses the ovalbumin (ova) antigen and SM1WT1 which expresses gp100 which are amenable to ACT such as OT-1 and pmel-1, respectively. The SM1WT1 cell line is derived from SM1 which is resistant to BRAF inhibitors by nature of a BRAF amplification and transversion thereby providing a suitable platform to study the response in the BRAFi resistance setting [6,22]. Whereas YOVAL1.1 harbours a BRAF^{V600E} mutation that is susceptible to BRAFi treatment. Importantly both YOVAL1.1 and SM1WT1 exhibit a *CDKN2A* deletion which encodes the tumor suppressor p16 which is an inhibitor of CDK4/6 and thus the cell cycle pathway. Hence both cell lines provide a mechanistic rationale for the addition of CDK4/6 inhibitor in melanoma.

2. Materials and Methods

2.1. Cell Culture and Drugs

The SM1WT1 cell line was derived at Peter MacCallum Cancer Centre from the SM1 cell line [22]. The YOVAL1.1 cell line was derived in our laboratory from YUMM1.1 [23]. SM1WT1 was maintained in Roswell Park Memorial Institute (RPMI) media supplemented with 10% (*v/v*) fetal bovine serum (FBS) and Glutamax (35050-061, Life Technologies, Carlsbad, CA, USA). YOVAL1.1 cells were maintained in RPMI supplemented with 10% (*v/v*) fetal bovine serum (FBS), glutamax, 1 mM sodium pyruvate, 1 mM MEM Non-Essential Amino Acids, and 0.1% 2-mercaptoethanol. Dabrafenib and trametinib were purchased from Ark Pharm (catalog No. AK174048, Wuhan, Hubei, China) and Focus Bioscience (catalog No. HY-10999, Queensland, Australia), respectively, and palbociclib was from Pfizer Oncology (New York, NY, USA).

2.2. Cell Proliferation Assays

Cell proliferation assays were performed as previously described [15]. Plates were imaged using the Incucyte, with continuous live cell imaging (Essen Bioscience, Ann Arbor, MI, USA) every 12 h. Cell confluence was calculated as a marker of proliferation from 4 fields per well.

2.3. Gene Expression Analysis

Total RNA was isolated using the RNeasy Mini kit (Qiagen, Hilden, Germany) following the manufacturer's instructions. Purity and concentration of RNA was assessed using the Nanodrop ND1000 spectrophotometer (Thermo Scientific, Waltam, MA, USA). Complementary DNA (cDNA) was generated using the High Capacity cDNA Reverse Transcription Kit (Life Technologies). Quantitative real-time PCR using Mastermix Lightcycler SBR Green Master Mix (Roche, Basel, Switzerland) was performed on a Lightcycler 480 (Roche). NONO RNA was plotted as relative expression values. H2K1 (Biorad PrimePCR Assay H2K1, Catalog 10025636), and TAP1 (Biorad PrimePCR Assay Tap1, Catalog 10025636) were sourced from Biorad (Richmond, CA, USA). The primer sequences are as follows:

B2M-Forward: TTCACCCCCACTGAG
B2M-Reverse: GTCTTGGGCTCGGCC
NONO-Forward: TATCAGGGGGAAGATTGCCC
NONO-Reverse: GCCAGAATGAAGGCTTGACT

2.4. Animal Work

All in vivo mice experiments were approved by the Animal Ethics Committee of Peter MacCallum Cancer Centre (Protocol E569). Male C57Bl/6 mice aged between 5 and 6 weeks were purchased from Walter and Eliza Hall Institute (Melbourne, Australia). Mice were housed in pathogen free conditions at the Peter MacCallum Cancer Centre Animal Hold facility.

Briefly mice were shaved on the right flank the day prior to implantation and were anaesthetized using inhaled isoflurane and then injected with freshly harvested 1×10^6 tumor cells in 0.1 mL of sterile PBS. For the SM1WT1 model only, male C57/Bl6 mice aged 12–16 weeks of age were exposed to 4 Gy radiation using the XRAD 320 irradiator immediately prior to tumor establishment. Tumor measurements commenced 5 days after implantation and were performed two or three times weekly using digital calipers. Tumor volume was calculated by the formula 0.5 × length × width squared. Mice were sacrificed when tumor volume reached 1200 mm^3.

Dabrafenib-trametinib was prepared daily for administration in an aqueous solution of 0.5% hydroxypropyl methylcellulose and 0.2% Tween 80 (Sigma-Aldrich, St. Louis, MO, USA). Palbociclib was suspended in sodium lactate 50 mM. All mice were weighed prior to oral gavage. Dabrafenib and trametinib was administered at 30 mg/kg and 0.3 mg/kg, respectively, once daily. Palbociclib was dosed at 80 mg/kg once daily.

2.5. T Cell Expansion and Adoptive Cell Transfer

Male pmel-1 C57/Bl6 were euthanized and spleens dissected and placed into cold phosphate buffered saline (PBS) [24]. Spleens were minced and then incubated with ammonium-chloride-potassium lysis buffer for 1 min. Splenocytes were washed and filtered through a 70 micron filter twice prior to a manual cell count. Cell suspended to a concentration of 1 million cells/mL and supplemented with gp100 peptide, IL-2, and IL-7 at final concentrations of 0.1 μg/mL, 50 IU/mL, 0.2 ng/mL, respectively. Splenocytes were then incubated at 37 °C 5% CO_2. Cells were inspected every 2 or 3 days and split in a 1:1 ratio and supplemented with IL-2 at final concentration of 50 IU/mL. The pmel-1 cells were injected via tail vein on day 6 of cell culture. IL-2 (5×10^5 IU) was injected intraperitoneally twice daily for 3 days commencing on the day of pmel-1 injection.

Male OT-1 mice were subjected to the same red cell lysis and washing procedures as above, however each spleen was placed into 100 mL of media supplemented with sinfekel, IL-2, and IL-7 at final concentrations of (1 μL per 50 mL), 100 IU/mL, and 0.2 ng/mL, respectively, incubated at 37 °C in 5% CO_2. Three days later the splenocyte cultures were counted then resuspended to a concentration of 4×10^6 cells/mL in fresh media replenished with IL-2 and IL-7. Cells were incubated for a further 3 days until tail vein injection into the recipient mice.

2.6. Flow Cytometry

Samples were blocked with 2% normal mouse serum. Fixable yellow (L34959, Invitrogen, Carlsbad, CA, USA) or 7AAD (Cat 00699350, eBioscience, Waltham, MA, USA) was used to stain live/dead cells. Anti-mouse antibodies used were CD3 (17A2, eBioscience), CD4 (GK1.5, BioLegend, San Diego, CA, USA), TCR Vα2 (KB5-C20, BD Pharmingen), CD8a (53-6.7, BioLegend), CD44 (IM7, Biolegend), CD62L (MEL-14, eBioscience), H-2Db (KH95, BD Pharmingen), H-2Kb (AF6–88.5, BD Pharmingen), PD-L1 (MIH5, eBioscience). Anti-human antibodies used were HLA ABC (W6/32, Biolegend), PD-L1 (29E.283, Biolegend), anti-mouse IgG2a K Isotype (Biolegend), and anti-mouse IgG2b K (Biolegend).

Fluorescence was measured on BD LSR Fortessa X-20 or BD FACSVerse flow cytometer (BD Biosciences, North Ryde, NSW, Australia) and data analyzed using the FlowJo, LLC software (BD Biosciences, Franklin Lakes, NJ, USA).

2.7. IFN-γ Release Assay

SM1WT1 or SM1 were co-cultured with IFN-γ (2 ng/mK) or control for 24 h. SM1WT1 cells were then trypsinized and washed twice prior to pulsing with gp100 peptide (1 ng/mL) for 30 min and then washed twice prior to incubation with pmel-1 cells for 4 h. Supernatants were transferred to a second 96 well plate and frozen at −20 °C until IFN-γ enzyme-linked-immunosorbant assay (ELISA) was performed as previously described [25].

2.8. Chromium Release Assay

Target cells were labelled with 250 μCi/mL Chromium-51 (51Cr; Perkin Elmer, VIC Australia) for 45 min prior to culturing with effector cells at 37 °C. Supernatant was collected and 51Cr was measured by a gamma counter (Wallac Wizard). 51Cr release due to effector-mediated killing was calculated as %Release = [(51CrSAMPLE − 51Cr-SPONT)/(51CrTOTAL − 51CrSPONT)] × 100; where 51CrSPONT is spontaneous 51Cr release from target cells cultured without effector cells, and 51CrTOTAL is total chromium release from cells lysed with 10% Triton X-100.

2.9. Statistical Analysis

All statistical analyses were performed with the GraphPad Prism version 8 software (GraphPad Software Inc, La Jolla, CA, USA). As indicated comparison between two groups were analyzed using Student's *t*-test. Multiple comparisons were analyzed using one-way analysis of variance (ANOVA). A *p*-value of <0.05 was considered significant.

3. Results

3.1. YOVAL1.1 but Not SM1WT1 Mouse Melanoma Cells Are Highly Sensitive to Combination BRAF-MEKi and the Addition of Palbociclib Enhances Inhibition of SM1WT1 Proliferation

We assessed the sensitivity of the YOVAL1.1 and SM1WT1 cell lines to dabrafenib (BRAFi), trametinib (MEKi), and palbociclib (CDK4/6i) (Figure 1A). YOVAL1.1 harbors a $BRAF^{V600E}$ mutation, while in contrast SM1WT1 possesses a BRAF amplification rendering it resistant to BRAFi. YOVAL1.1 cells were sensitive to dabrafenib, trametinib, and moderately sensitive to palbociclib having GI50's (dose required to inhibit growth by 50%) of 4.5 ± 1.3 nM, 0.5 ± 0.1 nM, and 623 ± 147 nM, respectively. In comparison, SM1WT1 cells were relatively resistant to both dabrafenib and trametinib but moderately sensitive to palbociclib, exhibiting GI50's of 519 ± 29.4 nM, 11 ± 3.2 nM, and 490 ± 52 nM, respectively. To assess the activity of BRAFi, MEKi, and CDK4/6i combination therapy, cell proliferation over time was assessed (Figure 1B). Combination dabrafenib and trametinib (DT) at relatively low concentrations (10 nM and 1 nM, respectively) robustly inhibited cell proliferation in YOVAL1.1 cells, and palbociclib alone partially inhibited proliferation. In contrast, SM1WT1 cells exhibited resistance to both dabrafenib and trametinib at very high concentrations of 1 μM and 30 nM, respectively which only partially inhibited cell proliferation. However, the addition of palbociclib to DT elicited a more robust response.

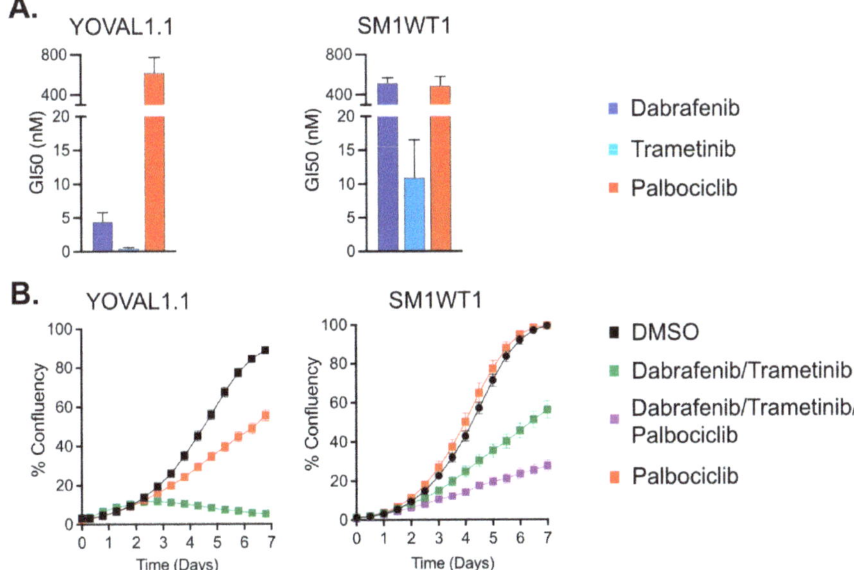

Figure 1. Sensitivity of mouse melanoma cell lines to targeted therapy. (**A**) Dose response assays were performed, and the concentration of drug required to inhibit proliferation by 50% (GI50) was determined. Bar graph represents mean ± SEM of 3–7 independent dose response experiments. For YOVAL1.1, a significant difference (*p* < 0.0001) in GI50's was observed between palbociclib (623 ± 147 nM) and both dabrafenib (4.5 ± 1.3 nM) and trametinb (0.5 ± 0.1 nM). For SM1WT1, a significant difference (*p* < 0.0002) in GI50's was observed between the trametinib (11.0 ± 3.2 nM) and both dabrafenib (519.0 ± 29.4 nM) and palbociclib (490 ± 52.0 nM). There was no difference in mean GI50 between the other groups within a cell line. One-way ANOVA was used to determine statistical significance. (**B**) To assess cell proliferation, cells were treated for 7 days, and percent confluency was analyzed over time using an IncuCyte. For YOVAL1.1, cells doses for dabrafenib, trametinib and palbociclib were 10 nM, 1 nM, and 2 μM, respectively. For SM1WT1, doses were 1 μM, 30 nM, and 1 μM, respectively. Mean ± SEM of 5 technical replicates.

3.2. Combination BRAF-MEK-CDK4/6i ± OT1 Is Highly Efficacious against YOVAL1.1

Earlier in vivo studies in our laboratory have shown the triplet combination of BRAF-MEK-CDK4/6i leads to robust responses in YOVAL1.1 tumors that far exceed the response to combination of BRAF-MEKi [16]. We therefore assessed the impact of the addition of CDK4/6 inhibitor (palbociclib) in the BRAFi sensitive YOVAL1.1 cell line in conjunction with OT-1 ACT (Figure 2A). Syngeneic C57BL/6 mice were inoculated with YOVAL1.1 subcutaneously. When tumors were at a target size of 50 mm^3, 5×10^6 OT-1 cells were injected via tail vein and daily gavages of dabrafenib-trametinib-palbociclib (DTP) commenced. Administration of OT-1 cells alone led to an anti-tumor response; however, by day 26 tumors re-emerged. The triplet combination of DTP led to a robust and sustained YOVAL1.1 tumor regression compared to OT-1 cells alone. When OT-1 ACT was combined with DTP a similar robust and sustained response was observed. Given some tumors in both DTP arms were impalpable, oral gavages of the targeted therapy were ceased at day 44, which led to subsequent regrowth of all tumors. However, a significant difference ($p < 0.03$) in median survival was demonstrated between DTP (65 days) and DTP plus OT-1 (85 days).

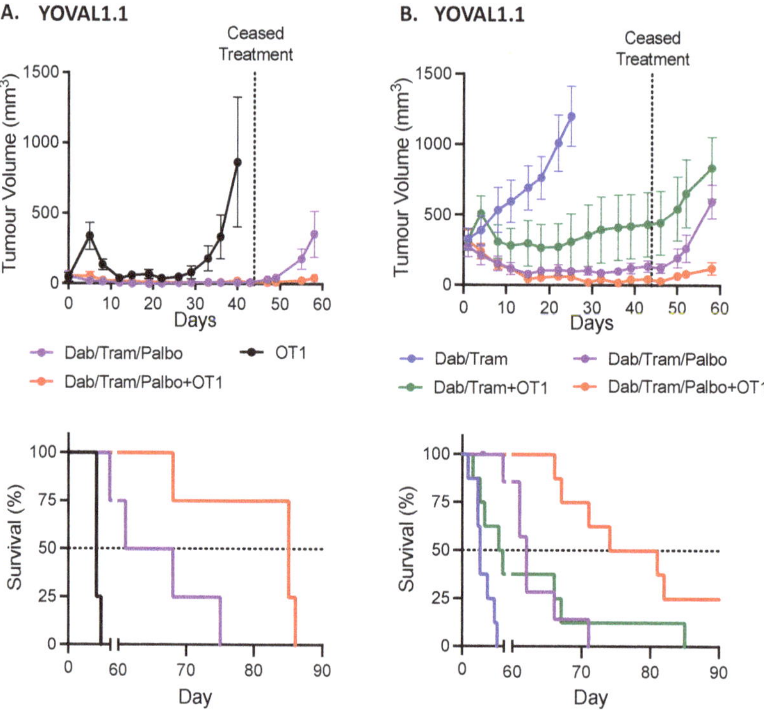

Figure 2. YOVAL1.1 tumor response to targeted and ACT. (**A**) In vivo YOVAL1.1 tumor volume growth and Kaplan–Meier overall survival curves of dabrafenib-trametinib-palbociclib (DTP ± OT-1 ACT with 4 mice per group (mean ± SEM). Gavages of DT ceased at day 44. Median overall survival (OS) for OT-1, DTP and DTP + OT-1 was 40, 64.5, and 85 days, respectively. OS hazard ratio (HR) for OT-1 versus DTP was 0.270, $p = 0.006$. OS HR of DTP versus DTP + OT-1 was 0.300, $p = 0.03$. (**B**) In vivo YOVAL1.1 tumor volume growth curve and Kaplan–Meier overall survival curves of dabrafenib-trametinib ± OT-1 ACT or dabrafenib-trametinib-palbociclib ± OT-1 ACT (mean ± SEM) with groups of 8 mice per each arm. Gavages of DT ceased at day 46. Median OS for DT, DTP, DT + OT-1 and DTP + OT-1 was 25, 62, 55, and 77.5 days, respectively. OS HR for DT versus DTP was 0.340, $p = 0.02$. OS HR for DTP versus DT + OT-1 was 1.154, $p = 0.76$. OS HR for DTP versus DTP + OT-1 was 0.250, $p = 0.001$. Hazard ratios determined with log-rank (Mantel-Cox).

In a second experiment (Figure 2B), we compared dabrafenib-trametinib (DT) or DTP with OT-1 for treating large tumors. DT alone did not induce tumor regression with median survival of 25 days. In contrast, DT + OT-1, DTP, DTP + OT1, and all led to strong anti-tumor responses that plateaued at day 15 in all groups, with mean volumes of 298 ± 163.0, 90 ± 28, and 46 ± 16 mm^3 respectively. Again, due to the deep regressions observed with DTP, oral gavages of DT and DTP were ceased at day 46 and all but one tumor in the OT1 + DTP group displayed regrowth. Median survival of DTP + OT1 was 78 days which was superior to DT + OT-1 (55 days, $p < 0.02$). DTP was highly efficacious and superior to both DT alone and DT + OT-1. Similar to the previous experiment, there was significant additional anti-tumor activity, when OT-1 was combined with DTP compared to DTP alone (median survival of 77.5 days versus 62 days, $p < 0.001$). Between both experiments the DTP arms led to average weight loss of between 2.3% to 4.3% in the first 15 days of treatment which then returned to their mean baseline between day 23 and 46.

3.3. In the Therapy Resistant SM1WT1 Model, ACT Does Not Enhance Response to Combination BRAF-MEKi ± CDK4/6i

Given the YOVAL1.1 in vivo results, we then sought to assess whether the addition of palbociclib to combination BRAF-MEKi and pmel-1 ACT would further enhance anti-tumor activity against the BRAFi resistant SM1WT1 tumors. Syngeneic C57BL/6 mice were subjected to 4 Gy radiation and then immediately inoculated with SM1WT1 subcutaneously. When tumors were at least 50 mm^3, the mice received 1×10^7 pmel-1 cells via tail vein injection or mock ACT both with 5×10^5 IU of IL-2 intraperitoneal injection (control). Dabrafenib-trametinib ± palbociclib gavages were also commenced. There was no difference in the tumor growth curves between the control and pmel-1 ACT arms (Figure 3). The two DT containing arms exhibited slower growth compared to control and this was enhanced by the addition of palbociclib. Surprisingly, pmel-1 ACT did not enhance either DT or DTP responses. Median survival (Figure 2) was improved substantially with both DT and DTP compared to control ($p < 0.01$ and $p < 0.001$, respectively) and DTP improved survival compared to DT ($p < 0.03$).

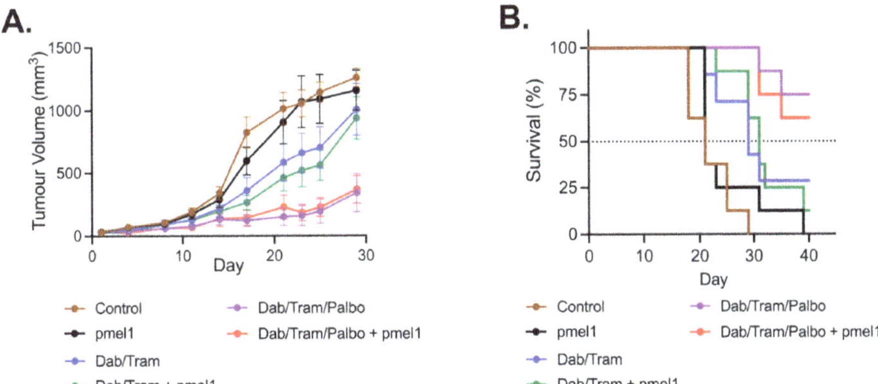

Figure 3. SM1WT1 tumor response to targeted therapy and ACT. (**A**) SM1WT1 tumor volume growth curves of dabrafenib-trametinib (DT) ± palbociclib (P) and pmel-1 adoptive cell transfer (ACT) with 8 mice per group (mean ± SEM). (**B**) Kaplan–Meier overall survival (OS) curves of data shown in (**A**). Median OS for control, pmel-1, DT, DT + pmel-1, DTP, and DTP + pmel-1 was 21, 21, 29, 31, not attained, and not attained, respectively. OS hazard ratio (HR) for control versus pmel-1 was 1.57, $p = 0.32$. OS HR for DT versus DT + pmel-1 was 0.995, $p > 0.99$. OS HR for DTP versus DTP + pmel-1 was 0.627, $p = 0.58$. OS HR for DT versus DTP was 4.695, $p = 0.03$. Hazard ratios determined with log-rank (Mantel-Cox).

3.4. Pmel-1 T Cells Kills SM1WT1 In Vitro Only with gp100 Stimulation

To investigate the lack of response in the SM1WT1-pmel-1 system, pmel ACT cells were further assessed. Flow cytometry of the injected pmel-1 ACT cells showed a highly activated phenotype (Figure S1) with a high proportion of CD3, CD8, CD44^{hi}, and CD62L^{hi} positive cells indicating a central memory phenotype. Chromium release assays were also performed to determine if pmel cells were effective at recognizing and killing SM1WT1 cells. Pmel-1 cells were able to kill approximately 80% of the highly immunogenic MC38 cells pulsed with gp100 and 40% SM1WT1 pulsed with gp100 with an effector:target ratio of 40:1 (Figure 4A). IFN-γ release assays (Figure 4B) showed low IFN-γ concentrations with pmel-1 and SM1WT co-cultures compared to pmel-1 and SM1WT cells pulsed with the gp100 peptide. These findings are surprising given we originally considered the melanoma SM1WT1 cells to express the classic gp100 melanoma peptide. To determine if SM1WT1 cells have a low expression of gp100 by MHC Class I, SM1WT1 cells were pre-incubated with IFN-γ for 24 h, to increase MHC Class I expression. Cells were washed extensively and then incubated with pmel-1 cells. Only upon pulsing IFN-γ stimulated SM1WT1 with gp100 peptide were high IFN-γ titers achieved; indicating low expression of this antigen as the likely cause for the poor activity of pmel-1 cells against SM1WT1 in vitro and potentially in vivo.

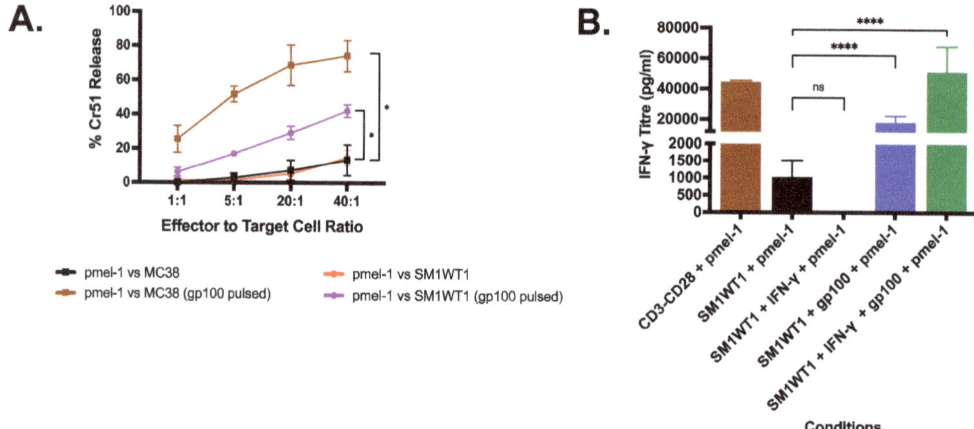

Figure 4. SM1WT1 tumor response to targeted and ACT. (**A**) Chromium release assay of MC38 and SM1WT1 vs. pmel-1 (mean ± SEM of 3 independent experiments). (**B**) SM1WT1-pmel-1 IFN-γ Release Assay (mean ± SEM of 3 independent experiments). SM1WT1 + pmel-1 were incubated for 16 h. To ensure MHC Class I expression, SM1WT1 cells were also pre-incubated with IFN-γ (2 ng/mL) for 24 h and washed twice prior to incubation with pmel-1 (SM1WT1 + IFN-γ + pmel-1). SM1WT1 was pulsed with gp100 peptide (1 ng/mL) for 30 min and washed twice prior to incubation with pmel-1 (SM1WT1 + gp100 + pmel-1). * $p < 0.05$, **** $p < 0.0001$.

3.5. BRAF-MEKi Upregulates MHC Class I and PD-L1 in SM1WT1 and YOVAL1.1 In Vitro

MHC Class I is a pre-requisite for responses to T cells including TIL ACT [26] and the loss of antigen presentation machinery is an important resistance mechanism of anti-PD1 therapy [27,28]. Inhibition of BRAF is associated with up-regulation of MHC Class I and presentation of antigen [29]. We therefore investigated if the addition of CDK4/6 inhibitor to BRAF-MEKi could further enhance MHC Class I expression in our models. Dabrafenib-trametinib led to a significant 2.4-fold upregulation of both H2Db and H2Kb over control in SM1WT1 (Figure 5A,B: $p \leq 0.01$). Similarly, dabrafenib-trametinib upregulated both H2Db and H2Kb by 3.6-fold over DMSO in YOVAL1.1 (Figure 5D,E: $p \leq 0.05$) and there was no significant difference with the addition of palbociclib in either cell line. Palbociclib itself did not alter YOVAL1.1 expression of MHC Class I (Figure 5F), while SM1WT1 H2Db and H2Kb expression increased by approximately 33% (Figure 5A,B). Representative FACS plots are shown in Figures S2 and S3.

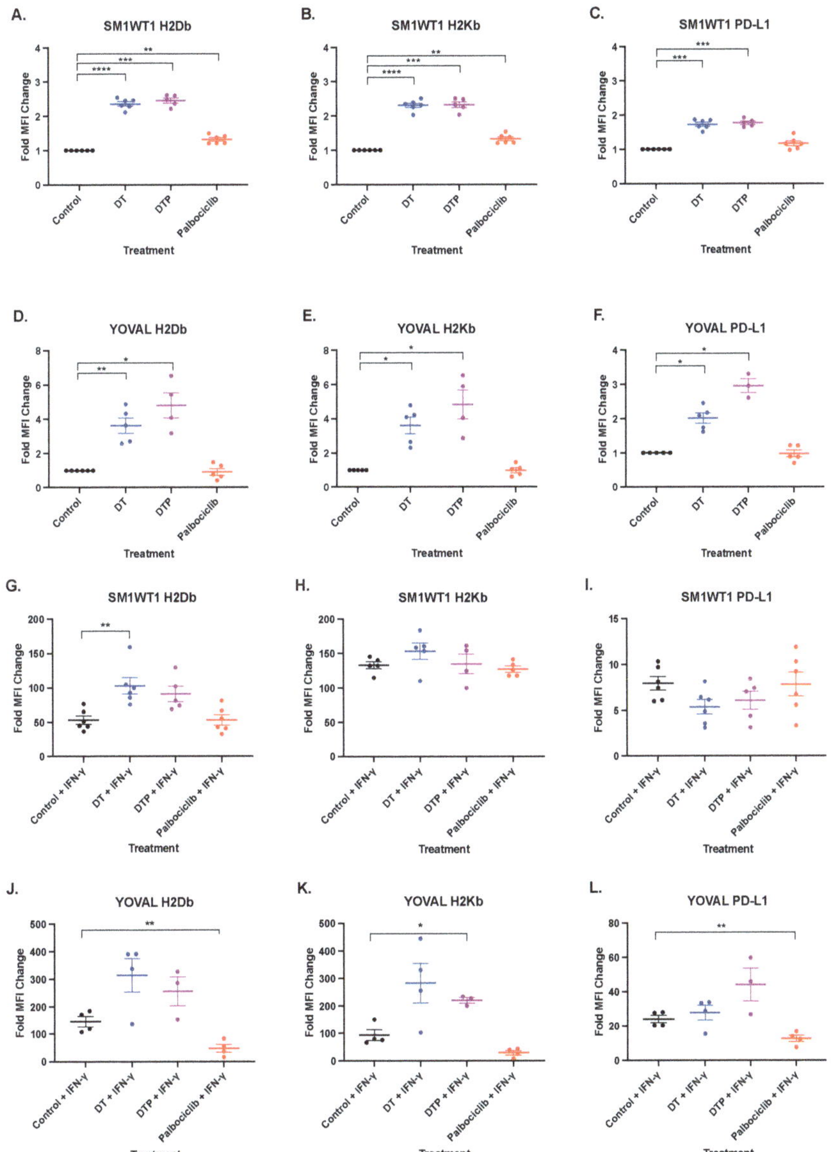

Figure 5. SM1WT1 and YOVAL1.1 MHC Class I and PD-L1 Expression. Samples analyzed using FACS for H2Db (**A,D,G,J**), H2Kb (**B,E,H,K**), and PD-L1 (**C,F,I,L**). SM1WT1 and YOVAL1.1 were treated with dabrafenib-trametinib (DT), dabrafenib-trametinib-palbociclib (DTP), or palbociclib alone. Median fluorescent intensity of the respective treatment group was normalized back to controls and expressed as fold MFI change. Mean $\pm$ SEM. n = 3–5. Statistical significance was determined using a one-way ANOVA * $p < 0.05$, ** $p < 0.01$, *** $p < 0.001$, **** $p < 0.0001$.

Although BRAF-MEKi upregulates MHC Class I expression, it can also enhance PD-L1 expression thereby potentially counteracting immune responses. SM1WT1 PD-L1 expression was increased by 1.7-fold over DMSO control by both DT and DTP treatment ($p < 0.002$) (Figure 5C). YOVAL1.1 expression of PD-L1 was increased by 2.0-fold ($p < 0.006$) and 2.9-fold ($p \leq 0.016$) with DT and DTP treatment, respectively (Figure 5F). Palbociclib itself did not alter expression of PD-L1 in either cell line (Figure 5C,F) indicating BRAF-MEKi was responsible for upregulation in the DTP treatment group.

In parallel with these experiments, we also assessed MHC Class I and PD-L1 expression in response to targeted therapy in the presence of IFN-γ. (Figure 5G–L). Under these conditions, DT and DTP treatment did not consistently increase H2Db and H2Kb expression compared to IFN-γ alone. Surprisingly, palbociclib treatment in the presence of IFN-γ reduced YOVAL1.1 H2Db expression (0.66-fold decrease, $p < 0.0018$) with a similar trend observed with H2Kb (0.674-fold decrease, $p < 0.099$). YOVAL1.1 PD-L1 expression was also inhibited with palbociclib plus IFN-γ treatment compared to IFN-γ control (0.474 decrease, $p < 0.006$). However, palbociclib did not alter MHC Class I expression in the human BRAF^{V600} mutant melanoma cell lines A375, HT144, SKMEL-28, and WM266-4 cell lines even in the presence of IFN-γ (Figure S4). Palbociclib enhanced PD-L1 expression in A375 in particularly with IFN-γ (Figure S5).

In order to explore the potential mechanism of MHC Class I upregulation induced by dabrafenib-trametinib $\pm$ palbociclib, real-time PCR of H2K1, Transport associated with Antigen Processing-1 (TAP1) and Beta-2-Microglobulin (β_2M) was performed (Figures 6 and S6). Dabrafenib-trametinib $\pm$ palbociclib upregulated TAP1 (approx. 6–7-fold) and β_2M (approx. 4-fold) mRNA expression in SM1WT1. H2K1 was also upregulated by dabrafenib-trametinib $\pm$ palbociclib although the increase observed by the drug triplet did not meet statistical significance. In contrast, palbociclib monotherapy down regulated H2K1 gene expression by 50% ($p < 0.05$: Figure 5A). In YOVAL1.1 cells, TAP1 appeared to be upregulated by dabrafenib-trametinib $\pm$ palbociclib although only the BRAF-MEKi group attained statistical significance ($p < 0.001$). Overall, there was no effect by BRAF-MEKi nor CDK4/6i on YOVAL1.1 H2K1 or β_2M expression.

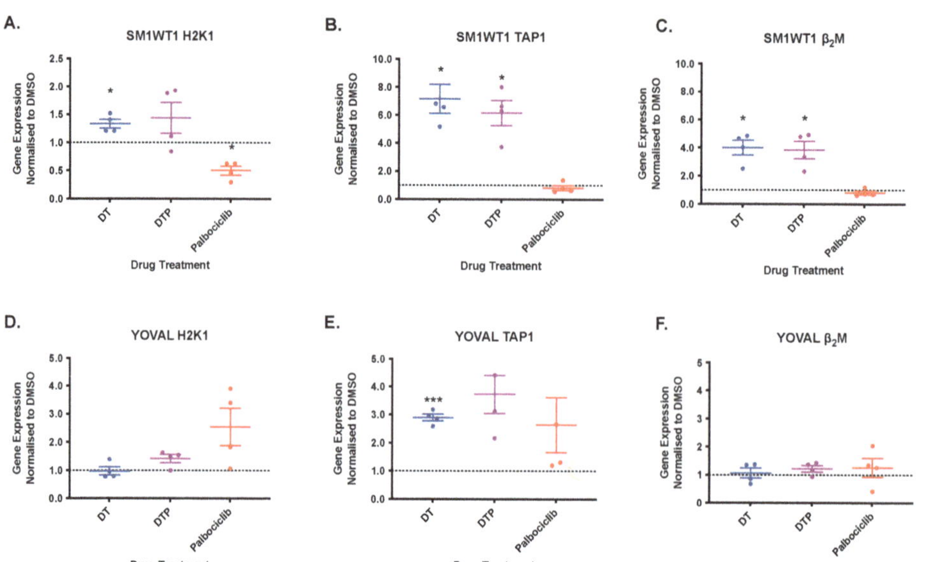

Figure 6. SM1WT1 and YOVAL1.1 gene expression of H2K1, TAP1 and β_2M. SM1WT1 and YOVAL1.1 treated with control (DMSO), dabrafenib-trametinib (DT), dabrafenib-trametinib-palbociclib (DTP), and palbociclib monotherapy. Samples analyzed using real time PCR for H2K1 (**A,D**), TAP1 (**B,E**), and β_2M (**C,F**). Mean $\pm$ SEM, $n = 4$. Gene expression normalized to DMSO control. Statistical significance was determined using one way ANOVA * $p < 0.05$, *** $p < 0.001$.

4. Discussion

The primary aim of this study was to assess whether the addition of palbociclib could augment anti-tumor responses in combination with adoptive cell transfer and BRAF-MEKi. Combination BRAF-MEKi can shape the tumor microenvironment by reducing immunosuppressive factors such as vascular endothelial growth factor, IL-6, IL-10, and TGF-β which corresponds with increasing tumor infiltrating lymphocytes [11,30]. Given the potential immunomodulation observed in previous studies, it is therefore logical to combine CDK4/6i with BRAF-MEKi. Previously we have shown that DTP elicited a robust anti-tumor response against YOVAL1.1 in vivo with overall survival of beyond 100 days compared to approximately 70 days for BRAF-MEKi [16]. Combination DTP increased T cell and CD8 infiltration in the tumor microenvironment while Treg populations were reduced compared to both controls and DT treated mice [16]. Critically DTP reduced CD103$^+$ dendritic cell (DC) populations in the tumor microenvironment which accounted for resistance to combination anti-CTLA-4 and anti-PD1 antibodies after progression of the targeted therapy triplet [16]. Given this observation, we reasoned that DTP could also antagonize ACT, however in BRAFi sensitive YOVAL1.1 tumors combined DTP and OT-1 ACT further enhanced the durability and depth of response compared to either treatment alone.

CDK4/6 inhibitors have been shown to enhance the immunogenicity of cancer and modulate the tumor microenvironment. Goel et al. demonstrated CDK4/6i upregulated MHC Class I expression via upregulation of HLA-A, HLA-C, B$_2$M and mRNA in breast cancer cell lines [17]. Similar upregulation of MHC Class I by CDK4/6i was also demonstrated in the murine melanoma cell line B16-OVA with co-culture experiments showing enhanced IFN-γ and TNF-α release when treated with OT-1 T cells [17]. Contrary to these prior studies, neither SM1WT1 nor YOVAL1.1 MHC Class I expression was altered by palbociclib monotherapy. BRAF-MEKi in both cell lines did enhance MHC Class I expression but there was no additional contribution with the addition of CDK4/6i. Furthermore, we did not observe changes of MHC Class I expression in several human melanoma cell lines which indicates the response to CDK4/6i is not universal.

CDK4/6i can also enhance inhibitory immune checkpoints namely PD-L1. Treatment with CDK4/6i inhibits speckle-type POZ protein (SPOP), a cullin E3 ubiquitin ligase protein that stimulates proteasome-mediated degradation of PD-L1 [20]. In this key paper, Zhang et al. demonstrated palbociclib upregulated PD-L1 in B16F10 in vivo. Additionally, they showed fluctuation of PD-L1 expression during cell cycle progression and palbociclib treatment consistently upregulated this immune checkpoint in a variety of different tissues such as brain, liver and colon. In our work we did not identify enhancement of PD-L1 expression in vitro with palbociclib or in combination with BRAF-MEKi in our melanoma models.

While we did not show palbociclib enhancement of either YOVAL1.1 or SM1WT1 MHC Class I expression, CDK4/6i itself can potentially enhance T cell and ACT activity. Palbociclib treatment is associated with upregulation of nuclear factor of activated T-cells (NFAT) in Jurkat cells with subsequent higher IL-2 and GM-CSF production [18]. Using a CRISPR/CAS9 screen on Jurkat T cells, retinoblastoma protein was also shown to be necessary for CDK4/6i upregulation of CD62L expression and skew TIL populations towards memory differentiation [21]. These studies also showed significantly enhanced CAR-T cell persistence and anti-tumor efficacy with palbociclib treatment indicating a potential role for CDK4/6i in ACT [21].

In the clinic, the targeted therapy triplet of BRAF-MEK-CDK4/6i could be employed in combination with TIL ACT. BRAFi have been combined with TIL ACT in small pilot studies with encouraging activity and safety [31–33]. In two trials, the BRAFi vemurafenib was commenced after excision of melanoma metastases for ACT production and briefly withheld during the pre-conditioning chemotherapy regimen for five days [32,33]. Objective responses were observed in 7 of 11 patients which included 2 participants with complete responses [33]. In a second trial, 6 of 16 patients (38%) exhibited objective responses at the 12 month mark with prolonged overall survival in responders varying from 38 to 66 months [32]. Importantly vemurafenib was able to prevent clinical progression during the three to six-week ACT manufacturing period which is a key limitation of this therapy. The BRAF-MEK-CDK4/6i combined with ACT might be of particular benefit for patients with poor prognostic features such as those with high volume disease or elevated lactate dehydrogenase (LDH) where both immune checkpoint inhibitors and combination BRAF-MEKi have substantially reduced efficacy [1,34]. Five-year progression free survival of patients with normal versus elevated LDH was 41% and 28%, respectively in patients treated with ipilimumab-nivolumab [1]. Moreover, only 8% of patients with elevated LDH treated with first line dabrafenib-trametinib had ongoing responses at the same time point indicating a critical need for new treatments in this poor prognostic group [2]. The rapid onset of responses with BRAF-MEKi and ACT might serve as useful treatments for these poor prognostic patients.

We acknowledge a limitation of this work is the use of murine melanoma rather than human ACT models. However, xenograft ACT models require immunodeficient mice which may confound outcomes. Furthermore, it would limit the ability to assess if depletion of tumor associated proinflammatory macrophages and cross-priming $CD103^+$ dendritic cells which we have previously observed with BRAF-MEK-CDK4/6i treatment would limit the efficacy of concurrent ACT treatment [16]. Although CDK4/6i induces neutropaenia, which may bring safety concerns with pre-conditioning chemotherapy required for TIL ACT, the potential for CDK4/6i to modulate T cell populations to a memory phenotype might also be advantageous for ACT. Clinical data on the potential additive benefit of palbociclib with BRAF-MEKi is pending with the phase Ib CELEBRATE trial (NCT04720768) which investigates the addition of palbociclib to encorafenib-binimetinib. This eagerly awaited study might provide an additional targeted therapy regimen that could set the stage for future trials in combination with adoptive cell transfer.

5. Conclusions

Overall our findings indicate the BRAF-MEK-CDK4/6i can be employed in combination with ACT and provides additional evidence that supports clinical studies of CDK4/6i in combination with BRAF-MEKi in advanced melanoma. We did not find that CDK4/6i alone or in combination with BRAF-MEKi enhanced MHC Class I in YOVAL1.1 or SM1WT1. Consistent with other studies BRAF-MEK-CDK4/6i led to robust anti-tumor activity in both BRAFi resistant SM1WT1 and BRAFi sensitive YOVAL1.1 models and importantly did not adversely affect the response to ACT. This data supports the use of this novel triplet targeted therapy with adoptive cell transfer.

Supplementary Materials: The following are available online at https://www.mdpi.com/article/ 10.3390/cancers13246342/s1, Figure S1: FACS plots of pmel-1 adoptive cell transfer, Figure S2: Representative FACS plots of SM1WT1 treated with DMSO, Dabrafenib-Trametinib (DT), Dabrafenib-Trametinib-Palbociclib (DTP) and Palbociclib for 72 h, Figure S3: Representative FACS plots of YOVAL1.1 treated with DMSO, Dabrafenib-Trametinib (DT), Dabrafenib-Trametinib-Palbociclib (DTP) and Palbociclib for 72 h, Figure S4: Human melanoma cell lines and HLA-A, -B, -C expression with palbociclib, Figure S5: Human melanoma cell lines and PD-L1 expression with palbociclib, Figure S6: SM1WT1 and YOVAL1.1 gene expression of H2K1, TAP1 and β_2M with Targeted Therapy IFN-γ Treatment.

Author Contributions: Conceptualization, P.K.H.L., C.C., C.Y.S., G.A.M. and K.E.S.; methodology, P.K.H.L., C.C., C.Y.S., L.K. and R.P.P.; formal analysis, P.K.H.L. and L.K.S.; investigation, P.K.H.L., C.C., S.J., R.W., B.v.S., L.K.S., A.S., L.K., R.P.P., C.Y.S., G.A.M. and K.E.S.; resources, P.K.H.L., C.C., C.Y.S., G.A.M. and K.E.S.; data curation, P.K.H.L., L.K.S., C.Y.S., L.K. and R.P.P.; original draft preparation, P.K.H.L., C.Y.S. and K.E.S.; review and editing, P.K.H.L., C.Y.S., G.A.M. and K.E.S.; supervision, C.C., C.Y.S., G.A.M. and K.E.S.; funding acquisition, G.A.M. and K.E.S. All authors have read and agreed to the published version of the manuscript.

Funding: This research was funded by National Health and Medical Research Council project grant to G.A. McArthur and K.E. Sheppard (1100189), and Melbourne University Research Scholarship to Peter Kar Han Lau.

Institutional Review Board Statement: The study was conducted according to the guidelines of the Declaration of Helsinki, and approved by the Animal Experimentation Ethics Committee of Peter MacCallum Cancer Centre (protocol code E569 and date of approval 14 September 2016).

Informed Consent Statement: Not applicable.

Data Availability Statement: The data is contained within the article or supplementary material.

Acknowledgments: The authors would like to acknowledge Emily Lelliott for her technical assistance in this project.

Conflicts of Interest: P.K.H. Lau reports personal fees from Pfizer (honoraria) outside the submitted work. G.A. McArthur reports grants from National Health and Medical Research Council during the conduct of the study, as well as other from Roche/Genentech (clinical trial reimbursement of costs) and Array/Pfizer (clinical trial reimbursement of costs) outside the submitted work. K.E. Sheppard reports grants from National Health and Medical Research Council and nonfinancial support from Pfizer Oncology (supply of palbociclib) during the conduct of the study, as well as nonfinancial support from GlaxoSmithKline (supply of therapeutics not used in this study) outside the submitted work. No disclosures were reported by the other authors.

References

1. Larkin, J.; Chiarion-Sileni, V.; Gonzalez, R.; Grob, J.-J.; Rutkowski, P.; Lao, C.D.; Cowey, C.L.; Schadendorf, D.; Wagstaff, J.; Dummer, R.; et al. Five-year survival with combined nivolumab and ipilimumab in advanced melanoma. *N. Engl. J. Med.* **2019**, *381*, 1535–1546. [CrossRef]
2. Robert, C.; Grob, J.J.; Stroyakovskiy, D.; Karaszewska, B.; Hauschild, A.; Levchenko, E.; Sileni, V.C.; Schachter, J.; Garbe, C.; Bondarenko, I.; et al. Five-year outcomes with dabrafenib plus trametinib in metastatic melanoma. *N. Engl. J. Med.* **2019**, *381*, 626–636. [CrossRef]
3. Rosenberg, S.A.; Yang, J.C.; Sherry, R.M.; Kammula, U.S.; Hughes, M.S.; Phan, G.Q.; Citrin, D.; Restifo, N.P.; Robbins, P.F.; Wunderlich, J.R.; et al. Durable complete responses in heavily pretreated patients with metastatic melanoma using T-cell transfer immunotherapy. *Clin. Cancer Res. Off. J. Am. Assoc. Cancer Res.* **2011**, *17*, 4550–4557. [CrossRef] [PubMed]
4. Rosenberg, S.A.; Packard, B.S.; Aebersold, P.M.; Solomon, D.; Topalian, S.L.; Toy, S.T.; Simon, P.; Lotze, M.T.; Yang, J.C.-H.; Seipp, C.A.; et al. Use of tumor-infiltrating lymphocytes and interleukin-2 in the immunotherapy of patients with metastatic melanoma. A preliminary report. *N. Engl. J. Med.* **1988**, *319*, 1676–1680. [CrossRef] [PubMed]
5. Sarnaik, A.A.; Hamid, O.; Khushalani, N.I.; Lewis, K.D.; Medina, T.; Kluger, H.M.; Thomas, S.S.; Domingo-Musibay, E.; Pavlick, A.C.; Whitman, E.D.; et al. Lifileucel, a tumor-infiltrating lymphocyte therapy, in metastatic melanoma. *J. Clin. Oncol. Off. J. Am. Soc. Clin. Oncol.* **2021**, *39*, 2656–2666. [CrossRef]
6. Koya, R.C.; Mok, S.; Otte, N.; Blacketor, K.J.; Comin-Anduix, B.; Tumeh, P.C.; Minasyan, A.; Graham, N.A.; Graeber, T.; Chodon, T.; et al. braf inhibitor vemurafenib improves the antitumor activity of adoptive cell immunotherapy. *Cancer Res.* **2012**, *72*, 3928–3937. [CrossRef] [PubMed]
7. Hu-Lieskovan, S.; Mok, S.; Moreno, B.H.; Tsoi, J.; Robert, L.; Goedert, L.; Pinheiro, E.M.; Koya, R.C.; Graeber, T.G.; Comin-Anduix, B.; et al. Improved antitumor activity of immunotherapy with BRAF and MEK inhibitors in BRAF V600E melanoma. *Sci. Transl. Med.* **2015**, *7*, 279ra241. [CrossRef]
8. Lau, P.K.H.; Ascierto, P.A.; McArthur, G. Melanoma: The intersection of molecular targeted therapy and immune checkpoint inhibition. *Curr. Opin. Immunol.* **2016**, *39*, 30–38. [CrossRef] [PubMed]
9. Boni, A.; Cogdill, A.; Dang, P.; Udayakumar, D.; Njauw, C.-N.J.; Sloss, C.M.; Ferrone, C.R.; Flaherty, K.T.; Lawrence, D.P.; Fisher, D.E.; et al. Selective BRAFV600E inhibition enhances T-cell recognition of melanoma without affecting lymphocyte function. *Cancer Res.* **2010**, *70*, 5213–5219. [CrossRef]
10. Bradley, S.; Chen, Z.; Melendez, B.; Talukder, A.; Khalili, J.S.; Rodriguez-Cruz, T.; Liu, S.; Whittington, M.; Deng, W.; Li, F.; et al. BRAFV600E co-opts a conserved MHC class I internalization pathway to diminish antigen presentation and CD8+ T-cell recognition of melanoma. *Cancer Immunol. Res.* **2015**, *3*, 602–609. [CrossRef] [PubMed]
11. Frederick, D.T.; Piris, A.; Cogdill, A.; Cooper, Z.; Lezcano, C.; Ferrone, C.R.; Mitra, D.; Boni, A.; Newton, L.P.; Liu, C.; et al. BRAF inhibition is associated with enhanced melanoma antigen expression and a more favorable tumor microenvironment in patients with metastatic melanoma. *Clin. Cancer Res. Off. J. Am. Assoc. Cancer Res.* **2013**, *19*, 1225–1231. [CrossRef] [PubMed]
12. Finn, R.S.; Crown, J.P.; Ettl, J.; Schmidt, M.; Bondarenko, I.; Lang, I.; Pinter, T.; Boer, K.; Patel, R.; Randolph, S.; et al. Efficacy and safety of palbociclib in combination with letrozole as first-line treatment of ER-positive, HER2-negative, advanced breast cancer: Expanded analyses of subgroups from the randomized pivotal trial PALOMA-1/TRIO-18. *Breast Cancer Res.* **2016**, *18*, 67. [CrossRef]

13. Hortobagyi, G.N.; Stemmer, S.M.; Burris, H.A.; Yap, Y.-S.; Sonke, G.S.; Paluch-Shimon, S.; Campone, M.; Blackwell, K.L.; Andre, F.; Winer, E.P.; et al. Ribociclib as first-line therapy for HR-positive, advanced breast cancer. *N. Engl. J. Med.* **2016**, *375*, 1738–1748. [CrossRef] [PubMed]

14. Young, R.J.; Waldeck, K.; Martin, C.; Foo, J.H.; Cameron, D.P.; Kirby, L.; Do, H.; Mitchell, C.; Cullinane, C.; Liu, W.; et al. Loss ofCDKN2A expression is a frequent event in primary invasive melanoma and correlates with sensitivity to the CDK4/6 inhibitor PD0332991 in melanoma cell lines. *Pigment. Cell Melanoma Res.* **2014**, *27*, 590–600. [CrossRef]

15. Martin, C.A.; Cullinane, C.; Kirby, L.; Abuhammad, S.; Lelliott, E.J.; Waldeck, K.; Young, R.J.; Brajanovski, N.; Cameron, D.P.; Walker, R.; et al. Palbociclib synergizes with BRAF and MEK inhibitors in treatment naïve melanoma but not after the development of BRAF inhibitor resistance. *Int. J. Cancer* **2018**, *142*, 2139–2152. [CrossRef]

16. Lelliott, E.J.; Mangiola, S.; Ramsbottom, K.M.; Zethoven, M.; Lim, L.; Lau, P.K.H.; Oliver, A.J.; Martelotto, L.G.; Kirby, L.; Martin, C.; et al. Combined BRAF, MEK, and CDK4/6 inhibition depletes intratumoral immune-potentiating myeloid populations in melanoma. *Cancer Immunol. Res.* **2021**, *9*, 136–146. [CrossRef]

17. Goel, S.; DeCristo, M.J.; Watt, A.C.; BrinJones, H.; Sceneay, J.; Li, B.B.; Khan, N.; Ubellacker, J.M.; Xie, S.; Metzger-Filho, O.; et al. CDK4/6 inhibition triggers anti-tumour immunity. *Nature* **2017**, *548*, 471–475. [CrossRef] [PubMed]

18. Deng, J.; Wang, E.S.; Jenkins, R.W.; Li, S.; Dries, R.; Yates, K.; Chhabra, S.; Huang, W.; Liu, H.; Aref, A.R.; et al. CDK4/6 inhibition augments antitumor immunity by enhancing T-cell activation. *Cancer Discov.* **2017**, *8*, 216–233. [CrossRef] [PubMed]

19. Jin, X.; Ding, D.; Yan, Y.; Li, H.; Wang, B.; Ma, L.; Ye, Z.; Ma, T.; Wu, Q.; Rodrigues, D.N.; et al. Phosphorylated RB promotes cancer immunity by inhibiting NF-kappaB activation and PD-L1 expression. *Mol. Cell* **2019**, *73*, 22–35.e6. [CrossRef]

20. Zhang, J.; Bu, X.; Wang, H.; Zhu, Y.; Geng, Y.; Nihira, N.T.; Tan, Y.; Ci, Y.; Wu, F.; Dai, X.; et al. Cyclin D–CDK4 kinase destabilizes PD-L1 via cullin 3–SPOP to control cancer immune surveillance. *Nature* **2018**, *553*, 91–95. [CrossRef] [PubMed]

21. Lelliott, E.J.; Kong, I.Y.; Zethoven, M.; Ramsbottom, K.M.; Martelotto, L.G.; Meyran, D.; Jiang Zhu, J.; Costacurta, M.; Kirby, L.; Sandow, J.J.; et al. CDK4/6 inhibition promotes anti-tumor immunity through the induction of T cell memory. *Cancer Discov.* **2021**, *11*, 2582–2601. [CrossRef]

22. Knight, D.A.; Ngiow, S.F.; Li, M.; Parmenter, T.J.; Mok, S.; Cass, A.; Haynes, N.M.; Kinross, K.M.; Yagita, H.; Koya, R.C.; et al. Host immunity contributes to the anti-melanoma activity of BRAF inhibitors. *J. Clin. Investig.* **2013**, *123*, 1371–1381. [CrossRef] [PubMed]

23. Lelliott, E.J.; Cullinane, C.; Martin, C.A.; Walker, R.; Ramsbottom, K.M.; Souza-Fonseca-Guimaraes, F.; AbuHammad, S.; Michie, J.; Kirby, L.; Young, R.J.; et al. A novel immunogenic mouse model of melanoma for the preclinical assessment of combination targeted and immune-based therapy. *Sci. Rep.* **2019**, *9*, 1225. [CrossRef]

24. Overwijk, W.W.; Theoret, M.R.; Finkelstein, S.E.; Surman, D.R.; De Jong, L.A.; Vyth-Dreese, F.A.; Dellemijn, T.A.; Antony, P.A.; Spiess, P.J.; Palmer, D.; et al. Tumor regression and autoimmunity after reversal of a functionally tolerant state of self-reactive CD8+ T cells. *J. Exp. Med.* **2003**, *198*, 569–580. [CrossRef]

25. Von Scheidt, B.; Wang, M.; Oliver, A.J.; Chan, J.D.; Jana, M.K.; Ali, A.I.; Clow, F.; Fraser, J.D.; Quinn, K.; Darcy, P.K.; et al. Enterotoxins can support CAR T cells against solid tumors. *Proc. Natl. Acad. Sci. USA* **2019**, *116*, 25229–25235. [CrossRef]

26. Kirtane, K.; Elmariah, H.; Chung, C.H.; Abate-Daga, D. Adoptive cellular therapy in solid tumor malignancies: Review of the literature and challenges ahead. *J. Immunother. Cancer* **2021**, *9*, e002723. [CrossRef]

27. Lee, J.; Shklovskaya, E.; Lim, S.Y.; Carlino, M.S.; Menzies, A.M.; Stewart, A.; Pedersen, B.; Irvine, M.; Alavi, S.; Yang, J.Y.H.; et al. Transcriptional downregulation of MHC class I and melanoma de- differentiation in resistance to PD-1 inhibition. *Nat. Commun.* **2020**, *11*, 1897. [CrossRef]

28. Zaretsky, J.M.; Garcia-Diaz, A.; Shin, D.S.; Escuin-Ordinas, H.; Hugo, W.; Hu-Lieskovan, S.; Torrejon, D.Y.; Abril-Rodriguez, G.; Sandoval, S.; Barthly, L.; et al. Mutations associated with acquired resistance to PD-1 blockade in melanoma. *N. Engl. J. Med.* **2016**, *375*, 819–829. [CrossRef]

29. Sapkota, B.; Hill, C.E.; Pollack, B.P. Vemurafenib enhances MHC induction inBRAFV600E homozygous melanoma cells. *OncoImmunology* **2013**, *2*, e22890. [CrossRef] [PubMed]

30. Sumimoto, H.; Imabayashi, F.; Iwata, T.; Kawakami, Y. The BRAF–MAPK signaling pathway is essential for cancer-immune evasion in human melanoma cells. *J. Exp. Med.* **2006**, *203*, 1651–1656. [CrossRef]

31. Borch, T.H.; Harbst, K.; Rana, A.H.; Andersen, R.; Martinenaite, E.; Kongsted, P.; Pedersen, M.; Nielsen, M.; Kjeldsen, J.W.; Kverneland, A.H.; et al. Clinical efficacy of T-cell therapy after short-term BRAF-inhibitor priming in patients with checkpoint inhibitor-resistant metastatic melanoma. *J. Immunother. Cancer* **2021**, *9*, e002703. [CrossRef] [PubMed]

32. Atay, C.; Kwak, T.; Lavilla-Alonso, S.; Donthireddy, L.; Richards, A.D.; Moberg, V.; Pilon-Thomas, S.; Schell, M.J.; Messina, J.L.; Rebecca, V.W.; et al. BRAF targeting sensitizes resistant melanoma to cytotoxic T cells. *Clin. Cancer Res. Off. J. Am. Assoc. Cancer Res.* **2019**, *25*, 2783–2794. [CrossRef] [PubMed]

33. Deniger, D.C.; Kwong, M.L.M.; Pasetto, A.; Dudley, M.E.; Wunderlich, J.R.; Langhan, M.M.; Lee, C.-C.; Rosenberg, S.A. A pilot trial of the combination of vemurafenib with adoptive cell therapy in patients with metastatic melanoma. *Clin. Cancer Res. Off. J. Am. Assoc. Cancer Res.* **2017**, *23*, 351–362. [CrossRef] [PubMed]

34. Schadendorf, D.; Long, G.; Stroyakovskiy, D.; Karaszewska, B.; Hauschild, A.; Levchenko, E.; Sileni, V.C.; Schachter, J.; Garbe, C.; Dutriaux, C.; et al. Three-year pooled analysis of factors associated with clinical outcomes across dabrafenib and trametinib combination therapy phase 3 randomised trials. *Eur. J. Cancer* **2017**, *82*, 45–55. [CrossRef] [PubMed]

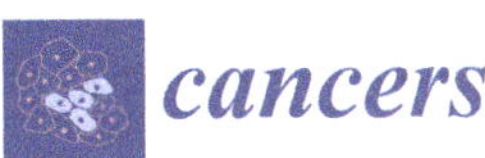 *cancers*

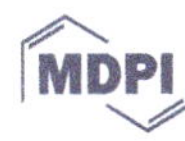

Article

Ropporin-1 and 1B Are Widely Expressed in Human Melanoma and Evoke Strong Humoral Immune Responses

Jessica Da Gama Duarte [1,2], Katherine Woods [1,2], Luke T. Quigley [1,2], Cyril Deceneux [1,2], Candani Tutuka [1,2], Tom Witkowski [1,2], Simone Ostrouska [1,2], Chris Hudson [1,2], Simon Chang-Hao Tsao [1,2], Anupama Pasam [1,2], Alexander Dobrovic [1,2,3], Jonathan M. Blackburn [4,5], Jonathan Cebon [1,2,6] and Andreas Behren [1,2,7,*]

[1] Olivia Newton-John Cancer Research Institute, Heidelberg, VIC 3084, Australia; jessica.duarte@onjcri.org.au (J.D.G.D.); katherine@nrlquality.org.au (K.W.); luke.quigley@onjcri.org.au (L.T.Q.); cyril.deceneux@rmit.edu.au (C.D.); dtutuka@akoyabio.com (C.T.); tom.witkowski@onjcri.org.au (T.W.); simone.ostrouska@onjcri.org.au (S.O.); chudson@phcn.vic.gov.au (C.H.); simon.tsao@svha.org.au (S.C.-H.T.); anu.pasam@petermac.org (A.P.); alexander.dobrovic@unimelb.edu.au (A.D.); j.cebon@onjcri.org.au (J.C.)

[2] School of Cancer Medicine, La Trobe University, Bundoora, VIC 3086, Australia

[3] Department of Clinical Pathology, Melbourne Medical School, University of Melbourne, Parkville, VIC 3010, Australia

[4] Department of Integrative Biomedical Sciences, Faculty of Health Sciences, University of Cape Town, Cape Town 7925, South Africa; jonathan.blackburn@uct.ac.za

[5] Institute for Infectious Disease and Molecular Medicine, University of Cape Town, Cape Town 7925, South Africa

[6] Medical Oncology Unit, Austin Health, Heidelberg, VIC 3084, Australia

[7] Department of Medicine—Austin, Melbourne Medical School, University of Melbourne, Parkville, VIC 3010, Australia

* Correspondence: andreas.behren@onjcri.org.au; Tel.: +61-3-9496-5837

Citation: Da Gama Duarte, J.; Woods, K.; Quigley, L.T.; Deceneux, C.; Tutuka, C.; Witkowski, T.; Ostrouska, S.; Hudson, C.; Tsao, S.C.-H.; Pasam, A.; et al. Ropporin-1 and 1B Are Widely Expressed in Human Melanoma and Evoke Strong Humoral Immune Responses. *Cancers* **2021**, *13*, 1805. https://doi.org/10.3390/cancers13081805

Academic Editor: Eduardo Nagore

Received: 22 March 2021
Accepted: 7 April 2021
Published: 9 April 2021

Publisher's Note: MDPI stays neutral with regard to jurisdictional claims in published maps and institutional affiliations.

Simple Summary: Despite the unprecedented clinical benefit of immunotherapy in melanoma, some patients still do not respond to treatment, arguing the need for novel therapeutic targets. The aim of this study was to investigate the therapeutic potential of two understudied proteins, Ropporin-1 (ROPN1) and 1B (ROPN1B). We confirmed that these proteins are widely expressed in melanoma patients using gene data derived from public datasets, and protein data derived from 61 patient tumours. Moreover, these proteins were able to evoke strong immune responses in 104 melanoma patients. These findings therefore suggest that ROPN1 and ROPN1B may be valuable targets for immunotherapy, alone or in combination with existing treatments.

Abstract: Antibodies that block immune regulatory checkpoints (programmed cell death 1, PD-1 and cytotoxic T-lymphocyte-associated antigen 4, CTLA-4) to mobilise immunity have shown unprecedented clinical efficacy against cancer, demonstrating the importance of antigen-specific tumour recognition. Despite this, many patients still fail to benefit from these treatments and additional approaches are being sought. These include mechanisms that boost antigen-specific immunity either by vaccination or adoptive transfer of effector cells. Other than neoantigens, epigenetically regulated and shared antigens such as NY-ESO-1 are attractive targets; however, tissue expression is often heterogeneous and weak. Therefore, peptide-specific therapies combining multiple antigens rationally selected to give additive anti-cancer benefits are necessary to achieve optimal outcomes. Here, we show that Ropporin-1 (ROPN1) and 1B (ROPN1B), cancer restricted antigens, are highly expressed and immunogenic, inducing humoral immunity in patients with advanced metastatic melanoma. By multispectral immunohistochemistry, 88.5% of melanoma patients tested ($n = 54/61$) showed ROPN1B expression in at least 1 of 2/3 tumour cores in tissue microarrays. Antibody responses against ROPN1A and ROPN1B were detected in 71.2% of melanoma patients tested ($n = 74/104$), with increased reactivity seen with more advanced disease stages. Thus, ROPN1A and ROPN1B may indeed be viable targets for cancer immunotherapy, alone or in combination with other cancer antigens, and could be combined with additional therapies such as immune checkpoint blockade.

Keywords: melanoma; tumour antigens; Ropporin-1; ROPN1; Ropporin-1B; ROPN1B

1. Introduction

Immune checkpoint blockade (ICB) targeting programmed cell death 1 (PD-1) and cytotoxic T-lymphocyte-associated antigen 4 (CTLA-4) has revolutionised the treatment of melanoma, with clinical benefit seen in up to 70% of patients when compared to either PD-1 (54%) or CTLA-4 blockade (41%) alone [1]. This is mediated by the induction or reactivation of antigen-specific effector T lymphocytes. There is considerable evidence that the peptide products of mutated genes [2] or aberrant post-translational changes are important immune targets in cancer [3]. These neoantigens have been correlated with patient responses to ICB. Additionally, a study in melanoma demonstrated immunogenicity of personalised neoantigen vaccines, designed to selectively target the mutated antigens of each patient [4]. However, next-generation sequencing and algorithms for human leukocyte antigen (HLA) binding indicate that as many as two thirds of human cancers do not generate mutational neoantigens at sufficiently high frequencies to ensure immune recognition [5,6]. Clearly, approaches that extend options for immunotherapy need to also account for tumours with low numbers or absent mutated antigens. Indeed, there is abundant evidence in pre-clinical models and in human clinical trials, indicating that ICB can be highly effective if combined with vaccines or adoptive cell transfer (ACT) of effector T lymphocytes, even in tumour models with few mutations [7–9]. Thus, combinations with antigen-specific therapeutic approaches are amendable for increasing the scope of ICB as long as appropriate antigens with optimal characteristics can be identified.

For practical purposes, vaccines that utilise shared antigens are attractive since this avoids the complexity and expense of generating customised products for individual patients. For such vaccines, the epigenetically-regulated cancer-testis antigens (CTAgs) can be considered as immune-neoantigens, since their expression is newly acquired as part of the malignant phenotype. A variety of CTAgs have been widely studied for their use as vaccine antigens or for ACT [10–13]. Arguably, the prototype CTAg is NY-ESO-1 (*CTAG1A* or identical gene copy *CTAG1B*), which induces spontaneous cellular and humoral immune responses in melanoma and other cancers [14–16]. However, while CTAgs have the distinct advantage of being tumour-specific, expression is often heterogeneous, patchy or weak [17]. To overcome this, cancer vaccines have been designed using several immunogenic epitopes from different CTAgs in combination [18–20]. To date, success with these treatment types has been limited. However, peptide vaccines are currently being reconsidered as combination treatments with ICB and ACT to boost immunity and broaden the cohort of responders [21–23]. Thus, identification of novel tumour-specific antigens continues to be of importance in the development of effective anti-cancer therapies. The ideal antigen would be one that is immunogenic and expressed in a large percentage of cancer patients, while limited in any normal tissue expression. Here, we describe and characterise ropporin-1 (ROPN1) and 1B (ROPN1B, 96% sequence homology with ROPN1) as antigens with the aforementioned properties. Based on studies of tissue distribution, CTAgs have been broadly classified as testis-restricted, testis/brain-restricted, and testis-selective, with ROPN1 being classified as the latter [24]. Despite this, the testis is an immune-privileged site that is protected from systemic immune attack, and hence ROPN1 or ROPN1B-specific therapeutic approaches should not result in testicular toxicity [25]. Hence, although poorly studied, we propose they represent promising targets for further clinical development.

Ropporin was firstly described in 1999 as a testis-restricted, rhophilin-binding protein by Fujita et al., using a yeast two hybrid screen on a mouse testis cDNA library [26]. Human ropporin has been shown to directly interact with and bind to A-kinase anchoring proteins (AKAPs) [27], predominantly AKAP110. While the exact function of ropporin remains elusive, its localization in sperm cells and expression data from patients with asthenozoospermia suggested a potential role in sperm motility [28]. The expression pattern of human ropporin is tissue-restricted, with the majority of expression detected in testis and foetal liver, as well as a variety of hematologic malignancies [29] and breast cancers [30].

A recent study using triple negative breast cancer cells suggests that ROPN1 activates RhoA signalling via rhophilin-1 (RHPN1), promoting cell migration, invasion and metastatic potential [30]. It was shown to be overexpressed in triple negative breast cancer cell lines and tissue, with high levels predictive of a poor prognosis [30]. Ropporin was identified as a potential target for immunotherapy in multiple myeloma, where its expression was detected in 44% of cases and its immunogenic potential was confirmed by the presence of antibodies and cytotoxic lymphocytes [31]. We therefore hypothesised that this may also be the case in melanoma and aimed to investigate the expression and immunogenicity of ROPN1 and ROPN1B. Here, we found that both ROPN1A and ROPN1B have favourable features as tumour antigens based on distribution and immunogenicity.

2. Results

2.1. Ropporin-1 (ROPN1) and Ropporin-1B (ROPN1B) Genes Are Expressed in Melanoma Samples and Correlated with Melanoma Differentiation Antigens

We tested the gene expression levels of *ROPN1* and *ROPN1B* (96% sequence homology with *ROPN1)* in a panel of melanoma cell lines generated in-house [32] (Table 1). In 45 out of 55 (81.8%) cell lines, we detected *ROPN1* gene expression compared to 46 out of 55 (83.6%) with *ROPN1B* expression (Figure 1A). For the purposes of comparison with a well-validated CTAg, we also determined the gene expression of *CTAG1A* (identical gene copy to *CTAG1B*) in the same cohort of cell lines. *CTAG1A* expression was detected in 20 out of 55 (36.4%) cell lines (Figure 1A), with 14 cell lines showing expression of both CTAgs. Expression of either *ROPN1/ROPN1B* or *CTAG1A* was observed in 52 out of 55 cell lines (94.5%).

Table 1. Summary of patient characteristics across all cohorts. This includes sample numbers, age, gender and disease stage. Cohort 1 was used to generate gene expression data (GEO dataset ID GSE89438) from 55 in-house generated melanoma cell lines derived from 52 patients [32]. Cohort 2 was used to generate gene expression data from 472 melanoma patient tumours derived from the TCGA Skin Cutaneous Melanoma Firehose Legacy dataset with 469 patients. Cohort 3 was used to generate protein expression data from 61 melanoma patient tumours across 2 TMAs (ME1002b, US Biomax, Derwood, MD, USA and 07 TMA Mel 1.8, in-house) derived from 61 patients. Cohort 4 was used to generate circulating antibody data from 104 melanoma patient serum or plasma. Gene Expression Omnibus, GEO; TCGA, The Cancer Genome Atlas; TMAs, tissue microarrays; yr, years.

	Cohort 1 (*n* = 52)	Cohort 2 (*n* = 469)	Cohort 3 (*n* = 61)	Cohort 4 (*n* = 104)
Sample Type	Cell lines	Tumours	Tumours	Serum or Plasma
Used to Determine	Gene Expression	Gene Expression	Protein Expression	Circulating Antibodies
Age–yr				
Median	56	58	53	54
Range	25–83	15–90	21–88	21–87
Gender–no. (%)				
Unknown	0 (0)	0 (0)	0 (0)	1 (0.9)
Male	33 (63.5)	289 (61.6)	35 (57.4)	63 (60.6)
Female	19 (36.5)	180 (38.4)	26 (42.6)	40 (38.5)
Stage–no. (%)				
Unknown	9 (17.3)	59 (12.6)	6 (9.8)	7 (6.7)
I	0 (0)	77 (16.4)	5 (8.2)	2 (1.9)
II	1 (1.9)	140 (29.9)	21 (34.4)	9 (8.7)
III	22 (42.3)	170 (36.2)	4 (6.6)	35 (33.7)
IV	20 (38.5)	23 (4.9)	25 (41.0)	51 (49.0)

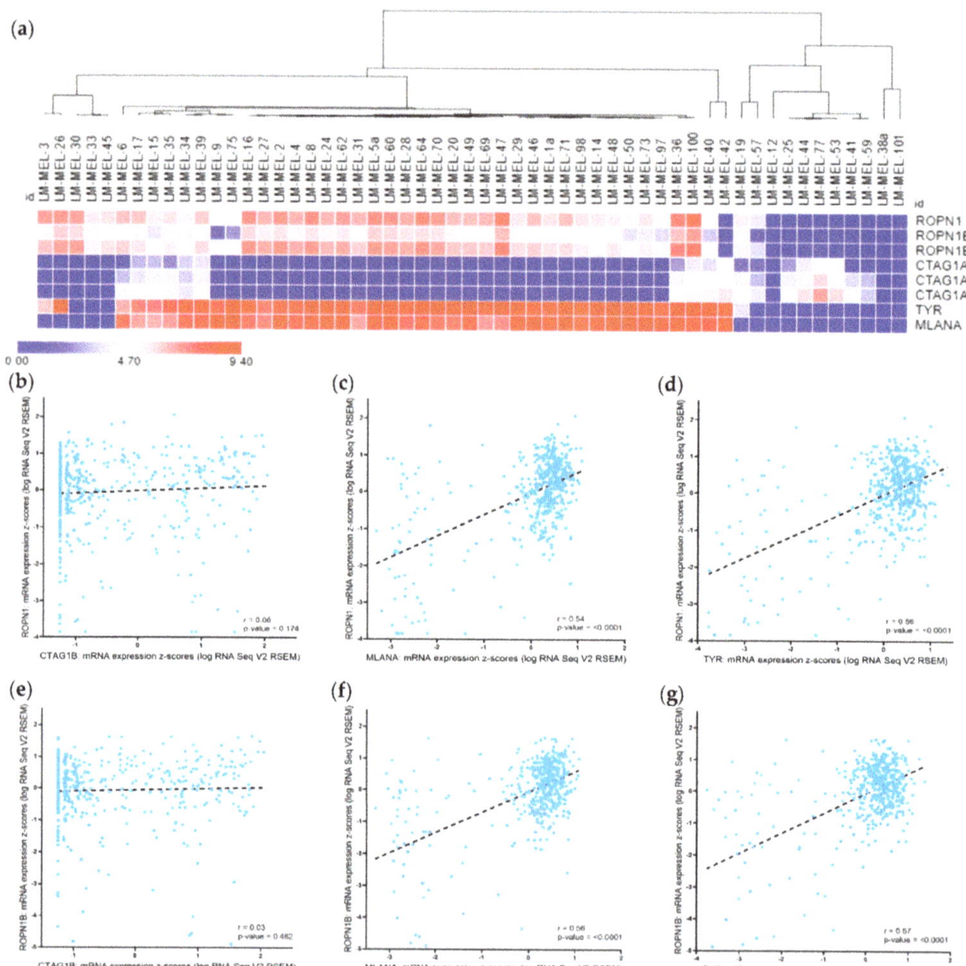

Figure 1. Gene expression of *ROPN1*, *ROPN1B*, *CTAG1A/B*, *TYR* and *MLANA* in melanoma cell lines and tumours. (**a**) Heat map representing the hierarchical clustering by Pearson correlation of *ROPN1*, *ROPN1B*, *CTAG1A*, *TYR* and *MLANA* gene expression in 55 in-house generated melanoma cell lines derived from 52 patients [32]. Each row shows absolute level of expression results for one specific probe for the respective gene. The full gene expression dataset can be found under GEO dataset ID GSE89438. (**b**) mRNA co-expression plots for *ROPN1* and *CTAG1B* ($r = -0.06$, *p*-value = 0.174), or (**c**) *TYR* ($r = 0.56$, *p*-value < 0.0001) or (**d**) *MLANA* ($r = 0.54$, *p*-value < 0.0001); and (**e**) mRNA co-expression plots for *ROPN1B* and *CTAG1B* ($r = 0.03$, *p*-value = 0.482), or (**f**) *TYR* ($r = 0.57$, *p*-value < 0.0001) or (**g**) *MLANA* ($r = 0.56$, *p*-value < 0.0001) in 472 TCGA melanoma patient samples (469 patients). mRNA expression is shown as z-scores relative to all samples (log RNA Seq V2 RSEM), and correlation is analysed using the Pearson correlation. Gene Expression Omnibus, GEO; TCGA, The Cancer Genome Atlas.

The expression of differentiation antigens that are commonly present and have been previously used as immunological targets in melanoma, namely, *TYR* (tyrosinase) and *MLANA* (Melan-A/MART1) [20,33], were compared with *CTAG1A* and *ROPN1* or *ROPN1B* in our panel of melanoma cell lines. We found a strong correlation in the expression of both *TYR* and *MLANA* with *ROPN1* and *ROPN1B* among our cell line panel (Figure 1A, *TYR* vs. *ROPN1*: $r = 0.73$, *p*-value < 0.0001; *TYR* vs. *ROPN1B*: $r = 0.73$, *p*-value < 0.0001; *MLANA* vs. *ROPN1*: $r = 0.61$, *p*-value < 0.0001; *MLANA* vs. *ROPN1B*: $r = 0.61$, *p*-value < 0.0001). In contrast, *CTAG1A* expression was found in more differentiated cell lines with high *TYR* and/or *MLANA* expression, and in less differentiated ones without *TYR* and/or *MLANA* expression (Figure 1A).

We further evaluated the gene expression levels of *ROPN1, ROPN1B, CTAG1B* (identical gene copy to *CTAG1A* for which no gene expression data is available), *TYR* and *MLANA* in 472 additional melanoma samples using data accessible via The Cancer Genome Atlas (TCGA) (Table 1). As expected, expression of *ROPN1* and its paralog *ROPN1B* was highly correlated ($r = 0.86$, *p*-value $= 8.71 \times 10^{-141}$). *ROPN1* and *ROPN1B* were expressed at transcript level in nearly all melanomas (*ROPN1*: $n = 467/472$, 98.9%, *ROPN1B*: $n = 466/472$, 98.7%), more frequently than *CTAG1B* ($n = 322/472$, 68.2%), and sometimes exclusively (Figure 1B, *ROPN1*: $r = 0.06$, *p*-value$=0.174$; Figure 1E, *ROPN1B*: $r = 0.03$, *p*-value $= 0.482$). As expected, *TYR* ($n = 469/472$, 99.4%) and *MLANA* ($n = 471/472$, 99.8%) were commonly expressed. We further demonstrated co-expression of *ROPN1/ROPN1B* and *TYR* (*ROPN1*: $r = 0.56$, *p*-value < 0.0001; *ROPN1B*: $r = 0.57$, *p*-value < 0.0001) or *MLANA* (*ROPN1*: $r = 0.54$, *p*-value < 0.0001; *ROPN1B*: $r = 0.56$, *p*-value < 0.0001) in the majority of patient samples (Figure 1C, 1F and 1D, 1G, respectively), and found no correlation between differentiation antigens and *CTAG1B* expression (Figure S1, *TYR*: $r = -0.06$, *p*-value$=0.165$, *MLANA*: $r = -0.05$, *p*-value $= 0.268$), reflecting the results of our cell line analysis.

We further investigated *ROPN1, ROPN1B* and *CTAG1B* gene expression across different stages of disease and genders in melanoma. *ROPN1, ROPN1B* and *CTAG1B* were expressed across all AJCC disease stages, without apparent differences (Figure S2, *ROPN1*: *p*-value $= 0.179$; *ROPN1B*: *p*-value $= 0.140$; *CTAG1B*: *p*-value $= 0.338$). Similarly, no difference was observed between males and females (Figure S3, *ROPN1*: *p*-value $= 0.944$; *ROPN1B*: *p*-value $= 0.362$; *CTAG1B*: *p*-value $= 0.829$).

2.2. Ropporin-1B (ROPN1B) Protein Is Expressed in Melanoma Tumours

We assessed expression of ROPN1B, NY-ESO-1 (single protein from *CTAG1A* or *CTAG1B* genes), MLANA and SOX10 (used here as a melanoma tumour marker) at the protein level by multispectral immunohistochemistry on melanoma tissue microarrays (TMAs) comprising two or three cores from 61 patient tumours (Table 1). Protein expression levels were at times heterogeneous amongst patient cores, and lack of expression was only reported in cases where all cores per patient were assessable. ROPN1B cytoplasmic expression was observed in 88.5% ($n = 54/61$) of patient samples, while cytoplasmic NY-ESO-1 was observed in 16.4% ($n = 10/61$) of samples (Figure S4). Expression of both ROPN1B and NY-ESO-1 was seen in 9 cases ($n = 9/61$, 14.8%), where tumour cells within cores showed instances of co-expression or exclusive expression of ROPN1B and/or NY-ESO-1 (Figures 2 and 3). Moreover, ROPN1B expression was often detected ubiquitously, whereas NY-ESO-1 appeared more scattered and diffuse throughout tumour cores (Figure S5). In patient samples with expression of both ROPN1B and NY-ESO-1, cells with exclusive ROPN1B positivity increased tumour cell coverage by 29.3% on average (range from 9.0% to 73.0%, Figure 3). Nuclear SOX10 ($n = 60/61$) or cytoplasmic MLANA ($n = 60/61$) expression was detected in nearly all tumour cores, as expected (Figure 2 and Figure S5).

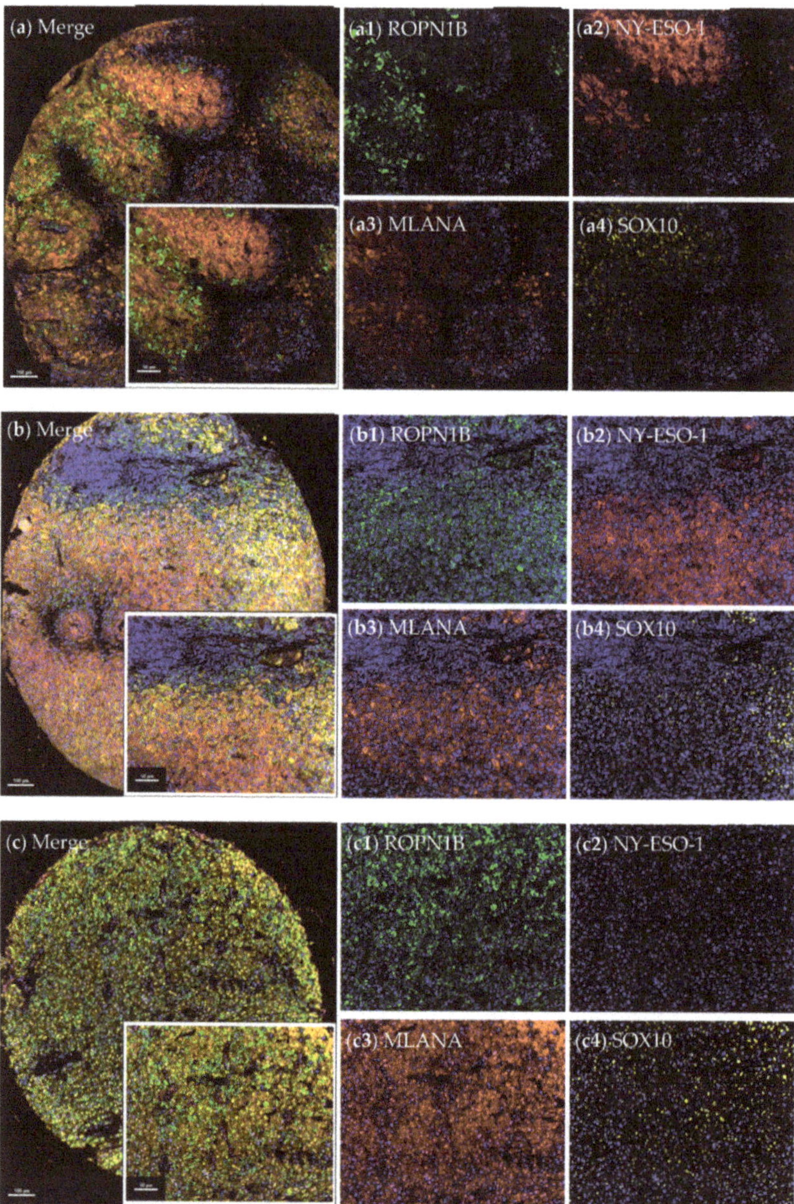

Figure 2. Patterns of ROPN1B and NY-ESO-1 expression in melanoma tumours. Multispectral immunohistochemistry of melanoma tumour cores showing staining for ROPN1B, NY-ESO-1, MLANA and SOX10. Representative cores showing ROPN1B and NY-ESO-1 co-expression in discreet (**a**) or shared (**b**) tumour regions, as well as exclusive (**c**) ROPN1B expression. Tissue microarrays were stained with anti-ROPN1B (green), anti-NY-ESO-1 (red), anti-MLANA (orange) and anti-SOX10 (yellow) antibodies with DAPI (blue) counterstain, and are displayed as merge (**a,b,c**) and single colour (**a1–a4,b1–b4, c1–c4**) cores. Whole tumour cores with more than 2% of the tissue cells staining for the target proteins were considered positive. All images were taken using a 20× objective, and scale bars indicate 100 μm (core) or 50 μm (region of interest).

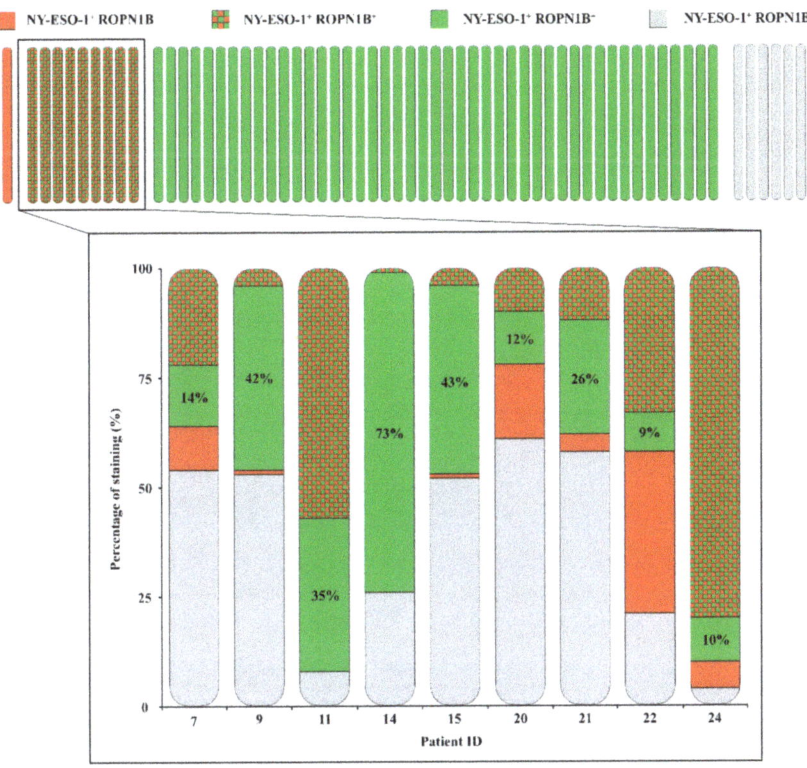

Figure 3. Tumour cell coverage of ROPN1B and NY-ESO-1 expression in investigated melanoma tumours. Upper panel indicates number of tumours with any expression of NY-ESO-1 alone (red), NY-ESO-1 and ROPN1B (chequered red and green), ROPN1B alone (green) or neither (grey) across the cohort. Magnified panel depicts quantitative distribution of NY-ESO-1 and ROPN1B staining relative to SOX10+ melanoma cells across patients displaying both NY-ESO-1 and ROPN1B expression. Percentages on bars show ROPN1B expression alone.

ROPN1B expression was seen in both early (I and II, n = 19/26, 73.1%) and late stages (III and IV, n = 29/29, 100.0%) of disease, more so than NY-ESO-1 (n = 1/26, 3.8% vs. n = 9/29, 31.0%, respectively). Nonetheless, expression was more predominant in advanced disease (ROPN1B: chi-square p-value = 0.003; NY-ESO-1: chi-square p-value = 0.009), with evidence of more abundant melanoma cell expression in tumour cores, in contrast to sparse, dispersed cells commonly identified in early-stage disease. ROPN1B (females: 88.5%, n = 23/26 vs. males: 88.6%, n = 31/35, chi-square p-value = 0.989) and NY-ESO-1 (females: 11.5%, n = 3/26 vs. males: 20.0%, n = 7/35, chi-square p-value = 0.377) protein expression did not differ between genders.

2.3. Ropporin-1A (ROPN1A) and Ropporin-1B (ROPN1B) Are Immunogenic Antigens in Melanoma

To explore the immunogenic potential of ROPN1A and ROPN1B, we screened sera or plasma from 104 melanoma patients (Table 1). These were tested for the presence and titre of antibodies against ROPN1A/B, NY-ESO-1, MLANA and TYR (Table S2). Antibodies were detected above noise threshold against ROPN1A/B in 71.2% (n = 74/104) of patients, and against NY-ESO-1 in 63.5% (n = 66/104) of patients. Although there were instances where reactivity was exclusive to either ROPN1A/B (19.2%, n = 20/104) or NY-ESO-1 (11.6%, n = 12/104), co-reactivity was seen in many cases (51.9%, n = 54/104) (Figure 4). Alternatively, a small subset of patients had reactivity to neither (17.3%, n = 18/104). In addition, co-reactivity against both ROPN1A/B and TYR (39.4%, $n = 41/104$) or ROPN1A/B and MLANA (31.7%, $n = 33/104$) was also seen, although to a lesser degree. Only 10.6% ($n = 11/104$) of the patient cohort had no antibody reactivity to any of these antigens.

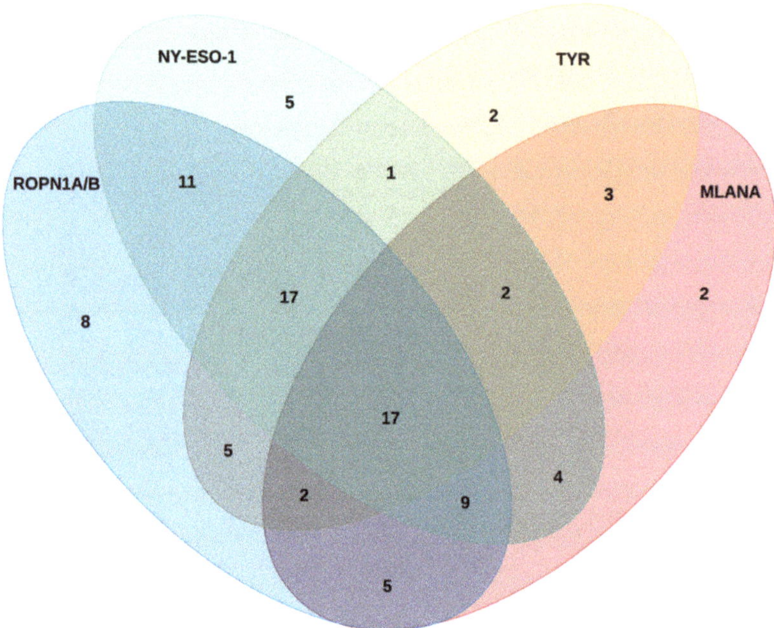

Figure 4. Venn diagram displaying predominance of ROPN1A/B, NY-ESO-1, TYR and MLANA-specific antibodies in melanoma patients. Antibody titres were measured in 104 melanoma patients using a custom protein microarray platform, and all resulting intensities above 500 RFU (defined noise threshold) were considered positive signals and plotted using a 4-way Venn diagram. RFU, relative fluorescent units.

This cohort consisted predominately of stage III and IV melanoma patients, with 74.4% ($n = 64/86$) of these seropositive for ROPN1A/B, and 62.8% ($n = 54/86$) seropositive for NY-ESO-1. Furthermore, it included 60.6% males and 38.8% females, with no gender-related differences seen for ROPN1A/B (females: 75.0%, $n = 30/40$ vs. males: 69.8%, $n = 44/63$, chi-square p-value = 0.571) or NY-ESO-1 antibody reactivity (females: 62.5%, $n = 25/40$ vs. males: 63.5%, $n = 40/63$ chi-square p-value = 0.919) (Figure S6).

3. Discussion

Neoantigens that arise from somatic mutations can play an important role in immune tumour rejection [34] but generally differ from tumour to tumour. In order to create personalised vaccines against these targets, individual therapies need to be tailored on a patient-by-patient basis, requiring gene sequencing and manufacturing of antigens. This approach has limitations for routine clinical use across hospitals both in terms of the associated costs and extensive timeframes. Nevertheless, a small study in melanoma designed personalised neoantigen-based peptide vaccines for six patients, which led to the generation of tumour-specific CD4[+] and CD8[+] T lymphocyte responses and clinical benefit (four out of six patients remaining cancer free at a 25-month follow up) [4]. One reason cited for the failure of prior therapies in melanoma, including cancer vaccine- based treatments, has been the considerable heterogeneity of melanoma cells [35,36]. Phenotypic plasticity and differentiation/de-differentiation is a likely contributor to this heterogeneity as it has been known to result in antigen down-regulation. Indeed, epithelial to mesenchymal transition-like phenotype switching has been implicated as an escape mechanism following vaccination or ACT [37,38]. CTAgs comprise a large group of antigens, many of which are expressed following de-repression of epigenetic silencing in cancer [39]. In contrast to the unique products of mutations, their expression is shared between tumours and restricted normal tissues, mostly at immune-privileged sites. Therefore, they are able to stimulate potent immune responses [40] and many have been widely trialled as vaccine antigens [39]. Namely, an NY-ESO-1 vaccine was able to induce antigen-specific cellular and humoral responses but did not affect overall survival, possibly due to its limited tumour expression [41].

In this study, gene-expression profiling of a large panel of early-passage melanoma cell lines [32] identified *ROPN1* and *ROPN1B* as being highly expressed in melanoma tumour samples (*ROPN1*: 81.8%, *ROPN1B*: 83.6%), more so than *CTAG1* (36.4%). Similarly, gene expression of *ROPN1* and *ROPN1B* was also commonly detected in a melanoma patient cohort accessed via the TCGA (*ROPN1*: 98.9%, *ROPN1B*: 98.7% vs. *CTAG1B*: 68.2%). When investigating melanoma TMAs, 88.5% of patient tumours expressed ROPN1B, a much larger proportion compared to NY-ESO-1 (16.4%). Even in instances of tumours expressing both NY-ESO-1 and ROPN1B (14.8%), the addition of ROPN1B increased the tumour cell coverage substantially.

The role of antibodies against tumour antigens in melanoma is unclear [42–44], and while an antibody response is not necessarily accompanied by cellular immunity, these often go hand-in-hand [45,46]. Antibody profiling using a custom protein array [47] detected high-titre antibodies against ROPN1A/B in the serum or plasma of a large cohort of melanoma patients (71.2%), more so when compared to NY-ESO-1 (63.5%). NY-ESO-1 antibodies were more commonly detected than expected, based on the above gene and protein expression studies. In previous studies that assessed the frequency of NY-ESO-1 antibody responses, reports have described NY-ESO-1-specific antibodies in ~10% [15] to 45% [48] of patients. However, the protein array used here is more sensitive than ELISA [47], which would contribute to a higher percentage of patients with detectable anti-NY-ESO-1 and/or anti-ROPN1A/B antibody responses when compared to historical data. Alternatively, NY-ESO-1 is known to be highly immunogenic, and hence it is possible that the detected circulating antibodies may be a result of earlier NY-ESO-1$^+$ cell eradication. Similarly, the prevalence of detectable antibodies against MLANA and TYR were below expected levels, particularly when considering the above gene expression data, arguing for inferior humoral immunogenicity when compared to ROPN1A/B and NY-ESO-1. Furthermore, a trend towards increasing ROPN1A/B and NY-ESO-1 antibody reactivity was seen with progression of disease stage. For example, 54.5% of Stage I/II had antibody responses to ROPN1A/B, compared with 74.4% of stage III/IV patients. The number of stage I and II patients screened here (n = 11) was too small to allow us to draw definitive conclusions, however, prior studies have also demonstrated a correlative increase in the proportion of NY-ESO-1 seropositivity with disease stage [17,49]. In addition, we observed that ROPN1A/B reactivity was slightly increased in females, albeit not significantly. This observation was also noted in a recent study where antibody responses to ROPN1 were significantly higher in female multiple myeloma patients [50]. An increased humoral response in females may explain the reduced melanoma incidence and the increased survival benefit independent of disease stage reported in women [51,52]. Together, these data show that (i) NY-ESO-1, ROPN1 and ROPN1B are highly immunogenic; and (ii) patients who have no evidence of NY-ESO-1 immunity can have antibody titres against other CTAgs, including ROPN1A and ROPN1B, thereby validating that the addition of ROPN1A and ROPN1B as target antigens can potentially enlarge the population of eligible patients who might benefit from a combined vaccine approach.

Ongoing immune editing occurring over the course of disease allows cancer escape from immune targeting of individual antigens [53]. For these reasons, the potential to achieve increased tumour coverage by targeting NY-ESO-1, ROPN1A and ROPN1B combined makes these immunogenic CTAgs highly compatible for combination in a cancer vaccine with the potential to generate synergistic immune responses to the tumour. It is tempting to speculate that further immunogenic tumour antigens could also be incorporated, leading to the design of a cancer vaccine that "covers all bases" in terms of heterogeneity and plasticity. As strategies are being pursued to widen the applicability of cancer immunotherapy, vaccination is now being proposed and trialled (NCT03092453) in combination with other immunotherapies, such as ICB [22,54,55]. Our study indicates that ROPN1A and ROPN1B may serve as promising candidates for such antigen-specific approaches, and therefore further studies are warranted and should be pursued to explore this.

4. Materials and Methods

4.1. Human Ethics Approval

Blood samples used in this study were derived from patients who provided written informed consent to participate in a clinical research protocol approved by the Austin Health Human Research Ethics Committee (HREC/14/Austin/425, approved on 6 November 2014) (Table 1).

4.2. Melanoma Cell Lines and Cell Culture

Establishment and characterisation of the melanoma cell lines used has been previously described [32]. Cells were cultured in RPMI 1640, 2 mM Glutamax, 100 U/mL Penicillin, 100 µg/mL Streptomycin and 10% foetal calf serum (RF10) (all Invitrogen, Carlsbad, CA, USA).

4.3. Cell Pellet DNA Extraction

DNA was extracted from pelleted cells using a DNeasy® Blood and Tissue kit (Qiagen, Hilden, Germany) as per the manufacturer's instructions. Briefly, pellets were suspended in 200 µL of PBS with 36 µL of Proteinase K (600 mAU/mL, Scimar, Templestowe, VIC, Australia) and 200µL AL buffer (Qiagen, Hilden, Germany), then incubated at 56 °C overnight. Clean-up was as per the manufacturer's instructions and samples were eluted in 50 µL of AE buffer (Qiagen, Hilden, Germany).

4.4. Gene Expression—Cell Lines

The gene expression array method and analysis have been previously described (Gene Expression Omnibus, GEO dataset ID GSE89438) [32,56]. Briefly, genomic DNA was purified from 55 melanoma cell lines originating from 52 patients (Qiagen AllPrep kit, Hilden, Germany) and assayed using Illumina standard protocols. Samples were subjected to whole-genome expression arrays (Illumina HT12, San Diego, CA, USA), and hierarchical clustering by Pearson correlation of *ROPN1* (probe ID: 5420739), *ROPN1B* (probe IDs: 730521 and 460291; 96% sequence homology with *ROPN1*), *CTAG1A* (probe IDs: 6770332, 1430215 and 1070577; identical gene copy to *CTAG1B*), *TYR* (probe ID: 5260253) and *MLANA* (probe ID: 7330367) was performed using the Morpheus software (https://software.broadinstitute.org/morpheus/index.html, Broad Institute, Cambridge, MA, USA). Absolute values were used to determine level of expression across cell lines, with any level above 0.3 considered "positive" for expression.

4.5. Gene Expression—The Cancer Genome Atlas (TCGA)

The gene expression data of *ROPN1*, *ROPN1B*, *CTAG1B* (identical gene copy to *CTAG1A* for which no gene expression data is available), *TYR* and *MLANA* in melanoma tumour samples was accessible via TCGA research network (http://cancergenome.nih.gov/) and analysed using the cBioPortal [57,58]. The TCGA dataset used was the Skin Cutaneous Melanoma, TCGA, Firehose Legacy, consisting of 472 samples (469 patients). Absolute mRNA transcript values were used to determine level of expression across TCGA patient samples, with any transcript level above zero considered "positive" for expression. mRNA expression of the respective genes is shown as z-scores (RNA Seq V2 RSEM) and represented in a log2 scale. Co-expression of mRNA is analysed using the Pearson correlation.

4.6. Multispectral Immunohistochemistry

Two (ME1002b, US Biomax, Derwood, MD, USA and 07 TMA Mel 1.8, in-house) melanoma TMAs containing two or three cores for 61 melanoma patient tumours (59 patients) were baked at 65 °C for 2 h, dewaxed in xylene three times for 10 min, rehydrated in ethanol twice for 10 min and manually stained. The staining included initial blocking of endogenous peroxidases using 3% hydrogen peroxide for 30 min, followed by sequential 15 min rounds of heat-induced epitope retrieval (microwave at 20% power); 10 min blocking of non-specific binding sites; 30 min primary (anti-NY-ESO-1 (single protein from *CTAG1A* or *CTAG1B* genes); ROPN1B, MLANA or SOX10); 10 min secondary (anti-mouse and anti-rabbit Opal™ horseradish peroxidase) antibody incubation; and 10 min fluorophore-tyramide signal amplification using Opal™ 520, 570, 620 and 690 fluorophores labelling target proteins, respectively (Akoya Biosciences®, Marlborough, MA, USA) (Table S1). Slides were counterstained with spectral DAPI, and tissue cores were scanned using the Vectra 3 Automated Quantitative Pathology Imaging System (Akoya Biosciences®, Marlborough, MA, USA) where target proteins were detected and imaged using the FITC, Cy3, Texas red and Cy5 filter cubes. Images were spectrally unmixed and analysed using inForm® Cell Analysis software version 3.0.5 or HALO™ Image Analysis Software version 3.2 (Akoya Biosciences®, Marlborough, MA, USA) with the assistance of a pathologist. Whole tumour cores with more than 2% of the tissue cells staining for the target proteins in at least one out of two or three cores per patient tumour were considered positive. Staining pattern of localization was defined as nuclear (if co-localised with DAPI) or cytoplasmic. Cytoplasmic staining was distinguished from membranous staining by performing immunohistochemistry using anti-MHC class I antibody (membranous expression on melanoma cells that have not experienced MHC class I loss, as well as stromal cells) with either anti-ROPN1B, anti-NY-ESO-1 or anti-MLANA antibodies, along with DAPI counterstain in melanoma tumours.

4.7. Antibody Profiling

Serum or plasma from melanoma patients was used to measure antibody titres towards ROPN1A/B, NY-ESO-1, MLANA and TYR using a custom tumour antigen protein microarray platform [47]. Blood samples originated from melanoma patients without available matched tumour tissue. Following the printing of previously expressed biotinylated antigens to a streptavidin-coated microarray slide using a QArray2 robotic arrayer (Genetix, Berkshire, UK), slides were immersed in blocking buffer (50 µM biotin in PBST) and incubated on ice in a plastic chamber protected from light for 1 h. Slides were then washed three times for 5 min in PBST and dried. Individual arrays were incubated with a unique serum or plasma sample (100 µL at 1:800 or 1:400 dilution, respectively) for 1 h at RT, washed in PBST and dH$_2$O, and incubated with 100 µL of 20 µg/mL Alexa Fluor 647 Goat anti-Human IgG (H + L) (Invitrogen, Carlsbad, CA, USA, 1:100 dilution in PBST) for 30 min at RT. The individual arrays were then washed, dried and scanned using a Tecan LS Reloaded fluorescence microarray scanner (Tecan Group Ltd., Männedorf, Switzerland) in automatic gain control (AGC) mode. All liquid handling steps were performed using QuadChambers on a Tecan HS4800 Pro automated hybridization station (Tecan Group Ltd., Männedorf, Switzerland). The resulting arrays were viewed using the ArrayPro Analyzer software Version 6.3 (Media Cybernetics, Rockville, MD, USA), and raw data was extracted. Finally, these data were processed using a custom bioinformatic tool for protein microarray data processing and normalisation, and the resulting data were analysed accordingly [59].

5. Conclusions

In this study, we have identified ROPN1 and ROPN1B as compelling novel therapeutic antigen targets for further clinical evaluation. Features include frequent humoral immunogenicity and abundance, with virtually universal tumour-specific expression across all melanomas tested.

Supplementary Materials: The following are available online at https://www.mdpi.com/article/10.3390/cancers13081805/s1, Figure S1: Gene expression of *CTAG1B* and differentiation antigens *TYR* and *MLANA* in melanoma tumours, Figure S2: Gene expression of *ROPN1, ROPN1B* and *CTAG1B* by AJCC disease stage codes in melanoma tumours, Figure S3: Gene expression of *ROPN1, ROPN1B* and *CTAG1B* by gender in melanoma tumours, Figure S4: Cytoplasmic expression of ROPN1B, NY-ESO-1 and MLANA in melanoma tumours, Figure S5: Variability seen between concentrated ROPN1B and diffuse NY-ESO-1 staining patterns in melanoma tumours, Figure S6: Venn diagram displaying predominance of ROPN1A/B and NY-ESO-1-specific antibodies in melanoma patients by gender, Table S1: Specifications of antibodies and conditions used for multispectral immunohistochemistry, Table S2: ROPN1A, ROPN1B, NY-ESO-1, MLANA and TYR-specific antibodies in melanoma patients.

Author Contributions: Conceptualization, J.D.G.D., K.W., A.D., J.M.B., J.C. and A.B.; methodology, J.D.G.D., K.W., L.T.Q., C.D., C.T., T.W., S.O., C.H., S.C.-H.T., A.P. and A.B.; formal analysis, J.D.G.D., K.W., L.T.Q., C.D., C.T., T.W., S.O., C.H., S.C.-H.T. and A.P.; investigation, J.D.G.D., K.W., L.T.Q., C.D., C.T., T.W., S.O., C.H., S.C.-H.T., A.P.; resources, A.D., J.M.B., J.C. and A.B.; data curation, J.D.G.D., K.W., L.T.Q., C.D., C.T., T.W., S.O., C.H., S.C.-H.T. and A.P.; writing—original draft preparation, J.D.G.D., K.W., and A.B.; writing—review and editing, J.D.G.D., K.W., L.T.Q., and A.B.; supervision, J.D.G.D., K.W., A.D., J.M.B., J.C. and A.B.; funding acquisition, A.D., J.M.B., J.C. and A.B. All authors have read and agreed to the published version of the manuscript.

Funding: This project was partially funded by a Clinical and Laboratory Integration Program (CLIP) grant from the Cancer Research Institute (CRI). This project was also funded in part by the Ludwig Institute for Cancer Research, Melanoma Research Alliance (MRA) and the Melbourne Research Victoria (MRV). The Olivia Newton-John Cancer Research Institute acknowledges the support of the Victorian Government Operational Infrastructure Support Program and the Ian Potter Foundation for providing funds to purchase the Vectra System. The contents of the published material are solely the responsibility of La Trobe University and do not reflect the views of Cancer Australia. J.D.G.D. is supported by Cure Cancer Australia through the Cancer Australia Priority-driven Cancer Research Scheme (#1187815). J.M.B. is supported by a research chair from the National Research Foundation (South Africa). A.B. is supported by a fellowship from the Department of Health and Human Services acting through the Victorian Cancer Agency (VCA).

Institutional Review Board Statement: Clinical research protocol approved on 6 November 2014 by the Austin Health Human Research Ethics Committee (HREC/14/Austin/425).

Informed Consent Statement: Informed consent was obtained from all subjects involved in the study.

Data Availability Statement: Publicly available datasets were analysed in this study. This data can be found here: https://www.ncbi.nlm.nih.gov/geo/query/acc.cgi?acc=GSE89438; and here: http://www.cbioportal.org/study/summary?id=skcm_tcga. The remaining data presented in this study are available within the article or in the supplementary material.

Acknowledgments: The authors would like to thank Ryan Farid and Nektaria Dimopoulous for their technical support.

Conflicts of Interest: The authors declare no conflict of interest. The funders had no role in the design of the study; in the collection, analyses, or interpretation of data; in the writing of the manuscript; or in the decision to publish the results.

References

1. Larkin, J.; Chiarion-Sileni, V.; Gonzalez, R.; Grob, J.J.; Rutkowski, P.; Lao, C.D.; Cowey, C.L.; Schadendorf, D.; Wagstaff, J.; Dummer, R.; et al. Five-year survival with combined nivolumab and ipilimumab in advanced melanoma. *N. Engl. J. Med.* **2019**, *381*, 1535–1546. [CrossRef] [PubMed]
2. Rizvi, N.A.; Hellmann, M.D.; Snyder, A.; Kvistborg, P.; Makarov, V.; Havel, J.J.; Lee, W.; Yuan, J.; Wong, P.; Ho, T.S.; et al. Cancer immunology. Mutational landscape determines sensitivity to PD-1 blockade in non-small cell lung cancer. *Science* **2015**, *348*, 124–128. [CrossRef] [PubMed]

3. Malaker, S.A.; Penny, S.A.; Steadman, L.G.; Myers, P.T.; Loke, J.C.; Raghavan, M.; Bai, D.L.; Shabanowitz, J.; Hunt, D.F.; Cobbold, M. Identification of Glycopeptides as Posttranslationally Modified Neoantigens in Leukemia. *Cancer Immunol. Res.* **2017**, *5*, 376–384. [CrossRef] [PubMed]

4. Ott, P.A.; Hu, Z.; Keskin, D.B.; Shukla, S.A.; Sun, J.; Bozym, D.J.; Zhang, W.; Luoma, A.; Giobbie-Hurder, A.; Peter, L.; et al. An immunogenic personal neoantigen vaccine for patients with melanoma. *Nature* **2017**, *547*, 217–221. [CrossRef] [PubMed]

5. Alexandrov, L.B.; Nik-Zainal, S.; Wedge, D.C.; Aparicio, S.A.J.R.; Behjati, S.; Biankin, A.V.; Bignell, G.R.; Bolli, N.; Borg, A.; Børresen-Dale, A.L.; et al. Signatures of mutational processes in human cancer. *Nature* **2013**, *500*, 415–421. [CrossRef]

6. Chalmers, Z.R.; Connelly, C.F.; Fabrizio, D.; Gay, L.; Ali, S.M.; Ennis, R.; Schrock, A.; Campbell, B.; Shlien, A.; Chmielecki, J.; et al. Analysis of 100,000 human cancer genomes reveals the landscape of tumor mutational burden. *Genome Med.* **2017**, *9*, 1–14. [CrossRef] [PubMed]

7. Fourcade, J.; Sun, Z.; Pagliano, O.; Chauvin, J.-M.; Sander, C.; Janjic, B.; Tarhini, A.A.; Tawbi, H.A.; Kirkwood, J.M.; Moschos, S.; et al. PD-1 and Tim-3 regulate the expansion of tumor antigen-specific CD8$^+$ T cells induced by melanoma vaccines. *Cancer Res.* **2014**, *74*, 1045–1055. [CrossRef] [PubMed]

8. Mahvi, D.A.; Meyers, J.V.; Tatar, A.J.; Contreras, A.; Suresh, M.; Leverson, G.E.; Sen, S.; Cho, C.S. Ctla-4 blockade plus adoptive T-cell transfer promotes optimal melanoma immunity in mice. *J. Immunother.* **2015**, *38*, 54–61. [CrossRef]

9. Kuramitsu, S.; Yamamichi, A.; Ohka, F.; Motomura, K.; Hara, M.; Natsume, A. Adoptive immunotherapy for the treatment of glioblastoma: Progress and possibilities. *Immunotherapy* **2016**, *8*, 1393–1404. [CrossRef]

10. Davis, I.D.; Chen, W.; Jackson, H.; Parente, P.; Shackleton, M.; Hopkins, W.; Chen, Q.; Dimopoulos, N.; Luke, T.; Murphy, R.; et al. Recombinant NY-ESO-1 protein with ISCOMATRIX adjuvant induces broad integrated antibody and CD4(+) and CD8(+) T cell responses in humans. *Proc. Natl. Acad. Sci. USA* **2004**, *101*, 10697–10702. [CrossRef]

11. Maraskovsky, E. NY-ESO-1 Protein Formulated in ISCOMATRIX Adjuvant Is a Potent Anticancer Vaccine Inducing Both Humoral and CD8+ T-Cell-Mediated Immunity and Protection against NY-ESO-1+ Tumors. *Clin. Cancer Res.* **2004**, *10*, 2879–2890. [CrossRef]

12. Phan, G.Q.; Rosenberg, S.A. Adoptive cell transfer for patients with metastatic melanoma: The potential and promise of cancer immunotherapy. *Cancer Control* **2013**, *20*, 289–297. [CrossRef]

13. Geldmacher, A.; Freier, A.; Losch, F.O.; Walden, P. Therapeutic vaccination for cancer immunotherapy: Antigen selection and clinical responses. *Hum. Vaccin.* **2011**, *7*, 115–119. [CrossRef]

14. Jackson, H.; Dimopoulos, N.; Mifsud, N.A.; Tai, T.Y.; Chen, Q.; Svobodova, S.; Browning, J.; Luescher, I.; Stockert, L.; Old, L.J.; et al. Striking immunodominance hierarchy of naturally occurring CD8+ and CD4+ T cell responses to tumor antigen NY-ESO-1. *J. Immunol.* **2006**, *176*, 5908–5917. [CrossRef]

15. Stockert, E.; Jäger, E.; Chen, Y.T.; Scanlan, M.J.; Gout, I.; Karbach, J.; Arand, M.; Knuth, A.; Old, L.J. A survey of the humoral immune response of cancer patients to a panel of human tumor antigens. *J. Exp. Med.* **1998**, *187*, 1349–1354. [CrossRef]

16. Knights, A.J.; Nuber, N.; Thomson, C.W.; De La Rosa, O.; Jäger, E.; Tiercy, J.M.; Van Den Broek, M.; Pascolo, S.; Knuth, A.; Zippelius, A. Modified tumour antigen-encoding mRNA facilitates the analysis of naturally occurring and vaccine-induced CD4 and CD8 T cells in cancer patients. *Cancer Immunol. Immunother.* **2009**, *58*, 325–338. [CrossRef]

17. Barrow, C.; Browning, J.; MacGregor, D.; Davis, I.D.; Sturrock, S.; Jungbluth, A.A.; Cebon, J. Tumor antigen expression in melanoma varies according to antigen and stage. *Clin. Cancer Res.* **2006**, *12*, 764–771. [CrossRef]

18. Filipazzi, P.; Pilla, L.; Mariani, L.; Patuzzo, R.; Castelli, C.; Camisaschi, C.; Maurichi, A.; Cova, A.; Rigamonti, G.; Giardino, F.; et al. Limited induction of tumor cross-reactive T cells without a measurable clinical benefit in early melanoma patients vaccinated with human leukocyte antigen class I-modified peptides. *Clin. Cancer Res.* **2012**, *18*, 6485–6496. [CrossRef]

19. Slingluff, C.L. The present and future of peptide vaccines for cancer: Single or multiple, long or short, alone or in combination? *Cancer J.* **2011**, *17*, 343–350. [CrossRef]

20. Slingluff, C.L.; Petroni, G.R.; Yamshchikov, G.V.; Hibbitts, S.; Grosh, W.W.; Chianese-Bullock, K.A.; Bissonette, E.A.; Barnd, D.L.; Deacon, D.H.; Patterson, J.W.; et al. Immunologic and clinical outcomes of vaccination with a multiepitope melanoma peptide vaccine plus low-dose interleukin-2 administered either concurrently or on a delayed schedule. *J. Clin. Oncol.* **2004**, *22*, 4474–4485. [CrossRef]

21. Kumai, T.; Fan, A.; Harabuchi, Y.; Celis, E. Cancer immunotherapy: Moving forward with peptide T cell vaccines. *Curr. Opin. Immunol.* **2017**, *47*, 57–63. [CrossRef] [PubMed]

22. Hersey, P.; Gallagher, S.J.; Kirkwood, J.M.; Cebon, J. Melanoma Vaccines. In *Cutaneous Melanoma*; Balch, C.M., Atkins, M.B., Garbe, C., Gershenwald, J.E., Halpern, A.C., Kirkwood, J.M., McArthur, G.A., Thompson, J.F., Sober, A.J., Eds.; Springer International Publishing: Cham, Switzerland, 2020; pp. 1243–1265. ISBN 978-3-030-05070-2.

23. Grenier, J.M.; Yeung, S.T.; Qiu, Z.; Jellison, E.R. Combining Adoptive Cell Therapy with Cytomegalovirus-Based Vaccine Is Protective against Solid Skin Tumors. *Front. Immunol.* **2017**, *8*, 1–10. [CrossRef] [PubMed]

24. Hofmann, O.; Caballero, O.L.; Stevenson, B.J.; Chen, Y.-T.Y.; Cohen, T.; Chua, R.; Maher, C.A.; Panji, S.; Schaefer, U.; Kruger, A.; et al. Genome-wide analysis of cancer/testis gene expression. *Proc. Natl. Acad. Sci. USA* **2008**, *105*, 20422–20427. [CrossRef] [PubMed]

25. Zhao, S.; Zhu, W.; Xue, S.; Han, D. Testicular defense systems: Immune privilege and innate immunity. *Cell. Mol. Immunol.* **2014**, *11*, 428–437. [CrossRef]

26. Fujita, A.; Nakamura, K.I.; Kato, T.; Watanabe, N.; Ishizaki, T.; Kimura, K.; Mizoguchi, A.; Narumiya, S. Ropporin, a sperm-specific binding protein of rhophilin, that is localized in the fibrous sheath of sperm flagella. *J. Cell Sci.* **2000**, *113*, 103–112.

27. Carr, D.W.; Fujita, A.; Stentz, C.L.; Liberty, G.A.; Olson, G.E.; Narumiya, S. Identification of Sperm-specific Proteins that Interact with A-kinase Anchoring Proteins in a Manner Similar to the Type II Regulatory Subunit of PKA. *J. Biol. Chem.* **2001**, *276*, 17332–17338. [CrossRef]

28. Chen, J.; Wang, Y.; Wei, B.; Lai, Y.; Yan, Q.; Gui, Y.; Cai, Z. Functional expression of ropporin in human testis and ejaculated spermatozoa. *J. Androl.* **2011**, *32*, 26–32. [CrossRef]

29. Li, Z.; Li, W.; Meklat, F.; Wang, Z.; Zhang, J.; Zhang, Y.; Lim, S.H. A yeast two-hybrid system using Sp17 identified Ropporin as a novel cancer-testis antigen in hematologic malignancies. *Int. J. Cancer* **2007**, *121*, 1507–1511. [CrossRef]

30. Liu, Q.; Huang, X.; Li, Q.; He, L.; Li, S.; Chen, X.; Ouyang, Y.; Wang, X.; Lin, C. Rhophilin-associated tail protein 1 promotes migration and metastasis in triple negative breast cancer via activation of RhoA. *FASEB J.* **2020**, *34*, 9959–9971. [CrossRef]

31. Chiriva-Internati, M.; Mirandola, L.; Yu, Y.; Jenkins, M.R.; Gornati, R.; Bernardini, G.; Gioia, M.; Chiaramonte, R.; Cannon, M.J.; Kast, W.M.; et al. Cancer testis antigen, ropporin, is a potential target for multiple myeloma immunotherapy. *J. Immunother.* **2011**, *34*, 490–499. [CrossRef]

32. Behren, A.; Anaka, M.; Lo, P.-H.; Vella, L.J.; Davis, I.D.; Catimel, J.; Cardwell, T.; Gedye, C.; Hudson, C.; Stan, R.; et al. The Ludwig institute for cancer research Melbourne melanoma cell line panel. *Pigment. Cell Melanoma Res.* **2013**, *26*, 597–600. [CrossRef]

33. Tarhini, A.A.; Leng, S.; Moschos, S.J.; Yin, Y.; Sander, C.; Lin, Y.; Gooding, W.E.; Kirkwood, J.M. Safety and immunogenicity of vaccination with MART-1 (26-35, 27L), gp100 (209-217, 210M), and tyrosinase (368-376, 370D) in adjuvant with PF-3512676 and GM-CSF in metastatic melanoma. *J. Immunother.* **2012**, *35*, 359–366. [CrossRef]

34. Schumacher, T.N.; Schreiber, R.D. Realising the Promise: Neoantigens in cancer immunotherapy. *Sci. Mag.* **2015**, *348*.

35. Roesch, A. Tumor heterogeneity and plasticity as elusive drivers for resistance to MAPK pathway inhibition in melanoma. *Oncogene* **2015**, *34*, 2951–2957. [CrossRef]

36. Monjazeb, A.M.; Zamora, A.E.; Grossenbacher, S.K.; Mirsoian, A.; Sckisel, G.D.; Murphy, W.J. Immunoediting and antigen loss: Overcoming the Achilles heel of immunotherapy with antigen non-specific therapies. *Front. Oncol.* **2013**, *3*, 1–10. [CrossRef]

37. Landsberg, J.; Kohlmeyer, J.; Renn, M.; Bald, T.; Rogava, M.; Cron, M.; Fatho, M.; Lennerz, V.; Wölfel, T.; Hölzel, M.; et al. Melanomas resist T-cell therapy through inflammation-induced reversible dedifferentiation. *Nature* **2012**, *490*, 412–416. [CrossRef]

38. Woods, K.; Pasam, A.; Jayachandran, A.; Andrews, M.C.; Cebon, J. Effects of epithelial to mesenchymal transition on t cell targeting of melanoma cells. *Front. Oncol.* **2014**, *4*, 1–7. [CrossRef]

39. Cebon, J.; Caballero, O.; John, T.; Klein, O. Cancer Testis Antigens. In *Tumor-Associated Antigens*; Gires, O., Seliger, B., Eds.; Wiley-VCH Verlag GmbH & Co. KGaA: Weinheim, Germany, 2009; pp. 161–177. ISBN 9783527320844.

40. Scanlan, M.J.; Gure, A.O.; Jungbluth, A.A.; Old, L.J.; Chen, Y. Cancer/testis antigens: An expanding family of targets for cancer immunotherapy. *Immunol. Rev.* **2002**, *188*, 22–32. [CrossRef]

41. Cebon, J.S.; Gore, M.; Thompson, J.F.; Davis, I.D.; McArthur, G.A.; Walpole, E.; Smithers, M.; Cerundolo, V.; Dunbar, P.R.; MacGregor, D.; et al. Results of a randomized, double-blind phase II clinical trial of NY-ESO-1 vaccine with ISCOMATRIX adjuvant versus ISCOMATRIX alone in participants with high-risk resected melanoma. *J. Immunother. Cancer* **2020**, *8*, 1–11. [CrossRef]

42. Maire, C.; Vercambre-Darras, S.; Devos, P.; D'Herbomez, M.; Dubucquoi, S.; Mortier, L. Metastatic melanoma: Spontaneous occurrence of auto antibodies is a good prognosis factor in a prospective cohort. *J. Eur. Acad. Dermatol. Venereol.* **2013**, *27*, 92–96. [CrossRef]

43. Kupsch, J.M.; Tidman, N.H.; Kang, N.V.; Truman, H.; Hamilton, S.; Patel, N.; Bishop, J.A.N.; Leigh, I.M.; Crowe, J.S. Isolation of human tumor-specific antibodies by selection of an antibody phage library on melanoma cells. *Clin. Cancer Res.* **1999**, *5*, 925–931.

44. Ohue, Y.; Wada, H.; Oka, M.; Nakayama, E. Antibody response to cancer/testis (CT) antigens: A prognostic marker in cancer patients. *Oncoimmunology* **2014**, *3*, e970032-1–e970032-3. [CrossRef]

45. Casadevall, A.; Pirofski, L. Antibody-mediated regulation of cellular immunity and the inflammatory response. *Trends Immunol.* **2003**, *24*, 474–478. [CrossRef]

46. Jäger, E.; Chen, Y.T.; Drijfhout, J.W.; Karbach, J.; Ringhoffer, M.; Jäger, D.; Arand, M.; Wada, H.; Noguchi, Y.; Stockert, E.; et al. Simultaneous humoral and cellular immune response against cancer-testis antigen NY-ESO-1: Definition of human histocompatibility leukocyte antigen (HLA)-A2-binding peptide epitopes. *J. Exp. Med.* **1998**, *187*, 265–270. [CrossRef]

47. Beeton-Kempen, N.; Duarte, J.; Shoko, A.; Serufuri, J.-M.; John, T.; Cebon, J.; Blackburn, J. Development of a novel, quantitative protein microarray platform for the multiplexed serological analysis of autoantibodies to cancer-testis antigens. *Int. J. Cancer* **2014**, *135*, 1842–1851. [CrossRef]

48. Gnjatic, S.; Atanackovic, D.; Jäger, E.; Matsuo, M.; Selvakumar, A.; Altorki, N.K.; Maki, R.G.; Dupont, B.; Ritter, G.; Chen, Y.-T.; et al. Survey of naturally occurring CD4+ T cell responses against NY-ESO-1 in cancer patients: Correlation with antibody responses. *Proc. Natl. Acad. Sci. USA* **2003**, *100*, 8862–8867. [CrossRef]

49. Svobodová, S.; Browning, J.; MacGregor, D.; Pollara, G.; Scolyer, R.A.; Murali, R.; Thompson, J.F.; Deb, S.; Azad, A.; Davis, I.D.; et al. Cancer-testis antigen expression in primary cutaneous melanoma has independent prognostic value comparable to that of Breslow thickness, ulceration and mitotic rate. *Eur. J. Cancer* **2011**, *47*, 460–469. [CrossRef]

50. Mirandola, L.; Wade, R.; Verma, R.; Pena, C.; Hosiriluck, N.; Figueroa, J.A.; Cobos, E.; Jenkins, M.R.; Chiriva-Internati, M. Sex-Driven Differences in Immunological Responses: Challenges and Opportunities for the Immunotherapies of the Third Millennium. *Int. Rev. Immunol.* **2015**, *34*, 134–142. [CrossRef]

51. Joosse, A.; Collette, S.; Suciu, S.; Nijsten, T.; Lejeune, F.; Kleeberg, U.R.; Coebergh, J.W.W.; Eggermont, A.M.M.; de Vries, E. Superior outcome of women with stage I/II cutaneous melanoma: Pooled analysis of four European Organisation for Research and Treatment of Cancer phase III trials. *J. Clin. Oncol.* **2012**, *30*, 2240–2247. [CrossRef]
52. Joosse, A.; Collette, S.; Suciu, S.; Nijsten, T.; Patel, P.M.; Keilholz, U.; Eggermont, A.M.M.; Coebergh, J.W.W.; de Vries, E. Sex is an independent prognostic indicator for survival and relapse/progression-free survival in metastasized stage III to IV melanoma: A pooled analysis of five European organisation for research and treatment of cancer randomized controlled trials. *J. Clin. Oncol.* **2013**, *31*, 2337–2346. [CrossRef]
53. Mittal, D.; Gubin, M.M.; Schreiber, R.D.; Smyth, M.J. New insights into cancer immunoediting and its three component phases–elimination, equilibrium and escape. *Curr. Opin. Immunol.* **2014**, *27*, 16–25. [CrossRef] [PubMed]
54. Ott, P.A.; Hodi, F.S.; Kaufman, H.L.; Wigginton, J.M.; Wolchok, J.D. Combination immunotherapy: A road map. *J. Immunother. Cancer* **2017**, *5*, 1–15. [CrossRef] [PubMed]
55. Gjerstorff, M.F.; Andersen, M.H.; Ditzel, H.J. Oncogenic cancer/testis antigens: Prime candidates for immunotherapy. *Oncotarget* **2015**, *6*, 15772–15787. [CrossRef] [PubMed]
56. Anaka, M.; Freyer, C.; Gedye, C.; Caballero, O.; Davis, I.D.; Behren, A.; Cebon, J. Stem cell media culture of melanoma results in the induction of a nonrepresentative neural expression profile. *Stem Cells* **2012**, *30*, 336–343. [CrossRef]
57. Cerami, E.; Gao, J.; Dogrusoz, U.; Gross, B.E.; Sumer, S.O.; Aksoy, B.A.; Jacobsen, A.; Byrne, C.J.; Heuer, M.L.; Larsson, E.; et al. The cBio Cancer Genomics Portal: An open platform for exploring multidimensional cancer genomics data. *Cancer Discov.* **2012**, *2*, 401–404. [CrossRef]
58. Gao, J.; Aksoy, B.A.; Dogrusoz, U.; Dresdner, G.; Gross, B.; Sumer, S.O.; Sun, Y.; Jacobsen, A.; Sinha, R.; Larsson, E.; et al. Integrative analysis of complex cancer genomics and clinical profiles using the cBioPortal. *Sci. Signal.* **2013**, *6*, pl1. [CrossRef]
59. Da Gama Duarte, J.; Goosen, R.W.; Lawry, P.J.; Blackburn, J.M. PMA: Protein Microarray Analyser, a user-friendly tool for data processing and normalization. *BMC Res. Notes* **2018**, *11*, 156. [CrossRef]

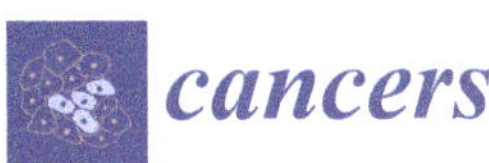

Article

Myxoma Virus Expressing LIGHT (TNFSF14) Pre-Loaded into Adipose-Derived Mesenchymal Stem Cells Is Effective Treatment for Murine Pancreatic Adenocarcinoma

Joanna Jazowiecka-Rakus [1,*], Agata Hadrys [1,2], Masmudur M. Rahman [3], Grant McFadden [3], Wojciech Fidyk [4], Ewa Chmielik [5], Marlena Pazdzior [1,2], Maciej Grajek [6], Violetta Kozik [2] and Aleksander Sochanik [1]

[1] Center for Translational Research and Molecular Biology of Cancer, Maria Sklodowska-Curie National Research Institute of Oncology, Gliwice Branch, Wybrzeze AK 15, 44-102 Gliwice, Poland; Agata.Hadrys@io.gliwice.pl (A.H.); Marlena.Pazdzior@io.gliwice.pl (M.P.); Aleksander.Sochanik@io.gliwice.pl (A.S.)

[2] Institute of Chemistry, University of Silesia, Szkolna 9, 40-007 Katowice, Poland; violetta.kozik@us.edu.pl

[3] Biodesign Institute, Arizona State University, Tempe, AZ 85287, USA; Masmudur.Rahman@asu.edu (M.M.R.); grantmcf@asu.edu (G.M.)

[4] Department of Bone Marrow Transplantation and Hematology-Oncology, Maria Sklodowska-Curie National Research Institute of Oncology, Gliwice Branch, Wybrzeze AK 15, 44-102 Gliwice, Poland; Wojciech.Fidyk@io.gliwice.pl

[5] Tumor Pathology Department, Maria Sklodowska-Curie National Research Institute of Oncology, Gliwice Branch, Wybrzeze AK 15, 44-102 Gliwice, Poland; Ewa.Chmielik@io.gliwice.pl

[6] Oncological and Reconstructive Surgery Department, Maria Sklodowska-Curie National Research Institute of Oncology, Gliwice Branch, Wybrzeze AK 15, 44-102 Gliwice, Poland; Maciej.Grajek@io.gliwice.pl

* Correspondence: Joanna.Jazowiecka@io.gliwice.pl; Tel.: +48-32-278-9844

Citation: Jazowiecka-Rakus, J.; Hadrys, A.; Rahman, M.M.; McFadden, G.; Fidyk, W.; Chmielik, E.; Pazdzior, M.; Grajek, M.; Kozik, V.; Sochanik, A. Myxoma Virus Expressing LIGHT (TNFSF14) Pre-Loaded into Adipose-Derived Mesenchymal Stem Cells Is Effective Treatment for Murine Pancreatic Adenocarcinoma. *Cancers* **2021**, *13*, 1394. https://doi.org/10.3390/cancers13061394

Academic Editors: Michael Kershaw and Clare Slaney

Received: 5 February 2021
Accepted: 17 March 2021
Published: 19 March 2021

Publisher's Note: MDPI stays neutral with regard to jurisdictional claims in published maps and institutional affiliations.

Simple Summary: Pancreatic cancer is a deadly disease with no effective therapy. Oncolytic viruses such as myxoma (MYXV) have revealed great potential to treat malignancies, due to dual anti-cancer effects—oncolytic and immune-stimulating effects. We aimed to verify whether adipose-derived mesenchymal stem cells (ADSCs) pre-loaded ex vivo with transgene-armed myxoma construct would be useful for transferring the virus to murine pancreatic lesions and whether this would reduce tumor burden. We confirmed that the carrier cells remained viable after infection, in contrast to pancreatic cancer cells, which were destroyed. Intraperitoneal (IP) administration of the shielded virus (ADSCs/MYXV) revealed localization in the pancreas, decreased tumor burden and an adaptive anti-tumor immune response. We conclude that ADSCs pre-loaded with recombinant MYXV and administered IP allowed for the ferrying of the virus to pancreatic cancer lesions, followed by tumor regression and extended survival in the treated mice. This therapeutic approach has excellent potential for treating pancreatic cancer.

Abstract: Pancreatic ductal adenocarcinoma (PDAC) is a weakly immunogenic fatal neoplasm. Oncolytic viruses with dual anti-cancer properties—oncolytic and immune response-boosting effects—have great potential for PDAC management. Adipose-derived stem cells (ADSCs) of mesenchymal origin were infected ex vivo with recombinant myxoma virus (MYXV), which encodes murine LIGHT, also called tumor necrosis factor ligand superfamily member 14 (TNFSF14). The viability and proliferation of ADSCs were not remarkably decreased (1–2 days) following MYXV infection, in sharp contrast to cells of pancreatic carcinoma lines studied, which were rapidly killed by the infection. Comparison of the intraperitoneal (IP) vs. the intravenous (IV) route of ADSC/MYXV administration revealed more pancreas-targeted distribution of the virus when ADSCs were delivered IP to mice bearing orthotopically injected PDAC. The biodistribution, tumor burden reduction and anti-tumor adaptive immune response were examined. Bioluminescence data, used to assess the presence of the luciferase-tagged virus after IP injection, indicated enhanced trafficking into the pancreata of mice bearing orthotopically-induced PDAC, as compared to tumor-free animals, resulting in extended survival of the treated PDAC-seeded animals and in the boosted expression of key adaptive immune response markers. We conclude that ADSCs pre-loaded with transgene-armed MYXV and

---

administered IP allow for the effective ferrying of the oncolytic virus to sites of PDAC and mediate improved tumor regression.

Keywords: adipose tissue-derived stem cells (ADSCs); mesenchymal stem cells; oncolytic virus; myxoma virus; oncolytic virotherapy; pancreatic ductal adenocarcinoma

1. Introduction

The incidence of pancreatic ductal adenocarcinoma (PDAC) has risen in the last 50 years and it is forecasted to be the second leading cause of cancer deaths within a decade. The dismal prognosis results from lack of specific early symptoms and early diagnostic methods. Patients usually present in the advanced stage of the disease and experience the failure of traditional anticancer therapies. Long-term disease-free survival is possible but the majority of diagnoses are unresectable cases, with an expected survival of less than 6 months. Modest curative benefits are offered only by early surgery with subsequent adjuvant therapy. Systemic recurrence after treatment suggests early metastasis in the course of pancreatic tumorigenesis, long before disease diagnosis [1].

The therapeutic failure in PDAC can be attributed to specific tumor cell biology, as well as features of the tumor milieu, both contributing to the high malignancy of this cancer. The tumor microenvironment of PDAC indeed presents a formidable challenge to therapy. Considerable desmoplastic stroma can constitute up to 90% of the tumor volume and are believed to originate from cancer-associated fibroblasts (CAFs) [2]. These are accountable for the chemoresistance of pancreatic tumors, by creating physical barriers that shield tumor cells from systemically injected therapeutic compounds. The heavy extracellular matrix within pancreatic cancer distorts tissue architecture and causes an abnormal structure of blood and lymphatic vasculature. The ensuing hypoxia is another hallmark of the PDAC microenvironment, associated with desmoplasia. It originates from desmoplasia-associated hypovascularization and, vice versa, favors desmoplastic progression by activating pancreatic stellate cells [3–5]. Desmoplasia and hypoxia are also barriers to the infiltration of both regulatory and effector lymphocytes, as well as to T cell activation [6–8]. Macrophages that are recruited adopt an immunosuppressive, pro-angiogenic M2-like state, block CD4+ T cell entry into the PDAC microenvironment, support PDAC progression, and thus are a marker of negative clinical prognosis [5,9,10].

The repertoire of treatment strategies in PDAC has been expanding in the last decades to include novel approaches such as targeted drugs, non-coding RNAs (miRNAs) and immunotherapy [11]. However, targeted chemotherapeutics have only moderately improved PDAC outcomes and have not altered 5-year survival. Gemcitabine and erlotinib, used to treat advanced disease, both yield only a modest clinical benefit. The development of chemoresistance and the pro-metastatic propensity of pancreatic cancer are related to the transition from epithelial to mesenchymal cells (EMT) [12,13]. Gene expression data have demonstrated the contribution of EMT cells to chemoresistance in PDAC [13,14].

Overall, the prevailing notion is that dense stroma, multiple genetic mutations, compensatory alternative pathways and aggressive metastatic spread cause PDAC chemoresistance, even to multidrug regimens. These factors are also at the root of the moderate success in targeting cancer-associated molecular pathways and the adverse effects linked to activated downstream effectors [11].

The ineffective nature of existing treatments for PDAC has stimulated the search for innovative therapeutic strategies. Oncolytic virotherapy is becoming increasingly sought-after for the treatment of many different neoplasms, including pancreatic cancer. The therapeutic effectiveness of oncolytic viruses (OVs) is the result of direct oncolysis, virus spread to adjacent cancer cells, and the elicited anti-tumor immune response.

Oncolytic viruses (OVs) are replication-competent and selectively target tumor cells, but they are not able to bind and/or productively replicate in most normal somatic cells.

OVs can be genetically engineered to express inserted foreign transgenes to induce cancer cell death in a fashion that can stimulate anti-tumor immune responses [15]. OV replication in cancer cells yields infectious progeny that may further spread and reduce tumor burden [16].

Myxoma virus (MYXV) is a poxvirus with attractive safety profile for oncolytic therapy. MYXV infects and produces symptoms only in rabbits. Although MYXV is nonpathogenic to humans and mice, the virus exhibits natural tropism for a wide spectrum of human cancers [17]. MYXV has a 160-kb double-stranded DNA genome that has the capacity to accept numerous transgenes and is easy to manipulate. In this study, we armed oncolytic MYXV with the murine Light gene, encoding mouse tumor necrosis factor ligand superfamily member 14 (TNFSF14, synonym: LIGHT), which was designed to promote the influx of T lymphocytes into the tumor and thus intensify the immune response directed against the tumor. This ought to help stimulate the transformation of the "cold" tumor microenvironment, with a small number of effector immune cells, into a "hot" environment, with increased infiltration of other immune cells and cytokines. LIGHT is an inducible lymphotoxin which competes with HSV glycoprotein D for binding to a herpesvirus entry mediator (HVEM) expressed on T lymphocytes. LIGHT is expressed on activated T cells, natural killer (NK) cells, immature dendritic cells (DCs) and on the tumor and in the stroma [18]. LIGHT is an immune stimulator that contributes to the anti-tumor immune response, and its expression in the TME is associated with improved overall survival and relapse-free survival [19]. LIGHT–HVEM interaction has been shown to induce apoptosis of several tumor cell lines directly [20]. Therefore, LIGHT is a promising biotherapeutic adjuvant agent for cancer immunotherapy with OVs [21].

Systemic delivery represents the desired route to reach poorly accessible sites or disseminated metastatic lesions. IV administration of naked OVs is, however, a very inefficient strategy for delivery. Rapid elimination from the bloodstream by antiviral defense mechanisms is the major obstacle to achieving the effective transfer of the viral cargo to distant tumor sites. IV delivery of a viral construct to tumor sites can be improved by exploiting protective carrier cells, e.g., [22]. Adipose-derived stem cells (ADSCs) of mesenchymal origin provide a unique cell carrier platform, where the virus can be at least partly protected from immune clearance pathways before delivery to the tumor site. In addition, ADSCs show natural chemotactic tropism for cancer tissues. However, in cases where IV delivery of cell-protected OV would not be effective (due to the "first pass" effect in the lungs) [23], the transfer of oncovirus cargo to a defined and identifiable tumor site can be accomplished through locoregional injection. In this study, we investigated whether carrier cells could also be beneficial for the delivery of OVs to PDAC via the intraperitoneal (IP) route. IP administration remains an interesting alternative when targeting OVs to abdominal-area cancer targets. Comparison of the two modes of OV delivery using a peritoneal murine tumor model revealed [24] that IP was associated with narrower biodistribution (a reduced frequency of virus detected in the kidney, lung and heart), decreased toxicity and greater therapeutic efficacy against peritoneal metastases. Tumor burden was more effectively reduced with IP, compared with IV administration. Median survival following IP administration was approximately twice that observed with IV administration.

Wennier et al. tested the use of unarmed recombinant vMyx-tdTr to treat disseminated pancreatic adenocarcinoma in the peritoneal cavity of immunocompetent mice. They showed that oncolytic therapy, followed by gemcitabine, could decisively improve animal survival [25]. In our study, we assessed the usefulness of the novel armed MYXV construct (vMyx-mLIGHT-Fluc/tdTr) in experimental therapy on orthotopically-induced murine PDAC via IP delivery of the viral cargo using the mesenchymal ADSC platform.

2. Materials and Methods

2.1. Recombinant Viruses

Recombinant MYXV constructs (vMyx-EGFP, vMyx-EGFP/tdTr and vMyx-mLIGHT/ FLuc/tdTr) derived from the wild-type Lausanne strain of myxoma virus (vMyx-WT) were used. The recombination cassettes were inserted in the intergenic region between the M135 and M136 open reading frames (ORFs). vMyx-EGFP expresses EGFP from the early/late promoter; the vMyx-EGFP/tdTr tandem system allows the expression of EGFP at both early and late infection stages (early/late promoter), whereas tdTr is expressed at the late infection stage (poxvirus p11 late promoter) [26]. The vMyx-mLIGHT-FLuc/tdTr construct expresses mouse LIGHT and firefly luciferase at both the early and late infection stages (early/late promoter) and tdTr under a synthetic poxvirus late promoter. vMyx-mLIGHT-FLuc/tdTr was constructed by inserting a DNA cassette containing the coding sequences of murine LIGHT (TNFSF14, see Supplementary Materials for the nucleotide sequence and Figure S1), firefly luciferase and tdTr at an intergenic location between the M135 and M136 genes in the wild-type MYXV strain Lausanne genome. A recombinant plasmid was constructed using the Gateway System (Thermo Fisher Scientific, Waltham, MA, USA) [17]. The sequence encoding murine LIGHT was PCR-amplified using gene-specific primers with the forward primer containing the synthetic early/late (sE/L) promoter sequence. The resultant sE/L-LIGHT fragment was PCR-ligated to another PCR fragment containing the MYXV M135 gene. The resultant attB1-M135-sE/L-LIGHT-attB4 PCR fragment was recombined into the pDONR221-P1P4 plasmid (Invitrogen, Waltham, MA, USA) using the BP clonase enzyme mix (Invitrogen). The construction of the plasmid having tdTr (attB4r-p11tdTr-attB3r) and another plasmid having FLuc and the MYXV M136 gene (attB3-sE/L-FLuc-M136-attB2) was described previously [27]. All three plasmids, along with the pDEST40 destination plasmid (Invitrogen) were then subjected to an LR recombination reaction using LR clonase II (Invitrogen) to generate the final plasmid construct. The recombinant virus was then created using the method described previously for making recombinant MYXV [17].

2.2. Virus Purification and Titration

MYXVs were produced in RK13 cells (at multiplicity of infection /MOI/ = 0.1). When the cytopathic effect was visible (ca. 72 h; $\pm 80\%$ confluency), cells were harvested, centrifuged (1500 rpm, 10 min, 4 °C), resuspended in 10 mM Tris–HCl (pH = 8), and subjected to three freeze/thaw cycles and cup sonication (5 × 1 min). Cell debris was removed by centrifugation. Homogenates containing the virus were layered onto the 36% sucrose cushion and ultracentrifuged ($10^5 \times$ g/1 h, 4 °C). The supernatant was removed, and the pellet resuspended in 10 mM Tris–HCl (pH = 8). The quantity of infectious viral particles was determined by titration on RK13 cells (4 × 10^5/well; 6-well plate). After 3–4 days, fluorescent foci were counted using an inverted microscope (Leica Microsystems, Mannheim Germany). Viral titer (focus-forming units per milliliter (FFU)/mL) was calculated as the number of foci multiplied by the dilution.

2.3. Cell Lines

Human (Panc–1, AsPC–1) and murine (Pan02) pancreatic ductal adenocarcinoma cell lines were used. The human lines were from ATCC; the murine line was a gift from GMF. Rabbit RK13 kidney epithelial cell line (ATCC) was used to propagate MYXV constructs. Cells were maintained in DMEM (RK13, Panc-1 and Pan02) or RPMI-1640 (AsPC–1) media, both supplemented with 10% FBS (EURx) and 1% penicillin-streptomycin (Sigma-Aldrich, Poznan, Poland) Cultures were grown in a humidified 5% CO_2 incubator at 37 °C and were routinely tested for mycoplasma contamination.

2.4. ADSCs Isolation and Culture

Fragments of adipose tissue obtained on-site (MSC National Research Institute of Oncology) from human donors (Table S1) were washed with PBS⁻ (Gibco™, ThermoFisher

Scientific, Warsaw, Poland) containing 1% FBS (EURx) to remove contaminating hematopoietic cells. The tissue was cut into small pieces and digested using collagenase type I solution (200 U/mL, Gibco) and shaking (1 h/37 °C/180 rpm). Cell suspensions were centrifuged (1500 rpm/10 min), filtered through 70-µm and 40-µm strainers and seeded in culture flasks using MEM (Sigma-Aldrich, Poznan, Poland) supplemented with 10% human platelet lysate (Sigma), heparin (2 U/mL, Polfa), 1% non-essential amino acids (Gibco) and 1% penicillin–streptomycin (Sigma). After 72 h, cultures were washed with PBS⁻ to remove non-adherent cells and rinsed with fresh culture medium. Sub-confluent cultures were split at a 1:3 ratio. Differentiation into adipocytes, osteocytes and chondrocytes was analyzed (passage 3) using the Human Mesenchymal Stem Cell Functional Identification Kit (SC006, R&D Systems), containing Goat Anti-Mouse FABP-4 Antigen Affinity-purified Polyclonal Antibody (adipocyte marker), a Mouse Anti-Human Osteocalcin Monoclonal Antibody (osteocyte marker) and Goat Anti-Human Aggrecan Antigen Affinity-purified Polyclonal Antibody (chondrocyte marker). Cells were stained with Biotinylated Rabbit Anti-Goat IgG (immunoglobulin G) Antibody (H + L), Texas Red Streptavidin (Vector Laboratories, BA-5000 and SA-5006, respectively) or Goat Anti-Mouse Alexa Fluor Plus 488 secondary antibody (Thermo Fisher Scientific, No. A32723). Nuclei were counterstained with DAPI (Thermo Fisher Scientific, No. 62248). The morphology of adipose-derived stem cells was inspected using the Zeiss LSM 710 confocal microscope system.

2.5. Flow Cytometry Analysis of ADSC Phenotype

To confirm the phenotype of ADSCs, cultured cells were incubated with appropriate antibodies (20 min/RT), rinsed with and resuspended in Cell Wash Buffer (BD Biosciences). Analysis was performed using a BD FACS Canto II flow cytometer (Becton-Dickinson). The phenotype of both uninfected and infected ADSCs (vMyx-WT; MOI = 5) was analyzed. The positive cell population gates were set using isotype IgG controls. The presence of ADSC-associated surface markers (CD73, CD90, and CD105) and the co-occurring absence of blood cell-lineage-specific markers (CD11b, CD19, CD34, CD45 and HLA-DR) was examined using the Human MSC Analysis Kit (BD Biosciences, No. 562245).

2.6. Infectiveness of RK13, ADSC and Pancreatic Cell Lines to MYXV

ADSCs, RK13 and three pancreatic adenocarcinoma cell lines (murine Pan02, human Panc-1 and AsPC-1) were tested for susceptibility to MYXV infection. Cultured cells (2×10^5 cells/well; 6-well plate) infected with vMyx-EGFP (MOI = 5) were collected (24, 48 and 72 h p.i.), centrifuged (2000 rpm/2 min), washed twice and resuspended in PBS⁻ (200 µL). Cell aliquots were incubated with 7-aminoactinomycin D (7-AAD; 5 µL) for 2 min to determine viability and analyzed for enhanced GFP expression using flow cytometry (BD FACS Canto II). 7-AAD emission was detected using a long-pass filter (670 nm), and a region for live cells was defined. Non-infected cells were used as a control.

2.7. Expression of Early and Late MYXV Genes

To visualize early and late gene expression, ADSCs, RK13 and three pancreatic adenocarcinoma cell lines (murine Pan02, human Panc-1 and AsPC-1) were infected with vMyx-EGFP/tdTr (MOI = 5). Cells were plated into 4-well chamber slides (5×10^4 cells/well). After 24 h p.i., cells were washed with PBS⁻ and fixed in paraformaldehyde (4%) for 10 min at room temperature (RT). Cell nuclei were stained with DAPI Counterstain (Life Technologies™, ThermoFisher Scientific, Warsaw, Poland). Infection was evaluated using fluorescence microscopy (Zeiss LSM 710 confocal workstation).

2.8. Single-Step Growth Analysis of Viral Replication in Cell Cultures

Cultures (5×10^4 cells/well; 24-well plate) of ADSCs, RK13 and three pancreatic cancer cells lines (murine Pan02, human Panc-1 and AsPC-1) were infected (in triplicate) with vMyx-mLIGHT/Fluc/tdTr (MOI = 5). The inoculum was removed at 90 min post-infection and cells were further incubated (5% CO_2, 37 °C) with fresh medium. Next, cells were trypsinized and collected (at 3-, 6-, 12- and 24-h time points). Following centrifugation (2000 rpm/2 min), cells were resuspended in 200 μL hypotonic swelling buffer (5 mL of 1M Tris-HCl (pH = 8.0) and 1 mL of 1M MgCl$_2$) and frozen at $-80\ ^{\circ}$C. Before titration, cells were thawed and sonicated (2 × 1 min) to disaggregate virus complexes. Samples from the examined time points were titrated back onto RK13 cells (4 × 10^5 cells/well; 6-well plate) by serial dilution. Foci were counted using an inverted fluorescent microscope (Leica Microsystems). Titers (FFU/mL) were calculated (number of foci multiplied by the dilution factor).

2.9. Cytotoxicity of MYXV for ADSCs, RK13 and Pancreatic Cancer Cell Lines

To assess cytotoxic effects of MYXV infection on ADSCs, RK13 and three pancreatic cancer cell lines (murine Pan02, human Panc-1 and AsPC-1) cell cultures (1 × 10^4 cells/well; 96-well plate) were infected with vMyx-mLIGHT/Fluc/tdTr at increasing MOIs (0.1, 1, 5 and 10). After 24 and 48 h, cell viability was evaluated using an MTS assay (CellTiter 96$^{\circledR}$ AQueous Non-Radioactive Cell Proliferation Assay kit; Promega) and a Biotek plate reader (490 nm).

2.10. Animal Care

All animal procedures were performed in accordance with European Union (EU) law, after approval by the Local Ethics Committee, Medical University of Silesia, Katowice, Poland. Six-to-eight-week-old C57Bl/6NCrl female mice (total n = 235; Charles River Laboratories) were used. Animals (18–22 g) were housed in HEPA-filtered IVC System cages (Allentown Caging Equipment) under a controlled dark/light cycle (12 h/12 h) and were fed a pathogen-free standard diet (Altromin 1314) and water ad libitum. All efforts were made to minimize animal suffering.

2.11. Orthotopic Tumor Implantation

For orthotopic tumor implantation, C57Bl/6NCrl female mice (subtotal n = 163) were anesthetized with isoflurane (1–3% vol.) and injected with carprofen (5 mg/kg, ScanVet) into the nape of the neck. The surgical field was sterilized with iodine and a ca. 1-cm-long incision was made beside the splenic silhouette. With the entire pancreas and spleen exposed, Pan02 cancer cell suspension was slowly injected into the pancreatic head area using a 27G needle, following which the pancreas and spleen were pushed slightly back into the abdominal cavity and the abdominal muscle layer was closed with a single continuous 4-0 polysorb suture. The skin incision was finally closed with an autoclip wound closing system and buprenorphine (0.03 mg/mL) was administered to assist recovery. Animal health was monitored daily. Only single animals from control groups reached termination criteria. Euthanasia was conducted by means of cervical dislocation.

2.12. Orthotopic Injection of Pan02-luc Cells with Simultaneous Administration of ADSCs Pre-Infected with MYXV

C57Bl/6NCrl mice (n = 6/group) were orthotopically injected with the Pan02 cells (1 × 10^6 cells/25 μL PBS$^-$), followed by immediate administration of ADSCs (5 × 10^5 cells/25 μL PBS$^-$) pre-infected (MOI = 5) with vMyx-mLIGHT/Fluc/tdTr. As controls, non-infected ADSCs, unshielded vMyx-mLIGHT/Fluc/tdTr (5 × 10^5 FFU/25 μL PBS$^-$) or PBS$^-$ alone were used. After 21 days, the mice were sacrificed, and pancreata and spleens were excised, weighed and measured for size.

2.13. Bioluminescence Imaging (BLI) of MYXV Distribution Following Administration to Mice

C57Bl/6NCrl mice (n = 3/group) were orthotopically implanted (day 0) with Pan02 cells (1 × 10^6/30 μL PBS$^-$) (designated the +Pan02 group), or with 30 μL PBS$^-$ for un-challenged mice (referred to as the −Pan02 group). Seven days after implantation, the mice were injected intraperitoneally (IP) with either a single dose of ADSCs previously infected (MOI = 5) for 24 h with vMyx-mLIGHT-Fluc/tdTr (5 × 10^5 cells/100 μL PBS$^-$), or with unshielded vMyx-mLIGHT-Fluc/tdTr (5 × 10^5 FFU/100 μL PBS$^-$). Bioluminescence imaging (BLI) was performed using the Lumina IVIS Imaging System (PerkinElmer). At various time points (3–96 h) after delivery of luciferase gene-carrying MYXV, the mice were injected IP with 1.5 mg D-luciferin (Promega). BLI data were acquired and regions of interest (ROIs) determined in both intact animals and dissected organs (pancreas, spleen, liver, lungs, heart and leg muscle).

2.14. Therapy of Immunocompetent Mice Bearing Orthotopic Pancreatic Tumors

Pancreatic tumors were established in recipient C57Bl/6NCrl mice ($n = 10$–11/group) (day 0) by orthotopic implantation of 1×10^6 Pan02 cells/30 µL PBS$^-$. For five-dose treatment regimens (days 4, 8, 12, 16 and 20), mice were injected IP with ADSCs infected (MOI = 5) for 24 h with vMyx-mLIGHT-Fluc/tdTr (5×10^5 cells/100 µL PBS$^-$) or with unshielded vMyx-mLIGHT-Fluc/tdTr (5×10^5 FFU/100 µL PBS$^-$) or 100 µL PBS$^-$ (control). After 21 days, mice ($n = 3$/group) were sacrificed, peripheral blood was collected, and the pancreas, spleen and liver were excised, weighed and measured for size. Peripheral blood and pancreatic tissue were used for flow cytometry studies, whereas pancreas, spleen and liver tissues were formalin-fixed and used for histological assessments. The remaining treated mice ($n = 7$–8/group) were monitored for survival.

2.15. Histological Assessments

Formalin-fixed and paraffin-embedded pancreas, spleen and liver sections (5 µm-thick) were H&E stained, scanned and analyzed microscopically using a digital slide scanner and CaseViewer software (3D HISTECH, Budapest, Hungary) by an experienced pathologist. Masson's staining was performed to assess the amount and localization of connective tissue in the tumor structure. Mitotic Index [28] was rated under $400\times$ magnification (40×10) for 10 high power fields (HPF; field number 26.5).

2.16. Flow-Cytometry Analysis of CD4, CD8, CD3 Tumor-Infiltrating Lymphocytes

Pancreatic tumors were established orthotopically, and five-dose treatment conducted as described earlier. After 21 days, mice ($n = 3$) were sacrificed, peripheral blood samples were collected in EDTA-coated tubes, and pancreata were excised. Blood samples were treated with Red Blood Cell Lysis Buffer (BD Biosciences). Single-cell suspensions derived from pancreas tissue were obtained using a digestion mix containing 250 U/mL collagenase Type I (Gibco), 0.2 mg/mL hyaluronidase type IV-S (Sigma-Aldrich) and 0.02 mg/mL DNase I (Worthington) in DMEM + 10% fetal bovine serum (EURx). The digested samples were mashed through a sterile 70-µm nylon mesh cell strainer into ice-cold PBS$^-$ containing 1% FBS. Red blood cells in pancreatic digests were lysed (3 min) on ice using ACK Lysis Buffer (Lonza) and passed through a 40-µm nylon mesh cell strainer. To quantify percentages of CD4+, and CD8+ populations in pancreas and blood, the generated samples were treated with antibodies (20 min/RT). After fluorescent labeling, 4×10^4 cells were washed and analyzed using flow cytometry (BD FACS Canto II). The following monoclonal antibodies were used according to the manufacturer's instructions: PerCP/Cyanine5.5 anti-mouse CD45 (clone 30-F11; BioLegend, San Diego, CA, USA), phycoerythrin (PE) anti-mouse CD3 (clone 17A2; BioLegend), fluorescein isothiocyanate (FITC) anti-mouse CD4 (clone GK1.5; BioLegend) and APC/Cyanine7 anti-mouse CD8a (clone 53-6.7; BioLegend).

2.17. Statistical Analysis

Graphs were plotted using GraphPad Prism 7 (GraphPad Software, San Diego, CA, USA) Statistical differences were determined using a one-way ANOVA test, followed by Tukey's multiple comparisons test or two-way ANOVA with Tukey's multiple comparisons test. Bartlett's test was performed to ensure the suitability of the data for parametric significance tests. Kaplan–Meier survival curves were compared statistically using a log-rank test (Mantel–Cox). Data are presented as bars indicating means ($\pm$SD). The significance levels are indicated with asterisks: * $p \leq 0.05$; ** $p \leq 0.01$; *** $p \leq 0.001$; **** $p \leq 0.0001$. p-values < 0.05 were considered statistically significant.

3. Results

3.1. Identity of Human Mesenchymal Adipose Tissue-Derived Stem Cells (ADSCs)

The isolated primary human cultured ADSCs were characterized (Figure 1a–c) by morphology, multipotency and the combination of positive as well as negative surface markers. ADSCs showed fibroblast-like morphology and their ability to differentiate into mature cells of other tissue types, specifically adipocytes, osteocytes and chondrocytes, was confirmed (Figure 1a). Using an MSC Functional Identification Kit and flow cytometry, the immunophenotype of virus-uninfected ADSCs (Figure 1b) or unarmed wild-type MYXV (vMyx-WT)-infected ADSCs (Figure 1c) was investigated and confirmed the presence of CD73, CD90 and CD105 (human ADSC-associated surface markers), and the concomitant absence of CD11b, CD19, CD34 and CD45 (blood cell lineage-specific markers), as well as the lack of HLA-DR (MHC Class II receptor). We also confirmed the expression of MYXV-encoded LIGHT in ADSCs infected with vMyx-mLIGHT-Fluc/tdTr construct and the absence of its expression in ADSCs infected with vMyx-WT and non-infected (Figure S2). The Light gene transcript was measured using RT-qPCR and expression was rendered as a ratio of the target gene (Light) vs. the reference gene (glyceraldehyde 3-phosphate dehydrogenase/GAPDH/). The distribution of the LIGHT protein in cells infected with vMyx-mLIGHT-Fluc/tdTr was also confirmed in the cytoplasm and cell surface (Figure S3).

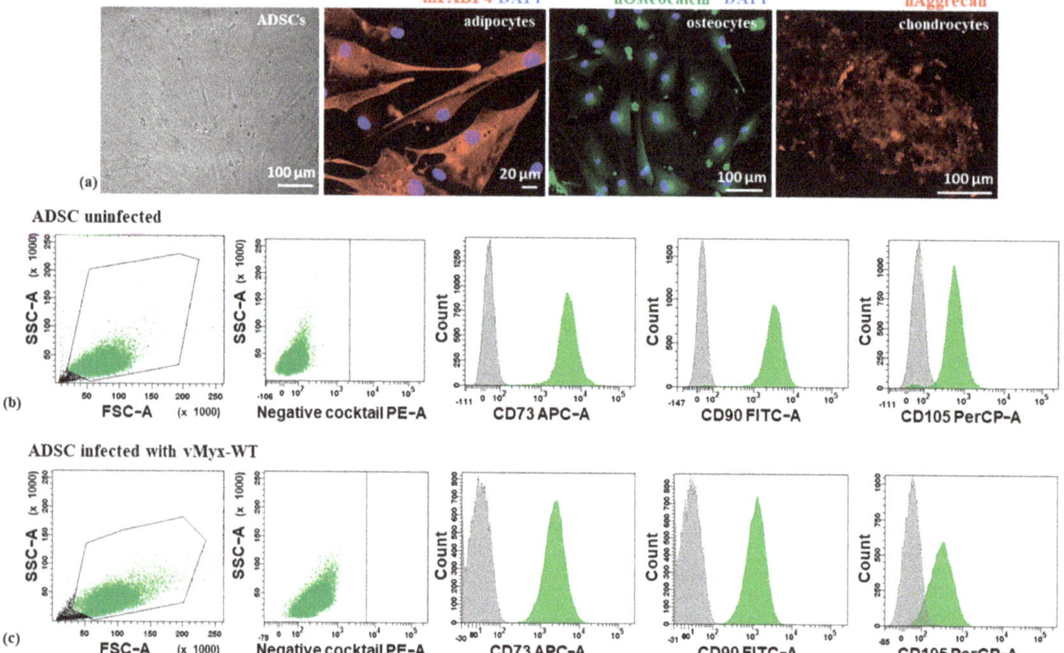

Figure 1. Characterization of adipose tissue-derived stem cell ADSC (**a**) morphology (far left) and differentiation of ADSCs into adipocytes (anti-mFABP4 antibody), osteocytes (anti-hOsteocalcin antibody) and chondrocytes (anti-hAggrecan antibody, red); DAPI-counterstained nuclei (magn. 40×; scale bar = 20 µm for adipocytes; magn. 20×; scale bar = 100 µm for osteocytes and chondrocytes). Flow cytometry plots of uninfected ADSCs (**b**) or ADSCs infected (**c**) with vMyx-WT (MOI = 10) confirming the presence of CD73, CD90 and CD105 and the concomitant absence of CD11b, CD19, CD34, CD45 or HLA-DR markers; gray: isotype control; green: viable ADSCs. Gating parameters based on the signal of isotype IgG control probes.

3.2. In Vitro Infection and Replication of MYXV in Pancreatic Ductal Adenocarcinoma Is Cell-Type-Dependent

MYXV is a potential OV candidate for the treatment of many human cancers. A panel of cell lines was tested for permissiveness to infection with unarmed vMyx-EGFP/tdTr, vMyx-EGFP (Figure 2a,b). Three pancreatic ductal adenocarcinoma cell lines (murine Pan02, human Panc-1, human AsPC-1), as well as primary human mesenchymal ADSC carrier cells and RK13 cells of rabbit origin used to propagate the virus were tested (positive control). Panc-1 and AsPC-1 harbor the mutant K-Ras gene, which is involved in the EGFR pathway. Pan02 is a non-metastatic murine line that is highly sensitive to gemcitabine, a drug widely used in pancreatic cancer treatment.

In order to better understand the permissiveness to MYXV infection in these cells, we compared the ability of the vMyx-EGFP/tdTr reporter construct expressing EGFP (enhanced green fluorescent protein; early/late expression) and tdTr (tandem dimer tomato red fluorescent protein; late expression only) or the vMyx-EGFP construct expressing only EGFP to infect and spread in different cell types from the tested panel. Cells were infected with the recombinant virus (MOI = 5) and evaluated by means of fluorescence microscopy (Figure 2a) or flow cytometry (Figure 2b). We observed significant differences in infection progression by the virus between the tested cell types. In RK13, ADSC and Pan02 cell lines, the MYXV construct appeared to initiate a permissive infection and underwent normal cell-to-cell spread. Fluorescence microscopy analysis revealed the expression of both EGFP and tdTr from vMyx-EGFP/tdTr and flow cytometry showed an increase in the percentage of infected EGFP-positive cells (Figure 2b). There was less MYXV infection observed in AsPc-1 and Panc-1 cell lines, which can be considered either semi-permissive or non-permissive for MYXV replication, although they did permit at least detectable levels of viral gene expression from early promoters. Flow cytometry showed a decreased percentage of infected EGFP-positive cells after 72 h p.i. (30% and 6%, respectively).

However, single-step growth curves showed that the recombinant vMyx-mLIGHT-Fluc/tdTr construct (LIGHT and Fluc—early/late expression; tdT—late expression only) used for the infection of AsPC-1 and Panc-1 cells did not produce new infectious virions, whereas the infection of RK13, ADSC and Pan02 cells with the same recombinant produced significantly more progeny virions (Figure 2c). The most notable differences were observed in Panc-1 cells, which did not support productive MYXV replication, as reported previously [29], despite allowing early gene expression in the initially infected cells (Figure 2c). Of note, human ADSCs and murine Pan02 cells showed the highest viral titers, an approximately 3.6-log and 3.2-log increase, respectively, at 24 h p.i. when compared to other tested cell lines. In rabbit RK-13 cells, the MYXV construct achieved a 1.7-log increase in titer. Of the panel of cell lines tested, human pancreatic cancer cell lines (AsPC-1 and Panc-1) were the least susceptible, with viral titers achieving approximately 0.17-log and 0.12-log increases, respectively, at 24 h p.i. Taken together, these results show that different types of pancreatic cancer cells were variably permissive for the MYXV construct tested, although all were capable of supporting at least detectable levels of early virus gene expression.

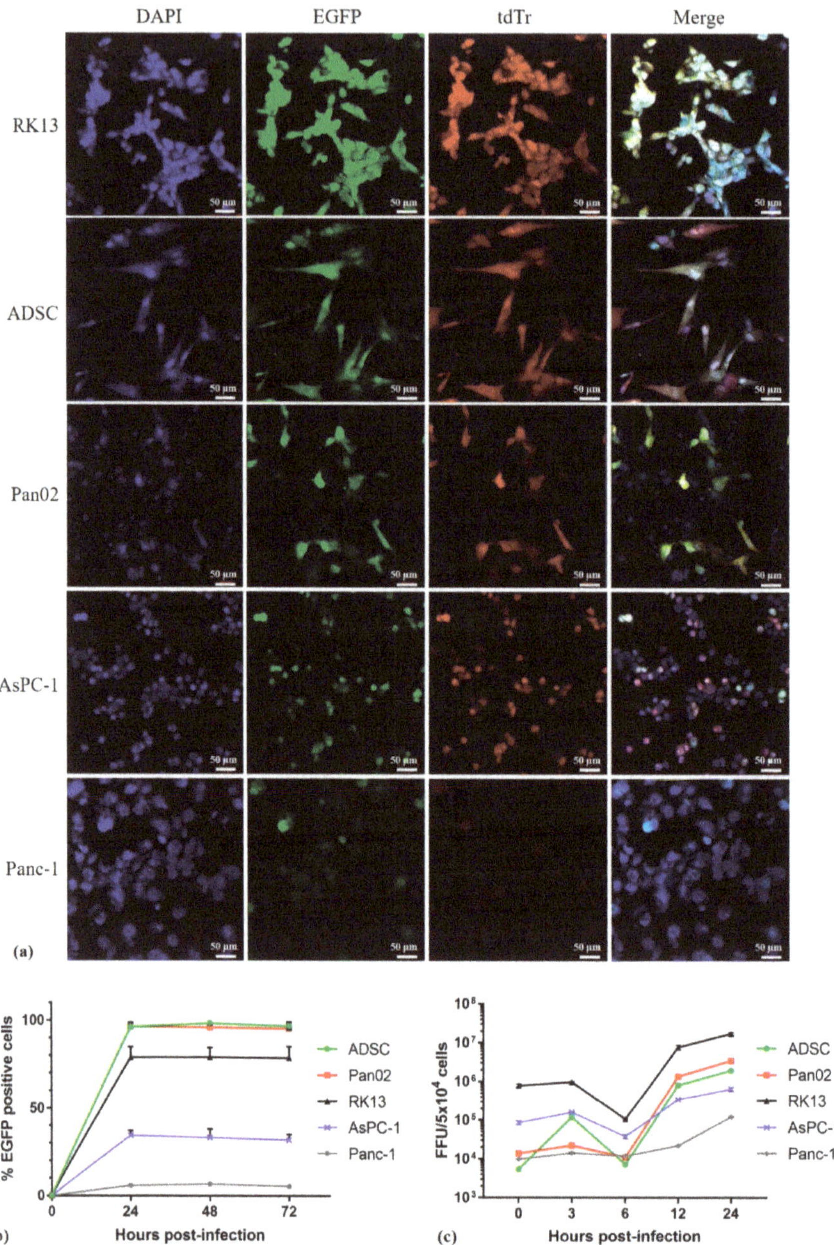

Figure 2. MYXV infection and replication in pancreatic cancer cells, RK13 and ADSC. Cultures of ADSCs, Pan02, RK13, AsPC-1 and Panc-1 cells were infected: (**a**) with vMyx-EGFP/tdTr (MOI = 5). At 24 h post infection (p.i.) the infection was visualized by fluorescence microscopy (magn. 20×; scale bar = 50 μm; Zeiss LSM 710 confocal Workstation); blue: DAPI staining (nuclei); green: EGFP fluorescence; red: tdTr fluorescence; (**b**) with vMyx-EGFP (MOI = 5), collected at the indicated time points and analyzed by means of flow cytometry to determine the percentage of infected EGFP-positive cells; (**c**) with vMyx-mLIGHT-Fluc/tdTr (MOI = 5) to generate single-step growth curves. Cells were collected at the indicated time points and lysed to determine viral titers. Titers for each sample were performed in triplicate; error bars shown are means ± SD.

3.3. MYXV Infection Reduces the Viability of Pancreatic Cancer Cells In Vitro

The MTS cell viability assay was used (Figure 3a,b) to determine if infection with oncolytic MYXV construct vMyx-mLIGHT-FLuc/tdTr at different MOIs (0.1–10) would result in reduced viability in cultures of cells from the tested panel at 24 and 48 h p.i. Primary human ADSCs remained the most viable, irrespective of increasing values of MOI, as compared to other cell lines at both time points tested (almost 90% at 24 h and 77% at 48 h/MOI = 5). On the other hand, the highly MYXV-susceptible RK13 cells showed viability reduced to 41% at 24 h, and to 20% at 48 h at the MOI = 10. The murine Pan02 cancer cell line, as well as the human AsPC-1 cancer line, were only 54% viable already at 24 h at the MOI = 10, and 24 h later only 39% and 45% cells, respectively, remained viable. Human Panc-1 cells were the least susceptible to the cytotoxic effects of vMyx-mLIGHT-FLuc/tdTr infection and retained 82% viability at 24 h and 67% at 48 h/MOI = 5). Thus, the infection of cultured pancreatic adenocarcinoma cells with the vMyx-mLIGHT-FLuc/tdTr construct leads to a marked-to-significant reduction in cell viability, suggesting that oncolytic treatment of even the semi- and non-permissive types of cancers may provide sizeable therapeutic benefits in vivo, as well as still delivering therapeutic proteins such as LIGHT, if expressed under early virus promoter control. ADSCs seem to fulfill the criteria for an effective viral cargo carrier that is also capable of supporting viral replication and potentially delivering either parental or progeny virus into cancer sites.

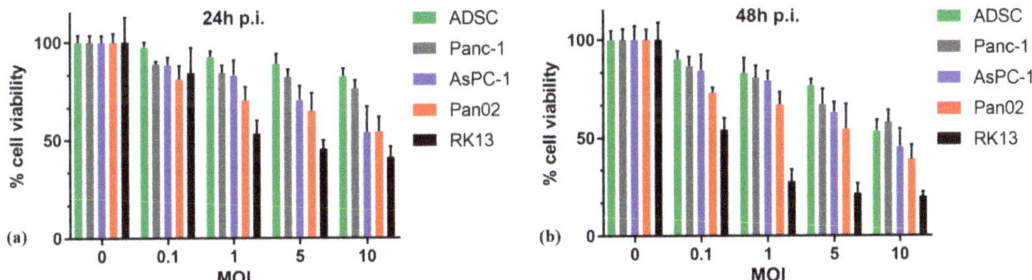

Figure 3. MYXV infection reduces the viability of pancreatic cancer cells. Pancreatic cancer cell (Panc-1, AsPC-1 and Pan02) ADSCs, as well as RK13 (1×10^4 cells/well), were infected with vMyx-mLIGHT-FLuc/tdTr at four various MOIs (0.1; 1; 5 and 10) and analyzed for cell viability using the MTS assay at (**a**) 24 h and (**b**) 48 h post-infection. The assays were performed in triplicate; error bars shown are means ± SD.

3.4. Orthotopic Injection of Pan02 Cells with ADSCs Pre-Infected Ex Vivo with MYXV Inhibits Establishment and Growth of Pancreatic Cancer

We examined if the oncolytic properties of MYXV could prevent the growth of pancreatic adenocarcinoma in mice following the orthotopic injection of murine cancer cells, under conditions in which the virus is co-delivered with the cancer cells (Figure 4). To do so, naïve immunocompetent mice were implanted orthotopically with Pan02 adenocarcinoma cells and then immediately treated by orthotopic injection of LIGHT-encoding MYXV construct (vMyx-mLIGHT-Fluc/tdTr), either unshielded or shielded by ADSC carrier cells (ADSCs that had been previously infected ex vivo with the vMyx-mLIGHT-Fluc/tdTr). As controls, ADSCs or PBS⁻ were used. Twenty-one days after this co-implantation procedure, the dissected pancreata were macroscopically inspected and both size and mass were recorded. The experiment revealed (Figure 4a) no tumor presence and no organ size increase if vMyx-mLIGHT-Fluc/tdTr constructs were injected (i.e., either ADSC-shielded or unshielded). Statistically significant differences were revealed (Figure 4b) between the masses of pancreata from control mice and pancreata from both virus-recipient mouse groups.

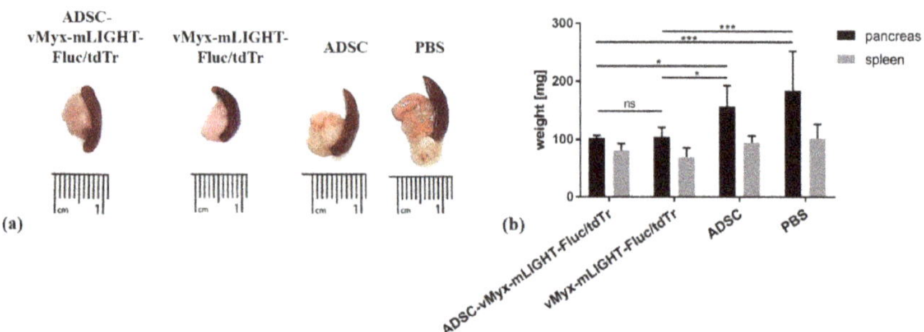

Figure 4. Inhibition of pancreatic adenocarcinoma formation after orthotopic implantation of Pan02 cells and consecutive injection of ADSC-shielded MYXV construct (vMyx-mLIGHT-Fluc/tdTr) or unshielded MYXV. (**a**) Macroscopic appearance of pancreas and spleen upon necropsy; (**b**) mass of pancreata and spleen (*n* = 6) after orthotopic injection (21 days). The data show means ± SD of two independent experiments. (* $p \leq 0.05$; *** $p \leq 0.001$; ns—not significant).

3.5. ADSC-Enhanced Biodistribution and Tumor Targeting of MYXV in Pancreatic Cancer-Bearing Mice after Intraperitoneal Injection

Comparison of the intraperitoneal (IP) versus intravenous (IV) route of ADSC/MYXV administration revealed pancreas-targeted distribution of the virus when ADSCs were delivered IP to mice bearing orthotopically injected PDAC (Figure S4). Bioluminescence (BLI) data were acquired using IVIS (Figure 5) to assess the distribution of the ADSC-shielded or unshielded vMyx-mLIGHT-Fluc/tdTr construct, administered intraperitoneally after 7 days (single IP injection) into recipient mice either harboring tumor lesions (+Pan02) or free from tumor lesions (−Pan02). Intact animals (Figure 5a) and dissected organs (Figure 5b) were examined. Following injection, bioluminescence signals for both shielded and unshielded MYXV peaked within three hours in the pancreas, but were also present in the spleen and liver. The shielded virus was detected throughout the examined time span (96 h post-injection); later, it faded away. In contrast, no bioluminescence signal from the unshielded MYXV construct was detected in the pancreas after 48 h. No bioluminescence signal was observed in the lungs, heart or muscle tissue from any tested group.

The analysis of total photon flux data (Figure 5c) from intact mice bearing tumors (+Pan02) revealed that after 24 h p.i., the signal from the shielded virus was 200-fold stronger than that from its unshielded counterpart. However, after a further 24 h (48-h time point) the signal from the shielded virus decreased 100-fold, indicating either some transfer event following the release of the construct from ADSCs, or simply viral clearance. This signal, however, was still high at 72 h, contrary to that in unshielded MYXV which, at 72 h, was undetectable. The persistence of the shielded virus signal suggests a different fate of the actively expressing virus after its probable release from ADSCs, or possibly a source of signals other than the pancreas. In tumor-free mice (−Pan02) there was no essential difference in the kinetics of signal quenching between the shielded and unshielded virus, except that absolute signal values were generally somewhat lower for the unshielded construct. In these tumor-free mice, the signal from the shielded virus at 24 h was 100-fold higher than that of its unshielded counterpart, similar to tumor-burdened animals, again showing the protective nature of ADSCs. When signals from tumor-bearing and tumor-free mice were compared at the 24-h time point, a 4-fold difference was seen in favor of the shielded virus, suggesting increased targeting, perhaps due to the inflammatory nature of tumor foci, which attract ADSCs. The decrease of the shielded virus signal in tumor-free mice, occurring between 24 and 48 h, was similar to that seen in tumor-bearing mice and again suggests a gene expression-related event following the virus release in the tumor bed. However, the decrease was 50-fold, twice as small as that seen in tumor-bearing mice, and this difference could be ascribed to the presence/absence of tumor lesions. Analysis of total photon flux data for the dissected pancreata (Figure 5d) shows the kinetics of the signal decrease in tumor-bearing mice (+Pan02) to be generally similar to that in intact animals (Figure 5c), except that the signal for the shielded virus after 72 h was lower. This points to the presence of some other source of the signal (in addition to the pancreas) in intact animals, at least at this time point. The exceptionally large difference between shielded and unshielded virus signals from pancreata of tumor-bearing mice at 24-h time point (more than three orders of magnitude) demonstrates the effective shielding of the viral construct delivered by ADSCs to adenocarcinoma lesions. Finally, the comparison of signals from the shielded construct at the 48-h time point between pancreata dissected from tumor-bearing and tumor-free mice, shows a ca. 10-fold higher signal from the former; this further corroborates the virus-protective and tumor-targeting capacities of ADSC carrier cells.

3.6. LIGHT-Encoding MYXV Shielded by ADSC Enhances Anti-Tumor Immune Response and Improves Survival of Mice Bearing Orthotopic Adenocarcinoma Lesions

The endurance of human ADSCs infected with therapeutic MYXV following IP injection into immunocompetent mice was deemed sufficient to allow the survival of virus during bloodstream transit and its delivery to PDAC lesions before immune clearance. We thus examined the therapeutic effect of the LIGHT-expressing oncolytic MYXV construct (vMyx-mLIGHT-Fluc/tdTr) using immunocompetent mice (Figure 6). The animals were first engrafted orthotopically with murine Pan02 cells. Four days later, the mice received IP injections of vMyx-mLIGHT-Fluc/tdTr, either in unshielded or ADSC-shielded form. Control mice received PBS$^-$ only. In total, five doses of the therapeutics were delivered (every 4 days), spanning three weeks of treatment (Figure 6a).

At the end of the therapeutic intervention (21st day) some animals were sacrificed and their pancreata and spleens inspected macroscopically for size and organ weight (Figure 6b,c). Pancreata from mice treated with ADSC-shielded MYXV revealed smaller sizes (Figure 6b), as well as reduced weight (Figure 6c) when compared to mice receiving unshielded MYXV or PBS$^-$ (ca. 25% and 50%, respectively), suggesting a positive response to ADSC-mediated oncolytic therapy.

Samples of pancreatic tissue and blood were also examined by means of flow cytometry (Figure 6d–f) for signs of an adaptive anti-tumor immune response after the conclusion of therapy. The percentage of CD4+ helper cells (Figure 6d) among CD3+ lymphocytes for both pancreata and blood decreased following treatment with shielded and unshielded virus, but was not statistically significant. The percentage of CD8+ cells (Figure 6e) in murine blood increased following delivery of both shielded or unshielded virus, but not significantly either. Contrarily, the increase of CD8+ in pancreatic samples was significant for the shielded ($p < 0.01$) as well as the unshielded ($p < 0.05$) virus when compared to the PBS$^-$ group. Changes in the CD4+/CD8+ ratio (Figure 6f) were only significant for pancreatic tissue samples and the shielded virus group ($p < 0.05$). Taken together, these changes suggest an enhanced immune response triggered by the oncolytic viral construct used and benefiting from using ADSCs as carrier cells.

H&E-stained tissue specimens (pancreas, spleen, liver) from both treatment groups and controls were microscopically evaluated by an experienced histopathologist. In pancreatic specimens from the group treated with unshielded MYXV, only minimal lymphocytic influx was usually present around the edge of tumor (Figure 6g, center panel). In contrast, pancreatic specimens treated with ADSC-shielded MYXV showed stronger lymphocytic infiltrates, especially in the peripancreatic adipose tissue (Figure 6g, right panel). Liver specimens revealed no pathology in the tissue architecture in any group.

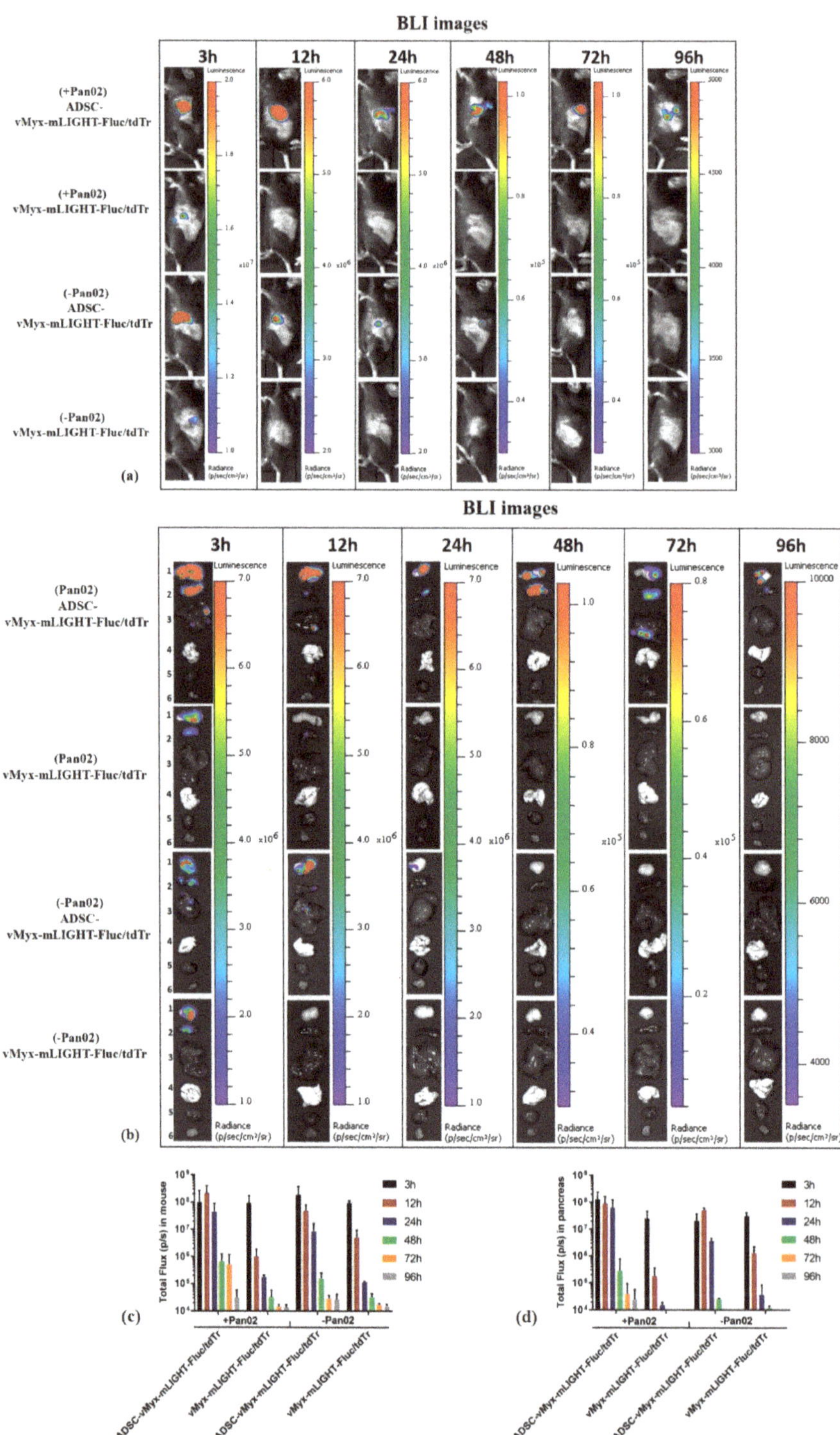

Figure 5. Effect of intraperitoneal injection of MYXV construct (vMyx-mLIGHT-Fluc/tdTr) on biodistribution in mice. Bioluminescence (BLI) images were acquired either in unchallenged (−Pan02) mice injected IP with PBS⁻ only, and in

challenged (+Pan02) orthotopic pancreatic adenocarcinoma-bearing mice at various time points (3 h, 12 h, 24 h, 48 h, 72 h and 96 h) post-injection of ADSC-shielded or unshielded MYXV construct (vMyx-mLIGHT-Fluc/tdTr); (**a**) intact mice; (**b**) dissected organs (1-pancreas, 2-spleen, 3-liver, 4-lungs, 5-heart and 6-muscle). Region of interest (ROI)-based analysis of total photon flux in (**c**) intact animals and (**d**) dissected pancreata. BLI is expressed as radiance (photons/sec/cm^2/sr). Different radiance scales are shown to cover the whole span of bioluminescence. The data show means $\pm$ SD of two independent experiments (n = 3).

The panels in Figure S5 (see Supplementary Materials) show additional micrographs of pancreatic and spleen sections from mice subjected to the therapeutic intervention with unshielded or shielded armed MYXV. Pancreata from animals treated with unshielded MYXV revealed spindle cell tumors, making up 25–60%; in the ADSC-shielded MYXV group the cellularity of tumor regions did not exceed 25% (panel 3). Both treated groups displayed large nuclear pleomorphism; oval, blunt-ended cell nuclei; no distinct nucleoli and fine-grained chromatin (panels 5–6). The unshielded MYXV group featured more atypical mitoses and spindle cells, with a hyperchromatic nucleus (panel 1). In the shielded MYXV group only single atypical mitoses and singly dispersed spindle cells were seen with a focal hyperchromatic nucleus (panel 6). The control group (PBS$^-$) showed pancreas sections that featured spindle cell tumors invading acinar cells and surrounding interlobular ducts, large nuclear pleomorphism, oval blunt-ended cell nuclei, no distinct nucleoli, fine-grained chromatin and sinusoidal blood vessels (panels 1,4 and 10). In turn, micrographs of the spleen specimens from the group treated with unshielded MYXV showed spindle cell tumors covering the spleen (panel 14), whereas in the group treated with shielded MYXV only cancer cells with hyperchromatic nuclei between collagen fibers were visible, along with thickened capsules, inflammatory lymphocytes, as well as eosinophils (panel 15). Spleen specimens from the control group (PBS$^-$) showed infiltration of spindle cell tumors adjacent to the spleen capsule (panel 13), whereas giant cells were scattered in the spleen parenchyma in all groups.

The mitotic index data (Figure 6h) for the pancreatic specimens show significantly decreased numbers of mitoses in the shielded MYXV group when compared to the PBS$^-$ control group ($p < 0.0001$) and to the virus-treated group ($p < 0.001$).

The remaining mice from the therapeutic experiment were monitored and compared for survival with controls. The difference in survival (Figure 6i) between controls and mice that received five doses of unshielded MYXV was 42.8%, whereas that for ADSC-shielded MYXV was 88% ($p = 0.0015$). On the 54th day, 50% of animals which received ADSC-shielded MYXV were alive, compared to none in the unshielded construct group.

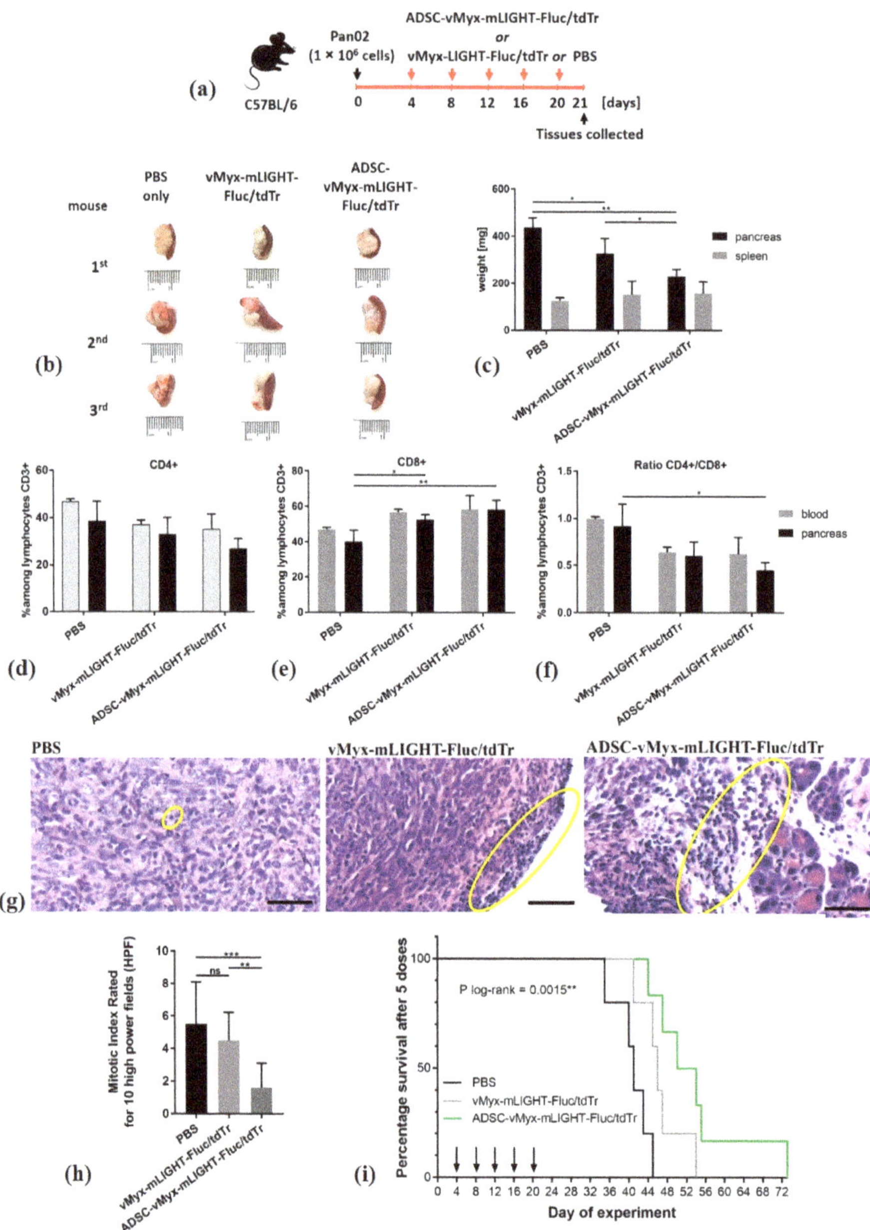

Figure 6. Therapy of experimental pancreatic adenocarcinoma using armed MYXV construct. C57Bl/6NCrl mice (*n* = 10–11) with induced orthotopic lesions were injected IP (days 4, 8, 12, 16 and 20) with LIGHT-expressing vMyx-mLIGHT-Fluc/tdTr, either ADSC-shielded or unshielded, or with PBS⁻; (**a**) timeline of experiment; (**b**) size of pancreata, 21st day; (**c**) weight of pancreata and spleen, 21st day; (**d**–**f**) flow cytometry data showing CD4+ and CD8+ cell percentages among CD3+ lymphocytes in the blood and pancreas; (**g**) histological appearance of representative H&E-stained sections (scale bars: 50 µm, magn. 48×): lymphocytic infiltrates: yellow ellipses, (**h**) mitotic index rated under 400× magnification for 10 high power fields (HPF); (**i**) mouse survival (*n* = 7–8): log-rank (Mantel–Cox) test; *p* = 0.0015. The data (mean ± SD) were analyzed with one-way ANOVA; statistically significant differences are indicated (* $p \leq 0.05$; ** $p \leq 0.01$; *** $p \leq 0.001$; ns – not significant).

4. Discussion

PDAC presents a formidable challenge for oncological researchers, as the overall outcome of PDAC patients remains desperately poor. The characteristic feature of PDAC is its resistance against practically any treatment [30–32].

Oncolytic virotherapy represents a promising approach to augmenting the PDAC therapeutic repertoire. In the current manuscript, we report the results of an experimental therapy targeting orthotopically-induced PDAC lesions in immunocompetent mice using recombinant oncolytic MYXV encoding mouse tumor necrosis factor ligand superfamily member 14 (also called LIGHT), designed to boost the anti-tumor immune response induced by the virotherapy. The vMyx-mLIGHT-Fluc/tdTr construct was pre-adsorbed ex vivo onto adipose tissue-derived stem cells (ADSCs) of mesenchymal origin and subsequently infused into the peritoneal cavity of experimental animals that had been pre-seeded orthotopically with murine PDAC into the pancreas.

We show that the cultured human ADSCs had correct morphology and multipotency. In-vitro-expanded ADSC cells were shown to differentiate into adult cells of the expected downstream lineages. The phenotype of ADSCs, as assessed by characteristic surface markers and migratory properties, was also shown to remain unchanged between MYXV-infected ADSCs and uninfected ADSCs, at least in the 1–2 day interval post-infection. We confirmed the level of permissiveness of ADSCs and three tested pancreatic cancer cell lines to MYXV. We observed significant differences between these pancreatic cancer cell lines concerning the level of infection and replication of MYXV. In general, cancer cells can be either fully permissive (i.e., produce in excess of 10 infectious progeny virus units per cell), semi-permissive (i.e., produce the progeny virus at a level below 10 infectious units/cell) or non-permissive (no detectable progeny virus) to MYXV. All three categories of cells can nevertheless express MYXV-encoded transgenes controlled by early virus promoters, but only the first two types can also express transgenes under late viral promoter control. The in vitro results indicated that MYXV productively infects the murine pancreatic cancer cell line (Pan02) with evidence of a cytopathic effect, complete viral replication and increased cell death. However, levels of productive MYXV replication in human pancreatic cancer cell lines (AsPC-1 and Panc-1) showed that they were less susceptible to infection, and we define them as semi-permissive or nonpermissive for MYXV, respectively. ADSCs remained the most viable after MYXV infection, whereas RK13 (the control rabbit cell line used to propagate the virus) was highly MYXV-susceptible.

Despite the variable levels of progeny virus generated, infection of all cultured pancreatic adenocarcinoma cells with vMyx-mLIGHT-FLuc/tdTr led to a marked-to-significant reduction in cell viability. ADSCs, in contrast, support viral infection without rapid cell death, making this viral cell carrier useful for in vivo experiments where cell viability and taxis need only be maintained for a brief period in order to ferry the virus into cancerous sites, likely hours or less. The ability of cultured ADSCs to support MYXV replication is similar to that observed with bone marrow-derived mesenchymal stem cells [23]. This is a key feature of ADSCs, allowing the successful transfer of the virus into adjacent tumor cells via cell–cell contact. ADSCs thus seem to fulfill the criteria for an effective viral cargo carrier that is capable of transferring both the input (parental) and progeny virus to tumor cells, yielding sizeable therapeutic benefits in vivo.

We first showed that ADSCs infected with MYXV could effectively prevent the outgrowth of experimentally induced PDAC lesions when the cancer cells were co-implanted with MYXV or with ADSCs pre-infected ex vivo with MYXV. On the other hand, control tumors were rapidly induced in the absence of the virus. This pre-treatment experiment indicated that MYXV can be highly therapeutic against PDAC if the virus delivery to cancer cells in situ can be optimized. Thus, the model is a sensitive indicator of the efficiency of delivery of an OV to tumor cells at the pancreatic site of PDAC. Essentially similar outcomes seen with co-implantation of cancer cells and therapeutic constructs provide evidence of viral construct transfer from infected MSCs to cancer cells under in vivo conditions [23].

OV-mediated systemic therapy, for example after IV infusion of the unshielded virus, faces rapid and efficient anti-viral immune host responses, as well as other clearance obstacles. During bloodstream transit, the viral cargo is largely cleared in organs like the liver and spleen, although protective carrier cells can mitigate against this [22]. Whether IP administration of the tested therapeutic recombinant MYXV would be contingent upon, or benefit from, shielding by a protective cell carrier like ADSCs was an open question that we approached in this study. We report that IP administration of the protected viral therapeutic cargo by pre-loading onto ADSCs ex vivo yielded desirable pancreas-restricted distribution as compared to more standard IV administration. The significance of pre-loading carrier cells with oncolytic virus cannot be overestimated. Our data highlight the outcome of delivering such pre-loaded ADSCs. IVIS-generated images tracking the distribution of the viral construct (vMyx-mLIGHT-Fluc/tdTr) in PDAC-bearing mice following IP injection clearly demonstrate the delivery of the virus into the pancreas. The unshielded recombinant MYXV was rather rapidly cleared from the body after IP administration, as opposed to the virus shielded by ADSCs. The existing dogma postulates that anti-OV immune responses restrict viral replication and spread, and thus reduce direct OV-mediated killing of cancer cells. Therefore, the anti-tumor activity of the unshielded virus, although present, is likely not optimal therapeutically. This point is also illustrated by the difference in survival between the two therapeutic groups (MYXV only vs. ADSC-MYXV).

Photon flux IVIS data from intact mice demonstrate the advantage of shielding the virus using ADSCs and temporal signal changes suggest the release and transfer of the virus from carrier cells into target pancreatic cancer cells. The persistence of the signal from virus that had been pre-shielded with ADSCs implies either a different fate of the virus transferred from ADSCs or a source of the signal other than pancreas. Comparison of the signal between tumor-bearing and tumor-free control mice also confirms the protective benefits of ADSC pre-shielding and increased targeting in favor of tumor bearing mice, perhaps due to the inflammatory nature of tumor foci. Temporal differences in the signal are also suggestive of virus release and de novo infection of cancer cells, and signal differences between tumor-bearing and tumor-free animals could be ascribed to the presence or absence of tumor lesions. Total photon flux data, showing exceptionally large differences between shielded vs. unshielded virus signals from pancreata of tumor-bearing mice (several orders of magnitude), point to effective delivery and transfer of the viral construct to cancer cells within the pancreas. The potential ability of ADSCs to seek out pancreatic cancer cells and deliver oncolytic MYXV from an IP injection could be of great therapeutic value, especially when other delivery strategies are ineffective.

Ex-vivo-expanded hypoimmunogenic human adipose-derived stem cells (ADSCs) represent a unique delivery platform for OVs. They combine a natural capacity to home to inflammatory sites with a tumor tropism that is coupled with potent amplification of the OV load and transient suppression of anti-viral innate immunity, which hinders OVs from colonizing the tumor site and infecting cancer cells [33]. Importantly, IFNγ, which is involved in the induction of an anti-viral state, also modulates immunosuppressive features of ADSCs, counteracting anti-viral immunity. Thus, the dual capacity of ADSCs to offset the innate and adaptive arms of anti-viral immunity and to allow viral load amplification potential is conducive for the success of oncolytic virotherapy. In studies involving mice and repetitive treatment in which the access route is challenging, IP delivery remains an alternative to IV when the latter strategy is clearly ineffective, as it generally is for PDAC. Targeting the pancreas with an OV using mesenchymal stem cells as carriers is not nearly as effective via IV delivery, for the same reason that targeting lung neoplasias in this manner is ineffective—the "first pass" effect [23]. Although IP administration of pharmacological agents is minimally used in the clinic (mostly for the treatment of peritoneal cancers), in experimental animals it is a justifiable route for proof-of-concept studies where the goal is to evaluate the effect(s) of target engagement rather than the properties of a drug formulation and/or its pharmacokinetics for clinical translation [34].

Following the postulated release of the virus from ADSCs at the targeted tumor site, some intratumoral antiviral events occur, resulting in a "cold" to "hot" transition, reversal of immunosuppression and recruitment of immune cells. Cancer cell death-associated signals further contribute to the development of a tumor-specific adaptive immune response. Overall, antiviral innate and adaptive responses targeting virus replication sites target cancer cells since OVs preferentially infect cancer cells [35]. A decisive factor in successful immunotherapy is the presence of T cells and the reactivation of their anti-tumor properties. Even though T cells are rather low in PDAC, some data suggest that the tumor microenvironment (TME) mainly consists of various cellular components and the extracellular matrix and is highly immunosuppressive. Tumor-infiltrating lymphocytes are one of the crucial players in the TME of pancreatic cancer. On the other hand, although numbers of T cells in PDAC appear low [36], the tumor-reactive T-cell repertoire was found to be similar to that in melanoma, in which immunotherapy does show a therapeutic impact [37]. Since strong intra-tumoral CD8+ T cell infiltration is associated with prolonged survival, induction of anti-tumor T cell responses can indeed be a promising approach for PDAC [38–40].

In a previous study, we showed that the therapy targeting experimentally induced lung melanoma in mice with IL-15-encoding MYXV construct (vMyx-IL15Rα-tdTr) delivered by MSCs was effective and was able to reduce the tumor burden as well as triggering the inflow of CD8+ cells [33]. Here, we demonstrate another ADSC-shielded recombinant MYXV that expresses LIGHT protein, used to extend the survival of treated mice and to increase the influx of T lymphocytes into the tumor.

Following a five-dose therapy of orthotopic PDAC lesions with ADSC-vMyx-mLIGHT-Fluc/tdTr, we have been able to show a reduced tumor burden effect, suggesting a positive response to treatment. At the end of the therapeutic intervention (21st day), some animals were thoroughly inspected post-mortem for any signs of macroscopic pathologies and none were found, except for remaining tumor lesions. Scars surgically-induced at the onset of the experiment were healed.

An adaptive anti-tumor immune response was evidenced by the slightly decreased percentage of CD4+ helper cells among CD3+ lymphocytes, both in the blood and in the pancreas, but concurrent with a statistically significant increase in the percentage of CD8+ cells in the pancreas. Changes in the CD4+/CD8+ ratio suggest an enhanced immune response triggered by ADSC-assisted oncolytic therapy. Analysis of H&E-stained tissue specimens from all treatment groups showed that a five-dose therapy appears to be safe for the animals as no pathology was revealed in the livers. Cancer cell infiltrations in the pancreas and spleen were evidenced in the PBS$^-$ control groups, whereas high lymphocyte infiltrates were present in specimens from the group treated with the ADSC-shielded virus; and minimal lymphocyte infiltrates were present in specimens from virus-treated group. The virus-treated groups revealed fibrotic strands suggestive of the eradication of cancer cells, further supported by the decreased mitotic index. Taken together, the results of flow cytometry and microscopic analysis suggest that vMyx-mLIGHT-Fluc/tdTr delivered by ADSCs was able to modulate the immune microenviroment in PDAC tissues and contribute to the prolonged survival of mice treated with the five-dose strategy.

We show in this proof-of concept study that the recombinant MYXV used, a therapeutic agent with a dual mode of action (as a tumor oncolytic agent and an elicitor of an acquired immune response) can be an efficient component of a multi-pronged approach to PDAC therapy. ADSC-mediated IP delivery of MYXV to treat orthotopic experimental PDAC lesions in mice proved to be highly effective. Our results demonstrated increased survival of animals bearing orthotopic PDAC tumor lesions following monotherapy with an engineered recombinant MYXV delivered by ADSC; they also showed increased numbers of T cells in pancreata dissected from the treated mice. This enables a more advanced approach to virus- and ADSC-based therapies.

The levels of productive MYXV replication in two human pancreatic cancer cell lines tested (AsPC-1 and Panc-1) showed lower susceptibility to infection yet marked-to-significant reductions in cell viability. This may obviously be a disadvantage in clinical oncology. Combinatory therapeutic approaches involving more advanced armed OVs triggering enhanced adaptive immunity effects, as well as agents targeting desmoplasia, should offset this drawback. Single-agent approaches seem insufficient to improve the therapeutic outcomes of PDAC [41].

Intelligent combinatorial therapies appear to be required to achieve significant synergism in PDAC treatment. For example, modern radiation techniques, eliciting abscopal effects via reconditioning of the tumor microenvironment, reprogramming tumor-infiltrating macrophages towards an M1-like phenotype and favoring the recruitment of adoptively transferred T cells [42] or activating cytosolic DNA sensors, such as STING, are on the horizon [43]. Another example are early phase clinical trials combining recombinant human hyaluronidase, gemcitabine and nab-paclitaxel, which have revealed promising results, particularly in those patients whose tumors were characterized by high levels of hyaluronan [44]. The rationale for all these approaches is to outcompete therapy resistance; this might be challenging, however, as combined modality treatments are frequently associated with higher toxicity levels [45]. Immunotherapy is another hope for novel strategies against pancreatic cancer, even though this deadly cancer has been so far resistant to immune checkpoint blockade and chimeric antigen receptor (CAR) T-cell therapies. Research involving the use of CAR T cells in pancreatic cancer therapy is rapidly developing, in combination with other treatments as well [46].

Overall, the successful strategies against PDAC should thus involve combinations of modern "classical" treatments with different immunotherapeutic approaches and, hopefully, with oncovirotherapy.

5. Conclusions

To sum up, we have shown that oncolytic monotherapy with adipose-derived mesenchymal stem cells loaded with LIGHT-expressing MYXV delivered IP to experimental orthotopic PDAC lesion-bearing mice resulted in increased animal survival and boosted the immune response.

Supplementary Materials: The following are available online at https://www.mdpi.com/2072-6694/13/6/1394/s1, Figure S1: Schematic design showing the organization and recombination region of vMyx-mLIGHT-Fluc/tdTr, Figure S2: Constitutive expression of Light in infected and non-infected ADSCs, Figure S3: Expression and localization of murine LIGHT in the vMyx-mLIGHT-FLuc/tdTr-infected cells, Figure S4: Effect of intraperitoneally vs. intravenously injected MYXV construct (vMyx-mLIGHT-Fluc/tdTr) on biodistribution in mice, Figure S5: Histological appearance of representative H&E-stained tissue sections, Table S1: The source of adipose tissue-derived mesenchymal stem cells.

Author Contributions: Conceptualization, J.J.-R. and A.S.; design and source of MYXV recombinants, G.M. and M.M.R.; adipose tissue source, M.G.; flow cytometry, W.F.; in vitro studies, J.J.-R., A.H. and M.P.; in vivo studies, J.J.-R. and A.S.; histological analysis, E.C.; validation and formal analysis, J.J.-R. and V.K.; writing—original draft preparation, J.J.-R. and A.S.; writing—review and editing, J.J.-R., A.S., V.K., M.M.R. and G.M.; visualization, supervision, project administration, and funding acquisition, J.J.-R. and A.S. All authors have read and agreed to the published version of the manuscript.

Funding: This research was funded by National Science Centre, Poland, grant number 2016/22/M/NZ6/00418. The construction of vMyx-mLIGHT-Fluc/tdTr was funded by a Sponsored Research Agreement (SRA) from DNAtrix.

Institutional Review Board Statement: All procedures involving human adipose-derived mesenchymal stem cells (ADSCs) were conducted according to the guidelines of the Declaration of Helsinki, and approved by the Bioethics Committee of the MSC National Research Institute of Oncology, Warsaw, Poland (Approval No. 63/2017). All animal procedures were performed in accordance with European Union (EU) law, after approval by the Local Ethics Committee, Medical University of Silesia, Katowice, Poland (Approval No. 20/2020).

Informed Consent Statement: Not applicable.

Data Availability Statement: Data sharing not applicable.

Acknowledgments: The Authors thank Gabriela Kramer-Marek for training in orthotopic animal surgery procedures; Krzysztof Rakus for discussion and Miriam Mojżesz for technical assistance with gene expression analysis. The Graphical Abstract was created with BioRender.com (accessed on February 2021, Toronto, ON, Canada).

Conflicts of Interest: G.M. is a co-founder and equity holder of OncoMyx Therapeutics, devoted to the clinical development of MYXV vectors for cancer. M.M.R. is a consultant for OncoMyx Therapeutics.

References

1. Rhim, A.D.; Mirek, E.T.; Aiello, N.M.; Maitra, A.; Bailey, J.M.; McAllister, F.; Reichert, M.; Beatty, G.L.; Rustgi, A.K.; Vonderheide, R.H.; et al. EMT and dissemination precede pancreatic tumor formation. *Cell* **2012**, *148*, 349–361. [CrossRef] [PubMed]
2. Dougan, S.K. The Pancreatic Cancer Microenvironment. *Cancer J.* **2017**, *23*, 321–325. [CrossRef] [PubMed]
3. Erkan, M.; Kurtoglu, M.; Kleeff, J. The role of hypoxia in pancreatic cancer: A potential therapeutic target? *Expert. Rev. Gastroenterol. Hepatol.* **2016**, *10*, 301–316. [CrossRef]
4. Heinemann, V.; Reni, M.; Ychou, M.; Richel, D.J.; Macarulla, T.; Ducreux, M. Tumour-stroma interactions in pancreatic ductal adenocarcinoma: Rationale and current evidence for new therapeutic strategies. *Cancer Treat. Rev.* **2014**, *40*, 118–128. [CrossRef]
5. Li, N.; Li, Y.; Li, Z.; Huang, C.; Yang, Y.; Lang, M.; Cao, J.; Jiang, W.; Xu, Y.; Dong, J.; et al. Hypoxia Inducible Factor 1 (HIF-1) Recruits Macrophage to Activate Pancreatic Stellate Cells in Pancreatic Ductal Adenocarcinoma. *Int. J. Mol. Sci.* **2016**, *17*, 799. [CrossRef] [PubMed]
6. Ene-Obong, A.; Clear, A.J.; Watt, J.; Wang, J.; Fatah, R.; Riches, J.C.; Marshall, J.F.; Chin-Aleong, J.; Chelala, C.; Gribben, J.G.; et al. Activated pancreatic stellate cells sequester CD8+ T cells to reduce their infiltration of the juxtatumoral compartment of pancreatic ductal adenocarcinoma. *Gastroenterology* **2013**, *145*, 1121–1132. [CrossRef] [PubMed]
7. Ozdemir, B.C.; Pentcheva-Hoang, T.; Carstens, J.L.; Zheng, X.; Wu, C.C.; Simpson, T.R.; Laklai, H.; Sugimoto, H.; Kahlert, C.; Novitskiy, S.V.; et al. Depletion of carcinomaassociated fibroblasts and fibrosis induces immunosuppression and accelerates pancreas cancer with reduced survival. *Cancer Cell* **2014**, *25*, 719–734. [CrossRef] [PubMed]
8. Daniel, S.K.; Sullivan, K.M.; Labadie, K.P.; Pillarisetty, V.G. Hypoxia as a barrier to immunotherapy in pancreatic adenocarcinoma. *Clin. Transl. Med.* **2019**, *8*, 10. [CrossRef]
9. Mitchem, J.B.; Brennan, D.J.; Knolhoff, B.L.; Belt, B.A.; Zhu, Y.; Sanford, D.E.; Belaygorod, L.; Carpenter, D.; Collins, L.; Piwnica-Worms, D.; et al. Targeting tumor-infiltrating macrophages decreases tumor-initiating cells, relieves immunosuppression, and improves chemotherapeutic responses. *Cancer Res.* **2013**, *73*, 1128–1141. [CrossRef]
10. Hu, H.; Hang, J.J.; Han, T.; Zhuo, M.; Jiao, F.; Wang, L.W. The M2 phenotype of tumor-associated macrophages in the stroma confers a poor prognosis in pancreatic cancer. *Tumour Biol.* **2016**, *37*, 8657–8664. [CrossRef]
11. Adamska, A.; Domenichini, A.; Falasca, M. Pancreatic Ductal Adenocarcinoma: Current and Evolving Therapies. *Int. J. Mol. Sci.* **2017**, *18*, 1338. [CrossRef]
12. Shah, A.N.; Summy, J.M.; Zhang, J.; Park, S.I.; Parikh, N.U.; Gallick, G.E. Development and characterization of gemcitabine-resistant pancreatic tumor cells. *Ann. Surg. Oncol.* **2007**, *14*, 3629–3637. [CrossRef]
13. Wang, Z.; Li, Y.; Kong, D.; Banerjee, S.; Ahmad, A.; Azmi, A.S.; Ali, S.; Abbruzzese, J.L.; Gallick, G.E.; Sarkar, F.H. Acquisition of epithelial-mesenchymal transition phenotype of gemcitabine-resistant pancreatic cancer cells is linked with activation of the notch signaling pathway. *Cancer Res.* **2009**, *69*, 2400–2407. [CrossRef] [PubMed]
14. Yang, A.D.; Camp, E.R.; Fan, F.; Shen, L.; Gray, M.J.; Liu, W.; Somcio, R.; Bauer, T.W.; Wu, Y.; Hicklin, D.J.; et al. Vascular endothelial growth factor receptor-1 activation mediates epithelial to mesenchymal transition in human pancreatic carcinoma cells. *Cancer Res.* **2006**, *66*, 46–51. [CrossRef] [PubMed]
15. Vacchelli, E.; Eggermont, A.; Sautès-Fridman, C.; Galon, J.; Zitvogel, L.; Kroemer, G.; Galluzzi, L. Trial watch: Oncolytic viruses for cancer therapy. *Oncoimmunology* **2013**, *2*, e24612. [CrossRef]
16. Zeyaullah, M.; Patro, M.; Ahmad, I.; Ibraheem, K.; Sultan, P.; Nehal, M.; Ali, A. Oncolytic viruses in the treatment of cancer: A review of current strategies. *Pathol. Oncol. Res.* **2012**, *18*, 771–781. [CrossRef] [PubMed]
17. Torres-Domínguez, L.E.; de Matos, A.L.; Rahman, M.M.; McFadden, G. Methods for the Construction of Recombinant Oncolytic Myxoma Viruses. *Methods Mol. Biol.* **2021**, *2225*, 63–75. [PubMed]
18. Pasero, C.; Barbarat, B.; Just-Landi, S.; Bernard, A.; Aurran-Schleinitz, T.; Rey, J.; Eldering, E.; Truneh, A.; Costello, R.T.; Olive, D. A role for HVEM, but not lymphotoxin-beta receptor, in LIGHT-induced tumor cell death and chemokine production. *Eur. J. Immunol.* **2009**, *39*, 2502–2514. [CrossRef]
19. Maker, A.V. Precise identification of immunotherapeutic targets for solid malignancies using clues within the tumor microenvironment-evidence to turn on the LIGHT. *Oncoimmunology* **2016**, *5*, e1069937. [CrossRef]
20. Šedý, J.R.; Ramezani-Rad, P. HVEM network signaling in cancer. *Adv. Cancer Res.* **2019**, *142*, 145–186.

21. Dai, S.; Lv, Y.; Xu, W.; Yang, Y.; Liu, C.; Dong, X.; Zhang, H.; Prabhakar, B.S.; Maker, A.V.; Seth, P.; et al. Oncolytic adenovirus encoding LIGHT (TNFSF14) inhibits tumor growth via activating anti-tumor immune responses in 4T1 mouse mammary tumor model in immune competent syngeneic mice. *Cancer Gene Ther.* **2020**, *27*, 923–933. [CrossRef]

22. Hadryś, A.; Sochanik, A.; McFadden, G.; Jazowiecka-Rakus, J. Mesenchymal stem cells as carriers for systemic delivery of oncolytic viruses. *Eur. J. Pharmacol.* **2020**, *874*, 172991. [CrossRef]

23. Jazowiecka-Rakus, J.; Sochanik, A.; Rusin, A.; Hadryś, A.; Fidyk, W.; Villa, N.; Rahman, M.M.; Chmielik, E.; Franco, L.S.; McFadden, G. Myxoma Virus-Loaded Mesenchymal Stem Cells in Experimental Oncolytic Therapy of Murine Pulmonary Melanoma. *Mol. Ther. Oncol.* **2020**, *6*, 335–350. [CrossRef]

24. Kulu, Y.; Dorfman, J.D.; Kuruppu, D.; Fuchs, B.C.; Goodwin, J.M.; Fujii, T.; Kuroda, T.; Lanuti, M.; Tanabe, K.K. Comparison of intravenous versus intraperitoneal administration of oncolytic herpes simplex virus 1 for peritoneal carcinomatosis in mice. *Cancer Gene Ther.* **2009**, *16*, 291–297. [CrossRef] [PubMed]

25. Wennier, S.T.; Liu, J.; Li, S.; Rahman, M.M.; Mona, M.; McFadden, G. Myxoma virus sensitizes cancer cells to gemcitabine and is an effective oncolytic virotherapeutic in models of disseminated pancreatic cancer. *Mol. Ther.* **2012**, *20*, 759–768. [CrossRef]

26. Bartee, E.; Mohamed, M.R.; Lopez, M.C.; Baker, H.V.; McFadden, G. The addition of tumor necrosis factor plus beta interferon induces a novel synergistic antiviral state against poxviruses in primary human fibroblasts. *J. Virol.* **2009**, *83*, 498–511. [CrossRef] [PubMed]

27. Zemp, F.J.; Lun, X.; McKenzie, B.A.; Zhou, H.; Maxwell, L.; Sun, B.; Kelly, J.J.; Stechishin, O.; Luchman, A.; Weiss, S.; et al. Treating brain tumor-initiating cells using a combination of myxoma virus and rapamycin. *Neuro. Oncol.* **2013**, *15*, 904–920. [CrossRef] [PubMed]

28. Matsuda, Y.; Yoshimura, H.; Ishiwata, T.; Sumiyoshi, H.; Matsushita, A.; Nakamura, Y.; Aida, J.; Uchida, E.; Takubo, K.; Arai, T. Mitotic index and multipolar mitosis in routine histologic sections as prognostic markers of pancreatic cancers: A clinicopathological study. *Pancreatology* **2016**, *16*, 127–132. [CrossRef] [PubMed]

29. Rahman, M.M.; Bagdassarian, E.; Ali, M.A.M.; McFadden, G. Identification of host DEAD-box RNA helicases that regulate cellular tropism of oncolytic Myxoma virus in human cancer cells. *Sci. Rep.* **2017**, *16*, 15710. [CrossRef]

30. Amrutkar, M.; Gladhaug, I.P. Pancreatic Cancer Chemoresistance to Gemcitabine. *Cancers* **2017**, *9*, 157. [CrossRef]

31. Grasso, C.; Jansen, G.; Giovannetti, E. Drug resistance in pancreatic cancer: Impact of altered energy metabolism. *Crit. Rev. Oncol. Hematol.* **2017**, *114*, 139–152. [CrossRef]

32. Morrison, A.H.; Byrne, K.T.; Vonderheide, R.H. Immunotherapy and Prevention of Pancreatic Cancer. *Trends Cancer* **2018**, *4*, 418–428. [CrossRef] [PubMed]

33. Draganov, D.D.; Santidrian, A.F.; Minev, I.; Nguyen, D.; Kilinc, M.O.; Petrov, I.; Vyalkova, A.; Lander, E.; Berman, M.; Minev, B.; et al. Delivery of oncolytic vaccinia virus by matched allogeneic stem cells overcomes critical innate and adaptive immune barriers. *J. Transl. Med.* **2019**, *17*, 100. [CrossRef]

34. Shoyaib, A.A.; Archie, S.R.; Karamyan, W.T. Intraperitoneal Route of Drug Administration: Should it Be Used in Experimental Animal Studies. *Pharm. Res.* **2019**, *37*, 12. [CrossRef]

35. Gujar, S.; Pol, J.G.; Kim, Y.; Lee, P.W. Kroemer, G. Antitumor Benefits of Antiviral Immunity: An Underappreciated Aspect of Oncolytic Virotherapies. *Trends Immunol.* **2018**, *39*, 209–221. [CrossRef] [PubMed]

36. Stromnes, I.M.; Hulbert, A.; Pierce, R.H.; Greenberg, P.D.; Hingorani, S.R. T-cell Localization, Activation, and Clonal Expansion in Human Pancreatic Ductal Adenocarcinoma. *Cancer Immunol. Res.* **2017**, *5*, 978–991. [CrossRef] [PubMed]

37. Poschke, I.; Faryna, M.; Bergmann, F.; Flossdorf, M.; Lauenstein, C.; Hermes, J.; Hinz, U.; Hank, T.; Ehrenberg, R.; Volkmar, M.; et al. Identification of a tumor-reactive T-cell repertoire in the immune infiltrate of patients with resectable pancreatic ductal adenocarcinoma. *Oncoimmunology* **2016**, *5*, e1240859. [CrossRef] [PubMed]

38. Connor, A.A.; Denroche, R.E.; Jang, G.H.; Timms, L.; Kalimuthu, S.N.; Selander, I.; McPherson, T.; Wilson, G.W.; Chan-Seng-Yue, M.A.; Borozan, I.; et al. Association of Distinct Mutational Signatures with Correlates of Increased Immune Activity in Pancreatic Ductal Adenocarcinoma. *JAMA Oncol.* **2017**, *3*, 774–783. [CrossRef]

39. Balachandran, V.P.; Luksza, M.; Zhao, J.N.; Makarov, V.; Moral, J.A.; Remark, R.; Herbst, B.; Askan, G.; Bhanot, U.; Senbabaoglu, Y.; et al. Identification of unique neoantigen qualities in long-term survivors of pancreatic cancer. *Nature* **2017**, *551*, 512–516. [CrossRef]

40. Werner, J.; Combs, S.E.; Springfeld, C.; Hartwig, W.; Hackert, T.; Buchler, M.W. Advanced-stage pancreatic cancer: Therapy options. *Nat. Rev. Clin. Oncol.* **2013**, *10*, 323–333. [CrossRef]

41. Orth, M.; Metzger, P.; Gerum, S.; Mayerle, J.; Schneider, G.; Belka, C.; Schnurr, M.; Lauber, K. Pancreatic ductal adenocarcinoma: Biological hallmarks, current status, and future perspectives of combined modality treatment approaches. *Radiat. Oncol.* **2019**, *14*, 141. [CrossRef]

42. Klug, F.; Prakash, H.; Huber, P.E.; Seibel, T.; Bender, N.; Halama, N.; Pfirschke, C.; Voss, R.H.; Timke, C.; Umansky, L.; et al. Low-dose irradiation programs macrophage differentiation to an iNOS(+)/M1 phenotype that orchestrates effective T cell immunotherapy. *Cancer Cell* **2013**, *24*, 589–602. [CrossRef] [PubMed]

43. Baird, J.R.; Friedman, D.; Cottam, B.; Dubensky, T.W., Jr.; Kanne, D.B.; Bambina, S.; Bahjat, K.; Crittenden, M.R.; Gough, M.J. Radiotherapy Combined with Novel STING-Targeting Oligonucleotides Results in Regression of Established Tumors. *Cancer Res.* **2016**, *76*, 50–61. [CrossRef] [PubMed]
44. Hingorani, S.R.; Zheng, L.; Bullock, A.J.; Seery, T.E.; Harris, W.P.; Sigal, D.S.; Braiteh, F.; Ritch, P.S.; Zalupski, M.M.; Bahary, N.; et al. HALO 202: Randomized Phase II Study of PEGPH20 Plus Nab-Paclitaxel/Gemcitabine Versus Nab-Paclitaxel/ Gemcitabine in Patients with Untreated, Metastatic Pancreatic Ductal Adenocarcinoma. *J. Clin. Oncol.* **2018**, *36*, 359–366. [CrossRef] [PubMed]
45. Niyazi, M.; Maihoefer, C.; Krause, M.; Rodel, C.; Budach, W.; Belka, C. Radiotherapy and "new" drugs-new side effects? *Radiat. Oncol.* **2011**, *6*, 177. [CrossRef] [PubMed]
46. Ali, A.I.; Oliver, A.J.; Samiei, T.; Chan, J.D.; Kershaw, M.H.; Slaney, C.Y. Genetic Redirection of T Cells for the Treatment of Pancreatic Cancer. *Front. Oncol.* **2019**, *9*, 56. [CrossRef] [PubMed]

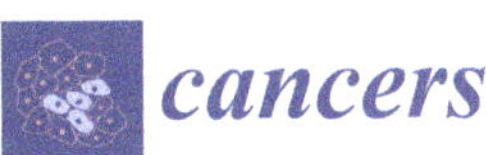
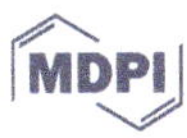

Article

Targeting CAR to the Peptide-MHC Complex Reveals Distinct Signaling Compared to That of TCR in a Jurkat T Cell Model

Ling Wu [1,2], Joanna Brzostek [1,2], Shvetha Sankaran [1,2], Qianru Wei [2], Jiawei Yap [1,2], Triscilla Y.Y. Tan [2], Junyun Lai [1,2], Paul A. MacAry [1,2,3,4] and Nicholas R. J. Gascoigne [1,2,3,*]

[1] Translational Immunology Research Programme, Yong Loo Lin School of Medicine, National University of Singapore, Singapore 119228, Singapore; ling.wu@u.nus.edu (L.W.); joanna.brzostek@biologie.uni-freiburg.de (J.B.); shvetha_sankaran@gis.a-star.edu.sg (S.S.); micyapj@nus.edu.sg (J.Y.); junyunlai@u.nus.edu (J.L.); micpam@nus.edu.sg (P.A.M.)

[2] Department of Microbiology and Immunology, Yong Loo Lin School of Medicine, National University of Singapore, 5 Science Drive 2, Singapore 117545, Singapore; qiw4003@med.cornell.edu (Q.W.); triscilla.tan@u.nus.edu (T.Y.Y.T.)

[3] Translational Cancer Research Programme, Yong Loo Lin School of Medicine, National University of Singapore, Singapore 119228, Singapore

[4] Life Sciences Institute, National University of Singapore, Singapore 117456, Singapore

[*] Correspondence: micnrjg@nus.edu.sg

Citation: Wu, L.; Brzostek, J.; Sankaran, S.; Wei, Q.; Yap, J.; Tan, T.Y.Y.; Lai, J.; MacAry, P.A.; Gascoigne, N.R.J. Targeting CAR to the Peptide-MHC Complex Reveals Distinct Signaling Compared to That of TCR in a Jurkat T Cell Model. *Cancers* **2021**, *13*, 867. https://doi.org/10.3390/cancers13040867

Academic Editors: Michael Kershaw and Clare Slaney

Received: 26 January 2021
Accepted: 16 February 2021
Published: 18 February 2021

Publisher's Note: MDPI stays neutral with regard to jurisdictional claims in published maps and institutional affiliations.

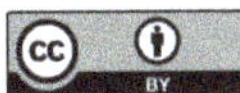

Simple Summary: Chimeric antigen receptors (CARs) redirect T cells without the need for major histocompatibility complex (MHC) restriction. CARs are designed based on T cell receptor (TCR) signaling and the recognition specificities of antibodies. This technology has achieved great clinical success in combatting cancers. Despite these successes, the mechanism of CAR signaling in the T cell and how this can impact function is not fully understood. To enhance our understanding and to identify the characteristics of CAR signaling, we designed a CAR to target a peptide-MHC complex, similar to the TCR. This allowed us to compare CAR and TCR head-to-head, such that novel traits of CAR signaling could be discovered. We found that CAR has distinct signaling characteristics compared to TCR, including the molecules that facilitate signal transduction. These findings offer explanations for the clinical behavior of CAR T cells (CAR-T) therapy and avenues to optimize the technology.

Abstract: Chimeric antigen receptor T cells (CAR-T) utilize T cell receptor (TCR) signaling cascades and the recognition functions of antibodies. This allows T cells, normally restricted by the major histocompatibility complex (MHC), to be redirected to target cells by their surface antigens, such as tumor associated antigens (TAAs). CAR-T technology has achieved significant successes in treatment of certain cancers, primarily liquid cancers. Nonetheless, many challenges hinder development of this therapy, such as cytokine release syndrome (CRS) and the efficacy of CAR-T treatments for solid tumors. These challenges show our inadequate understanding of this technology, particularly regarding CAR signaling, which has been less studied. To dissect CAR signaling, we designed a CAR that targets an epitope from latent membrane protein 2 A (LMP2 A) of the Epstein–Barr virus (EBV) presented on HLA*A02:01. Because of this, CAR and TCR signaling can be compared directly, allowing us to study the involvement of other signaling molecules, such as coreceptors. This comparison revealed that CAR was sufficient to bind monomeric antigens due to its high affinity but required oligomeric antigens for its activation. CAR sustained the transduced signal significantly longer, but at a lower magnitude, than did TCR. CD8 coreceptor was recruited to the CAR synapse but played a negligible role in signaling, unlike for TCR signaling. The distinct CAR signaling processes could provide explanations for clinical behavior of CAR-T therapy and suggest ways to improve the technology.

Keywords: T cell receptor; chimeric antigen receptor (CAR) T cell (CAR-T); signal transduction; CD8 coreceptor; signaling kinetics; oligomerization

1. Introduction

Chimeric antigen receptor T cell (CAR-T) technology takes advantage of the specificity of an antibody (Ab) and the signaling of a T cell receptor (TCR), such that a T cell can be redirected to target cells in a non-major histocompatibility complex (MHC) restricted manner. CAR-T technology has achieved significant clinical success in recent years, with two commercial products available, Kymriah® (tisagenlecleucel; Novartis, Basel, Switzerland) and Yescarta® (axicabtagene ciloleucel; Gilead, Foster City, CA, USA), with many more coming down the pipeline [1–3]. A typical CAR construct comprises an extracellular recognition domain, generally a single chain variable fragment (scFv) of an Ab, hinge region, transmembrane, co-stimulatory domain, and signal activation domain. The latter is typically from CD3 z, but other variants, such as CD3 e or CD3 z mutants, have also been shown to have enhanced functionality compared with CD3 z [3]. Each part of the design plays an important role in determining the downstream signaling, but the parameters are not fully understood at this time [3,4].

Understanding CAR signaling is critical to explain the different clinical behavior of each CAR-T therapy and to facilitate rational design of CAR constructs. Taking cytokine release syndrome (CRS) as an example [5], one of the most severe side effects is caused by the strength of CAR signaling while killing the cancer cells. The Gasdermin E (GSDME) signal pathway is activated, leading to pyroptosis of cancer cells and increased expression of damage-associated molecular pattern molecules (DAMPs), which in turn activate macrophages to release CRS-related cytokines [6]. Moreover, CD28-CAR-T and CD137-CAR-T have distinct in vitro and in vivo clinical performance. CD28-CAR-T cells were shown to have a higher cytotoxic activity and antigen sensitivity in vitro and in vivo than did CD137-CAR-T cells [7,8]. The less potent CD137-CAR signaling was later demonstrated to be caused by the recruitment of the negative signaling molecular complex THEMIS-SHP1 [9], which is important in integrating T cell signal strength [10]. Overexpression of LCK countered this negative regulation and led to enhanced CD137-CAR-T therapy [9].

Several studies have been performed to understand intracellular CAR signaling networks [11–13]. CAR signaling was found to have a different magnitude and different kinetics of phosphorylation events compared to those of TCR signaling. Some novel protein interactions, such as capsule synthesis 1 domain containing 1 (CASD1), butyrophilin-like 3 (BTNL3), and an additional form of CD3ζ, p21, have been found to be associated with CAR signaling [13]. Nevertheless, the mechanism and impact of these interactions are poorly understood. To better decipher CAR signaling and its mechanism, it is important to compare CAR and TCR head-to-head, such that the divergence of CAR signaling from TCR signaling can be delineated. However, most of the studies thus far have been based on tumor associated antigens (TAAs), such as CD19, that may omit important molecules involved in TCR signaling, such as coreceptors. Therefore, a CAR designed to target the peptide-MHC (pMHC) complex can offer a better comparison between CAR and TCR. Only a few studies using this comparison have been done so far, where CAR was predicted to have a distinct signaling by mathematical modelling, but such a distinct signaling patten has not yet been substantiated [14,15].

To this end, we designed a CAR based on a "TCR-like" Ab that targets a peptide from latent membrane protein 2 A (LMP2 A) protein of the Epstein–Barr virus (EBV) presented by HLA-A*02:01. The affinity of the TCR-like Ab is in the nanomolar range, whereas TCRs are typically micromolar [16]. These affinities are within the normal ranges for Ab and TCR so that they imitate the real situation. In this study, we found that CAR signal activation requires clustering—since the pMHC monomer would not initiate the CAR signaling—and that CAR signaling produces more sustained calcium signaling kinetics compared with TCR. We observed recruitment of the CD8 coreceptor into the CAR signaling synapse, but the CD8 coreceptor did not elevate the CAR signaling, unlike the case with TCR signaling. These findings are important for our understanding of how CAR initiates signaling and how it differs from TCR signaling, and could potentially explain differences in clinical behavior of CAR-T from other adoptive T cell therapies.

2. Results

2.1. CAR Signal Initiation Requires Clustering

A TCR-like Ab targeting the peptide LMP2 $A_{426-434}$ ("L2"; sequence CLGGLLTMV) from EBV presented by HLA-A*02:01 was utilized to generate first and second generation CARs containing CD28 costimulatory domain [17,18] (Figure S1A). These were stained with pMHC (A*02:01) tetramers. The CAR-1 or CAR-2-transduced Jurkat cells showed strong binding to the L2-tetramer, but no binding to an irrelevant M1-tetramer, which presented $M1_{58-66}$ (GILGFVFTL) from the influenza A virus (Figure 1A). Besides tetramer binding capacity, the CAR protein also showed significant binding to the L2-A*02:01 monomer. This monomer-binding capacity was comparable to the Ab staining of the CAR protein (Figure 1B) and tetramer (Figure 1C). In comparison, TCR showed binding capacity only to the tetramer (Figure 1B,C). Nevertheless, the monomer-binding ability of CAR did not result in activation (Figure 1D). The CAR signal was transduced when the monomers were clustered with the tetramer, as was the case for TCR. However, as seen by Western blotting, the size of CAR-1 and CAR-2 without dithiothreitol (DTT) appeared to be two times bigger than the reduced samples (Figure S1C). This indicates that CAR exists as a covalently linked dimer in the cells.

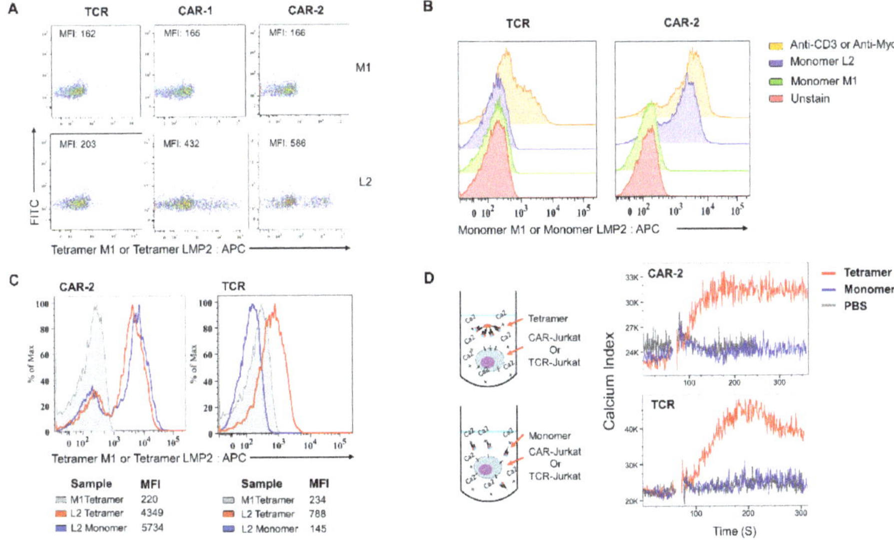

Figure 1. Monomer or tetramer binding and activation to the chimeric antigen receptor (CAR) and T cell receptor (TCR). (**A**) TCR and CAR binding to the specific peptide-major histocompatibility complex (pMHC) tetramer. CAR-1 and CAR-2 refer to first and second generation of CAR design, respectively. L2 and M1 represents the antigenic LMP2 $A_{426-434}$ (CLGGLLTMV) and irrelevant $M1_{58-66}$ (GILGFVFTL) peptide tetramer, respectively. The tetramer was formed by loading monomers with antigen presenting cell (APC)-streptavidin. Overall mean fluorescent intensity is labeled in the graph. (**B**) Monomer binding to CAR and TCR. The monomer binding was detected by using anti-B2 M APC. Anti-CD3-APC and Anti-Myc-APC were used to measure the expression of TCR and CAR on the surface, respectively. (**C**) Comparison of monomer and tetramer binding to CAR and TCR. (**D**) CAR and TCR activation upon monomer and tetramer binding. The schematic graph is shown at the left panel, the tetramer and monomer activation groups contained equal amounts of monomer. The Ca^{2+} index was calculated by the ratio of the mean fluorescence intensity (MFI) of BUV395 to the MFI of Indo-1 (Bv421). The cells were stabilized for 1 to 1.5 min, followed by addition of the tetramer or monomer. The calcium flux was recorded for an additional 3–4 min. All data are representative of at least three independent experiments.

2.2. CAR Transduces a Sustained but Lower Signaling Compared with TCR

A difference in Ca^{2+} signaling kinetics between CAR and TCR was observed (Figure 1D), where CAR signaling reached and sustained a plateau, but TCR signaling waned after reaching a peak. We therefore extended the duration for Ca^{2+} flux detection from 3–4 min to 10 min, to test whether the sustained Ca^{2+} flux would last over a longer period. CAR signaling was more sustained than was TCR signaling (Figure 2A). Moreover, the sustained CAR signaling was not attributable to the costimulatory domain, since the first generation CAR-1 also showed signal transduction in a sustained manner (Figure S2). The phosphorylation of downstream signaling molecules, such as ERK, was also shown to be consistent with the distinct CAR signaling kinetics (Figure 2C). Though more sustained compared with TCR signaling, the magnitude of CAR signaling was much lower than that of TCR signaling, both in Ca^{2+} flux (Figure 2A,B) and in the phosphorylation of downstream molecules (Figure 2C,D).

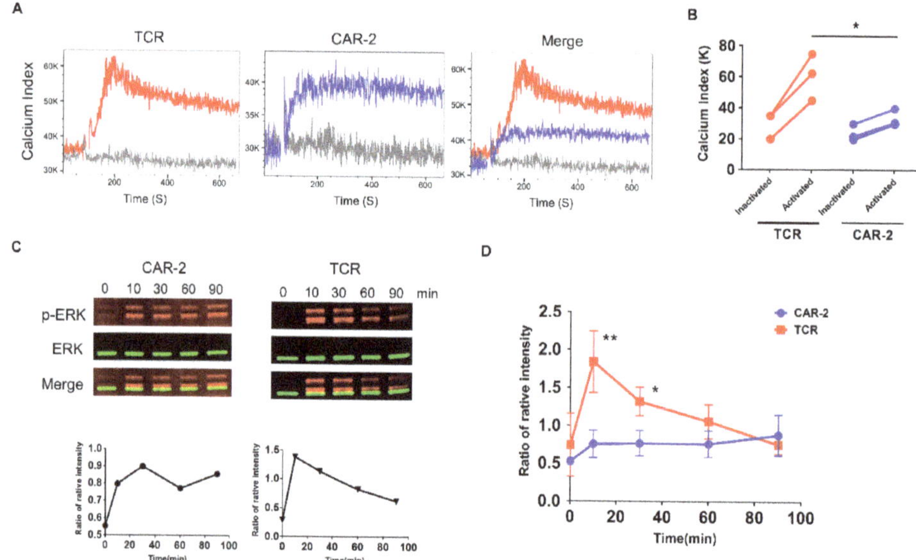

Figure 2. Sustained CAR and TCR signaling kinetics by Ca^{2+} flux and downstream phosphorylation. (**A**) Long-term Ca^{2+} flux of CAR and TCR signaling. The Ca^{2+} flux was recorded for 10 min after the tetramer was added. Calcium index was calculated as the ratio of BUV395/Indo-1 (UV). The negative control, shown in grey, was from after adding PBS. (**B**) Quantification data of TCR and CAR Ca^{2+} flux. Activated data dots indicate the highest value of the Ca^{2+} flux from TCR or CAR samples. (**C**) Phosphorylation of the ERK molecule of CAR and TCR after stimulation at different timepoints. Phosphorylation strength of pERK1/2 was calculated by comparing the intensity of p-ERK to that of total ERK. The two graphs are then grouped to compare their intensity strength; Uncropped Western Blots are available in Figure S3. (**D**) Quantification data of p-ERK of TCR and CAR-Jurkat cells after activation. All data are representative of at least three independent experiments. Student's *t* test, two-tailed, was used to measure the significance; * $p < 0.05$, ** $p < 0.01$.

2.3. Distinct CAR Signaling Is Reflected by IL-2 Production Upon Activation by Antigen-Presenting Cells

IL-2 production represents a downstream result of TCR signaling. We therefore tested and identified the difference in IL-2 production patterns between CAR-Jurkat and TCR-Jurkat cells. To this end, an artificial antigen presenting cell (APC) was constructed based on Chinese hamster ovary (CHO) cells. A single chain version of HLA-A*02:01 tethered to the L2 peptide was generated (Figure S4A). The transduced CHO-APC expressed the antigenic peptide-MHC (pMHC) complex, which was specifically recognized by the anti-HLA-A*02:01-L2 TCR-like Ab (Figure 3A). The scFv version of this TCR-like Ab was also shown to specifically bind to CHO cells expressing HLA-A*02:01-L2 (Figure S4B). The CAR-T and TCR-T cells were then incubated with the CHO-APCs. As seen in Figure 3B, TCR-T cells produced IL-2 in 3 phases within 24 h, with acceleration, stable, and then deceleration phases. The first phase started from 0 to 4 h, the second from 4 to 10 h, then the third from 10 to 24 h. In marked distinction, the CAR-T cells produced IL-2 only in a stable and consistent manner, in agreement with our previous observations, shown in Figure 2. Around 90% of the IL-2 production by TCR-Jurkat cells was finished by 10 h, yet only around 35% of IL-2 of CAR-T cells were produced by that timepoint (Figure 3B).

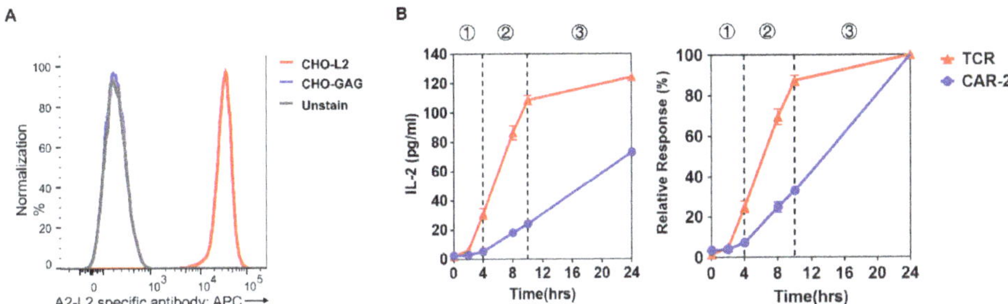

Figure 3. IL-2 production kinetics of CAR and TCR. (**A**) Expression of HLA*A02:01-L2 by CHO-APC. The TCR-like antibody was used to detect the expression and specificity. CHO-L2 and CHO-GAG refers to CHO-APC presented antigenic LMP2 A peptide and irrelevant GAG peptide, respectively. (**B**) IL-2 production of CAR-T and TCR-T upon stimulation by CHO-APC. The IL-2 production of TCR is separated by 3 phases, labeled as 1, 2, 3 in the graph, representing the acceleration, stable, and deceleration phases, respectively. The amount of IL-2 production in the left panel is calculated as a percentage and shown in the right panel. Data are representative of at least three independent experiments, plotted as mean ± SD of technical triplicates.

2.4. CD8 Coreceptor Is Recruited by TCR-Like CAR but Does Not Enhance Activation

Since L2-specific TCR-like CAR has similar specificity for pMHC as does the TCR, we tested the contribution of the CD8 coreceptor to CAR-T cell activation. CD8α was expressed as a fusion with the fluorescent protein mCherry (Figure S5A). We first showed that CD8 could be recruited to the immunological synapse (IS) by CAR-T cells, as is found in TCR-T cells [19,20], using total internal reflection fluorescence microscopy (TIRFM) to detect events at the contact surface (Figure 4A). A supported lipid bilayer with ICAM1, with or without pMHC was made. CAR-T or TCR-T cells were added onto the bilayer for 10 min. Mean fluorescence intensity (MFI) at the IS significantly increased in both CAR-T and TCR-T cells on bilayers containing pMHC, with clear clustering of CD8α-mCherry (Figure 4B, Figure S5B). We also calculated the MFI ratio inside/outside of the IS upon interaction between CAR-T or TCR-T cells with CHO-L2 cells using widefield fluorescent microscopy (Figure S5C). No significant difference was detected between CAR-T and TCR-T with CD8α-mCherry upon contact with CHO-APC, and both MFI ratios exceeded our cut-off ratio definition for IS formation of 1.5. These data show that that CD8α-mCherry was recruited in both CAR-T and TCR-T if cognate pMHC was present.

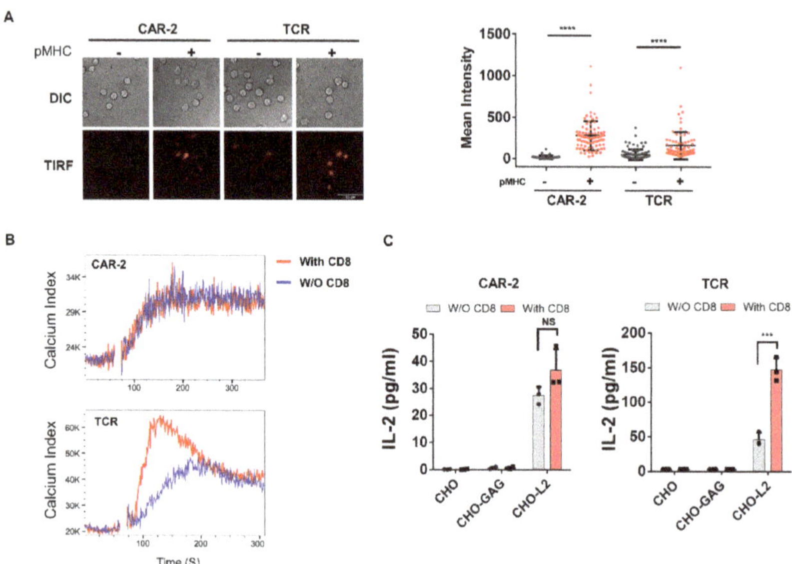

Figure 4. Interaction of TCR-like CAR CD8 coreceptor. (**A**) CD8 recruitment using TIRFM visualizing CD8α-mCherry. Left: representative images, scale bar is at 50 μm. Right: background-corrected mean fluorescence intensity of cell contact surface (*n* > 80 cells). (**B**) Ca^{2+} flux of CAR-T and TCR-T ± CD8. (**C**) CAR and TCR responsiveness ± CD8 to antigenic CHO-L2 or irrelevant CHO-GAG. Data are representative of at least three independent experiments, plotted as mean ± SD of technical triplicates. *** $p < 0.001$, **** $p < 0.0001$; NS: not significant at $p > 0.05$, by Student's *t*-test.

We next sought to identify whether CD8 would contribute to CAR-T functionally, since it was recruited to the CAR-T cell IS. After CD8α and β were co-transduced into both CAR-T and TCR-T cells, and expressions were shown to be similar (Figure S5D,E), reactivity of TCR-T bearing the CD8αβ coreceptor was significantly increased. As expected, CD8$^+$ TCR-T showed faster and stronger Ca^{2+} flux and IL-2 production was nearly 3-fold higher than CD8$^-$ TCR-T (Figure 4B,C). However, reactivity of CAR-T-bearing CD8 was not enhanced over CD8$^-$ CAR-T. These data show that CD8 does not enhance CAR signaling, even though the CAR-recognized pMHC and CD8 were recruited to the IS of CAR-T cells.

3. Material and Methods

3.1. Plasmids and Sequences

The lentiviral vector, pLv, and its associated packaging plasmids, bearing Gag/Pol, Rev and VSV-G, respectively, were purchased from Vectorbuilder (Chicago, IL, USA). Chimeric antigen receptors with or without CD28 costimulatory sequences were synthesized and cloned into a lentiviral vector by Vectorbuilder. Human *CD8 A* and *CD8 B* genes were cloned from a human cDNA library in-house. The scFv construct for TCR-like Abs [17] was produced in P.A.M.'s lab (National University of Singapore, Singapore), and TCR construct specific for HLA-A*02:01 with peptide LMP2 A$_{426-434}$ (from EBV) was a generous gift from Hans Stauss (University College London, London, United Kingdom). Single-chain trimer HLA-A*02:01-GAG was a gift from Keith Gould (Imperial College London, London, United Kingdom). Peptide mutagenesis: GAG (SLYNTVATL) to LMP2 A$_{426-434}$ ("L2": CLGGLLTMV) was done by using a Q5 mutagenesis Kit (New England Biolabs, Ipswich, MA, USA). All the molecular cloning work was done by using an In-Fusion HD cloning kit (Clontech, Mountain View, CA, USA), and single-chain trimer MHC constructs were cloned into pLv to generate artificial antigen-presenting CHO cells [21–23].

3.2. Cell Lines and Cell Culture

Endogenous TCR and coreceptor-deficient Jurkat76 was a kind gift from Heemskerk et al. [24]. Jurkat cells were maintained in complement RPMI-1640 media (Hyclone, Marlborough, MA, USA), supplemented with 10% fetal bovine serum (Hyclone), 2 mM L-glutamine (Gibco, Waltham, MA, USA), and MEM non-essential amino acid (Gibco) in a humidified 5% CO_2 incubator at 37 °C. Human embryonic kidney epithelial cells (HEK293) were cultured in complete DMEM (Hyclone), which was supplemented with 10% fetal bovine serum (Hyclone), 2 mM L-glutamine (Gibco), and MEM non-essential amino acids (Gibco). The tetracycline-regulated expression (T-REx) CHO cell line was purchased from Invitrogen (Waltham, MA, USA) and used for the generation of artificial APC, which were single-cell sorted after transfection with single-chain MHC construct (scMHC). The CHO and CHO-APC cells were cultured in complete Ham's F-12 (Gibco) medium, supplemented with 10% fetal bovine serum (Hyclone) and MEM non-essential amino acid (Gibco). The pMHC complex expression was checked regularly by flow cytometry.

3.3. Antibodies and Chemicals

The following antibodies were used in this study: Myc-Tag mouse mAb Alexa Fluor 647 (9 B11), anti-p44/42 ERK1/2, anti-ERK1/2 (all from Cell Signaling Technology, Danvers, MA, USA); anti-human CD3 APC and anti-B2 M APC (purchased from Biolegend, San Diego, CA, USA); anti-human CD8 A APC and anti-human CD8 B PE-Cy7 (all from eBioscience, San Diego, CA, USA); goat anti-mouse IgG (H + L) secondary antibody Alexa Fluor 647 (Thermo Fisher Scientific, Waltham, MA, USA); anti-Myc-Tag clone 4 A6 (Millipore, Burlington, MA, USA) was used for Western blotting; and specific HLA-A*02:01-L2 TCR-like antibodies were produced as described [17]. The scFv was produced by BL21 (DE3) (Novagen, Burlington, MA, USA) at 30 °C overnight, and the protein expression was induced by IPTG when OD_{600} reached 0.7. The bacteria were then pelleted and ultrasound sonicated. The scFv was purified through Ni-NTA beads (Thermo Fisher Scientific) and AKTA FPLC (GE) by size exclusion column and ion exchange column (MonoS, Sigma-Aldrich, St. Louis, MI, USA).

3.4. Lentivirus Production and Transduction

A total of 6.5×10^5 HEK293 cells per well were seeded onto 6-well plates one day before transfection and incubated at 37 °C with 5% CO_2. The cells were then transfected with packaging plasmid and lentiviral vector using polyethylenimine (PEI), and the medium was replaced after 12 h. The viral supernatant was harvested twice in the following two days. The collected viral supernatant was titered, filtered by a 0.45 mm membrane filter (Millipore), and concentrated by a 100 K ultracentrifuge tube (Millipore). For lentivirus transductions, polybrene and HEPES were added at 8–10 mg/mL and 10 mM, respectively, with Jurkat cells at 1×10^6 per well in 1 mL, followed by spinoculation at $1200 \times g$, for 2 h. For CHO cell transduction, the viral solution was directly added with the cell without spinoculation. After 24 h, cells and viral solutions were separated, and cells were cultured in the maintenance medium. After an additional 48 h culture period, flow cytometry analysis was performed to check the expression of the constructs.

3.5. Calcium Flux Assay

The Ca^{2+} flux assay was performed as previously described [25]. In brief, cell samples were suspended at a density of 10^7 cells per ml in phosphate-buffered saline (PBS) and loaded with 2 mM Indo-1 AM (acetoxymethyl) for 30 min at 37 °C, followed by washing twice with culture RPMI. Cells were pre-warmed to 37 °C for 10 min before analysis and were kept at 37 °C in culture RPMI during the event collection. For cell stimulation, an HLA-A*02:01-L2 monomer was pre-refolded, biotinylated [26], and crosslinked with streptavidin Alexa 647 (Thermo Fisher Scientific) to form the antigen tetramer. Cells were then stimulated with monomers or tetramers. The mean fluorescence ratio of Indo-1 high to Indo-1 low was calculated using FlowJo (Version 10) kinetics program.

3.6. Western Blotting and Immunoprecipitation

A total of 10^6 cells were lysed by NP-40 lysis buffer. Cell debris was pelleted at $13,000 \times g$ for 15 min at 4 °C, and the supernatant was collected and heated with reduced protein loading buffer (Nacalai-Tesque, Kyoto, Japan) or nonreduced loading buffer (without DTT). To detect phosphorylation after stimulation, 10^5 CHO-APC cells were seeded per well in a 12-well plate one day before stimulation. Then, 10^6 CAR-T or TCR-T cells were added into each well and incubated at 37 °C and 5% CO_2 for the designated duration. The stimulated CAR-T or TCR-T cells were collected and prepared as above. All samples were loaded in a 4–12% Bis-Tris gradient gel (NuPAGE, Invitrogen, Waltham, MA, USA) and transferred to a PVDF membrane (Immobilon-FL Transfer Membrane, Millipore). The membrane was then blocked using blocking buffer (Odyssey, LI-COR, Lincoln, NE, USA) for 1 h at room temperature. Subsequently, the membrane was probed with different primary antibodies. The secondary antibodies used were IRDye 800 CW Goat anti-Mouse (926–32210, LI-COR) and IRDye 680 LT Goat anti-Rabbit (926–68021, LI-COR). Visualization and quantification of the blot was by the LI-COR Odyssey infrared imaging system.

3.7. T Cell Stimulation and Cytokine Secretion Assay

This was performed largely as described [22,23]. Artificial antigen presenting CHO cells (CHO-APC) were seeded onto a 96-well, flat-bottom plate at $2–3 \times 10^4$ per well one day before the assay. Each CAR-T or TCR T cell sample was counted and suspended at a concentration of 10^6 per mL in culturing RPMI medium. Then, 200 mL per well of suspended cell solution was added into the APC-CHO pre-seeded plate. Technical triplicates were performed for all experiments. The cells were incubated at 37 °C and 5% CO_2 for 18 h or to designated timepoints. After incubation, the supernatant was collected for human IL-2 ELISA assay, which was performed according to the manufacturer's protocol (Invitrogen).

3.8. Imaging

For total internal reflection fluorescence microscopy (TIRFM), lipid bilayers containing specific pMHC and other anchoring proteins were prepared as previously described [22,27]. In short, 0.2 mol% liposomes were used, evaporated by N_2 at 37 °C and sonicated to prepare 4 mM lipid stock. Before adding the lipid, 6 M NaOH was used to clean glass 8-well chamber LabTekII chamber slides (Thermo Fisher Scientific) for 2 h and then they were rinsed with distilled H_2O. The 4 mM lipid stock was diluted 10 times in PBS then added to the cleaned chamber slides and incubated for 30 min at room temperature. Then, 12 mL PBS was applied to wash away excess liposomes after incubation, and 2 mg/mL BSA was added to block the bilayers for 30 min, followed by the addition of 5 μg/mL streptavidin and incubation for 30 min. Biotinylated HLA-A*02:01-L2 monomer (produced as previously described [26]), recombinant human ICAM1 Protein, and hIgG1-Fc.His Tag (Thermo Fisher Scientific), after another wash for excess streptavidin, were added to the bilayers for 30 min. After washing, the bilayers loaded with specific pMHC were ready to be used. We prepared 10^6 cells per mL of CAR-Jurkat or TCR-Jurkat with CD8α-mCherry and 100 mL of cells were added onto one well of the chamber at 37 °C for 10 min. Then, 100 μL of 8% paraformaldehyde was directly added to fix the cell and stop the stimulation. TIRF microscopy was later performed on an Olympus IX83 inverted microscope fitted with a four-laser TIRF module. Images were acquired using a 100×/1.49 NA oil-immersion lens. Fluorescence excited within the 100-nm evanescent field was recorded with a Hamamatsu ORCA Flash 4.0 camera. For regular fluorescent imaging, 10^5 cells of CAR-Jurkat or TCR-Jurkat with CD8α-mCherry were mixed with 10^5 cells specific CHO-APC in 100 μL RPMI medium for 10 min on one well of the chamber, followed by adding 100 μL of 8% paraformaldehyde. CD8 recruitment was later detected on an Olympus IX83 inverted microscope in the normal module. Images were acquired using a 20–40×/1.49 NA oil-immersion lens.

3.9. Flow Cytometry and Cell Sorting

BD LSR Fortessa X-20 (Becton Dickinson, Franklin Lakes, NJ, USA) was regularly used to detect the expression of the protein transduced and for conducting flow cytometry experiments. Mo-Flo XDP (Beckman Coulter, Inc., Brea, CA, USA) or SY3200 (Sony Biotechnology Inc., San Jose, CA, USA), in the Flow Cytometry Laboratory, Immunology Program, National University of Singapore, were used to purify transduced cells and perform single-cell sorting. All flow data analysis was performed in FlowJo (Version 10).

3.10. Statistical Information and Data Analysis

The two-tailed Student's *t*-test was used to test the significance between different sample groups throughout the study in GraphPad Prism (Version 7). Variance was considered similar in different sample groups. The significance cut-off (p value) was 0.05.

4. Discussion

TCR signaling has been studied for several decades. Though incompletely understood, three main mechanisms have been proposed regarding how TCR signaling is triggered: receptor clustering; mechanosensing, in which the TCR complex experiences a conformational change [28]; and size-dependent protein segregation, where large cell surface proteins, including the phosphatase CD45, are excluded so that phosphorylation is then triggered by kinases [29]. We took advantage of the ability to make pMHC molecules into monomeric or tetrameric forms to study the receptor clustering effects of CAR signal triggering. Compared with antigens presented by cells [30], soluble antigens will not form immunological synapses. Therefore, the soluble pMHC, either monomeric or tetrameric form, would provide a better way to study the cluster effect for the triggering of signals at the molecular level. We found that only the tetrameric form of the antigen was able to trigger CAR signaling, but not the monomeric form, even though pMHC monomer had been shown to bind strongly to the CAR. This indicated that receptor clustering is important for CAR signal triggering. The results are consistent with other findings using dimerized GFP and TGF-b as the antigens for CAR [31]. On the other hand, TCR also showed a requirement for antigen clustering to trigger the signal. However, monomeric antigen has been demonstrated as sufficient to initiate TCR signaling [32,33]. The disparate observations could be due to other signaling molecules such as the CD8 coreceptor, which were deliberately not involved in this model, that has been shown to facilitate monomer activation for TCR [34]. Therefore, without facilitation from these molecules, oligomerization would still be important for TCR signal triggering. In our experiments, the tetramer formed through the interaction between biotin and streptavidin was not homogenous, as shown in the supplemental data. CAR-1 and CAR-2 were also detected to be dimers bound by covalent disulfate bonds. To what degree the CAR needs to be clustered is not known under this circumstance. However, a study done by Chang et al. suggests that a dimeric form of the antigen would suffice to trigger CAR signaling [31].

While Ca^{2+} flux was activated by the pMHC tetramer, we observed distinct signaling kinetics between CAR and TCR, where CAR seemed to sustain the Ca^{2+} flux but TCR signaling waned after quickly reaching a peak. To our surprise, the Ca^{2+} flux of CAR continued even 10 min after activation. The strength of the sustained CAR signal was much weaker than the peak of TCR signal, but close to that of TCR signal after 10 min. To rule out the impact of the costimulatory domain of the second generation CAR, we demonstrated, by using the first generation CAR, that the sustained CAR signaling could be attributed to the basic CAR design (the recognition the scFv domain, stalk, transmembrane region, and CD3 z domains) and not to the costimulatory domain. Besides, the activation curves shown by TCR and CAR are reminiscent of the binding profiles of TCR and the antibody tested by surface plasmon resonance (SPR), where the antibody has a dramatically longer K_{off} than that of TCR [17]. This similarity may infer that it is the affinity profile of each recognition domain, i.e., scFv or the variable domains of TCR, that makes their signaling kinetics distinct. It is plausible that as long as CAR is conjugated with an antigen and clustered, the signal activation would last. The prolonged and high affinity contact with the surface antigen may also contribute to trogocytosis, which contributes to the antigen escape of cancer cells [8]. Another point worth noting is the lower magnitude of CAR signaling compared to that of TCR signaling. This may be due to each TCR complex comprising 6 CD3 subunits with 10 immunoreceptor tyrosine-based activation motifs (ITAMs), whereas each CAR only has 3 ITAMS. Thus, CAR activates a long but low downstream signal contrast with TCR, which activates a short but high downstream signal.

IL-2 production represents a culmination of signaling cascades, requiring activation of all three signaling pathways downstream of TCR signaling [35]. We examined the distinct signal kinetics based on IL-2 production. Consistent with the sustained CAR signaling detected, we observed that IL-2 production by CAR-T cells is more stable than that of TCR where TCR produced IL-2 in three phases within 18 h, but CAR-T cells produced IL-2 in a relatively linear manner. This CAR signaling pattern may also potentially explain why CAR-T cells could activate the GSDME signaling pathway of cancer cells, since CAR activation could be accumulated in the long-term, leading to enhanced killing functions.

We investigated a CAR with TCR-like specificity to enable comparison to conventional TCR and to test whether certain canonical signaling molecules, such as CD8, are involved in CAR signaling. We tested whether TCR-like CAR would use assistance from the CD8 coreceptor to enhance CAR-T activation, in a similar manner to that of TCR. However, no significant augmentation of either immediate calcium flux or later IL-2 production was observed, even though we found CD8 recruitment to the IS on CAR-T. We previously showed that CD8 can be concentrated into the IS, so long as MHC-I is available on the APC, even in the absence of TCR [19,20]. The CD8 coreceptor enhances the sensitivity of TCR through its interaction with LCK and stabilizes its binding with the antigenic pMHC complex [36] or non-antigenic, co-agonist pMHCs [21,22]. The inability of the CD8 coreceptor to enhance CAR signaling could potentially be explained by extracellular and intracellular effects. Since CAR has a significantly higher affinity than that of TCR, the stabilization effects from CD8 to TCR may not be required for CAR, which have been partly demonstrated by its capacity for monomer binding. On the other hand, because CD8 binds to a non-polymorphic part of the MHC-I a3 domain, and TCR binds in a conserved orientation to the pMHC, it ensures that the CD8-associated LCK is recruited in a particular orientation to the complex of TCR-CD3 and pMHC [37]. The orientation of the TCR-like CAR recognizing pMHC-I is not subject to such constraints, so that CD8 recruiting LCK to the pMHC is unlikely to force it into a suitable orientation to start signaling through the CD3 z subunit of the CAR. Intracellularly, LCK is better able to bind and phosphorylate CD3 e rather than CD3 z to initiate the cascade [38], so this may also be a factor in the lack of a CD8 requirement to initiate the CAR signaling.

In our study, we compared CAR with TCR signaling using Jurkat T cells. Although studies on Jurkat T cells have produced many seminal findings on T cell signaling [39], using Jurkat as a model system has limitations. Jurkat cells are deficient in tumor suppressor phosphatase PTEN, which dephosphorylates phosphatidylinositol (3,4,5)-trisphosphate (PIP3) to phosphatidylinositol (4,5)-trisphosphate PIP2. This deficiency causes a constitutive activation of AKT [40,41]. The study we report here involves early signal triggering and extracellular molecular interactions, which are not directly involved in PTEN-AKT signaling, suggesting that similar results would be obtained in primary cells, although this remains to be directly demonstrated.

5. Conclusions

We constructed a CAR with the same specificity as the TCR construct targeting peptide-MHC with the aim to understand the CAR signal triggering and activation patterns. CAR signal triggering was demonstrated to require receptor clustering. In addition, CAR transduces the signaling in a more sustained manner while in a lower magnitude compared with that of TCR. Furthermore, the CD8 coreceptors, though recruited by TCR-like CAR, play a limited role in enhancing the CAR signaling, at least for CD28-CAR.

Supplementary Materials: The following are available online at https://www.mdpi.com/2072-6694/13/4/867/s1, Figure S1: CAR constructs and pMHC tetramer, Figure S2: Ca^{2+} flux of first generation CAR in long-term activation, Figure S3: Uncropped Western Blots of Figure 2C and Figure S1, Figure S4: Artificial CHO antigen-presenting cells, Figure S5: CD8 recruitment to the IS and functional impact of CD8 for CAR-T and TCR-T.

Author Contributions: L.W. designed and conducted the experiments and analyzed the data; J.B. and N.R.J.G. provided discussion and co-designed the experiments; S.S. and Q.W. aided with imaging experiments; J.Y. and T.Y.Y.T. provided technical help; J.L. and P.A.M. provided antibody sequences and reagents; L.W. and N.R.J.G. wrote the paper, with input and final approval from all authors. All authors have read and agreed to the published version of the manuscript.

Funding: Singapore Ministry of Health's National Medical Research Council, OFIRG19 nov-0066, Ministry of Education, NUHSRO/2020/110/T1/SEED-MAR/06. L.W., Q.W. and J.L. were supported by research scholarships from Yong Loo Lin School of Medicine.

Institutional Review Board Statement: Not applicable.

Informed Consent Statement: Not applicable.

Data Availability Statement: The datasets generated during and/or analyzed during the current study are available from the corresponding author on request. The data are not publicly available due to no relevant data to upload to a database.

Acknowledgments: We are grateful to Paul Hutchinson and Guohui Teo, Flow Cytometry Laboratory, Immunology Program, National University of Singapore, for cell sorting. We also thank Hans Stauss (UCL) and Keith Gould (Imperial College, London) for providing TCR and single chain HLA constructs.

Conflicts of Interest: The authors declare no conflict of interests.

References

1. Porter, D.L.; Levine, B.L.; Kalos, M.; Bagg, A.; June, C.H. Chimeric Antigen Receptor–Modified T Cells in Chronic Lymphoid Leukemia. *N. Engl. J. Med.* **2011**, *365*, 725–733. [CrossRef] [PubMed]

2. Maude, S.L.; Laetsch, T.W.; Buechner, J.; Rives, S.; Boyer, M.; Bittencourt, H.; Bader, P.; Verneris, M.R.; Stefanski, H.E.; Myers, G.D.; et al. Tisagenlecleucel in Children and Young Adults with B-Cell Lymphoblastic Leukemia. *N. Engl. J. Med.* **2018**, *378*, 439–448. [CrossRef]

3. Wu, L.; Wei, Q.; Brzostek, J.; Gascoigne, N.R.J. Signaling from T cell receptors (TCRs) and chimeric antigen receptors (CARs) on T cells. *Cell. Mol. Immunol.* **2020**, *17*, 600–612. [CrossRef]

4. Dwivedi, A.; Karulkar, A.; Ghosh, S.; Rafiq, A.; Purwar, R. Lymphocytes in Cellular Therapy: Functional Regulation of CAR T Cells. *Front. Immunol.* **2019**, *9*, 3180. [CrossRef] [PubMed]

5. Grupp, S.A.; Kalos, M.; Barrett, D.; Aplenc, R.; Porter, D.L.; Rheingold, S.R.; Teachey, D.T.; Chew, A.; Hauck, B.; Wright, J.F.; et al. Chimeric Antigen Receptor–Modified T Cells for Acute Lymphoid Leukemia. *N. Engl. J. Med.* **2013**, *368*, 1509–1518. [CrossRef] [PubMed]

6. Liu, Y.; Fang, Y.; Chen, X.; Wang, Z.; Liang, X.; Zhang, T.; Liu, M.; Zhou, N.; Lv, J.; Tang, K.; et al. Gasdermin E–mediated target cell pyroptosis by CAR T cells triggers cytokine release syndrome. *Sci. Immunol.* **2020**, *5*, eaax7969. [CrossRef] [PubMed]

7. Cheng, Z.; Wei, R.; Ma, Q.; Shi, L.; He, F.; Shi, Z.; Jin, T.; Xie, R.; Wei, B.; Chen, J.; et al. In Vivo Expansion and Antitumor Activity of Coinfused CD28- and 4-1BB-Engineered CAR-T Cells in Patients with B Cell Leukemia. *Mol. Ther.* **2018**, *26*, 976–985. [CrossRef]

8. Hamieh, M.; Dobrin, A.; Cabriolu, A.; Van Der Stegen, S.J.C.; Giavridis, T.; Mansilla-Soto, J.; Eyquem, J.; Zhao, Z.; Whitlock, B.M.; Miele, M.M.; et al. CAR T cell trogocytosis and cooperative killing regulate tumour antigen escape. *Nat. Cell Biol.* **2019**, *568*, 112–116. [CrossRef]

9. Sun, C.; Shou, P.; Du, H.; Hirabayashi, K.; Chen, Y.; Herring, L.E.; Ahn, S.; Xu, Y.; Suzuki, K.; Li, G.; et al. THEMIS-SHP1 Recruitment by 4-1BB Tunes LCK-Mediated Priming of Chimeric Antigen Receptor-Redirected T Cells. *Cancer Cell* **2020**, *37*, 216–225.e6. [CrossRef]

10. Brzostek, J.; Gautam, N.; Zhao, X.; Chen, E.W.; Mehta, M.; Tung, D.W.H.; Chua, Y.L.; Yap, J.; Cho, S.H.; Sankaran, S.; et al. T cell receptor and cytokine signal integration in CD8+ T cells is mediated by the protein Themis. *Nat. Immunol.* **2020**, *21*, 186–198. [CrossRef]

11. Salter, A.I.; Ivey, R.G.; Kennedy, J.J.; Voillet, V.; Rajan, A.; Alderman, E.J.; Voytovich, U.J.; Lin, C.; Sommermeyer, D.; Liu, L.; et al. Phosphoproteomic analysis of chimeric antigen receptor signaling reveals kinetic and quantitative differences that affect cell function. *Sci. Signal.* **2018**, *11*, eaat6753. [CrossRef]

12. Karlsson, H.; Svensson, E.; Gigg, C.; Jarvius, M.; Olsson-Strömberg, U.; Savoldo, B.; Dotti, G.; Loskog, A. Evaluation of Intracellular Signaling Downstream Chimeric Antigen Receptors. *PLoS ONE* **2015**, *10*, e0144787. [CrossRef] [PubMed]

13. Ramello, M.C.; Benzaïd, I.; Kuenzi, B.M.; Lienlaf-Moreno, M.; Kandell, W.M.; Santiago, D.N.; Pabón-Saldaña, M.; Darville, L.; Fang, B.; Rix, U.; et al. An immunoproteomic approach to characterize the CAR interactome and signalosome. *Sci. Signal.* **2019**, *12*, eaap9777. [CrossRef]
14. Harris, D.T.; Hager, M.V.; Smith, S.N.; Cai, Q.; Stone, J.D.; Kruger, P.; Lever, M.; Dushek, O.; Schmitt, T.M.; Greenberg, P.D.; et al. Comparison of T Cell Activities Mediated by Human TCRs and CARs That Use the Same Recognition Domains. *J. Immunol.* **2018**, *200*, 1088–1100. [CrossRef] [PubMed]
15. Oren, R.; Hod-Marco, M.; Haus-Cohen, M.; Thomas, S.; Blat, D.; Duvshani, N.; Denkberg, G.; Elbaz, Y.; Benchetrit, F.; Eshhar, Z.; et al. Functional Comparison of Engineered T Cells Carrying a Native TCR versus TCR-like Antibody–Based Chimeric Antigen Receptors Indicates Affinity/Avidity Thresholds. *J. Immunol.* **2014**, *193*, 5733–5743. [CrossRef]
16. Watanabe, K.; Kuramitsu, S.; Posey, A.D.J.; June, C.H. Expanding the Therapeutic Window for CAR T Cell Therapy in Solid Tumors: The Knowns and Unknowns of CAR T Cell Biology. *Front. Immunol.* **2018**, *9*, 2486. [CrossRef]
17. Sim, A.C.N.; Too, C.T.; Oo, M.Z.; Lai, J.; Eio, M.Y.; Song, Z.; Srinivasan, N.; Tan, D.A.L.; Pang, S.W.; Gan, S.U.; et al. Defining the expression hierarchy of latent T-cell epitopes in Epstein-Barr virus infection with TCR-like antibodies. *Sci. Rep.* **2013**, *3*, 3232. [CrossRef] [PubMed]
18. Lai, J.; Tan, W.J.; Too, C.T.; Choo, J.A.L.; Wong, L.H.; Mustafa, F.B.; Srinivasan, N.; Lim, A.P.C.; Zhong, Y.; Gascoigne, N.R.J.; et al. Targeting Epstein-Barr virus–transformed B lymphoblastoid cells using antibodies with T-cell receptor–like specificities. *Blood* **2016**, *128*, 1396–1407. [CrossRef]
19. Yachi, P.P.; Ampudia, J.; Gascoigne, N.R.; Zal, T. Nonstimulatory peptides contribute to antigen-induced CD8–T cell receptor interaction at the immunological synapse. *Nat. Immunol.* **2005**, *6*, 785–792. [CrossRef]
20. Rybakin, V.; Clamme, J.-P.; Ampudia, J.; Yachi, P.P.; Gascoigne, N.R.J. CD8$\alpha\alpha$ and -$\alpha\beta$ isotypes are equally recruited to the immunological synapse through their ability to bind to MHC class I. *EMBO Rep.* **2011**, *12*, 1251–1256. [CrossRef] [PubMed]
21. Hoerter, J.A.; Brzostek, J.; Artyomov, M.N.; Abel, S.M.; Casas, J.; Rybakin, V.; Ampudia, J.; Lotz, C.; Connolly, J.M.; Chakraborty, A.K.; et al. Coreceptor affinity for MHC defines peptide specificity requirements for TCR interaction with coagonist peptide–MHC. *J. Exp. Med.* **2013**, *210*, 1807–1821. [CrossRef]
22. Zhao, X.; Sankaran, S.; Yap, J.; Too, C.T.; Ho, Z.Z.; Dolton, G.; Legut, M.; Ren, E.C.; Sewell, A.K.; Bertoletti, A.; et al. Nonstimulatory peptide-MHC enhances human T-cell antigen-specific responses by amplifying proximal TCR signaling. *Nat. Commun.* **2018**, *9*, 2716. [CrossRef] [PubMed]
23. Zhao, X.; Hamidinia, M.; Choo, J.A.L.; Too, C.T.; Ho, Z.Z.; Ren, E.C.; Bertoletti, A.; Macary, P.A.; Gould, K.G.; Brzostek, J.; et al. Use of Single Chain MHC Technology to Investigate Co-agonism in Human CD8+ T Cell Activation. *J. Vis. Exp.* **2019**, *10*, e59126. [CrossRef] [PubMed]
24. Heemskerk, M.H.M.; Hoogeboom, M.; De Paus, R.A.; Kester, M.G.D.; Van Der Hoorn, M.A.W.G.; Goulmy, E.A.J.M.; Willemze, R.; Falkenburg, J.H.F. Redirection of antileukemic reactivity of peripheral T lymphocytes using gene transfer of minor histocompatibility antigen HA-2-specific T-cell receptor complexes expressing a conserved alpha joining region. *Blood* **2003**, *102*, 3530–3540. [CrossRef]
25. Fu, G.; Gascoigne, N.R. Multiplexed labeling of samples with cell tracking dyes facilitates rapid and accurate internally controlled calcium flux measurement by flow cytometry. *J. Immunol. Methods* **2009**, *350*, 194–199. [CrossRef]
26. Choo, J.A.L.; Thong, S.Y.; Yap, J.; Van Esch, W.J.E.; Raida, M.; Meijers, R.; Lescar, J.; Verhelst, S.H.L.; Grotenbreg, G.M. Bioorthogonal Cleavage and Exchange of Major Histocompatibility Complex Ligands by Employing Azobenzene-Containing Peptides. *Angew. Chem. Int. Ed.* **2014**, *53*, 13390–13394. [CrossRef]
27. Vardhana, S.; Dustin, M. Supported Planar Bilayers for the Formation of Study of Immunological Synapses and Kinapse. *J. Vis. Exp.* **2008**, e947. [CrossRef]
28. Feng, Y.; Reinherz, E.L.; Lang, M.J. $\alpha\beta$ T Cell Receptor Mechanosensing Forces out Serial Engagement. *Trends Immunol.* **2018**, *39*, 596–609. [CrossRef]
29. Van Der Merwe, P.A.; Dushek, O. Mechanisms for T cell receptor triggering. *Nat. Rev. Immunol.* **2010**, *11*, 47–55. [CrossRef]
30. Salzer, B.; Schueller, C.M.; Zajc, C.U.; Peters, T.; Schoeber, M.A.; Kovacic, B.; Buri, M.C.; Lobner, E.; Dushek, O.; Huppa, J.B.; et al. Engineering AvidCARs for combinatorial antigen recognition and reversible control of CAR function. *Nat. Commun.* **2020**, *11*, 1–16. [CrossRef] [PubMed]
31. Chang, Z.L.; Lorenzini, M.H.; Chen, X.; Tran, U.; Bangayan, N.J.; Chen, Y.Y. Rewiring T-cell responses to soluble factors with chimeric antigen receptors. *Nat. Chem. Biol.* **2018**, *14*, 317–324. [CrossRef] [PubMed]
32. Brameshuber, M.; Kellner, F.; Rossboth, B.K.; Ta, H.; Alge, K.; Sevcsik, E.; Göhring, J.; Axmann, M.; Baumgart, F.; Gascoigne, N.R.J.; et al. Monomeric TCRs drive T cell antigen recognition. *Nat. Immunol.* **2018**, *19*, 487–496. [CrossRef]
33. Huang, J.; Brameshuber, M.; Zeng, X.; Xie, J.; Li, Q.-J.; Chien, Y.-H.; Valitutti, S.; Davis, M.M. A Single Peptide-Major Histocompatibility Complex Ligand Triggers Digital Cytokine Secretion in CD4+ T Cells. *Immunity* **2013**, *39*, 846–857. [CrossRef]
34. Delon, J.; Grégoire, C.; Malissen, B.; Darche, S.; Lemaître, F.; Kourilsky, P.; Abastado, J.-P.; Trautmann, A. CD8 Expression Allows T Cell Signaling by Monomeric Peptide-MHC Complexes. *Immunity* **1998**, *9*, 467–473. [CrossRef]
35. Moulton, V.R.; Tsokos, G.C. Abnormalities of T cell signaling in systemic lupus erythematosus. *Arthritis Res.* **2011**, *13*, 207. [CrossRef] [PubMed]

36. Laugel, B.; Cole, D.K.; Clement, M.; Wooldridge, L.; Price, D.A.; Sewell, A.K. The multiple roles of the CD8 coreceptor in T cell biology: Opportunities for the selective modulation of self-reactive cytotoxic T cells. *J. Leukoc. Biol.* **2011**, *90*, 1089–1099. [CrossRef]
37. La Gruta, N.L.; Gras, S.; Daley, S.R.; Thomas, P.G.; Rossjohn, J. Understanding the drivers of MHC restriction of T cell receptors. *Nat. Rev. Immunol.* **2018**, *18*, 467–478. [CrossRef]
38. Li, L.; Guo, X.; Shi, X.; Li, C.; Wu, W.; Yan, C.; Wang, H.; Li, H.; Xu, C. Ionic CD3−Lck interaction regulates the initiation of T-cell receptor signaling. *Proc. Natl. Acad. Sci. USA* **2017**, *114*, E5891–E5899. [CrossRef]
39. Abraham, R.T.; Weiss, A. Jurkat T cells and development of the T-cell receptor signalling paradigm. *Nat. Rev. Immunol.* **2004**, *4*, 301–308. [CrossRef]
40. Shan, X.; Czar, M.J.; Bunnell, S.C.; Liu, P.; Liu, Y.; Schwartzberg, P.L.; Wange, R.L. Deficiency of PTEN in Jurkat T Cells Causes Constitutive Localization of Itk to the Plasma Membrane and Hyperresponsiveness to CD3 Stimulation. *Mol. Cell. Biol.* **2000**, *20*, 6945–6957. [CrossRef]
41. Astoul, E. PI 3-K and T-cell activation: Limitations of T-leukemic cell lines as signaling models. *Trends Immunol.* **2001**, *22*, 490–496. [CrossRef]

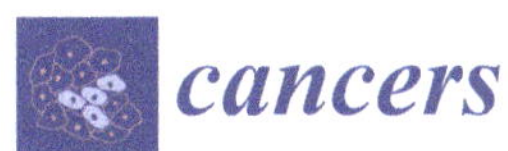

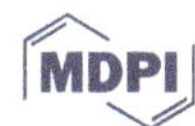

Article

Real-World Experience of Pembrolizumab Monotherapy in Patients with Recurrent or Persistent Cervical Cancer: A Korean Multi-Center Retrospective Study (KGOG1041)

Min Chul Choi [1,*,†], Yong-Man Kim [2,†], Jeong-Won Lee [3,*], Yong Jae Lee [4], Dong Hoon Suh [5], Sung Jong Lee [6], Taek Sang Lee [7], Maria Lee [8], Dong Choon Park [9], Min Kyu Kim [10], Jong-Min Lee [11], Seung-Hyuk Shim [12], Seob Jeon [13], Kyung Jin Min [14], Mi Kyung Kim [15], Bo Wook Kim [16], Jeong Yeol Park [2], Byoung-Gie Kim [3], Dae Yeon Kim [2], Moon-Hong Kim [17], Hyun-Soo Kim [18] and Jung-Yun Lee [4]

1   Comprehensive Gynecologic Cancer Center, CHA Bundang Medical Center, CHA University, Seongnam-si, Gyeonggi-do 13496, Korea
2   Department of Obstetrics and Gynecology, University of Ulsan College of Medicine, Asan Medical Center, Seoul 05505, Korea; ymkim@amc.seoul.kr (Y.-M.K.); obgyjypark@amc.seoul.kr (J.Y.P.); kdyog@amc.seoul.kr (D.Y.K.)
3   Department of Obstetrics and Gynecology, Samsung Medical Center, Sungkyunkwan University School of Medicine, Seoul 06351, Korea; bgkim@skku.edu
4   Department of Obstetrics and Gynecology, Yonsei University College of Medicine, Seoul 03722, Korea; SVASS@yuhs.ac (Y.J.L.); jungyunlee@yuhs.ac (J.-Y.L.)
5   Department of Obstetrics and Gynecology, Seoul National University Bundang Hospital, Seongnam 13620, Korea; sdhwcj@snubh.org
6   Department of Obstetrics and Gynecology, Seoul St. Mary's Hospital, College of Medicine, The Catholic University of Korea, Seoul 06591, Korea; orlando@catholic.ac.kr
7   Department of Obstetrics and Gynecology, SMG-SNU Boramae Medical Center, Seoul 07061, Korea; tslee70@snu.ac.kr
8   Department of Obstetrics and Gynecology, Seoul National University College of Medicine, Seoul 03080, Korea; marialee@snu.ac.kr
9   Department of Obstetrics and Gynecology, St. Vincent's Hospital, The Catholic University of Korea, Suwon 16247, Korea; dcpark@catholic.ac.kr
10   Division of Gynecologic Oncology, Department of Obstetrics and Gynecology, Samsung Changwon Hospital, Sungkyunkwan University School of Medicine, Changwon 51353, Korea; minkyukim@skku.edu
11   Department of Obstetrics and Gynecology, Kyung Hee University Hospital at Gangdong, Seoul 05278, Korea; jmleemd@khu.ac.kr
12   Department of Obstetrics and Gynecology, Research Institute of Medical Science, Konkuk University School of Medicine, Seoul 05030, Korea; 20130131@kuh.ac.kr
13   Department of Obstetrics and Gynecology, Soonchunhyang University College of Medicine, Cheonan 31151, Korea; sjeon@schmc.ac.kr
14   Department of Obstetrics and Gynecology, Korea University Medical Center, Korea University College of Medicine, Seoul 15355, Korea; mikji97@korea.ac.kr
15   Department of Obstetrics and Gynecology, Ewha Womans University College of Medicine, Seoul 07985, Korea; asterik79@ewha.ac.kr
16   Department of Obstetrics and Gynecology, International St. Mary's Hospital, Catholic Kwandong University College of Medicine, Incheon 22711, Korea; kimbw@ish.ac.kr
17   Department of Obstetrics and Gynecology, Korea Cancer Center Hospital, Korea Institute of Radiological & Medical Sciences, Seoul 01812, Korea; garymh@kcch.re.kr
18   Department of Pathology and Translational Genomics, Samsung Medical Center, Sungkyunkwan University School of Medicine, Seoul 06351, Korea; hyun-soo.kim@samsung.com
*   Correspondence: oursk79@cha.ac.kr (M.C.C.); garden.lee@samsung.com (J.-W.L.); Tel.: +82-31-780-6191 (M.C.C.); +82-2-3410-1382 (J.-W.L.); Fax: +82-31-780-6194 (M.C.C.); +82-2-3410-0630 (J.-W.L.)

† These authors contributed equally to this study.

Received: 29 September 2020; Accepted: 26 October 2020; Published: 29 October 2020

Simple Summary: Immune checkpoint inhibitors have received considerable interest because of their ability to generate durable response in many intractable malignant solid tumors. The therapeutic results of immune checkpoint inhibitors in recurrent or advanced uterine cervical cancer, which associated with persistent infection with human papillomavirus, from several well-designed clinical trials are reported. However real-world experiences are not yet provided. In this study, we retrospectively assessed the efficacy and safety of pembrolizumab, one of the immune checkpoint inhibitors, in real-world practice among patients in Korea with recurrent or persistent cervical cancers. The results of this study show modest antitumor activity comparable to that found in previously reported clinical trials. Although in patients with favorable performance status, pembrolizumab showed effective antitumor activity. Some safety profiles should be carefully monitored during treatment.

Abstract: This study investigated the antitumor activity and safety of pembrolizumab in patients with recurrent cervical cancer in real-world practice. We conducted a multi-center retrospective study of patients with recurrent or persistent cervical cancer treated with pembrolizumab at sixteen institutions in Korea between January 2016 and March 2020. The primary endpoints were the objective response rate (ORR) and safety. Data were available for 117 patients. The median age was 53 years (range, 28–79). Sixty-four (54.7%) patients had an Eastern Cooperative Oncology Group (ECOG) performance status of ≥2. Forty-nine (41.9%) patients were stage ≥III at diagnosis. Eighty-eight (75.2%) patients had squamous cell carcinoma. The median number of prior chemotherapy lines was two (range, 1–6). During the median follow-up of 4.9 months (range, 0.2–35.3), the ORR was 9.4%, with three complete responses and eight partial responses. The median time to response was 2.8 months (range 1.3–13.1), and the median duration of response (DOR) was not reached. In the population of patients with favorable performance status (ECOG ≤1) ($n = 53$), the ORR was 18.9%, and the median DOR was 8.9 months (range, 7.3–10.4). Adverse events occurred in 55 (47.0%) patients, including eight (6.8%) patients who experienced grade ≥3 events, and two of them were suspicious treatment-related deaths. Pembrolizumab had modest antitumor activity in patients with recurrent cervical cancer comparable to that found in previously reported clinical trials. However, in patients with favorable performance status, pembrolizumab showed effective antitumor activity. Some safety profiles should be carefully monitored during treatment.

Keywords: cervical cancer; immune checkpoint inhibitor; pembrolizumab; recurrence

---

1. Introduction

Uterine cervical cancer is one of the most common gynecologic cancers and the fourth leading cause of cancer-related death in women worldwide. More than 569,847 women were diagnosed with cervical cancer in 2018, resulting in more than 311,365 deaths [1]. It is estimated that 3148 new cases of cervical cancer and 801 cancer-related deaths will occur in Korea in 2020 [2]. For recurrent or metastatic cervical cancer, bevacizumab in combination with cisplatin-based chemotherapy is currently the standard treatment, and this approach provides a median survival of approximately 17 months [3]. Therapeutic options are limited for patients who progress after initial therapy to recurrent or metastatic cervical cancer.

It has been established that persistent infection with human papillomavirus (HPV) is associated with the carcinogenesis of cervical cancer [4] and HPV infections account for as much as 86% of the worldwide incidence of cervical cancer [5]. Two viral oncogenes, E6 and E7, play a major role in the malignant transformation of HPV-infected cervical cells. These viral antigens are consistently expressed in HPV-induced neoplasm and might represent attractive targets for cancer immunotherapy [6,7]. Cancer cells can induce immune evasion by immune checkpoints such as cytotoxic T-lymphocyte antigen 4 or programmed death-1 (PD-1), allowing them to escape from the tumor-specific T-cell response [8]. These negative signals in several solid tumors have been shown to be provided mainly by PD-1, and programmed death-ligand 1 (PD-L1) expression was recently identified in more than half of cervical cancers [9,10]. Therefore, using a monoclonal antibody to inhibit PD-1/PD-L1 co-inhibitory pathways might be an effective therapeutic approach to reverse immune suppression and to activate a cancer-specific immune response in cervical cancer patients.

Several clinical trials have been conducted to explore the application of PD-1 inhibitors to cervical cancer. The objective response rate to these PD-1 inhibitors (i.e., pembrolizumab and nivolumab) in patients with advanced or recurrent cervical cancer was reported to be 4%–26% [11–14]. Based on these results, the U.S. Food and Drug Administration approved pembrolizumab in June 2018 for the treatment of patients with PD-L1-positive recurrent or metastatic cervical cancer. However, real-world efficacy data are limited.

In Korea, pembrolizumab can be offered off-label to patients with recurrent squamous cell cervical cancer and PD-L1-positive recurrent cervical cancer. In this study, we retrospectively assessed the efficacy and safety of pembrolizumab in real-world practice among patients in Korea with recurrent or persistent cervical cancers.

2. Materials and Methods

2.1. Study Design and Patients

We conducted a multi-center, retrospective study at sixteen institutions affiliated with the Korean Gynecologic Oncology Group (KGOG). We reviewed the clinicopathologic and radiologic records of women diagnosed with recurrent or persistent uterine cervical cancer who were treated with pembrolizumab between January 2016 and March 2020. The inclusion criteria were as follows: (1) histologically confirmed cervical cancer; (2) tumor progression during or after the use of one or more lines of chemotherapy with measurable disease, irrespective of Eastern Cooperative Oncology Group (ECOG) performance status; (3) use of pembrolizumab for at least one treatment cycle. Patients were administered 200 mg of pembrolizumab as 30-min intravenous infusions every 3 weeks until disease progression, unacceptable toxicity, or patient withdrawal occurred. This study was approved by the Institutional Review Board at each participating institution (CHA IRB 2019-11-003) and adhered to the principles in the Declaration of Helsinki.

Pathologic information, including histology and results of PD-L1 staining, was collected, and some institutions additionally performed a PD-L1 test. Tumor PD-L1 expression was analyzed using the PD-L1 IHC 22C3 antibody (Dako, Santa Clara, CA) to determine the tumor proportion score (TPS), defined as the percentage of viable tumor cells, or using the PD-L1 IHC 22C3 pharmDx assay (Agilent Technologies, Carpinteria, CA) to determine the combined positive score (CPS), defined as the ratio of PD-L1-positive cells (tumor cells, lymphocytes, and macrophages) to the total number of viable tumor cells multiplied by 100. PD-L1 positivity was defined as a TPS $\geq$1% or a CPS >1.

The datasets supporting the conclusions of this article are included within the article and its additional images. Raw data are available from the corresponding author upon reasonable request.

2.2. Assessments

Tumor imaging was basically performed by abdomino-pelvic and/or chest computed tomography (CT) every 9 weeks. If clinical symptoms were deteriorated, image studies were performed immediately at the clinician's discretion. Pelvic magnetic resonance imaging, whole body bone scan, or positron emission tomography/CT scans were performed when indicated. The tumor response assessment was performed according to the Response Evaluation Criteria in Solid Tumors (RECIST) version 1.1 by gynecologic oncologists. Safety was assessed by retrospective chart review of laboratory tests and physical examinations were performed before each treatment cycle to detect any possible adverse events (AEs), which were evaluated according to the Common Terminology Criteria for Adverse Events version 4.03. (http://www.oncology.tv/SymptomManagement/NationalCancerInstituteUpdatesCTCAEtov403.aspx).

2.3. Primary and Secondary Objectives

The primary endpoints were the objective response rate (ORR), defined as the proportion of patients with a complete response (CR) or a partial response (PR), as assessed by RECIST version 1.1, and the rate of any AEs. The secondary endpoints were the duration of response, defined as the time from the response to tumor progression or death, whichever occurred first; progression-free survival (PFS), defined as the time from the start of pembrolizumab to tumor progression or death; overall survival (OS), defined as the time from the start of treatment to death from any cause. An additional efficacy analysis was conducted in the subgroup of patients with favorable performance status (ECOG ≤ 1).

ORR point estimates, accompanied by 95% confidence intervals (CIs), were calculated using the Clopper–Pearson exact method. Patients without response data were considered to be non-responders. Duration of response, PFS, and OS were estimated using the Kaplan–Meier method. To identify factors affecting the ORR, univariate logistic regression analyses were performed. A further multivariate logistic regression analysis was intended to use factors with a significance level of less than 0.1 in the univariate analyses.

3. Results

3.1. Patients

Information for 117 patients treated with pembrolizumab was collected from 16 sites affiliated with KGOG. One patient diagnosed with vaginal cancer and two duplicate patients were excluded (Table S1). The clinicopathologic characteristics of the patients are listed in Table 1. The median age was 53.0 years (range, 28–79 years). Of the patients, 45.3% (53/117) had an ECOG performance status (PS) of ≤1, and 41.9% (49/117) had stage III or IV at diagnosis. The HPV test was done in 71 patients (60.7%), of whom 57 (80.3%) were HPV-positive. PD-L1 expression was tested in 72 patients (61.5%), of whom 60 (83.3%) were PD-L1-positive by TPS or CPS. Eighty-eight (75.2%) patients had squamous cell carcinoma histology. Fifty patients (42.7%) had received previous radiotherapy, and 62 patients (53.0%) had received previous surgery. The median number of prior chemotherapy lines, including neoadjuvant chemotherapy, was two (range, 1–6). As of 31 March, 2020, the data cutoff, the median follow-up time was 4.9 months (range, 0.2–35.3 months). Ninety-nine patients (84.6%) had discontinued pembrolizumab, most commonly due to disease progression (57.3%; *n* = 67) (Figure 1). The median number of pembrolizumab cycles was three (range, 1–24 cycles).

Table 1. Clinico-pathologic characteristics of the patients (*n* = 117).

Characteristic	No. (%)
Age, Years Median, range	53 (28–79)
ECOG performance status	
0	16 (13.7%)
1	37 (31.6%)
2	45 (38.5%)
3	16 (13.7%)
4	3 (2.6%)

Table 1. *Cont.*

Characteristic	No. (%)
FIGO stage at diagnosis	
I	31 (26.5%)
II	34 (29.1%)
III	22 (18.8%)
IV	27 (23.1%)
Unknown	3 (2.6%)
HPV test result	
Positive [^]	57 (48.7%)
Negative	14 (12.0%)
Unknown	46 (39.3%)
PD-L1 expression [*]	
1≤	60 (51.3%)
1>	12 (10.3%)
Unknown	45 (38.5%)
Histology	
Squamous cell carcinoma	88 (75.2%)
Adenocarcinoma	19 (16.2%)
Adenosquamous cell carcinoma	4 (3.4%)
Neuroendocrine cell carcinoma	4 (3.4%)
Glassy cell carcinoma	1 (0.9%)
Basaloid squamous cell carcinoma	1 (0.9%)
Target lesion size, mm [#]	
Median, range	67 (10–529)
Previous radiation therapy	50 (42.7%)
(CC)RTx	38 (76.0%)
(CC)RTx + hysterectomy	12 (24.0%) [@]
Previous surgery	62 (53.0%)
RH	17 (27.4%) [%]
RH + (CC)RTx	45 (72.6%) [&]
Number of previous lines of chemotherapy	
1	38 (32.5%)
2	43 (36.8%)
3	24 (20.5%)
4	8 (6.8%)
≥5	4 (3.4%)

ECOG, Eastern Cooperative Oncology Group; FIGO, International Federation of Gynecology and Obstetrics; HPV, human papillomavirus; N/A, non-available; PD-L1, programmed death-ligand 1; (CC)RTx, concurrent chemoradiation or radiation therapy; RH, radical hysterectomy. [^] presence of any type of high-risk human papillomavirus regardless of test type. [*] determined by either the tumor proportion score (TPS) or the combined positive score (CPS). [#] sum of the target lesions. [@] including 2 cases of pelvic exenteration. [%] including 2 cases of radical trachelectomy. [&] including 2 cases of pelvic exenteration followed by radiation.

3.2. Antitumor Activity

In the total population, three patients (2.6%) achieved a CR and eight (6.8%) achieved a PR, resulting in an ORR of 9.4% (95% CI, 4.8–16.2) (Table 2). A clinical summary of the 11 responders is provided in Table S2. Ten of the 11 responders had squamous cell carcinoma (one, BCHA013, had adenosquamous histology) and 10 had favorable ECOG PS (one, BCHA006, had a PS of 3). The median time to response was 2.8 months (range, 1.3–13.1 months) and the median duration of response was not reached (range, 8.9–not reached). Eight of the 11 responders were still receiving pembrolizumab at the data cutoff date (Figure 2A). In the population of patients (*n* = 53) with favorable PS, the ORR was 18.9% (95% CI, 9.4–32.0) (Table 2). The median time to response in that group was 3.0 months (range, 1.3–13.1 months), and their median duration of response was 8.9 months (range, 7.3–10.4 months).

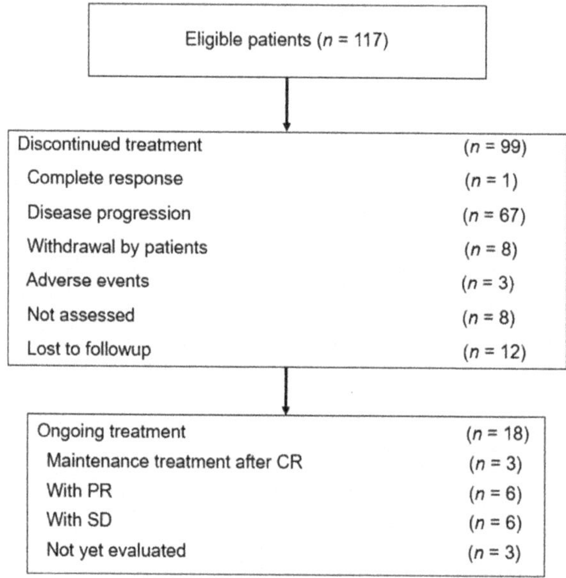

Figure 1. Patient disposition. CR, complete response; PR, partial response; SD, stable disease.

Table 2. Tumor responses assessed by RECIST v.1.1 (n = 117).

Anti-Tumor Activity	Total Population	Favorable PS Group (ECOG $\leq$1)
	n = 117	n =53
Best overall response		
CR	3 (2.6%)	3 (5.7%)
PR	8 (6.8%)	7 (13.2%)
SD	28 (23.9%)	14 (26.4%)
PD	67 (57.3%)	26 (49.1%)
Not able to be assessed	11 (9.4%)	3 (5.7%)
Objective response rate	11 (9.4%)	10 (18.9%)
95% CI	4.8 to 16.2	9.4 to 32.0
Disease control rate	39 (33.3%)	24 (45.3%)
95% CI	24.9 to 42.6	31.6 to 59.6
Time to response, months [#]		
Median (range)	2.8 (1.3–13.1)	3.0 (1.3–13.1)
Duration of response, months [#,&]		
Median (range)	NR (8.9–NR)	8.9 (7.3–10.4)
Duration of response, months [#,*]	(n = 11)	(n = 10)
$\geq$6	6 (54.5%)	5 (50.0%)
$\geq$9	4 (36.4%)	3 (30.0%)
$\geq$12	2 (18.2%)	1 (10.0%)

CR, complete response; PR, partial response; SD, stable disease; PD, progressive disease; CI, confidence interval; NR, not reached; PS, performance status. [#] Evaluated in patients who had a response (n = 11 for total population, n = 10 for favorable PS group). [&] Estimated using Kaplan-Meier method. [*] Percentages as a fraction of the number of responders.

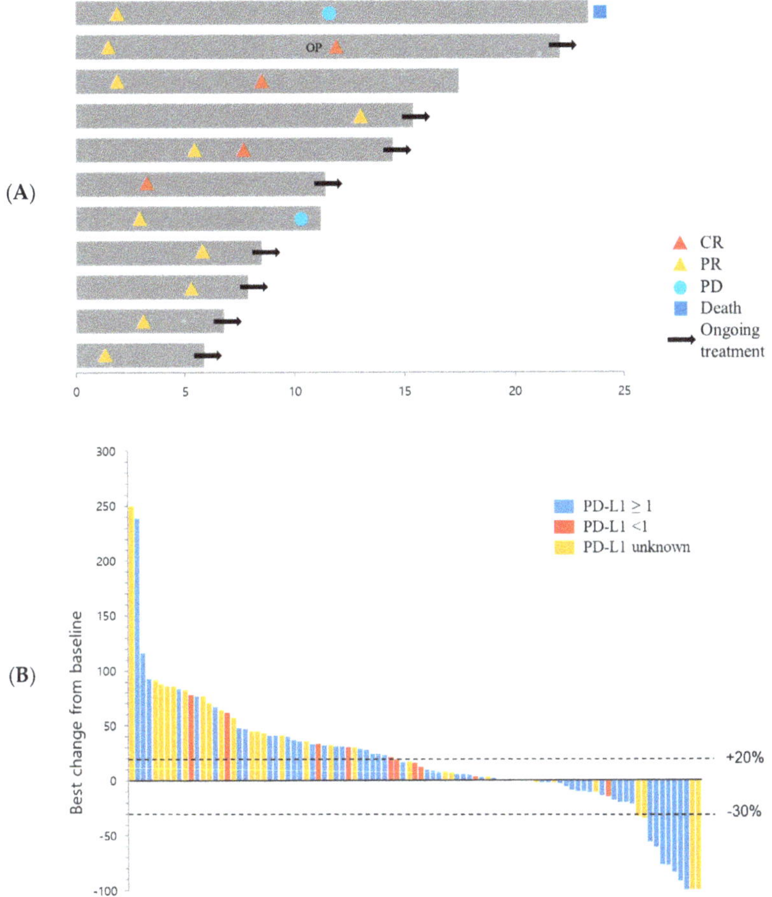

Figure 2. Antitumor activity of pembrolizumab. (**A**) Time to and duration of response in patients whose best overall response was CR or PR (*n* = 11). The length of bars represents the time to the last image assessment. (**B**) Waterfall plot showing the distribution of the best percentage change in the sum of the target lesion size from baseline according to Response Evaluation Criteria in Solid Tumors (RECIST) version 1.1 (*n* = 95). OP, operation; CR, complete response; PR, partial response; PD, progressive disease; PD-L1, programmed death-ligand 1.

Twenty-eight patients (23.9%) in the total population and 14 patients (26.4%) in the favorable PS group showed stable disease, leading to disease control rates of 33.3% (95% CI, 24.9–42.6) and 45.3% (95% CI, 31.6–59.6), respectively (Table 2). The best percentage change in target lesion from baseline among the 95 patients with one or more evaluable post-baseline imaging assessments is shown in Figure 2B.

At the time of data cutoff, 81 (69.2%) patients in the total population had experienced disease progression or death. The median PFS was 2.7 months (95% CI, 2.3–3.1 months), and the estimated PFS rates at six and 12 months were 29.6% and 16.6%, respectively (Figure 3A). In the favorable PS group, which had 32 patients with disease progression (60.4%), the median PFS was 4.5 months (95% CI, 1.8–7.2 months; Figure S1A). A total of 53 patients (45.3%) in the total population and 15 (28.3%) in the favorable PS group had died. The median OS was 8.8 months (95% CI, 5.6–12.1 months) in the total population (Figure 3B) and 19.1 months (95% CI, 2.5–35.6 months) in the favorable PS group

(Figure S1B). The six-month estimates of OS were 58.6% and 84.1%, respectively, and the 12-month estimates were 41.1% and 57.3%, respectively. One of the 11 responders (BCHA010) expired due to cancer progression (Table S2).

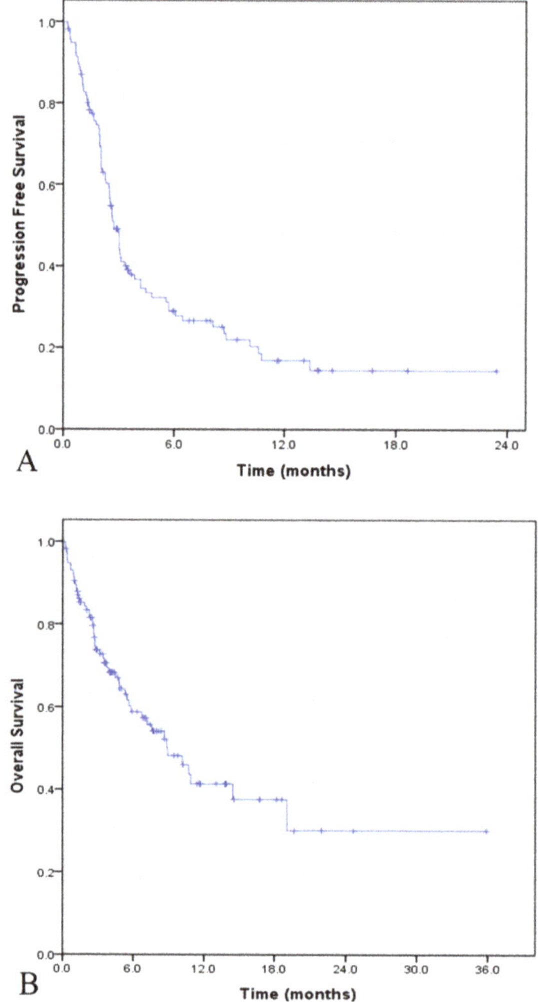

Figure 3. Kaplan–Meier estimates of survival in the total study population (*n* = 117). (**A**) Progression-free survival; (**B**) overall survival.

3.3. Safety

A total of 55 patients (47.0%) experienced one or more adverse events, including eight (6.8%) patients who experienced grade ≥3 events (Table 3). Three patients (2.6%) discontinued pembrolizumab due to AEs, including two whose deaths were suspected to have resulted from treatment-related AEs. One of these patients, who suddenly developed pneumonitis with pulmonary edema 20 days after the first cycle, refused further management for the AE, and expired the day after symptom manifestation. The second patient, who had grade 4 colitis after three cycles, also refused further management for the AE, and died 10 days later. The third patient discontinued treatment due to the occurrence of grade 3 Guillain–Barré syndrome; the patient recovered from these symptoms, but received no further pembrolizumab. The most common AEs for any grade were hypothyroidism (7.7%), fatigue (4.3%), and skin rash (4.3%).

Table 3. Treatment-related adverse events in the total population ($n = 117$).

Adverse Event	Any Grade	Grade 3/4
Any AE	55 (47.0%)	8 (6.8%)
Hypothyroidism	9 (7.7%)	0
Fatigue	5 (4.3%)	0
Skin rash	5 (4.3%)	2 (1.7%)
Anemia	4 (3.4%)	1 (0.9%)
AST/ALT elevated	3 (2.6%)	1 (0.9%)
Nausea	3 (2.6%)	0
Abdominal pain	3 (2.6%)	0
Dyspnea	3 (2.6%)	0
Colitis	2 (1.7%)	1 (0.9%)
Neutropenia	2 (1.7%)	1 (0.9%)
Thrombocytopenia	2 (1.7%)	0
Hyperphosphatemia	2 (1.7%)	0
Hypoalbuminemia	2 (1.7%)	0
Renal insufficiency	2 (1.7%)	0
Cough	2 (1.7%)	0
Hyperthyroidism	1 (0.9%)	0
Pneumonitis with pulmonary edema	1 (0.9%)	1 (0.9%)
Constipation	1 (0.9%)	0
Vomiting	1 (0.9%)	0
Dizziness	1 (0.9%)	0
Guillain-Barré syndrome	1 (0.9%)	1 (0.9%)
Any AE leading to discontinuation		
Guillain-Barre syndrome	1	1
Colitis	1	1
Pneumonitis with pulmonary edema	1	1

AE, adverse events; AST, aspartate aminotransferase; ALT, alanine aminotransferase.

3.4. Prognostic Factors

Analyses examining how HPV positivity, histology, the number of previous lines of chemotherapy, ECOG status, PD-L1 positivity, and burden of tumor affected ORR were performed using logistic regressions (Table 4). Favorable ECOG PS ($\leq$1) was the only significant factor in the univariate regression analyses (odds ratio, 14.651; 95% CI, 1.809–118.675; $p = 0.012$), so no further multivariate regression analysis was done.

Table 4. Logistic regression analysis of predictive factors for the objective response rate.

Predictive Factors	Univariate Analysis	
	OR (95% CI)	*p*-Value
HPV test result		
Negative	1	
Positive	1.529 (0.169–13.842)	0.705
Histology		
Non-SqCC	1	
SqCC	3.590 (0.439–29.329)	0.233

Table 4. *Cont.*

Predictive Factors	Univariate Analysis	
	OR (95% CI)	*p*-Value
Number of prior lines of chemotherapy		
≤2	1	
≥3	1.315 (0.328–5.263)	0.699
ECOG performance status		
≥2	1	
≤1	14.651 (1.809–118.675)	0.012
PD-L1 expression		
<20	1	
≥20	2.133 (0.440–10.338)	0.347
Burden of tumor [#]		0.120
<2cm	1	
2cm≤ <5cm	1.429 (0.244–8.375)	
5cm≤ <10cm	0.270 (0.34–2.165)	
≥10cm	0.192 (0.016–2.363)	

OR, odds ratio; HPV, human papillomavirus; SqCC, squamous cell carcinoma; ECOG, Eastern Cooperative Oncology Group; PD-L1, programmed death-ligand 1. [#] sum of the target lesion.

4. Discussion

4.1. Antitumor Activity

The results of this study show modest antitumor activity for pembrolizumab in patients with recurrent or persistent cervical cancer. The ORR was 9.4%, with three patients achieving a CR and eight patients a PR. The median PFS was 2.7 months, and the estimated PFS rate at six months was 29.6%. The median OS was 8.8 months, and the six- and 12-month estimates for OS were 58.6% and 41.1%, respectively. The therapeutic results from PD-1 inhibitors monotherapy in recurrent or advanced cervical cancer are summarized in Table 5 [11–14]. Although it is difficult to directly compare our results with those from well-designed clinical trials, they are generally consistent. As in a previous report, when we analyzed the 88 patients with squamous cell carcinoma, which is known to have a relatively favorable prognosis, their ORR was 11.4% (Table S3). The results from prospective clinical trials and our results from this retrospective study differ in some points. The prospective studies could only enroll patients with a favorable PS (ECOG ≤1), but in real-world practice, patients with poor general condition (ECOG ≥2) are also treated. In the real world, immune checkpoint inhibitors (ICIs) tend to be tried as a last attempt for heavily treated patients in poor general condition. In this study, more than half (54.7%, 64/117) of the patients had an ECOG ≥2 (Table 1), which well reflects real-world clinical circumstances.

Table 5. Therapeutic results of PD-1 inhibitors monotherapy in recurrent or advanced cervical cancer patients.

Study	Keynote028	Keynote158	Checkmate358	NRG-GY002	Present Study	
					Total population	Favorable PS group
Phase	IB	II	I/II	II	Retro	Retro
Drug	Pembrolizumab 10mg/kg q2w	Pembrolizumab 200mg q3w	Nivolumab 240mg q2w	Nivolumab 3mg/kg q2w	Pembrolizumab 200mg q3w	Pembrolizumab 200mg q3w
N	24	98	19	25	117	53
Age, median (age)	42	46	51	45	53	52
Histology of SqCC	23 (96%)	92 (94%)	19 (100%)	15 (60%)	88 (75%)	42 (79%)
ECOG $\leq$1	24 (100%)	98 (100%)	18 (95%)	25(100%)	53 (45%)	53 (100%)
Prior lines CTx $\geq$3	9 (38%)	30 (31%)	0	N/A	36(31%)	15 (28%)
Positive PD–L1 expression	24 (100%) [*]	82 (84%) [#]	10 (53%) [%]	17(77%) [#]	57(49%) [$]	30 (57%) [$]
BOR						
CR	0	3 (3%)	3 (16%)	0	3 (3%)	3 (6%)
PR	4 (17%)	9 (8%)	2 (10%)	1 (4%)	8 (7%)	7 (13%)
SD	3 (13%)	18 (18%)	8 (42%)	9 (36%)	28 (24%)	14 (26%)
PD	16 (67%)	55 (56%)	6 (32%)	11 (44%)	67 (57%)	26 (49%)
Not evaluable	1 (4%)	13 (13%)	0	4 (16%)	11 (0%)	3 (6%)
ORR	4 (17%)	12(12%)	5 (26%)	1 (4%)	11 (9%)	10 (19%)
DCR	7 (29%)	30 (31%)	13 (68%)	10 (40%)	39 (33%)	24 (45%)
Time to response, months Median (range)	1.9 (1.7–8.2)	2.1(1.6–4.1)	1.7 (1.6–1.9)	N/A	2.8 (1.4–13.4)	3.0 (1.4–13.4)
Duration of response, monthsMedian (range)	5.4 (4.1–7.5)	NR ($\geq$3.7–$\geq$18.6)	NR (23.3–29.5)	3.8	NR (8.9-NR)	8.9 (7.3–10.4)
AE $\geq$3	5 (21%)	12 (12%)	4(21%)	6 (24%)	8 (7%)	3 (6%)
PFS at 6m	21%	25%	36%	16%	30%	44%
OS at 6m, 12m	67%, 40%	75%, 41%	89%, 78%	78%	59%, 41%	84%, 57%

PS, performance status; Retro, retrospective study; SqCC, squamous cell carcinoma; ECOG, Eastern Cooperative Oncology Group; PD-L1, programmed death-ligand 1; CTx, chemotherapy; BOR, best overall response; CR, complete response; PR, partial response; SD, stable disease; PD, progressive disease; ORR, objective response rate; DCR, disease control rate; AE, adverse events; PFS, progression-free survival; OS, overall survival; N/A, non-available. [*] $\geq$1% of modified proportion score, [#] $\geq$1 of combined positive score (CPS), [%] $\geq$1% of tumor proportion score (TPS), [$] TPS $\geq$ 1% or CPS $\geq$ 1.

In this context, the promising antitumor activity of pembrolizumab could be assessed by analyzing the treatment response in only the favorable PS group in this study. The ORR in this group (*n* = 53) was 18.9%, and their disease control rate was 45.3% (Table 2). Furthermore, their median PFS was 4.5 months (95% CI, 1.8–7.2 months), with an estimated PFS rate of 44% at six months. Their median OS was 19.1 months (95% CI, 2.5–35.6 months), and the estimated six- and 12-month estimates of OS were 84.1% and 57.3%, respectively (Table 5). These results indicate that pembrolizumab has antitumor activity that is somewhat better than that reported in the KEYNOTE-158 study [14], which used the same dose of pembrolizumab. Therefore, the results of this real-world study indicate that among patients with recurrent or persistent cervical cancer, pembrolizumab treatment showed better antitumor activity in patients with favorable PS.

In addition, as in the results of the CheckMate 358 trial [12] of nivolumab, patients treated with less than two previous chemotherapy lines had an ORR of 26% (Table 5), suggesting that a low number of prior treatments improved the response. As previously suggested by Tewari [15], treatment with ICIs could be a second-line therapeutic option for patients with progressed cervical cancer who have failed with standard therapy after confirmation of PD-L1 expression. An ongoing phase III randomized trial is investigating chemotherapy with ICIs as a first-line treatment for chemo-naïve patients with persistent, recurrent, or metastatic cervical cancer [16,17].

4.2. Adverse Events

According to a recent meta-analysis [18], AEs of any grade occurred in 65.8% of patients receiving an ICI, and 16.6% of patients experienced grade ≥3 AEs. Treatment discontinuation due to AEs occurred in 6.4% of patients, and treatment-related death (TRD) was less common in patients treated with ICIs (0.9%) than in patients treated with chemotherapy (1.3%). To date, TRD has not been reported in studies of cervical cancer patients [11–14]. In the present study, an AE occurred in 47.0% of patients, and 6.8% of patients experienced grade ≥3 AEs. Treatment discontinuation due to AEs occurred in 2.6% of patients, and suspicious TRD occurred in two (1.5%) patients.

Compared to the reported clinical trials, the frequency of AEs in this study was relatively low, which is likely due to the limitations of a retrospective study conducted using chart reviews, because minor AEs might not have been recorded. In contrast, 1.5% (*n* = 2) of patients were suspected of TRD. These patients might not have died if they had been adequately managed for their AEs. Furthermore, it was difficult to identify the accurate cause of death in these patients because no autopsy or additional investigation was conducted. The most commonly reported causes of TRD are known to be immune-related pneumonitis and intestinal perforation/colitis [18]; therefore, clinicians have to be fully aware of these risks when prescribing ICIs.

4.3. Prognostic Marker

Microsatellite instability-high and/or deficient DNA mismatch repair (MSI-H/MMRd) has been identified as a potential predictive marker for response to ICIs [19–21]. Regardless of the type of cancer, solid tumors showing MSI-H/MMRd are known to have a favorable response to pembrolizumab, with an ORR of 34%–53% [19,21]. However, tumors with MSI-H/MMRd represent only 2%–4% of all diagnosed cancers [22,23]. In gynecologic cancers, MSI-H/MMRd tumors are found in 22%–33% of all endometrial cancers, and only 10% of all ovarian and cervical cancers [19,20]. Therefore, other prognostic markers, such as PD-L1 expression, tumor mutational burden, and clinical biomarkers, have been studied. Of them, PD-L1 expression on either tumor or immune cells has emerged as an alternative predictive biomarker. The ORR was higher in patients with PD-L1-positive cervical cancers than in the overall population (14.6% vs. 12.2%, respectively) in a previous clinical trial [14]. PD-L1 positivity was confirmed in 60 (83.3%) of the 72 patients in our study based on the test results (Table 1), and their ORR was 11.7% (7/60) (data not provided). However, the role of PD-L1 expression has not been clarified, so it currently has limited value as a predictive biomarker [24].

HPV infection in cervical cancer is also considered to be a possible prognostic marker of ICI response, although the role of HPV infection has not yet been clarified. Cervical cancer is known to be an HPV-induced neoplasm, and several researchers have found that HPV positivity is positively correlated with increased PD-L1 expression in cervical cancer [10,25]. However, as previously described, because the role of PD-L1 expression as a prognostic marker is unclear, additional investigation is required to elucidate the specific contribution of HPV-induced cervical carcinogenesis.

In the present study, we examined the effect of several factors on ORR: HPV positivity, histology (squamous vs. non-squamous), number of prior lines of chemotherapy, ECOG status, PD-L1 positivity, and burden of tumor. Only an ECOG ≤1 showed a significant difference in the univariate analyses (OR, 14.651; 95% CI, 1.809–118.675; p = 0.012). The other factors showed no statistically significant differences (Table 4). In non-small cell lung cancer patients, poor PS (ECOG ≥2) has been suggested as a negative predictive factor for ICIs treatment [26] or not [27]. Studies on the treatment response according to PS have not been reported in cervical cancer patients, and prospective clinical trials are needed. MSI-H/MMRd data could be obtained for only 28 patients, so this factor was not analyzed in the present study.

4.4. Limitations

The limitations of this study stem mainly from its retrospective design and short follow-up time. The lack of an independent central radiologic and pathologic review could also be a confounding factor. Because the central pathologic review was not conducted, the MSI-H/MMRd and PD-L1 information of tumor was not obtained from all patients. Furthermore, the response assessment could not be centralized by an independent central radiologic review. We did not perform an evaluation based on immune RECIST or immune-related RECIST to assess the immune response. The AE evaluation was also conducted retrospectively based on chart review, which is probably why the frequency of AEs reported here was low compared to prospective clinical trials that evaluated AEs using strict criteria.

Nevertheless, to the best of our knowledge, this retrospective study of a relatively large, mainly Asian cohort is the first to evaluate the effectiveness and safety of pembrolizumab treatment in patients with recurrent cervical cancer in a real-world setting.

5. Conclusions

In summary, the present study showed that pembrolizumab treatment has modest antitumor activity in patients with recurrent or persistent cervical cancer, including effective activity especially in patients with favorable performance status, in real-world practice. Further studies are warranted to identify predictive biomarkers for immune checkpoint inhibitors in cervical cancer.

Supplementary Materials: The following are available online at http://www.mdpi.com/2072-6694/12/11/3188/s1, Figure S1. Kaplan-Meier estimates of survival in the favorable performance status group (n = 53). (A) Progression-free survival, (B) Overall survival, Table S1. Participating institutions (n = 16), Table S2. Clinical summary of patients whose best overall response was complete or partial response (n = 11), Table S3. Tumor responses in patients with squamous cell carcinoma histology (n = 88).

Author Contributions: Conceptualization, M.C.C., Y.-M.K. and J.-W.L.; Data curation, all authors; Formal analysis, M.C.C., S.-H.S. and J.-W.L.; Investigation, M.C.C., Y.-M.K., J.-W.L., Y.J.L., D.H.S., S.J.L., T.S.L., M.L., D.C.P., M.K.K., J.-M.L., S.-H.S., S.J., K.J.M., M.K.K., B.W.K., J.Y.P., B.-G.K., D.Y.K., M.-H.K., H.-S.K. and J.-Y.L.; Writing—original draft preparation, M.C.C. and J.-W.L.; Writing—review and editing, M.C.C., Y.-M.K., J.-W.L., Y.J.L., D.H.S., S.J.L., T.S.L., M.L., D.C.P., M.K.K., J.-M.L., S.-H.S., S.J., K.J.M., M.K.K., B.W.K., J.Y.P., B.-G.K., D.Y.K., M.-H.K., H.-S.K. and J.-Y.L.; Project administration, M.C.C., Y.-M.K. and J.-W.L.; Funding acquisition, M.C.C. All authors have read and agreed to the published version of the manuscript.

Funding: This research received no external funding.

Acknowledgments: This research was supported by research grants from Hanmi Healthcare Co., Inc. The authors would like to thank to the following bioinformatician for statistical advices; Sohyun Hwang, Department of pathology and Department of Biomedical Science, CHA Bundang Medical Center, CHA University, Seongnam, Korea.

Conflicts of Interest: The authors have no conflicts of interest to declare.

References

1. Bray, F.; Me, J.F.; Soerjomataram, I.; Siegel, R.L.; Torre, L.A.; Jemal, A. Global cancer statistics 2018: GLOBOCAN estimates of incidence and mortality worldwide for 36 cancers in 185 countries. *CA A Cancer J. Clin.* **2018**, *68*, 394–424. [CrossRef] [PubMed]
2. Jung, K.-W.; Won, Y.-J.; Hong, S.; Kong, H.-J.; Lee, E.S. Prediction of Cancer Incidence and Mortality in Korea, 2020. *Cancer Res. Treat.* **2020**, *52*, 351–358. [CrossRef] [PubMed]
3. Tewari, K.S.; Sill, M.W.; Long, H.J., 3rd; Penson, R.T.; Huang, H.; Ramondetta, L.M.; Landrum, L.M.; Oaknin, A.; Reid, T.J.; Leitao, M.M.; et al. Improved survival with bevacizumab in advanced cervical cancer. *N. Engl. J. Med.* **2014**, *370*, 734–743. [CrossRef] [PubMed]
4. Radley, D.; Saah, A.; Stanley, M. Persistent infection with human papillomavirus 16 or 18 is strongly linked with high-grade cervical disease. *Hum. Vaccines Immunother.* **2015**, *12*, 768–772. [CrossRef] [PubMed]
5. Alemany, L.; De Sanjosé, S.; Tous, S.; Quint, W.; Vallejos, C.; Shin, H.-R.; Santaella-Tenorio, J.; Alonso, P.; Lima, M.A.; Guimerà, N.; et al. Time trends of human papillomavirus types in invasive cervical cancer, from 1940 to 2007. *Int. J. Cancer* **2013**, *135*, 88–95. [CrossRef] [PubMed]
6. Tashiro, H.; Brenner, M.K. Immunotherapy against cancer-related viruses. *Cell Res.* **2016**, *27*, 59–73. [CrossRef] [PubMed]
7. Santin, A.D.; Bellone, S.; Gokden, M.; Cannon, M.J.; Parham, G.P. Vaccination with HPV-18 E7–Pulsed Dendritic Cells in a Patient with Metastatic Cervical Cancer. *New Engl. J. Med.* **2002**, *346*, 1752–1753. [CrossRef]
8. Pardoll, D.M. The blockade of immune checkpoints in cancer immunotherapy. *Nat. Rev. Cancer* **2012**, *12*, 252–264. [CrossRef]
9. Heeren, A.M.; Punt, S.; Bleeker, M.C.G.; Gaarenstroom, K.N.; Van Der Velden, J.; Kenter, G.G.; De Gruijl, T.D.; Jordanova, E.S. Prognostic effect of different PD-L1 expression patterns in squamous cell carcinoma and adenocarcinoma of the cervix. *Mod. Pathol.* **2016**, *29*, 753–763. [CrossRef]
10. Meng, Y.; Liang, H.; Hu, J.; Liu, S.; Hao, X.; Wong, M.S.K.; Li, X.; Hu, L. PD-L1 Expression Correlates With Tumor Infiltrating Lymphocytes And Response To Neoadjuvant Chemotherapy In Cervical Cancer. *J. Cancer* **2018**, *9*, 2938–2945. [CrossRef]
11. Frenel, J.-S.; Le Tourneau, C.; O'Neil, B.; Ott, P.A.; Piha-Paul, S.A.; Gomez-Roca, C.; Van Brummelen, E.M.; Rugo, H.S.; Thomas, S.; Saraf, S.; et al. Safety and Efficacy of Pembrolizumab in Advanced, Programmed Death Ligand 1–Positive Cervical Cancer: Results From the Phase Ib KEYNOTE-028 Trial. *J. Clin. Oncol.* **2017**, *35*, 4035–4041. [CrossRef] [PubMed]
12. Naumann, R.W.; Hollebecque, A.; Meyer, T.; Devlin, M.-J.; Oaknin, A.; Kerger, J.; López-Picazo, J.M.; Machiels, J.-P.; Delord, J.-P.; Evans, T.R.J.; et al. Safety and Efficacy of Nivolumab Monotherapy in Recurrent or Metastatic Cervical, Vaginal, or Vulvar Carcinoma: Results From the Phase I/II CheckMate 358 Trial. *J. Clin. Oncol.* **2019**, *37*, 2825–2834. [CrossRef] [PubMed]
13. Santin, A.D.; Deng, W.; Frumovitz, M.; Buza, N.; Bellone, S.; Huh, W.; Khleif, S.; Lankes, H.A.; Ratner, E.S.; O'Cearbhaill, R.E.; et al. Phase II evaluation of nivolumab in the treatment of persistent or recurrent cervical cancer (NCT02257528/NRG-GY002). *Gynecol. Oncol.* **2020**, *157*, 161–166. [CrossRef]
14. Chung, H.C.; Ros, W.; Delord, J.-P.; Perets, R.; Italiano, A.; Shapira-Frommer, R.; Manzuk, L.; Piha-Paul, S.A.; Xu, L.; Zeigenfuss, S.; et al. Efficacy and Safety of Pembrolizumab in Previously Treated Advanced Cervical Cancer: Results From the Phase II KEYNOTE-158 Study. *J. Clin. Oncol.* **2019**, *37*, 1470–1478. [CrossRef] [PubMed]
15. Tewari, K.S. Immune Checkpoint Blockade in PD-L1–Positive Platinum-Refractory Cervical Carcinoma. *J. Clin. Oncol.* **2019**, *37*, 1449–1454. [CrossRef] [PubMed]
16. Grau, J.F.; Farinas-Madrid, L.; Oaknin, A. A randomized phase III trial of platinum chemotherapy plus paclitaxel with bevacizumab and atezolizumab versus platinum chemotherapy plus paclitaxel and bevacizumab in metastatic (stage IVB), persistent, or recurrent carcinoma of the cervix: The BEATcc study (ENGOT-Cx10/GEICO 68-C/JGOG1084/GOG-3030). *Int. J. Gynecol. Cancer* **2019**, *30*, 139–143. [CrossRef]
17. Tewari, K.; Shapira-Frommer, R. KEYNOTE-826: A Phase 3, Randomized, Double-blind, Placebo-Controlled Study of Pembrolizumab Plus Chemotherapy for First-line Treatment of Persistent, Recurrent, or Metastatic Cervical Cancer. *J. Clin. Oncol.* **2019**, *37*. [CrossRef]

18. Magee, D.; Hird, A.; Klaassen, Z.; Sridhar, S.; Nam, R.; Wallis, C.; Kulkarni, G.S. Adverse event profile for immunotherapy agents compared with chemotherapy in solid organ tumors: A systematic review and meta-analysis of randomized clinical trials. *Ann. Oncol.* **2020**, *31*, 50–60. [CrossRef]

19. Le, D.T.; Durham, J.N.; Smith, K.N.; Wang, H.; Bartlett, B.R.; Aulakh, L.K.; Lu, S.; Kemberling, H.; Wilt, C.; Luber, B.S.; et al. Mismatch repair deficiency predicts response of solid tumors to PD-1 blockade. *Science* **2017**, *357*, 409–413. [CrossRef]

20. Dudley, J.C.; Lin, M.-T.; Le, D.T.; Eshleman, J.R. Microsatellite Instability as a Biomarker for PD-1 Blockade. *Clin. Cancer Res.* **2016**, *22*, 813–820. [CrossRef]

21. Marabelle, A.; Le, D.T.; Ascierto, P.A.; Di Giacomo, A.M.; De Jesus-Acosta, A.; Delord, J.-P.; Geva, R.; Gottfried, M.; Penel, N.; Hansen, A.R.; et al. Efficacy of Pembrolizumab in Patients With Noncolorectal High Microsatellite Instability/Mismatch Repair–Deficient Cancer: Results From the Phase II KEYNOTE-158 Study. *J. Clin. Oncol.* **2020**, *38*, 1–10. [CrossRef] [PubMed]

22. Latham, A.; Srinivasan, P.; Kemel, Y.; Shia, J.; Bandlamudi, C.; Mandelker, D.; Middha, S.; Hechtman, J.; Zehir, A.; Dubard-Gault, M.; et al. Microsatellite Instability Is Associated With the Presence of Lynch Syndrome Pan-Cancer. *J. Clin. Oncol.* **2019**, *37*, 286–295. [CrossRef] [PubMed]

23. Cortes-Ciriano, I.; Lee, S.; Park, W.-Y.; Kim, T.-M.; Park, P.J. A molecular portrait of microsatellite instability across multiple cancers. *Nat. Commun.* **2017**, *8*, 15180. [CrossRef]

24. Davis, A.A.; Patel, V.G. The role of PD-L1 expression as a predictive biomarker: An analysis of all US Food and Drug Administration (FDA) approvals of immune checkpoint inhibitors. *J. Immunother. Cancer* **2019**, *7*, 1–8. [CrossRef]

25. Mezache, L.; Paniccia, B.; Nyinawabera, A.; Nuovo, G.J. Enhanced expression of PD L1 in cervical intraepithelial neoplasia and cervical cancers. *Mod. Pathol.* **2015**, *28*, 1594–1602. [CrossRef] [PubMed]

26. Spigel, D.R.; McCleod, M.; Jotte, R.M.; Einhorn, L.; Horn, L.; Waterhouse, D.M.; Creelan, B.; Babu, S.; Leighl, N.B.; Chandler, J.C.; et al. Safety, Efficacy, and Patient-Reported Health-Related Quality of Life and Symptom Burden with Nivolumab in Patients with Advanced Non–Small Cell Lung Cancer, Including Patients Aged 70 Years or Older or with Poor Performance Status (CheckMate 153). *J. Thorac. Oncol.* **2019**, *14*, 1628–1639. [CrossRef]

27. Middleton, G.W.; Brock, K.; Savage, J.; Mant, R.; Summers, Y.; Connibear, J.; Shah, R.; Ottensmeier, C.; Shaw, P.; Lee, S.-M.; et al. Pembrolizumab in patients with non-small-cell lung cancer of performance status 2 (PePS2): A single arm, phase 2 trial. *Lancet Respir. Med.* **2020**, *8*, 895–904. [CrossRef]

Publisher's Note: MDPI stays neutral with regard to jurisdictional claims in published maps and institutional affiliations.

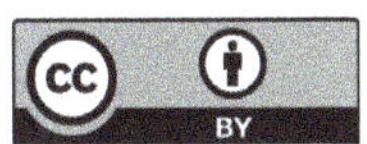

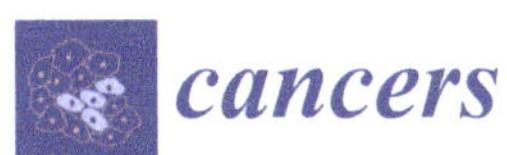 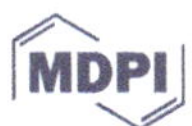

Article

The Oncoprotein SKI Acts as A Suppressor of NK Cell-Mediated Immunosurveillance in PDAC

Viviane Ponath [1], Miriam Frech [2,†], Mathis Bittermann [1,†], Reem Al Khayer [1,†], Andreas Neubauer [2], Cornelia Brendel [2] and Elke Pogge von Strandmann [1,*]

[1] Institute for Tumor Immunology, Clinic for Hematology, Oncology and Immunology, Philipps University of Marburg, Hans-Meerwein-Strasse 3, 35043 Marburg, Germany; viviane.ponath@staff.uni-marburg.de (V.P.); ms.bittermann@web.de (M.B.); reem.alkhayer@imt.uni-marburg.de (R.A.K.)

[2] Clinic for Hematology, Oncology, Immunology and Center for Tumor Biology and Immunology, Philipps University of Marburg, Baldingerstrasse, 35037 Marburg, Germany; frechm@staff.uni-marburg.de (M.F.); neubauer@staff.uni-marburg.de (A.N.); brendelc@staff.uni-marburg.de (C.B.)

[*] Correspondence: poggevon@staff.uni-marburg.de or poggevonstrandmann@staff.uni-marburg.de; Tel.: +49-6421-2821640; Fax: +49-64212868923

[†] These authors contributed equally to this work.

Received: 3 September 2020; Accepted: 29 September 2020; Published: 3 October 2020

Simple Summary: Pancreatic ductal adeno carcinoma is one of the most lethal solid tumors and the survival rate has not improved significantly over the past decades. The disease is characterized by an immune-suppressive tumor microenvironment, which promotes the limited response to novel immunotherapies. The aim of our study was to contribute to a better understanding of the diminished Natural Killer (NK) cell-activity in pancreatic cancer. We showed that oncoprotein SKI, which is involved in CBP/p300-mediated acetylation, diminished the expression of activating ligands for the cytotoxicity receptor NKG2D on tumor cells, thereby counteracting NK cell-dependent cytotoxicity. Treatment of tumor cells with histone deacetylase inhibitors (HDACi) induced the expression of these ligands and improved NK cell-dependent killing. Thus, we unraveled a so far unknown role of SKI in NK cell-mediated immunosurveillance. Our results suggest that the combination of HDACi with NK cell-based immunotherapies may be beneficial for pancreatic cancer patients.

Abstract: Drugs targeting epigenetic mechanisms such as histone deacetylase inhibitors (HDACi) suppress tumor growth. HDACi also induce the expression of ligands for the cytotoxicity receptor NKG2D rendering tumors more susceptible to natural killer (NK) cell-dependent killing. The major acetylases responsible for the expression of NKG2D ligands (NKG2D-L) are CBP and p300. The role of the oncogene and transcriptional repressor SKI, an essential part of an HDAC-recruiting co-repressor complex, which competes with CBP/p300 for binding to SMAD3 in TGFβ signaling, is unknown. Here we show that the siRNA-mediated downregulation of *SKI* in the pancreatic cancer cell lines Panc-1 and Patu8988t leads to an increased target cell killing by primary NK cells. However, the higher cytotoxicity of NK cells did not correlate with the induction of NKG2D-L. Of note, the expression of NKG2D-L and consequently NK cell-dependent killing could be induced upon LBH589 (LBH, panobinostat) or valproic acid (VPA) treatment irrespective of the SKI expression level but was significantly higher in pancreatic cancer cells upon genetic ablation of *SKI*. These data suggest that SKI represses the inducible expression of NKG2D-L. The combination of HDACi with NK cell-based immunotherapy is an attractive treatment option for pancreatic tumors, specifically for patients with high SKI protein levels.

Keywords: pancreatic tumor; NK cell immunosurveillance; NKG2D; histon (de)acetylation

---

1. Introduction

Pancreatic ductal adenocarcinoma (PDAC) represents 85% of all pancreatic cancers and exhibits the poorest prognosis of all solid tumors. Incidence rates in the industrialized world are steadily increasing and the 5-year survival rate is below 10% with a median survival of 6 months [1–3]. Reasons for the poor prognosis include delayed diagnosis associated with non-resectable locally advanced or metastatic disease and chemo-resistance. One component which critically contributes to drug resistance is the peritumoral desmoplasia, which impairs intra-tumoral drug delivery [4]. PDAC is moreover characterized by an immune-suppressive tumor microenvironment (TME) producing TGFβ and other factors to counteract immunosurveillance, while promoting tumor growth and metastasis for example, through the recruitment of tumor supporting macrophages [5]. Thus, the response of patients with PDAC to immunotherapy is overall limited [6]. However increasing pieces of evidence suggest that the restoration of NK cell activity in the tumor microenvironment (TME) may interfere with PDAC progression [7,8] exerting direct cytotoxicity and orchestrating the anti-tumor immune response.

One of the major NK cell receptors involved in the recognition and killing of transformed cells is the cytotoxic receptor NKG2D [9]. NKG2D is expressed on NK cells, CD8+ T cells, some γδ T cells and possibly also some CD4+ T cells [10] and known as a sensor for damaged or dangerous cells. In humans, NKG2D is engaged by several ligands, namely MHC class I polypeptide-related sequence A and B (MICA and MICB) [9] and the UL16-binding proteins 1-6 (ULBP1-6) [11–14]. Not surprisingly, tumor cells develop mechanisms to escape the innate immune surveillance and these strategies include the release of soluble NKG2D-L to render target cells invisible for an NKG2D-dependent NK cell-attack. Soluble ligands for NKG2D do not only passively block receptor activation but moreover cause a downregulation of receptor surface expression [15].

While NKG2D-L are not expressed on healthy cells, they are upregulated on tumor cells. Their expression is regulated by transcriptional, translational and posttranslational mechanisms [16], although the transcription factors involved are not yet entirely defined. A better understanding of the factors that direct NKG2D-L on the surface of target cells will allow the development of novel therapeutic strategies aiming at an increased NKG2D-L expression on tumor cells and thus a potential killing by NK cells.

Previously we showed that the major acetyltransferases CBP and p300 have a robust, mandatory and general impact on the up-regulation of mouse and human NKG2D-L in response to cellular stress signals or upon HDAC inhibition [17]. These acetyltransferases interact with the oncogene and transcriptional repressor Sloan-Kettering Institute (SKI), for example, by binding to SMAD3 to modulate TGFβ signaling [18].

Thus, SKI inhibits SMAD association with the p300/CBP coactivators and facilitates the recruitment of histone deacetylases to repress gene transcription [19]. SKI is known to promote pancreatic cancer cell proliferation and SKI overexpression is significantly associated with a decreased patients' survival time [20,21]. Given that HDAC inhibitors (HDACi) induce surface expression of NKG2D-ligands on tumor cells in a CBP/p300-dependent manner [17] we hypothesize that SKI suppresses NKG2D-ligands on pancreatic cancer cells supporting immune evasion.

2. Results and Discussion

The effect of HDACi is reported to induce NKG2D-L on the surface of tumor cells, which promotes tumor cell recognition and killing by NK cells supporting an anti-tumor immune response. The cellular responses and the affected ligands vary depending on the HDACi applied and the tumor type. Data for pancreatic cancer cells are rare, however the upregulation of MICA/B upon treatment of tumor cell lines with VPA (an HDACi originally developed for the treatment of epilepsy) through the induction of the PI3K/AKT signaling pathway was described [22]. Treatment of the pancreatic cancer cell lines PaTu8988t and Panc-1 with the pan-HDACi panobinostat (LBH589) and subsequent qRT-PCR analysis established that LBH induced the transcription of the ligands *MICA* and *ULBP2* (Figure 1A,B). Induced transcription was most pronounced after 16 h treatment and declined after 48 h and 72 h. The up-regulation of the mRNAs was in line with the enhanced surface expression of ligands for NKG2D measured by flow cytometry (Figure 1C). Here, a similar efficacy for LBH and VPA both used in sublethal concentrations was observed, although the induction efficacy of LBH for MICA and ULBP2 was more robust under the conditions used (Figure S1).

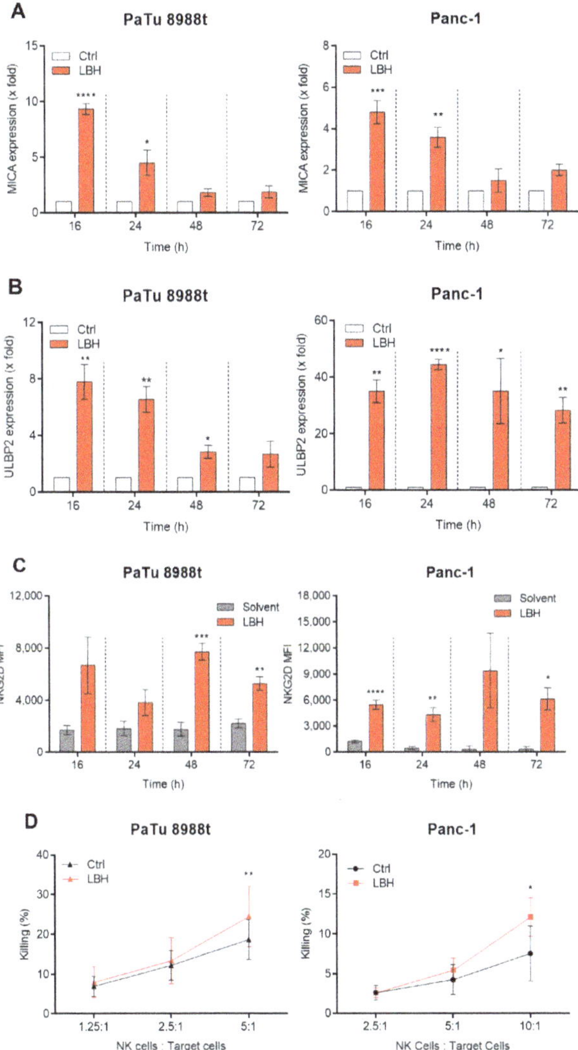

Figure 1. NKG2D ligand expression in PaTu 8988t and Panc-1 cells after treatment with HDACi LBH589. The mRNA of NKG2D ligands (**A**) MICA and (**B**) ULBP2 was measured in PaTu 8988t (left panel) and Panc-1 (right panel) 16, 24, 48 and 72 h after treatment with 100 nM LBH58th 25 nM LBH for up to 72 h and NKG2D-L and the mean fluorescence intensity (MFI) was measured by flow cytometry using recombinant human NKG2D Fc chimera protein. (**D**) Tumor cells were treated with 100 nM LBH589 for 16 h before they were co-cultured with primary NK cells for 3 h and NK cell-mediated killing of target cells was measured by flow cytometry. Data are the mean of three (**A**,**B**,**D**) or four to five independent experiments (**C**) ± SEM. Statistical significance between treated and untreated samples of the individual time points was calculated using Student's *t*-test (* $p < 0.05$, ** $p < 0.01$, *** $p < 0.001$, **** $p < 0.0001$).

To test, whether the HDACi-mediated NKG2D ligand induction actually is of biological significance, flow cytometry (FC)-based NK cell killing assays using primary NK cells were performed. Indeed, NK cells were significantly more potent in lysing LBH-treated pancreatic cell lines compared to untreated controls (Figure 1D), manifesting functional relevance of LBH-induced NKG2D ligand upregulation.

We and others showed that enhanced expression of NKG2D-L results in increased in vitro NK cell killing activity (Figure 1D, [23–25]. Xenograft mouse models moreover demonstrated that the pharmacological increase in NKG2D ligand expression also results in enhanced NK cell-mediated tumor surveillance [23–25]. The same holds true for syngeneic mouse models where NKG2D ligand induction enables NK cells to reject MHC class I-bearing tumors [26]. Moreover, bifunctional recombinant proteins which are applied to retarget NK cells to tumor cells triggering NKG2D activation reveal potent anti-tumor activity in vivo and in vitro [27]. These observations highlight the promising role of the NKG2D-NKG2D-L axis as a therapeutic target to overcome NK cell anergy in tumor patients.

Having demonstrated that HDACi can induce NKG2D-L and trigger NK cell cytotoxicity we analyzed whether the oncoprotein SKI was involved in NKG2D-ligand regulation. siRNA targeting *SKI* was used to effectively down-regulate SKI in PaTu8988t (upper panel Figure 2A) and Panc-1 (upper panel Figure 2B) pancreatic adenocarcinoma cells and the expression level was determined using Western blotting (Figure 2, see Figure S2 for quantification) and qRT-PCR (lower panel, Figure 2A,B).

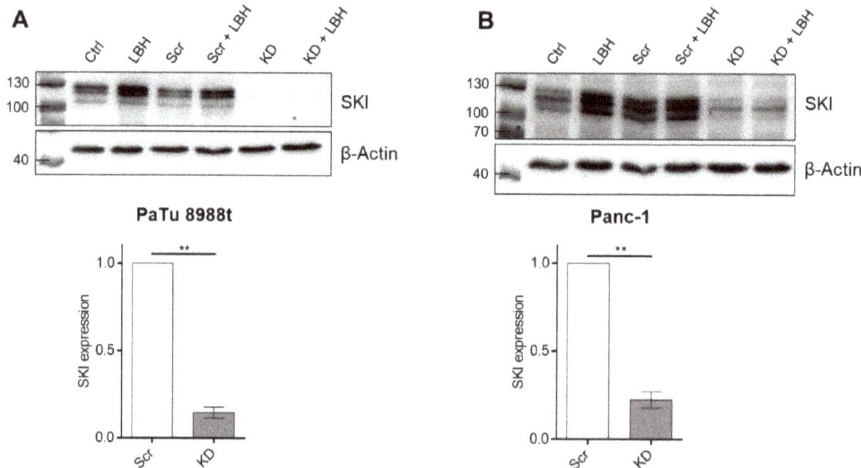

Figure 2. siRNA-mediated knockdown (KD) of SKI. (**A**) PaTu8988t and (**B**) Panc-1 cells were treated with siRNA for SKI knockdown for 24 h followed by 16 h of 100 nM LBH589 treatment before the knockdown was quantified by Western Blot analysis. Ctrl: non treated, scr: scrambled siRNA. The lower panel depicts the quantification of qRT-PCR data for scrambled siRNA-treated sample and siRNA treated samples. Data are the mean of three independent experiments ± SEM. Statistical significance was calculated using Student's *t*-test (** *p* < 0.01). KD = knockdown, Scr = scrambled.

Of note, a cytotoxicity assay using primary purified NK cells from healthy donors as effector cells showed that the knockdown of SKI was associated with a significantly better killing efficacy (Figure 3A). The analysis of NKG2D-L expression revealed that *MICA* and *ULBP2* were significantly higher expressed in PaTu8988t cells with diminished SKI expression (Figure 3B), whereas the ligand expression in Panc-1 cells was not affected. We conclude that the increased expression of *MICA* and *ULBP2* in PaTu8988t cells upon SKI knockdown may contribute to a better NK cell-mediated killing but SKI seems to suppress susceptibility against NK cell-mediated killing also by additional, not yet defined mechanisms. In this regard, we found in acute myeloid leukemia (AML) cells that SKI acts rather as a transcriptional repressor and inhibits target genes associated with inflammatory response, immune cell differentiation as well as TNFα signaling via NFκB [28]. Hence, SKI-expressing tumor cells may evade NK cell-killing via inhibition of pro-inflammatory factors like TNFα. In line with the contribution of SKI to *MICA* gene regulation, ChIPseq analyses of the AML cell line HL60 revealed an enrichment of SKI in the promoter region of *MICA*, which was diminished upon SKI knockdown, confirming specificity (Figure 3C).

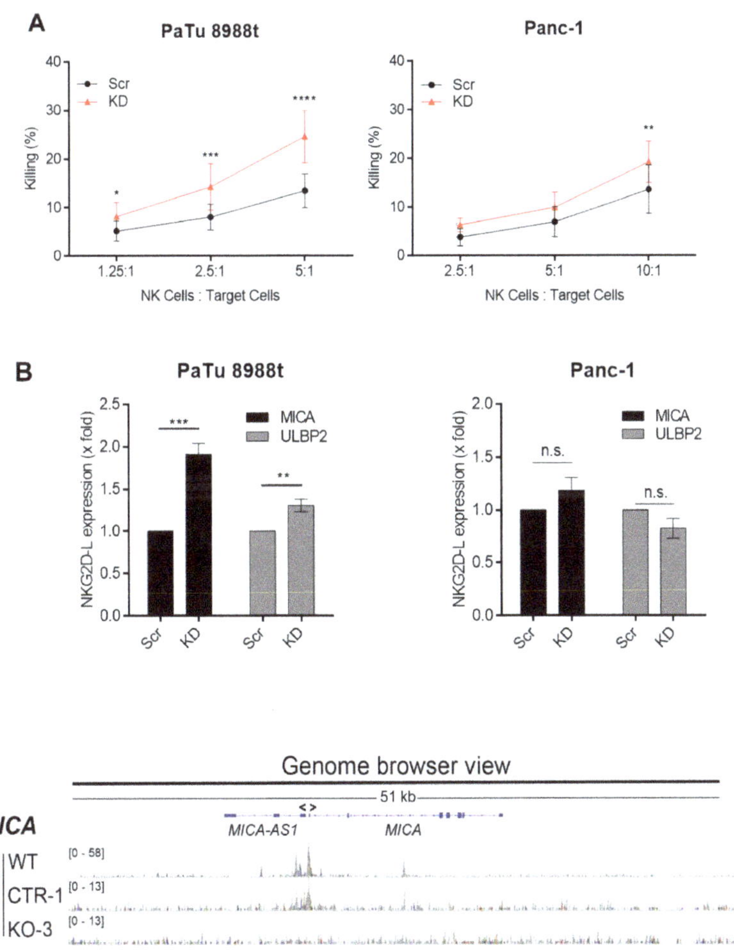

Figure 3. Effect of SKI knockdown on NK cell-mediated killing of target cells and expression of NKG2D-L. (**A**) SKI knockdown was performed in PaTu89888t (left panel) and Panc-1 (right panel) cells for 24 h. Then, cells were co-cultured with primary NK cells for 3 h before target cell killing was measured by flow cytometry. (**B**) The mRNA expression of NKG2D-L *MICA* and *ULBP2* was measured in SKI knockdown cells. Data are the mean of four (**3B**) to five (**3A**) independent experiments ± SEM. Statistical significance was calculated using 2-way ANOVA and Sidak's multiple comparisons test (**3A**) and Student's *t*-test (**3B**) (* $p < 0.05$, ** $p < 0.01$, *** $p < 0.001$, **** $p < 0.0001$, n.s.: not significant). (**C**) Genome browser view of the *MICA* genomic region of the SKI ChIPseq analyses of the cell line HL60 (WT), HL60 control cells (CTR-1, CRISPR-Cas9) and HL60-SKI deficient cells (KO-3, CRISPR-Cas9).

Next, both SKI wildtype and SKI knockdown cells were treated with LBH and the impact on the inducible expression of *MICA* and *ULBP2* was analyzed by qRT-PCR. Interestingly, we observed in knockdown cell lines a significantly higher induction of *ULBP2* transcription, which was in line with enhanced NK cell-dependent killing of PaTu8988t cells (Figure 4A,B). These data suggest that SKI interferes with the HDACi-dependent *ULBP2* upregulation on these pancreatic cancer cells. However, the HDACi-dependent induction of *MICA* remained unaltered in SKI wildtype cells and upon knockdown (Figure 4A). LBH-treated SKI-deficient Panc-1 cells were more efficiently killed than wildtype cells. However, no significant upregulation of *ULBP2* or *MICA* could be detected, suggesting that SKI suppresses NK cell immunosurveillance also by NKG2D/NKG2D-L-independent mechanisms.

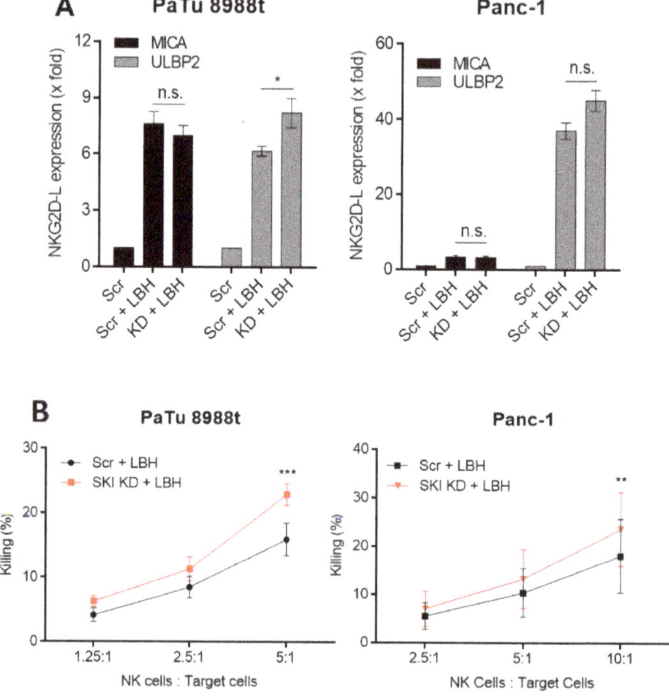

Figure 4. Effect of SKI knockdown and LBH treatment on NKG2D-L expression and NK cell-mediated killing. (**A**) siRNA-mediated SKI knockdown was performed for 24 h followed by 100 nM LBH589 and *MICA* and *ULBP2* were measured in PaTu8988t (**left panel**) and Panc-1 (**right panel**) by qRT-PCR. (**B**) 24 h after SKI knockdown and LBH treatment, NK cell-mediated killing of tumor cells was measured by flow cytometry. Data are the mean of three to five independent experiments ± SEM. Statistical significance was calculated using 1-way and 2-way ANOVA analyses (* $p < 0.05$, ** $p < 0.01$, *** $p < 0.001$, n.s.: not significant).

In conclusion the combination of HDACi with NK cell-based immunotherapy is an attractive treatment option for pancreatic tumors. Therapy may be further improved by additional inhibition of SKI oncogenic activity, for example, via re-expression of NKG2D-L or pro-inflammatory factors leading to an improved recruitment and activation of NK cells to the TME. Further studies are needed to identify the crucial factors mediating the SKI repressive function in NK cell-killing.

Recent approaches to treat PDAC patients with NK cell-based immunotherapy showed promising results. One example is the adoptive transfer of ex vivo-expanded and antibody-activated NK cells resulting in IFNγ secretion and significant anti-tumor activity against pancreatic cancer cells [29].

Clinical trials have illustrated that the combination of allogeneic NK cell immunotherapy with percutaneous irreversible electroporation enhances the progression-free survival and overall survival in stage III PDAC and extends the overall survival in stage IV PDAC [30]. Recently, it was shown using a PDAC mouse model that the anti-tumor activity of gemcitabine chemotherapy was mediated through an increase of tumor-infiltrating NK cells and the decrease of myeloid-derived suppressor cells [31]. Interestingly, it was reported that gemcitabine, like HDACi, also modulates the expression of NKG2D-L on tumor cells further supporting NK cell-mediated anti-tumor effects.

HDACi may also impact directly on NK cells, for example, via up-regulation of NKG2D and stimulation of IFNg release and toxicity in NK-tumor cell co-cultures [32]. However, HDACi monotherapy was already tested in clinical trials but received rather disappointing results [33]. Our data suggest that the combination of HDACi with NK cell-based immunotherapy, such as adoptive NK cell transfer may be beneficial for PDAC patients. Strategies including the combination of epigenetic approaches or radiation with immune therapy are under investigation [34].Thus, HDACi may be used to change the immunosuppressive TME and demask the tumor cells for immunotherapeutic approaches for example, with activated transferred NK cells. However, a better understanding and strategies to overcome the immunosuppressive TME diminishing NK cell activity for example, via targeting the oncoprotein SKI, is mandatory for further studies. Taken together, there is evidence for the potential of NK cell-based therapies for PDAC. However the complex interactions of NK cells with the immunosuppressive TME of PDAC are only poorly understood and require further research.

3. Material and Methods

3.1. Isolation of Primary NK Cells and Culture of Tumor Cell Lines

Cell lines: The human pancreatic cancer cell lines Panc-1 and PaTu8988t cells were purchased from ATCC. The cells were cultured in DMEM with 10% FCS and 1% P/S at 37 °C and 5% CO_2.

NK cells: Leukocytes from leukoreduction system chambers of healthy donors were provided by the blood bank of the University Hospital of Giessen and Marburg. Peripheral blood mononuclear cells (PBMCs) were purified by ficoll density centrifugation followed by a centrifugation step at 10 g for 5 min to deplete the sample of monocytes. NK cells were then isolated using a negative selection NK cell isolation kit (Miltenyi Biotec, Bergisch Gladbach, Germany). Isolated NK cells were cultured in IMDM medium with 10% FCS, 1% P/S, 100 ng/mL IL-15 and 200 U/mL IL-2 and rested at 37 °C overnight before killing assays were performed.

3.2. Killing Assay

For killing assays, target cells were stained with 5 µM CellTracker^{TM} Violet BMQC (Invitrogen, Carlsbad, CA, USA) fluorescent dye in serum-free medium at 37 °C for 45 min. Then, cells were washed twice in complete medium and seeded accordingly in IMDM medium with 10% FCS and 1% P/S in U-shaped 96-well plates. NK cells were added to the target cells in ratios ranging from 1.25:1 to 10:1. The cells were co-cultured for 3 h before they were harvested and centrifuged at 300 g for 5 min. The supernatant was discarded and the cells were resuspended in 200 µL PBS before they were stained with 100 ng 7-AAD (Biolegend, San Diego CA, USA). Cell death was measured by flow cytometry using a FACS Canto II cytometer (BD Bioscience, Heidelberg, Germany) and analyzed by FACS Diva software and FlowJo (version 10.6.1, (BD Bioscience, Heidelberg, Germany).

3.3. Detection of NKG2D-L on Tumor Cells

Tumor cells were treated with 25 nM LBH589 (Selleckchem, München, Germany), 2.5 mM VPA (Sigma-Aldrich, Darmstadt, Germany) or solvent DMSO (Sigma-Aldrich, Darmstadt, Germany) for 16 to 72 h before they were collected. The cells were centrifuged at 300 g for 5 min, the supernatant was discarded and the cells were resuspended in 200 µL PBS. Samples were then split in two and one half was incubated with 10 ng/100 µL sample anti-ULBP-2/5/6 PE-conjugated antibody (R&D

Systems, Wiesbaden, Germany) and the other half with the corresponding IgG2a control (Biolegend, Koblenz, Germany) for 30 min on ice in the dark. The cells were washed with PBS and then analyzed by flow cytometry. Alternatively, cells were incubated with 0.15 μg/100 μL sample recombinant human NKG2D Fc chimera protein (R&D systems) or corresponding recombinant IgG1 Fc protein (R&D Systems, Wiesbaden, Germany) for 30 min on ice. Cells were washed with PBS and then incubated with AF647-coupled anti-human IgG Fc antibody for 25 min. Cells were washed with PBS and then analyzed by flow cytometry. Data were analyzed using FloJo software (BD Bioscience, Heidelberg, Germany).

3.4. Quantitative Real-Time PCR (qRT-PCR) of NKG2D-L

Tumor cells were treated with 100 nM LBH589 for 16 to 72 h before cells were harvested and mRNA was isolated using the NucleoSpin RNA isolation kit according to the manufacturer's instructions (Macherey-Nagel). Absolute SYBR Green Mix (ThermoFisher Scientific, Schwerte, Germany) was used with the following primers: ULBP2_for 5′-GCCGCTACCAAGATCCTTCT-3′, ULBP2_rev 5′-GCAAAGAGAGTGAGGGTCGG-3′, MICA_for 5′-CTGCAGGAACTACGGCGATA-3′, MICA_rev 5′-CCCTCTGAGGCCTCGCT-3′, L27_for 5′-AAAGCTGTCATCGTGAAGAAC-3′ and L27_rev 5′-GCTGTCACTTTGCGGGGGTAG-3′. The qPCR reactions were run in technical triplicates in a Thermo Cycler Mx3005P (Stratagen) using the following protocol: Initial step of 95 °C for 15 min, then 40 cycles of 95 °C for 15 s, 60 °C for 20 s and 72 °C for 15 s, followed by a denaturation step at 95 °C for 60 s and a melting curve analysis. The relative expression level of genes of interest was calculated by the ΔΔCt-method, with each target normalized to L27. Biological replicates were used to calculate standard deviations.

3.5. SKI Knockdown Using siRNA and ChIP-Seq

4×10^5 Panc-1 or PaTu8988t cells were seeded in 6-well plates. The next day, cells were transfected with 100 pmol siRNA using Lipofectamine according to the manufacturer's instructions (Thermo Fisher Scientific, Schwerte, Germany) and were harvested 24 h later. Human siGENOME SKI siRNA SMARTpool (M-003927-02-0005) and non-targeting siRNA #5 (D-001210-05) were purchased from Horizon Discovery (Waterbach, UK). ChIP-seq data were collected [28] and bioinformatical analysis are described there in the Materials & Methods section.

3.6. Western Blot Analysis

For cell lysis, cells were pelleted and then lysed in RIPA buffer (50 mM Tris-Base, pH 7.4; 150 mM NaCl; 1 mM EDTA; 1% NP-40; 0.25% sodium deoxycholate and protease inhibitors (Roche, Rotkreutz, Germany) for 30 min on ice. The samples were centrifuged at 13,000 g at 4 °C for 15 min and the supernatant was collected for SDS-PAGE and immunoblotting. The following antibodies were used: anti-SKI (G8, sc-33693, Santa Cruz Biotechnology, CA, USA) in 10% Blocking Reagent (11096176001, Roche) and anti-β-Actin (a1978, Sigma-Aldrich, Taufkirchen, Germany). Detection was performed with horseradish peroxidase-conjugated secondary antibodies (DAKO, Hamburg, Germany) using Amersham ECL Plus (GE Healthcare, Freiburg, Germany).

3.7. Statistical Analysis

Statistical significance was calculated using GraphPad Prism Software (GraphPad, La Jolla, CA, USA). 1-way and 2-way ANOVA, Sidak's multiple comparisons test and Student's *t*-test were applied as indicated in the figure legends.

4. Conclusions

In conclusion, the combination of HDACi with NK cell-based immunotherapy is an attractive treatment option for pancreatic tumors, specifically for patients with high SKI protein levels to overcome SKI-mediated immune evasion.

Supplementary Materials: The following are available online at http://www.mdpi.com/2072-6694/12/10/2857/s1, Figure S1: NKG2D-L (A) and ULBP2/5/6 (B) expression on tumor cells after treatment with LBH589 and VPA; Figure S2: Western blots of SKI/ß-ACTIN detection in PaTu899t lysate and Panc-1 lysate.

Author Contributions: Conceptualization, E.P.v.S.; methodology, E.P.v.S. and V.P.; software, V.P., M.B. and M.F.; validation, V.P.; formal analysis, E.P.v.S. and V.P.; investigation, M.B., R.A.K., V.P. and M.F.; resources, M.F., A.N., C.B. and E.P.v.S.; writing—original draft preparation, E.P.v.S.; writing—review and editing, A.N., C.B., V.P., M.F. and M.B.; supervision, E.P.v.S., V.P. and R.A.K.; project administration, E.P.v.S.; funding acquisition, E.P.v.S. All authors have read and agreed to the published version of the manuscript.

Funding: This research was funded by the Deutsche Forschungsgemeinschaft grant numbers KFO325, GRK2573 and PO1408/13-1.

Conflicts of Interest: The authors declare no conflict of interest.

References

1. Ying, H.; Dey, P.; Yao, W.; Kimmelman, A.C.; Draetta, G.F.; Maitra, A.; Depinho, R.A. Genetics and biology of pancreatic ductal adenocarcinoma. *Genes Dev.* **2016**, *30*, 355–385. [CrossRef] [PubMed]

2. Siegel, R.L.; Miller, K.D.; Jemal, A. Cancer Statistics. *CA Cancer J. Clin.* **2016**, *66*, 7–30. [CrossRef] [PubMed]

3. Sperb, N.; Tsesmelis, M.; Wirth, T. Crosstalk between Tumor and Stromal Cells in Pancreatic Ductal Adenocarcinoma. *Int. J. Mol. Sci.* **2020**, *21*, 5486. [CrossRef]

4. Schober, M.; Jesenofsky, R.; Faissner, R.; Weidenauer, C.; Hagmann, W.; Michl, P.; Heuchel, R.L.; Haas, S.L.; Löhr, J.-M. Desmoplasia and Chemoresistance in Pancreatic Cancer. *Cancers* **2014**, *6*, 2137–2154. [CrossRef]

5. Griesmann, H.; Drexel, C.; Milosevic, N.; Sipos, B.; Rosendahl, J.; Gress, T.M.; Michl, P. Pharmacological macrophage inhibition decreases metastasis formation in a genetic model of pancreatic cancer. *Gut* **2016**, *66*, 1278–1285. [CrossRef] [PubMed]

6. Sunami, Y.; Kleeff, J. Immunotherapy of pancreatic cancer. *Prog. Mol. Biol. Transl. Sci.* **2019**, *164*, 189–216.

7. Lim, S.A.; Kim, J.; Jeon, S.; Shin, M.H.; Kwon, J.; Kim, T.-J.; Im, K.; Han, Y.; Kwon, W.; Kim, S.-W.; et al. Defective Localization With Impaired Tumor Cytotoxicity Contributes to the Immune Escape of NK Cells in Pancreatic Cancer Patients. *Front. Immunol.* **2019**, *10*, 496. [CrossRef]

8. Lin, X.; Huang, M.; Xie, F.; Zhou, H.; Yang, J.; Huang, Q. Gemcitabine inhibits immune escape of pancreatic cancer by down regulating the soluble ULBP2 protein. *Oncotarget* **2016**, *7*, 70092–70099. [CrossRef]

9. Bauer, S. Activation of NK Cells and T Cells by NKG2D, a Receptor for Stress-Inducible MICA. *Science* **1999**, *285*, 727–729. [CrossRef]

10. Raulet, D.H.; Gasser, S.; Gowen, B.G.; Deng, W.; Jung, H. Regulation of Ligands for the NKG2D Activating Receptor. *Annu. Rev. Immunol.* **2013**, *31*, 413–441. [CrossRef]

11. Cosman, D.; Müllberg, J.; Sutherland, C.L.; Chin, W.; Armitage, R.; Fanslow, W.; Kubin, M.; Chalupny, N.J. ULBPs, novel MHC class I-related molecules, bind to CMV glycoprotein UL16 and stimulate NK cytotoxicity through the NKG2D receptor. *Immunity* **2001**, *14*, 123–333. [CrossRef]

12. Eagle, R.A.; Traherne, J.A.; Hair, J.R.; Jafferji, I.; Trowsdale, J. ULBP6/RAET1L is an additional human NKG2D ligand. *Eur. J. Immunol.* **2009**, *39*, 3207–3216. [CrossRef] [PubMed]

13. Eagle, R.A.; Flack, G.; Warford, A.; Martinez-Borra, J.; Jafferji, I.; Traherne, J.A.; Ohashi, M.; Boyle, L.H.; Barrow, A.D.; Caillat-Zucman, S.; et al. Cellular expression, trafficking, and function of two isoforms of human ULBP5/RAET1G. *PLoS ONE* **2009**, *4*, e4503. [CrossRef] [PubMed]

14. Chalupny, N.J.; Sutherland, C.L.; Lawrence, W.A.; Rein-Weston, A.; Cosman, D. ULBP4 is a novel ligand for human NKG2D. *Biochem. Biophys. Res. Commun.* **2003**, *305*, 129–135. [CrossRef]

15. Champsaur, M.; Lanier, L.L. Effect of NKG2D ligand expression on host immune responses. *Immunol. Rev.* **2010**, *235*, 267–285. [CrossRef]

16. Lanier, L.L. NKG2D Receptor and Its Ligands in Host Defense. *Cancer Immunol. Res.* **2015**, *3*, 575–582. [CrossRef]

17. Sauer, M.; Schuldner, M.; Hoffmann, N.; Cetintas, A.; Reiners, K.S.; Shatnyeva, O.; Hallek, M.; Hansen, H.P.; Gasser, S.; Von Strandmann, E.P. CBP/p300 acetyltransferases regulate the expression of NKG2D ligands on tumor cells. *Oncogene* **2016**, *36*, 933–941. [CrossRef]

18. Chen, W.; Lam, S.S.; Srinath, H.; Schiffer, C.A.; Royer, W.E.; Lin, K. Competition between Ski and CREB-binding Protein for Binding to Smad Proteins in Transforming Growth Factor-beta Signaling. *J. Boil. Chem.* **2007**, *282*, 11365–11376. [CrossRef]

19. Tecalco-Cruz, A.C.; Rios-Lopez, D.G.; Vazquez-Victorio, G.; Rosales-Alvarez, R.E.; Marcias-Silva, M. Transcriptional cofactors Ski and SnoN are major regulators of the TGF-beta/Smad signaling pathway in health and disease. *Signal Transduct. Target Ther.* **2018**, *3*, 15. [CrossRef]

20. Heider, T.R.; Lyman, S.; Schoonhoven, R.; Behrns, K.E. Ski Promotes Tumor Growth Through Abrogation of Transforming Growth Factor-?? Signaling in Pancreatic Cancer. *Ann. Surg.* **2007**, *246*, 61–68. [CrossRef]

21. Wang, P.; Chen, Z.; Meng, Z.; Fan, J.; Luo, J.-M.; Liang, W.; Lin, J.-H.; Zhou, Z.-H.; Chen, H.; Wang, K.; et al. Dual role of Ski in pancreatic cancer cells: Tumor-promoting versus metastasis-suppressive function. *Carcinogenesis* **2009**, *30*, 1497–1506. [CrossRef] [PubMed]

22. Shi, P.; Yin, T.; Zhou, F.; Cui, P.; Gou, S.; Wang, C.-Y. Valproic acid sensitizes pancreatic cancer cells to natural killer cell-mediated lysis by upregulating MICA and MICB via the PI3K/Akt signaling pathway. *BMC Cancer* **2014**, *14*, 370. [CrossRef] [PubMed]

23. Boll, B.; Eltaib, F.; Reiners, K.S.; von Tresckow, B.; Tawadros, S.; Simhadri, V.R.; Burrows, F.; Lundgren, K.; Hansen, H.; Engert, A.; et al. Heat shock protein 90 inhibitor BIIB021 (CNF2024) depletes NF-kappaB and sensitizes Hodgkin's lymphoma cells for natural killer cell-mediated cytotoxicity. *Clin. Cancer Res.* **2009**, *15*, 5108–5116. [CrossRef] [PubMed]

24. Höring, E.; Podlech, O.; Silkenstedt, B.; Rota, I.A.; Adamopoulou, E.; Naumann, U. The histone deacetylase inhibitor trichostatin a promotes apoptosis and antitumor immunity in glioblastoma cells. *Anticancer. Res.* **2013**, *33*, 1351–1360. [PubMed]

25. Huang, B.; Sikorski, R.; Sampath, P.; Thorne, S.H.; Thorne, S.H. Modulation of NKG2D-ligand Cell Surface Expression Enhances Immune Cell Therapy of Cancer. *J. Immunother.* **2011**, *34*, 289–296. [CrossRef]

26. Cerwenka, A.; Baron, J.L.; Lanier, L.L. Ectopic expression of retinoic acid early inducible-1 gene (RAE-1) permits natural killer cell-mediated rejection of a MHC class I-bearing tumor in vivo. *Proc. Natl. Acad. Sci. USA* **2001**, *98*, 11521–11526. [CrossRef]

27. Vyas, M.; Schneider, A.-C.; Shatnyeva, O.; Reiners, K.S.; Tawadros, S.; Kloess, S.; Köhl, U.; Hallek, M.; Hansen, H.P.; Von Strandmann, E.P. Mono- and dual-targeting triplebodies activate natural killer cells and have anti-tumor activity in vitro and in vivo against chronic lymphocytic leukemia. *OncoImmunology* **2016**, *5*, e1211220. [CrossRef]

28. Feld, C.; Sahu, P.; Frech, M.; Finkernagel, F.; Nist, A.; Stiewe, T.; Bauer, U.-M.; Neubauer, A. Combined cistrome and transcriptome analysis of SKI in AML cells identifies SKI as a co-repressor for RUNX1. *Nucleic Acids Res.* **2018**, *46*, 3412–3428. [CrossRef]

29. Masuyama, J.; Murakami, T.; Iwamoto, S.; Fujita, S. Ex vivo expansion of natural killer cells from human peripheral blood mononuclear cells co-stimulated with anti-CD3 and anti-CD52 monoclonal antibodies. *Cytotherapy* **2016**, *18*, 80–90. [CrossRef]

30. Lin, M.; Liang, S.; Wang, X.; Liang, Y.; Zhang, M.; Chen, J.; Niu, L.; Xu, K. Percutaneous irreversible electroporation combined with allogeneic natural killer cell immunotherapy for patients with unresectable (stage III/IV) pancreatic cancer: A promising treatment. *J. Cancer Res. Clin. Oncol.* **2017**, *143*, 2607–2618. [CrossRef]

31. Gürlevik, E.; Fleischmann-Mundt, B.; Brooks, J.; Demir, I.E.; Steiger, K.; Ribback, S.; Yevsa, T.; Woller, N.; Kloos, A.; Ostroumov, D.; et al. Administration of Gemcitabine After Pancreatic Tumor Resection in Mice Induces an Antitumor Immune Response Mediated by Natural Killer Cells. *Gastroenterology* **2016**, *151*, 338–350.e7.

32. Idso, J.M.; Lao, S.; Schloemer, N.J.; Knipstein, J.; Burns, R.; Thakar, M.S.; Malarkannan, S. Entinostat augments NK cell functions via epigenetic upregulation of IFIT1-STING-STAT4 pathway. *Oncotarget* **2020**, *11*, 1799–1815. [CrossRef] [PubMed]

33. Hessmann, E.; Johnsen, S.A.; Siveke, J.T.; Ellenrieder, V. Epigenetic treatment of pancreatic cancer: Is there a therapeutic perspective on the horizon? *Gut* **2016**, *66*, 168–179. [CrossRef] [PubMed]

34. Gómez, V.; Mustapha, R.; Ng, K.; Ng, T. Radiation therapy and the innate immune response: Clinical implications for immunotherapy approaches. *Br. J. Clin. Pharmacol.* **2020**, *86*, 1726–1735. [CrossRef]

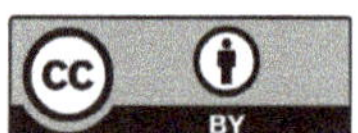

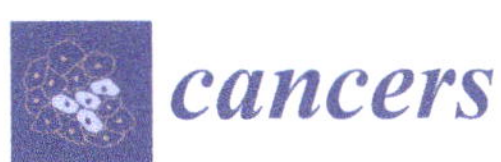 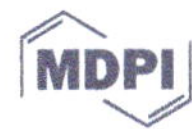

Article

Interleukin-15 after Near-Infrared Photoimmunotherapy (NIR-PIT) Enhances T Cell Response against Syngeneic Mouse Tumors

Yasuhiro Maruoka, Aki Furusawa, Ryuhei Okada, Fuyuki Inagaki, Hiroaki Wakiyama, Takuya Kato, Tadanobu Nagaya, Peter L. Choyke and Hisataka Kobayashi *

Molecular Imaging Program, Center for Cancer Research, National Cancer Institute, NIH, Bethesda, MD 20892, USA; ymaruoka@med.kyushu-u.ac.jp (Y.M.); Aki.Furusawa@nih.gov (A.F.); Ryuhei.Okada@nih.gov (R.O.); Fuyuki.Inagaki@nih.gov (F.I.); Hiroaki.Wakiyama@nih.gov (H.W.); Takuya.Kato@nih.gov (T.K.); nagaya@shinshu-u.ac.jp (T.N.); pchoyke@mail.nih.gov (P.L.C.)
* Correspondence: kobayash@mail.nih.gov

Received: 13 August 2020; Accepted: 6 September 2020; Published: 10 September 2020

Simple Summary: Near infrared photoimmunotherapy is a newly developed and highly selective cancer treatment that employs a monoclonal antibody conjugated to a photo-absorber dye, IRDye700DX, which is activated by 690 nm light. Cancer cell-targeted near infrared photoimmunotherapy selectively induces rapid necrotic/immunogenic cell death only on target cancer cells and this induces antitumor host immunity including re-priming and proliferation of multi-chronal T-cells that can react with cancer-specific antigens. Interleukin-15 is a type-I cytokine that activates natural killer-, B- and T-cells while having minimal effect on regulatory T-cells that lack the interleukin-15 receptor. Therefore, interleukin-15 administration combined with cancer cell-targeted near infrared photoimmunotherapy could further inhibit tumor growth by increasing antitumor host immunity. In tumor-bearing immunocompetent mice receiving this combination therapy, significant tumor growth inhibition and prolonged survival was demonstrated compared with either single therapy alone, and tumor infiltrating CD8+ T-cells increased in number in combination-treated mice. Interleukin-15 enhances therapeutic effects of cancer-targeted near infrared photoimmunotherapy.

Abstract: Near infrared photoimmunotherapy (NIR-PIT) is a newly developed and highly selective cancer treatment that employs a monoclonal antibody (mAb) conjugated to a photo-absorber dye, IRDye700DX, which is activated by 690 nm light. Cancer cell-targeted NIR-PIT induces rapid necrotic/immunogenic cell death (ICD) that induces antitumor host immunity including re-priming and proliferation of T cells. Interleukin-15 (IL-15) is a cytokine that activates natural killer (NK)-, B- and T-cells while having minimal effect on regulatory T cells (Tregs) that lack the IL-15 receptor. Here, we hypothesized that IL-15 administration with cancer cell-targeted NIR-PIT could further inhibit tumor growth by increasing antitumor host immunity. Three syngeneic mouse tumor models, MC38-luc, LL/2, and MOC1, underwent combined CD44-targeted NIR-PIT and short-term IL-15 administration with appropriate controls. Comparing with the single-agent therapy, the combination therapy of IL-15 after NIR-PIT inhibited tumor growth, prolonged survival, and increased tumor infiltrating CD8+ T cells more efficiently in tumor-bearing mice. IL-15 appears to enhance the therapeutic effect of cancer-targeted NIR-PIT.

Keywords: near infrared photoimmunotherapy; monoclonal antibodies; CD44; interleukin-15; cancer

---

1. Introduction

Near infrared photoimmunotherapy (NIR-PIT), which is a new type of cancer therapy that induces highly selective cell death on targeted cells only in NIR light exposed tumor beds, by employing a monoclonal antibody (mAb) conjugated to a silica-phthalocyanine photoabsorbing dye, (IRDye700DX: IR700) [1,2]. The antibody-IR700 conjugate is administered intravenously, followed by exposure to 690 nm NIR light which activates the IR700 dye. Tumor cells treated with NIR-PIT experience nearly immediate cell membrane damage and impaired cell function [3,4]. Treated cells show rapid volume expansion, followed by cell membrane rupture and extrusion of the cell contents into the extracellular space [3,5–8]. Unlike most other therapies that induce apoptotic cell death, NIR-PIT induces highly selective necrotic and immunogenic cell death of tumors with minimal damage to adjacent normal cells including immune cells in the tumor microenvironment (TME) [3,4]. NIR-PIT has shown to be effective clinically and a global phase III clinical trial of NIR-PIT using the EGFR-targeted antibody-IR700 conjugate, cetuximab-IR700 (ASP-1929) in patients with recurrent head and neck cancer is underway (https://clinicaltrials.gov/ct2/show/NCT03769506). Both the US Food and Drug Administration (FDA) and the Pharmaceuticals and Medical Devices Agency (PMDA) in Japan have given fast track status to this agent.

In this study, we sought to augment the effects of tumor targeted NIR-PIT using interleukin-15 (IL-15). We employed CD44 as a tumor target, which is a well-known marker of cancer stem cells [9] and is expressed on the cell membrane of several cancers [10]. High expression of CD44 is associated with tumor aggressiveness, drug resistance, and poor treatment outcome [11,12]. NIR-PIT using anti-CD44-mAb-IR700 induces effective tumor killing in CD44-expressing syngeneic mouse models [13–16]. Cell membrane rupture after NIR-PIT releases tumor-specific antigens into the TME and promotes dendritic cell (DC) maturation, resulting in presentation of cancer-specific antigens on DCs to naive T cells for priming [14,15,17]. Thus, NIR-PIT causes both direct cell killing and indirect cell killing by antitumor immunity.

IL-15 has recently emerged as a candidate immune-activator for the treatment of cancer [18]. IL-15 induces adaptive immune responses that include T-cell proliferation, the generation of cytotoxic T lymphocytes (CTL), stimulation of immunoglobulin synthesis by B cells, and the generation and persistence of natural killer (NK) cells. Some of its functions are shared with IL-2 [19]. However, IL-15 is not required for the maintenance of regulatory T cells (Tregs) that suppress antitumor immune responses, unlike IL-2 [20]. Therefore, IL-15 can induce protective effects against cancer development with minimal effects on Tregs. In preclinical studies, the administration of IL-15 has antitumor effects in several mouse tumor models [21–23]. We hypothesized that IL-15 administration following cancer-antigen targeted NIR-PIT could enhance tumor growth inhibition. The purpose of this study was to investigate the in vivo therapeutic efficacy of CD44-targted NIR-PIT and IL-15 treatment in syngeneic mouse models of cancer compared to either therapy alone.

2. Results

2.1. Efficacy of CD44-Targeted NIR-PIT Combined with IL-15 Administration for MC38-luc Tumor

In vitro and in vivo CD44 expression in all three tumor models (Figure S1) and cytotoxic effects of CD44 targeted NIR-PIT have been previously reported [24]. The NIR-PIT regimen and imaging protocol are depicted in Figure 1A. In the NIR-PIT treated group, 1 day after injection of anti-CD44-mAb-IR700, the tumors were exposed to 50 J/cm^2 of NIR light on day 0. IR700 fluorescence signal in tumors decreased due to dispersion of fluorophore from dying cells and partial photo-bleaching in all cases (Figure 1B). To investigate tumor-killing efficacy after NIR-PIT, bioluminescence imaging was performed before and after treatment up to day 7 (Figure 1C). In most mice treated with NIR-PIT, luciferase activity decreased initially after NIR-PIT due to cell killing and then gradually increased as the tumor regrew (Figure 1C). In all treated groups luciferase activity was significantly lower at 2, 3, 4, 5, 6, and 7 days in the treatment groups than in the control group ($p < 0.05$, Tukey-Kramer test) (Figure 1D). CD44-targeted

NIR-PIT combined with IL-15 treatment showed significantly lower luciferase activity compared with CD44-targeted NIR-PIT alone at 5, 6, and 7 days after NIR-PIT, with IL-15 ($p < 0.05$, Tukey–Kramer test) (Figure 1D). Tumor volume in all treated groups was significantly less at 5, 7, and 10 days compared with controls ($p < 0.05$, Tukey–Kramer test) (Figure 1E). The combination group showed significantly greater tumor reduction compared with IL-15 treatment or CD44-targeted NIR-PIT groups at 5, 7, and 10 days ($p < 0.05$, Tukey–Kramer test) (Figure 1E). These data demonstrate that CD44-targeted NIR-PIT combined with IL-15 resulted in the slowest rate of tumor regrowth compared with other groups. The combined therapy also was associated with significantly prolonged survival compared with IL-15 treatment alone or CD44-targeted NIR-PIT alone ($p < 0.05$, log-rank test) (Figure 1F). Thus, our results demonstrate that CD44-targeted NIR-PIT combined with IL-15 administration produced superior in vivo therapeutic results compared with the other two monotherapies for MC38-luc tumors.

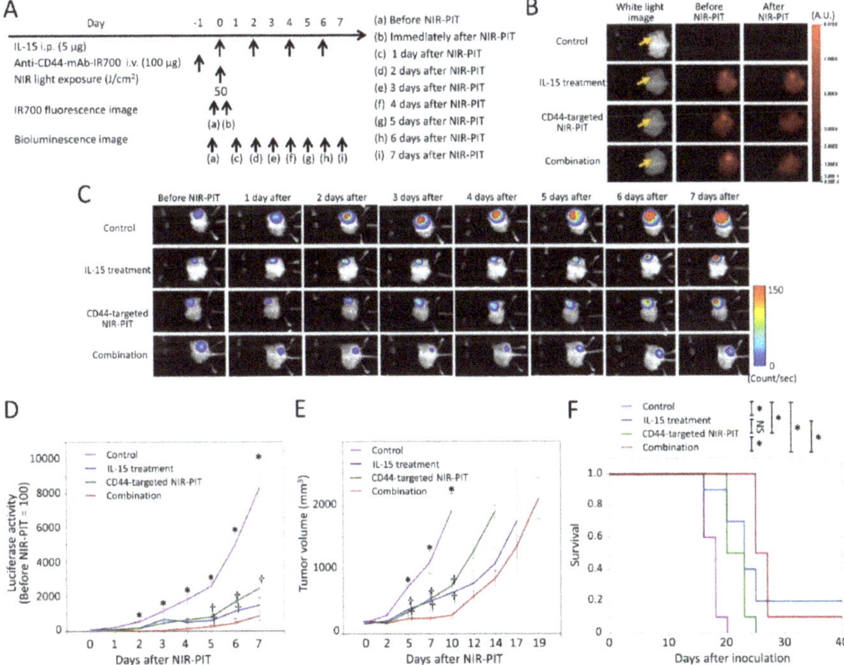

Figure 1. In vivo effect of CD44-targeted near infrared photoimmunotherapy (NIR-PIT) and interleukin-15 (IL-15) administration for MC38-luc tumor model. (**A**) NIR-PIT regimen. Bioluminescence and fluorescence images were obtained at each time point as indicated. i.p., intraperitoneal injection; i.v., intravenous injection. (**B**) Real-time in vivo IR700 fluorescence imaging of tumor-bearing mice before and approximately 10 min after NIR-PIT. The yellow arrows indicate the tumor locations. (**C**) In vivo bioluminescence imaging of tumor-bearing mice before and after treatment at the indicated timepoints. (**D**) Quantitative analysis of luciferase activity before and after treatment in tumor-bearing mice. $n = 10$/group, mean ± SEM; *, $p < 0.05$, vs. the other groups; †, $p < 0.05$, vs. combination group; Tukey–Kramer test. (**E**) Tumor growth in control and treated groups. $n = 10$/group, mean ± SEM; *, $p < 0.05$, vs. the other groups; †, $p < 0.05$, vs. combination group; Tukey–Kramer test. (**F**) Survival curves for control and treated groups. $n = 10$/group; *, $p < 0.05$; NS, not significant; log-rank test with Bonferroni correction.

2.2. Augmented CD8+ T Cells Infiltration in MC38-luc Tumors after CD44-Targeted NIR-PIT Combined with IL-15 Administration

In order to assess the density of tumor infiltrating T cells, an important indicator of antitumor immune activity, multiplex immunohistochemistry (IHC) was performed in MC38-luc tumors (Figure 2, also see Figure S2). With IL-15 administration, the cell density of CD8 T cells within tumors significantly increased at day 4, however, this augmentation of CD8 T cells was less prominent at day 7, suggesting that the CD8 T-cell population seen at day 4 was short-lived. On the other hand, in the tumors treated with the combination therapy, the augmentation of CD8 T-cell infiltration was not observed at day 4. This result could be attributed to the cytotoxic effect of CD44-targeted PIT against activated immune cells which express CD44. However, the cell density of CD8 T cells inside the tumor tissue dramatically increased 7 days after the combination therapy. The infiltration of CD4 T cells also increased 7 days after the combination therapy. CD44 targeted NIR-PIT alone did not induce the increase of T cell population. These results indicated that only CD44-targeted NIR-PIT combined with IL-15 administration resulted in newly activated T cells within the tumor microenvironment.

The cell density of Tregs significantly increased in stroma 7 days after IL-15 administration and combination therapy. This was thought to be a secondary effect in response to the rapid increase of CD8 T cells.

We also tested the distribution of Granzyme B (Gzmb) expressing cytotoxic cells. With the combination of IL-15 and CD44-targeted NIR-PIT, the number of Gzmb-positive CD8 T cells in the tumor tissue significantly increased at day 7 after the therapy (Figure S3A,C). With IL-15 administration alone, we observed the increase of Gzmb-positive CD8 T cells was less significant. This result indicates that the combination therapy successfully increased the tumor-infiltration of fully differentiated effector T cells. In addition to CD8 T cells, after IL-15 administration or combination of IL-15 and CD44-targeted NIR-PIT, we also observed increased number of another Gzmb positive cytotoxic cells, which were not CD8- or CD4-positive, namely non-T cytotoxic cells (Figure S3A,B,D). Such non-T cytotoxic cells including NK cells were more prominent in day 4 than day 7, suggesting that IL-15 stimulates the cytotoxic activity of T and non-T cell population at acute and subacute phase of tumor rejection.

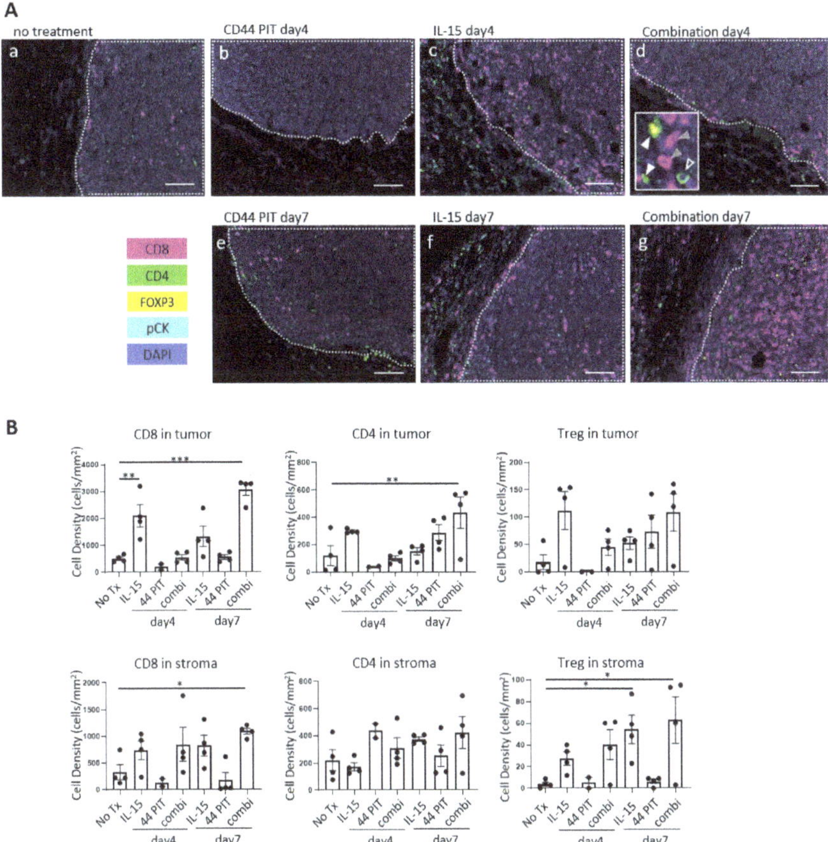

Figure 2. Immunohistochemical analysis after CD44-targeted NIR-PIT and/or IL-15 treatment in MC38-luc tumor model. (**A**) Representative multiplex immunohistochemistry (IHC) images in MC38-luc tumors 4 or 7 days after the treatments indicated. Antibody staining of CD8, CD4, FOXP3, and pan-Cytokeratin (pCK) are shown in magenta, green, yellow, and cyan respectively. Nucleus are stained with DAPI and shown in blue. Tumor areas are indicated in white dotted line. The inset in window d shows examples of CD8 T cell (gray filled arrowhead), CD4 T cell (open arrowhead), and Tregs (white filled arrowhead). Scale bar = 100 μm. (**B**) Cell density of CD8 T cells, CD4 T cells and Tregs in tumor and stroma calculated from IHC images. No Tx, no treatment; IL-15, IL-15 administration only; 44 PIT, CD44-targeted PIT only; combi, combination therapy of CD44-targeted PIT and IL-15 administration. Bars represent mean, dots represent individual samples, and error bars represent SEM. $n = 4$/group except $n = 2$ for CD44 day 4. **, $p < 0.05$, **, $p < 0.01$ ***, $p < 0.0001$; one-way ANOVA (followed by Dunnett's multiple comparison test, vs. no Tx).

2.3. Efficacy of CD44-Targeted NIR-PIT Combined with IL-15 Administration for LL/2 Tumor

The NIR-PIT regimen and imaging protocol are depicted in Figure 3A. In the NIR-PIT treated group, 1 day after injection of anti-CD44-mAb-IR700, the tumors were exposed to 50 J/cm² of NIR light on day 0. IR700 tumor fluorescence signal decreased due to dispersion of fluorophore from dying cells and partial photo-bleaching (Figure 3B). Tumor volumes in the treated groups were significantly reduced at all time points after treatment compared to the control group ($p < 0.05$, Tukey–Kramer test) (Figure 3C). The combination group showed significantly greater tumor reduction compared with the IL-15 treatment group at 2, 5, 7, 10, and 12 days after NIR-PIT ($p < 0.05$, Tukey–Kramer test)

(Figure 3C), and showed significantly greater tumor reduction compared with CD44-targeted NIR-PIT group at 5, 7, 10, and 12 days after NIR-PIT ($p < 0.05$, Tukey–Kramer test) (Figure 3C). In the long-term follow-up, the combination group had significantly prolonged survival after NIR-PIT compared with IL-15 treatment or CD44-targeted NIR-PIT group ($p < 0.05$, log-rank test) (Figure 4D). This combined therapy was superior therapeutically to the other two types of monotherapies in LL/2 tumors.

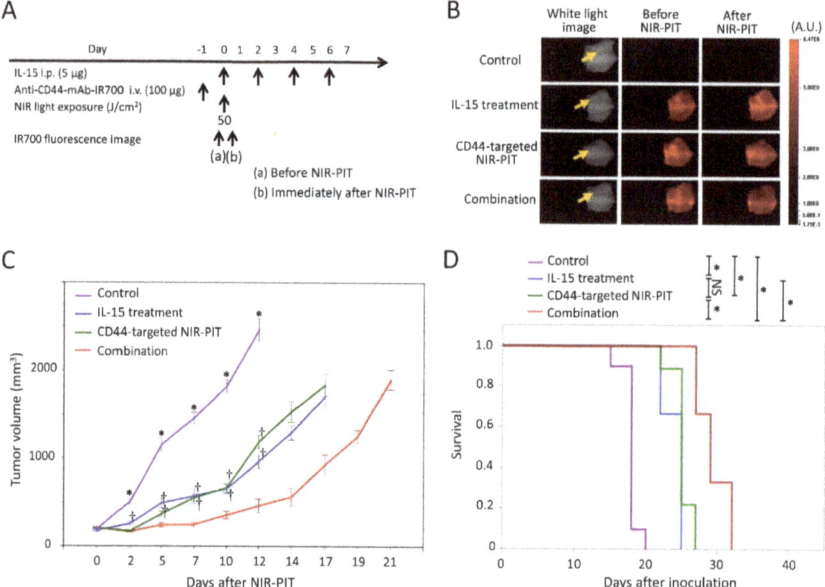

Figure 3. In vivo effect of CD44-targeted NIR-PIT and/or IL-15 administration in LL/2 tumor model. (**A**) NIR-PIT regimen. IR700 fluorescence images were obtained at each time point as indicated. i.p., intraperitoneal injection; i.v., intravenous injection. (**B**) Real-time in vivo IR700 fluorescence imaging of tumor-bearing mice before and approximately 10 min after NIR-PIT. The yellow arrows indicate the tumor locations. (**C**) Tumor growth in control and treated groups. $n = 9$/group, mean ± SEM; *, $p < 0.05$, vs. the other groups; †, $p < 0.05$, vs. combination group; Tukey–Kramer test. (**D**) Survival curves for control and treated groups. $n = 9$/group; *, $p < 0.05$; NS, not significant; log-rank test with Bonferroni correction.

2.4. Efficacy of CD44-Targeted NIR-PIT Combined with IL-15 Administration for MOC1 Tumor

Our previous study showed MOC1 tumor has low and more heterogeneous CD44 expression and CD44-targeted NIR-PIT was less effective against this type of tumor [13]. The NIR-PIT regimen and imaging protocol are depicted in Figure 4A. In the NIR-PIT treated group, 1 day after injection of anti-CD44-mAb-IR700, the tumors were exposed to 50 J/cm² of NIR light on day 0. IR700 tumor fluorescence signal decreased due to dispersion of fluorophore from dying cells and partial photo-bleaching. (Figure 4B). The tumor volume in all treated groups was significantly reduced 4, 7, 11, 14, 21, 24, 28, and 31 days after NIR-PIT compared to the control group ($p < 0.05$, Tukey–Kramer test) (Figure 4C). The combination group showed significantly greater tumor reduction 17, 28, and 31 days after NIR-PIT compared to CD44-targeted NIR-PIT group ($p < 0.05$, Tukey–Kramer test). The combination therapy showed significantly prolonged survival compared to CD44-targeted NIR-PIT group, although IL-15 treatment group had no significant difference in survival compared to CD44-targeted NIR-PIT group ($p < 0.05$, log-rank test) (Figure 4D). This combined therapy was superior therapeutically to the other two types of single therapies in MOC1 tumors.

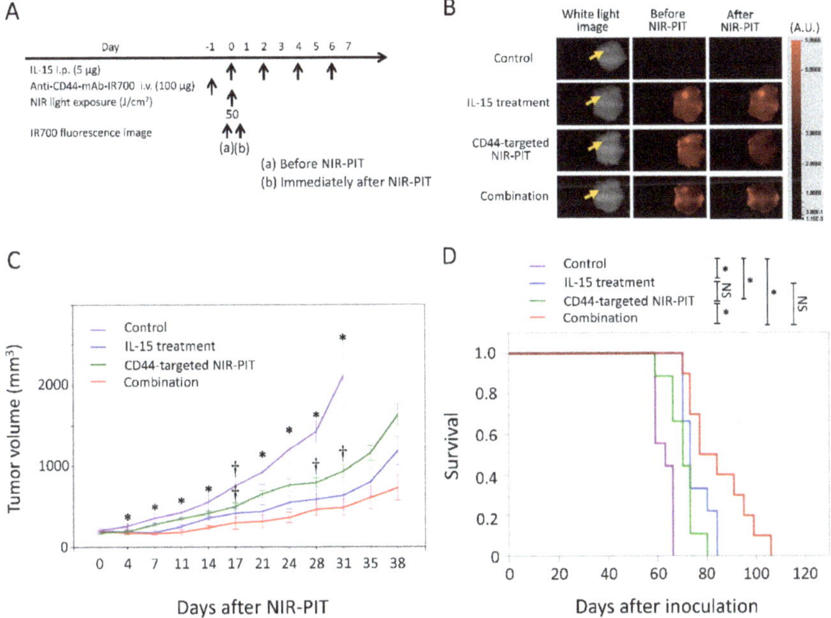

Figure 4. In vivo effect of CD44-targeted NIR-PIT and/or IL-15 administration in the MOC1 tumor model. (**A**) NIR-PIT regimen. IR700 fluorescence images were obtained at each time point as indicated. i.p., intraperitoneal injection; i.v., intravenous injection. (**B**) Real-time in vivo IR700 fluorescence imaging of tumor-bearing mice before and approximately 10 min after NIR-PIT. The yellow arrows indicate the tumor locations. (**C**) Tumor growth in control and treated groups. n = 10/group, mean ± SEM; *, $p < 0.05$, vs. the other groups; †, $p < 0.05$, vs. combination group; Tukey–Kramer test. (**D**) Survival curves for control and treated groups. n = 10/group; *, $p < 0.05$; NS, not significant; log-rank test with Bonferroni correction.

3. Discussion

The combination of IL-15 administration and CD44-targeted NIR-PIT showed superiority in survival to IL-15 treatment alone in all three tumor types tested here. IL-15 binds and sends signals through a heterotrimeric receptor composed of the IL-15-specific IL-15Rα, shared IL-2R/IL-15Rβ (CD122) with the IL-2 receptor, and the common type I cytokine receptor γ-chain (γc, CD132; [25,26]). IL-15 is highly bound through trans-presentation by IL-15Rα expressed on activated DCs or monocytes to the IL-2R/IL-15Rβ and γc on effector T, B, and NK cells [27]. When IL-15 binds its receptor, DCs can cause potent activation of the immune response [18,27]. Immunogenic cell death of cancer cells shortly after NIR-PIT releases damage-associated signals such as ATP, calreticulin, and high-mobility group box 1, which promotes DC maturation and subsequent effector T-cell activation mediated by IL-15 [3,14]. Thus, NIR-PIT and IL-15 administration trigger an immune response that is greater than either therapy alone.

In all tumor types used in this study, MC38-luc, LL/2, and MOC1, infiltration of Tregs was observed within the TME [24]. Tregs tend to attenuate antitumor activity and are, therefore, not necessarily a desired outcome. However, IL-15 may be a safer choice of cytokine than IL-2 because the former does not stimulate Tregs while the latter is required for Treg maintenance [20]. In our study, significant increases in stromal Tregs were observed after IL-15 administration and the combination therapy, which was likely to be a secondary effect in response to the rapid increase of CD8 T cells in the TME. Our results showed that CD44-targeted NIR-PIT combined with short-term IL-15 treatment increased the infiltration of fully differentiated CD8+ effector T-cells which contributed to significantly prolonged survival compared to

CD44-targeted NIR-PIT alone in all three types of tumors. Considering that administration of IL-15 alone only induced short-lived CD8 T cells, and CD44-targeted NIR-PIT alone did not increase the infiltration of T cells, the superior therapeutic effect of the combination therapy was thought to be the result of IL-15 mediated reinforcement of NIR-PIT-induced antitumor immune activation.

In addition to CD8 T cells, we observed increasing number of Gzmb-high non-T cytotoxic cells within a few days after IL-15 administration or the combination therapy. Since IL-15 is known to stimulate the cytotoxic function on both CD8 T and NK cells, these cells were most likely to be NK cells. Therefore, the combination therapy of CD44-targeted NIR-PIT and IL-15 administration demonstrate its therapeutic efficacy probably by stimulating both the NK-mediated innate immunity and T-cell mediated adoptive immunity.

This report represents an extension of previous studies which attempt to augment the immune response initiated by NIR-PIT. For instance, a previous study demonstrated that the combination of CD44-targeted NIR-PIT and either immune checkpoint blockade or Treg-targeted NIR-PIT showed inconsistent therapeutic efficacy among these three tumor models [13,14,24]. CD44-targeted NIR-PIT in combination with other therapies showed promising results in MC38-luc and LL/2 but was less effective against MOC1 tumor which has low CD44 expression and fewer CD44 positive tumor cells compared to MC38-luc and LL/2. On the other hand, in this study, the combination with IL-15 therapy was effective in all three tumor models including MOC1. Even though the release of damage-associated signals after NIR-PIT is likely to have been lower in MOC1 cells, IL-15 administration following NIR-PIT nevertheless contributed to enhancement of antitumor host immunity by activating tumor-attacking T and NK cells making this combination therapy similarly effective for all tumors. Further combination therapy of cancer-targeting NIR-PIT with both IL-15 and an immune-checkpoint blockade or Treg-targeting NIR-PIT could theoretically enhance tumor immunity. However, such therapies need to be designed cautiously since excessively enhanced immunity might induce cytokine storm as an adverse effect. Photodynamic therapy (PDT) is another therapeutic approach that utilizes light to treat cancer [28]. However, NIR-PIT is different from PDT in several aspects. Porphyrin-based photosensitizers used in conventional PDT do not selectively target cancer cells, resulting in damage to surrounding normal cells in organs or vasculatures. In contrast, because NIR-PIT induces selective immunogenic cell death only on targeted cancer cells in NIR light exposing tumor beds, it spares the normal cells including all immune cells in the TME allowing them to play a role in immune activation [3]. Therefore, rapid and effective activation of antitumor host immunity is induced by NIR-PIT [14], whereas such effects are not generally induced by nonselective cell killing with PDT.

This study had several limitations. First, we used subcutaneously implanted tumor models, whereas an orthotopic or transgenic mouse model would be considered as a superior clinically relevant animal model [29]. However, in the present study, it was technically important to obtain a consistent size, shape, and location of each tumor in order to fairly compare tumor growth between tested groups. The orthotopic model could produce variable results depending on surgical procedure for implanting tumor within the organ. Second, although CD44 is expressed on these syngeneic cancer cells, CD44 is also expressed on activated immune cells. CD44-targeted NIR-PIT could thus damage effector immune cells. Indeed, counts of all kinds of T cells decreased 4 days after CD44-targeted NIR-PIT alone. Thus, CD44 is not ideal as a tumor target. Since NIR-PIT is applicable to any antibody that targets tumor cell surface antigens [30], NIR-PIT using an anti-mouse EGFR antibody, the target molecule in NIR-PIT clinical trials, would have been preferable. However, there is no thoroughly established EGFR+ mouse tumor model, and commercially available anti-mouse EGFR Abs are too expensive for experimental cancer therapy studies. Further investigation is required to clarify the degree of enhancement of antitumor host immunity through NIR-PIT. Third, we may not have optimized the dosing of IL-15. IL-15 has a circulation half-life of around 1 h [31] that is longer than IL-2 (15 min), and only 5 µg of IL-15 was administered i.p. up to 1 week after CD44-targeted NIR-PIT. A more prolonged administration of IL-15 might have induced greater therapeutic effects albeit balanced by an increased risk of lymphoproliferative disorder or lymphoma, either of which was seen in the

IL-15 transgenic mouse [32]. In a previous article, Yu et al. reported that administration of IL-15 alone simultaneously activated both immune-system and negative regulatory checkpoints that might weaken the antitumor immune response [22]. To elucidate the reason why the treatment regimen of this combined NIR-PIT therapy with IL-15 was difficult to cure tumors, further investigation of the T cell status such as exhaustion, activation, and memory differentiation would be required.

4. Materials and Methods

4.1. Cell Culture

MC38 cells (murine colon cancer), which were generously provided by Dr. Thomas Waldmann, NIH [33] stably expressing luciferase (MC38-luc, generated via stable transduction with RediFect Red-Fluc lentivirus from PerkinElmer per manufacturer recommendations), which was purchased from ATCC (Rockville, MD, USA), LL/2 cells (murine Lewis lung carcinoma), which was purchased from ATCC (Rockville, MD, USA), and MOC1 cells (murine oral carcinoma), which were produced and generously provided by Dr. Clint Allen, NIH [34] were used in this study. Luciferase expression on the MC38-luc cells was confirmed through 10 passages. MC38-luc and LL/2 cells were cultured in RPMI1640 supplemented with 10% FBS and 1% penicillin–streptomycin (all Gibco brand, ThermoFisher Scientific, Waltman, MA, USA) in tissue culture flasks (182 cm^2; CELLTREAT Scientific Products, Pepperell, MA, USA) in a humidified incubator at 37 °C in an atmosphere of 95% air and 5% carbon dioxide. MOC1 cells were cultured in HyClone Iscove's modified Dulbecco's medium (Crytiva, Marlborough, MA, USA)/HyClone Ham's Nutrient Mixture F12 (Crytiva, Marlborough, MA, USA) at a 2:1 mixture with 5% FBS, 1% penicillin/streptomycin, 3.5 ng/mL EGF (MilliporeSigma, Burlington, MA, USA), 40 ng/mL hydrocortisone (MilliporeSigma, Burlington, MA, USA), and 5 ng/mL insulin (MilliporeSigma, Burlington, MA, USA) in the tissue culture flasks in a humidified incubator at 37 °C in an atmosphere of 95% air and 5% carbon dioxide. Cells were authenticated via in vitro growth characteristics.

4.2. Reagents

Water soluble, silica-phthalocyanine derivative, IRDye700DX NHS ester was obtained from LI-COR Bioscience (Lincoln, NE, USA). An anti-mouse/human CD44 mAb (IM7) was purchased from Bio X Cell (Lebanon, NH, USA). All other chemicals were of reagent grade.

4.3. Synthesis of IR700-Conjugated Anti-CD44 mAb

Briefly, anti-CD44-IgG (1 mg, 6.7 nmol/L) was incubated with IR700 NHS ester (65.1 µg, 33.3 nmol, 10 mmol/L in DMSO) and 0.1 mol/L Na2HPO4 (pH 8.5) at room temperature for 1 h. The mixture was purified with a gel filtration column (Sephadex G 25 column, PD-10, Crytiva, Marlborough, MA, USA). The protein concentration was measured with Coomassie Plus protein assay kit (Thermo Fisher Scientific Inc, Waltman, MA, USA) by determining absorption at 595 nm with a UV-Vis spectroscopy system (8453 Value System; Agilent Technologies, Santa Clara, CA, USA). We abbreviate IR700-conjugated anti-CD44 mAb as anti-CD44-mAb-IR700.

4.4. Animal Model

All procedures were performed in compliance with the Guide for the Care and Use of Laboratory Animals and approved by the local Animal Care and Use Committee on 12-02-2019 (MIP-003). Six- to eight-week-old female C57BL/6 mice (strain #000664) were purchased from the Jackson laboratory (Bar Harbor, ME, USA). The lower part of the body of the mice was shaved as fur can interfere with light activation of the conjugate and bioluminescence imaging. Mice with tumors reaching approximately 150 mm^3 in volume were used for the experiments. Tumor volumes were calculated from the greatest longitudinal diameter (length) and the greatest transverse diameter (width) using the following formula; tumor volume = length × $width^2$ × 0.5, based on caliper measurements. Mice were monitored each day and tumor volumes were measured three times a week for MC38-luc and LL/2 tumors and twice a week for MOC1 tumors until the tumor volume reached 2000 mm^3, whereupon the mice were euthanized by inhalation of carbon dioxide gas.

4.5. In Vivo NIR-PIT

MC38-luc cells (8 million), LL/2 cells (8 million), and MOC1 cells (4 million) were subcutaneously injected in the dorsum of mice. Once tumors reached volumes of approximately 150 mm^3 mice were divided randomly into one of the following four experimental groups: (1) no treatment (control); (2) intraperitoneal injection of 5 µg murine IL-15 (PeproTech, Rocky Hill, NJ, USA) on days 0, 2, 4, and 6 following intravenous injection of 100 µg anti-CD44-mAb-IR700 (IL-15 treatment); (3) intravenous injection of 100 µg anti-CD44-mAb-IR700 followed by external NIR light irradiation at 50 J/cm^2 on day 0 (CD44-targeted NIR-PIT); (4) intravenous injection of 100 µg anti-CD44-mAb-IR700 followed by external NIR light irradiation at 50 J/cm^2 on day 0 and 100 J/cm^2 on day 1 with intraperitoneal injection of 5 µg murine IL-15 on days 0, 2, 4, and 6 (combination). For the mice with MC38-luc tumor, LL/2 tumor, and MOC1 tumor in the NIR-PIT treated groups, intravenous injection of the anti-CD44-mAb-IR700 was performed 5, 5, and 28 days after tumor inoculation, respectively. NIR light was administered to tumor-bearing mice using a red-light emitting diode (LED), which emits light in the range of 670–710 nm wavelength (L690-66-60; Marubeni America Co., New York, NY, USA) at a power density of 50 mW/cm^2 as measured with an optical power meter (PM 100, Thorlabs, Newton, NJ, USA). IR700 absorbs light at approximately 690 nm. IR700 fluorescence images were obtained before and after therapy.

4.6. In Vivo Bioluminescence Imaging and IR700 Fluorescence Imaging

To obtain bioluminescence images in MC38-luc tumor-bearing mice, D-luciferin (15 mg/mL, 150 mL; Goldbio, St Louis, MO, USA) was intraperitoneally injected. Luciferase activity was analyzed with a bioluminescence imaging system (Photon Imager; Biospace Lab, Nesles la Vallée, FRANCE) using units of relative light units (RLU). Regions of interests (ROIs) were placed over the entire tumor. The counts per minute of RLUs were calculated using M3 Vision Software (Biospace Lab) and converted to a percentage ratio based on the following formula: [(RLU after treatment)/(RLU before treatment) × 100 (%); [35]]. Bioluminescence imaging was performed before and after NIR-PIT (protocol below) on day 0 to day 7. In vivo IR700 fluorescence images were obtained with a Pearl Imager (LI-COR Biosciences, Lincoln, NE, USA) using the 700-nm fluorescence channel.

4.7. Multicolor Immunofluorescence

Multicolor immunofluorescence was performed using Opal 7-Color Automation immunohistochemistry staining Kit (Akoya Bioscience, Menlo Park, CA, USA) and BOND RXm auto stainer (Leica Biosystems, Wetzlar, Germany). The following antibodies were used: anti-CD44 (clone IM7; 1:5000 dilution; Bio X Cell, Lebanon, NH, USA), anti-CD8 (clone EPR20305; 1:500 dilution; Abcam, Cambridge, MA, USA), anti-CD4 (clone EPR19514; 1:1000 dilution; Abcam), anti-FOXP3 (clone 1054C; 1:1000 dilution; Novus Biologicals, Littleton, CO, USA), anti-pan cytokeratin (rabbit poly; 1:500 dilution, Bioss, Woburn, MA, USA), anti-CD45 (clone D3F8Q, 1:500 dilution, Cell Signaling Technology, Danvers, MA, USA), and anti-Granzyme B (rabbit poly; 1:500 dilution, Abcam). The staining was performed according to the Opal 7 color protocol provided by manufacturer with following modification: (i) antigen retrieval was performed using BOND ER2 solution (Leica Biosystems, Wetzlar, Germany) for 20 min and (ii) the ImmPRESS HRP anti-Rabbit IgG (Peroxidase) Polymer Detection Kit (Vector Laboratories, Burlingame, CA, USA) was used instead of anti-mouse/human secondary antibody provided in the kit. Stained slides were mounted with VECTASHIELD Hardset Antifade Mounting Medium (Vector Laboratories) and then imaged using Mantra Quantitative Pathology Workstation (Akoya Biosciences). Images were analyzed with inForm software (Akoya Biosciences). inForm software was trained to detect tissues and cell phenotypes according to following criteria: areas with pan-cytokeratin expression = tumor, other areas = stroma, CD4+FOXP3+ cells = Tregs, CD4+FOXP3− = CD4 T cells,

CD8+ = CD8+ T cells, respectively. At least five images were taken from each tumor sample, areas for each tissue phenotype and cell count of each phenotype were combined to calculate the cell density. As for Gzmb expression analysis, cell phenotyping (CD8+/CD45+ = CD8+ T cells, CD4+/CD45+ = CD4+ T cells, Gzmb+/CD8−/CD4− = non-T-cell cytotoxic cells) and Gzmb expression analysis (Gzmb + and other) were performed separately using inForm for the same set of images, then cell segmentation data were consolidated and analyzed using phenoptrReports and phenoptr (Akoya Biosciences) to calculate the density of Gzmb+CD8 T cells.

4.8. Statistical Analysis

Quantitative data were expressed as means ± SEM. The Mann–Whitney U test was used to compare differences between two groups. For multiple comparisons (≥3 groups), a one-way analysis of variance (ANOVA) followed by the Tukey–Kramer test or Dunnett's multiple comparison test was used. The cumulative survival was analyzed by the Kaplan–Meier survival curve analysis, and the differences between tested groups were compared using the log-rank test followed by Bonferroni correction. Statistical analysis was performed with JMP 13 software (SAS Institute, Cary, NC, USA). A p value of less than 0.05 was granted significant.

5. Conclusions

CD44-targeted NIR-PIT combined with IL-15 treatment showed superior in vivo therapeutic efficacy to either CD44-targeted NIR-PIT or IL-15 treatment alone in colon, lung, and oral cancer models. IL-15 might have potential to become a versatile adjuvant after cancer NIR-PIT.

Supplementary Materials: The following are available online at http://www.mdpi.com/2072-6694/12/9/2575/s1, Figure S1: CD44 expression within MC38-luc (A), LL/2 (B), and MOC1 (C) tumors, Figure S2: Tissue and cell phenotyping based on the multiplex immunohistochemistry (IHC), Figure S3: Distribution of Granzyme B (Gzmb) expressing cytotoxic cells within the treated tumors.

Author Contributions: Y.M. mainly designed and conducted experiments, performed analysis, and wrote the manuscript; A.F., R.O., F.I., H.W., T.K., and T.N. performed experiments and analysis; P.L.C. wrote the manuscript and supervised the project; and H.K. planned and initiated the project, designed and conducted experiments, wrote the manuscript, and supervised the entire project. All authors have read and agreed to the published version of the manuscript.

Funding: This research was supported by the Intramural Research Program of the National Institutes of Health, National Cancer Institute, Center for Cancer Research (ZIA BC011513).

Acknowledgments: This research was supported by the Intramural Research Program of the National Institutes of Health, National Cancer Institute, Center for Cancer Research (ZIA BC011513). FI was also supported with a grant from National Center for Global Health and Medicine Research Institute, Tokyo, Japan.

Conflicts of Interest: The authors declare no conflict of interest. The funders had no role in the design of the study; in the collection, analyses, or interpretation of data; in the writing of the manuscript, or in the decision to publish the results.

References

1. Kobayashi, H.; Choyke, P.L. Near-Infrared Photoimmunotherapy of Cancer. *Acc. Chem. Res.* **2019**, *52*, 2332–2339. [CrossRef]
2. Mitsunaga, M.; Ogawa, M.; Kosaka, N.; Rosenblum, L.T.; Choyke, P.L.; Kobayashi, H. Cancer cell-selective in vivo near infrared photoimmunotherapy targeting specific membrane molecules. *Nat. Med.* **2011**, *17*, 1685–1691. [CrossRef] [PubMed]
3. Ogawa, M.; Tomita, Y.; Nakamura, Y.; Lee, M.J.; Lee, S.; Tomita, S.; Nagaya, T.; Sato, K.; Yamauchi, T.; Iwai, H.; et al. Immunogenic cancer cell death selectively induced by near infrared photoimmunotherapy initiates host tumor immunity. *Oncotarget* **2017**, *8*, 10425–10436. [CrossRef] [PubMed]
4. Sato, K.; Ando, K.; Okuyama, S.; Moriguchi, S.; Ogura, T.; Totoki, S.; Hanaoka, H.; Nagaya, T.; Kokawa, R.; Takakura, H.; et al. Photoinduced Ligand Release from a Silicon Phthalocyanine Dye Conjugated with Monoclonal Antibodies: A Mechanism of Cancer Cell Cytotoxicity after Near-Infrared Photoimmunotherapy. *ACS Cent. Sci.* **2018**, *4*, 1559–1569. [CrossRef] [PubMed]

5. Mitsunaga, M.; Nakajima, T.; Sano, K.; Kramer-Marek, G.; Choyke, P.L.; Kobayashi, H. Immediate in vivo target-specific cancer cell death after near infrared photoimmunotherapy. *BMC Cancer* **2012**, *12*, 345. [CrossRef]

6. Nakamura, Y.; Bernardo, M.; Nagaya, T.; Sato, K.; Harada, T.; Choyke, P.L.; Kobayashi, H. MR imaging biomarkers for evaluating therapeutic effects shortly after near infrared photoimmunotherapy. *Oncotarget* **2016**, *7*, 17254–17264. [CrossRef]

7. Sato, K.; Nagaya, T.; Choyke, P.L.; Kobayashi, H. Near infrared photoimmunotherapy in the treatment of pleural disseminated NSCLC: Preclinical experience. *Theranostics* **2015**, *5*, 698–709. [CrossRef]

8. Sato, K.; Nakajima, T.; Choyke, P.L.; Kobayashi, H. Selective cell elimination in vitro and in vivo from tissues and tumors using antibodies conjugated with a near infrared phthalocyanine. *RSC Adv.* **2015**, *5*, 25105–25114. [CrossRef]

9. Ponta, H.; Sherman, L.; Herrlich, P.A. CD44: From adhesion molecules to signalling regulators. *Nat. Rev. Mol. Cell. Biol.* **2003**, *4*, 33–45. [CrossRef]

10. Naor, D.; Nedvetzki, S.; Golan, I.; Melnik, L.; Faitelson, Y. CD44 in cancer. *Crit. Rev. Clin. Lab. Sci.* **2002**, *39*, 527–579. [CrossRef]

11. Chen, J.; Zhou, J.; Lu, J.; Xiong, H.; Shi, X.; Gong, L. Significance of CD44 expression in head and neck cancer: A systemic review and meta-analysis. *BMC Cancer* **2014**, *14*, 15. [CrossRef]

12. de Jong, M.C.; Pramana, J.; van der Wal, J.E.; Lacko, M.; Peutz-Kootstra, C.J.; de Jong, J.M.; Takes, R.P.; Kaanders, J.H.; van der Laan, B.F.; Wachters, J.; et al. CD44 expression predicts local recurrence after radiotherapy in larynx cancer. *Clin. Cancer Res.* **2010**, *16*, 5329–5338. [CrossRef]

13. Maruoka, Y.; Furusawa, A.; Okada, R.; Inagaki, F.; Fujimura, D.; Wakiyama, H.; Kato, T.; Nagaya, T.; Choyke, P.L.; Kobayashi, H. Combined CD44- and CD25-Targeted Near-Infrared Photoimmunotherapy Selectively Kills Cancer and Regulatory T Cells in Syngeneic Mouse Cancer Models. *Cancer Immunol. Res.* **2020**, *8*, 345–355. [CrossRef] [PubMed]

14. Nagaya, T.; Friedman, J.; Maruoka, Y.; Ogata, F.; Okuyama, S.; Clavijo, P.E.; Choyke, P.L.; Allen, C.; Kobayashi, H. Host Immunity Following Near-Infrared Photoimmunotherapy Is Enhanced with PD-1 Checkpoint Blockade to Eradicate Established Antigenic Tumors. *Cancer Immunol. Res.* **2019**, *7*, 401–413. [CrossRef]

15. Nagaya, T.; Nakamura, Y.; Okuyama, S.; Ogata, F.; Maruoka, Y.; Choyke, P.L.; Allen, C.; Kobayashi, H. Syngeneic Mouse Models of Oral Cancer Are Effectively Targeted by Anti-CD44-Based NIR-PIT. *Mol. Cancer Res. MCR* **2017**, *15*, 1667–1677. [CrossRef] [PubMed]

16. Okada, R.; Maruoka, Y.; Furusawa, A.; Inagaki, F.; Nagaya, T.; Fujimura, D.; Choyke, P.L.; Kobayashi, H. The Effect of Antibody Fragments on CD25 Targeted Regulatory T Cell Near-Infrared Photoimmunotherapy. *Bioconjug. Chem.* **2019**, *30*, 2624–2633. [CrossRef] [PubMed]

17. Inoue, H.; Tani, K. Multimodal immunogenic cancer cell death as a consequence of anticancer cytotoxic treatments. *Cell Death Differ.* **2014**, *21*, 39–49. [CrossRef] [PubMed]

18. Steel, J.C.; Waldmann, T.A.; Morris, J.C. Interleukin-15 biology and its therapeutic implications in cancer. *Trends Pharmacol. Sci.* **2012**, *33*, 35–41. [CrossRef]

19. Waldmann, T.A.; Tagaya, Y. The multifaceted regulation of interleukin-15 expression and the role of this cytokine in NK cell differentiation and host response to intracellular pathogens. *Annu. Rev. Immunol.* **1999**, *17*, 19–49. [CrossRef]

20. Berger, C.; Berger, M.; Hackman, R.C.; Gough, M.; Elliott, C.; Jensen, M.C.; Riddell, S.R. Safety and immunologic effects of IL-15 administration in nonhuman primates. *Blood* **2009**, *114*, 2417–2426. [CrossRef]

21. Oh, S.; Berzofsky, J.A.; Burke, D.S.; Waldmann, T.A.; Perera, L.P. Coadministration of HIV vaccine vectors with vaccinia viruses expressing IL-15 but not IL-2 induces long-lasting cellular immunity. *Proc. Natl. Acad. Sci. USA* **2003**, *100*, 3392–3397. [CrossRef] [PubMed]

22. Yu, P.; Steel, J.C.; Zhang, M.; Morris, J.C.; Waldmann, T.A. Simultaneous blockade of multiple immune system inhibitory checkpoints enhances antitumor activity mediated by interleukin-15 in a murine metastatic colon carcinoma model. *Clin. Cancer Res.* **2010**, *16*, 6019–6028. [CrossRef] [PubMed]

23. Zhang, M.; Yao, Z.; Dubois, S.; Ju, W.; Muller, J.R.; Waldmann, T.A. Interleukin-15 combined with an anti-CD40 antibody provides enhanced therapeutic efficacy for murine models of colon cancer. *Proc. Natl. Acad. Sci. USA* **2009**, *106*, 7513–7518. [CrossRef] [PubMed]

24. Maruoka, Y.; Furusawa, A.; Okada, R.; Inagaki, F.; Fujimura, D.; Wakiyama, H.; Kato, T.; Nagaya, T.; Choyke, P.L.; Kobayashi, H. Near-infrared photoimmunotherapy combined with CTLA4 checkpoint blockade in syngeneic mouse cancer models. *Vaccines* **2020**. (under review)

25. Giri, J.G.; Ahdieh, M.; Eisenman, J.; Shanebeck, K.; Grabstein, K.; Kumaki, S.; Namen, A.; Park, L.S.; Cosman, D.; Anderson, D. Utilization of the beta and gamma chains of the IL-2 receptor by the novel cytokine IL-15. *EMBO J.* **1994**, *13*, 2822–2830. [CrossRef]

26. Giri, J.G.; Kumaki, S.; Ahdieh, M.; Friend, D.J.; Loomis, A.; Shanebeck, K.; DuBose, R.; Cosman, D.; Park, L.S.; Anderson, D.M. Identification and cloning of a novel IL-15 binding protein that is structurally related to the alpha chain of the IL-2 receptor. *EMBO J.* **1995**, *14*, 3654–3663. [CrossRef] [PubMed]

27. Dubois, S.; Mariner, J.; Waldmann, T.A.; Tagaya, Y. IL-15Ralpha recycles and presents IL-15 In trans to neighboring cells. *Immunity* **2002**, *17*, 537–547. [CrossRef]

28. Mroz, P.; Hashmi, J.T.; Huang, Y.Y.; Lange, N.; Hamblin, M.R. Stimulation of anti-tumor immunity by photodynamic therapy. *Expert Rev. Clin. Immunol.* **2011**, *7*, 75–91. [CrossRef]

29. Hoffman, R.M. Patient-derived orthotopic xenografts: Better mimic of metastasis than subcutaneous xenografts. *Nat. Rev. Cancer* **2015**, *15*, 451–452. [CrossRef]

30. Kobayashi, H.; Griffiths, G.L.; Choyke, P.L. Near-Infrared Photoimmunotherapy: Photoactivatable Antibody-Drug Conjugates (ADCs). *Bioconjug. Chem.* **2020**, *31*, 28–36. [CrossRef]

31. Kobayashi, H.; Carrasquillo, J.A.; Paik, C.H.; Waldmann, T.A.; Tagaya, Y. Differences of biodistribution, pharmacokinetics, and tumor targeting between interleukins 2 and 15. *Cancer Res.* **2000**, *60*, 3577–3583. [PubMed]

32. Kobayashi, H.; Dubois, S.; Sato, N.; Sabzevari, H.; Sakai, Y.; Waldmann, T.A.; Tagaya, Y. Role of trans-cellular IL-15 presentation in the activation of NK cell-mediated killing, which leads to enhanced tumor immunosurveillance. *Blood* **2005**, *105*, 721–727. [CrossRef] [PubMed]

33. Robbins, P.F.; Kantor, J.A.; Salgaller, M.; Hand, P.H.; Fernsten, P.D.; Schlom, J. Transduction and expression of the human carcinoembryonic antigen gene in a murine colon carcinoma cell line. *Cancer Res.* **1991**, *51*, 3657–3662. [PubMed]

34. Judd, N.P.; Allen, C.T.; Winkler, A.E.; Uppaluri, R. Comparative analysis of tumor-infiltrating lymphocytes in a syngeneic mouse model of oral cancer. *Otolaryngol. Head Neck Surg.* **2012**, *147*, 493–500. [CrossRef] [PubMed]

35. Maruoka, Y.; Nagaya, T.; Nakamura, Y.; Sato, K.; Ogata, F.; Okuyama, S.; Choyke, P.L.; Kobayashi, H. Evaluation of Early Therapeutic Effects after Near-Infrared Photoimmunotherapy (NIR-PIT) Using Luciferase-Luciferin Photon-Counting and Fluorescence Imaging. *Mol. Pharm.* **2017**, *14*, 4628–4635. [CrossRef] [PubMed]

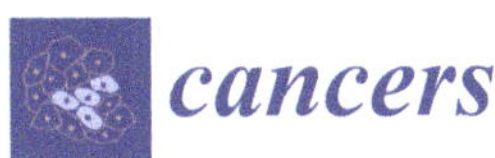

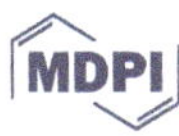

Review

Nonreplicating Adenoviral Vectors: Improving Tropism and Delivery of Cancer Gene Therapy

Nayara Gusmão Tessarollo, Ana Carolina M. Domingues, Fernanda Antunes , Jean Carlos dos Santos da Luz, Otavio Augusto Rodrigues, Otto Luiz Dutra Cerqueira and Bryan E. Strauss *

Viral Vector Laboratory, Center for Translational Investigation in Oncology, Cancer Institute of São Paulo/LIM24, University of São Paulo School of Medicine, São Paulo 01246-000, Brazil; nayara.tessarollo@hc.fm.usp.br (N.G.T.); ana.domingues@fm.usp.br (A.C.M.D.); fernanda.antunes@hc.fm.usp.br (F.A.); jc.santosluz@usp.br (J.C.d.S.d.L.); otavio.rodrigues@hc.fm.usp.br (O.A.R.); ottoluix@usp.br (O.L.D.C.)
* Correspondence: bstrauss@usp.br or bryan.strauss@hc.fm.usp.br

Simple Summary: The treatment of cancer has progressed greatly with the advent of immunotherapy and gene therapy, including the use of nonreplicating adenoviral vectors to deliver genes with antitumor activity for cancer gene therapy. Even so, the successful application of these vectors may benefit from modifications in their design, including their molecular structure, so that specificity for the target cell is increased and off-target effects are minimized. With such improvements, we may find new opportunities for systemic administration of adenoviral vectors as well as the delivery of strategic antigen targets of an antitumor immune response. We propose that the improvement of nonreplicating adenoviral vectors will allow them to continue to hold a key position in cancer gene therapy and immunotherapy.

Citation: Tessarollo, N.G.; Domingues, A.C.M.; Antunes, F.; Luz, J.C.d.S.d.; Rodrigues, O.A.; Cerqueira, O.L.D.; Strauss, B.E. Nonreplicating Adenoviral Vectors: Improving Tropism and Delivery of Cancer Gene Therapy. *Cancers* **2021**, *13*, 1863. https://doi.org/10.3390/cancers13081863

Academic Editors: Michael Kershaw and Clare Slaney

Received: 26 February 2021
Accepted: 6 April 2021
Published: 14 April 2021

Publisher's Note: MDPI stays neutral with regard to jurisdictional claims in published maps and institutional affiliations.

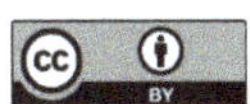

Abstract: Recent preclinical and clinical studies have used viral vectors in gene therapy research, especially nonreplicating adenovirus encoding strategic therapeutic genes for cancer treatment. Adenoviruses were the first DNA viruses to go into therapeutic development, mainly due to well-known biological features: stability in vivo, ease of manufacture, and efficient gene delivery to dividing and nondividing cells. However, there are some limitations for gene therapy using adenoviral vectors, such as nonspecific transduction of normal cells and liver sequestration and neutralization by antibodies, especially when administered systemically. On the other hand, adenoviral vectors are amenable to strategies for the modification of their biological structures, including genetic manipulation of viral proteins, pseudotyping, and conjugation with polymers or biological membranes. Such modifications provide greater specificity to the target cell and better safety in systemic administration; thus, a reduction of antiviral host responses would favor the use of adenoviral vectors in cancer immunotherapy. In this review, we describe the structural and molecular features of nonreplicating adenoviral vectors, the current limitations to their use, and strategies to modify adenoviral tropism, highlighting the approaches that may allow for the systemic administration of gene therapy.

Keywords: nonreplicating adenovirus vector; cancer; gene therapy; routes of delivery; virus coated with cancer cell membrane

1. Overview: Structural and Molecular Features of Nonreplicating Adenoviral Vectors

Adenoviruses (Ads) are one of the most well-studied and widely used viral vectors, representing 17.5% ($n = 573$) of vectors used in gene therapy clinical trials [1]. The first gene therapy was approved in 2003 by the China Food and Drug Administration. Gendicine is a recombinant nonreplicating adenovirus encoding human p53 and, despite more than 17 years of commercial use, it has only been tested in clinical trials in China for the treatment of hepatocellular, nasopharyngeal, gastric, liver, lung, breast, prostate, ovarian, and head and neck cancer, either alone or in combination with radio- or chemotherapy [2]. This therapy serves to illustrate the potential for using nonreplicating adenoviral vectors as part of effective cancer treatment.

Recently, nonreplicating adenoviral vectors have gained attention due to their use in the development of vaccines, especially to combat SARS-CoV-2, the novel coronavirus. These vaccines include those based on recombinant adenovirus serotypes, such as human adenovirus vector 5 [3–7], chimpanzee adenovirus vector ChAdOx1 [8,9], and combined human serotypes vectors 5 and 26 [10,11]. The Ad vectors can elicit robust and durable cellular and humoral immune responses [12]. The induction of a balanced innate immune response makes the Ad vectors good candidates for vaccine platforms, and they can also play a role in cancer gene therapy.

Replicating adenoviral vectors are used for the induction of oncolysis (also referred to as oncolytic adenovirus or virotherapy), and these vectors have played a major role in showing the potential of adenoviruses in cancer immunotherapy. The use of nonreplicating adenoviral vectors also deserves particular attention. We argue that nonreplicating vectors perform quite well and may even offer advantages when compared to the use of their replicating counterparts, especially concerning the delivery of proimmune but antiviral transgenes. While we do not discount oncolytic viruses, we do support the continued development of nonreplicating adenoviral vectors for cancer immunotherapy. As shown in Table 1, many clinical trials that are underway involve the use of nonreplicating adenoviral vectors for cancer gene therapy. In this review, we focus on nonreplicating adenoviral vectors, discussing vector biology and current barriers to cancer gene therapy. We also propose some strategies that enhance vector performance, especially in terms of virus delivery and targeting, thus supporting the use of nonreplicating adenoviruses for cancer immunotherapy.

Table 1. Clinical trials using nonreplicating adenoviral vectors for cancer gene therapy.

Vector	Transgene	Cancer	Mechanism	Therapy	Phase	Clinical Trial/ Reference	Status
Ad5-SGE-REIC/Dkk3	REIC/Dkk3	Localized prostate cancer	Cancer cell death induction and anticancer immunity	Neoadjuvant	I/II	NCT01931046 [13] #	Active, not recruiting
Ad5-SGE-REIC/Dkk3 (MTG201)	REIC/Dkk3	Relapsed malignant pleural mesothelioma	Cancer cell death induction and anticancer immunity	Combination with nivolumab	II	NCT04013334 [14] #	Active, recruiting
AdHSV-tk /GCV	HSV-tk Ad-hCMV-Flt3L	High-grade malignant gliomas	TK: direct tumor cell killing Flt3L: immunostimulating effects		I/II	NCT01811992 [15] #	Active, not recruiting
Adv/tk (GMCI)	HSV-tk	Advanced nonmetastatic pancreatic adenocarcinoma	TK: direct tumor cell killing	Neoadjuvant plus chemora-diation	II	NCT02446093	Active, not recruiting
Adv/tk	HSV-tk	Advanced hepatocellular carcinoma	TK: direct tumor cell killing	Liver trans-plantation	III	NCT03313596 [16] #	Active, recruiting
Adv/tk (GMCI)	Adv-tk	Pediatric brain tumors	Direct tumor cell killing	Combination with radiation therapy	I	NCT00634231 [17] #	Active, not recruiting
Adv/RSV-tk	HSV-tk	Recurrent prostate cancer	Direct tumor cell killing	Combination with brachytherapy	I/II	NCT01913106	Active, recruiting

Table 1. *Cont.*

Vector	Transgene	Cancer	Mechanism	Therapy	Phase	Clinical Trial/ Reference	Status
Adv/HSV-tk	HSV-tk	Metastatic nonsmall cell lung carcinoma and uveal melanoma	Direct tumor cell killing	Combination with stereotactic body radiation therapy or nivolumab	II	NCT02831933	Terminated (Lack of funding)
Ad/PNP + fludarabine	PNP	Head and neck squamous cell carcinoma	PNP protein actives the second component of the therapy fludarabine phosphate		I	NCT01310179 [18]	Completed
rAd-IFN/Syn-3 (Instiladrin)	IFN α-2b	High-grade nonmuscle invasive bladder cancer	Immunoregulatory effects		III	NCT02773849 [19] #	Active, not recruiting
BG00001	IFN-β	Pleural mesothelioma	Immunoregulatory effects		I	NCT00299962 [20]	Completed
Ad-RTS-hIL-12	IL-12	Advanced or metastatic breast cancer	Proinflammatory cytokine, enhances the cytotoxic activity of T-lymphocytes and resting natural killer cells	Combination with VELEDIMEX	Ib/II	NCT02423902	Unknown
Ad-RTS-hIL-12	IL-12	Recurrent or progressive glioblastoma	Proinflammatory cytokine, enhances the cytotoxic activity of T-lymphocytes and resting natural killer cells	Ad-RTS-hIL-12 + Veledimex in combination with Cemiplimab	II	NCT04006119	Active, not recruiting
Ad-RTS-hIL-12	IL-12	Glioblastoma or malignant glioma	Proinflammatory cytokine, enhances the cytotoxic activity of T-lymphocytes and resting natural killer cells	Combination with Veledimex	I	NCT02026271 [21] #	Active, not recruiting
SCH-58500	P53	Primary ovarian, fallopian tube, or peritoneal cancer	Tumor suppressor gene: antitumor effect by blocking cell cycle progression at the G1/S, activating DNA repair pathways		I	NCT00002960 [22]	Completed
Ad-p53	P53	Recurrent or metastatic head and neck squamous cell carcinoma	Tumor suppressor gene: antitumor effect by blocking cell cycle progression at the G1/S, activating DNA repair pathways	Adjuvant in combination with Anti-PD-1 or Anti-PD-L1 therapy	II	NCT03544723	Active, recruiting
ADVEXIN	P53	Squamous cell carcinoma of the oral cavity, oropharynx, hypopharynx, and larynx	Tumor suppressor gene: antitumor effect by blocking cell cycle progression at the G1/S, activating DNA repair pathways		I/II	NCT00064103 [23]	Completed

partial outcomes.

Human adenoviruses (HAds) are subdivided into seven species (A–G) and >50 serotypes based on serological properties, DNA homology, genome organization, and oncogenicity [24]. More than 100 types of human adenovirus and >200 nonhuman Ad serotypes have been identified to date [25].

Ads carry a linear double-stranded DNA genome (26 to 46 kb in length) and core proteins inside an icosahedral capsid [26]. The Ad DNA genome contains two inverted terminal repeats (100–140 bp) and can be divided into five early genes and five late genes. The capsid facets are formed by structural proteins, mainly composed of hexons, and each vertex contains a penton base that anchors the trimeric protein fiber, divided into the fiber knob and shaft. The viral particles have around one million amino acid residues (weight around 150 MDa) and an average size of 90–100 nm [27]. In the infection process, the knob interacts with cell surface receptors such as the coxsackievirus and adenovirus receptor (CAR), CD46, CD80/86, and desmoglein 2 (DSG2) [28,29]. This interaction leads to viral particle immobilization, which facilitates the interaction between the penton base and integrins [30] and, thus, virion internalization. The DNA and some core proteins are transported through the microtubular complexes to the nuclear pore and are introduced into the cell's nucleus [31]. Inside the nucleus, the viral DNA remains episomal, and the expression of the early genes (E1A, E1B, E2, E3, and E4) suppresses transcription from the host genome, thus favoring adenovirus protein synthesis and replication. Then, the late genes (L1–L5) are expressed, leading to virus encapsulation and viral particle maturation in the nucleus during the completion of the lytic cycle. Nuclear and cytoplasmatic membranes are disrupted, and new virions are released from permissive cells 48–72 h after infection [32,33].

Many characteristics of adenoviruses, such as their safety, broad cell tropism, and ability to stimulate a robust immune response, favor their use as a viral vector platform employed as a gene delivery tool in gene therapy, as an oncolytic cancer treatment, and in the development of vaccines [12,32]. Moreover, the genome of Ads is well characterized, genetically stable, and does not integrate into the host's genome but remains as episomal DNA in the cell nucleus. In addition, adenoviral vectors are modified to control viral replication, have a large cloning capacity (up to 37 kb), can transduce both dividing and quiescent cells, and have high in vivo transduction efficiency [34–36]. Human adenovirus type 5 (HAd5) is the most frequently used adenovirus for the development of gene therapy vectors, which promote the expression of transgenes in the target cells yet have impaired replication and, hence, prevent unwanted virus spread. There are three generations of nonreplicating adenoviral vectors used in gene therapy. In the first generation, E1 and E3 early genes were deleted, rendering vector replication defective but maintaining the ability to transduce host cells without killing them and liberating ~8 kb of space in the genome for the genetic payload (transgene(s) plus regulatory sequences) [37,38]. Since the E1 region is essential for virus replication, E1A proteins induce the transcription of Ad genes, and E1B proteins inhibit cellular apoptosis. Vector production requires that the E1 gene be supplied by transcomplementation, using cell lines (such as HEK293 or PERC.6) that were modified to incorporate the viral E1 region [39,40]. For the second-generation adenoviral vectors, beyond E1/E3 deletions, E2 or E4 regions have also been removed, providing additional space for cargo sequences (~10.5 kb). Third-generation adenoviral vectors were generated after deletion of almost all viral sequences except for the ITRs, the packaging signal, and minimal sequences required for genome replication and encapsulation during vector production [41].

Therefore, nonreplicating adenoviral vectors, different from their replicating counterparts, do not provoke the same cellular responses due to their lack of viral protein expression, absence of viral genome replication, and deficiency in the ability to induce cytopathic effects.

2. Current Applications of Nonreplicating Adenoviral Vectors in Cancer Immunotherapy

There are two main routes to delivering gene therapy vectors: ex vivo and in vivo. In vivo gene transfer raises concerns related to the specificity of vector transduction and transgene transcription in the intended target cells in order to achieve the desired therapeutic outcome, a goal that may be compromised by off-target effects. Ex vivo gene transfer occurs outside the body, where the patient's cells are modified and reinfused. Here, we focus on the in vivo route, particularly the challenges associated with the antiviral immune response.

In general, gene therapy approaches that overcome the immunosuppressive tumor microenvironment (TME) and activate an antitumor immune response are expected to function as cancer immunotherapies. To this end, adenoviral vectors have been modified with a variety of immune-stimulating genes, such as cytokines, costimulatory molecules, tumor-associated antigens, and tumor-suppressor genes [42]. The purpose is not only the direct killing of tumor cells but also the activation of immune cells to attack the tumor. Thus, gene therapy may induce immunogenic cell death and/or the liberation of factors that will then go on to promote the immune response.

The adenoviral vector itself is expected to participate in the activation of an antiviral response that may be both an asset and a complication for gene therapy since attracting the immune response to the tumor site is desirable but the inhibition of viral activity may thwart treatment. After viral entry, pathogen-associated molecular patterns (PAMPs), including viral nucleic acids and viral capsids, are recognized by pattern recognition receptors (PRRs) and activate antiviral immune responses that result in the production of type-I interferons (IFNs), proinflammatory cytokines, and chemokines.

Another important signaling cascade stimulated by the interaction of the virus with CAR and αv integrins is nuclear factor-kB (NF-kB), which mediates the expression of chemokines and interleukin (IL)-1 [43]. Inside the cell, viral DNA is sensed by several cytosolic PRRs such as Toll-like receptor (TLR)-9 [44], DNA-dependent activator of IFN-regulatory factors (DAIs) [45], cytosolic inflammasomes (NALP3) [46], and nucleotide-binding oligomerization domain-like receptors (NOD-like receptors (NLRs)) [47]. As a result, a signaling cascade is initiated, either dependent or independent of myeloid differentiation primary response gene 88 (MyD88), which culminates in the transcription factor (NF-kB, IRF3, IRF7)-mediated expression of IFN-α, IFN-β, and IL-6, among other proinflammatory cytokines and chemokines. In turn, the immunosuppressive TME is modulated to facilitate the recruitment of antigen-presenting cells (APCs) and helper and cytotoxic T-cells. Adenoviral vectors can be especially useful in the treatment of cold tumors [48], which lack immune infiltrate, although the increase in immune cell infiltration may not be enough for the eradication of the tumor [49]. Thus, the approach may be improved if the vector is armed with additional immune-stimulating factors.

Replication-deficient adenoviral vectors have been employed as vaccines and in cancer gene therapy due to strong humoral and T-cell responses to transgenes expressed by the vector [50]. Tatsis et al. (2007) showed that the application of replication-defective adenoviral vectors resulted in sustained levels of CD8$^+$ T-cells specific for the transgene product and persistent levels of transcriptionally active adenoviral vector genomes at the site of inoculation in the liver and lymphatic tissues [51]. In comparisson, replicating adenoviral vectors mimic natural virus infection, resulting in the induction of cytokines and costimulatory molecules that provide a potent adjuvant effect [52]. Both nonreplicating and replicating Ad vectors have been shown to activate effector CD8$^+$ T-cells and central memory T-cells in treated mice. For this, Osada et al. [53] compared Ad5[E1+]CEA, a replicating adenoviral vector carrying the carcinoembryonic antigen (CEA) with two nonreplicating vectors, Ad5[E1−] and Ad5[E1−, E2b−]. When used for the ex vivo transduction of human dendritic cells (DCs), they found that all three vectors yielded similar infectivity and temporal dynamics of transgene expression. In addition, replicating Ad5[E1+]CEA showed toxicity to DCs, eliciting less maturation of DCs and greater clearance by NK cells.

Moreover, Ad5[E1−] and Ad5[E1−, E2b−] were superior to Ad5[E1+] in their capacity to induce and expand antigen-specific T-cell responses. The results suggest that increased replication of an Ad vector may result in diminished efficacy in this scenario, and the deletion of E1, E2, and E3 genes promoted a superior generation of CEA-specific T-cell responses in mice with pre-existing Ad5 immunity.

In the following discussion, we highlight some of the strategies for using nonreplicating adenoviral vectors as cancer immunotherapies in preclinical and clinical assays.

For example, preclinical outcomes in a prostate cancer model have revealed the benefit of immunotherapy based on a heterologous prime-boost, where the virus is injected as a vaccine with concomitant administration of a PD-1-blocking antibody. Similarly, a ChAdOx1–MVA vaccination strategy (a simian adenovirus, ChAdOx1, with the modified vaccinia Ankara virus, MVA) induced CD8$^+$ T-cell responses to the tumor-specific self-antigen of prostate 1 (STEAP1) in murine models. The combination with the anti-PD-1 antibody improved the survival of the animals since tumors were abolished in 80% of the mice [54].

Our laboratory has developed an adenoviral vector, AdRGD-PG, with improved tropism and transgene expression. By including the RGD motif in the fiber knob, transduction no longer relies on CAR but instead uses integrins, which are more widely distributed. The use of a p53-responsive promoter (called PG) to control transgene expression resulted in high-level expression in the presence of wild-type p53 [55,56]. When used to deliver p19Arf (a functional partner of p53) and IFN-β, we observed cooperation between these genes for the induction of cell death in vitro and in vivo using the mouse model of melanoma, B16–F10 [56,57]. Moreover, only combined gene transfers conferred the emission of immunogenic cell death markers ATP, calreticulin, and HMGB1 [56]. The combination of p19Arf and IFN-β proved to be an effective immunotherapy since we confirmed the participation of natural killer (NK) cells and CD4$^+$ and CD8$^+$ T-lymphocytes in immune protection against B16-F10 tumor progression [58]. Other assays showed that the gene transfer of p19Arf and IFN-β using our nonreplicating Ad vector in the LLC1 mouse model of lung carcinoma was able to induce markers of immunogenic cell death. In situ gene therapy with IFN-β, either alone or in combination with p19Arf, could retard tumor progression, but only the combination approach limited the progression of challenge tumors, thus acting as an in situ vaccine [59]. Thus, the p19Arf + IFN-β gene transfer approach induces oncolysis and immune activation even in the absence of viral replication, functioning as a cancer vaccine and immunotherapy, at least in mice [60,61].

We have taken great care to use different models to demonstrate the functionality of our approach since it involves IFN-β, which is known to have species-specific activities [62]. To examine our approach in human melanoma cell lines, we used the AdRGD-PG backbone to construct vectors encoding the human cDNAs p14ARF and hIFN-β and showed immunogenic cell death characterized by the emission of critical markers in vitro as well as successful ex vivo priming of human T-cells [63].

Most of the clinical trials using nonreplicating Ads are in Phase I/II (Table 1). Kumon et al. [13] have demonstrated in preclinical and clinical data the benefit of in situ Ad-REIC (adenoviral vector carrying the human *REIC/Dkk-3* gene) treatment. In preclinical data, they showed that Ad-REIC induces selective toxicity in response to endoplasmic reticulum stress and IL-7 overproduction by infected normal cells, including cells of the TME. These cells can activate innate immunity, especially NK cells, as well as cytotoxic T-lymphocytes (CTLs). In addition, DCs induced by secreted REIC proteins can present cancer antigens from apoptotic cancer cells and induce tumor-associated antigen-specific CD8$^+$ CTLs. In clinical settings, preliminary outcomes have shown cytopathic effects and tumor-infiltrating lymphocytes in patients with high-risk localized prostate cancer, undergoing radical prostatectomy, who received two ultrasound-guided intratumoral injections at 2-week intervals, followed by surgery six weeks after the second injection.

Another interesting approach is gene-mediated cytotoxic immunotherapy (GMCI), which uses an adenoviral vector expressing the herpes simplex virus (HSV) thymidine kinase (TK) gene (ADV/HSV-TK), followed by an antiherpetic prodrug. The HSV-TK protein has two principal functions: (1) nucleotide analog products of prodrug phosphorylation lead to the death of dividing cancer cells, and (2) TK is a superantigen that stimulates a potent immune reaction [64]. GMCI activates the stimulator of interferon genes (STING) pathway, enhancing the production of proinflammatory cytokines such as IFNs and promoting T-cell activation. The first study using ADV/HSV-TK plus ganciclovir for the treatment of human prostate cancer was conducted by Herman et al. [65]. The patients received a single injection of the vector (10^8 to 10^{11} vector particles) into the prostate gland in the region with the greatest concentration of tumor cells. Not only did the regimen prove safe, with minimal toxicity, but three patients that received 10^9–10^{11} viral particles had a decrease of more than 50% in serum prostate-specific antigen (PSA) levels for periods ranging from 45 to 330 days. The safety and efficacy of GMCI to convert the TME from cold to hot have been noted for studies in different tumor types, including glioma [66], retinoblastoma [67], and mesothelioma [68].

A promising Phase III clinical trial is being conducted on patients with BCG refractory nonmuscle invasive bladder cancer (NMIBC). This disease is an early form of bladder cancer, and the recommended treatment for these patients is the use of intravesical Bacillus Calmette-Guérin (BCG). However, data has shown that around 30% to 50% of cases will recur. The outcomes of BCG-unresponsive patients are poor, and total cystectomy (complete removal of the bladder) is the standard of care for patients who are operative candidates [69].

Alternatively, patients with bladder cancer are treated with nadofaragene firadenovec (rAd–IFN-α2b/Syn3), a replication-deficient recombinant Ad carrying the interferon-α gene, which can have both TRAIL- and non-TRAIL-mediated cytotoxic effects. The patients receive the treatment directly into the bladder using a catheter every three months, and there is elevated interferon production and, consequently, increased exposure to urothelium-enhanced cytotoxic activity. Among 157 patients with carcinoma in situ, 53% of patients achieved a complete response in as early as three months, and about 24% of patients remained free of high-grade recurrence at one year. The outcomes are encouraging and currently awaiting Food and Drug Administration (FDA) approval [70].

As mentioned before, replication-defective Ads are also used as cancer vaccine strategies. GVAX, a GM-CSF gene-modified tumor vaccine, was developed by transducing autologous tumor cells with E1/E3-deleted Ad vectors encoding GM-CSF in autologous tumor cells extracted from each patient. In a phase I/II trial, 33 patients with NSCLCs that were refractory to standard treatment received the GVAX vaccine consisting of 5–100×10^6 irradiated tumor cells per dose, every 2 weeks. This strategy was shown to be safe, and three patients had radiologically complete responses that lasted for more than six months [71].

Nonreplicating Ads have also been exploited as delivery vehicles in dendritic cells (DCs). Briefly, viral particles processed via proteasome result in the presentation of self and foreign antigens by MHCI and MHCII molecules to both CD8$^+$ and CD4$^+$ T-cells, inducing protective humoral and cellular immunity [72]. A phase I/II clinical trial tested the immune response against a vaccine consisting of autologous DCs obtained from patients, transduced ex vivo with Ads encoding the full-length melanoma antigen MART-1/Melan-A. This study pointed to an increase in CD8$^+$ and CD4$^+$ T-cells in 6/11 and 2/4 metastatic melanoma patients, respectively [73].

Another phase I clinical trial performed on patients with advanced NSCLC showed the induction of systemic tumor antigen-specific immune responses with enhanced CD8$^+$ T-cell infiltration of tumors in 7/13 of patients. The treatment consisted of two intradermal injections of autologous DCs, transduced ex vivo with an Ad vector expressing the CCL21 gene [74]. Similar outcomes have been observed in small cell lung cancer, where 41.8% of patients presented specific anti-p53 immune responses when treated with a vaccine consisting of DCs transduced with an Ad encoding p53 [75]. These positive outcomes are not limited to solid tumors. In a phase II study, acute myeloid leukemia (AML) patients with early molecular relapse received a modified DC vaccine. The DCs were modified with two tumor-associated antigens (TAAs), survivin and MUC1, plus secretory bacterial flagellin for DC maturation and RNA interference to suppress SOCS1. The complete remission rate was 83% among all relapsed AML patients [76].

TAAs are usually expressed in normal tissues at low levels but overexpressed in tumor cells. Many TAAs have been identified as targets for tumor-reactive T-cells and can be isolated from tumor-infiltrating lymphocytes (TILs) [77]. In contrast, tumor-specific antigens (TSAs) are only encoded in cancer cells as a consequence of somatic mutations that alter the amino acid sequence, resulting in foreign proteins that can be presented to the immune system. Therefore, the neoantigens are less susceptible to the mechanisms of immunological tolerance, comprising an interesting target for vaccination [78]. Thus, gene-based vaccination using Ad vectors as a delivery agent is emerging as one of the most promising approaches for loading antigens (TAA or TSA) onto DCs. Important advantages of this modified DC approach include persistent expression of the antigen that results in activation of CD4$^+$ and CD8$^+$ T-cells and the induction of antibody responses and the natural adjuvant stimulating effect that Ads mediate, which contributes to DC maturation [79].

As mentioned above, ex vivo modification of DCs followed by the reintroduction of these cells in the patient is a standard strategy for these vaccines. Even so, in situ targeting of DCs has been explored using either human or murine cells, though it can often be limited by the patient's pre-existing immunity against the adenovirus [80].

3. Challenges of Using Adenoviral Vectors

Even though the use of nonreplicating adenoviral vectors has shown great promise for cancer immunotherapy, several aspects of the virus and its delivery present barriers to its effectiveness. Ideally, the vector should transfer the gene to the intended cell type without causing undue antiviral host responses. In the following discussion, we present the molecular basis for Ad tropism, the anti-Ad immune responses, and the issues surrounding the systemic administration of Ad vectors. With a thorough understanding of these mechanisms, we can then explore solutions for the challenges that they pose.

3.1. Tissue Tropism

As mentioned previously, most human adenovirus serotypes use CAR as their primary receptor, which is expressed on several cell types, including hepatocytes, myocardiocytes, myoblasts, and epithelial and endothelial cells [51] (Table 2). Additionally, some Ads can bind to CD46, a complement regulatory protein that is present on most nucleated human cells, including hematopoietic stem cells and dendritic cells, as well as the costimulatory molecules CD80 and CD86, present on antigen-presenting cells [81–83]. Different primary receptors such as integrin $\alpha v \beta 5$, heparin sulfate proteoglycans, sialic acid, and DSG2 and GD1a glycans have also been reported to support adenovirus internalization [81,84,85], with different primary receptors influencing the route of intracellular viral traffic [86].

Table 2. Classification and tropism of human adenoviruses.

Classification and Tropism of Human Adenoviruses			
Subgroup	Serotypes	Identified Receptors	Tropism
A	12, 18, 31, 61	CAR	Enteric, respiratory
B	3, 7, 11, 14, 16, 21, 34, 35, 50, 55, 66,68, 76–79	CD46, DSG2, CD80, CD86	Renal, ocular, respiratory
C	1, 2, 5, 6, 57, 89	CAR, VCAM-1, HSPG, MHC1-a2, SR	Ocular, lymphoid, respiratory, hepatic
D	8–10, 13, 15, 17, 19, 20, 22–30, 32, 33, 36–39, 42–49, 51, 53, 54, 56, 58–60, 62–65, 67, 69–75, 80–88, 90–103	SA, CD46, CAR, GD1a	Ocular, enteric
E	4	CAR	Ocular, respiratory
F	40, 41	CAR	Enteric
G	52	CAR, AS	Enteric

CAR: coxsackie adenovirus receptor. DSG2: desmoglein-2. GD1a: GD1a ganglioside. HSPG, heparin sulfate proteoglycans. MHC1-a2: major histocompatibility complex-a2. SA: sialic acid. SR: scavenger receptor. VCAM-1, vascular cell adhesion molecule-1. Adapted from [85,87].

Engineered HAd can transduce target cells and are internalized in a similar way to wild-type adenovirus infection. The internalization can be augmented by interactions between an arginine-glycine-aspartate (RGD) motif found in the penton base and integrins. Upon attaching to CAR, the fiber knob disassociates from the capsid, and the exposed penton base interacts with a secondary receptor, usually membrane integrins $\alpha v \beta 3$ or $\alpha v \beta 5$, responsible for virus internalization [86,88], followed by virion endocytosis via integrin-mediated signaling [86,89].

Different subgroups of adenovirus can use different types of integrins as receptors, reinforcing their characteristic cell tropism [89,90]. The virus enters the cell by a clathrin-coated vesicle and is transported in endosomes, where capsid disassembly occurs due to endosome acidity. The virion escapes the endosome and traffics to the nucleus by microtubular complexes, where replication occurs [31,85]. After 2 h, about 40% of the internalized wild-type virions arrive in the nucleus, ready to be transcribed due to their double-stranded genome. Additionally, 48–72 h after infection, nuclear and cytoplasmatic membranes are disrupted, and around 10,000 new virions are released [32].

Different serotypes may favor particular receptors; for example, HAd5 from subgroup C has been shown to utilize CAR for facilitating entry into cells [91], while HAd11 and HAd35 from subgroup B utilize CD46 as their primary receptor [83]. As mentioned, the adenoviral vectors may be chosen due to their inherent tissue-specificity and compatibility with the intended route of administration. For example, when the virus is injected into the brain, tropism for specific cell populations depends on the interaction with CAR, and lower transduction is observed with vectors that bind neither to CAR nor integrins [92]. Even so, HAd5 has been shown to enter cells by CAR-independent mechanisms, including via a hexon–lactoferrin bridge [93,94]

The native tropism of Ads for CAR on the cell surface and the interaction of viral vectors with nontarget tissues can result in toxicity and poor therapeutic efficacy. Thus, viral proteins can be genetically tailored to expand or restrict viral replication, and vector replication machinery can even be modified to augment or restrict viral replication in target cells [49]. Beyond that, nonhuman adenoviruses, such as canine (CAd2), bovine (BAd3), chimpanzee (ChAd1-7, ChAd68), and ovine (OAd7), can also be used to overcome the pre-existing immunity in human patients [95].

3.2. Pre-Existing Immunity in the Host

Due to the growing application of adenoviral vectors in gene therapy and vaccines, studies of seroprevalence in global populations are important. However, these studies may be limited by the lack of data from South America, Australasia, and most African countries [96]. Moreover, predominant HAdV types can change over time within a region [97], and transmission of new strains across continents appears to be frequent. A recent study conducted by Mennechet et al. [96] showed that HAdV-D26 seroprevalence appears to be relatively high in Africa and Asia and low in North America and Europe, while HAdV-B35 seroprevalence is low worldwide. HAdV-C5 is the most common serotype that infects humans, particularly in developing countries [98,99], and it is one the most commonly used adenoviral vectors; thus, the limitations on the applicability of the HadV-C5 vector, due to pre-existing immunity, have led to the construction of novel vectors derived from rare Ad serotypes [100].

HAd serotypes are often associated with specific diseases. For instance, serotypes 2–5, 7, and 21 commonly infect the respiratory tract of individuals [101–104], while serotypes 8, 19, and 37 are responsible for keratoconjunctivitis outbreaks [105–107]. Pharyngoconjunctivitis is often associated with serotypes 3, 4, and 7 [108,109] and acute gastroenteritis with serotypes 40 and 41 [110,111]. Likewise, neurological disorders and obesity seem to have some correlation with adenoviral infections [112–114]. Due to this frequent occurrence of these infections worldwide, humans have extensive preexisting immunity to adenoviruses [115–119].

HAd capsid proteins are very immunogenic, especially the hexon protein [120]. The host's adaptive immunity arm detects the hypervariable regions (HVRs) in the hexon protein and releases serotype-specific neutralizing antibodies (NAs) that appear to block a postentry step [121,122]. Thus, at second contact with the same adenovirus serotype, the host NAs may rapidly neutralize it. Interestingly, at the same time, coagulation factor X (FX) in the blood binds to the hexon protein and activates complements (C4 and C4BP in the classical and alternative complement pathways) against the adenoviruses. In a fair number of tested individuals, it also protected the virions from neutralization by serum components [123]. The HAd5 vector interacts with FX, which, in turn, binds cell surface heparan sulfate proteoglycans on hepatocytes; thus, FX is essential for intravenously injected Ad5 vectors to transduce the liver [124].

Even with FX binding the hexon proteins, anti-knob fiber and anti-penton base antibodies can also prevent the adenovirus from transducing cells [125]. Nevertheless, the HAd species C knob and penton base proteins have also been shown to induce serotype-specific NAs [126].

Beyond antibodies, strong and sustained CD8$^+$ T-cell responses follow adenoviral infections [127]. Up to one-third of circulating T-cells against HAd have been reported to be CD4$^+$ T-cells specific for a hexon epitope conserved between HAd serotypes. Hence, the host's preexisting CD4$^+$ T-lymphocytes might promptly respond to various subsequent adenovirus serotypes in either blood or gut [128].

3.3. Different Administration Routes and Their Particularities

Although the administration of lower doses of Ads is well-tolerated, higher doses are known to overstimulate innate and adaptive immune responses, which might result in acute toxicity. For example, with HAd5 at the concentration 1×10^{11} PFU/kg, 70% of hepatocytes and 15% of Kupffer cells expressed transgene three days later [129]. Systemic delivery, which theoretically could solve the issue of reaching metastatic foci, is confounded by sequestration of the virus by the liver and the subsequent antiviral immune response as well as possible liver damage [130]. For example, at doses up to 4×10^{12} vp/kg of HAd5, approximately 98% of the injected virus was found in the liver 30 min after injection [131]. Thus, systemic delivery of adenoviral vectors is associated with dose-dependent toxicity and a high risk of hepatotoxicity. Several studies have shown that the delivery of adenoviral vectors to immunocompetent mice by different routes, such as intravenous [132], intraperitoneal and intratracheal [133] or via direct injection into the pancreas, resulted in the production of neutralizing antibodies, decreasing the effectiveness of a second administration [134].

The relationship between the route of administration and viral load on CD8$^+$ T-cell populations has already been studied. Holst et al. [135] administered adenoviral vectors encoding β-galactosidase by intravenous or subcutaneous routes and then examined transgene-specific CD8$^+$ T-cells. Independently of the route of administration, doses above 10^9 particles were disseminated systemically. In moderate doses, both routes induced a transient peak of IFN-γ produced by CD8$^+$ T-cells 2 to 3 weeks postinfection. However, with intravenous administration, these cells were only detected in the liver. Additionally, after 2 to 4 months, the systemic immunization created dysfunctional transgene-specific CD8$^+$ T-cells impaired in both cytokine production and in vivo effector functions as well as the accumulation of specific CD8$^+$ T-cells in the spleen. Thus, the most important influence of adenovirus administration on CD8$^+$ T cell response is the route of injection and not the total antigen load [135].

In another study, the intralymphnodal administration of a nonreplicating recombinant adenoviral vector encoding the LacZ reporter gene in canine lymphosarcoma was found to be safe, with no relevant adverse effects. This finding presents the potential for its administration to lymph node metastases in both animal and human models [136]. The examples above demonstrate that efficient gene delivery using adenoviral vectors can be performed without hepatic injury or systemic immunogenicity if off-target effects are avoided. To this end, several strategies have been developed to minimize interactions of the adenoviral vector with the liver and to protect the virus from neutralizing antibodies. Some of these approaches, such as the engineering of adenovirus capsid, hexon, or fiber proteins, use of nonhuman serotypes, and nanoformulation-coated adenoviral vectors will be discussed in more detail below.

4. Strategies to Modify Adenovirus Tropism

Although Ads infect many different types of cells, low (or no) expression of CAR, especially in tumor cells, confounds the attachment step and represents one of the hurdles to gene therapy using adenoviral vectors. Several strategies have been employed to overcome this barrier and redirect the Ads to the intended recipient and, consequently, decrease off-target effects (Figure 1).

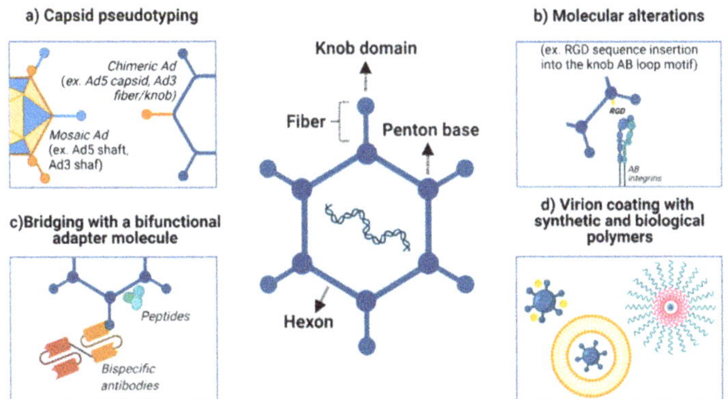

Figure 1. Improvements in vector delivery to and targeting of cancer cells. (**a**) Several approaches can be used to modify viral attachment and entry, such as inhibiting the binding to natural receptors (detargeting) and creating tropism for neoplasms and their metastatic foci (retargeting). (**b**) An alternative to CAR-mediated viral attachment is modifying the fiber (for example, incorporation of the RGD sequence into the knob AB-loop motif). (**c**) Ad structure permits retargeting through the incorporation of synthetic molecules and antibody fragments within the virus capsid. (**d**) Both biological (e.g., cell membrane, liposome) and chemical (e.g., gold, silver, PEG) approaches may be used to coat the virus and improved delivery, especially for the systemic route. PEG: polyethylene glycol. Created with BioRender.com.

4.1. Modifications in Viral Entry: Attachment Receptors and Virus Internalization

To explore the targeting of adenovirus particles to tumor cells, initial events related to infection/transduction must be modulated: (i) viral attachment and (ii) viral entry. This strategy can target tissues by inhibiting binding to natural receptors (detargeting) in normal liver cells, for example, and, simultaneously, creating tropism for neoplasms and their metastatic foci (retargeting) [137]. Another strategy is pseudotyping, the creation of variants by recombining their capsid proteins. Here, we detail works that have used a variety of strategies to modify tropism.

The tropism of HAd5 is predominantly mediated by the interaction of fiber/knob with CAR. As an alternative to CAR-mediated viral attachment, one of the classical fiber modifications is the incorporation of the RGD sequence into the knob AB-loop motif, which greatly expands the spectrum of cell types that may be transduced [138]. Even so, the genetic incorporation of an RGD-4C peptide into the HI loop or the C-terminal end of the HAd5 fiber knob modifies the Ad knob domain without ablating native CAR-binding [139]. Another possibility is the insertion of positively charged polylysine motifs [140]. This modification permits the virus to target the tumor cell's heparan sulfate proteoglycans, common constituents of the cell surface, and the extracellular matrix, overexpressed in several different cancer types, including cervical cancer [141].

On the other hand, directing transduction and expression of the transgenes to occur only in tumor cells (but not in normal cells) should minimize the adverse effects of the therapy. Wickham and coworkers [142] successfully used bispecific antibodies to promote the targeting of an adenoviral vector to endothelial and smooth muscle cells. However, the attempt to noncovalently associate antibodies or molecules with the surface of the viral particle may be hampered by the instability of this binding, especially if used in vivo. For this reason, the adenovirus fiber gene sequence can be edited and, thus, the peptide ligands can be incorporated directly into the protein sequence [137,143–145].

Taking cues from the phage display technique, adenovirus libraries can be generated with random peptide combinations and screened for their ability to transduce a particular cell type, thus refining specificity to tumor populations in a strict manner [146–148]. Joung et al. [148] devised a technique for producing adenovirus with modified fibers that involved cotransfecting a packaging cell with a plasmid encoding a genetically fiber-less adenovirus with a plasmid containing the open reading frames (ORFs) of the fiber of interest. Moreover, Yoshida et al. [144] developed a Cre-lox-mediated recombination system using a plasmid library encoding modified fiber and the adenoviral genome. Using this approach, these authors inserted unique peptides, each with seven random amino acids, into the AB-loop of the fiber, and, after screening, they were successful in targeting these viral vectors to glioma cells [143,149]. Although the idea seems highly promising, there are technical complications that hinder this approach. The compaction and self-assembly of the protein monomers to form the adenovirus particle is a very delicate process. The insertion of random peptides can compromise the final structure of the viral particle as well as virus production [150].

Even though two receptors are required for the adenovirus particle to penetrate the target cells, each interaction is a distinct step. While attachment receptors apparently only recognize the target cell, the HAd5 penton base–αv integrin interaction activates signaling pathways such as p38MAPK [151,152] and Rho GTPases [153], which then trigger changes in the cell cytoskeleton for endocytosis mediated by clathrin [153,154]. Interestingly, mutation of the penton base RGD sequence slows but does not impair virus internalization and infection, nor does it prevent liver tropism [86].

4.2. Pseudotyping the Capsid Using Components from Different Adenoviruses

Chimeric adenoviruses are usually based on HAd5 with the fiber or its knob domain replaced by that of another serotype [155]. This creates perspectives for the recombination of these subtypes and, thus, the modulation of targeting: a concept known as pseudotyping. However, the resulting range of tropisms will be restricted to the respective serotypes used in the construction and may not necessarily contemplate the range of existing receptors found in neoplasms. Table 3 summarizes important findings in studies that have employed adenovirus pseudotyping strategies.

Table 3. Different studies using adenovirus pseudotyping strategies.

Attachment Receptor	Tropism	Modification	Serotype Origin/ Subgroup	Results	Reference
CD46	Glioma	Fiber replacement	Ad35, Ad16, Ad50	Increased transduction of patient-derived cells	[156]
Adenovirus serotype 3 receptor	Ovarian cancer cells	Fiber knob replacement	Ad3 (modified)/B1	Enhanced gene transfer to various cancer cell lines and primary tumor tissues	[157]
Adenovirus serotype 3 receptor	Lung cancer (NSCLC primary tissue)	Fiber knob replacement	Ad3 (modified)/B1	Improved killing of NSCLC cells	[158]
Sialic acid, phage display for kidney	Renal cancer and detargeting the liver	Fiber knob replacement	Ad5 (modified)/19p (fiber)	Reduced liver tropism and improved gene transfer to renal cancer	[159]
Unidentified cellular receptor	Cancer cell lines of pancreatic, breast, lung, esophageal, and ovarian	Fiber knob replacement	Ad5 (modified)/D49	Efficiently transduced	[160]
CD46	Primary human cell cultures	Fiber replacement	Ad5PTD/F35	Increased transduction capacity of T-cells, monocytes, macrophages, dendritic cells, pancreatic islets, mesenchymal stem cells, and tumor-initiating cells	[161]

PTD: Tat-PTD hexon modification.

4.3. Encapsulation of Adenovirus Using Synthetic Polymers

Shielding the virus with nanoparticles allows the Ad to escape immune recognition and avoid the undesirable accumulation of the vector in the liver upon systemic delivery. Furthermore, this approach can enhance the specific targeting of tumor cells. Several studies have been conducted to evaluate the efficacy of encapsulation of negatively charged Ads with cationic liposomes or particles that aim to prevent virus clearance from circulation [162].

Some Ad features, such as regular geometries, well-characterized surface properties, and nanoscale dimensions, make it a biocompatible scaffold for a wide variety of inorganic and biological structures. The Ad capsid has free lysines, the majority of them located on hexon, penton, and fiber proteins, which can be covalently linked to other molecules such as polymers, sugars, biotin, and fluorophores [163]. Polymers offer a wide range of conjugation and encapsulation that make them a safe option for immunotherapy. The main biopolymers studied are polyethylene glycol (PEG) and hydroxylpropyl methacrylamide (pHPMA), the latter being covalently bound to capsid proteins; thus, it can efficiently transduce solid tumors after intravenous injection into mice [164]. The first study using this polymer demonstrated passive tumor targeting of polymer-coated adenoviruses administered by intravenous injection; the authors observed that the coated virus accumulated inside solid subcutaneous AB22 mesothelioma tumors 40 times more than the unmodified virus [164].

As mentioned, Ad structure permits retargeting through the incorporation of synthetic molecules and antibody fragments within the virus capsid. For instance, PEG is an uncharged, hydrophilic, nonimmunogenic, synthetic linear polymer (CH_2CH_2O repetitions) [165] that is frequently utilized in the biopharmaceutical industry and can be useful to protect therapeutic molecules from proteolysis as well as humoral and cellular immune responses [166]. According to Fisher et al. [164], one advantage of vector PEGylation is the retention of viability after storage at various temperatures compared to conventional Ads. Covalent attachment of PEG to the adenovirus capsid may be achieved by using PEG activation mechanisms. PEG presents hydroxyl groups (OH) that make PEG-protein bonds impossible; thus, it is necessary to use chemical activation before protein attachment. In the specific case of adenoviruses, activation can be achieved through the use of tresyl-monomethoxypolyethylene glycol (TMPEG), succinimidyl succinate-monomethoxypolyethylene glycol (SSPEG), or cyanuric chloride-monomethoxypolyethylene glycol (CCPEG), which react preferentially with lysine residues in the capsid, thus supporting the formation of covalent bonds with PEG [167].

In addition to the PEGylation of the virus particle, ligands can also bind to the opposite extremity of PEG, thus providing a specific ligand to retarget the virus to the corresponding cellular receptor.

Such approaches also aid the vector in reaching distant tumor sites, as found by Eto et al. [167]. They used a cationic liposome that was composed of (1, 2-dioleoyloxypropyl)-N, N, N-trimethy-lammonium chloride:cholesterol to encapsulate the Ad vectors carrying the antiangiogenic gene (pigment epithelium-derived factor (PEDF)). The results showed that systemic administration of Ad-PEDF/liposome was well tolerated and caused the suppression of tumor growth. The coated Ad-PEDF increased apoptosis compared to uncoated Ad in the B16-F10 melanoma cell line and inhibited murine pulmonary metastasis in vivo. Moreover, Ad-luciferase encapsulated with liposome exhibited decreased liver tropism and increased transduction in the lung. Additionally, the anti-Ad IgG level after administration of the Ad-PEDF/liposome was significantly lower compared to Ad-PEDF alone. Eto et al. [167] showed that positively charged 14-nm gold nanoparticles increased the efficiency of Ad infection in mesenchymal stem cells, usually refractory to Ad transduction, mainly because CAR expression is absent or downregulated. The strategies described here support future exploration of additional formulations for liposome-encapsulated adenoviruses and their ability to target cancer cells.

4.4. Cancer Cell Membrane-Coated Adenoviral Vectors

Nanoparticle-based delivery systems have been extensively explored for improving cancer treatment. Cell membranes, which can be obtained from a variety of source cells, including leukocytes, platelets, red blood cells, and cancer cells, are being employed to encapsulate particles such as liposomes, polymers, silica, and Ad vectors in order to improve tumor-targeted drug delivery in addition to prolonged circulation time, reduced interaction with macrophages, and decreased nanoparticle uptake in the liver [168]. The membrane-based functions of cancer-related cells include extravasation, chemotaxis, and cancer cell adhesion [169]. As a source of cell membranes, cancer cells offer certain advantages. They can be obtained from cell lines or patient samples and possess a wide range of membrane surface proteins, such as MHC, TAAs, and neoantigens, that can program the immune system to attack local and distant tumor sites [170], as represented in Figure 2.

Tumors frequently develop a variety of mechanisms to subvert immune attack, resulting in an immune-suppressive TME. Although tumor cells can stimulate a variety of cell types, including fibroblasts, immune-inflammatory cells, and endothelial cells, through the production and secretion of stimulatory growth factors and cytokines [171], the TME can be modulated by the tumor cells themselves and tumor-infiltrating leukocytes (including regulatory T-cells (Tregs)), myeloid-derived suppressor cells (MDSCs), and alternatively activated (type 2) macrophages (M2), cytokines (IL-10, TGF-β), expression of inhibitory receptors (such as cytotoxic T-lymphocyte antigen 4 (CTLA-4) and programmed death-ligand 1 (PD-L1)) or impediment of T-cell function, resulting in the reduced effectiveness of immunotherapy [172]. Although many TAAs have been identified, their immunogenicity is generally insufficient to elicit potent antitumor responses. Typically, when the tumor reaches the malignant stage, the most immunogenic tumor-specific antigens have been eliminated via negative selection. Frequently, the nanoparticles are associated with adjuvants, secretory cytokines, antibodies, and/or viral vectors to improve the immune response [173].

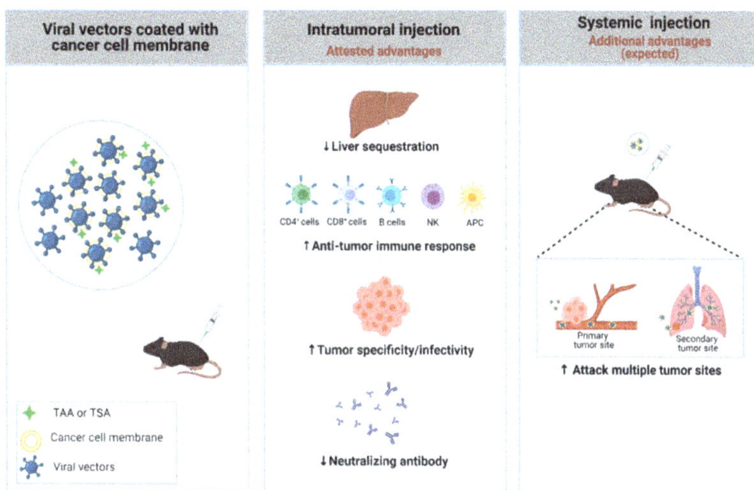

Figure 2. Strategy used to improve the specificity of adenoviral vectors. An adenovirus coated with a cancer cell membrane has some advantages, such as the presence of TSA and TAA, which aids the anti-tumor immune response. Additionally, the membrane can be engineered to present specific molecules/receptors, improving the power of interaction with the tumor. Moreover, the viral coating can offer several benefits, including suppression of liver toxicity, increase of specific infectivity to cancer cells, preferential antitumor (not antiviral) immune response, and escape from pre-existing neutralizing antibodies in both routes of delivery (intratumoral and systemic). Systemic administration using virus coated with membranes could offer a highly desirable outcome: targeting metastatic foci. TAA: tumor-associated antigens; TSA: tumor-specific antigens. Created with BioRender.com.

Coating polymeric nanoparticles with cancer cell membranes can be used for different types of cancer therapy. For anticancer drug delivery, Zhuang et al. [173] showed that polymeric nanoparticle cores made of poly(lactic-co-glycolic acid) (PLGA), a polymer coated in an MDA-MB-435 membrane, significantly increased cellular adhesion to the source cells compared to naked nanoparticles due to a homotypic binding mechanism. For cancer immunotherapy, the authors demonstrated that a polymer coated with a B16−F10 membrane, which creates a stabilized particle, facilitated the uptake of membrane-bound tumor antigens and, consequently, the presentation and maturation of DCs. Another approach using a biohybrid (tumor-membrane-coated) nanoparticle was also able to elicit an antitumor immune response in melanoma models, changing the microenvironment profile. The administration of the vaccine enhanced the activation of APCs and increased the priming of CD8⁺ T-cells. When combining the nanovaccine with a checkpoint inhibitor, 87.5% of the animals responded, including two complete remissions, when compared to the immune checkpoint inhibitor alone. These results point to opportunities for the association of nanoparticles and immunomodulators to enhance T-cell responses [174].

The effects from the association of polymers, cancer cell membranes, and adjuvants were also observed by Fontana et al. [175]. PLGA nanoparticles were loaded with the TLR7 agonist and then coated with membranes from B16-OVA cancer cells since the presentation of foreign peptide OVA permits the tracking of responses. The nanovaccine was able to enhance uptake by antigen-presenting cells and showed efficacy in delaying tumor growth as a preventative vaccine besides displaying activity against established tumors when coadministered with the anti-programmed death 1 (PD-1) monoclonal antibody.

In another study, CpG oligodeoxynucleotide (CpG) was used as an immunological adjuvant and encapsulated into PLGA nanoparticle cores coated with membranes derived from B16–F10 mouse melanoma cells. The effect of nanoformulation on DC maturation was observed by the upregulated expression of costimulatory markers CD40, CD80, CD86, and MHC-II. Both prophylactic and therapeutic vaccines presented positive results. In the prophylactic study using the poorly immunogenic wild-type B16–F10 model, tumor occurrence was prevented in 86% of mice 150 days after challenge with tumor cells. Interestingly, mice vaccinated with the CpG-nanoformulation alone had tumor growth comparable to the control group and a median survival of 22 days. This reinforces the role of the cancer cell membrane in targeting the elimination of malignant cells by the immune system. In the therapeutic model, mice challenged with B16–F10 cells and subsequently treated with the nanoformulation presented a modest ability to control tumor growth. However, the combination of nanoformulation and a checkpoint blockade cocktail (anti-CTLA4 and anti-PD1) significantly enhanced tumor growth control. As such, the results encourage further research into nanoparticle vaccine formulation and possible associations with other immunotherapies that modulate different aspects of immunity [176].

In a different strategy, Fusciello et al. [177] combined an oncolytic virus (due to its natural adjuvant properties) and cancer cell membranes carrying tumor antigens. They found that viral transduction was significantly increased with the coated virus, implying an uptake mechanism different than that utilized by the naked virus, which requires CAR, representing a significant advantage for transducing CAR-negative cell lines. Additionally, the coated virus was better able to control tumor growth compared to other treatments. The vaccination using coated viruses created a highly specific anticancer immune response, redirecting the immune response against the tumor [177]. Thus, personalized cancer vaccines can represent an alternative approach to target cancer even without determining specific antigens for each patient. We hypothesize that this approach will also be applicable to nonreplicating adenoviral vectors, though this has not yet been shown.

4.5. Association of Antibodies and Viral Structures

The incorporation of antibodies into the viral structure is another interesting option for creating specificity. Despite the obstacles to the use of conventional antibodies (human, murine, and goat), smaller molecules from other species, such as alpacas, can be added to the structure of the Ad capsid without disturbing its synthesis and assembly. For example, van Erp et al. [178] generated a single domain camelid antibody against the human carcinoembryonic antigen present in human colorectal adenocarcinoma cells. They incorporated this molecule into the adenovirus capsid, achieving a more specific tropism for tumor cells and reducing off-target toxicity. Although the strategy was developed to retarget oncolytic viruses, it can also be used to improve nonreplicative adenoviral vectors.

Despite the cited possibilities, the need to re-engineer vectors de novo for each novel target may be an unnecessary and costly effort. Since it is possible to combat different kinds of cancers through similar molecular mechanisms, such as the induction of immunogenic cell death, the development of adaptable platforms may allow the establishment of virus-based therapies in a more scalable and affordable way. Such approaches may, in the future, permit low-effort adaptation of pre-existing therapies to target different cellular markers and treat other tumors.

A viable alternative may be the use of adapter molecules. Bhatia et al. [179] developed an anti-CXCR4 bispecific adapter (sCAR-CXCL12). Chemokine receptor type 4 (CXCR4) is known to be overexpressed in a wide variety of cancers, such as melanoma [180] and breast cancer [181], and it is associated with metastasis and poor overall survival. Bhatia et al. [179] designed a recombinant adapter molecule composed of an ectodomain portion of the human CAR, followed by a 5-peptide linker (GGPGS) and a 6-His tag sequence, fused to the mature human chemokine CXCL12/SDF-1a sequence (CXCR4 ligand). According to the researchers, this bispecific adapter attenuated liver infection in vivo and a promoted a considerable increase in cancer cell infection, as observed in xenograft tumors in mice.

In another interesting work, Schmid et al. [182] achieved, simultaneously, the retargeting of type 5 adenovirus tropism to a specific cancer marker and the reduction of its liver sequestration. Unlike other adapter strategies, they utilized designed ankyrin repeat proteins (DARPins). Similar to antibodies, these proteins can bind to a target with rather good specificity. Moreover, these molecules can be engineered to target different antigens on the cell surface [183]. Schmid et al. [182] designed an adenovirus-antigen adapter composed of three monomers. Each monomer was made of a retargeting DARPin, a flexible linker, a knob-binding DARPin, and a trimerization motif [182,184]. The last component is responsible for the stability of the complex, allowing the coating of the adenovirus fiber knob and, consequently, impeding virus natural tropism. In addition, according to the researchers and some early works, the removal of CAR and integrin interactions may reduce liver tropism [185,186], an effect also observed when those capsid sites are blocked by DARPin adapters. Furthermore, this protein was able to hide the region responsible for adenovirus–liver interaction without disturbing the adenovirus–integrin interaction. Nonetheless, the researchers developed an adenovirus-binding molecule, named "shield", derived from humanized antihexon scFv, which was designed to bind to hexon proteins, effectively protecting them from neutralizing antibodies [182].

4.6. Genetic and Chemical Capsid Modifications and Association with Polymers

Other strategies have emerged that support the retargeting and detargeting of adenoviral vectors. For example, the CGKRK peptide mediates the targeting of tumor cells and tumor neovasculature and has been tested for its ability to retarget PEGylated adenoviral vectors: PEG molecules are conjugated to the surface of the viral vector; then, the peptide is attached via a chemical reaction, resulting in its conjugation to the functional group of PEG [187]. Moreover, Bonsted and colleagues demonstrated that a linker between the poly(2-(dimethylamino)ethyl methacrylate) (pDMAEMA) and the epidermal growth factor (EGF), commonly overexpressed in tumors, efficiently transduced CAR-deficient cells [188,189]. Additionally, an EGF mimetic peptide linked to the cationic PAMAM (polyamidoamine) dendrimer polymer through a PEG linker has been used to retarget dendrimer-coated Ad vectors; it has been shown to increase transgene expression in target cells compared with the untargeted vector [190].

Kreppel et al. [191] introduced a genetic–chemical concept for vector re- and detargeting. For that, the authors genetically modified the virus in order to present cysteine residues in the capsid, including the fiber HI-loop [191], protein IX [192], and hexon [193]. The cysteine residues were then covalently modified with thiol-reactive coupling moieties, including ligands, shielding polymers, carbohydrates, small molecules, and fluorescent dyes [194]. Kreppel et al. demonstrated that amine-based PEGylation and thiol-based coupling of transferrin to the fiber knob HI-loop successfully retargeted the modified Ad vectors to CAR-deficient cells [191].

These studies highlight the possibility of creating adenoviral vector platforms that need no further genetic modification; thus, a wide variety of target tissues may be explored with the aim of improving specificity and decreasing the neutralizing effects of preexisting antibodies.

5. Conclusions and Future Perspectives

Many features make Ads interesting vehicles for the delivery of foreign antigenic proteins or gene therapy: large cloning capacity, genetic stability, and high in vivo transduction capacity in both dividing and nondividing cells. The natural antiviral immune response can be useful to reprogram the tumor microenvironment from "cold" to "hot" by inducing T-cell-specific immune responses and proinflammatory cytokine expression [195]. The success of therapy depends on several other factors, such as the quality, intensity, specificity, and half-life of immune responses against the tumor. In this scenario, neoantigens have emerged as an attractive target for cancer therapy. Major advances in using the non-self-peptides are the absence of pre-existing central tolerance, potential strong immunogenicity, and lower risk of autoimmunity diseases [196]. We expect that continued refinement of Ad vector design and a deeper understanding of neoantigens will converge to provide an exceptional platform for cancer immunotherapy.

Even so, we point out some limitations for the use of neoantigens in personalized medicine: (1) neoantigens are limited by the diversity of somatic mutations in different tumor types and their individual specificity; (2) the probability that the neoantigens are shared between patients is very low; (3) identification and verification of neoantigens is still time-consuming and expensive [197]. In addition, the construction of adenoviral vectors encoding each neoantigen would be costly and time-consuming; thus, approaches that do not require vector construction may be preferable, including the use of peptides and membrane coatings.

Otherwise, the effectiveness in the use of neoantigens has already been observed in preclinical [198,199] and clinical data [200–202]. In addition, patients with high mutation burden tumors, like melanoma [203,204], non small-cell lung cancer [205], and bladder cancer [206], have had more clinical benefit from checkpoint-blockade therapy than those with lower mutation loads [196]. Moreover, the prediction of peptides binding to MHC molecules and, consequently, the identification of neoepitopes able to stimulate the immune response are emerging as novel approaches that could be associated with adenoviral vectors, reversing part of the tumor-induced immunosuppression.

Recently, D'Alise and collaborators [207] demonstrated the satisfactory benefits of genetic vaccines based on Ads derived from nonhuman great apes (GAd) encoding multiple neoantigens applied in the CT26 murine colon carcinoma model. Both prophylactic and early therapeutic vaccinations elicited strong and effective T-cell responses and controlled tumor growth in mice. The tumor-infiltrating T-cells were diversified in animals treated with GAd and anti-PD1 compared to anti-PD1 alone [207]. The big challenge of neoantigens is the complexity in identifying immunogenic antigens unique to each patient. However, more optimized sequencing platforms and bioinformatics tools are helping to make personalized therapy truly viable. All in all, the data presented here highlight new perspectives of cancer vaccines and gene therapy using modified nonreplicating adenoviruses and different strategies to turn the immune response against the tumor more specific and robust, contributing to local and distant control of tumor progression.

Although viral delivery systems are quite promising strategies in gene therapy, there are some limitations to their clinical application. The major barriers are host immune responses that result in the clearance of vectors, interaction with plasma proteins, liver sequestration, Ad CAR-dependence, and off-target effects [208]. Regarding these issues, a number of genetic manipulations have been exploited to redirect adenovirus binding to different cell surface receptors and, consequently, increase affinity for the target, with lower adverse effects [50].

In this scenario, different strategies using coated viruses have emerged in recent years, and both biological and chemical approaches can be used to coat the virus and improve delivery, especially for the systemic route. Since these strategies involve using cancer cell membranes that can be obtained directly from tumor cell lines, they provide greater biocompatibility with the tumor site and, consequently, specifically target these cells [209]. A growing body of evidence suggests that cancer cell membrane-coated viruses can be delivered by the systemic route, improving the targeting of metastases, with higher retention time, lower immune recognition, and decreased liver sequestration, toxicity, and accumulation in healthy tissues. The induction of immunogenic cell death by nonreplicating Ad vectors is associated with innate immune responses, antigen processing and presentation, and, finally, the activation of the cellular immune response. While few examples currently exist of using membrane-coated adenoviral vectors, we hypothesize that this approach will continue to be studied, including in nonreplicating vectors.

In summary, improvements in vector delivery and targeting will provide an even greater potential for the use of nonreplicating adenoviral vectors in cancer immunotherapy. In particular, we envision vectors adapted to support systemic delivery, achieve tumor specificity, induce tumor cell death and supply specific antigens to guide antitumor immune responses.

Author Contributions: N.G.T. conceived the review topic, wrote and edited the text, and prepared the figures; A.C.M.D. wrote and edited the text and prepared the figures, F.A., J.C.d.S.d.L., O.A.R., and O.L.D.C. wrote and edited the text; B.E.S. edited the text and provided funding. All authors have read and agreed to the published version of the manuscript.

Funding: This research was funded by the Sao Paulo Research Foundation (FAPESP; grant 15/26580-9 (B.E.S.) and fellowships 17/25290-2 (N.G.T.), 18/25555-9 (A.C.M.D.), 17/25284-2 (O.A.R.), and 17/23068-0 (O.L.D.C.)). Funding was also provided by the Conselho Nacional de Desenvolvimento Científico e Tecnológico (CNPq; fellowships 134305/2018-3 (J.C.d.S.d.L.) and 302888/2017/9 (B.E.S.)).

Data Availability Statement: No new data were created or analyzed in this study. Data sharing is not applicable to this article.

Conflicts of Interest: The authors declare no conflict of interest.

References

1. Ginn, S.L.; Amaya, A.K.; Alexander, I.E.; Edelstein, M.; Abedi, M.R. Gene therapy clinical trials worldwide to 2017: An update. *J. Gene Med.* **2018**, *20*, e3015. [CrossRef] [PubMed]
2. Zhang, W.-W.; Li, L.; Li, D.; Liu, J.; Li, X.; Li, W.; Xu, X.; Zhang, M.J.; Chandler, L.A.; Lin, H.; et al. The First Approved Gene Therapy Product for Cancer Ad- *P53* (Gendicine): 12 Years in the Clinic. *Hum. Gene Ther.* **2018**, *29*, 160–179. [CrossRef]
3. National Library of Medicine. A Phase II Clinical Trial to Evaluate the Recombinant Vaccine for COVID-19 (Adenovirus Vector). 2020. Available online: https://clinicaltrials.gov/ct2/show/NCT04341389 (accessed on 1 April 2021).
4. National Library of Medicine. ChiCTR2000030906. A Phase I Clinical Trial for Recombinant Novel Coronavirus (2019-COV) Vaccine (Adenoviral Vector). 2020. Available online: https://clinicaltrials.gov/ct2/show/NCT04313127 (accessed on 1 April 2021).
5. Chinese Clinical Trial Registry (ChiCTR). ChiCTR2000031781. A Randomized, Double-Blinded, Placebo-Controlled Phase II Clinical Trial for Recombinant Novel Coronavirus (2019-NCOV) Vaccine (Adenovirus Vector). 2020. Available online: http://www.chictr.org.cn/showprojen.aspx?proj=52006 (accessed on 1 April 2021).
6. National Library of Medicine. Phase I Clinical Trial of a COVID-19 Vaccine in 18–60 Healthy Adults. 2020. Available online: https://clinicaltrials.gov/ct2/show/NCT04313127 (accessed on 1 April 2021).
7. National Library of Medicine. Phase I/II Clinical Trial of Recombinant Novel Coronavirus Vaccine (Adenovirus Type 5 Vector) in Canada. 2020. Available online: https://www.clinicaltrials.gov/ct2/show/NCT04398147 (accessed on 1 April 2021).
8. National Library of Medicine. COVID-19 Vaccine (ChAdOx1 NCoV-19) Trial in South African Adults with and without HIV-Infection. 2020. Available online: https://clinicaltrials.gov/ct2/show/NCT04444674 (accessed on 1 April 2021).
9. National Library of Medicine. A Study of a Candidate COVID-19 Vaccine (COV001). 2020. Available online: https://clinicaltrials.gov/ct2/show/NCT04324606 (accessed on 1 April 2021).
10. National Library of Medicine. An Open Study of the Safety, Tolerability and Immunogenicity of "Gam-COVID-Vac Lyo" Vaccine Against COVID-19. 2020. Available online: https://clinicaltrials.gov/ct2/show/NCT04437875 (accessed on 1 April 2021).
11. Gamaleya Research Institute of Epidemiology and Microbiology. An Open Study of the Safety, Tolerability and Immunogenicity of the Drug "Gam-COVID-Vac" Vaccine against COVID-19. 2020. Available online: https://www.smartpatients.com/trials/NCT04437875 (accessed on 1 April 2021).
12. Coughlan, L. Factors Which Contribute to the Immunogenicity of Non-Replicating Adenoviral Vectored Vaccines. *Front. Immunol.* **2020**, *11*, 909. [CrossRef] [PubMed]
13. Kumon, H.; Ariyoshi, Y.; Sasaki, K.; Sadahira, T.; Araki, M.; Ebara, S.; Yanai, H.; Watanabe, M.; Nasu, Y. Adenovirus Vector Carrying REIC/DKK-3 Gene: Neoadjuvant Intraprostatic Injection for High-Risk Localized Prostate Cancer Undergoing Radical Prostatectomy. *Cancer Gene Ther.* **2016**, *23*, 400–409. [CrossRef] [PubMed]
14. Goto, Y.; Ohe, Y.; Kuribayashi, K.; Nakano, T.; Okada, M.; Toyooka, S.; Kumon, H.; Nakanishi, Y. P2.06-11 A Phase I/II Study of Intrapleural Ad-SGE-REIC Administration in Patients with Refractory Malignant Pleural Mesothelioma. *J. Thorac. Oncol.* **2018**, *13*, S746. [CrossRef]
15. Lowenstein, P.R.; Orringer, D.A.; Sagher, O.; Heth, J.; Hervey-Jumper, S.L.; Mammoser, A.G.; Junck, L.; Leung, D.; Umemura, Y.; Lawrence, T.S.; et al. First-in-Human Phase I Trial of the Combination of Two Adenoviral Vectors Expressing HSV1-TK and FLT3L for the Treatment of Newly Diagnosed Resectable Malignant Glioma: Initial Results from the Therapeutic Reprogramming of the Brain Immune System. *J. Clin. Oncol.* **2019**, *37*, 2019. [CrossRef]
16. Zhu, R.; Weng, D.; Lu, S.; Lin, D.; Wang, M.; Chen, D.; Lv, J.; Li, H.; Lv, F.; Xi, L.; et al. Double-Dose Adenovirus-Mediated Adjuvant Gene Therapy Improves Liver Transplantation Outcomes in Patients with Advanced Hepatocellular Carcinoma. *Hum. Gene Ther.* **2018**, *29*, 251–258. [CrossRef]
17. Kieran, M.W.; Goumnerova, L.; Manley, P.; Chi, S.N.; Marcus, K.J.; Manzanera, A.G.; Polanco, M.L.S.; Guzik, B.W.; Aguilar-Cordova, E.; Diaz-Montero, C.M.; et al. Phase I Study of Gene-Mediated Cytotoxic Immunotherapy with AdV-Tk as Adjuvant to Surgery and Radiation for Pediatric Malignant Glioma and Recurrent Ependymoma. *Neuro Oncol.* **2019**, *21*, 537–546. [CrossRef]
18. Behbahani, T.E.; Rosenthal, E.L.; Parker, W.B.; Sorscher, E.J. Intratumoral Generation of 2-fluoroadenine to Treat Solid Malignancies of the Head and Neck. *Head Neck* **2019**, *41*, 1979–1983. [CrossRef] [PubMed]

19. Shore, N.D.; Boorjian, S.A.; Canter, D.J.; Ogan, K.; Karsh, L.I.; Downs, T.M.; Gomella, L.G.; Kamat, A.M.; Lotan, Y.; Svatek, R.S.; et al. Intravesical RAd–IFNα/Syn3 for Patients with High-Grade, Bacillus Calmette-Guerin–Refractory or Relapsed Non–Muscle-Invasive Bladder Cancer: A Phase II Randomized Study. *J. Clin. Oncol.* **2017**, *35*, 3410–3416. [CrossRef]
20. Sterman, D.H.; Recio, A.; Haas, A.R.; Vachani, A.; Katz, S.I.; Gillespie, C.T.; Cheng, G.; Sun, J.; Moon, E.; Pereira, L.; et al. A Phase I Trial of Repeated Intrapleural Adenoviral-Mediated Interferon-β Gene Transfer for Mesothelioma and Metastatic Pleural Effusions. *Mol. Ther.* **2010**, *18*, 852–860. [CrossRef]
21. Chiocca, E.A.; Yu, J.S.; Lukas, R.V.; Solomon, I.H.; Ligon, K.L.; Nakashima, H.; Triggs, D.A.; Reardon, D.A.; Wen, P.; Stopa, B.M.; et al. Regulatable Interleukin-12 Gene Therapy in Patients with Recurrent High-Grade Glioma: Results of a Phase 1 Trial. *Sci. Transl. Med.* **2019**, *11*, eaaw5680. [CrossRef] [PubMed]
22. Buller, R.E.; Runnebaum, I.B.; Karlan, B.Y.; Horowitz, J.A.; Shahin, M.; Buekers, T.; Petrauskas, S.; Kreienberg, R.; Slamon, D.; Pegram, M. A Phase I/II Trial of RAd/P53 (SCH 58500) Gene Replacement in Recurrent Ovarian Cancer. *Cancer Gene Ther.* **2002**, *9*, 553–566. [CrossRef] [PubMed]
23. Yoo, G.H.; Moon, J.; LeBlanc, M.; Lonardo, F.; Urba, S.; Kim, H.; Hanna, E.; Tsue, T.; Valentino, J.; Ensley, J.; et al. A Phase 2 Trial of Surgery with Perioperative INGN 201 (Ad5CMV-P53) Gene Therapy Followed by Chemoradiotherapy for Advanced, Resectable Squamous Cell Carcinoma of the Oral Cavity, Oropharynx, Hypopharynx, and Larynx: Report of the Southwest Oncology Group. *Arch. Otolaryngol. Neck Surg.* **2009**, *135*, 869. [CrossRef] [PubMed]
24. Robinson, C.M.; Singh, G.; Lee, J.Y.; Dehghan, S.; Rajaiya, J.; Liu, E.B.; Yousuf, M.A.; Betensky, R.A.; Jones, M.S.; Dyer, D.W.; et al. Molecular Evolution of Human Adenoviruses. *Sci. Rep.* **2013**, *3*, 1812. [CrossRef]
25. HAdV Working Group. Available online: http://hadvwg.gmu.edu. (accessed on 22 June 2020).
26. San Martín, C. Latest Insights on Adenovirus Structure and Assembly. *Viruses* **2012**, *4*, 847–877. [CrossRef]
27. Russell, W.C. Adenoviruses: Update on Structure and Function. *J. Gen. Virol.* **2009**, *90*, 1–20. [CrossRef] [PubMed]
28. Baker, A.T.; Greenshields-Watson, A.; Coughlan, L.; Davies, J.A.; Uusi-Kerttula, H.; Cole, D.K.; Rizkallah, P.J.; Parker, A.L. Diversity within the Adenovirus Fiber Knob Hypervariable Loops Influences Primary Receptor Interactions. *Nat. Commun.* **2019**, *10*, 741. [CrossRef]
29. Loustalot, F.; Kremer, E.J.; Salinas, S. The Intracellular Domain of the Coxsackievirus and Adenovirus Receptor Differentially Influences Adenovirus Entry. *J. Virol.* **2015**, *89*, 9417–9426. [CrossRef] [PubMed]
30. Murakami, S.; Sakurai, F.; Kawabata, K.; Okada, N.; Fujita, T.; Yamamoto, A.; Hayakawa, T.; Mizuguchi, H. Interaction of Penton Base Arg-Gly-Asp Motifs with Integrins Is Crucial for Adenovirus Serotype 35 Vector Transduction in Human Hematopoietic Cells. *Gene Ther.* **2007**, *14*, 1525–1533. [CrossRef]
31. Strunze, S.; Engelke, M.F.; Wang, I.-H.; Puntener, D.; Boucke, K.; Schleich, S.; Way, M.; Schoenenberger, P.; Burckhardt, C.J.; Greber, U.F. Kinesin-1-Mediated Capsid Disassembly and Disruption of the Nuclear Pore Complex Promote Virus Infection. *Cell Host Microbe* **2011**, *10*, 210–223. [CrossRef]
32. Ricobaraza, A.; Gonzalez-Aparicio, M.; Mora-Jimenez, L.; Lumbreras, S.; Hernandez-Alcoceba, R. High-Capacity Adenoviral Vectors: Expanding the Scope of Gene Therapy. *Int. J. Mol. Sci.* **2020**, *21*, 3643. [CrossRef]
33. Khanal, S.; Ghimire, P.; Dhamoon, A. The Repertoire of Adenovirus in Human Disease: The Innocuous to the Deadly. *Biomedicines* **2018**, *6*, 30. [CrossRef]
34. Lee, C.S.; Bishop, E.S.; Zhang, R.; Yu, X.; Farina, E.M.; Yan, S.; Zhao, C.; Zeng, Z.; Shu, Y.; Wu, X.; et al. Adenovirus-Mediated Gene Delivery: Potential Applications for Gene and Cell-Based Therapies in the New Era of Personalized Medicine. *Genes Dis.* **2017**, *4*, 43–63. [CrossRef]
35. Crystal, R.G. Adenovirus: The First Effective In Vivo Gene Delivery Vector. *Hum. Gene Ther.* **2014**, *25*, 3–11. [CrossRef] [PubMed]
36. Gao, J.; Mese, K.; Bunz, O.; Ehrhardt, A. State-of-the-art Human Adenovirus Vectorology for Therapeutic Approaches. *FEBS Lett.* **2019**, *593*, 3609–3622. [CrossRef]
37. McGrory, W.J.; Bautista, D.S.; Graham, F.L. A Simple Technique for the Rescue of Early Region I Mutations into Infectious Human Adenovirus Type 5. *Virology* **1988**, *163*, 614–617. [CrossRef]
38. Bett, A.J.; Haddara, W.; Prevec, L.; Graham, F.L. An Efficient and Flexible System for Construction of Adenovirus Vectors with Insertions or Deletions in Early Regions 1 and 3. *Proc. Natl. Acad. Sci. USA* **1994**, *91*, 8802–8806. [CrossRef] [PubMed]
39. Kovesdi, I.; Hedley, S.J. Adenoviral Producer Cells. *Viruses* **2010**, *2*, 1681–1703. [CrossRef]
40. Graham, F.L.; Smiley, J.; Russell, W.C.; Nairn, R. Characteristics of a Human Cell Line Transformed by DNA from Human Adenovirus Type 5. *J. Gen. Virol.* **1977**, *36*, 59–72. [CrossRef] [PubMed]
41. Lusky, M.; Christ, M.; Rittner, K.; Dieterle, A.; Dreyer, D.; Mourot, B.; Schultz, H.; Stoeckel, F.; Pavirani, A.; Mehtali, M. In Vitro and In Vivo Biology of Recombinant Adenovirus Vectors with E1, E1/E2A, or E1/E4 Deleted. *J. Virol.* **1998**, *72*, 2022–2032. [CrossRef]
42. Seth, P. Vector-Mediated Cancer Gene Therapy: An Overview. *Cancer Biol. Ther.* **2005**, *4*, 512–517. [CrossRef] [PubMed]
43. Di Paolo, N.C.; Miao, E.A.; Iwakura, Y.; Murali-Krishna, K.; Aderem, A.; Flavell, R.A.; Papayannopoulou, T.; Shayakhmetov, D.M. Virus Binding to a Plasma Membrane Receptor Triggers Interleukin-1α-Mediated Proinflammatory Macrophage Response In Vivo. *Immunity* **2009**, *31*, 110–121. [CrossRef]
44. Zhu, J.; Huang, X.; Yang, Y. Innate Immune Response to Adenoviral Vectors Is Mediated by Both Toll-Like Receptor-Dependent and -Independent Pathways. *J. Virol.* **2007**, *81*, 3170–3180. [CrossRef] [PubMed]

45. Takaoka, A.; Wang, Z.; Choi, M.K.; Yanai, H.; Negishi, H.; Ban, T.; Lu, Y.; Miyagishi, M.; Kodama, T.; Honda, K.; et al. DAI (DLM-1/ZBP1) Is a Cytosolic DNA Sensor and an Activator of Innate Immune Response. *Nature* **2007**, *448*, 501–505. [CrossRef]
46. Muruve, D.A.; Pétrilli, V.; Zaiss, A.K.; White, L.R.; Clark, S.A.; Ross, P.J.; Parks, R.J.; Tschopp, J. The Inflammasome Recognizes Cytosolic Microbial and Host DNA and Triggers an Innate Immune Response. *Nature* **2008**, *452*, 103–107. [CrossRef]
47. Franchi, L.; Warner, N.; Viani, K.; Nuñez, G. Function of Nod-like Receptors in Microbial Recognition and Host Defense. *Immunol. Rev.* **2009**, *227*, 106–128. [CrossRef] [PubMed]
48. Binnewies, M.; Roberts, E.W.; Kersten, K.; Chan, V.; Fearon, D.F.; Merad, M.; Coussens, L.M.; Gabrilovich, D.I.; Ostrand-Rosenberg, S.; Hedrick, C.C.; et al. Understanding the Tumor Immune Microenvironment (TIME) for Effective Therapy. *Nat. Med.* **2018**, *24*, 541–550. [CrossRef]
49. Shaw, A.R.; Suzuki, M. Immunology of Adenoviral Vectors in Cancer Therapy. *Mol. Ther. Methods Clin. Dev.* **2019**, *15*, 418–429. [CrossRef] [PubMed]
50. Wold, W.S.M.; Toth, K. Adenovirus Vectors for Gene Therapy, Vaccination and Cancer Gene Therapy. *Curr. Gene Ther.* **2013**, *13*, 421–433. [CrossRef] [PubMed]
51. Tatsis, N.; Ertl, H.C.J. Adenoviruses as Vaccine Vectors. *Mol. Ther.* **2004**, *10*, 616–629. [CrossRef]
52. Robert-Guroff, M. Replicating and Non-Replicating Viral Vectors for Vaccine Development. *Curr. Opin. Biotechnol.* **2007**, *18*, 546–556. [CrossRef] [PubMed]
53. Osada, T.; Yang, X.Y.; Hartman, Z.C.; Glass, O.; Hodges, B.L.; Niedzwiecki, D.; Morse, M.A.; Lyerly, H.K.; Amalfitano, A.; Clay, T.M. Optimization of Vaccine Responses with an E1, E2b and E3-Deleted Ad5 Vector Circumvents Pre-Existing Anti-Vector Immunity. *Cancer Gene Ther.* **2009**, *16*, 673–682. [CrossRef]
54. Cappuccini, F.; Stribbling, S.; Pollock, E.; Hill, A.V.S.; Redchenko, I. Immunogenicity and Efficacy of the Novel Cancer Vaccine Based on Simian Adenovirus and MVA Vectors Alone and in Combination with PD-1 MAb in a Mouse Model of Prostate Cancer. *Cancer Immunol. Immunother.* **2016**, *65*, 701–713. [CrossRef]
55. Bajgelman, M.C.; Strauss, B.E. Development of an Adenoviral Vector with Robust Expression Driven by P53. *Virology* **2008**, *371*, 8–13. [CrossRef]
56. Hunger, A.; Medrano, R.F.; Zanatta, D.B.; Del Valle, P.R.; Merkel, C.A.; de Almeida Salles, T.; Ferrari, D.G.; Furuya, T.K.; Bustos, S.O.; de Freitas Saito, R.; et al. Reestablishment of P53/Arf and Interferon-β Pathways Mediated by a Novel Adenoviral Vector Potentiates Antiviral Response and Immunogenic Cell Death. *Cell Death Discov.* **2017**, *3*, 17017. [CrossRef] [PubMed]
57. Merkel, C.A.; da Silva Soares, R.B.; de Carvalho, A.C.V.; Zanatta, D.B.; Bajgelman, M.C.; Fratini, P.; Costanzi-Strauss, E.; Strauss, B.E. Activation of Endogenous P53 by Combined P19Arf Gene Transfer and Nutlin-3 Drug Treatment Modalities in the Murine Cell Lines B16 and C6. *BMC Cancer* **2010**, *10*, 316. [CrossRef]
58. Medrano, R.F.V.; Catani, J.P.P.; Ribeiro, A.H.; Tomaz, S.L.; Merkel, C.A.; Costanzi-Strauss, E.; Strauss, B.E. Vaccination Using Melanoma Cells Treated with P19arf and Interferon Beta Gene Transfer in a Mouse Model: A Novel Combination for Cancer Immunotherapy. *Cancer Immunol. Immunother.* **2016**, *65*, 371–382. [CrossRef] [PubMed]
59. Catani, J.P.P.; Medrano, R.F.V.; Hunger, A.; Del Valle, P.; Adjemian, S.; Zanatta, D.B.; Kroemer, G.; Costanzi-Strauss, E.; Strauss, B.E. Intratumoral Immunization by P19Arf and Interferon-β Gene Transfer in a Heterotopic Mouse Model of Lung Carcinoma. *Transl. Oncol.* **2016**, *9*, 565–574. [CrossRef]
60. Hunger, A.; Medrano, R.F.; Strauss, B.E. Harnessing Combined P19Arf and Interferon-Beta Gene Transfer as an Inducer of Immunogenic Cell Death and Mediator of Cancer Immunotherapy. *Cell Death Dis.* **2017**, *8*, e2784. [CrossRef]
61. Medrano, R.F.V.; Hunger, A.; Catani, J.P.P.; Strauss, B.E. Uncovering the Immunotherapeutic Cycle Initiated by P19Arf and Interferon-β Gene Transfer to Cancer Cells: An Inducer of Immunogenic Cell Death. *OncoImmunology* **2017**, e1329072. [CrossRef] [PubMed]
62. Qin, X.-Q.; Beckham, C.; Brown, J.L.; Lukashev, M.; Barsoum, J. Human and Mouse IFN-β Gene Therapy Exhibits Different Anti-Tumor Mechanisms in Mouse Models. *Mol. Ther.* **2001**, *4*, 356–364. [CrossRef]
63. Cerqueira, O.L.D.; Clavijo-Salomon, M.A.; Cardoso, E.C.; Citrangulo Tortelli Junior, T.; Mendonça, S.A.; Barbuto, J.A.M.; Strauss, B.E. Combined P14ARF and Interferon-β Gene Transfer to the Human Melanoma Cell Line SK-MEL-147 Promotes Oncolysis and Immune Activation. *Front. Immunol.* **2020**, *11*, 576658. [CrossRef]
64. Aguilar, L.K.; Shirley, L.A.; Chung, V.M.; Marsh, C.L.; Walker, J.; Coyle, W.; Marx, H.; Bekaii-Saab, T.; Lesinski, G.B.; Swanson, B.; et al. Gene-Mediated Cytotoxic Immunotherapy as Adjuvant to Surgery or Chemoradiation for Pancreatic Adenocarcinoma. *Cancer Immunol. Immunother.* **2015**, *64*, 727–736. [CrossRef]
65. Herman, J.R.; Adler, H.L.; Aguilar-Cordova, E.; Rojas-Martinez, A.; Woo, S.; Timme, T.L.; Wheeler, T.M.; Thompson, T.C.; Scardino, P.T. In Situ Gene Therapy for Adenocarcinoma of the Prostate: A Phase I Clinical Trial. *Hum. Gene Ther.* **1999**, *10*, 1239–1250. [CrossRef] [PubMed]
66. Maatta, A.-M.; Samaranayake, H.; Pikkarainen, J.; Wirth, T.; Yla-Herttuala, S. Adenovirus Mediated Herpes Simplex Virus-Thymidine Kinase/Ganciclovir Gene Therapy for Resectable Malignant Glioma. *Curr. Gene Ther.* **2009**, *9*, 356–367. [CrossRef]
67. Chévez-Barrios, P.; Chintagumpala, M.; Mieler, W.; Paysse, E.; Boniuk, M.; Kozinetz, C.; Hurwitz, M.Y.; Hurwitz, R.L. Response of Retinoblastoma with Vitreous Tumor Seeding to Adenovirus-Mediated Delivery of Thymidine Kinase Followed by Ganciclovir. *J. Clin. Oncol.* **2005**, *23*, 7927–7935. [CrossRef] [PubMed]

68. Sterman, D.H.; Recio, A.; Vachani, A.; Sun, J.; Cheung, L.; DeLong, P.; Amin, K.M.; Litzky, L.A.; Wilson, J.M.; Kaiser, L.R.; et al. Long-Term Follow-up of Patients with Malignant Pleural Mesothelioma Receiving High-Dose Adenovirus Herpes Simplex Thymidine Kinase/Ganciclovir Suicide Gene Therapy. *Clin. Cancer Res.* **2005**, *11*, 7444–7453. [CrossRef]

69. Siddiqui, M.R.; Grant, C.; Sanford, T.; Agarwal, P.K. Current Clinical Trials in Non–Muscle Invasive Bladder Cancer. *Urol. Oncol. Semin. Orig. Investig.* **2017**, *35*, 516–527. [CrossRef]

70. Boorjian, S.A.; Alemozaffar, M.; Konety, B.R.; Shore, N.D.; Gomella, L.G.; Kamat, A.M.; Bivalacqua, T.J.; Montgomery, J.S.; Lerner, S.P.; Busby, J.E.; et al. Intravesical Nadofaragene Firadenovec Gene Therapy for BCG-Unresponsive Non-Muscle-Invasive Bladder Cancer: A Single-Arm, Open-Label, Repeat-Dose Clinical Trial. *Lancet Oncol.* **2021**, *22*, 107–117. [CrossRef]

71. Nemunaitis, J. Vaccines in Cancer: GVAX®, a GM-CSF Gene Vaccine. *Expert Rev. Vaccines* **2005**, *4*, 259–274. [CrossRef]

72. Oosterhoff, D.; Sluijter, B.J.R.; Hangalapura, B.N.; de Gruijl, T.D. The Dermis as a Portal for Dendritic Cell-Targeted Immunotherapy of Cutaneous Melanoma. In *Intradermal Immunization*; Current Topics in Microbiology and Immunology; Teunissen, M.B.M., Ed.; Springer: Berlin/Heidelberg, Germany, 2011; Volume 351, pp. 181–220, ISBN 978-3-642-23689-1.

73. Butterfield, L.H.; Comin-Anduix, B.; Vujanovic, L.; Lee, Y.; Dissette, V.B.; Yang, J.-Q.; Vu, H.T.; Seja, E.; Oseguera, D.K.; Potter, D.M.; et al. Adenovirus MART-1–Engineered Autologous Dendritic Cell Vaccine for Metastatic Melanoma: *J. Immunother.* **2008**, *31*, 294–309. [CrossRef] [PubMed]

74. Lee, J.M.; Lee, M.-H.; Garon, E.; Goldman, J.W.; Salehi-Rad, R.; Baratelli, F.E.; Schaue, D.; Wang, G.; Rosen, F.; Yanagawa, J.; et al. Phase I Trial of Intratumoral Injection of *CCL21* Gene–Modified Dendritic Cells in Lung Cancer Elicits Tumor-Specific Immune Responses and CD8 $^+$ T-Cell Infiltration. *Clin. Cancer Res.* **2017**, *23*, 4556–4568. [CrossRef]

75. Chiappori, A.A.; Soliman, H.; Janssen, W.E.; Antonia, S.J.; Gabrilovich, D.I. INGN-225: A Dendritic Cell-Based P53 Vaccine (Ad.P53-DC) in Small Cell Lung Cancer: Observed Association between Immune Response and Enhanced Chemotherapy Effect. *Expert Opin. Biol. Ther.* **2010**, *10*, 983–991. [CrossRef]

76. Wang, D.; Huang, X.F.; Hong, B.; Song, X.-T.; Hu, L.; Jiang, M.; Zhang, B.; Ning, H.; Li, Y.; Xu, C.; et al. Efficacy of Intracellular Immune Checkpoint-Silenced DC Vaccine. *JCI Insight* **2018**, *3*, e98368. [CrossRef]

77. Lu, Y.-C.; Robbins, P.F. Cancer Immunotherapy Targeting Neoantigens. *Semin. Immunol.* **2016**, *28*, 22–27. [CrossRef] [PubMed]

78. Gubin, M.M.; Artyomov, M.N.; Mardis, E.R.; Schreiber, R.D. Tumor Neoantigens: Building a Framework for Personalized Cancer Immunotherapy. *J. Clin. Investig.* **2015**, *125*, 3413–3421. [CrossRef]

79. Basak, S.K.; Kiertscher, S.M.; Harui, A.; Roth, M.D. Modifying Adenoviral Vectors for Use as Gene-Based Cancer Vaccines. *Viral Immunol.* **2004**, *17*, 182–196. [CrossRef]

80. Goyvaerts, C.; Breckpot, K. The Journey of in Vivo Virus Engineered Dendritic Cells from Bench to Bedside: A Bumpy Road. *Front. Immunol.* **2018**, *9*, 2052. [CrossRef] [PubMed]

81. Singh, S.; Kumar, R.; Agrawal, B. Adenoviral Vector-Based Vaccines and Gene Therapies: Current Status and Future Prospects. In *Adenoviruses*; Desheva, Y., Ed.; IntechOpen: London, UK, 2019; ISBN 978-1-78984-990-5.

82. Short, J.J.; Vasu, C.; Holterman, M.J.; Curiel, D.T.; Pereboev, A. Members of Adenovirus Species B Utilize CD80 and CD86 as Cellular Attachment Receptors. *Virus Res.* **2006**, *122*, 144–153. [CrossRef]

83. Gaggar, A.; Shayakhmetov, D.M.; Lieber, A. CD46 Is a Cellular Receptor for Group B Adenoviruses. *Nat. Med.* **2003**, *9*, 1408–1412. [CrossRef] [PubMed]

84. Lyle, C.; McCormick, F. Integrin Avβ5 Is a Primary Receptor for Adenovirus in CAR-Negative Cells. *Virol. J.* **2010**, *7*, 148. [CrossRef]

85. Nemerow, G.; Flint, J. Lessons Learned from Adenovirus (1970–2019). *FEBS Lett.* **2019**, *593*, 3395–3418. [CrossRef]

86. Zhang, Y.; Bergelson, J.M. Adenovirus Receptors. *J. Virol.* **2005**, *79*, 12125–12131. [CrossRef]

87. Gao, J.; Zhang, W.; Ehrhardt, A. Expanding the Spectrum of Adenoviral Vectors for Cancer Therapy. *Cancers* **2020**, *12*, 1139. [CrossRef]

88. Moyer, C.L.; Wiethoff, C.M.; Maier, O.; Smith, J.G.; Nemerow, G.R. Functional Genetic and Biophysical Analyses of Membrane Disruption by Human Adenovirus. *J. Virol.* **2011**, *85*, 2631–2641. [CrossRef]

89. Stasiak, A.C.; Stehle, T. Human Adenovirus Binding to Host Cell Receptors: A Structural View. *Med. Microbiol. Immunol.* **2020**, *209*, 325–333. [CrossRef] [PubMed]

90. Meier, O.; Greber, U.F. Adenovirus Endocytosis. *J. Gene Med.* **2004**, *6*, S152–S163. [CrossRef] [PubMed]

91. Bergelson, J.M. Isolation of a Common Receptor for Coxsackie B Viruses and Adenoviruses 2 and 5. *Science* **1997**, *275*, 1320–1323. [CrossRef]

92. Thomas, C.E.; Edwards, P.; Wickham, T.J.; Castro, M.G.; Lowenstein, P.R. Adenovirus Binding to the Coxsackievirus and Adenovirus Receptor or Integrins Is Not Required to Elicit Brain Inflammation but Is Necessary to Transduce Specific Neural Cell Types. *J. Virol.* **2002**, *76*, 3452–3460. [CrossRef]

93. Zhang, N.-H.; Peng, R.-Q.; Ding, Y.; Zhang, X.-S. Rejection of Adenovirus Infection Is Independent of Coxsackie and Adenovirus Receptor Expression in Cisplatin-Resistant Human Lung Cancer Cells. *Oncol. Rep.* **2016**, *36*, 715–720. [CrossRef] [PubMed]

94. Persson, B.D.; Lenman, A.; Frängsmyr, L.; Schmid, M.; Ahlm, C.; Plückthun, A.; Jenssen, H.; Arnberg, N. Lactoferrin-Hexon Interactions Mediate CAR-Independent Adenovirus Infection of Human Respiratory Cells. *J. Virol.* **2020**, *94*, e00542-20. [CrossRef] [PubMed]

95. Bots, S.T.F.; Hoeben, R.C. Non-Human Primate-Derived Adenoviruses for Future Use as Oncolytic Agents? *Int. J. Mol. Sci.* **2020**, *21*, 4821. [CrossRef] [PubMed]

96. Mennechet, F.J.D.; Paris, O.; Ouoba, A.R.; Salazar Arenas, S.; Sirima, S.B.; Takoudjou Dzomo, G.R.; Diarra, A.; Traore, I.T.; Kania, D.; Eichholz, K.; et al. A Review of 65 Years of Human Adenovirus Seroprevalence. *Expert Rev. Vaccines* **2019**, *18*, 597–613. [CrossRef]

97. Lin, K.-H.; Lin, Y.-C.; Chen, H.-L.; Ke, G.-M.; Chiang, C.-J.; Hwang, K.-P.; Chu, P.-Y.; Lin, J.-H.; Liu, D.-P.; Chen, H.-Y. A Two Decade Survey of Respiratory Adenovirus in Taiwan: The Reemergence of Adenovirus Types 7 and 4. *J. Med. Virol.* **2004**, *73*, 274–279. [CrossRef]

98. Sumida, S.M.; Truitt, D.M.; Lemckert, A.A.C.; Vogels, R.; Custers, J.H.H.V.; Addo, M.M.; Lockman, S.; Peter, T.; Peyerl, F.W.; Kishko, M.G.; et al. Neutralizing Antibodies to Adenovirus Serotype 5 Vaccine Vectors Are Directed Primarily against the Adenovirus Hexon Protein. *J. Immunol.* **2005**, *174*, 7179–7185. [CrossRef]

99. Shiver, J.W.; Emini, E.A. Recent Advances in the Development of HIV-1 Vaccines Using Replication-Incompetent Adenovirus Vectors. *Annu. Rev. Med.* **2004**, *55*, 355–372. [CrossRef]

100. Abbink, P.; Lemckert, A.A.C.; Ewald, B.A.; Lynch, D.M.; Denholtz, M.; Smits, S.; Holterman, L.; Damen, I.; Vogels, R.; Thorner, A.R.; et al. Comparative Seroprevalence and Immunogenicity of Six Rare Serotype Recombinant Adenovirus Vaccine Vectors from Subgroups B and D. *J. Virol.* **2007**, *81*, 4654–4663. [CrossRef]

101. Abbas, K.Z.; Lombos, E.; Duvvuri, V.R.; Olsha, R.; Higgins, R.R.; Gubbay, J.B. Temporal Changes in Respiratory Adenovirus Serotypes Circulating in the Greater Toronto Area, Ontario, during December 2008 to April 2010. *Virol. J.* **2013**, *10*, 15. [CrossRef] [PubMed]

102. Heim, A.; Ebnet, C.; Harste, G.; Pring-Åkerblom, P. Rapid and Quantitative Detection of Human Adenovirus DNA by Real-Time PCR. *J. Med. Virol.* **2003**, *70*, 228–239. [CrossRef]

103. Lee, W.-J.; Jung, H.-D.; Cheong, H.-M.; Kim, K. Molecular Epidemiology of a Post-Influenza Pandemic Outbreak of Acute Respiratory Infections in Korea Caused by Human Adenovirus Type 3: Post-Influenza Pandemic Outbreak of Human Adenovirus Type 3. *J. Med. Virol.* **2015**, *87*, 10–17. [CrossRef] [PubMed]

104. Scott, M.K.; Chommanard, C.; Lu, X.; Appelgate, D.; Grenz, L.; Schneider, E.; Gerber, S.I.; Erdman, D.D.; Thomas, A. Human Adenovirus Associated with Severe Respiratory Infection, Oregon, USA, 2013–2014. *Emerg. Infect. Dis.* **2016**, *22*, 1044–1051. [CrossRef]

105. Richmond, S.; Burman, R.; Crosdale, E.; Cropper, L.; Longson, D.; Enoch, B.E.; Dodd, C.L. A Large Outbreak of Keratoconjunctivitis Due to Adenovirus Type 8. *J. Hyg.* **1984**, *93*, 285–291. [CrossRef]

106. Tanaka-Yokogui, K.; Itoh, N.; Usui, N.; Takeuchi, S.; Uchio, E.; Aoki, K.; Usui, M.; Ohno, S. New Genome Type of Adenovirus Serotype 19 Causing Nosocomial Infections of Epidemic Keratoconjunctivitis in Japan. *J. Med. Virol.* **2001**, *65*, 530–533. [CrossRef] [PubMed]

107. Jernigan, J.A.; Lowry, B.S.; Hayden, F.G.; Kyger, S.A.; Conway, B.P.; Groschel, D.H.M.; Farr, B.M. Adenovirus Type 8 Epidemic Keratoconjunctivitis in an Eye Clinic: Risk Factors and Control. *J. Infect. Dis.* **1993**, *167*, 1307–1313. [CrossRef]

108. Aronson, B.; Aronson, S.; Sobel, G.; Walker, D. Pharyngoconjunctival Fever; Report of an Epidemic Outbreak. *AMA J. Dis. Child.* **1956**, *92*, 596–612.

109. Harley, D.; Harrower, B.; Lyon, M.; Dick, A. A Primary School Outbreak of Pharyngoconjunctival Fever Caused by Adenovirus Type 3. *Commun. Dis. Intell.* **2001**, *25*, 9–12. [PubMed]

110. Qiu, F.; Shen, X.; Li, G.; Zhao, L.; Chen, C.; Duan, S.; Guo, J.; Zhao, M.; Yan, T.; Qi, J.-J.; et al. Adenovirus Associated with Acute Diarrhea: A Case-Control Study. *BMC Infect. Dis.* **2018**, *18*, 450. [CrossRef]

111. Uhnoo, I.; Wadell, G.; Svensson, L.; Johansson, M.E. Importance of Enteric Adenoviruses 40 and 41 in Acute Gastroenteritis in Infants and Young Children. *J. Clin. Microbiol.* **1984**, *20*, 365–372. [CrossRef] [PubMed]

112. Mitra, A.K.; Clarke, K. Viral Obesity: Fact or Fiction? *Obes. Rev.* **2010**, *11*, 289–296. [CrossRef]

113. Shang, Q.; Wang, H.; Song, Y.; Wei, L.; Lavebratt, C.; Zhang, F.; Gu, H. Serological Data Analyses Show That Adenovirus 36 Infection Is Associated with Obesity: A Meta-Analysis Involving 5739 Subjects: Ad36 Associated with Obesity by Meta-Analysis. *Obesity* **2014**, *22*, 895–900. [CrossRef] [PubMed]

114. Schwartz, K.L.; Richardson, S.E.; MacGregor, D.; Mahant, S.; Raghuram, K.; Bitnun, A. Adenovirus-Associated Central Nervous System Disease in Children. *J. Pediatr.* **2019**, *205*, 130–137. [CrossRef]

115. Xie, L.; Zhang, B.; Xiao, N.; Zhang, F.; Zhao, X.; Liu, Q.; Xie, Z.; Gao, H.; Duan, Z.; Zhong, L. Epidemiology of Human Adenovirus Infection in Children Hospitalized with Lower Respiratory Tract Infections in Hunan, China: XIE ET AL. *J. Med. Virol.* **2019**, *91*, 392–400. [CrossRef]

116. Lai, C.-Y.; Lee, C.-J.; Lu, C.-Y.; Lee, P.-I.; Shao, P.-L.; Wu, E.-T.; Wang, C.-C.; Tan, B.-F.; Chang, H.-Y.; Hsia, S.-H.; et al. Adenovirus Serotype 3 and 7 Infection with Acute Respiratory Failure in Children in Taiwan, 2010–2011. *PLoS ONE* **2013**, *8*, e53614. [CrossRef]

117. Binder, A.M.; Biggs, H.M.; Haynes, A.K.; Chommanard, C.; Lu, X.; Erdman, D.D.; Watson, J.T.; Gerber, S.I. Human Adenovirus Surveillance—United States, 2003–2016. *MMWR Morb. Mortal. Wkly. Rep.* **2017**, *66*, 1039–1042. [CrossRef] [PubMed]

118. Muñoz-Hernández, A.M.; Duquesroix, B.; Benítez-del-Castillo, J.M. ADenoVirus Initiative Study in Epidemiology (ADVISE): Resultados de un estudio epidemiológico multicéntrico en España. *Arch. Soc. Esp. Oftalmol.* **2018**, *93*, 113–118. [CrossRef] [PubMed]

119. Mayindou, G.; Ngokana, B.; Sidibé, A.; Moundélé, V.; Koukouikila-Koussounda, F.; Christevy Vouvoungui, J.; Kwedi Nolna, S.; Velavan, T.P.; Ntoumi, F. Molecular Epidemiology and Surveillance of Circulating Rotavirus and Adenovirus in Congolese

Children with Gastroenteritis: Rotavirus and Adenovirus in Congolese Children. *J. Med. Virol.* **2016**, *88*, 596–605. [CrossRef] [PubMed]

120. Krause, A.; Joh, J.H.; Hackett, N.R.; Roelvink, P.W.; Bruder, J.T.; Wickham, T.J.; Kovesdi, I.; Crystal, R.G.; Worgall, S. Epitopes Expressed in Different Adenovirus Capsid Proteins Induce Different Levels of Epitope-Specific Immunity. *J. Virol.* **2006**, *80*, 5523–5530. [CrossRef] [PubMed]

121. Bradley, R.R.; Maxfield, L.F.; Lynch, D.M.; Iampietro, M.J.; Borducchi, E.N.; Barouch, D.H. Adenovirus Serotype 5-Specific Neutralizing Antibodies Target Multiple Hexon Hypervariable Regions. *J. Virol.* **2012**, *86*, 1267–1272. [CrossRef] [PubMed]

122. Smith, J.G.; Cassany, A.; Gerace, L.; Ralston, R.; Nemerow, G.R. Neutralizing Antibody Blocks Adenovirus Infection by Arresting Microtubule-Dependent Cytoplasmic Transport. *J. Virol.* **2008**, *82*, 6492–6500. [CrossRef]

123. Duffy, M.R.; Doszpoly, A.; Turner, G.; Nicklin, S.A.; Baker, A.H. The Relevance of Coagulation Factor X Protection of Adenoviruses in Human Sera. *Gene Ther.* **2016**, *23*, 592–596. [CrossRef]

124. Xu, Z.; Qiu, Q.; Tian, J.; Smith, J.S.; Conenello, G.M.; Morita, T.; Byrnes, A.P. Coagulation Factor X Shields Adenovirus Type 5 from Attack by Natural Antibodies and Complement. *Nat. Med.* **2013**, *19*, 452–457. [CrossRef] [PubMed]

125. Tomita, K.; Sakurai, F.; Iizuka, S.; Hemmi, M.; Wakabayashi, K.; Machitani, M.; Tachibana, M.; Katayama, K.; Kamada, H.; Mizuguchi, H. Antibodies against Adenovirus Fiber and Penton Base Proteins Inhibit Adenovirus Vector-Mediated Transduction in the Liver Following Systemic Administration. *Sci. Rep.* **2018**, *8*, 12315. [CrossRef] [PubMed]

126. Yu, B.; Dong, J.; Wang, C.; Zhan, Y.; Zhang, H.; Wu, J.; Kong, W.; Yu, X. Characteristics of Neutralizing Antibodies to Adenovirus Capsid Proteins in Human and Animal Sera. *Virology* **2013**, *437*, 118–123. [CrossRef]

127. Yang, T.C.; Dayball, K.; Wan, Y.H.; Bramson, J. Detailed Analysis of the CD8+ T-Cell Response Following Adenovirus Vaccination. *J. Virol.* **2003**, *77*, 13407–13411. [CrossRef] [PubMed]

128. Olive, M.; Eisenlohr, L.; Flomenberg, N.; Hsu, S.; Flomenberg, P. The Adenovirus Capsid Protein Hexon Contains a Highly Conserved Human CD4 $^+$ T-Cell Epitope. *Hum. Gene Ther.* **2002**, *13*, 1167–1178. [CrossRef] [PubMed]

129. Wheeler, M.D.; Yamashina, S.; Froh, M.; Rusyn, I.; Thurman, R.G. Adenoviral Gene Delivery Can Inactivate Kupffer Cells: Role of Oxidants in NF-κB Activation and Cytokine Production. *J. Leukoc. Biol.* **2011**, *69*, 622–630.

130. Khare, R.; Chen, Y.C.; Weaver, A.E.; Barry, A.M. Advances and Future Challenges in Adenoviral Vector Pharmacology and Targeting. *Curr. Gene Ther.* **2011**, *11*, 241–258. [CrossRef]

131. Green, N.K.; Herbert, C.W.; Hale, S.J.; Hale, A.B.; Mautner, V.; Harkins, R.; Hermiston, T.; Ulbrich, K.; Fisher, K.D.; Seymour, L.W. Extended Plasma Circulation Time and Decreased Toxicity of Polymer-Coated Adenovirus. *Gene Ther.* **2004**, *11*, 1256–1263. [CrossRef]

132. Barr, D.; Tubb, J.; Ferguson, D.; Scaria, A.; Lieber, A.; Wilson, C.; Perkins, J.; Kay, M.A. Strain Related Variations in Adenovirally Mediated Transgene Expression from Mouse Hepatocytes in Vivo: Comparisons between Immunocompetent and Immunodeficient Inbred Strains. *Gene Ther.* **1995**, *2*, 151–155.

133. Yang, Y.; Jooss, K.U.; Su, Q.; Ertl, H.C.; Wilson, J.M. Immune Responses to Viral Antigens versus Transgene Product in the Elimination of Recombinant Adenovirus-Infected Hepatocytes in Vivo. *Gene Ther.* **1996**, *3*, 137–144.

134. Chen, P.; Kovesdi, I.; Bruder, J.T. Effective Repeat Administration with Adenovirus Vectors to the Muscle. *Gene Ther.* **2000**, *7*, 587–595. [CrossRef] [PubMed]

135. Holst, P.J.; Ørskov, C.; Thomsen, A.R.; Christensen, J.P. Quality of the Transgene-Specific CD8 + T Cell Response Induced by Adenoviral Vector Immunization Is Critically Influenced by Virus Dose and Route of Vaccination. *J. Immunol.* **2010**, *184*, 4431–4439. [CrossRef] [PubMed]

136. Núñez-Ochoa, L.; Madrid-Marina, V.; Gutiérrez-López, A. Evaluation of Adverse Events in Dogs with Adenoviral Therapy by Intralymphonodal Administration in Canine Spontaneous Multicentric Lymphosarcoma. *Clin. Oncol.* **2017**, *2*, 1–8.

137. Yamamoto, Y.; Nagasato, M.; Yoshida, T.; Aoki, K. Recent Advances in Genetic Modification of Adenovirus Vectors for Cancer Treatment. *Cancer Sci.* **2017**, *108*, 831–837. [CrossRef] [PubMed]

138. Beatty, M.S.; Curiel, D.T. Adenovirus Strategies for Tissue-Specific Targeting. In *Advances in Cancer Research*; Elsevier: Amsterdam, The Netherlands, 2012; Volume 115, pp. 39–67, ISBN 978-0-12-398342-8.

139. Dmitriev, I.; Krasnykh, V.; Miller, C.R.; Wang, M.; Kashentseva, E.; Mikheeva, G.; Belousova, N.; Curiel, D.T. An Adenovirus Vector with Genetically Modified Fibers Demonstrates Expanded Tropism via Utilization of a Coxsackievirus and Adenovirus Receptor-Independent Cell Entry Mechanism. *J. Virol.* **1998**, *72*, 9706–9713. [CrossRef]

140. Wickham, T.J.; Roelvink, P.W.; Brough, D.E.; Kovesdi, I. Adenovirus Targeted to Heparan-Containing Receptors Increases Its Gene Delivery Efficiency to Multiple Cell Types. *Nat. Biotechnol.* **1996**, *14*, 1570–1573. [CrossRef] [PubMed]

141. Blackhall, F.H.; Merry, C.L.R.; Davies, E.J.; Jayson, G.C. Heparan Sulfate Proteoglycans and Cancer. *Br. J. Cancer* **2001**, *85*, 1094–1098. [CrossRef] [PubMed]

142. Wickham, T.J.; Segal, D.M.; Roelvink, P.W.; Carrion, M.E.; Lizonova, A.; Lee, G.M.; Kovesdi, I. Targeted Adenovirus Gene Transfer to Endothelial and Smooth Muscle Cells by Using Bispecific Antibodies. *J. Virol.* **1996**, *70*, 6831–6838. [CrossRef]

143. Miura, Y.; Yoshida, K.; Nishimoto, T.; Hatanaka, K.; Ohnami, S.; Asaka, M.; Douglas, J.T.; Curiel, D.T.; Yoshida, T.; Aoki, K. Direct Selection of Targeted Adenovirus Vectors by Random Peptide Display on the Fiber Knob. *Gene Ther.* **2007**, *14*, 1448–1460. [CrossRef] [PubMed]

144. Yoshida, Y.; Sadata, A.; Zhang, W.; Saito, K.; Shinoura, N.; Hamada, H. Generation of Fiber-Mutant Recombinant Adenoviruses for Gene Therapy of Malignant Glioma. *Hum. Gene Ther.* **1998**, *9*, 2503–2515. [CrossRef]

145. Krasnykh, V.; Dmitriev, I.; Mikheeva, G.; Miller, C.R.; Belousova, N.; Curiel, D.T. Characterization of an Adenovirus Vector Containing a Heterologous Peptide Epitope in the HI Loop of the Fiber Knob. *J. Virol.* **1998**, *72*, 1844–1852. [CrossRef]
146. Nicklin, S.A.; Von Seggern, D.J.; Work, L.M.; Pek, D.C.K.; Dominiczak, A.F.; Nemerow, G.R.; Baker, A.H. Ablating Adenovirus Type 5 Fiber–CAR Binding and HI Loop Insertion of the SIGYPLP Peptide Generate an Endothelial Cell-Selective Adenovirus. *Mol. Ther.* **2001**, *4*, 534–542. [CrossRef]
147. Nicklin, S.A.; White, S.J.; Nicol, C.G.; Von Seggern, D.J.; Baker, A.H. In Vitro Andin Vivo Characterisation of Endothelial Cell Selective Adenoviral Vectors. *J. Gene Med.* **2004**, *6*, 300–308. [CrossRef] [PubMed]
148. Joung, I.; Harber, G.; Gerecke, K.M.; Carroll, S.L.; Collawn, J.F.; Engler, J.A. Improved Gene Delivery into Neuroglial Cells Using a Fiber-Modified Adenovirus Vector. *Biochem. Biophys. Res. Commun.* **2005**, *328*, 1182–1187. [CrossRef] [PubMed]
149. Miura, Y.; Yamasaki, S.; Davydova, J.; Brown, E.; Aoki, K.; Vickers, S.; Yamamoto, M. Infectivity-Selective Oncolytic Adenovirus Developed by High-Throughput Screening of Adenovirus-Formatted Library. *Mol. Ther.* **2013**, *21*, 139–148. [CrossRef] [PubMed]
150. Müller, O.J.; Kaul, F.; Weitzman, M.D.; Pasqualini, R.; Arap, W.; Kleinschmidt, J.A.; Trepel, M. Random Peptide Libraries Displayed on Adeno-Associated Virus to Select for Targeted Gene Therapy Vectors. *Nat. Biotechnol.* **2003**, *21*, 1040–1046. [CrossRef] [PubMed]
151. Bhat, N.R.; Fan, F. Adenovirus Infection Induces Microglial Activation: Involvement of Mitogen-Activated Protein Kinase Pathways. *Brain Res.* **2002**, *948*, 93–101. [CrossRef]
152. Tibbles, L.A.; Spurrell, J.C.L.; Bowen, G.P.; Liu, Q.; Lam, M.; Zaiss, A.K.; Robbins, S.M.; Hollenberg, M.D.; Wickham, T.J.; Muruve, D.A. Activation of P38 and ERK Signaling during Adenovirus Vector Cell Entry Lead to Expression of the C-X-C Chemokine IP-10. *J. Virol.* **2002**, *76*, 1559–1568. [CrossRef]
153. Li, E.; Stupack, D.; Bokoch, G.M.; Nemerow, G.R. Adenovirus Endocytosis Requires Actin Cytoskeleton Reorganization Mediated by Rho Family GTPases. *J. Virol.* **1998**, *72*, 8806–8812. [CrossRef]
154. Wickham, T.J.; Mathias, P.; Cheresh, D.A.; Nemerow, G.R. Integrins Avβ3 and Avβ5 Promote Adenovirus Internalization but Not Virus Attachment. *Cell* **1993**, *73*, 309–319. [CrossRef]
155. Ranki, T.; Hemminki, A. Serotype Chimeric Human Adenoviruses for Cancer GeneTherapy. *Viruses* **2010**, *2*, 2196–2212. [CrossRef] [PubMed]
156. Brouwer, E.; Havenga, M.J.; Ophorst, O.; de Leeuw, B.; Gijsbers, L.; Gillissen, G.; Hoeben, R.C.; ter Horst, M.; Nanda, D.; Dirven, C.; et al. Human Adenovirus Type 35 Vector for Gene Therapy of Brain Cancer: Improved Transduction and Bypass of Pre-Existing Anti-Vector Immunity in Cancer Patients. *Cancer Gene Ther.* **2007**, *14*, 211–219. [CrossRef]
157. Kanerva, A.; Mikheeva, G.V.; Krasnykh, V.; Coolidge, C.J.; Lam, J.T.; Mahasreshti, P.J.; Shannon, D.B.; Barker, S.D. Targeting Adenovirus to the Serotype 3 Receptor Increases Gene Transfer Efficiency to Ovarian Cancer Cells. *Clin. Cancer Res. Off. J. Am. Assoc. Cancer Res.* **2002**, *8*, 275–280.
158. Sarkioja, M.; Kanerva, A.; Salo, J.; Kangasniemi, L.; Eriksson, M.; Raki, M.; Ranki, T.; Hakkarainen, T.; Hemminki, A. Noninvasive Imaging for Evaluation of the Systemic Delivery of Capsid-Modified Adenoviruses in an Orthotopic Model of Advanced Lung Cancer. *Cancer* **2006**, *107*, 1578–1588. [CrossRef]
159. Diaconu, I.; Denby, L.; Pesonen, S.; Cerullo, V.; Bauerschmitz, G.J.; Guse, K.; Rajecki, M.; Dias, J.D.; Taari, K.; Kanerva, A.; et al. Serotype Chimeric and Fiber-Mutated Adenovirus Ad5/19p-HIT for Targeting Renal Cancer and Untargeting the Liver. *Hum. Gene Ther.* **2009**, *20*, 611–620. [CrossRef] [PubMed]
160. Baker, A.T.; Davies, J.A.; Bates, E.A.; Moses, E.; Mundy, R.M.; Marlow, G.; Cole, D.K.; Bliss, C.M.; Rizkallah, P.J.; Parker, A.L. The Fiber Knob Protein of Human Adenovirus Type 49 Mediates Highly Efficient and Promiscuous Infection of Cancer Cell Lines Using a Novel Cell Entry Mechanism. *J. Virol.* **2020**, *95*, e01849-20. [CrossRef] [PubMed]
161. Yu, D.; Jin, C.; Ramachandran, M.; Xu, J.; Nilsson, B.; Korsgren, O.; Le Blanc, K.; Uhrbom, L.; Forsberg-Nilsson, K.; Westermark, B.; et al. Adenovirus Serotype 5 Vectors with Tat-PTD Modified Hexon and Serotype 35 Fiber Show Greatly Enhanced Transduction Capacity of Primary Cell Cultures. *PLoS ONE* **2013**, *8*, e54952. [CrossRef] [PubMed]
162. Ishida, T.; Harashima, H.; Kiwada, H. Liposome Clearance. *Biosci. Rep.* **2002**, *22*, 197–224. [CrossRef]
163. Singh, R.; Kostarelos, K. Designer Adenoviruses for Nanomedicine and Nanodiagnostics. *Trends Biotechnol.* **2009**, *27*, 220–229. [CrossRef]
164. Fisher, K.D.; Green, N.K.; Hale, A.; Subr, V.; Ulbrich, K.; Seymour, L.W. Passive Tumour Targeting of Polymer-Coated Adenovirus for Cancer Gene Therapy. *J. Drug Target.* **2007**, *15*, 546–551. [CrossRef]
165. Kreppel, F.; Kochanek, S. Modification of Adenovirus Gene Transfer Vectors With Synthetic Polymers: A Scientific Review and Technical Guide. *Mol. Ther.* **2008**, *16*, 16–29. [CrossRef] [PubMed]
166. Harris, J.M.; Chess, R.B. Effect of Pegylation on Pharmaceuticals. *Nat. Rev. Drug Discov.* **2003**, *2*, 214–221. [CrossRef] [PubMed]
167. Eto, Y.; Yoshioka, Y.; Mukai, Y.; Okada, N.; Nakagawa, S. Development of PEGylated Adenovirus Vector with Targeting Ligand. *Int. J. Pharm.* **2008**, *354*, 3–8. [CrossRef] [PubMed]
168. Fontana, F.; Shahbazi, M.-A.; Liu, D.; Zhang, H.; Mäkilä, E.; Salonen, J.; Hirvonen, J.T.; Santos, H.A. Multistaged Nanovaccines Based on Porous Silicon@Acetalated Dextran@Cancer Cell Membrane for Cancer Immunotherapy. *Adv. Mater.* **2017**, *29*, 1603239. [CrossRef]
169. Li, R.; He, Y.; Zhang, S.; Qin, J.; Wang, J. Cell Membrane-Based Nanoparticles: A New Biomimetic Platform for Tumor Diagnosis and Treatment. *Acta Pharm. Sin. B* **2018**, *8*, 14–22. [CrossRef]

170. Yang, F.; Shi, K.; Jia, Y.; Hao, Y.; Peng, J.; Qian, Z. Advanced Biomaterials for Cancer Immunotherapy. *Acta Pharmacol. Sin.* **2020**, *41*, 911–927. [CrossRef]
171. Kerkar, S.P.; Restifo, N.P. Cellular Constituents of Immune Escape within the Tumor Microenvironment: Figure 1. *Cancer Res.* **2012**, *72*, 3125–3130. [CrossRef]
172. Devaud, C.; John, L.B.; Westwood, J.A.; Darcy, P.K.; Kershaw, M.H. Immune Modulation of the Tumor Microenvironment for Enhancing Cancer Immunotherapy. *OncoImmunology* **2013**, *2*, e25961. [CrossRef]
173. Zhuang, J.; Holay, M.; Park, J.H.; Fang, R.H.; Zhang, J.; Zhang, L. Nanoparticle Delivery of Immunostimulatory Agents for Cancer Immunotherapy. *Theranostics* **2019**, *9*, 7826–7848. [CrossRef]
174. Fang, R.H.; Hu, C.-M.J.; Luk, B.T.; Gao, W.; Copp, J.A.; Tai, Y.; O'Connor, D.E.; Zhang, L. Cancer Cell Membrane-Coated Nanoparticles for Anticancer Vaccination and Drug Delivery. *Nano Lett.* **2014**, *14*, 2181–2188. [CrossRef] [PubMed]
175. Fontana, F.; Fusciello, M.; Groeneveldt, C.; Capasso, C.; Chiaro, J.; Feola, S.; Liu, Z.; Mäkilä, E.M.; Salonen, J.J.; Hirvonen, J.T.; et al. Biohybrid Vaccines for Improved Treatment of Aggressive Melanoma with Checkpoint Inhibitor. *ACS Nano* **2019**, *13*, 6477–6490. [CrossRef] [PubMed]
176. Kroll, A.V.; Fang, R.H.; Jiang, Y.; Zhou, J.; Wei, X.; Yu, C.L.; Gao, J.; Luk, B.T.; Dehaini, D.; Gao, W.; et al. Nanoparticulate Delivery of Cancer Cell Membrane Elicits Multiantigenic Antitumor Immunity. *Adv. Mater.* **2017**, *29*, 1703969. [CrossRef]
177. Fusciello, M.; Fontana, F.; Tähtinen, S.; Capasso, C.; Feola, S.; Martins, B.; Chiaro, J.; Peltonen, K.; Ylösmäki, L.; Ylösmäki, E.; et al. Artificially Cloaked Viral Nanovaccine for Cancer Immunotherapy. *Nat. Commun.* **2019**, *10*, 5747. [CrossRef] [PubMed]
178. van Erp, E.A.; Kaliberova, L.N.; Kaliberov, S.A.; Curiel, D.T. Retargeted Oncolytic Adenovirus Displaying a Single Variable Domain of Camelid Heavy-Chain-Only Antibody in a Fiber Protein. *Mol. Ther. Oncolytics* **2015**, *2*, 15001. [CrossRef]
179. Bhatia, S.; O'Bryan, S.M.; Rivera, A.A.; Curiel, D.T.; Mathis, J.M. CXCL12 Retargeting of an Adenovirus Vector to Cancer Cells Using a Bispecific Adapter. *Oncolytic Virother.* **2016**, *5*, 99–113. [CrossRef] [PubMed]
180. Mitchell, B.; Mahalingam, M. The CXCR4/CXCL12 Axis in Cutaneous Malignancies with an Emphasis on Melanoma. *Histol. Histopathol.* **2014**, 1539–1546. [CrossRef]
181. Zhang, Z.; Ni, C.; Chen, W.; Wu, P.; Wang, Z.; Yin, J.; Huang, J.; Qiu, F. Expression of CXCR4 and Breast Cancer Prognosis: A Systematic Review and Meta-Analysis. *BMC Cancer* **2014**, *14*, 49. [CrossRef]
182. Schmid, M.; Ernst, P.; Honegger, A.; Suomalainen, M.; Zimmermann, M.; Braun, L.; Stauffer, S.; Thom, C.; Dreier, B.; Eibauer, M.; et al. Adenoviral Vector with Shield and Adapter Increases Tumor Specificity and Escapes Liver and Immune Control. *Nat. Commun.* **2018**, *9*, 450. [CrossRef]
183. Stumpp, M.T.; Binz, H.K.; Amstutz, P. DARPins: A New Generation of Protein Therapeutics. *Drug Discov. Today* **2008**, *13*, 695–701. [CrossRef]
184. Dreier, B.; Honegger, A.; Hess, C.; Nagy-Davidescu, G.; Mittl, P.R.E.; Grutter, M.G.; Belousova, N.; Mikheeva, G.; Krasnykh, V.; Pluckthun, A. Development of a Generic Adenovirus Delivery System Based on Structure-Guided Design of Bispecific Trimeric DARPin Adapters. *Proc. Natl. Acad. Sci. USA* **2013**, *110*, E869–E877. [CrossRef]
185. Einfeld, D.A.; Schroeder, R.; Roelvink, P.W.; Lizonova, A.; King, C.R.; Kovesdi, I.; Wickham, T.J. Reducing the Native Tropism of Adenovirus Vectors Requires Removal of Both CAR and Integrin Interactions. *J. Virol.* **2001**, *75*, 11284–11291. [CrossRef]
186. Koizumi, N.; Mizuguchi, H.; Sakurai, F.; Yamaguchi, T.; Watanabe, Y.; Hayakawa, T. Reduction of Natural Adenovirus Tropism to Mouse Liverby Fiber-Shaft Exchange in Combination with Both CAR- Andαv Integrin-BindingAblation. *J. Virol.* **2003**, *77*, 13062–13072. [CrossRef]
187. Yao, X.-L.; Yoshioka, Y.; Ruan, G.-X.; Chen, Y.-Z.; Mizuguchi, H.; Mukai, Y.; Okada, N.; Gao, J.-Q.; Nakagawa, S. Optimization and Internalization Mechanisms of PEGylated Adenovirus Vector with Targeting Peptide for Cancer Gene Therapy. *Biomacromolecules* **2012**, *13*, 2402–2409. [CrossRef]
188. Black, P.C.; Agarwal, P.K.; Dinney, C.P.N. Targeted Therapies in Bladder Cancer—An Update. *Urol. Oncol. Semin. Orig. Investig.* **2007**, *25*, 433–438. [CrossRef]
189. Bonsted, A.; Engesæter, B.Ø.; Høgset, A.; Mælandsmo, G.M.; Prasmickaite, L.; D'Oliveira, C.; Hennink, W.E.; van Steenis, J.H.; Berg, K. Photochemically Enhanced Transduction of Polymer-Complexed Adenovirus Targeted to the Epidermal Growth Factor Receptor. *J. Gene Med.* **2006**, *8*, 286–297. [CrossRef] [PubMed]
190. Vetter, A.; Virdi, K.S.; Espenlaub, S.; Rödl, W.; Wagner, E.; Holm, P.S.; Scheu, C.; Kreppel, F.; Spitzweg, C.; Ogris, M. Adenoviral Vectors Coated with PAMAM Dendrimer Conjugates Allow CAR Independent Virus Uptake and Targeting to the EGF Receptor. *Mol. Pharm.* **2013**, *10*, 606–618. [CrossRef]
191. Kreppel, F.; Gackowski, J.; Schmidt, E.; Kochanek, S. Combined Genetic and Chemical Capsid Modifications Enable Flexible and Efficient De- and Retargeting of Adenovirus Vectors. *Mol. Ther.* **2005**, *12*, 107–117. [CrossRef] [PubMed]
192. Corjon, S.; Wortmann, A.; Engler, T.; van Rooijen, N.; Kochanek, S.; Kreppel, F. Targeting of Adenovirus Vectors to the LRP Receptor Family with the High-Affinity Ligand RAP via Combined Genetic and Chemical Modification of the PIX Capsomere. *Mol. Ther.* **2008**, *16*, 1813–1824. [CrossRef] [PubMed]
193. Prill, J.-M.; Espenlaub, S.; Samen, U.; Engler, T.; Schmidt, E.; Vetrini, F.; Rosewell, A.; Grove, N.; Palmer, D.; Ng, P.; et al. Modifications of Adenovirus Hexon Allow for Either Hepatocyte Detargeting or Targeting with Potential Evasion From Kupffer Cells. *Mol. Ther.* **2011**, *19*, 83–92. [CrossRef] [PubMed]
194. Jönsson, F.; Hagedorn, C.; Kreppel, F. Combined Genetic and Chemical Capsid Modifications of Adenovirus-Based Gene Transfer Vectors for Shielding and Targeting. *J. Vis. Exp.* **2018**, 58480. [CrossRef]

195. Gujar, S.; Pol, J.G.; Kroemer, G. Heating It up: Oncolytic Viruses Make Tumors 'Hot' and Suitable for Checkpoint Blockade Immunotherapies. *OncoImmunology* **2018**, e1442169. [CrossRef]

196. Tran, E.; Robbins, P.F.; Rosenberg, S.A. "Final Common Pathway" of Human Cancer Immunotherapy: Targeting Random Somatic Mutations. *Nat. Immunol.* **2017**, *18*, 255–262. [CrossRef] [PubMed]

197. Peng, M.; Mo, Y.; Wang, Y.; Wu, P.; Zhang, Y.; Xiong, F.; Guo, C.; Wu, X.; Li, Y.; Li, X.; et al. Neoantigen Vaccine: An Emerging Tumor Immunotherapy. *Mol. Cancer* **2019**, *18*, 128. [CrossRef]

198. Beck-Engeser, G.B.; Monach, P.A.; Mumberg, D.; Yang, F.; Wanderling, S.; Schreiber, K.; Espinosa, R.; Le Beau, M.M.; Meredith, S.C.; Schreiber, H. Point Mutation in Essential Genes with Loss or Mutation of the Second Allele. *J. Exp. Med.* **2001**, *194*, 285–300. [CrossRef] [PubMed]

199. Sato-Dahlman, M.; LaRocca, C.J.; Yanagiba, C.; Yamamoto, M. Adenovirus and Immunotherapy: Advancing Cancer Treatment by Combination. *Cancers* **2020**, *12*, 1295. [CrossRef] [PubMed]

200. Cohen, C.J.; Gartner, J.J.; Horovitz-Fried, M.; Shamalov, K.; Trebska-McGowan, K.; Bliskovsky, V.V.; Parkhurst, M.R.; Ankri, C.; Prickett, Toddd, D.; Crystal, J.S.; et al. Isolation of Neoantigen-Specific T Cells from Tumor and Peripheral Lymphocytes. *J. Clin. Investig.* **2015**, *125*, 3981–3991. [CrossRef]

201. Prickett, T.D.; Crystal, J.S.; Cohen, C.J.; Pasetto, A.; Parkhurst, M.R.; Gartner, J.J.; Yao, X.; Wang, R.; Gros, A.; Li, Y.F.; et al. Durable Complete Response from Metastatic Melanoma after Transfer of Autologous T Cells Recognizing 10 Mutated Tumor Antigens. *Cancer Immunol. Res.* **2016**, *4*, 669–678. [CrossRef]

202. Lu, Y.-C.; Yao, X.; Crystal, J.S.; Li, Y.F.; El-Gamil, M.; Gross, C.; Davis, L.; Dudley, M.E.; Yang, J.C.; Samuels, Y.; et al. Efficient Identification of Mutated Cancer Antigens Recognized by T Cells Associated with Durable Tumor Regressions. *Clin. Cancer Res.* **2014**, *20*, 3401–3410. [CrossRef]

203. Snyder, A.; Makarov, V.; Merghoub, T.; Yuan, J.; Zaretsky, J.M.; Desrichard, A.; Walsh, L.A.; Postow, M.A.; Wong, P.; Ho, T.S.; et al. Genetic Basis for Clinical Response to CTLA-4 Blockade in Melanoma. *N. Engl. J. Med.* **2014**, *371*, 2189–2199. [CrossRef] [PubMed]

204. Hugo, W.; Zaretsky, J.M.; Sun, L.; Song, C.; Moreno, B.H.; Hu-Lieskovan, S.; Berent-Maoz, B.; Pang, J.; Chmielowski, B.; Cherry, G.; et al. Genomic and Transcriptomic Features of Response to Anti-PD-1 Therapy in Metastatic Melanoma. *Cell* **2016**, *165*, 35–44. [CrossRef] [PubMed]

205. Rizvi, N.A.; Hellmann, M.D.; Snyder, A.; Kvistborg, P.; Makarov, V.; Havel, J.J.; Lee, W.; Yuan, J.; Wong, P.; Ho, T.S.; et al. Mutational Landscape Determines Sensitivity to PD-1 Blockade in Non–Small Cell Lung Cancer. *Science* **2015**, *348*, 124–128. [CrossRef] [PubMed]

206. Powles, T.; Eder, J.P.; Fine, G.D.; Braiteh, F.S.; Loriot, Y.; Cruz, C.; Bellmunt, J.; Burris, H.A.; Petrylak, D.P.; Teng, S.; et al. MPDL3280A (Anti-PD-L1) Treatment Leads to Clinical Activity in Metastatic Bladder Cancer. *Nature* **2014**, *515*, 558–562. [CrossRef] [PubMed]

207. D'Alise, A.M.; Leoni, G.; Cotugno, G.; Troise, F.; Langone, F.; Fichera, I.; De Lucia, M.; Avalle, L.; Vitale, R.; Leuzzi, A.; et al. Adenoviral Vaccine Targeting Multiple Neoantigens as Strategy to Eradicate Large Tumors Combined with Checkpoint Blockade. *Nat. Commun.* **2019**, *10*, 2688. [CrossRef]

208. Yoon, A.-R.; Hong, J.; Kim, S.W.; Yun, C.-O. Redirecting Adenovirus Tropism by Genetic, Chemical, and Mechanical Modification of the Adenovirus Surface for Cancer Gene Therapy. *Expert Opin. Drug Deliv.* **2016**, *13*, 843–858. [CrossRef] [PubMed]

209. Harris, J.C.; Scully, M.A.; Day, E.S. Cancer Cell Membrane-Coated Nanoparticles for Cancer Management. *Cancers* **2019**, *11*, 1836. [CrossRef] [PubMed]

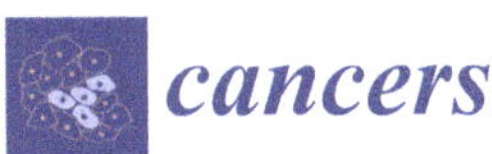

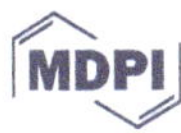

Review

The Flt3L/Flt3 Axis in Dendritic Cell Biology and Cancer Immunotherapy

Francisco J. Cueto * and David Sancho *

Centro Nacional de Investigaciones Cardiovasculares (CNIC), 28029 Madrid, Spain
* Correspondence: fjcueto@cnic.es (F.J.C.); dsancho@cnic.es (D.S.)

Simple Summary: Cancer immunotherapy is currently focused mainly on the enhancement of the effector function of T cells. However, dendritic cells (DCs) are needed to prime T cells, suggesting that DCs can be an attractive target for immunotherapy. Flt3L/Flt3 is an essential pathway for DC development and function, although its potential in cancer immunotherapy is not yet clearly established. Herein, we will review the current evidence which suggests that the stimulation of DCs through the Flt3/Flt3L axis may contribute to improved cancer immunotherapy.

Abstract: Dendritic cells (DCs) prime anti-tumor T cell responses in tumor-draining lymph nodes and can restimulate T effector responses in the tumor site. Thus, in addition to unleashing T cell effector activity, current immunotherapies should be directed to boost DC function. Herein, we review the potential function of Flt3L as a tool for cancer immunotherapy. Flt3L is a growth factor that acts in Flt3-expressing multipotent progenitors and common lymphoid progenitors. Despite the broad expression of Flt3 in the hematopoietic progenitors, the main effect of the Flt3/Flt3L axis, revealed by the characterization of mice deficient in these genes, is the generation of conventional DCs (cDCs) and plasmacytoid DCs (pDCs). However, Flt3 signaling through PI3K and mTOR may also affect the function of mature DCs. We recapitulate the use of Flt3L in preclinical studies either as a single agent or in combination with other cancer therapies. We also analyze the use of Flt3L in clinical trials. The strong correlation between type 1 cDC (cDC1) infiltration of human cancers with overall survival in many cancer types suggests the potential use of Flt3L to boost expansion of this DC subset. However, this may need the combination of Flt3L with other immunomodulatory agents to boost cancer immunotherapy.

Keywords: Flt3; Flt3L; dendritic cells; cancer immunotherapy

Citation: Cueto, F.J.; Sancho, D. The Flt3L/Flt3 Axis in Dendritic Cell Biology and Cancer Immunotherapy. *Cancers* **2021**, *13*, 1525. https://doi.org/10.3390/cancers13071525

Academic Editors: Michael Kershaw and Clare Slaney

Received: 28 February 2021
Accepted: 23 March 2021
Published: 26 March 2021

Publisher's Note: MDPI stays neutral with regard to jurisdictional claims in published maps and institutional affiliations.

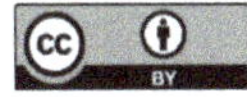

1. Introduction

The development and refinement of immunotherapy constitutes a revolution in the treatment of cancer. Most of the current immunotherapies target and unleash the effector function of lymphocytes. However, lymphocyte functions depend on their previous activation by antigen-presenting cells, among which dendritic cells (DCs) stand out. DCs were initially characterized according to their morphology and the expression of major histocompatibility complex class II and CD11c [1,2]. DCs continuously sample their microenvironment, where they can take up antigens and present them to T cells [3,4]. The outcome of the DC–T cell interaction can lead to immunity or tolerance depending on costimulatory signals present during the priming phase. Thus, DCs act as decision nodes in the initiation of T cell responses [3,4].

DCs derive from hematopoietic stem cells in the bone marrow (Figure 1) [5]. These can give rise to $Lin^-IL7Ra^-Sca1^-cKit^+FcgR^{lo}CD34^+$ common myeloid progenitors (CMPs), which can further differentiate into $Lin^-CX3CR1^+CD11b^-CSF1R^+cKit^+Flt3^+$ macrophage/DC progenitors (MDPs). MDPs can differentiate into $Lin^-CSF1R^+cKit^{lo}Flt3^+$ common DC progenitors (CDPs) which are completely committed to the DC lineage. CDPs can give rise to type 1 and type 2 conventional DCs (cDC1s and cDC2s) and plasmacytoid DCs (pDCs) [6].

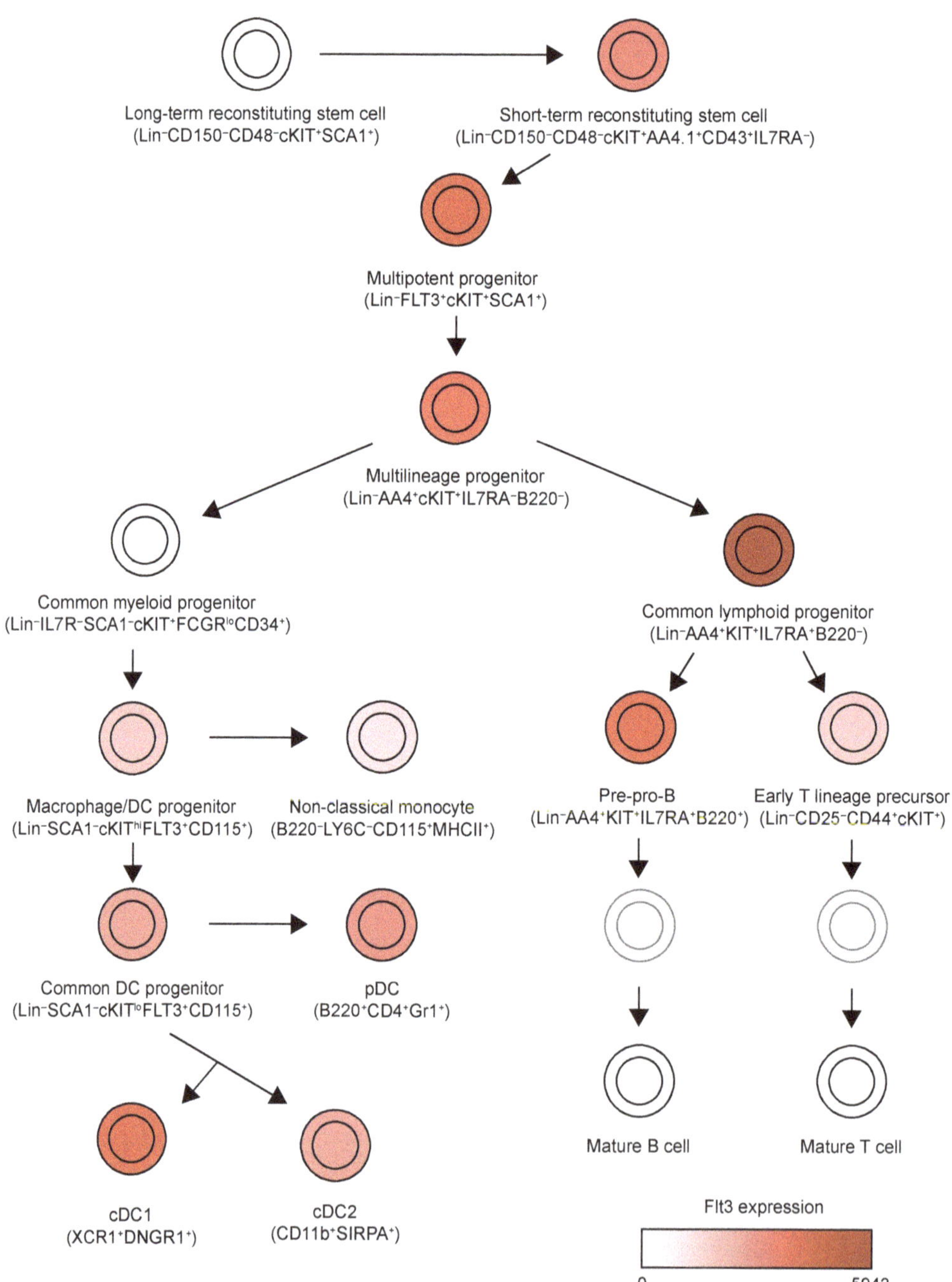

Figure 1. Expression pattern of Flt3 across mouse hematopoietic lineages. We have simplified the lineage tree generated by Jojic et al. [5]. This tree includes all cell populations identified by the first project of ImmGen to express high levels of *Flt3* (relative expression > 1000). In the case of mature cDC1s, cDC2s and pDCs, an average of Flt3 expression has been used to color them, because different populations from different organs were characterized in this consortium.

cDC1 depends on basic leucine zipper ATF-like transcription factor 3 (BATF3) and interferon regulatory factor 8 (IRF8) and expresses X-C motif chemokine receptor 1 (XCR1) and dendritic cell natural killer lectin group receptor 1 (DNGR1; CLEC9A) in humans and mice, and BDCA3 (thrombomodulin; CD141) within the $MHCII^+CD11c^+$ population in humans. In mice, two cDC1 populations can be identified: a lymphoid tissue-resident population characterized by the expression of $CD8\alpha$, and a peripheral population that expresses CD103. cDC1s stand out among other DC populations in their capacity to cross-present antigens and their production of IL12, which drives CD8 T cell responses, but are also key in CD4 T cell priming [7]. $Batf3^{-/-}$ mice cannot generate peripheral cDC1s and the cell-associated cross-presentation by their resident cDC1s is impaired. These $Batf3^{-/-}$ mice fail at controlling the development of highly immunogenic tumors, similar to $Rag1^{-/-}$ mice that lack mature lymphocytes [8].

On the other hand, cDC2s constitute a group of cells that rely on V-rel reticuloendotheliosis viral oncogene homolog B (RELB), interferon regulatory factor 4 (IRF4), and zinc finger E-box-binding homeobox 2 (ZEB2) [9]. cDC2s express CD11b and signal regulatory protein alpha (SIRPα; CD172a) in mice, and BDCA1 (CD1c) in humans. Single-cell RNA sequencing technologies have enabled discrimination od a number of subsets within cDC2s [10,11]. These findings raise new questions about their differential developmental origin and their relevance in disease. Of note, a subset that expresses macrophage galactose N-acetyl-galactosamine specific lectin 2 (MGL2) displays outstanding antitumor capacities [11].

CDPs can also give rise to at least part of the pDCs, which can also derive from other lymphoid progenitors. pDCs are characterized by the expression of IL3 receptor alpha (IL3RA; CD123) and B220 in humans and mice, respectively. E2-2 and IRF8 are the main transcription factors involved in the development of pDCs. While pDCs are important producers of IFN-I during viral infections and IFN-I may have antitumor effects [12,13], cancers can disrupt the production of IFN-I by pDCs [14–16]. Furthermore, infiltration of pDCs within human tumors associates with poor prognosis [15,17].

The roles of the different DC subsets in orchestrating adaptive immune responses make them a very attractive target to boost antitumor immunity. Different strategies have been developed and evaluated in an effort to mobilize these populations, such as the administration of GM-CSF or the adoptive transfer of cells generated or stimulated in vitro. Among those efforts, we will focus this review on the use of Flt3L to enhance antitumor immunity.

2. Expression Pattern of Flt3 and Flt3L

The Fms-like tyrosine kinase receptor 3 (Flt3) was discovered as a surface protein intensely expressed on hematopoietic stem cells (HSCs) [18] (Figure 1). However, the improvements in the characterization of different hematopoietic progenitors identified CMPs and MDPs as the main expressors of Flt3 [19]. It should be noted that Flt3 expression is preserved in terminally differentiated cDCs and pDCs [20], which suggests that Flt3 signaling might have a functional impact on mature DCs. On the other hand, Flt3 is also expressed in some lymphoid progenitors. Although its function in this ontogeny branch has not been explored as profoundly, it plays a role in the early differentiation of B cells [21] and is re-expressed by B cells in the germinal center [22]. Moreover, new data indicate that the Flt3L/Flt3 axis is necessary for the development of NK and type 2 and 3 innate lymphoid cells [23] and their progenitors [24].

Flt3 belongs to the class III of tyrosine kinase receptors, characterized by a five immunoglobulin-domain extracellular region and a split tyrosine kinase domain. Class III tyrosine kinase receptors also include CSF1R, PDGFR, KIT and FMS [25,26]. Flt3 is encoded in chromosomes 13 in human and 5 in mice, encoding for 1000 and 993 aminoacid-long proteins, respectively [27].

$Flt3^{-/-}$ mice show decreased numbers of pre-DCs ($CD11c^{int}CD45RA^{lo}CD43^{int}$ SIRP $\alpha^{int}CD4^-CD8^-MHCII^-$), cDCs, and pDCs in their spleens [19], as well as a clear drop in peripheral CD103$^+$ cDC1s, but not CD11b$^+$ cDC2s [20]. However, Flt3$^{-/-}$ mice bear normal numbers of MDPs, indicating that Flt3 signaling is not required until the developmental stage of MDPs [19].

Two years after the discovery of Flt3, Lyman et al. identified a murine protein that could bind a soluble form of Flt3 [28]. This Flt3 ligand (Flt3L) promotes the expansion of Flt3$^+$ primitive hematopoietic stem cells [28]. Soon afterwards, the human homolog of Flt3L (FLT3LG) was cloned, and a soluble version comprising its extracellular domain (amino acids 27 through 179) was found to induce proliferation in human CD34$^+$ HSCs [29]. In the organism, Flt3L is expressed by multiple cell types, including stromal bone marrow and thymic cells [30,31], activated T lymphocytes [32], and NK cells [33], among others. Of note, blood levels of Flt3L are highly elevated in patients with aplastic anemia or receiving bone marrow-damaging chemotherapy or radiotherapy [34,35], and return to normal levels within three months from successful bone marrow transplantation [34].

In mice, three main isoforms have been reported [36]. Two of them contain a plasma membrane-spanning region and are tethered to the membrane [36]. The first one contains a cytoplasmic tail and its ectodomain can be cleaved to act as a soluble form [36]. The second membrane-bound isoform results from the retention of an intron during splicing, which limits the proteolytic release of the ectodomain [36]. TNFα-converting enzyme (TACE) mediates the shedding of the ectodomain of membrane-bound forms, which releases Flt3L ectodomain [37]. Accordingly, Tace$^{-/-}$ mice display reduced levels of Flt3L in serum [37]. A third isoform lacks the membrane-spanning region and can be directly released from the cell [36]. In humans, the complete and the soluble isoforms have been identified, although not the one lacking the cytoplasmic domain [36].

Mice deficient in Flt3L show a dramatic absence of cDC1s, cDC2s and pDCs in both lymphoid and nonlymphoid tissues [20,38]. Flt3L$^{-/-}$ mice also bear fewer CDPs and common lymphoid progenitors (CLPs, c-Kit^{int}Flt3$^+$CSF1R^{lo}IL7Rα^+) in their bone marrows [38]. Thus, the deficiency in the DC lineage in Flt3L$^{-/-}$ mice is more profound than in Flt3$^{-/-}$ mice, which has been attributed to a compensatory mechanism in Flt3$^{-/-}$ mice, where DC progenitors become more sensitive to CSF1R signaling, which can compensate for Flt3 deficiency and promote DC development [39]. Under physiological conditions, NK cells, as well as other lymphocytes, have been identified as an important source of Flt3L within the tumor microenvironment (TME) [33]. The use of tumors that overexpress Flt3L has been extensively used to expand systemic cDC1s [40], but also tumor-infiltrating cDC1s [41]. Of note, several reports could not reproduce the expansion of cDC1s within the TME with systemic administration of Flt3L [42,43], which raises the possibility of some tumors becoming impervious to circulating Flt3L.

3. Flt3 Signaling in Response to Its Ligand

One of the main driving mutations in acute myeloid and acute lymphoid leukemias occurs in Flt3. This genetic alteration consists of internal tandem duplication sequences and is associated with poor prognosis in leukemia patients. Therefore, signaling pathways downstream of Flt3 have been extensively studied in the context of leukemia. However, physiological signaling through Flt3 in the context of DC generation remains largely unexplored. In the context of DCpoiesis, we will focus on homeostatic Flt3L signaling through Flt3.

As in most tyrosine kinase receptors, unstimulated Flt3 is thought to appear as a monomer on the plasma membrane, which renders its tyrosine kinase domain inactive [44]. Human Flt3L promotes the dimerization of Flt3 after binding through a compact binding domain fitting with the lock-and-key model [45,46]. Upon binding, Flt3L promotes the internalization of Flt3 receptors, which can be detected as soon as five minutes after the addition of Flt3L [46]. The internalized receptors are processed, and the products of their degradation can be observed around 20 min after the engagement of Flt3 and its ligand. The interaction of Flt3 with its ligand promotes the autophosphorylation of Flt3 tyrosine residues [47].

The first studies on the signaling cascade downstream of FLT3 used chimeric receptors composed of the extracellular domain of CSF1R and the transmembrane and cytoplasmic modules of FLT3 [48,49]. Upon the engagement of CSF1, the cytoplasmic domain of these chimeric receptors was found to bind phospholipase C gamma 1 (PLCγ1), the p85 subunit of phosphatidyl inositol 3'-kinase (PI3K), growth factor receptor-bound protein 2 (Grb2), and SHC1 [48,49]. This led to the phosphorylation of Ras GTPase-activating protein (GAP), Vav, Nck, Signal transducer and activator of transcription 5a (STAT5a), and SH2 domain-containing inositol phosphatase 1 (SHIP1), but no direct interaction with these proteins has been found [48–51]. Additionally, tyrosine residues in Gab1 and Gab2 become phosphorylated upon the FLT3/FLT3L engagement, which may act as adaptor proteins for Src homology region 2 domain-containing phosphatase 2 (SHP2), Grb2 and phosphatidylinositol 3 kinase (PI3K) [47]. Besides, Src homology 2 domain-containing transforming protein 1 (SHC) can interact and phosphorylate SHIP through its amino-terminal phosphotyrosine binding domain [50]. While most of the proteins identified downstream of Flt3 could potentially mediate its signaling, the phosphatases SHP2 and SHIP might act as negative regulators of the process.

Despite the great efforts directed to elucidating the signaling cascade triggered by Flt3, it has to be noted that most were performed in different cell lines that do not lead to the generation of mature DCs. The work in this context is more limited. Of note, Flt3L induces the phosphorylation of STAT3 during the generation of pDCs from bone marrow HSCs [52–54]. Accordingly, in mice, STAT3 is required for the development of pDCs, and its deficiency cannot be overcome by Flt3L administration [52].

Whether PI3K directly interacts or not with FLT3, the PI3K/mammalian target of the rapamycin (mTOR) cascade is clearly required for the generation of cDCs and pDCs by Flt3L [55]. In fact, CD11c-specific deletion of phosphatase and tensin homolog (PTEN), an Akt inhibitor that blocks the PI3K/mTOR pathway, expands the cDCs and pDCs [55]. In CD11cΔPten mice, both lymphoid-resident CD8α^+ and peripheral CD103$^+$ cDC1s display a stronger expansion than CD11b$^+$ cDC2s, which can be reverted by rapamycin [55].

4. Expansion of DCs with Flt3L

Flt3L fosters the expansion of granulocyte-macrophage colony-forming units (CFU-GM) and granulocyte, erythrocyte, monocyte, megakaryocyte colony-forming units (CFU-GEMM) [56], which ultimately reinforces the generation of DCs [57]. Especially, Flt3L was found to strongly expand a splenic DC population characterized by the co-expression of MHCII, CD11c, DEC205 and CD8α [57]. Flt3L can drive the expansion of various bone marrow progenitor populations, which results in the differentiation of B cells, NK cells, monocytes, red pulp macrophages, granulocytes, and innate lymphoid cells [23,38,56,58,59]. However, Flt3 expression is only conserved in mature cDCs and pDCs; not on B cells, monocytes, neutrophils, NK cells, or other innate lymphoid cells. In fact, the expansive effect of Flt3L has been reported to rely on the trans-presentation of IL15 by expanded DCs [60]. Focusing on the DC lineage, the administration of Flt3L promotes the expansion of MDPs in mice, which contributes to the expansion of both cDCs and pDCs [19]. Similarly, Flt3L can expand the amount of blood pre-DCs (CD11c$^-$IL3Rα^+ or SSC^{lo}CD117$^+$CD116$^+$CD135$^+$CD45RA$^+$ CD115$^-$) and CD141$^+$ cDC1s, CD1c$^+$ cDC2s and CD303$^+$ pDCs in human volunteers, which can increase their frequencies even more than one order of magnitude [61,62].

The lymphoproliferative effects of Flt3L, together with the described mutations of the Flt3 receptor in different leukemias, suggest that its administration might promote lymphoproliferative malignancies. In mice, one report indicated this might be the case in mice inoculated with Flt3L-expressing retroviral vectors [63]. However, such effects have not been observed in the multiple studies where Flt3L was used for immunotherapeutic purposes. This might be caused by chronicity of the exposure to supraphysiologic levels of Flt3L and/or the use of irradiated mice and retroviral vectors, which can be tumorigenic on their own, or because of the local expression of Flt3L in the bone marrow. To the best of our knowledge, no clinical trial where Flt3L has been administered to patients or volunteers has reported the promotion of lymphoproliferative malignancies.

Addition of Flt3L to culture media drives the differentiation of bone marrow cell suspensions into the DC lineage [64]. Bone marrow cell cultures in the presence of Flt3L lead to mixtures of both cDC1s and cDC2s [64], with an important population of CD11c$^+$B220$^+$ pDCs that can produce IFN-I [65]. Flt3L culture-derived cDC1s resemble naturally occurring lymphoid tissue-resident cDC1s, but they lack the bona fide cDC1 markers CD8α and DEC205 [64,66]. Addition of Notch ligand Delta-like 1 to the standard Flt3L-supplemented media facilitates the generation of CD8α^+DEC205$^+$CD103$^+$ cells, with capacity to migrate through CCR7 [67]. In addition, culturing CD34$^+$ human cells with Flt3L required Notch signaling for full cDC1 generation, with granulocyte-macrophage colony-stimulating factor (GM-CSF) providing a synergistic effect [68]. Indeed, Flt3L can be used in combination with GM-CSF to generate CD103$^+$ cDC1s from bone marrow cultures [69]. These CD103$^+$ cDC1s are responsive to TLR stimulation, which drives the expression of activation markers such as CCR7, CD80 or CD86 [69].

5. Preclinical Studies Involving Flt3L

DCs are central to inducing T cell responses that might prevent cancer growth; therefore, Marakovsky et al. suggested that Flt3L might induce powerful antitumor immune responses [57]. Among the immune populations expanded by Flt3L, cDC1s stand out, whose infiltration within the TME has been extensively associated with patient survival. Flt3L did not affect the activation state of tumor-infiltrating cDC1s, because it did not affect the levels of CD40, CD86 or MHCII in tumor-infiltrating cDC1s [70]. However, it enhanced the proliferation of tumor-specific CD8 T cells at the tumor-draining lymph node [70], possibly by increasing the number of cross-presenting dendritic cells, especially cDC1s [41,71], although an effect of Flt3L on other immunomodulatory genes cannot be ruled out. Despite the frequent identification of cDC1s as the main cross-presenting DC population, other DC populations can promote antitumor CD8 T cell responses [41,71]. In fact, cDC1s express a cluster of BATF3-dependent genes, independent of IRF8-stabilization and cross-presentation, which are required for efficient antitumor immunity [72].

Indeed, administration of Flt3L as a single agent was demonstrated to delay or revert the growth of methylcholanthrene-induced fibrosarcomas [73], C3L5 breast tumors [74], B16 melanomas, and EL4 thymomas [75]. In these cases, the protection provided by Flt3L was associated with an expansion of DCs in both lymphoid and peripheral tissues, together with tumor antigen-specific T cell responses [73–75]. This observation has been recapitulated with tumor cell lines that stably express Flt3L, which regress after initial establishment [76]. However, some studies could not reproduce the protective effect of Flt3L as a single agent. An Flt3L-encoding adenovirus injected intravenously did not show any therapeutic effect on the cl-66 mammary tumor model [42]. Despite expanding DCs and other immune populations in spleen, this Flt3L-encoding adenovirus failed at promoting the infiltration of immune cells within tumors [42]. In this line, intraperitoneal administration of human recombinant Flt3L to mice failed at controlling the growth of CT26 and B16 tumors [43]. Once again, the administration of Flt3L did not increase the amount of MHCII$^+$CD11c$^+$ cells, which might include macrophages, within the TME, despite an intense increase in the number of circulating MHCII$^+$CD11c$^+$ DCs (up to 50-fold) [43]. In another study from the same laboratory, intraperitoneal administration of Flt3L enriched tumor-infiltrating cDC1s, but not cDC2s, within an ovalbumin-expressing B16 cell line [70]. The disparity of results obtained from preclinical models treated with Flt3L can be ascribed to differences in cancer models, Flt3L administration strategies, and dosage.

As with combination chemotherapy [77], a rational combination of immunotherapeutic strategies can synergize and provide increased protection against cancer [78]. In this case, it had been suggested that, by increasing the number of DCs, Flt3L might successfully synergize with other therapies that augment the availability of tumor antigens. Accordingly, Flt3L successfully increased survival after local radiation therapy in a metastasis model of Lewis lung carcinoma, which relied on antitumor T cell responses [79]. cDC1s are required for the abscopal (out-of-field) effect of radiation therapy, supporting that this might explain these benefits [80]. Additionally, recombinant human Flt3L has been administered to mice in combination with immunostimulatory DNA and tumor antigens to raise efficient antitumor immune responses that rely on $CD8^+$ T cells and NK cells [81].

In the context of immune checkpoint blockades, tumor-infiltrating cDC1s have also been identified to play a pivotal role. Mice deficient in cDC1s do not respond to immunotherapy with anti-CTLA4 blocking antibodies [82]. Accordingly, in B16 melanomas and TRAMP prostate adenocarcinomas, anti-CTLA4 therapy can be improved by the inoculation of an Flt3L-expressing Vaccinia virus administered either intratumorally or subcutaneously in the opposite flank [83]. cDC1s are also required for other immune checkpoint therapies targeting PD1, PDL1 or 41BB [33,70,71]. cDC1-deficient mice displayed a reduced expression of PD1 in their tumor-infiltrating CD8 T cells [71], suggesting that cDC1s are required for a basal activation of cytotoxic immune responses. Besides cross-presentation, cDC1s excel at producing IL12 in the TME [41,84]. IL12 is necessary for immune checkpoint therapy [85], but not sufficient to restore responsiveness to immune checkpoint therapy in cDC1-deficient mice [71]. In several studies, a synergistic effect of Flt3L with polyI:C has been shown, whereby the cross-presentation of tumor antigens and tumor control is improved [70,71,86]. Here, a combination of Flt3L with TLR3 agonists improved the efficacy of anti-PDL1, anti-PD1 and anti-41BB [70,71,86]. However, in these reports, the precise contribution of Flt3L to the combination with immune checkpoint therapy is difficult to discern, because the antitumor effects of polyI:C do not rely on cDC1s [87]. Finally, Batf3-dependent cDC1s are also required for efficacious adoptive T cell transfer therapy [88,89]. Thus, adoptive transfer of Flt3L-secreting CD8 T cells expands tumor-infiltrating cDC1s and potentiates immunotherapy with polyI:C and 41BB-activating antibodies [76]. Overall, Flt3L constitutes a potential therapeutic agent for the treatment of cancer; multiple studies indicate that it improves antitumor immunity and restricts tumor growth. However, a better understanding of its mechanism of action might help prevent undesired interactions with other cancer therapies.

6. Flt3L in the Clinic

The potential therapeutic effect of Flt3L has given it access to several clinical trials (Table 1). In patients with metastatic colon cancer, pre-resection administration of Flt3L expanded both blood and perilesional DCs, but not tumor-infiltrating DCs [90]. In that study, Flt3L administration was associated with enhanced T cell immunity, shown by the increased sensitivity to recall antigens, but no objective response to Flt3L was observed [90]. Moreover, Fong et al. [91] reported that subcutaneous administration of recombinant Flt3L expands circulating DCs ($HLADR^+CD3^-CD14^-CD19^-CD56^-$) in carcinoembryonic antigen $(CEA)^+$ cancer patients. The increase in blood DCs for the generation of a leukapheresis product was loaded with CEA and reinfused into the patient [91]. Fong et al. allowed a two-day gap where they kept the DCs in culture to promote the upregulation of the costimulatory molecules CD80, CD86, CD40, CD83 and CMRF-44 and the chemokine receptor CCR7 [91]. Out of 12 patients, two showed tumor regression, one showed a mixed response, and in two the disease stabilized for at least three months, which associated with an enhanced cytotoxic potential from their peripheral blood mononuclear cells [91]. In another phase I clinical trial, Flt3L was administered for 14 consecutive days monthly to patients with human epidermal growth factor receptor 2 $(HER-2/neu)^+$ breast and ovarian cancers [92]. Flt3L boosted the efficacy of a vaccine based on HER-2/neu peptides administered with GM-CSF [92].

Among its concerning adverse effects, Flt3L was suggested to drive lymphoproliferative malignancies [63]. Flt3L might promote the proliferation of Flt3L-dependent/-addict cancers, which is a frequent feature of acute myeloid leukemia. However, even some acute myeloid leukemia models can benefit from the immunostimulatory effects of Flt3L [93]. Thus, caution should be taken when administrating Flt3L to immune cell malignancies.

Among the reported unwanted consequences, inflammatory effects stand out. Pre-resection administration of Flt3L to patients with metastatic colon cancers, only local symptoms such as erythematous nodules with no arthralgia, myalgia or fever were reported [90]. Fong et al. indicated that Flt3L administration only caused minor adverse effects, while DC reinfusion caused self-limited low-grade rigors and diarrhea [91]. In their study with gynecological cancer patients, Disis et al. [92] indicated that only one out of five patients receiving Flt3L alone developed a low-grade rash. Here, two out of five patients receiving Flt3L and GM-CSF developed serological alterations, with one of them suffering Sicca syndrome [92]. This study also reported the development of transient nonspecific autoimmune adverse effects in some patients [92]. As mentioned before, Bhardwaj and colleagues [94] tested the effect of Flt3L on patients receiving polyICLC, and described several low-grade local and systemic side effects, and even some high-grade effects such as anemia, hypophosphatemia, syncope, skin ulceration and sepsis. However, these are compatible with the administration of polyICLC [94]. Therefore, despite the concerns on the tumorigenic potential of Flt3L, all its adverse effects are associated with inflammatory disorders. However, all these reports agree that Flt3L was well tolerated, and no dose-limiting toxicity was observed.

Table 1. Clinical Trials targeting the Flt3 receptor. Clinical trials registered in ClinicalTrials.gov where FLT3L has been used with immunostimulatory ends. This table includes clinical trials reported by 24 November 2020. Note that FLT3L is often used in a cytokine cocktail to expand hematopoietic precursors to improve the efficacy of bone marrow transplantation [95], but those have been excluded. s.c.: subcutaneous * Estimated accrual.

Identifier	Title	Indication	Therapeutic Strategy	Accrual	Clinical Trial Phase
Status: Completed					
NCT00006223	Flt3L in Treating Patients With Acute Myeloid Leukemia	Acute myeloid leukemia in remission	S.c. recombinant FLT3L vs. observation alone	139 *	III
NCT00003431	Flt3L in Treating Patients With Metastatic Colorectal Cancer	Metastatic colorectal cancer	S.c. recombinant FLT3L before resection of hepatic metastases	12 *	I
NCT00019396	Flt3L With or Without Vaccine Therapy in Treating Patients With Metastatic Melanoma or Renal Cell Cancer	Stage IV melanoma, stage IV renal cell cancer, recurrent renal cell cancer and recurrent melanoma	S.c. recombinant FLT3L alone or with melanoma-associated peptides	54–96 *	II
NCT00020540	Biological Therapy in Treating Patients With Metastatic Melanoma or Metastatic Kidney Cancer	Metastatic skin melanoma and metastatic kidney cancer	S.c. recombinant FLT3L with s.c. recombinant CD40L	5 *	I
NCT01465139	A Study to Evaluate CDX-301 (rhuFlt3L) in Healthy Volunteers	Healthy volunteers	Escalating doses of s.c. recombinant FLT3L (CDX-301)	30	I
NCT01484470	Umbilical Cord Transplantation for the Elderly Population	Multiple hematologic malignancies	Biological: StemEx	18	II
NCT02139267	Dose-finding, Safety Study of Plasmid DNA Therapeutic Vaccine to Treat Cervical Intraepithelial Neoplasia	Cervical intraepithelial neoplasia	Electroporation of DNA vaccine encoding for FLT3L and shuffled E6 and E7 genes of HPV type 16/18 (GX-188E)	72	II

Table 1. *Cont.*

Identifier	Title	Indication	Therapeutic Strategy	Accrual	Clinical Trial Phase
Status: Active, not Recruiting					
NCT02839265	FLT3 Ligand Immunotherapy and Stereotactic Radiotherapy for Advanced Non-small Cell Lung Cancer	Advanced non-small cell lung cancer	S.c. recombinant FLT3L (CDX-301) with stereotactic body radiotherapy	29	II
NCT01811992	Combined Cytotoxic and Immune-Stimulatory Therapy for Glioma	Malignant glioma and glioblastoma multiforme	Dose escalation of adenovirus gene transfer that drives direct tumor killing and FLT3L expression	19	I
NCT02129075	CDX-1401 and Poly-ICLC Vaccine Therapy With or Without CDX-301 in Treating Patients With Stage IIB-IV Melanoma	Stage IIB-IV melanoma	S.c. recombinant FLT3L (CDX-301), s.c. or i.d. DEC-205/NY-ESO-1 fusion protein (CDX-1401) and s.c. poly-ICLC	60	II
Status: Recruiting					
NCT03789097	Vaccination With Flt3L, Radiation, and Poly-ICLC	Non-Hodgkin's lymphoma, metastatic breast cancer and head and neck squamous cell carcinoma	In situ recombinant FLT3L, radiation and Poly ICLC with pembrolizumab	56 *	I/II
NCT01976585	In Situ Vaccine for Low-Grade Lymphoma: Combination of Intratumoral Flt3L and Poly-ICLC With Low-Dose Radiotherapy	Low-grade B-cell lymphoma	In situ recombinant FLT3L (CDX-301) and poly-ICLC	30 *	I/II
NCT03329950	A Study of CDX-1140 (CD40) as Monotherapy or in Combination in Patients With Advanced Malignancies	Multiple cancer types	CD40 agonist antibody (CDX-1140) alone vs. combination with recombinant FLT3L (CDX-301) vs. combination with pembrolizumab vs. combination with chemotherapy	260 *	I
Status: not yet Recruiting					
NCT04491084	FLT3 Ligand, CD40 Agonist Antibody, and Stereotactic Radiotherapy	Non-small cell lung cancer	FLT3L (CDX-301) with CD40 agonist antibody (CDX-1140) and stereotactic radiotherapy vs. stereotactic radiotherapy alone	46 *	I/II
NCT04616248	Radio-immunotherapy (CDX-301, Radiotherapy, CDX-1140 and Poly-ICLC) for the Treatment of Unresectable or Metastatic Breast Cancer Patients	Unresectable and metastatic breast cancer	In situ FLT3L, CD40 agonist antibody (CDX-1140), poly ICLC and radiation therapy vs. addition of i.v. CDX-1140	36 *	I

Table 1. *Cont.*

Identifier	Title	Indication	Therapeutic Strategy	Accrual	Clinical Trial Phase
		Status: Unknown			
NCT03206138	Safety and Efficacy of GX-188E Administered Via EP Plus GX-I7 or Imiquimod.	Cervical intraepithelial neoplasia 3	GX-188E with GX-I7 vs. GX-188E with imiquimod	50 *	
NCT02411019	Safety and Efficacy of GX-188E DNA Therapeutic Vaccine Administered by Electroporation After Observation	Cervical intraepithelial neoplasia 3	GX-188E	72	II

In a recent study, in situ vaccination based on local administration of Flt3L, radiation therapy and the TLR3 ligand polyICLC showed increased CD8$^+$ T cell responses in patients suffering indolent non-Hodgkin's lymphoma [86]. This study reported systemic tumor regression in some patients, but not in those that had not responded to previous treatments [86]. These studies show strong evidence for a role for Flt3L in boosting antitumor immune responses, but it is important to note that trials which prove its clinical efficacy are still lacking.

7. Conclusions and Future Perspective

Due to the importance of DCs in antigen-(cross-)presenting populations, and the association of their infiltration within cancer with a positive prognosis, different compounds that drive the expansion of these populations has been actively pursued in the last years. To that aim, Flt3L is currently being evaluated in multiple clinical trials (e.g., NCT03789097, NCT02839265, NCT01976585) [86], but no clear therapeutic benefit has been reported.

Different results may rely on the administration route and dosage. In several reports, the administration of intravenous Flt3L did not show a therapeutic effect, but that might be due to the lack of DC expansion observed in those trials. It might be possible that a greater systemic dosage obtains an efficacious expansion of tumor-infiltrating cDC1s, while Flt3L expression in the TME, whether by tumor cells or adoptively transferred cells, might bring up the availability of Flt3L in situ.

In another line, Flt3L is a growth factor that is induced upon acute damage to the bone marrow. It has been shown that the seral levels of Flt3L are increased in patients with low blood cell counts, caused by aplastic anemia, chemotherapy, or radiation [34,35]. The success of bone marrow transplantation can also be tracked by determining the seral levels of Flt3L, which return to normal about three months after the procedure [34]. If chemotherapeutic drugs can drive the augmentation of Flt3L levels, the utility of exogenous Flt3L might be in the spotlight when combined with these therapies. However, it has been suggested that Flt3L can help overcome the toxicity of these therapies, similar to GM-CSF derivates.

Another aspect that remains unexplored is the effect of Flt3L on mature DC subsets, which maintain Flt3 expression. According to Cohen et al., STAT3 activation downstream of Flt3 is necessary for the efficient generation of cDC1s [96], although STAT3 signaling becomes a burden in differentiated cDC1s challenged with tumor-conditioned culture media [97]. Reviewing the significance of most of these studies is complicated, because they were carried out before a clear classification of DC had been established, and we have a better idea of which DC subsets are preferable to boost.

Another key factor that remains to be explored in depth is the impact of Flt3L in the expansion of tumor-infiltrating pDCs. Contrary to cDC1s, whose infiltration associates with good prognosis [41,82,84,98], and cDC2s, whose role in antitumor immunity is not clear [11], infiltration of human cancers by pDCs associates with poor prognosis [17].

Despite their potential as IFN-I producers, pDC functionality is impaired in the TME and instead drives Th2 and Treg immune responses through OX40L and ICOSL [15]. It is possible that Flt3L expands both cDC1s and pDCs with no net effect, but a rational combination of Flt3L with pDC-mediated immune checkpoints.

The relevance of DCs in driving antitumor immune responses, especially the strong association between cDC1 infiltration of human cancers with positive outcomes, maintain great expectation on the clinical utility of Flt3L. Despite the lack of positive results from clinical trials, designing rational therapeutic approaches through the combination of Flt3L with other immunomodulatory agents could have an impact in the war against cancer.

Author Contributions: Conceptualization, F.J.C. and D.S.; writing—original draft preparation, F.J.C.; writing—review and editing, F.J.C. and D.S.; supervision, D.S.; funding acquisition, D.S. Both authors have read and agreed to the published version of the manuscript.

Funding: Work in the D.S. laboratory is funded by the CNIC; by the European Research Council (ERC-2016-Consolidator Grant 725091); by Agencia Estatal de Investigación (PID2019-108157RB); by Comunidad de Madrid (B2017/BMD-3733 Immunothercan-CM); by Fondo Solidario Juntos (Banco Santander); and by Fundació La Marató de TV3 (201723). The CNIC is supported by the Instituto de Salud Carlos III (ISCIII), the MICINN and the Pro CNIC Foundation.

Acknowledgments: We are grateful to D.S. lab members for discussions.

Conflicts of Interest: The authors declare no conflict of interest.

References

1. Guilliams, M.; Ginhoux, F.; Jakubzick, C.; Naik, S.H.; Onai, N.; Schraml, B.U.; Segura, E.; Tussiwand, R.; Yona, S. Dendritic cells, monocytes and macrophages: A unified nomenclature based on ontogeny. *Nat. Rev. Immunol.* **2014**, *14*, 571–578. [CrossRef]
2. Merad, M.; Sathe, P.; Helft, J.; Miller, J.; Mortha, A. The Dendritic Cell Lineage: Ontogeny and Function of Dendritic Cells and Their Subsets in the Steady State and the Inflamed Setting. *Annu. Rev. Immunol.* **2013**, *31*, 563–604. [CrossRef]
3. Banchereau, J.; Steinman, R.M. Dendritic cells and the control of immunity. *Nature* **1998**, *392*, 245–252. [CrossRef] [PubMed]
4. Steinman, R.M.; Hawiger, D.; Nussenzweig, M.C. Tolerogenic Dendritic Cells. *Annu. Rev. Immunol.* **2003**, *21*, 685–711. [CrossRef] [PubMed]
5. Jojic, V.; Shay, T.; Sylvia, K.; Zuk, O.; Sun, X.; Kang, J.; Regev, A.; Koller, D.; Best, A.J.; Knell, J.; et al. Identification of transcriptional regulators in the mouse immune system. *Nat. Immunol.* **2013**, *14*, 633–643. [CrossRef] [PubMed]
6. Schraml, B.U.; Van Blijswijk, J.; Zelenay, S.; Whitney, P.G.; Filby, A.; Acton, S.E.; Rogers, N.C.; Moncaut, N.; Carvajal, J.J.; Reis, E.; et al. Genetic tracing via DNGR-1 expression history defines dendritic cells as a hematopoietic lineage. *Cell* **2013**, *154*, 843–858. [CrossRef] [PubMed]
7. Ferris, S.T.; Durai, V.; Wu, R.; Theisen, D.J.; Ward, J.P.; Bern, M.D.; Davidson, J.T.; Bagadia, P.; Liu, T.; Briseño, C.G.; et al. cDC1 prime and are licensed by CD4+ T cells to induce anti-tumour immunity. *Nature* **2020**, *584*, 624–629. [CrossRef]
8. Hildner, K.; Edelson, B.T.; Purtha, W.E.; Diamond, M.; Matsushita, H.; Kohyama, M.; Calderon, B.; Schraml, B.U.; Unanue, E.R.; Diamond, M.S.; et al. Batf3 deficiency reveals a critical role for CD8alpha+ dendritic cells in cytotoxic T cell immunity. *Science* **2008**, *322*, 1097–1100. [CrossRef]
9. Böttcher, J.P.; Reis e Sousa, C. The Role of Type 1 Conventional Dendritic Cells in Cancer Immunity. *Trends Cancer* **2018**, *4*, 784–792. [CrossRef]
10. Villani, A.-C.; Satija, R.; Reynolds, G.; Sarkizova, S.; Shekhar, K.; Fletcher, J.; Griesbeck, M.; Butler, A.; Zheng, S.; Lazo, S.; et al. Single-cell RNA-seq reveals new types of human blood dendritic cells, monocytes, and progenitors. *Science* **2017**, *356*, eaah4573. [CrossRef] [PubMed]
11. Binnewies, M.; Mujal, A.M.; Pollack, J.L.; Combes, A.J.; Hardison, E.A.; Barry, K.C.; Tsui, J.; Ruhland, M.K.; Kersten, K.; Abushawish, M.A.; et al. Unleashing Type-2 Dendritic Cells to Drive Protective Antitumor CD4+ T Cell Immunity. *Cell* **2019**, *177*, 556–571.e16. [CrossRef] [PubMed]
12. Kirkwood, J.M.; Ibrahim, J.G.; Sosman, J.A.; Sondak, V.K.; Agarwala, S.S.; Ernstoff, M.S.; Rao, U. High-Dose Interferon Alfa-2b Significantly Prolongs Relapse-Free and Overall Survival Compared with the GM2-KLH/QS-21 Vaccine in Patients With Resected Stage IIB-III Melanoma: Results of Intergroup Trial E1694/S9512/C509801. *J. Clin. Oncol.* **2001**, *19*, 2370–2380. [CrossRef]
13. Tarhini, A.A.; Cherian, J.; Moschos, S.J.; Tawbi, H.A.; Shuai, Y.; Gooding, W.E.; Sander, C.; Kirkwood, J.M. Safety and Efficacy of Combination Immunotherapy With Interferon Alfa-2b and Tremelimumab in Patients with Stage IV Melanoma. *J. Clin. Oncol.* **2011**, *30*, 322–328. [CrossRef]
14. Conrad, C.; Gregorio, J.; Wang, Y.-H.; Ito, T.; Meller, S.; Hanabuchi, S.; Anderson, S.; Atkinson, N.; Ramirez, P.T.; Liu, Y.-J.; et al. Plasmacytoid dendritic cells promote immunosuppression in ovarian cancer via ICOS costimulation of Foxp3(+) T-regulatory cells. *Cancer Res.* **2012**, *72*, 5240–5249. [CrossRef]

15. Aspord, C.; Leccia, M.-T.; Charles, J.; Plumas, J. Plasmacytoid Dendritic Cells Support Melanoma Progression by Promoting Th2 and Regulatory Immunity through OX40L and ICOSL. *Cancer Immunol. Res.* **2013**, *1*, 402–415. [CrossRef]
16. Combes, A.; Camosseto, V.; N'Guessan, P.; Argüello, R.J.; Mussard, J.; Caux, C.; Bendriss-Vermare, N.; Pierre, P.; Gatti, E. BAD-LAMP controls TLR9 trafficking and signalling in human plasmacytoid dendritic cells. *Nat. Commun.* **2017**, *8*, 913. [CrossRef]
17. Demoulin, S.; Herfs, M.; Delvenne, P.; Hubert, P. Tumor microenvironment converts plasmacytoid dendritic cells into immunosuppressive/tolerogenic cells: Insight into the molecular mechanisms. *J. Leukoc. Biol.* **2013**, *93*, 343–352. [CrossRef] [PubMed]
18. Matthews, W.; Jordan, C.T.; Wiegand, G.W.; Pardoll, D.; Lemischka, I.R. A receptor tyrosine kinase specific to hematopoietic stem and progenitor cell-enriched populations. *Cell* **1991**, *65*, 1143–1152. [CrossRef]
19. Waskow, C.; Liu, K.; Darrasse-Jèze, G.; Guermonprez, P.; Ginhoux, F.; Merad, M.; Shengelia, T.; Yao, K.; Nussenzweig, M. The receptor tyrosine kinase Flt3 is required for dendritic cell development in peripheral lymphoid tissues. *Nat. Immunol.* **2008**, *9*, 676–683. [CrossRef]
20. Ginhoux, F.; Liu, K.; Helft, J.; Bogunovic, M.; Greter, M.; Hashimoto, D.; Price, J.; Yin, N.; Bromberg, J.; Lira, S.A.; et al. The origin and development of nonlymphoid tissue CD103 + DCs. *J. Exp. Med.* **2009**, *206*, 3115–3130. [CrossRef]
21. Ray, R.J.; Paige, C.J.; Furlonger, C.; Lyman, S.D.; Rottapel, R. Flt3 ligand supports the differentiation of early B cell progenitors in the presence of interleukin-11 and interleukin-7. *Eur. J. Immunol.* **1996**, *26*, 1504–1510. [CrossRef] [PubMed]
22. Svensson, M.N.D.; Andersson, K.M.E.; Wasén, C.; Erlandsson, M.C.; Nurkkala-Karlsson, M.; Jonsson, I.M.; Brisslert, M.; Bemark, M.; Bokarewa, M.I. Murine germinal center B cells require functional fms-like tyrosine kinase 3 signaling for IgG1 class-switch recombination. *Proc. Natl. Acad. Sci. USA* **2015**, *112*, E6644–E6653. [CrossRef]
23. Baerenwaldt, A.; von Burg, N.; Kreuzaler, M.; Sitte, S.; Horvath, E.; Peter, A.; Voehringer, D.; Rolink, A.G.; Finke, D. Flt3 Ligand Regulates the Development of Innate Lymphoid Cells in Fetal and Adult Mice. *J. Immunol.* **2016**, *196*, 2561–2571. [CrossRef]
24. Parigi, S.M.; Czarnewski, P.; Das, S.; Steeg, C.; Brockmann, L.; Fernandez-Gaitero, S.; Yman, V.; Forkel, M.; Höög, C.; Mjösberg, J.; et al. Flt3 ligand expands bona fide innate lymphoid cell precursors in vivo. *Sci. Rep.* **2018**, *8*, 1–12. [CrossRef]
25. Agnès, F.; Shamoon, B.; Dina, C.; Rosnet, O.; Birnbaum, D.; Galibert, F. Genomic structure of the downstream part of the human FLT3 gene: Exon/intron structure conservation among genes encoding receptor tyrosine kinases (RTK) of subclass III. *Gene* **1994**, *145*, 283–288. [CrossRef]
26. Rosnet, O.; Birnbaum, D. Hematopoietic receptors of class III receptor-type tyrosine kinases. *Crit. Rev. Oncog.* **1993**, *4*, 595–613. [PubMed]
27. Gary Gilliland, D.; Griffin, J.D. The roles of FLT3 in hematopoiesis and leukemia. *Blood* **2002**, *100*, 1532–1542. [CrossRef]
28. Lyman, S.D.; James, L.; Bos, T.V.; de Vries, P.; Brasel, K.; Gliniak, B.; Hollingsworth, L.T.; Picha, K.S.; McKenna, H.J.; Splett, R.R.; et al. Molecular cloning of a ligand for the flt3 flk-2 tyrosine kinase receptor: A proliferative factor for primitive hematopoietic cells. *Cell* **1993**, *75*, 1157–1167. [CrossRef]
29. Lyman, S.D.; James, L.; Johnson, L.; Brasel, K.; de Vries, P.; Escobar, S.S.; Downey, H.; Splett, R.R.; Beckmann, M.P.; McKenna, H.J. Cloning of the human homologue of the murine flt3 ligand: A growth factor for early hematopoietic progenitor cells. *Blood* **1994**, *83*, 2795–2801. [CrossRef] [PubMed]
30. Hannum, C.; Culpepper, J.; Campbell, D.; McClanahan, T.; Zurawski, S.; Kastelein, R.; Bazan, J.F.; Hudak, S.; Wagner, J.; Mattson, J.; et al. Ligand for FLT3/FLK2 receptor tyrosine kinase regulates growth of haematopoietic stem cells and is encoded by variant RNAs. *Nature* **1994**, *368*, 643–648. [CrossRef] [PubMed]
31. Lisovsky, M.; Braun, S.E.; Ge, Y.; Takahira, H.; Lu, L.; Savchenko, V.G.; Lyman, S.D.; Broxmeyer, H.E. Flt3-ligand production by human bone marrow stromal cells. *Leukemia* **1996**, *10*, 1012–1018.
32. Chklovskaia, E.; Nissen, C.; Landmann, L.; Rahner, C.; Pfister, O.; Wodnar-Filipowicz, A. Cell-surface trafficking and release of flt3 ligand from T lymphocytes is induced by common cytokine receptor gamma-chain signaling and inhibited by cyclosporin A. *Blood* **2001**, *97*, 1027–1034. [CrossRef]
33. Barry, K.C.; Hsu, J.; Broz, M.L.; Cueto, F.J.; Binnewies, M.; Combes, A.J.; Nelson, A.E.; Loo, K.; Kumar, R.; Rosenblum, M.D.; et al. A natural killer–dendritic cell axis defines checkpoint therapy–responsive tumor microenvironments. *Nat. Med.* **2018**, *24*, 1178–1191. [CrossRef]
34. Wodnar-Filipowicz, A.; Lyman, S.D.; Gratwohl, A.; Tichelli, A.; Speck, B.; Nissen, C. Flt3 ligand level reflects hematopoietic progenitor cell function in aplastic anemia and chemotherapy-induced bone marrow aplasia. *Blood* **1996**, *88*, 4493–4499. [CrossRef]
35. Balog, R.P.; Bacher, R.; Chang, P.; Greenstein, M.; Jammalamadaka, S.; Javitz, H.; Knox, S.J.; Lee, S.; Lin, H.; Shaler, T.; et al. Development of a biodosimeter for radiation triage using novel blood protein biomarker panels in humans and non-human primates. *Int. J. Radiat. Biol.* **2019**, *3*, 1–13. [CrossRef] [PubMed]
36. Lyman, S.; James, L.; Escobar, S.; Downey, H.; de Vries, P.; Brasel, K.; Stocking, K.; Beckmann, M.; Copeland, N.; Cleveland, L. Identification of soluble and membrane-bound isoforms of the murine flt3 ligand generated by alternative splicing of mRNAs. *Oncogene* **1995**, *10*, 149–157. [PubMed]
37. Horiuchi, K.; Morioka, H.; Takaishi, H.; Akiyama, H.; Blobel, C.P.; Toyama, Y. Ectodomain Shedding of FLT3 Ligand Is Mediated by TNF-α Converting Enzyme. *J. Immunol.* **2009**, *182*, 7408–7414. [CrossRef]
38. Kingston, D.; Schmid, M.A.; Onai, N.; Obata-Onai, A.; Baumjohann, D.; Manz, M.G. The concerted action of GM-CSF and Flt3-ligand on in vivo dendritic cell homeostasis. *Blood* **2009**, *114*, 835–843. [CrossRef]

39. Durai, V.; Bagadia, P.; Briseño, C.G.; Theisen, D.J.; Iwata, A.; Davidson, J.T.; Gargaro, M.; Fremont, D.H.; Murphy, T.L.; Murphy, K.M. Altered compensatory cytokine signaling underlies the discrepancy between *Flt3*$^{-/-}$ and *Flt3l*$^{-/-}$ mice. *J. Exp. Med.* **2018**, *215*, 1417–1435. [CrossRef]

40. Wculek, S.K.; Amores-Iniesta, J.; Conde-Garrosa, R.; Khouili, S.C.; Melero, I.; Sancho, D. Effective cancer immunotherapy by natural mouse conventional type-1 dendritic cells bearing dead tumor antigen. *J. Immunother. Cancer* **2019**, *7*, 100. [CrossRef] [PubMed]

41. Broz, M.L.; Binnewies, M.; Boldajipour, B.; Nelson, A.E.; Pollack, J.L.; Erle, D.J.; Barczak, A.; Rosenblum, M.D.; Daud, A.; Barber, D.L.; et al. Dissecting the Tumor Myeloid Compartment Reveals Rare Activating Antigen-Presenting Cells Critical for T Cell Immunity. *Cancer Cell* **2014**, *26*, 638–652. [CrossRef]

42. Solheim, J.C.; Reber, A.J.; Ashour, A.E.; Robinson, S.; Futakuchi, M.; Kurz, S.G.; Hood, K.; Fields, R.R.; Shafer, L.R.; Cornell, D.; et al. Spleen but not tumor infiltration by dendritic and T cells is increased by intravenous adenovirus-Flt3 ligand injection. *Cancer Gene.* **2007**, *14*, 364–371. [CrossRef] [PubMed]

43. Furumoto, K.; Soares, L.; Engleman, E.G.; Merad, M. Induction of potent antitumor immunity by in situ targeting of intratumoral DCs. *J. Clin. Investig.* **2004**, *113*, 774–783. [CrossRef]

44. Stirewalt, D.L.; Radich, J.P. The role of FLT3 in haematopoietic malignancies. *Nat. Rev. Cancer* **2003**, *3*, 650–665. [CrossRef] [PubMed]

45. Verstraete, K.; Vandriessche, G.; Januar, M.; Elegheert, J.; Shkumatov, A.V.; Desfosses, A.; Van Craenenbroeck, K.; Svergun, D.I.; Gutsche, I.; Vergauwen, B.; et al. Structural insights into the extracellular assembly of the hematopoietic Flt3 signaling complex. *Blood* **2011**, *118*, 60–68. [CrossRef] [PubMed]

46. Turner, A.M.; Lin, N.L.; Issarachai, S.; Lyman, S.D.; Broudy, V.C. FLT3 receptor expression on the surface of normal and malignant human hematopoietic cells. *Blood* **1996**, *88*, 3383–3390. [CrossRef]

47. Zhang, S.; Broxmeyer, H.E. Flt3 Ligand Induces Tyrosine Phosphorylation of Gab1 and Gab2 and Their Association with Shp-2, Grb2, and PI3 Kinase. *Biochem. Biophys. Res. Commun.* **2000**, *277*, 195–199. [CrossRef]

48. Dosil, M.; Wang, S.; Lemischka, I.R. Mitogenic signalling and substrate specificity of the Flk2/Flt3 receptor tyrosine kinase in fibroblasts and interleukin 3-dependent hematopoietic cells. *Mol. Cell. Biol.* **1993**, *13*, 6572–6585. [CrossRef]

49. Rottapel, R.; Turck, C.W.; Casteran, N.; Liu, X.; Birnbaum, D.; Pawson, T.; Dubreuil, P. Substrate specificities and identification of a putative binding site for PI3K in the carboxy tail of the murine Flt3 receptor tyrosine kinase. *Oncogene* **1994**, *9*, 1755–1765. [PubMed]

50. Marchetto, S.; Fournier, E.; Beslu, N.; Aurran-Schleinitz, T.; Dubreuil, P.; Borg, J.P.; Birnbaum, D.; Rosnet, O. SHC and SHIP phosphorylation and interaction in response to activation of the FLT3 receptor. *Leukemia* **1999**, *13*, 1374–1382. [CrossRef]

51. Zhang, S.; Fukuda, S.; Lee, Y.; Hangoc, G.; Cooper, S.; Spolski, R.; Leonard, W.J.; Broxmeyer, H.E. Essential Role of Signal Transducer and Activator of Transcription (Stat)5a but Not Stat5b for Flt3-Dependent Signaling. *J. Exp. Med.* **2000**, *192*, 719–728. [CrossRef]

52. Laouar, Y.; Welte, T.; Fu, X.-Y.; Flavell, R.A. STAT3 Is Required for Flt3L-Dependent Dendritic Cell Differentiation. *Immunity* **2003**, *19*, 903–912. [CrossRef]

53. Esashi, E.; Wang, Y.-H.; Perng, O.; Qin, X.-F.; Liu, Y.-J.; Watowich, S.S. The Signal Transducer STAT5 Inhibits Plasmacytoid Dendritic Cell Development by Suppressing Transcription Factor IRF8. *Immunity* **2008**, *28*, 509–520. [CrossRef] [PubMed]

54. Li, H.S.; Yang, C.Y.; Nallaparaju, K.C.; Zhang, H.; Liu, Y.J.; Goldrath, A.W.; Watowich, S.S. The signal transducers STAT5 and STAT3 control expression of Id2 and E2-2 during dendritic cell development. *Blood* **2012**, *120*, 4363–4373. [CrossRef] [PubMed]

55. Sathaliyawala, T.; O'Gorman, W.E.; Greter, M.; Bogunovic, M.; Konjufca, V.; Hou, Z.E.; Nolan, G.P.; Miller, M.J.; Merad, M.; Reizis, B. Mammalian Target of Rapamycin Controls Dendritic Cell Development Downstream of Flt3 Ligand Signaling. *Immunity* **2010**, *33*, 597–606. [CrossRef]

56. Brasel, K.; McKenna, H.J.; Morrissey, P.J.; Charrier, K.; Morris, A.E.; Lee, C.C.; Williams, D.E.; Lyman, S.D. Hematologic effects of flt3 ligand in vivo in mice. *Blood* **1996**, *88*, 2004–2012. [CrossRef] [PubMed]

57. Maraskovsky, E.; Brasel, K.; Teepe, M.; Roux, E.R.; Lyman, S.D.; Shortman, K.; McKenna, H.J. Dramatic increase in the numbers of functionally mature dendritic cells in Flt3 ligand-treated mice: Multiple dendritic cell subpopulations identified. *J. Exp. Med.* **1996**, *184*, 1953–1962. [CrossRef] [PubMed]

58. Jensen, C.T.; Kharazi, S.; Boiers, C.; Cheng, M.; Lubking, A.; Sitnicka, E.; Jacobsen, S.E.W. FLT3 ligand and not TSLP is the key regulator of IL-7-independent B-1 and B-2 B lymphopoiesis. *Blood* **2008**, *112*, 2297–2304. [CrossRef]

59. Karsunky, H.; Merad, M.; Cozzio, A.; Weissman, I.L.; Manz, M.G. Flt3 Ligand Regulates Dendritic Cell Development from Flt3 $^+$ Lymphoid and Myeloid-committed Progenitors to Flt3 $^+$ Dendritic Cells In Vivo. *J. Exp. Med.* **2003**, *198*, 305–313. [CrossRef]

60. Guimond, M.; Freud, A.G.; Mao, H.C.; Yu, J.; Blaser, B.W.; Leong, J.W.; Vandeusen, J.B.; Dorrance, A.; Zhang, J.; Mackall, C.L.; et al. In Vivo Role of Flt3 Ligand and Dendritic Cells in NK Cell Homeostasis. *J. Immunol.* **2010**, *184*, 2769–2775. [CrossRef]

61. Maraskovsky, E.; Daro, E.; Roux, E.; Teepe, M.; Maliszewski, C.R.; Hoek, J.; Caron, D.; Lebsack, M.E.; McKenna, H.J. In vivo generation of human dendritic cell subsets by Flt3 ligand. *Blood* **2000**, *96*, 878–884. [CrossRef]

62. Breton, G.; Lee, J.; Zhou, Y.J.; Schreiber, J.J.; Keler, T.; Puhr, S.; Anandasabapathy, N.; Schlesinger, S.; Caskey, M.; Liu, K.; et al. Circulating precursors of human CD1c $^+$ and CD141 $^+$ dendritic cells. *J. Exp. Med.* **2015**, *212*, 401–413. [CrossRef]

63. Hawley, T.S.; Fong, A.Z.C.; Griesser, H.; Lyman, S.D.; Hawley, R.G. Leukemic Predisposition of Mice Transplanted With Gene-Modified Hematopoietic Precursors Expressing flt3 Ligand. *Blood* **1998**, *92*, 2003–2011. [CrossRef] [PubMed]

64. Brasel, K.; De Smedt, T.; Smith, J.L.; Maliszewski, C.R. Generation of murine dendritic cells from flt3-ligand-supplemented bone marrow cultures. *Blood* **2000**, *96*, 3029–3039. [CrossRef]
65. Gilliet, M.; Boonstra, A.; Paturel, C.; Antonenko, S.; Xu, X.-L.; Trinchieri, G.; O'Garra, A.; Liu, Y.-J. The Development of Murine Plasmacytoid Dendritic Cell Precursors Is Differentially Regulated by FLT3-ligand and Granulocyte/Macrophage Colony-Stimulating Factor. *J. Exp. Med.* **2002**, *195*, 953–958. [CrossRef]
66. Helft, J.; Böttcher, J.; Chakravarty, P.; Zelenay, S.; Huotari, J.; Schraml, B.U.; Goubau, D.; Reise Sousa, C. GM-CSF Mouse Bone Marrow Cultures Comprise a Heterogeneous Population of CD11c+MHCII+ Macrophages and Dendritic Cells. *Immunity* **2015**, *42*, 1197–1211. [CrossRef] [PubMed]
67. Kirkling, M.E.; Cytlak, U.; Lau, C.M.; Lewis, K.L.; Resteu, A.; Khodadadi-Jamayran, A.; Siebel, C.W.; Salmon, H.; Merad, M.; Tsirigos, A.; et al. Notch Signaling Facilitates In Vitro Generation of Cross-Presenting Classical Dendritic Cells. *Cell Rep.* **2018**, *23*, 3658–3672.e6. [CrossRef] [PubMed]
68. Balan, S.; Arnold-Schrauf, C.; Abbas, A.; Couespel, N.; Savoret, J.; Imperatore, F.; Villani, A.C.; Vu Manh, T.P.; Bhardwaj, N.; Dalod, M. Large-Scale Human Dendritic Cell Differentiation Revealing Notch-Dependent Lineage Bifurcation and Heterogeneity. *Cell Rep.* **2018**, *24*, 1902–1915.e6. [CrossRef] [PubMed]
69. Mayer, C.T.; Ghorbani, P.; Nandan, A.; Dudek, M.; Arnold-Schrauf, C.; Hesse, C.; Berod, L.; Stüve, P.; Puttur, F.; Merad, M.; et al. Selective and efficient generation of functional Batf3-dependent CD103+ dendritic cells from mouse bone marrow. *Blood* **2014**, *124*, 3081–3091. [CrossRef]
70. Salmon, H.; Idoyaga, J.; Rahman, A.; Leboeuf, M.; Remark, R.; Jordan, S.; Casanova-Acebes, M.; Khudoynazarova, M.; Agudo, J.; Tung, N.; et al. Expansion and Activation of CD103+ Dendritic Cell Progenitors at the Tumor Site Enhances Tumor Responses to Therapeutic PD-L1 and BRAF Inhibition. *Immunity* **2016**, *44*, 924–938. [CrossRef]
71. Sanchez-Paulete, A.R.; Cueto, F.J.; Martinez-Lopez, M.; Labiano, S.; Morales-Kastresana, A.; Rodriguez-Ruiz, M.E.; Jure-Kunkel, M.; Azpilikueta, A.; Aznar, M.A.; Quetglas, J.I.; et al. Cancer immunotherapy with immunomodulatory anti-CD137 and anti–PD-1 monoclonal antibodies requires BATF3-dependent dendritic cells. *Cancer Discov.* **2016**, *6*, 71–79. [CrossRef]
72. Theisen, D.J.; Ferris, S.T.; Briseño, C.G.; Kretzer, N.; Iwata, A.; Murphy, K.M.; Murphy, T.L. Batf3-dependent genes control tumor rejection induced by dendritic cells independently of cross-presentation. *Cancer Immunol. Res.* **2019**, *7*, 29–39. [CrossRef] [PubMed]
73. Lynch, D.H.; Andreasen, A.; Maraskovsky, E.; Whitmore, J.; Miller, R.E.; Schuh, J.C.L. Flt3 ligand induces tumor regression and antitumor immune responses in vivo. *Nat. Med.* **1997**, *3*, 625–631. [CrossRef] [PubMed]
74. Chen, K.; Braun, S.; Lyman, S.; Fan, Y.; Traycoff, C.M.; Wiebke, E.A.; Gaddy, J.; Sledge, G.; Broxmeyer, H.E.; Cornetta, K. Antitumor activity and immunotherapeutic properties of Flt3-ligand in a murine breast cancer model. *Cancer Res.* **1997**, *57*, 3511–3516.
75. Esche, C.; Subbotin, V.M.; Maliszewski, C.; Lotze, M.T.; Shurin, M.R. FLT3 ligand administration inhibits tumor growth in murine melanoma and lymphoma. *Cancer Res.* **1998**, *58*, 380–383. [PubMed]
76. Lai, J.; Mardiana, S.; House, I.G.; Sek, K.; Henderson, M.A.; Giuffrida, L.; Chen, A.X.Y.; Todd, K.L.; Petley, E.V.; Chan, J.D.; et al. Adoptive cellular therapy with T cells expressing the dendritic cell growth factor Flt3L drives epitope spreading and antitumor immunity. *Nat. Immunol.* **2020**, *21*, 914–926. [CrossRef]
77. Frei, E.; Holland, J.F.; Schneidermann, M.A.; Pinkel, D.; Selkirk, G.; Freireich, E.J.; Silver, R.T.; Gold, G.L.; Regelson, W. A Comparative Study of Two Regimens of Combination Chemotherapy in Acute Leukemia. *Blood* **1958**, *13*, 1126–1148. [CrossRef]
78. Hailemichael, Y.; Woods, A.; Fu, T.; He, Q.; Nielsen, M.C.; Hasan, F.; Roszik, J.; Xiao, Z.; Vianden, C.; Khong, H.; et al. Cancer vaccine formulation dictates synergy with CTLA-4 and PD-L1 checkpoint blockade therapy. *J. Clin. Investig.* **2018**, *128*, 1338–1354. [CrossRef]
79. Chakravarty, P.K.; Alfieri, A.; Thomas, E.K.; Beri, V.; Tanaka, K.E.; Vikram, B.; Guha, C. Flt3-ligand administration after radiation therapy prolongs survival in a murine model of metastatic lung cancer. *Cancer Res.* **1999**, *59*, 6028–6032.
80. Rodriguez-Ruiz, M.E.; Rodriguez, I.; Garasa, S.; Barbes, B.; Solorzano, J.L.; Perez-Gracia, J.L.; Labiano, S.; Sanmamed, M.F.; Azpilikueta, A.; Bolaños, E.; et al. Abscopal effects of radiotherapy are enhanced by combined immunostimulatory mAbs and are dependent on CD8 T cells and crosspriming. *Cancer Res.* **2016**, *76*, 5994–6005. [CrossRef]
81. Merad, M.; Sugie, T.; Engleman, E.G.; Fong, L. In vivo manipulation of dendritic cells to induce therapeutic immunity. *Blood* **2002**, *99*, 1676–1682. [CrossRef]
82. Spranger, S.; Bao, R.; Gajewski, T.F. Melanoma-intrinsic β-catenin signalling prevents anti-tumour immunity. *Nature* **2015**, *523*, 231–235. [CrossRef]
83. Curran, M.A.; Allison, J.P. Tumor Vaccines Expressing Flt3 Ligand Synergize with CTLA-4 Blockade to Reject Preimplanted Tumors. *Cancer Res.* **2009**, *69*, 7747–7755. [CrossRef] [PubMed]
84. Ruffell, B.; Chang-Strachan, D.; Chan, V.; Rosenbusch, A.; Ho, C.M.T.; Pryer, N.; Daniel, D.; Hwang, E.S.; Rugo, H.S.; Coussens, L.M. Macrophage IL-10 Blocks CD8+ T Cell-Dependent Responses to Chemotherapy by Suppressing IL-12 Expression in Intratumoral Dendritic Cells. *Cancer Cell* **2014**, *26*, 623–637. [CrossRef] [PubMed]
85. Garris, C.S.; Arlauckas, S.P.; Kohler, R.H.; Trefny, M.P.; Garren, S.; Piot, C.; Engblom, C.; Pfirschke, C.; Siwicki, M.; Gungabeesoon, J.; et al. Successful Anti-PD-1 Cancer Immunotherapy Requires T Cell-Dendritic Cell Crosstalk Involving the Cytokines IFN-γ and IL-12. *Immunity* **2018**, *49*, 1148–1161.e7. [CrossRef] [PubMed]

86. Hammerich, L.; Marron, T.U.; Upadhyay, R.; Svensson-Arvelund, J.; Dhainaut, M.; Hussein, S.; Zhan, Y.; Ostrowski, D.; Yellin, M.; Marsh, H.; et al. Systemic clinical tumor regressions and potentiation of PD1 blockade with in situ vaccination. *Nat. Med.* **2019**, *25*, 814–824. [CrossRef] [PubMed]

87. Gilfillan, C.B.; Kuhn, S.; Baey, C.; Hyde, E.J.; Yang, J.; Ruedl, C.; Ronchese, F. Clec9A [+] Dendritic Cells Are Not Essential for Antitumor CD8 [+] T Cell Responses Induced by Poly I:C Immunotherapy. *J. Immunol.* **2018**, *200*, 2978–2986. [CrossRef]

88. Enamorado, M.; Iborra, S.; Priego, E.; Cueto, F.J.; Quintana, J.A.; Martínez-Cano, S.; Mejías-Pérez, E.; Esteban, M.; Melero, I.; Hidalgo, A.A.A.; et al. Enhanced anti-tumour immunity requires the interplay between resident and circulating memory CD8+ T cells. *Nat. Commun.* **2017**, *8*, 16073. [CrossRef]

89. Spranger, S.; Dai, D.; Horton, B.; Gajewski, T.F. Tumor-Residing Batf3 Dendritic Cells Are Required for Effector T Cell Trafficking and Adoptive T Cell Therapy. *Cancer Cell* **2017**, *31*, 711–723.e4. [CrossRef]

90. Morse, M.A.; Nair, S.; Fernandez-Casal, M.; Deng, Y.; St Peter, M.; Williams, R.; Hobeika, A.; Mosca, P.; Clay, T.; Cumming, R.I.; et al. Preoperative Mobilization of Circulating Dendritic Cells by Flt3 Ligand Administration to Patients with Metastatic Colon Cancer. *J. Clin. Oncol.* **2000**, *18*, 3883–3893. [CrossRef]

91. Fong, L.; Hou, Y.; Rivas, A.; Benike, C.; Yuen, A.; Fisher, G.A.; Davis, M.M.; Engleman, E.G. Altered peptide ligand vaccination with Flt3 ligand expanded dendritic cells for tumor immunotherapy. *Proc. Natl. Acad. Sci. USA* **2001**, *98*, 8809–8814. [CrossRef]

92. Disis, M.L.; Rinn, K.; Knutson, K.L.; Davis, D.; Caron, D.; dela Rosa, C.; Schiffman, K. Flt3 ligand as a vaccine adjuvant in association with HER-2/neu peptide-based vaccines in patients with HER-2/neu-overexpressing cancers. *Blood* **2002**, *99*, 2845–2850. [CrossRef]

93. Wang, A.; Braun, S.E.; Sonpavde, G.; Cornetta, K. Antileukemic activity of Flt3 ligand in murine leukemia. *Cancer Res.* **2000**, *60*, 1895–1900.

94. Bhardwaj, N.; Friedlander, P.A.; Pavlick, A.C.; Ernstoff, M.S.; Gastman, B.R.; Hanks, B.A.; Curti, B.D.; Albertini, M.R.; Luke, J.J.; Blazquez, A.B.; et al. Flt3 ligand augments immune responses to anti-DEC-205-NY-ESO-1 vaccine through expansion of dendritic cell subsets. *Nat. Cancer* **2020**, *1*, 1204–1217. [CrossRef]

95. He, S.; Chu, J.; Vasu, S.; Deng, Y.; Yuan, S.; Zhang, J.; Fan, Z.; Hofmeister, C.C.; He, X.; Marsh, H.C.; et al. FLT3L and plerixafor combination increases hematopoietic stem cell mobilization and leads to improved transplantation outcome. *Biol. Blood Marrow Transpl.* **2014**, *20*, 309–313. [CrossRef]

96. Cohen, P.A.; Koski, G.K.; Czerniecki, B.J.; Bunting, K.D.; Fu, X.-Y.; Wang, Z.; Zhang, W.-J.; Carter, C.S.; Awad, M.; Distel, C.A.; et al. STAT3- and STAT5-dependent pathways competitively regulate the pan-differentiation of CD34pos cells into tumor-competent dendritic cells. *Blood* **2008**, *112*, 1832–1843. [CrossRef] [PubMed]

97. Nefedova, Y.; Huang, M.; Kusmartsev, S.; Bhattacharya, R.; Cheng, P.; Salup, R.; Jove, R.; Gabrilovich, D. Hyperactivation of STAT3 is involved in abnormal differentiation of dendritic cells in cancer. *J. Immunol.* **2004**, *172*, 464–474. [CrossRef] [PubMed]

98. Zelenay, S.; van der Veen, A.G.; Böttcher, J.P.; Snelgrove, K.J.; Rogers, N.; Acton, S.E.; Chakravarty, P.; Girotti, M.R.; Marais, R.; Quezada, S.A.; et al. Cyclooxygenase-Dependent Tumor Growth through Evasion of Immunity. *Cell* **2015**, *162*, 1257–1270. [CrossRef] [PubMed]

Review

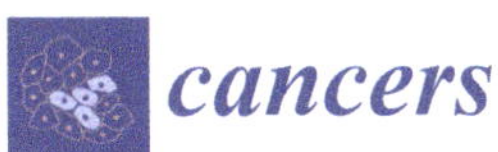

Metabolic and Mitochondrial Functioning in Chimeric Antigen Receptor (CAR)—T Cells

Ali Hosseini Rad S. M. [1,2,3,*,†], Joshua Colin Halpin [1,†], Mojtaba Mollaei [4,‡], Samuel W. J. Smith Bell [1,‡], Nattiya Hirankarn [2,3] and Alexander D. McLellan [1,*]

1   Department of Microbiology and Immunology, University of Otago, Dunedin 9010, Otago, New Zealand; josh.halpin@postgrad.otago.ac.nz (J.C.H.); smisa123@student.otago.ac.nz (S.W.J.S.B.)
2   Department of Microbiology, Faculty of Medicine, Chulalongkorn University, Bangkok 10330, Thailand; Nattiya.H@chula.ac.th
3   Center of Excellence in Immunology and Immune-Mediated Diseases, Chulalongkorn University, Bangkok 10330, Thailand
4   Department of Immunology, School of Medicine, Tarbiat Modares University, Tehran 14117-13116, Iran; mojtaba.mollaei@modares.ac.ir
*   Correspondence: ali.hosseinirad@otago.ac.nz (A.H.R.S.M.); alex.mclellan@otago.ac.nz (A.D.M.); Tel.: +64-3-479-7728 (A.H.R.S.M.); +64-3-479-7728 (A.D.M.)
†   These authors contributed equally to the work.
‡   These authors contributed equally to the work.

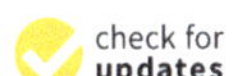

Citation: Rad S. M., A.H.; Halpin, J.C.; Mollaei, M.; Smith Bell, S.W.J.; Hirankarn, N.; McLellan, A.D. Metabolic and Mitochondrial Functioning in Chimeric Antigen Receptor (CAR)—T Cells. *Cancers* **2021**, *13*, 1229. https://doi.org/10.3390/cancers13061229

Academic Editors: Michael Kershaw and Clare Slaney

Received: 10 February 2021
Accepted: 5 March 2021
Published: 11 March 2021

Publisher's Note: MDPI stays neutral with regard to jurisdictional claims in published maps and institutional affiliations.

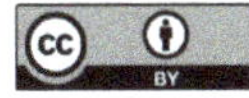

Simple Summary: We review the mechanisms of cellular metabolism and mitochondrial function that have potential to impact on the success of chimeric antigen receptor (CAR) T cell therapy. The review focuses readers on mitochondrial functions to allow a better understanding of the complexity of T cell metabolic pathways, energetics and apoptotic/antiapoptotic pathways occurring in CAR T cells. We highlight potential modifications of T cell metabolism and mitochondrial function for the benefit of improved adoptive cellular therapy. Reprogramming metabolism in CAR T cells is an attractive approach to improve antitumour functions, increase persistence and enable adaptation to the nutrient-restricted solid tumour environment.

Abstract: Chimeric antigen receptor (CAR) T-cell therapy has revolutionized adoptive cell therapy with impressive therapeutic outcomes of >80% complete remission (CR) rates in some haematological malignancies. Despite this, CAR T cell therapy for the treatment of solid tumours has invariably been unsuccessful in the clinic. Immunosuppressive factors and metabolic stresses in the tumour microenvironment (TME) result in the dysfunction and exhaustion of CAR T cells. A growing body of evidence demonstrates the importance of the mitochondrial and metabolic state of CAR T cells prior to infusion into patients. The different T cell subtypes utilise distinct metabolic pathways to fulfil their energy demands associated with their function. The reprogramming of CAR T cell metabolism is a viable approach to manufacture CAR T cells with superior antitumour functions and increased longevity, whilst also facilitating their adaptation to the nutrient restricted TME. This review discusses the mitochondrial and metabolic state of T cells, and describes the potential of the latest metabolic interventions to maximise CAR T cell efficacy for solid tumours.

Keywords: CAR T cell therapy; T cell metabolism; mitochondria; memory T cell; metabolic reprogramming

1. Introduction

Generally, a CAR is composed of both antibody and T cell receptor (TCR) components that can recognise tumour-associated antigen (TAA) in an MHC-independent manner [1]. Indeed, this is the most significant advantage of CAR T cells over other types of adoptive cell therapy (ACT), such as tumour-infiltrating lymphocytes (TILs) and TCR therapies, especially in cases where tumour cells lose or downregulate MHC expression [1]. Regardless of the generation of CAR, a CAR is composed of three main parts: the extracellular domain (antigen recognition domain and hinge), a transmembrane (TM) domain and intracellular domain(s). The antigen recognition domain is a single-chain variable fragment (scFV) consisting of variable light (VL) and heavy (VH) chain regions of a monoclonal antibody (mAb). A flexible linker, usually made of glycine and serine repeats, separates the VL and VH. The hinge and TM are commonly derived from CD28, CD8α or IgG. So far, five generations of CAR T cells have been developed utilizing a different combination of costimulatory domains in their intracellular domains (CD28, CD137, CD134, etc.). For more information about CAR T cell design, see the recent reviews [1,2].

CAR T cell therapy involves the isolation and transduction of patient or allogeneic donor-derived T cells with a cancer-specific CAR, followed by around two weeks ex vivo expansion prior to administration to the patient [3]. During this period, the patient is normally conditioned with lymphodepleting chemotherapeutic drugs to reduce competition from endogenous T cells to allow lymphopenic expansion of transfused CAR T cells [3,4]. Thus, ex vivo expansion of CAR T cells differs from physiologic T cells expansion occurring during physiological T cell responses in several aspects [3].

The efficacy of CAR T cell therapy has been most impressive in treating B-cell lymphoma expressing CD19. Recent studies have reported response rates for B-cell non-Hodgkin's lymphoma (B-NHL) and diffuse large B cell lymphoma (DLBCL) in the range of 50–80% [5–7]. The high rate of success in the treatment of B-cell lymphomas can be attributed to several reasons such as isolated antigen expression, manageable side effects and minimal impact of patient risk factors such as age, previous treatment or high international prognostic index (IPI) score used to determine patient risk group and prognosis for B-cell lymphomas [5–7]. Overall, this equates to CAR T cell therapy as an effective treatment of B cell lymphoma. However, this same efficacy has not been seen in CAR T cell clinical trials for solid malignancies (see Table 1) [8,9].

Table 1. List of recent clinical trials for CAR T cell therapy.

Clinical Trial Identifier	Phase of Study	Start Date	Target Cancer	Target Antigen	CAR Structure and Specification
NCT04697940	I/II	2020	Relapse and refractory B-cell NHL	CD19 and CD20	Tandem dual Specificity targeting CD19 and CD20 CARs
NCT04503980	I	2020	Colorectal cancer, Ovarian cancer	MSLN	MSLN-CAR-T cells secreting PD-1 nanobodies
NCT04185038	I	2019	Wide range of brain tumours	B7H3	Autologous T cells lentivirally transduced to express a 2nd generation B7H3 CAR and EGFRt
NCT03618381	I	2019	Wide range of brain tumours	EGFR806	Autologous T cells that are lentivirally transduced to express 2nd generation EGFR806 CAR and EGFRt
NCT03500991	I	2018	Wide range of brain tumours	HER2	Autologous T cells lentivirally transduced to express a 2nd generation HER2 CAR and EGFRt
NCT03198052	I	2017	Lung Cancer	HER2, MSLN, PSCA, MUC1, Lewis-Y, GPC3, AXL, EGFR, Claudin18.2 and B7-H3	3rd generation CAR-T cells targeting HER2, Mesothelin, PSCA, MUC1, Lewis-Y, GPC3, AXL, EGFR, Claudin18.2, or B7-H3

Table 1. *Cont.*

Clinical Trial Identifier	Phase of Study	Start Date	Target Cancer	Target Antigen	CAR Structure and Specification
NCT03618381	I	2019	Paediatric Solid Tumours	EGFR806, CD19 and HER22tG	Autologous T cells lentivirally transduced to express a 2nd generation EGFR806-EGFRt and a 2nd generation CD19-Her2tG
NCT03525782	II	2018	Non-small cell lung cancer	MUC1	Autologous anti-MUC1 CAR-T cells with PD-1 knockout
NCT04489862	Early I	2020	Non-small-cell lung cancer mesothelioma	MSLN	Autologous MSLN- CAR T cells secreting PD-1 nanobodies
NCT04581473	Ib/II	2020	Gastric adenocarcinoma/Pancreatic cancer/Gastroesophageal Junction Adenocarcinoma	Claudin18.2	2nd generation
NCT03356782	I/II	2017	Sarcoma/Osteoid Sarcoma/Ewing Sarcoma	CD133, GD2, MUC-1 and CD117	4th generation CAR T cell
NCT03916679	I/II	2020	Relapsed and refractory epithelial ovarian cancer	MSLN	CRISPR/Cas9 mediated PD-1 knocked-out
NCT03323944	I	2020	Pancreatic Cancer	MSLN	2nd generation/fully humanized/lentiviral transduced huCAR T-meso cells
NCT03198546	I	2019	Hepatocellular carcinoma	GPC3 and TGF-β	CD4$^+$ T cells are genetically engineered to express TGFβ-CAR and secret IL-7/CCL19 and/or scFvs against PD1/CTLA4/Tigit; CD8$^+$ T cells are constructed to express GPC3-DAP10-CAR with knockdown of PD1/HPK1
NCT02915445	I	2016	Nasopharyngeal carcinoma/Breast cancer	EpCAM	3rd generation
NCT01869166	I	2018	Unresectable/metastatic Cholangiocarcinoma	EGFR and CD133	2nd generation
NCT03198546	I	2017	Advanced hepatocellular carcinoma	GPC3 and TGF-β	3rd and 4th generation CART cells with/or without IL-7/CCL19 and/or scFv against PD1/CTLA4/Tigit in T cells knockdown of PD1/HPK1
NCT03818165	I	2019	Metastatic Pancreatic Carcinoma	CEA	Using pressure enhanced delivery device (PEDD) to increase the CAR T cell migration
NCT04650451	II	2018	HER2-positive Gastric cancer HER2-positive Breast cancer	HER2	Dual-switch using inducible coactivation domain MyD88/CD40 and an CaspaCIDe®safety switch

CAR, chimeric antigen receptor; NHL, non-Hodgkin lymphoma; MSLN, mesothelin; EGFRt, truncated epidermal growth factor receptor; HER2, human epidermal growth factor receptor 2; PSA, prostate-specific antigen; MUC1, mucin1; GPC3, glypican-3; scFv, single-chain variable fragment; PD1, programmed cell death protein 1; CTLA4, cytotoxic T-lymphocyte-associated protein 4; Tigit, T cell immunoglobulin and immunoreceptor tyrosine-based inhibitory motif (ITIM) domain; EPCAM, epithelial cell adhesion molecule; HPK1, hematopoietic progenitor kinase 1; CEA, carcinoembryonic antigen.

In contrast to bloodborne malignancies, solid tumours possess other properties that aid in tumorigenesis. Solid tumours develop an immunosuppressive microenvironment that antagonises the efficiency of the immune response. This occurs through physical factors such as low pH and immunosuppressive metabolites such as adenosine, but also through the increased expression of inhibitory ligands such as programmed cell death 1 (PD-1), cytotoxic T lymphocyte antigen 4 (CTLA-4) and lymphocyte activation gene 3 (LAG-3) [8,10]. In combination with the expression of inhibitory ligands, the extracellular environment is both highly acidic and hypoxic and being devoid of nutrients needed for cell survival and containing a high concentration of molecules that induce the recruitment and differentiation of immunoregulatory cell populations to maintain immune tolerance against the tumour [8,9,11]. For these reasons, current CAR T cell modalities have been ineffective in the treatment of solid tumours.

Therefore, several recent studies have focussed on ways to increase the efficiency of the T cell-mediated antitumour responses [9,12–16]. Effective antitumour responses require T cell infiltration to the TME, to allow T cell activation by tumour antigen recognition. T cell activation involves proliferation and differentiation, after which T cell subsets can carry out their various effector functions, which enable the destruction of malignant cells. Following rapid proliferation, T cells then undergo a contraction phase leaving long-lived memory T (T_M) cells to maintain long-term protection from relapse. Metabolic regulation is critical to enable effective response [12,17]. T cells undergo significant metabolic reprogramming throughout activation to ensure energy requirements are met and providing biosynthetic pathways with sufficient intermediates to enable macromolecule synthesis of necessary cellular components [12,17].

Mitochondria play a key role in the regulation of T cell metabolism within the TME. The role of the mitochondria in T cells is multifaceted, with key roles in energy generation, biosynthesis, migration, cell fate and programmed cell death, all of which impact on the elimination of cancer [18]. T cells are exquisitely dependent on nutrient availability to carry out their effector functions and nutrient-sensing by T cells regulates their effector functions in accordance with the availability of nutrients in the surrounding environment [19]. The metabolically flawed nature of the TME has consequently been shown to have a severe impact on the efficacy of CAR T cell treatment of solid tumours and, therefore, patient prognosis [8,12–14].

2. Mitochondria Regulates Cellular Metabolism and Biosynthesis

Adenosine triphosphate (ATP) is a key metabolite for energy expenditure in cells. Three macromolecules are used to produce ATP, carbohydrates (e.g., glucose), fatty acids and amino acids (e.g., glutamine) by catabolic metabolism. Resting cells such as naïve T (T_N) and T_M cells preferentially use this pathway to generate ATP [12,20]. Glucose catabolism initiates with glycolysis to generate two ATP and pyruvate.

The tricarboxylic acid cycle (TCA) is a cyclical series of reactions used to generate additional ATP. The initial reaction involves the combination of acetyl-CoA, generated through fatty acid, pyruvate or amino acid oxidation, with oxalacetate resulting in the six-carbon citrate molecule. Citrate is then converted into isocitrate that is decarboxylated and converted to α-ketoglutarate, and then further to succinyl-CoA releasing two CO_2 and one NADH molecule. Succinyl-CoA conversion to succinate is coupled with GTP synthesis, which can later be converted to ATP. Oxidation of succinate results in fumarate generation and the transfer of two H^+ molecules transferring to FAD to produce $FADH_2$. Fumarate is then converted to malate and further into oxalacetate to combine with acetyl-CoA to continue the cycle. NADH and $FADH_2$ generate thirty-four ATPs by passing through the electron transport chain (ETC) [12,17–21] (Figure 1).

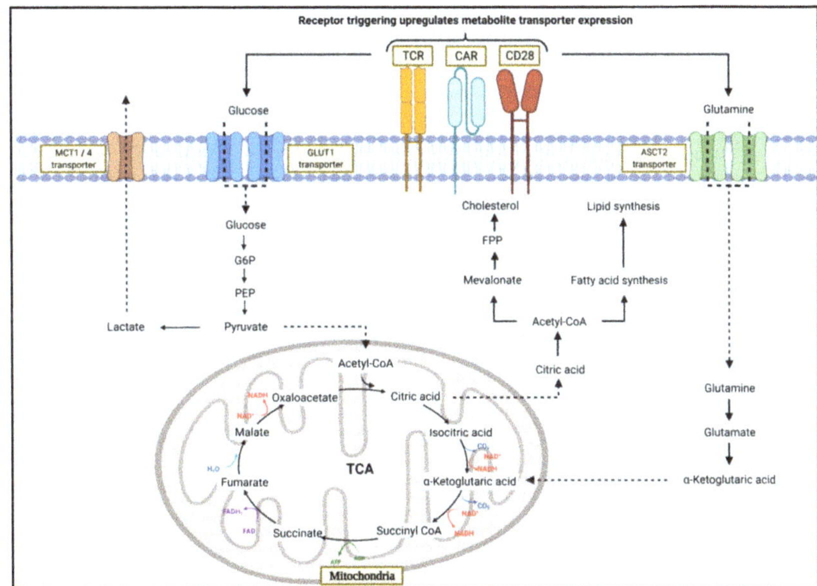

Figure 1. Schematic diagram of metabolic pathways in T cells. During T cell activation and rapid proliferation, glycolytic metabolism is enhanced by increases in glycolytic transporters such as GLUT-1. This increases glycolytically derived pyruvate conversion to acetyl-CoA, which is further converted to citrate within the TCA cycle. In the activated T cells, citrate is exported into the cytoplasm, where it is converted back to acetyl-CoA for use in the mevalonate pathway to synthesise cholesterol. To balance the export of citrate out of the TCA cycle, glutamine transporters are also upregulated. TCR, T-cell receptor; CAR, chimeric antigen receptor; MCT1, monocarboxylate transporter 1; GLUT1, glucose transporter 1; ASCT2, alanine-serine-cysteine transporter 2; G6P, glucose 6-phosphate; PEP, phosphoenolpyruvate; FPP, farnesyl diphosphate; TCA, Tricarboxylic acid cycle.

Rapidly proliferating cells such as effector T (T_{EFF}) cells use anabolic metabolism, a process to manufacture new molecules to meet the demand for newly synthesised DNA, proteins and phospholipids for cell membranes. Acetyl-CoA produced in the mitochondria can be exported to the cytosol for the synthesis of fatty acids needed for lipid biosynthesis. Similarly, other metabolic intermediates from the TCA can be used for macromolecular synthesis, in a process known as cataplerosis, utilising cholesterol, nucleotides and amino acids needed for cell proliferation. This comes at the cost of metabolite depletion, in which the mitochondria balances through anaplerosis where molecules are fed back into the cycle. Anabolic metabolism only produces two ATP in exchange for one glucose through glycolysis [12,17–21].

3. An Overview of Mitochondrial Dynamic in T Cells

Mitochondria exist in two morphologies within T cells, either short or long tubules formed through fission or fusion [18]. Mitochondrial fusion and fission allow control over mitochondrial mass and metabolism. The mitochondrial dynamic is controlled by external (e.g., growth factors and nutrients) and internal factors (e.g., transcription factors and reactive oxygen species) [22]. The induction of these processes can be triggered in response to T cell activation and changes in T cells transcriptome [22], and environmental factors such as decreased nutrient availability, such that is seen in the TME [19] (see Sections 5 and 6).

In addition to ATP production, mitochondria are involved in lipid synthesis, signalling, calcium regulation and cell cycle progression, which all together act in an anabolic manner providing fundamental materials for the activation, clonal expansion and differentiation of T cells [18,21]. The contribution of mitochondria to these events includes fission and fusion, which fulfil adapting their location, size and distribution. There is also an interaction between mitochondria and other organelles, especially the endoplasmic reticulum, to maintain its function during the procedures mentioned above. These organisational structures are known as mitochondria-associated membranes (MAMs) [23]. During T cell adaptation, mitochondria travel towards the immune synapse, where they serve as local-ATP generators and calcium-buffering infrastructures to facilitate intracellular signalling and intercellular communication for T cell activation, proliferation and differentiation [18] (Figure 2).

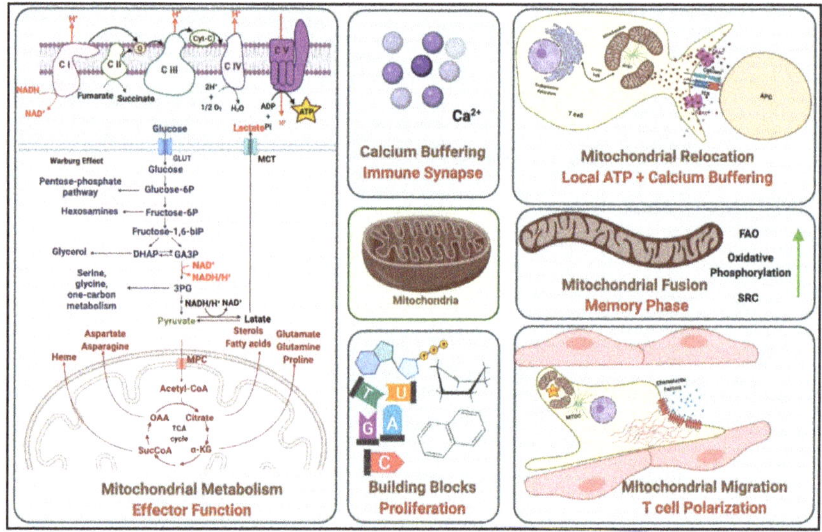

Figure 2. Mitochondrial functions in T cells. When T cells detect the chemotactic factors, mitochondria accumulate at the uropod to support the energy demand during T cell migration. Mitochondria take up calcium during stimulation and have a role in calcium homeostasis. Besides, mitochondria by anabolic metabolism provide ATP and energy for T cells, while by catabolic metabolism providing building blocks for cell proliferation. C I/II/III/IV/V, complex I/II/III/IV/V; MPC, mitochondrial pyruvate carrier; FAO, fatty acid oxidation; SRC, spare respiratory capacity.

The exact mechanisms of fusion and fission transition are poorly understood. In T cells, mitochondrial fission is triggered by T cell activation through the phosphorylation of dynamin-related protein 1 (Drp1) by protein kinase C. Drp1, a GTPase protein is translocated to the outer mitochondrial membrane (OMM) to fission sites by mitochondrial dynamic proteins, Mid49 and Mid51, and mitochondrial fission factor (MFF). Drp1 oligomerizes forming a belt around the mitochondria that constricts mitochondria through by GTP hydrolysis, splitting the inner- and outer-membranes [24,25].

Mitochondrial fusion involves three GTPases, mitofusion 1 and 2 (Mfn1 and Mfn2) and optic atrophy 1 (OPA1). During fusion, Mfn1/2 are localized at the OMM and form complexes between two adjacent mitochondria. C-terminal regions of Mfn1/2 contain hydrophobic heptad repeat region (HR2) that dimerizes with other Mfn1/2 proteins on the adjacent mitochondria bringing them into contact for fusion. OPA1 and cardiolipin are located within the mitochondria intermembrane space and are responsible for inner membrane fusion (IMM) [24,25].

Mitochondrial fusion increases cristae formation promoting increased oxidative phosphorylation (OXPHOS) and fatty acid oxidation (FAO); both pathways are essential for the survival of T_N cells and the formation of T_M cells [17,22]. In contrast, mitochondria fission promotes aerobic glycolysis within T_{EFF} cells, such as $CD8^+$ T cells. This switch to anabolic metabolism is necessary to support the production of molecules needed to carry out effector functions [17,22].

4. The Role of Mitochondria in Cell Death

Cell death encompasses a variety of processes ranging from the relatively disordered necrosis to the highly ordered, active process of apoptosis. Regulation of cell death is crucial for maintaining homeostasis, at both the tissue and system level. Antigen specific activation of T cells typically leads to clonal expansion followed by contraction, with a small population of long-lived memory cells persisting in circulation [3]. A lack of T cell contraction leads to debilitating or even fatal lymphoproliferative disorders. Apoptosis can proceed through two distinct pathways, the intrinsic and extrinsic pathways, each of which has a distinct set of apoptotic cascades triggered by both overlapping and unique induction stimuli [26]. While both apoptotic pathways are triggered by distinct stimuli and follow divergent signalling pathways, they converge at the mitochondria, where the maintenance of mitochondrial membrane integrity acts as the essential mediator of apoptotic fate. Mitochondrial membrane integrity is maintained through the complex interplay of the Bcl-2 family of proteins, consisting of both pro-apoptotic (Bax, Bak, Bok, Bid, Bim, Bad, Noxa and Puma) and antiapoptotic members (Bcl-2, Bcl-xL, Bcl-w, A1 and Mcl-1) [26].

Intrinsic apoptosis is triggered by a range of stimuli, such as DNA damage, oxidative stress or removal of homeostatic cytokines [27]. Under normal conditions, antiapoptotic members of the Bcl-2 family are able to sequester the function of the proapoptotic BH3-only family members. Apoptotic stimuli lead to increased BH-3-only protein activity, including the direct activation of apoptotic effector proteins and the suppression of Bl-2 family activity [28]. The stimuli-induced increase in activity is multifaceted, with evidence of transcriptional, post-transcriptional and post-translational modifications all shown to play a role in triggering intrinsic apoptotic cascade [29]. The activation of BH3-proteins leads to the dimerisation of Bak and Bax on the MOM mediating the cytosolic release of Cytochrome C (Cyto-C), Smac/DIABLO and the serine protease HtrA2/Omi [26,27]. Cytosolic Cyto-C then forms a multiprotein complex known as the apoptosome, consisting of Apaf-1 and the zymogenic procaspase 9. The formation of the apoptosome induces the autoproteolytic processing of procaspase 9, with the active caspase 9 then cleaving effector caspases downstream [26,30] (Figure 3).

The extrinsic apoptotic pathway is triggered through the interaction of death receptors belonging to the tumour necrosis factor (TNF) receptor superfamily, including CD95 (APO-1/Fas), TNF receptor 1 (TNFR1), TNF-related apoptosis-inducing ligand receptor 1 (TRAIL-R1) and TRAIL-R2, with their respective ligands. The prototypical receptor–ligand pair is CD95:CD95L, an important regulator of T cell contraction but also T cell activation [31]. The binding of CD95L induces a conformational change in the intracellular region of CD95 and subsequent formation of the death-inducing signalling complex (DISC). DISC is composed of Fas-associated death domain (FADD), the procaspase regulator c-FLIP, and the inactive caspase 8 and -10 zymogens. The oligomerisation of procaspase 8 leads to autoproteolytic processing, with active caspase 8 initiating the apoptotic cascade [26,30,32].

Of note, it is possible for cells to proceed through two distinct pathways following procaspase 8 activations, deemed type I and II, respectively [33]. Type I responses occur when the levels of active caspase 8 are sufficient to process caspase 3, leading to apoptosis directly. Alternatively, type II apoptotic responses involve the cleavage of the Bcl-2 family member Bib and subsequently leads to the dimerisation of Bak and Bax on the MOM, mitochondrial depolarisation and the release of Cyto-C into the cytosol [33,34] (Figure 3).

The impact of apoptosis on the maintenance of T cell function can depend on the nature of the immune response and the differentiation/activation state of the T cell [35]. Intrinsic apoptosis regulates both naïve and activated T cells; however, the nonapoptotic Bcl-2 family members play varying roles throughout T cell life. T_N cells express high levels of Bcl-2, with a rapid decrease upon TCR engagement, concurrent with a rapid increase in Mcl-1 expression [35,36]. While Mcl-1 has been shown to be critical for T cell survival at all stages of development, Bcl-2 and Bcl-xL are thought to serve distinct roles during T cell development [37].

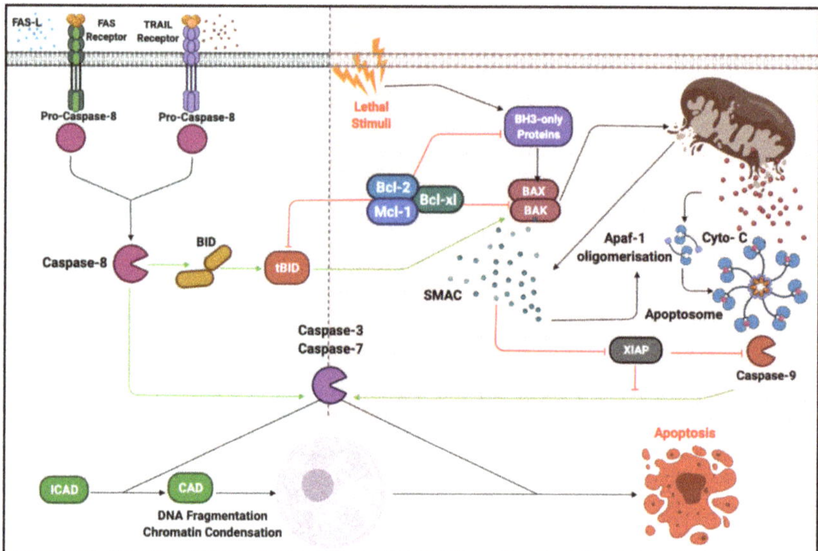

Figure 3. Mitochondrial pathways of cell death in T cells. Activation of CD95 or TNFR1 upon binding to CD95L results in the formation of DISC. Activation of caspase-8, in type I cells leads to direct activation of caspase-3 and then induction of apoptosis independent of mitochondria. In type II cells, caspase-8 cleaves the Bid proapoptotic protein to make truncated tBid. Next, tBid promote the oligomerisation of Bak/Bax complexes to form pores in the mitochondria outer membrane. Releasing Cyto-C in the cytosol activates caspase-9, which in turn activates caspase-3 to induce downstream events of apoptosis. TRAIL, TNF-related apoptosis inducing ligand; BID, BH3 interacting domain death agonist; CAD, caspase-activated DNase; ICAD, inhibitor of caspase-activated DNase; Bcl-2, B-cell lymphoma 2; Mcl-1, myeloid cell leukemia 1; Apaf1, apoptotic peptidase activating factor 1; Cyto-C, Cytochrome C; XIAP, X-linked inhibitor of apoptosis protein; TNFR1, tumor necrosis factor receptor 1; DISC, death inducing signaling complex.

Triggering of external apoptosis through CD95:CD95L interactions is critical in ensuring overactive T cells are removed from the circulation during a healthy immune function by activation-induced cell death (AICD). Intriguingly, ablation of the CD95:CD95L pathway has been shown to have little impact upon T cell contraction during acute infections but is instead essential for controlling T cell expansion in chronic antigen stimulation [38]. Constitutive exposure to CD95L also impairs DISC formation and leads to the appearance of CD95-resistant T cells with reduced AICD capacity [39].

CD95-induced apoptosis is one of the main ways that both CD4[+] and CD8[+] cytolytic T$_{EFF}$ kill transformed and virally infected cells [40]. Almost all human tumours express CD95 and CD95L on their cell surface [40]. Upregulation of CD95L along with downregulation of CD95 promote tumour progression. In the "tumour counterattack" theory, a high level of CD95L on the tumour cell surface activates AICD in TILs [40].

Tumour cells also benefit from nonapoptotic functions of CD95 signalling. Cancer cells upregulating CD95/CD95L express chemotactic factors such as IL-8 and MCP1 [41]. Chemotactic proteins increase the recruitment of proinflammatory cells and create an inflammatory environment supporting cancer growth [42]. Activation of CD95 in apoptosis-resistant tumour cells results in the induction of pathways or a set of genes with a variety of roles in tumour progression. For instance, activation of CD95 is an inducer for NF-κB and all three major mammalian target of rapamycin (MAPK) pathways: ERK1/2, p38 and JNK1/2 [43]. These pathways have implications for growth, invasion, metastasis, resistance to apoptosis and cell cycle progression [44]. Moreover, the vast majority of reports have shown that upregulation of CD95L by cancer cells is an adverse prognostic marker for many solid tumours [40], and the elimination of CD95 or CD95L in cancer cells induces "death induced by CD95 or CD95L" [45].

The implications of CD95:CD95L pathway has also been investigated in CAR T cell therapy. CAR T cells use CD95L to lysis CD95 positive target cells. Hong et al. showed that CD30-CAR T cells killed their CD30$^+$ target cells as well as CD30$^-$ surrounding cells via a cell–cell contact-dependent CD95:CD95L interaction [46]. In addition, it is well known that T$_M$ cells express CD95 as their marker, and high CD95 expression have been shown in T memory stem cells (T$_{SCM}$) [47]. In another study, Klebanoff et al. showed that stimulating CD95 signalling using soluble trimeric CD95L elevated memory CAR T cell differentiation [48].

Recent reports suggest that CD95:CD95L signalling may play a role in the limited long-term persistence of CAR T cells in treating solid tumours [49,50]. Blockade of the signalling pathway has been shown to both increase CAR T cell persistence and number without adverse effects [49–53]. Inhibiting the CD95:CD95L pathway enhanced the CAR T cell therapy in vitro and in vivo. For example, inhibition of CD95 or CD95L translation via siRNA increased the persistence of anti-CD171 CAR T cells [49]. Blockade of CD95:CD95L either with a dominant-negative form of FADD or mAb, increases the number of CAR T cells without causing autoimmunity [50,51,53]. However, due to the vital role of CD95:CD95L pathway in the development of memory CAR T cells, modulation of CAR T cells by ablating CD95 signalling must be investigated with an abundance of caution. We have recently shown that Her2-CAR T cells overexpressing Mcl-1 exhibit high resistance to AICD-mediated by CD95L [54]. Since Mcl-1 acts at a later stage of AICD, induction of Mcl-1 expression to overcome CAR T cell loss could be considered as a future approach. An additional advantage of modulating Mcl-1 expression is the ability of Mcl-1 to enhance mitochondrial and energetic dynamics and its potential role in the generation of T$_M$ cells [37,55].

5. Mitochondrial Function during T Cell Activation and Differentiation

The initiation of T cell activation results in the reprogramming of cellular metabolic processes in order to meet the bioenergetic and biosynthetic demand. Sustained TCR signalling, and costimulation, are required to initiate metabolic changes to facilitate proliferation, differentiation and production of effector molecules such as cytokines [56].

T cell activation results in a shift from OXPHOS and FAO with the promotion of the anabolic pathways of glycolysis and glutaminolysis within T cells [57,58]. This is facilitated through the engagement of the TCR to a recognised antigen; this engagement must be both high affinity and sustained to initiate downstream activation pathways [59]. The costimulation mediated by CD28 is also needed to avoid senescence, and drive the metabolic shift toward anabolic pathways needed for activation [57]. TCR engagement phosphorylates receptor-proximal tyrosine kinases that in turn activate phospholipase Cγ (PLC-γ). PLC-γ mediates two pathways, one through Ca$^+$ flux and the other through protein kinase C (PKC) activation. An increase of Ca$^+$ through its release from the endoplasmic reticulum stimulates the phosphatase calcineurin, which dephosphorylates the transcription factor NFAT. This allows for NFAT nuclear translocation to promote the expression of genes associated with T cell activation such as the (mTORC)-1 and mTORC2 [57,58]. PKC activates the mitogen-activated protein kinase MAPKs family, which also increases the rate of ribosomal synthesis within activated T cells [60].

The activation of mTORC2 activates AKT, which increases expression of GLUT1, a glucose transporter. Increased GLUT-1 expression increases glucose uptake to fuel glycolysis, thereby facilitating cell growth and proliferation [12,17,57]. Glycolytic impairment due to lower GLUT-1 expression in CD8$^+$ T cells obtained from chronic lymphocytic leukaemia (CLL) patients was suggested to contribute to dysfunctional CD8$^+$ T cells [61,62]. Increases in intracellular glucose levels further induce the differentiation of T helper 1 (Th1) and T follicular helper (Tfh) cells [63]. However, an increase in glycolytic metabolism results in an elevated level of glycolytic byproducts such as lactate. To compensate for increases in intracellular lactate concentrations, activated T cells increase expression of the monocarboxylate lactate transporters (MCTs), which regulates lactate influx and efflux [64]. Increases in cellular lactate can lead to inhibition of glycolysis in effector cells [65,66], whilst regulatory T (T$_{reg}$) cells are able to oxidize lactate to pyruvate, therefore, leading to an increase in T$_{reg}$ cells [67]. Inhibition of lactate dehydrogenase (LDH) was shown to increase the importation of pyruvate into the TCA, promoting metabolic programming in CD8$^+$ T cells with higher antitumour activity T$_{SCM}$ phenotypes [68]. Tumour cells also possess a highly glycolytic metabolism, exporting high levels of lactate into the TME, resulting in impairment of effector cell differentiation and function, whilst creating a favourable environment for T$_{reg}$ cells to further the immunosuppressive environment.

The increase of glycolysis also results in higher glycolytic intermediates such as pyruvate that is then converted to acetyl-CoA within the mitochondria via oxidation. Acetyl-CoA can then activate histone acetyltransferases (HATs), and act as an intermediate for the synthesis of fatty acids and amino acids [69].

mTOR activation results in glutamine anaplerosis via the upregulation of glutamine transporters such as ASCT2 [70]. Increases in cellular concentrations of glutamine result in fumarate accumulation, which has been shown to inhibit the action of histone demethylases that are involved in the differentiation of T cell subsets such as Th17 [71]. The ASCT2 transporter is highly overexpressed in many cancers such as melanoma [72], highlighting the competition for nutrients between malignant and immune cells within the TME. Therefore, glutamine metabolism may pose a serious therapeutic target not only for prevent tumour growth but also aiding in T$_{EFF}$ cell proliferation and function.

ERK-MAPK activation leads to an increase in ribosomal synthesis [60]. T cell activation results in large increases in the expression of genes GAR1, NHP2, RRS1, EBP2, NIP7, HRAMT and dyskerin, which have all been shown to regulate rRNA processing [60]. Similarly, TCR-triggered ERK activation results in the phosphorylation of transcription factors responsible for rRNA synthesis. Ribosomal synthesis is crucial for the production of proteins needed for effective immune function. Inhibitors of mitochondrial ribosomal pathways have been shown to decrease mitochondrial protein synthesis and cytokine production leading to impaired immune function [60].

Mitochondrial mass and mitochondrial DNA (mtDNA) also have been shown to substantially increase by the first hour of activation [58]. mtDNA encodes numerous components of the mitochondrial ETC. Mitochondrial transcription factor A (Tfam) plays a distinct role in the regulation of these genes, their transcription and the stability of mtDNA. Tfam blockage results in an impaired mitochondrial respiratory chain and mtDNA depletion, and Tfam-knocked-out T cells are less proliferative compared to wild-type T cells [73]. Similar effects have been seen in T cells with dysfunction in complexes I, II and III caused by silencing the apoptosis-inducing factor (AIF) [74]. In addition, T cells that lack stomatin-like protein 2 (SLP-2) lean toward glycolysis with decreased proliferation and IL-2 secretion due to changes in the IMM that impair the functionality of complexes I, II and III [75–77].

During T cell activation, newly synthesised mitochondria are metabolically redesigned and are dependent on a one-carbon metabolic pathway, which is comprised of three interlinked reactions: the folate cycle, the methionine cycle and the trans-sulfuration pathway. These reactions provide one-carbon methyl units needed for biosynthesis of amino acids, phospholipids and nucleotides but also involved in maintaining redox homeostasis. The conversion of folate to tetrahydrofolate (THF) is the key step of one-carbon metabolism. Addition of a one-carbon methyl unit to THF results in the generation of 5,10-methylene-THF, which is a central metabolite needed for the continuation of many metabolic pathways including the methionine and trans-sulfuration pathways. Generation of 5,10-methylene-THF is an NADPH dependent process and is facilitated by the enzyme SHMT2. This conversion is the most critical step of the one-carbon pathway, inhibition of SHMT2 activity has been shown to diminish T cell proliferation and lifespan [78]. To compensate for the high consumption of NADPH the one-carbon pathway also generates NADPH though conversion of 5,10-methylene-THF to 10-formyl-THF, resulting in the conversion of NADP$^+$ to NADPH.

NADPH is a key regulator of reactive oxygen species (ROS) and therefore the consumption and generation of NADPH/NADP$^+$ during metabolic processes such as OXPHOS and glycolysis must be balanced to maintain effective cell function and prevent ROS induced apoptosis [79]. To protect the cell from ROS generated during metabolism, glutathione (GSH), one of the most abundant antioxidants within cells, is produced [79]. Production of GSH is dependent on glutamate uptake into the cell where glutamate cysteine ligase combines glutamate, glycine and cysteine derived from the trans-sulfuration pathway to form GSH. The detoxification of ROS species by GSH results in the generation of glutathione disulphide (GSSG), a reversible reaction dependent on NADPH, highlighting its role in maintaining redox homeostasis [79,80].

Increased glutaminolysis during T cell activation, as mentioned previously, not only provides increased ATP generation but also provides essential precursor metabolites for biosynthetic pathways including the synthesis of GSH, which facilitates redox homeostasis during T cell activation. Previous research by Gaojian et al. [81] illustrated that glutamine derived glutamate was a key precursor in the de novo synthesis of GSH and furthermore that glutamine catabolism directed T cell lineage fate, in particular that glutamine deprivation skewed differentiation toward T$_{reg}$ phenotypes [82,83]. Decreased glutamine levels within the TME not only impacts T cell energy generation but also the ability for T cells to maintain redox homeostasis needed to ensure effective cytokine production and cell proliferation and lineage differentiation [83,84].

The rate of protein, nucleic acid and lipid biosynthesis is increased within activated T cells when compared to T$_N$ cells in order to maintain high levels of cell division. Increases in biosynthetic activities can be attributed to increases in glycolytic intermediates, a result of increased glycolysis within activated T cells as mentioned above. Hexokinase (HK) isoforms are mediators for the rate limiting step of glycolysis, the conversion of glucose to glucose-6-phoshpate (G6P) [58,85]. Upon T cell activation there is a significant increase in the levels of HK1 and HK2 isoforms, shown to have the highest level of catalytic activity [86]. G6P can be dehydrogenated in the pentose phosphate pathway (PPP) to produce NADH for use as both a reducing agent in the synthesis of fatty acids and a cofactor in the synthesis of nucleotides for DNA replication. Dwindling glycolysis capacity by blocking HK2 favours T cell expansion [58], without affecting CD8$^+$ T cell activation through TCR-CD28 stimulation [58,87]. HK2 knock-out causes a severe antitumour activity in CD8$^+$ T cells by overexpressing PD-1 and Tim3 [87]. Interestingly, HK2 deletion seems to be dispensable for CD4$^+$ T cell responses against viral infection [85,88] but not for CD8$^+$ responses [87]. However, the long-term efficacy of T cells that no longer possess a key metabolic gene is difficult to predict. It is difficult to elucidate whether the effects observed after deletion of HK2 are direct or indirect due to lack of HK2. Besides, it has been shown that HK1 could serve as a compensatory gene in the absence of HK2 [88]. Hence, further studies using small molecules or knockdown HK1/HK2 are needed to clarify the HKs function in T cells.

Mitochondrial-derived acetyl-CoA concentrations also increase during activation due to increased pyruvate levels; another glycolytic intermediate increased upon activation [57]. During proliferation, glycolysis-derived pyruvate feeds into the TCA, where it is converted to acetyl-CoA and then citrate within the mitochondria. This citrate is then exported to the cytosol, where it is catalysed to cytosolic acetyl-CoA used in fatty acid synthesis and made available for the mevalonate pathway [89]. Citrate export is an example of how the mitochondria maintain balance during T cell expansion, as without activation induced increases in glutamine oxidation and glycolysis, citrate export would result in TCA stalling [89]. Instead, imported glutamine can be converted into α-ketoglutarate to enter the TCA to compensate for the lack of citrate conversion. Interestingly studies have shown excess α-ketoglutarate can undergo reductive carboxylation within the cytoplasm to form citrate and subsequently acetyl-CoA to also feed the mevalonate pathway [90]. The mevalonate pathway involves the condensation of acetyl-CoA to hydroxy-3-methylglutaryl-CoA (HMG-CoA). Through a cascade of anabolic conversions, farnesyl pyrophosphate (FPP) is formed and is a substrate for the synthesis of cholesterol, steroids, dolichol and ubiquinone [89].

T cell activation increases the expression of the genes, which encode HMG-synthase and reductase, both of which are needed for the initiation of the mevalonate pathway [89]. The role of cholesterol in T cell activation and its relation to solid cancers has not been fully investigated. Studies have shown that inhibition of ACAT1, a cholesterol esterification enzyme, has led to increased cellular cholesterol that has, in turn, increased CD8$^+$ function through increased TCR clustering at the plasma membrane [91]. In contrast, other work has shown that increased cellular cholesterol has inhibited glycolysis, and increased expression of inhibitory markers resulting in exhaustion of TILs [92]. Thus, the exact role cholesterol metabolism has in T cell activation is not yet fully understood.

Overall mitochondrial metabolic pathways are reprogrammed during T cell activation away from OXPHOS and FAO and instead toward anabolic pathways such as glycolysis and glutaminolysis. The balance of intermediates produced within these pathways enables the biosynthesis of macromolecules needed for T cell activation. After antigen clearance, most T_{EFF} cells undergo contraction, while a small number of T cells differentiate to long-lived T_M cells. Activation of FAO metabolic program is necessary for T_M differentiation, long-term survival and enhanced response to the second antigen encounter [22]. It has been shown that the enhanced response in T_M cells compared to T_{EFF} cells is linked to the mitochondria mass, upregulation of genes involved in FAO and their higher spare respiratory capacity (SRC) [17,22]. The impact of the TME by disrupting and exploiting these processes promotes tumorigenesis by impeding immune metabolic pressures resulting in an inadequate immune response against the malignancy.

6. Mitochondrial State in TILs and Exhausted T Cells within TME

Solid tumours remain the greatest challenge to ACT, with limited responsiveness to a raft of currently available cellular therapies. In a large part, this is owing to the TME, which represents a highly immunosuppressive, physically obstructive and nutrient-depleted environment that severely limits the ability of ACT to generate effective antitumour responses. The TME also includes infiltrating immune cells, tumour stroma, blood vessels and soluble factors that all act to limit tumour immunity.

The presence of TILs within tumour masses is a known positive prognostic factor for the response to immunotherapy. However, certain TIL populations show a functionally exhausted phenotype and drastically reduced effector function, allowing for tumour escape. [11]. In addition to TIL, a range of T cell populations are present in the TME that suffer similar functional exhaustion that is thought to play a key role in the ability for malignant cells to outgrow and cause disease. As with the endogenous immune response, ACT approaches using CAR T cells for treating solid tumours face the same obstacles.

A range of studies has shown that this functional insufficiency and exhausted phenotype can be linked to mitochondrial dysfunction [93,94]. As previously described, a number of metabolic processes play important roles in maintaining REDOX balance within T cells [79,81,84]. Recent studies have indicated that tumour-localised T cells can show a loss of redox balance leading to the development of a functionally exhausted phenotype. Vardhana et al. showed that mitochondrial insufficiency in T cells exposed to chronic antigen leads to an increase in the NADH/NAD$^+$ ratio [94]. The increased oxidative stress was linked to the expression of T cell exhaustion genes and an inability of these cells to undergo proliferation or self-renewal [94]. While this study showed that treatment of exhausted T cells with antioxidants could partially restore functional capacity, studies examining the efficacy of anti-PD-1 therapy have shown contrary results when examining the role of ROS in improving therapeutic outcomes [95–97]. Alternatively, a CAR T cell construct coexpressing catalase was shown to reduce intracellular oxidative stress and outperform traditional CAR T cells [98]. These results indicate that the role that ROS play in the functioning of T cells within the TME is poorly understood and will remain an area of active research.

Tumour cells show augmented metabolism to fuel their rapid proliferation, leading to markedly lower levels of a range of crucial nutrients in the TME than healthy tissue. The nutrient restrictions faced by T cells within the TME contribute to reduced effector function, proliferation and differentiation. Glucose is an essential nutrient required for the rapid generation of ATP to support the rapid proliferation of activated T_{EFF}, and the production of cytokines for effective immune activity. Activation of tumour-specific T cells in glucose low concentration leads to hyporesponsiveness, with decreased expression of genes associated with cell cycle progression, effector function and cytokine production [8, 11,99]. Glycolytically active T cells may be pushed towards an unsustainable metabolic program in which the ability to produce ATP through glycolytic metabolism is unable to satisfy cellular requirements. Glucose-deprived $CD8^+$ T cells show an increased AMP:ATP ratio, leading to the activation of AMP-activated protein kinase (AMPK) and subsequent shift towards anabolic metabolism in an attempt to maintain viability and regulate energy homeostasis [12,17,21]. Additionally, the activation of AMPK in nutrient-poor conditions has been linked to the senescence of T cells. AMPK is known as the key element in the regulation of FAO [12,17,71,73,89]. In normal conditions, the differentiation toward T_M cells is partially linked to FAO, which is accomplished through AMPK and lipolysis.

In addition to glucose, glutamine is also scarce in the TME and serves as a key regulator of the function of activated T cells. Glutamine depletion reduces the ability of activated T cells to produce IL-2 or IFN-γ, and provoking a drastic reduction in activation mediated proliferation. Coupled with a loss in key effector functions, reduced glutamine impacts upon $CD4^+$ T cell differentiation and further potentiates the TME [70]. Deficiencies in the ASCT2 glutamine transporter blunt T_N cell differentiation from Th1 to Th17 cells, but still maintain T_{reg} differentiation. However, downregulation of glutaminolysis regulates the conversion of Th1 toward T_{reg} cells [70,90]. Therefore, a lack of glutamine prevents T cells functioning correctly in the TME, and stimulates the emergence of regulatory T cell subtypes [100]. Recently Leone et al. [82] developed an inert glutamine antagonist (JHU083), which is only activated upon cleavage of the prodrug through enriched enzymes in the TME. They showed that conditional activation of JHU083 suppresses tumour cell growth while boosting the $CD8^+$ T cell proliferation, activation and T_M differentiation. The combination of JHU083 with anti-PD-1 augmented the antitumour activity of TILs in vivo [82].

A hallmark of the TME is hypoxia generated by heterogeneous and ineffectual vascular networks and aberrant tumour cell metabolism. Hypoxia leads to a range of alterations in cellular function, including an increase in glycolytic metabolism and a decrease in proliferation [12,17,21]. The hypoxic response is mediated primarily through the action of the hypoxia inducible factor (HIF) family, with hypoxia leading to increased activity through stabilisation of HIFs. Hypoxia leads to the recruitment of T cells to the TME in addition to a vast array of potentially immunosuppressive cells to the TME including myeloid-derived suppressor cells (MDSCs) and macrophages [11,101]. The binding of HIF-1 to HIF regulatory elements induces the upregulation of PDL-1 in macrophages, MDSC and tumour cells [11,101]. Additionally, HIF signalling increases the expression of the coinhibitory receptor CTLA-4 on $CD8^+$ T cells [101]. The upregulation of these coreceptors negatively impacts the ability of activated T cells to undergo glycolysis, and instead switches metabolic function towards FAO and reduces IFN-γ production [101]. Increased HIF-1a expression and encouragement of FAO are vital processes that allow the survival of T_{reg} in the TME compared to alternative T cell subtypes that show high glycolytic commitment [101]. Irrespective of the evidence outlined above, HIF signalling has been shown in some circumstances to potentially increase the cytotoxic capacity of $CD8^+$ T cells [102]. However, these studies may not fully represent the encounter of $CD8^+$ T cells with tumour antigen in the context of TME hypoxia [103].

The range of inhibitory immune cells present within the TME, including T_{reg} cells, produce a milieu of soluble factors that serve to negatively regulate the function of TILs. At the centre of these suppressive factors is TGF-β, secreted by MDSCs, macrophages, T_{reg} and tumour cells within the TME [11]. The impact of TGF-β upon the T cell function is distinct in T_N and T_{EFF} cells, with T_N cell differentiation augmented while TEFF show impaired proliferation and cytokine expression [104]. Blockade of TGF-ß in a murine tumour model has been shown to improve tumour regression and enhance the function of cytotoxic lymphocytes [105]. Accordingly, CAR T cells have been engineered to allow for resistance or subversion of TGF-β signalling. CAR T cells harbouring a knockout of the endogenous TGF-β receptor showed improved effector function and increased tumour elimination [106]. Additionally, redirecting CAR T cells to recognise soluble TGF-β converted the immunosuppressive effect of TGF-β, whilst also allowing for neighbouring immune cells to be protected from TGF-β induced T_{reg} differentiation [106,107].

7. Strategies to Improve CAR T Cell Therapy by Metabolic Reprogramming

Increased interest in the metabolism's role in cancer progression and the impact on the effectiveness of immunotherapeutic treatments have led to the development of new therapies that aim to manipulate these metabolic processes increasing the efficacy of treatment. It is well-known that there is a tug of war between tumour cells and TILs for nutrition with a few exceptions, such as CLL, which lowers glucose uptake in TILs, not due to nutrition competition but instead, it was proposed to result from the lower expression of nutrition transporters on the cell surface of $CD8^+$ TILs [61,62].

In the last decade, strategies to overcome T cell hyporesponsiveness have mostly focused on the use of immune checkpoints (ICP) blockades such as anti-PD-1, anti-CTLA-4 and anti-LAG-3 [108]. Although using ICP blockade has shown promising results in clinical trials for the treatment of certain malignancies and adverse effects, termed immune-related adverse events (IRAEs), have also been reported [109,110]. In addition to cytokines (e.g., TGF-β and IL-10) and ICP, metabolic stresses on TILs confer a significant immunosuppressive effect on T cell function and differentiation. The disorganized vascular system within TME leads to low perfusion of nutrients and the accumulation of metabolic wastes such as adenosine, prostaglandin E2 (PGE2), lactate, vascular endothelial growth factor, phosphatidylserine, high extracellular K^+ levels, hypoxia and free radicals [13]. Therefore, manipulating the metabolic pathways that armoured CAR T cells to encounter such a hostile environment emerge as worthwhile therapeutic strategies (Figure 4).

7.1. Costimulatory Molecules

The inclusion of costimulatory domains within CAR T cell constructs was one of the initial approaches used it improve CAR T cell efficacy. CD137 (4-1BB) is a potent costimulator of T cell proliferation and expansion and can improve T cell mitochondrial biogenesis and metabolism. Second and third-generation CAR T cells with 4-1BB costimulatory domains have shown superior metabolic capacity, enhanced antitumour activity, persistence and a higher number of memory phenotypes [2,3,111,112]. The increased metabolic function because of 4-1BB inclusion can be attributed to improvement in mitochondrial mass, biogenesis, mitochondrial membrane potential (ΔΨm), fusion, activation of the p38-MAPK pathway [111] and depends on OPA-1 [112]. CAR T cells using 4-1BB costimulatory molecules have been shown to persist for four years in patients with acute lymphoblastic leukaemia (ALL) [113].

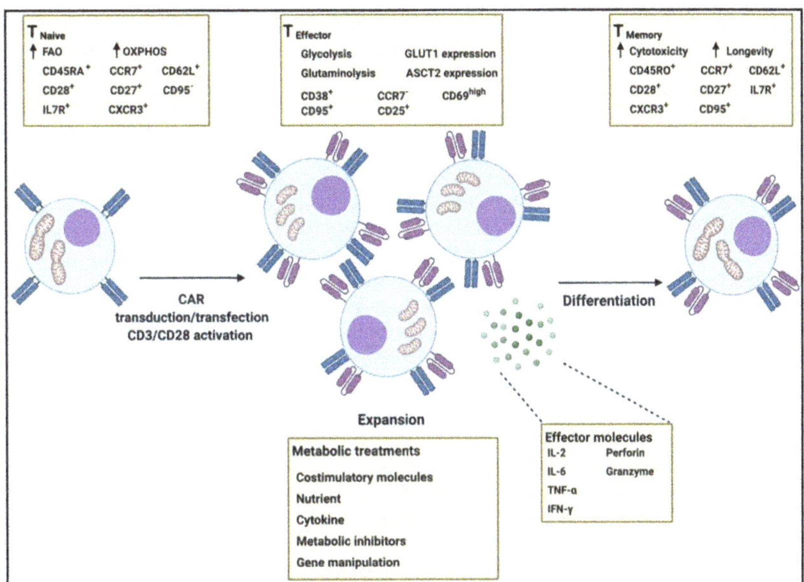

Figure 4. Metabolic interventions to reprogramme CAR T cell metabolism. T_N transduced/transfected with the CAR construct, following which they are stimulated with CD3/CD28 to generate T_{EFF} cells capable of tumour targeting and killing. In contrast to physiological T cells that undergo contraction after the expansion phase, CAR T cells are expanded for a period of around two weeks during which they can be metabolically reprogramed toward long-lived T_M cells or be acclimated to the nutrient profile of the TME.

CD28 is the most prevalent costimulatory domain used in CAR T cell therapy. It has been shown to be effective in the induction of glycolysis and differentiation toward effector memory phenotypes [114]. Dysfunctional TILs from CLL patients showed an impaired ability to induce glycolysis, the main metabolic program of TEFF cells [61]. A comparison of CD28 and 4-1BB costimulatory molecules showed that CAR T cells with 4-1BB have longer persistence as they tend to have a higher number of T_{CM} phenotypes [114]. However, such differences were not seen in patients with relapsed/refractory B cell leukaemia [115]. Moreover, it is worthwhile noting that the importance of CAR T cell persistence may also be cancer dependent [2,3]. Therefore, the type of cancer should be considered when choosing the costimulatory molecules in designing the CAR constructs.

Several strategies have been developed to convert the negative effects of immunosuppressive factors into the beneficial effects of costimulatory molecules. One approach involves the use of the chimeric costimulatory molecules termed "costimulatory converters" [116]. These are fusion proteins encompassing the extracellular domain that recognise immunosuppressive molecules, such as PD-1, fused to an intracellular domain of a costimulatory molecule such as CD28 or 4-1BB [117]. Another technology for the avoidance of CAR T cell immunosuppression uses bispecific T cell engagers (BiTEs). BiTEs are recombinant proteins consisting of two distinct scFvs coupled by a short flexible linker [118]. One of the scFv is specific to a TAA on the tumour surface, while the other recognises the CD3ε/γ heterodimer on T cells, enabling CAR T cells coexpressing the BiTE to engage with two antigens. This is of particular benefit when one of the TAA is heterogeneously expressed on the tumour surface [118].

7.2. Nutrition-Restricted Media

T cells are heterogeneous and plastic, facilitating the conversion to different subtypes and allowing adaptation to new environments. The plasticity enables them to respond to fluctuations of nutrients in the environment and adjust their metabolism accordingly. Shortly after T_N cells recognise an antigen, they differentiate to TEFF cells with specific metabolic characteristics and functional effects. Mimicking the TME metabolic stresses during the ex vivo expansion is a promising strategy to allow CAR T cells to adjust their metabolism to TME [14]. Evidence in favour of this approach includes studies that expand CAR T cells in restricted media. For instance, inhibition of glutamine metabolism via culturing T cells in glutamine-depleted medium or the addition of glutamine-metabolic inhibitors (e.g., AOA, L-Don EGCG) enhances the antitumour activity of $CD8^+$ T cells and their trafficking in mouse models [119]. Expanding the CAR T cells in glucose-restricted media augments the CAR T cell function and T_{CM} phenotypes [120]. To make this strategy clinically practical, a metabolic atlas for all human tumours need to be developed. Finally, the nutrient restriction concept also appears to contrast with well-documented data concerning the suppression of T cell function by nutrient starvation [121].

7.3. Cytokines

Generally, after transduction or transfection, CAR T cells will be expanded in media supplemented with one or two γ chain (γc) cytokine families to facilitate CAR T cell expansion, survival and differentiation. So far, γc cytokines that have been used in manufacturing CAR T cells include IL-2, IL-7, IL-15, IL-21 and IL-9 [122]. Aside from the biological functions, γc cytokines also impact the metabolism of CAR T cells [122]. IL-2 seems to encourage anabolic metabolism necessary for T_{EFF} development through activation of PI3K and mTOR signalling [12]. IL-7 promotes FAO metabolism in CAR T cells through increased expression of glycerol transporters and triglyceride (TAG) synthesis [123]. IL-15 also fosters FAO metabolism through upregulation carnitine palmitoyl transferase and uptake of fatty acid precursors [14]. Similar effects have been observed for CAR T cells treated with IL-21 and IL-9 with enhanced FAO metabolism and higher mitochondrial fitness [124].

Expanding CAR T cells in a combination of IL-7, IL-15 or IL-21 leads to metabolic reprogramming from aerobic glycolysis towards FAO and promotes mitochondrial fusion and fitness. It also reduces the expression of exhaustion markers and increases the number of $T_{SCM/CM}$ population. However, concentration, combination and duration of treatment should be carefully considered. CAR T cells grown solely in IL-15 had elevated mTORC1-p38 MAPK activity and higher T_{SCM} phenotypes compared to the combination of IL-7 and IL-15 [125]. Furthermore, continuous exposure to IL-15 can lead to NK cell exhaustion [126], although such an effect has not been reported in T cells. Moreover, continuous stimulation with IL-7 has been shown to induce "cytokine-induced cell death" (CICD) by elevating the level of active caspase-3, Fas, FasL and proapoptotic protein Bim [127].

7.4. Metabolic Inhibitors

The advantages of using metabolic inhibitors to reprogram metabolic pathways include the enzyme specificity and the ease at which concentration and time of exposure can be controlled. As mentioned before, the PI3K-AKT pathway increases glycolysis, leading to terminally differentiated and exhausted T_{EFF} cells [12]. Ex vivo culture of CAR T cells with 10 μM of LY294002 (PI3K inhibitor) yielded a higher number of $T_{SCM/CM}$ cells and dramatically improved the efficacy of CD33 CAR T cells in vivo [16]. Interestingly, anti-BCMA CAR T cells cultured in IL-7 and IL-15 failed to control tumour growth in vivo, while CAR T cells preconditioned with IL-2 and PI3K inhibitor demonstrated long-term and complete remission in the mouse model [128]. Similarly, Akt inhibition in CAR T cells promotes FAO metabolism, dampens glycolysis pathways, reduced glucose uptake, lactate production and downregulating pro-apoptotic genes (BAX and BAD), whilst encouraging T_{CM} differentiation [9,15,129]. Lastly, using inhibitors against glycolytic mediators such as HK isoforms also improves persistence, effector function, T_M development and CAR T cell efficacy in vivo [9,130,131]. Taken together, ex vivo supplementing CAR T cells with metabolic inhibitors is a feasible approach in manufacturing fitter CAR T cells for solid tumours.

7.5. Gene Manipulation

Advances in molecular biology have fuelled CAR T cell therapy, allowing more sophisticated genetic constructs to function or differentiate toward desire cell products. Up-/downregulation and knock-in/-out of target genes in CAR T cells have been widely used to improve CAR T cell performance. The expression of genes involved in a particular metabolic pathway can be modulated using constitutive or inducible systems. The constitutive expression can be achieved using dual-promoter systems [132], bidirectional promoters [133], 2A self-cleaving peptides [52] or adding internal ribosome entry site (IRES) sequences [134]. For controlled expression over gene-of-interest (GOI), tetracycline (Tet)-On/Off system [135] or endogenous inducible promoters (e.g., IL-2 minimal promoter) [136] can be employed. The use of base-editing using clustered regularly interspaced short palindromic repeats (CRISPR)-Cas-based technologies can introduce mutation(s) in the coding region of DNA, resulting in mutant enzymes that no longer bind to their natural ligand allowing for more precise control of genes with minimal side effects [137].

Amino acid uptake by tumour cells limits the availability of amino acids for TILs, which are vital for T cell function and survival. The manipulation of amino acid transporter expression can be used to increase uptake of critical nutrients whilst also allowing for removal of metabolites, which might otherwise inhibit effector function. T cells express a low level of arginosuccinate synthase (ASS) and ornithine transcarbamylase (OTC), making them vulnerable to arginine deprivation in TME. Exogenously overexpression of ASS and OTC enzymes in CAR T cells, using 2A self-cleaving peptides, significantly enhanced CAR T cell performance in vivo without negative impact on exhaustion and cytotoxicity of CAR T cells [99].

Adenosine is the final byproduct of ATP consumption. It has been shown to accumulate in TME and suppress TILs function [11]. Adenosine binds to adenosine 2a receptor (A2aR) on activated T cells, where it promotes production and accumulation of cytosolic cyclic AMP (cAMP), which dampens T cell activation and cytotoxicity [138]. Downregulation of A2aR transcripts using shRNA, enhanced cytotoxicity, cytokine production and in vivo activity of anti-mesothelin-CAR T cells [139]. In another approach, Newick et al. used a decoy peptide to block the activation of protein kinase A (PKA) signalling [140]. In this study expression of a small peptide called RAID (regulatory subunit I anchoring disruptor) was incorporated into CAR T cells and showed that CAR-RIAD T cells were resistant to the immunosuppressive effects of PGE2 and adenosine [140].

Overall, whilst there is great promise in incorporating gene manipulation in CAR T cell therapy there are also disadvantages that limit the feasibility of the approach. Firstly, although several tools have been used to control GOI expression, the basal expression or immunogenicity of transactivators in such systems restrain their performance [135,141]. Secondly, the expression patterns of genes within T cells are still largely unknown, and uncertainty surrounding the extent of the interactions between transgenes and their endogenous regulators. Continuous expression or inhibition of a gene may affect other pathways with unpredicted outcomes. Lastly, providing additional promoter or regulatory elements (e.g., IRES sequences) could negatively impact the viral packaging and transduction process, thereby reducing the efficiency of CAR T cell manufacturing and adding additional cost to an already expensive therapy. Therefore, whilst gene manipulation is a valuable approach for the study of metabolic pathways through the regulation of GOI within a CAR T cell system in vitro and in vivo, further understanding of the extent and control of metabolic processes is needed before it is a practical approach in the clinic.

8. Conclusions

Several factors in the TME restrain the potential application of CAR T cell therapy for solid tumours. To mount an effective and durable treatment, there have been substantial efforts to discover the metabolic properties of highly effective CAR T cells. CAR T cells from patients with sustained remission have higher $T_{N/SCM}$ and T_{CM} phenotypes with FAO/OXPHOS metabolism and higher mitochondrial mass. Numerous studies support the idea that reprogramming metabolic activity and mitochondria during expansion is a feasible approach to obtain better clinical outcomes. The time frame from the isolation of a patient's T cells, transduction with CAR construct, and ex vivo expansion prior to infusion into the patient provides a feasible metabolic intervention window. A variety of approaches can be used to reach this objective by utilising costimulatory domains, treatment with cytokines, pharmacological drugs and gene manipulation.

Funding: This research was funded by the Royal Society of New Zealand Marsden Fund, grant number UOO1806. A.H.R.S.M. was supported by the Second Century Fund (C2F) Chulalongkorn University.

Acknowledgments: All figures were created with BioRender.com. We thank Alinor Rose for preparing the graphic abstract.

References

1. Tokarew, N.; Ogonek, J.; Endres, S.; von Bergwelt-Baildon, M.; Kobold, S. Teaching an old dog new tricks: Next-generation CAR T cells. *Br. J. Cancer* **2019**, *120*, 26–37. [CrossRef]
2. Weinkove, R.; George, P.; Dasyam, N.; McLellan, A.D. Selecting costimulatory domains for chimeric antigen receptors: Functional and clinical considerations. *Clin. Transl. Immunol.* **2019**, *8*, e1049. [CrossRef]
3. McLellan, A.D.; Ali Hosseini Rad, S.M. Chimeric antigen receptor T cell persistence and memory cell formation. *Immunol. Cell Biol.* **2019**, *97*, 664–674. [CrossRef]
4. Boyiadzis, M.M.; Dhodapkar, M.V.; Brentjens, R.J.; Kochenderfer, J.N.; Neelapu, S.S.; Maus, M.V.; Porter, D.L.; Maloney, D.G.; Grupp, S.A.; Mackall, C.L. Chimeric antigen receptor (CAR) T therapies for the treatment of hematologic malignancies: Clinical perspective and significance. *J. Immunother. Cancer* **2018**, *6*, 1–12. [CrossRef]
5. Al-Mansour, M.; Al-Foheidi, M.; Ibrahim, E. Efficacy and safety of second-generation CAR T-cell therapy in diffuse large B-cell lymphoma: A meta-analysis. *Mol. Clin. Oncol.* **2020**, *13*, 1. [CrossRef]
6. Schuster, S.J.; Bishop, M.R.; Tam, C.S.; Waller, E.K.; Borchmann, P.; McGuirk, J.P.; Jäger, U.; Jaglowski, S.; Andreadis, C.; Westin, J.R. Tisagenlecleucel in adult relapsed or refractory diffuse large B-cell lymphoma. *N. Engl. J. Med.* **2019**, *380*, 45–56. [CrossRef] [PubMed]
7. Kochenderfer, J.N.; Somerville, R.P.; Lu, T.; Yang, J.C.; Sherry, R.M.; Feldman, S.A.; McIntyre, L.; Bot, A.; Rossi, J.; Lam, N. Long-duration complete remissions of diffuse large B cell lymphoma after anti-CD19 chimeric antigen receptor T cell therapy. *Mol. Ther.* **2017**, *25*, 2245–2253. [CrossRef]
8. Rodriguez-Garcia, A.; Palazon, A.; Noguera-Ortega, E.; Powell, D.J., Jr.; Guedan, S. CAR-T cells hit the tumor microenvironment: Strategies to overcome tumor escape. *Front. Immunol.* **2020**, *11*, 1109. [CrossRef]
9. Rostamian, H.; Fallah-Mehrjardi, K.; Khakpoor-Koosheh, M.; Pawelek, J.M.; Hadjati, J.; Brown, C.E.; Mirzaei, H.R. A metabolic switch to memory CAR T cells: Implications for cancer treatment. *Cancer Lett.* **2020**, *500*, 107–118. [CrossRef] [PubMed]
10. Rafiq, S.; Hackett, C.S.; Brentjens, R.J. Engineering strategies to overcome the current roadblocks in CAR T cell therapy. *Nat. Rev. Clin. Oncol.* **2020**, *17*, 147–167. [CrossRef] [PubMed]
11. Anderson, K.G.; Stromnes, I.M.; Greenberg, P.D. Obstacles posed by the tumor microenvironment to T cell activity: A case for synergistic therapies. *Cancer Cell* **2017**, *31*, 311–325. [CrossRef] [PubMed]
12. Saravia, J.; Raynor, J.L.; Chapman, N.M.; Lim, S.A.; Chi, H. Signaling networks in immunometabolism. *Cell Res.* **2020**, *30*, 328–342. [CrossRef] [PubMed]
13. Weinberg, S.E.; Chandel, N.S. Targeting mitochondria metabolism for cancer therapy. *Nat. Chem. Biol.* **2015**, *11*, 9. [CrossRef] [PubMed]
14. Xu, X.; Gnanaprakasam, J.; Sherman, J.; Wang, R. A metabolism toolbox for CAR T therapy. *Front. Oncol.* **2019**, *9*, 322. [CrossRef]
15. Zhang, Q.; Ding, J.; Sun, S.; Liu, H.; Lu, M.; Wei, X.; Gao, X.; Zhang, X.; Fu, Q.; Zheng, J. Akt inhibition at the initial stage of CAR-T preparation enhances the CAR-positive expression rate, memory phenotype and in vivo efficacy. *Am. J. Cancer Res.* **2019**, *9*, 2379.
16. Zheng, W.; Carol, E.; Alli, R.; Basham, J.H.; Abdelsamed, H.A.; Palmer, L.E.; Jones, L.L.; Youngblood, B.; Geiger, T.L. PI3K orchestration of the in vivo persistence of chimeric antigen receptor-modified T cells. *Leukemia* **2018**, *32*, 1157–1167. [CrossRef]
17. Buck, M.D.; O'sullivan, D.; Pearce, E.L. T cell metabolism drives immunity. *J. Exp. Med.* **2015**, *212*, 1345–1360. [CrossRef]

18. Desdín-Micó, G.; Soto-Heredero, G.; Mittelbrunn, M. Mitochondrial activity in T cells. *Mitochondrion* **2018**, *41*, 51–57. [CrossRef]

19. Wei, J.; Raynor, J.; Nguyen, T.-L.M.; Chi, H. Nutrient and metabolic sensing in T cell responses. *Front. Immunol.* **2017**, *8*, 247. [CrossRef]

20. Chao, T.; Wang, H.; Ho, P.-C. Mitochondrial control and guidance of cellular activities of T cells. *Front. Immunol.* **2017**, *8*, 473. [CrossRef]

21. Bantug, G.R.; Galluzzi, L.; Kroemer, G.; Hess, C. The spectrum of T cell metabolism in health and disease. *Nat. Rev. Immunol.* **2018**, *18*, 19. [CrossRef]

22. Buck, M.D.; O'Sullivan, D.; Geltink, R.I.K.; Curtis, J.D.; Chang, C.-H.; Sanin, D.E.; Qiu, J.; Kretz, O.; Braas, D.; van der Windt, G.J.; et al. Mitochondrial dynamics controls T cell fate through metabolic programming. *Cell* **2016**, *166*, 63–76. [CrossRef]

23. Missiroli, S.; Patergnani, S.; Caroccia, N.; Pedriali, G.; Perrone, M.; Previati, M.; Wieckowski, M.R.; Giorgi, C. Mitochondria-associated membranes (MAMs) and inflammation. *Cell Death Dis.* **2018**, *9*, 1–14. [CrossRef] [PubMed]

24. Chan, D.C. Mitochondrial fusion and fission in mammals. *Annu. Rev. Cell Dev. Biol.* **2006**, *22*, 79–99. [CrossRef] [PubMed]

25. Meyer, J.N.; Leuthner, T.C.; Luz, A.L. Mitochondrial fusion, fission, and mitochondrial toxicity. *Toxicology* **2017**, *391*, 42–53. [CrossRef] [PubMed]

26. Bock, F.J.; Tait, S.W. Mitochondria as multifaceted regulators of cell death. *Nat. Rev. Mol. Cell Biol.* **2020**, *21*, 85–100. [CrossRef]

27. Brenner, D.; Mak, T.W. Mitochondrial cell death effectors. *Curr. Opin. Cell Biol.* **2009**, *21*, 871–877. [CrossRef]

28. Kim, H.; Rafiuddin-Shah, M.; Tu, H.-C.; Jeffers, J.R.; Zambetti, G.P.; Hsieh, J.J.-D.; Cheng, E.H.-Y. Hierarchical regulation of mitochondrion-dependent apoptosis by BCL-2 subfamilies. *Nat. Cell Biol.* **2006**, *8*, 1348–1358. [CrossRef] [PubMed]

29. Cui, J.; Placzek, W.J. Post-transcriptional regulation of anti-apoptotic BCL2 family members. *Int. J. Mol. Sci.* **2018**, *19*, 308.

30. Baker, N.; Patel, J.; Khacho, M. Linking mitochondrial dynamics, cristae remodeling and supercomplex formation: How mitochondrial structure can regulate bioenergetics. *Mitochondrion* **2019**, *49*, 259–268. [CrossRef]

31. Paulsen, M.; Valentin, S.; Mathew, B.; Adam-Klages, S.; Bertsch, U.; Lavrik, I.; Krammer, P.H.; Kabelitz, D.; Janssen, O. Modulation of CD4+ T-cell activation by CD95 co-stimulation. *Cell Death Differ.* **2011**, *18*, 619–631. [CrossRef]

32. Chalah, A.; Khosravi-Far, R. The mitochondrial death pathway. *Program. Cell Death Cancer Progress. Ther.* **2008**, *615*, 25–45.

33. Özören, N.; El-Deiry, W.S. Defining characteristics of Types I and II apoptotic cells in response to TRAIL. *Neoplasia* **2002**, *4*, 551–557. [CrossRef] [PubMed]

34. Le Gallo, M.; Poissonnier, A.; Blanco, P.; Legembre, P. CD95/Fas, non-apoptotic signaling pathways, and kinases. *Front. Immunol.* **2017**, *8*, 1216. [CrossRef]

35. Dunkle, A.D. *The Roles of the Bcl-2 Family Proteins in T Lymphocyte Development and Homeostasis*; Duke University: Durham, NC, USA, 2011.

36. Rad, S.A.H.; Tan, G.M.Y.; Poudel, A.; He, K.; McLellan, A.D. Regulation of human Mcl-1 by a divergently-expressed antisense transcript. *Gene* **2020**, *762*, 145016.

37. Perciavalle, R.M.; Opferman, J.T. Delving deeper: MCL-1's contributions to normal and cancer biology. *Trends Cell Biol.* **2013**, *23*, 22–29. [CrossRef]

38. Ramaswamy, M.; Clel, S.Y.; Cruz, A.C.; Siegel, R.M. Many checkpoints on the road to cell death: Regulation of Fas–FasL interactions and Fas signaling in peripheral immune responses. *Death Recept. Cogn. Ligands Cancer* **2009**, *49*, 17–47.

39. Strauss, G.; Knape, I.; Melzner, I.; Debatin, K.-M. Constitutive caspase activation and impaired death-inducing signaling complex formation in CD95-resistant, long-term activated, antigen-specific T cells. *J. Immunol.* **2003**, *171*, 1172–1182. [CrossRef] [PubMed]

40. Peter, M.; Hadji, A.; Murmann, A.; Brockway, S.; Putzbach, W.; Pattanayak, A.; Ceppi, P. The role of CD95 and CD95 ligand in cancer. *Cell Death Differ.* **2015**, *22*, 549–559. [CrossRef]

41. Matsumoto, N.; Imamura, R.; Suda, T. Caspase-8-and JNK-dependent AP-1 activation is required for Fas ligand-induced IL-8 production. *FEBS J.* **2007**, *274*, 2376–2384. [CrossRef] [PubMed]

42. Peter, M.E.; Budd, R.C.; Desbarats, J.; Hedrick, S.M.; Hueber, A.-O.; Newell, M.K.; Owen, L.B.; Pope, R.M.; Tschopp, J.; Wajant, H. The CD95 receptor: Apoptosis revisited. *Cell* **2007**, *129*, 447–450. [CrossRef] [PubMed]

43. Barnhart, B.C.; Legembre, P.; Pietras, E.; Bubici, C.; Franzoso, G.; Peter, M.E. CD95 ligand induces motility and invasiveness of apoptosis-resistant tumor cells. *EMBO J.* **2004**, *23*, 3175–3185. [CrossRef] [PubMed]

44. Hanahan, D.; Weinberg, R.A. Hallmarks of cancer: The next generation. *Cell* **2011**, *144*, 646–674. [CrossRef]

45. Hadji, A.; Ceppi, P.; Murmann, A.E.; Brockway, S.; Pattanayak, A.; Bhinder, B.; Hau, A.; De Chant, S.; Parimi, V.; Kolesza, P. Death induced by CD95 or CD95 ligand elimination. *Cell Rep.* **2014**, *7*, 208–222. [CrossRef]

46. Hong, L.K.; Chen, Y.; Smith, C.C.; Montgomery, S.A.; Vincent, B.G.; Dotti, G.; Savoldo, B. CD30-Redirected chimeric antigen receptor T cells target CD30+ and CD30− embryonal Carcinoma via antigen-Dependent and Fas/FasL interactions. *Cancer Immunol. Res.* **2018**, *6*, 1274–1287. [CrossRef] [PubMed]

47. Gattinoni, L.; Lugli, E.; Ji, Y.; Pos, Z.; Paulos, C.M.; Quigley, M.F.; Almeida, J.R.; Gostick, E.; Yu, Z.; Carpenito, C.; et al. A human memory T cell subset with stem cell–like properties. *Nat. Med.* **2011**, *17*, 1290–1297. [CrossRef]

48. Klebanoff, C.A.; Scott, C.D.; Leonardi, A.J.; Yamamoto, T.N.; Cruz, A.C.; Ouyang, C.; Ramaswamy, M.; Roychoudhuri, R.; Ji, Y.; Eil, R.L.; et al. Memory T cell–driven differentiation of naive cells impairs adoptive immunotherapy. *J. Clin. Investig.* **2016**, *126*, 318–334. [CrossRef]

49. Künkele, A.; Johnson, A.J.; Rolczynski, L.S.; Chang, C.A.; Hoglund, V.; Kelly-Spratt, K.S.; Jensen, M.C. Functional tuning of CARs reveals signaling threshold above which CD8+ CTL antitumor potency is attenuated due to cell Fas–FasL-dependent AICD. *Cancer Immunol. Res.* **2015**, *3*, 368–379. [CrossRef] [PubMed]

50. Tschumi, B.O.; Dumauthioz, N.; Marti, B.; Zhang, L.; Schneider, P.; Mach, J.-P.; Romero, P.; Donda, A. CART cells are prone to Fas-and DR5-mediated cell death. *J. Immunother. Cancer* **2018**, *6*, 1–9.

51. He, B.; Wang, L.; Neuber, B.; Schmitt, A.; Kneisel, N.; Hoeger, T.; Mueller-Tidow, C.; Schmitt, M.; Hofmann, S. *Blockade of CD95/CD95L Death Signaling Enhances CAR T Cell Persistence and Antitumor Efficacy*; American Society of Hematology: Washington, DC, USA, 2019.

52. Rad SM, A.H.; Poudel, A.; Tan, G.M.Y.; McLellan, A.D. Promoter choice: Who should drive the CAR in T cells? *PLoS ONE* **2020**, *15*, e0232915.

53. Yamamoto, T.N.; Lee, P.-H.; Vodnala, S.K.; Gurusamy, D.; Kishton, R.J.; Yu, Z.; Eidizadeh, A.; Eil, R.; Fioravanti, J.; Gattinoni, L.; et al. T cells genetically engineered to overcome death signaling enhance adoptive cancer immunotherapy. *J. Clin. Investig.* **2019**, *129*, 1551–1565. [CrossRef] [PubMed]

54. Rad, A.H.; Tan, G.M.Y.; Poudel, A.; McLellan, A. P06. 02 Enhancing CAR T cell persistence and memory through modulating mitochondrial function. *BMJ Spec. J.* **2020**, *8*. [CrossRef]

55. Perciavalle, R.M.; Stewart, D.P.; Koss, B.; Lynch, J.; Milasta, S.; Bathina, M.; Temirov, J.; Cleland, M.M.; Pelletier, S.; Schuetz, J.D.; et al. Anti-apoptotic MCL-1 localizes to the mitochondrial matrix and couples mitochondrial fusion to respiration. *Nat. Cell Biol.* **2012**, *14*, 575–583. [CrossRef] [PubMed]

56. Malissen, B.; Bongrand, P. Early T cell activation: Integrating biochemical, structural, and biophysical cues. *Annu. Rev. Immunol.* **2015**, *33*, 539–561. [CrossRef]

57. Chapman, N.M.; Boothby, M.R.; Chi, H. Metabolic coordination of T cell quiescence and activation. *Nat. Rev. Immunol.* **2020**, *20*, 55–70. [CrossRef] [PubMed]

58. Tan, H.; Yang, K.; Li, Y.; Shaw, T.I.; Wang, Y.; Blanco, D.B.; Wang, X.; Cho, J.-H.; Wang, H.; Rankin, S.; et al. Integrative proteomics and phosphoproteomics profiling reveals dynamic signaling networks and bioenergetics pathways underlying T cell activation. *Immunity* **2017**, *46*, 488–503. [CrossRef] [PubMed]

59. Wülfing, C.; Rabinowitz, J.D.; Beeson, C.; Sjaastad, M.D.; McConnell, H.M.; Davis, M.M. Kinetics and extent of T cell activation as measured with the calcium signal. *J. Exp. Med.* **1997**, *185*, 1815–1825. [CrossRef] [PubMed]

60. Asmal, M.; Colgan, J.; Naef, F.; Yu, B.; Lee, Y.; Magnasco, M.; Luban, J. Production of ribosome components in effector CD4+ T cells is accelerated by TCR stimulation and coordinated by ERK-MAPK. *Immunity* **2003**, *19*, 535–548. [CrossRef]

61. Van Bruggen, J.A.; Martens, A.W.; Fraietta, J.A.; Hofland, T.; Tonino, S.H.; Eldering, E.; Levin, M.-D.; Siska, P.J.; Endstra, S.; Rathmell, J.C.; et al. Chronic lymphocytic leukemia cells impair mitochondrial fitness in CD8+ T cells and impede CAR T-cell efficacy. *Blood* **2019**, *134*, 44–58. [CrossRef]

62. Siska, P.J.; van der Windt, G.J.; Kishton, R.J.; Cohen, S.; Eisner, W.; MacIver, N.J.; Kater, A.P.; Weinberg, J.B.; Rathmell, J.C. Suppression of Glut1 and glucose metabolism by decreased Akt/mTORC1 signaling drives T cell impairment in B cell leukemia. *J. Immunol.* **2016**, *197*, 2532–2540. [CrossRef]

63. Zeng, H.; Cohen, S.; Guy, C.; Shrestha, S.; Neale, G.; Brown, S.A.; Cloer, C.; Kishton, R.J.; Gao, X.; Youngblood, B. mTORC1 and mTORC2 kinase signaling and glucose metabolism drive follicular helper T cell differentiation. *Immunity* **2016**, *45*, 540–554. [CrossRef] [PubMed]

64. Wu, H.; Estrella, V.; Beatty, M.; Abrahams, D.; El-Kenawi, A.; Russell, S.; Ibrahim-Hashim, A.; Longo, D.L.; Reshetnyak, Y.K.; Moshnikova, A.; et al. T-cells produce acidic niches in lymph nodes to suppress their own effector functions. *Nat. Commun.* **2020**, *11*, 1–13. [CrossRef] [PubMed]

65. Kirk, Á.; Wilson, M.; Heddle, C.; Brown, M.; Barclay, A.; Halestrap, A. CD147 is tightly associated with lactate transporters MCT1 and MCT4 and facilitates their cell surface expression. *EMBO J.* **2000**, *19*, 3896–3904. [CrossRef]

66. Brand, A.; Singer, K.; Koehl, G.E.; Kolitzus, M.; Schoenhammer, G.; Thiel, A.; Matos, C.; Bruss, C.; Klobuch, S.; Peter, K.; et al. LDHA-associated lactic acid production blunts tumor immunosurveillance by T and NK cells. *Cell Metab.* **2016**, *24*, 657–671. [CrossRef] [PubMed]

67. Comito, G.; Iscaro, A.; Bacci, M.; Morandi, A.; Ippolito, L.; Parri, M.; Montagnani, I.; Raspollini, M.; Serni, S.; Simeoni, L.; et al. Lactate modulates CD4+ T-cell polarization and induces an immunosuppressive environment, which sustains prostate carcinoma progression via TLR8/miR21 axis. *Oncogene* **2019**, *38*, 3681–3695. [CrossRef]

68. Hermans, D.; Gautam, S.; García-Cañaveras, J.C.; Gromer, D.; Mitra, S.; Spolski, R.; Li, P.; Christensen, S.; Nguyen, R.; Lin, J.-X.; et al. Lactate dehydrogenase inhibition synergizes with IL-21 to promote CD8+ T cell stemness and antitumor immunity. *Proc. Natl. Acad. Sci. USA* **2020**, *117*, 6047–6055. [CrossRef]

69. Cai, L.; Sutter, B.M.; Li, B.; Tu, B.P. Acetyl-CoA induces cell growth and proliferation by promoting the acetylation of histones at growth genes. *Mol. Cell* **2011**, *42*, 426–437. [CrossRef] [PubMed]

70. Nakaya, M.; Xiao, Y.; Zhou, X.; Chang, J.-H.; Chang, M.; Cheng, X.; Blonska, M.; Lin, X.; Sun, S.-C. Inflammatory T cell responses rely on amino acid transporter ASCT2 facilitation of glutamine uptake and mTORC1 kinase activation. *Immunity* **2014**, *40*, 692–705. [CrossRef]

71. Arts, R.J.; Novakovic, B.; Ter Horst, R.; Carvalho, A.; Bekkering, S.; Lachmandas, E.; Rodrigues, F.; Silvestre, R.; Cheng, S.-C.; Wang, S.-Y.; et al. Glutaminolysis and fumarate accumulation integrate immunometabolic and epigenetic programs in trained immunity. *Cell Metab.* **2016**, *24*, 807–819. [CrossRef] [PubMed]

72. Wang, Q.; Beaumont, K.A.; Otte, N.J.; Font, J.; Bailey, C.G.; van Geldermalsen, M.; Sharp, D.M.; Tiffen, J.C.; Ryan, R.M.; Jormakka, M.; et al. Targeting glutamine transport to suppress melanoma cell growth. *Int. J. Cancer* **2014**, *135*, 1060–1071. [CrossRef]

73. Baixauli, F.; Acín-Pérez, R.; Villarroya-Beltrí, C.; Mazzeo, C.; Nuñez-Andrade, N.; Gabandé-Rodriguez, E.; Ledesma, M.D.; Blázquez, A.; Martin, M.A.; Falcón-Pérez, J.M.; et al. Mitochondrial respiration controls lysosomal function during inflammatory T cell responses. *Cell Metab.* **2015**, *22*, 485–498. [CrossRef]

74. Johnson, M.O.; Rathmell, J.C. AIF is "Always in Fashion" for T Cells. *Immunity* **2016**, *44*, 11–13. [CrossRef] [PubMed]

75. Christie, D.A.; Mitsopoulos, P.; Blagih, J.; Dunn, S.D.; St-Pierre, J.; Jones, R.G.; Hatch, G.M.; Madrenas, J. Stomatin-like protein 2 deficiency in T cells is associated with altered mitochondrial respiration and defective CD4+ T cell responses. *J. Immunol.* **2012**, *189*, 4349–4360. [CrossRef]

76. Weinberg, S.E.; Singer, B.D.; Steinert, E.M.; Martinez, C.A.; Mehta, M.M.; Martínez-Reyes, I.; Gao, P.; Helmin, K.A.; Abdala-Valencia, H.; Sena, L.A.; et al. Mitochondrial complex III is essential for suppressive function of regulatory T cells. *Nature* **2019**, *565*, 495–499. [CrossRef] [PubMed]

77. Sena, L.A.; Li, S.; Jairaman, A.; Prakriya, M.; Ezponda, T.; Hildeman, D.A.; Wang, C.-R.; Schumacker, P.T.; Licht, J.D.; Perlman, H.; et al. Mitochondria are required for antigen-specific T cell activation through reactive oxygen species signaling. *Immunity* **2013**, *38*, 225–236. [CrossRef] [PubMed]

78. Ron-Harel, N.; Santos, D.; Ghergurovich, J.M.; Sage, P.T.; Reddy, A.; Lovitch, S.B.; Dephoure, N.; Satterstrom, F.K.; Sheffer, M.; Spinelli, J.B.; et al. Mitochondrial biogenesis and proteome remodeling promote one-carbon metabolism for T cell activation. *Cell Metab.* **2016**, *24*, 104–117. [CrossRef]

79. Ying, W. NAD+/NADH and NADP+/NADPH in cellular functions and cell death: Regulation and biological consequences. *Antioxid. Redox Signal.* **2008**, *10*, 179–206. [CrossRef] [PubMed]

80. Xiao, W.; Wang, R.-S.; Handy, D.E.; Loscalzo, J. NAD (H) and NADP (H) redox couples and cellular energy metabolism. *Antioxid. Redox Signal.* **2018**, *28*, 251–272. [CrossRef] [PubMed]

81. Lian, G.; Gnanaprakasam, J.R.; Wang, T.; Wu, R.; Chen, X.; Liu, L.; Shen, Y.; Yang, M.; Yang, J.; Chen, Y.; et al. Glutathione de novo synthesis but not recycling process coordinates with glutamine catabolism to control redox homeostasis and directs murine T cell differentiation. *eLife* **2018**, *7*, e36158. [CrossRef]

82. Leone, R.D.; Zhao, L.; Englert, J.M.; Sun, I.-M.; Oh, M.-H.; Sun, I.-H.; Arwood, M.L.; Bettencourt, I.A.; Patel, C.H.; Wen, J.; et al. Glutamine blockade induces divergent metabolic programs to overcome tumor immune evasion. *Science* **2019**, *366*, 1013–1021. [CrossRef] [PubMed]

83. Klysz, D.; Tai, X.; Robert, P.A.; Craveiro, M.; Cretenet, G.; Oburoglu, L.; Mongellaz, C.; Floess, S.; Fritz, V.; Matias, M.I.; et al. Glutamine-dependent α-ketoglutarate production regulates the balance between T helper 1 cell and regulatory T cell generation. *Sci. Signal.* **2015**, *8*, ra97. [CrossRef] [PubMed]

84. Cluntun, A.A.; Lukey, M.J.; Cerione, R.A.; Locasale, J.W. Glutamine metabolism in cancer: Understanding the heterogeneity. *Trends Cancer* **2017**, *3*, 169–180. [CrossRef]

85. Mehta, M.M.; Weinberg, S.E.; Steinert, E.M.; Chhiba, K.; Martinez, C.A.; Gao, P.; Perlman, H.R.; Bryce, P.; Hay, N.; Chandel, N.S.; et al. Hexokinase 2 is dispensable for T cell-dependent immunity. *Cancer Metab.* **2018**, *6*, 1–18. [CrossRef] [PubMed]

86. Ardehali, H.; Yano, Y.; Printz, R.L.; Koch, S.; Whitesell, R.R.; May, J.M.; Granner, D.K. Functional organization of mammalian hexokinase II: Retention of catalytic and regulatory functions in both the NH2-and COOH-terminal halves. *J. Biol. Chem.* **1996**, *271*, 1849–1852. [CrossRef]

87. Gu, M.; Zhou, X.; Sohn, J.H.; Zhu, L.; Jie, Z.; Yang, J.-Y.; Zheng, X.; Xie, X.; Yang, J.; Shi, Y.; et al. NF-κB-inducing kinase maintains T cell metabolic fitness in antitumor immunity. *Nat. Immunol.* **2021**, *22*, 193–204. [CrossRef]

88. Varanasi, S.K.; Jaggi, U.; Hay, N.; Rouse, B.T. Hexokinase II may be dispensable for CD4 T cell responses against a virus infection. *PLoS ONE* **2018**, *13*, e0191533. [CrossRef] [PubMed]

89. Thurnher, M.; Gruenbacher, G. T lymphocyte regulation by mevalonate metabolism. *Sci. Signal.* **2015**, *8*, re4. [CrossRef]

90. Metallo, C.M.; Gameiro, P.A.; Bell, E.L.; Mattaini, K.R.; Yang, J.; Hiller, K.; Jewell, C.M.; Johnson, Z.R.; Irvine, D.J.; Guarente, L.; et al. Reductive glutamine metabolism by IDH1 mediates lipogenesis under hypoxia. *Nature* **2012**, *481*, 380–384. [CrossRef]

91. Yang, W.; Bai, Y.; Xiong, Y.; Zhang, J.; Chen, S.; Zheng, X.; Meng, X.; Li, L.; Wang, J.; Xu, C.; et al. Potentiating the antitumour response of CD8+ T cells by modulating cholesterol metabolism. *Nature* **2016**, *531*, 651–655. [CrossRef]

92. Ma, X.; Bi, E.; Lu, Y.; Su, P.; Huang, C.; Liu, L.; Wang, Q.; Yang, M.; Kalady, M.F.; Qian, J.; et al. Cholesterol induces CD8+ T cell exhaustion in the tumor microenvironment. *Cell Metab.* **2019**, *30*, 143–156. [CrossRef]

93. Scharping, N.E.; Menk, A.V.; Moreci, R.S.; Whetstone, R.D.; Dadey, R.E.; Watkins, S.C.; Ferris, R.L.; Delgoffe, G.M. The tumor microenvironment represses T cell mitochondrial biogenesis to drive intratumoral T cell metabolic insufficiency and dysfunction. *Immunity* **2016**, *45*, 374–388. [CrossRef] [PubMed]

94. Vardhana, S.A.; Hwee, M.A.; Berisa, M.; Wells, D.K.; Yost, K.E.; King, B.; Smith, M.; Herrera, P.S.; Chang, H.Y.; Satpathy, A.T.; et al. Impaired mitochondrial oxidative phosphorylation limits the self-renewal of T cells exposed to persistent antigen. *Nat. Immunol.* **2020**, *21*, 1022–1033. [CrossRef] [PubMed]

95. Chamoto, K.; Chowdhury, P.S.; Kumar, A.; Sonomura, K.; Matsuda, F.; Fagarasan, S.; Honjo, T. Mitochondrial activation chemicals synergize with surface receptor PD-1 blockade for T cell-dependent antitumor activity. *Proc. Natl. Acad. Sci. USA* **2017**, *114*, E761–E770. [CrossRef]

96. Scharping, N.E.; Menk, A.V.; Whetstone, R.D.; Zeng, X.; Delgoffe, G.M. Efficacy of PD-1 blockade is potentiated by metformin-induced reduction of tumor hypoxia. *Cancer Immunol. Res.* **2017**, *5*, 9–16. [CrossRef]

97. Weinberg, F.; Ramnath, N.; Nagrath, D. Reactive oxygen species in the tumor microenvironment: An overview. *Cancers* **2019**, *11*, 1191. [CrossRef]

98. Ligtenberg, M.A.; Mougiakakos, D.; Mukhopadhyay, M.; Witt, K.; Lladser, A.; Chmielewski, M.; Riet, T.; Abken, H.; Kiessling, R. Coexpressed catalase protects chimeric antigen receptor–redirected T cells as well as bystander cells from oxidative stress–induced loss of antitumor activity. *J. Immunol.* **2016**, *196*, 759–766. [CrossRef]

99. Fultang, L.; Booth, S.; Yogev, O.; Martins da Costa, B.; Tubb, V.; Panetti, S.; Stavrou, V.; Scarpa, U.; Jankevics, A.; Lloyd, G. Metabolic engineering against the arginine microenvironment enhances CAR-T cell proliferation and therapeutic activity. *Blood J. Am. Soc. Hematol.* **2020**, *136*, 1155–1160.

100. Ren, W.; Liu, G.; Yin, J.; Tan, B.; Wu, G.; Bazer, F.W.; Peng, Y.; Yin, Y. Amino-acid transporters in T-cell activation and differentiation. *Cell Death Dis.* **2017**, *8*, e2655. [CrossRef] [PubMed]

101. Palazon, A.; Goldrath, A.W.; Nizet, V.; Johnson, R.S. HIF transcription factors, inflammation, and immunity. *Immunity* **2014**, *41*, 518–528. [CrossRef] [PubMed]

102. Vuillefroy de Silly, R.; Ducimetière, L.; Yacoub Maroun, C.; Dietrich, P.Y.; Derouazi, M.; Walker, P.R. Phenotypic switch of CD8+ T cells reactivated under hypoxia toward IL-10 secreting, poorly proliferative effector cells. *Eur. J. Immunol.* **2015**, *45*, 2263–2275. [CrossRef] [PubMed]

103. Vuillefroy de Silly, R.; Dietrich, P.-Y.; Walker, P.R. Hypoxia and antitumor CD8+ T cells: An incompatible alliance? *Oncoimmunology* **2016**, *5*, e1232236. [CrossRef]

104. Oh, S.A.; Li, M.O. TGF-β: Guardian of T cell function. *J. Immunol.* **2013**, *191*, 3973–3979. [CrossRef]

105. Gorelik, L.; Flavell, R.A. Immune-mediated eradication of tumors through the blockade of transforming growth factor-β signaling in T cells. *Nat. Med.* **2001**, *7*, 1118–1122. [CrossRef]

106. Tang, N.; Cheng, C.; Zhang, X.; Qiao, M.; Li, N.; Mu, W.; Wei, X.-F.; Han, W.; Wang, H. TGF-β inhibition via CRISPR promotes the long-term efficacy of CAR T cells against solid tumors. *JCI Insight* **2020**, *5*, e133977. [CrossRef] [PubMed]

107. Hartley, J.; Abken, H. Chimeric antigen receptors designed to overcome transforming growth factor-β-mediated repression in the adoptive T-cell therapy of solid tumors. *Clin. Transl. Immunol.* **2019**, *8*, e1064. [CrossRef] [PubMed]

108. Minn, A.J.; Wherry, E.J. Combination cancer therapies with immune checkpoint blockade: Convergence on interferon signaling. *Cell* **2016**, *165*, 272–275. [CrossRef]

109. Byun, D.J.; Wolchok, J.D.; Rosenberg, L.M.; Girotra, M. Cancer immunotherapy—immune checkpoint blockade and associated endocrinopathies. *Nat. Rev. Endocrinol.* **2017**, *13*, 195–207. [CrossRef] [PubMed]

110. Iglesias, P. Cancer immunotherapy-induced endocrinopathies: Clinical behavior and therapeutic approach. *Eur. J. Intern. Med.* **2018**, *47*, 6–13. [CrossRef] [PubMed]

111. Menk, A.V.; Scharping, N.E.; Rivadeneira, D.B.; Calderon, M.J.; Watson, M.J.; Dunstane, D.; Watkins, S.C.; Delgoffe, G.M. 4-1BB costimulation induces T cell mitochondrial function and biogenesis enabling cancer immunotherapeutic responses. *J. Exp. Med.* **2018**, *215*, 1091–1100. [CrossRef] [PubMed]

112. Teijeira, A.; Labiano, S.; Garasa, S.; Etxeberria, I.; Santamaría, E.; Rouzaut, A.; Enamorado, M.; Azpilikueta, A.; Inoges, S.; Bolaños, E. Mitochondrial morphological and functional reprogramming following CD137 (4-1BB) costimulation. *Cancer Immunol. Res.* **2018**, *6*, 798–811. [CrossRef] [PubMed]

113. Porter, D.L.; Hwang, W.-T.; Frey, N.V.; Lacey, S.F.; Shaw, P.A.; Loren, A.W.; Bagg, A.; Marcucci, K.T.; Shen, A.; Gonzalez, V. Chimeric antigen receptor T cells persist and induce sustained remissions in relapsed refractory chronic lymphocytic leukemia. *Sci. Transl. Med.* **2015**, *7*, ra139–ra303. [CrossRef]

114. Kawalekar, O.U.; O'Connor, R.S.; Fraietta, J.A.; Guo, L.; McGettigan, S.E.; Posey Jr, A.D.; Patel, P.R.; Guedan, S.; Scholler, J.; Keith, B.; et al. Distinct signaling of coreceptors regulates specific metabolism pathways and impacts memory development in CAR T cells. *Immunity* **2016**, *44*, 380–390. [CrossRef] [PubMed]

115. Cheng, Z.; Wei, R.; Ma, Q.; Shi, L.; He, F.; Shi, Z.; Jin, T.; Xie, R.; Wei, B.; Chen, J.; et al. In vivo expansion and antitumor activity of coinfused CD28-and 4-1BB-engineered CAR-T cells in patients with B cell leukemia. *Mol. Ther.* **2018**, *26*, 976–985. [CrossRef] [PubMed]

116. Ankri, C.; Cohen, C.J. Out of the bitter came forth sweet: Activating CD28-dependent co-stimulation via PD-1 ligands. *Oncoimmunology* **2014**, *3*, e27399. [CrossRef] [PubMed]

117. Ankri, C.; Shamalov, K.; Horovitz-Fried, M.; Mauer, S.; Cohen, C.J. Human T cells engineered to express a programmed death 1/28 costimulatory retargeting molecule display enhanced antitumor activity. *J. Immunol.* **2013**, *191*, 4121–4129. [CrossRef] [PubMed]

118. Slaney, C.Y.; Wang, P.; Darcy, P.K.; Kershaw, M.H. CARs versus biTEs: A comparison between T cell–redirection strategies for cancer treatment. *Cancer Discov.* **2018**, *8*, 924–934. [CrossRef]

119. Nabe, S.; Yamada, T.; Suzuki, J.; Toriyama, K.; Yasuoka, T.; Kuwahara, M.; Shiraishi, A.; Takenaka, K.; Yasukawa, M.; Yamashita, M.; et al. Reinforce the antitumor activity of CD 8+ T cells via glutamine restriction. *Cancer Sci.* **2018**, *109*, 3737–3750. [CrossRef]

120. Amini, A.; Veraitch, F. Glucose deprivation enriches for central memory T cells during chimeric antigen receptor-T cell expansion. *Cytotherapy* **2019**, *21*, S30–S31. [CrossRef]
121. Cohen, S.; Danzaki, K.; MacIver, N.J. Nutritional effects on T-cell immunometabolism. *Eur. J. Immunol.* **2017**, *47*, 225–235. [CrossRef]
122. Dwyer, C.J.; Knochelmann, H.M.; Smith, A.S.; Wyatt, M.M.; Rangel Rivera, G.O.; Arhontoulis, D.C.; Bartee, E.; Li, Z.; Rubinstein, M.P.; Paulos, C.M. Fueling cancer immunotherapy with common gamma chain cytokines. *Front. Immunol.* **2019**, *10*, 263. [CrossRef]
123. Cui, G.; Staron, M.M.; Gray, S.M.; Ho, P.-C.; Amezquita, R.A.; Wu, J.; Kaech, S.M. IL-7-induced glycerol transport and TAG synthesis promotes memory CD8+ T cell longevity. *Cell* **2015**, *161*, 750–761. [CrossRef]
124. Loschinski, R.; Böttcher, M.; Stoll, A.; Bruns, H.; Mackensen, A.; Mougiakakos, D. IL-21 modulates memory and exhaustion phenotype of T-cells in a fatty acid oxidation-dependent manner. *Oncotarget* **2018**, *9*, 13125. [CrossRef]
125. Battram, A.; Bachiller, M.; Urbano-Ispizua, Á.; Martin-Antonio, B. 104 BCMA-targeting CAR-T cells expanded in IL-15 have an improved phenotype for therapeutic use compared to those grown in IL-2 or IL-15/IL-7. *BMJ Spec. J.* **2020**, *8*, A115. [CrossRef]
126. Felices, M.; Lenvik, A.J.; McElmurry, R.; Chu, S.; Hinderlie, P.; Bendzick, L.; Geller, M.A.; Tolar, J.; Blazar, B.R.; Miller, J.S.; et al. Continuous treatment with IL-15 exhausts human NK cells via a metabolic defect. *JCI Insight* **2018**, *3*, e96219. [CrossRef]
127. Kimura, M.Y.; Pobezinsky, L.A.; Guinter, T.I.; Thomas, J.; Adams, A.; Park, J.-H.; Tai, X.; Singer, A. IL-7 signaling must be intermittent, not continuous, during CD8+ T cell homeostasis to promote cell survival instead of cell death. *Nat. Immunol.* **2013**, *14*, 143–151. [CrossRef]
128. Perkins, M.R.; Grande, S.; Hamel, A.; Horton, H.M.; Garrett, T.E.; Miller, S.M.; Latimer, H.J., IV; Horvath, C.J.; Kuczewski, M.; Friedman, K.M. *Manufacturing an Enhanced CAR T cell Product by Inhibition of the PI3K/Akt Pathway during T Cell Expansion Results in Improved In vivo Efficacy of Anti-BCMA CAR T Cells*; American Society of Hematology: Washington, DC, USA, 2015.
129. Klebanoff, C.A.; Crompton, J.G.; Leonardi, A.J.; Yamamoto, T.N.; Chandran, S.S.; Eil, R.L.; Sukumar, M.; Vodnala, S.K.; Hu, J.; Ji, Y.; et al. Inhibition of AKT signaling uncouples T cell differentiation from expansion for receptor-engineered adoptive immunotherapy. *JCI Insight* **2017**, *2*, e95103. [CrossRef] [PubMed]
130. Fraietta, J.A.; Lacey, S.F.; Orlando, E.J.; Pruteanu-Malinici, I.; Gohil, M.; Lundh, S.; Boesteanu, A.C.; Wang, Y.; O'Connor, R.S.; Hwang, W.-T.; et al. Determinants of response and resistance to CD19 chimeric antigen receptor (CAR) T cell therapy of chronic lymphocytic leukemia. *Nat. Med.* **2018**, *24*, 563–571. [CrossRef] [PubMed]
131. Sukumar, M.; Liu, J.; Ji, Y.; Subramanian, M.; Crompton, J.G.; Yu, Z.; Roychoudhuri, R.; Palmer, D.C.; Muranski, P.; Karoly, E.D.; et al. Inhibiting glycolytic metabolism enhances CD8+ T cell memory and antitumor function. *J. Clin. Investig.* **2013**, *123*, 4479–4488. [CrossRef] [PubMed]
132. Wei, J.; Luo, C.; Wang, Y.; Guo, Y.; Dai, H.; Tong, C.; Ti, D.; Wu, Z.; Han, W. PD-1 silencing impairs the anti-tumor function of chimeric antigen receptor modified T cells by inhibiting proliferation activity. *J. Immunother. Cancer* **2019**, *7*, 1–15. [CrossRef]
133. He, K.; Rad, S.; Poudel, A.; McLellan, A.D. Compact bidirectional promoters for dual-gene expression in a Sleeping Beauty transposon. *Int. J. Mol. Sci.* **2020**, *21*, 9256. [CrossRef]
134. Haran, K.P.; Hajduczki, A.; Pampusch, M.S.; Mwakalundwa, G.; Vargas-Inchaustegui, D.A.; Rakasz, E.G.; Connick, E.; Berger, E.A.; Skinner, P.J. Simian immunodeficiency virus (SIV)-specific chimeric antigen receptor-T cells engineered to target B cell follicles and suppress SIV replication. *Front. Immunol.* **2018**, *9*, 492. [CrossRef] [PubMed]
135. Rad, S.A.H.; Poudel, A.; Tan, G.M.Y.; McLellan, A.D. Optimisation of Tet-On inducible systems for Sleeping Beauty-based chimeric antigen receptor (CAR) applications. *Sci. Rep.* **2020**, *10*, 1–12.
136. Liu, Y.; Di, S.; Shi, B.; Zhang, H.; Wang, Y.; Wu, X.; Luo, H.; Wang, H.; Li, Z.; Jiang, H.; et al. Armored inducible expression of il-12 enhances antitumor activity of glypican-3–targeted chimeric antigen receptor–engineered T cells in hepatocellular carcinoma. *J. Immunol.* **2019**, *203*, 198–207. [CrossRef] [PubMed]
137. Kantor, A.; McClements, M.E.; MacLaren, R.E. CRISPR-Cas9 DNA base-editing and prime-editing. *Int. J. Mol. Sci.* **2020**, *21*, 6240. [CrossRef]
138. Ohta, A.; Gorelik, E.; Prasad, S.J.; Ronchese, F.; Lukashev, D.; Wong, M.K.; Huang, X.; Caldwell, S.; Liu, K.; Smith, P.; et al. A2A adenosine receptor protects tumors from antitumor T cells. *Proc. Natl. Acad. Sci. USA* **2006**, *103*, 13132–13137. [CrossRef] [PubMed]
139. Masoumi, E.; Jafarzadeh, L.; Mirzaei, H.R.; Alishah, K.; Fallah-Mehrjardi, K.; Rostamian, H.; Khakpoor-Koosheh, M.; Meshkani, R.; Noorbakhsh, F.; Hadjati, J.; et al. Genetic and pharmacological targeting of A2a receptor improves function of anti-mesothelin CAR T cells. *J. Exp. Clin. Cancer Res.* **2020**, *39*, 1–12. [CrossRef]
140. Newick, K.; O'Brien, S.; Sun, J.; Kapoor, V.; Maceyko, S.; Lo, A.; Puré, E.; Moon, E.; Albelda, S.M. Augmentation of CAR T-cell trafficking and antitumor efficacy by blocking protein kinase A localization. *Cancer Immunol. Res.* **2016**, *4*, 541–551. [CrossRef] [PubMed]
141. Latta-Mahieu, M.; Rolland, M.; Caillet, C.; Wang, M.; Kennel, P.; Mahfouz, I.; Loquet, I.; Dedieu, J.-F.; Mahfoudi, A.; Trannoy, E. Gene transfer of a chimeric trans-activator is immunogenic and results in short-lived transgene expression. *Hum. Gene Ther.* **2002**, *13*, 1611–1620. [CrossRef]

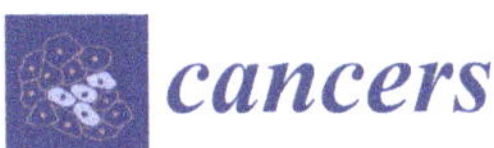

Review

TAM Receptor Inhibition–Implications for Cancer and the Immune System

Pia Aehnlich [1,*,†], **Richard Morgan Powell** [1,*,†], **Marlies J. W. Peeters** [1], **Anne Rahbech** [1] and **Per thor Straten** [1,2,*]

[1] National Center for Cancer Immune Therapy (CCIT-DK), Department of Oncology, Copenhagen University Hospital Herlev, 2730 Herlev, Denmark; marlies.peeters@regionh.dk (M.J.W.P.); anne.rahbech@regionh.dk (A.R.)

[2] Department of Immunology and Microbiology, Faculty of Health and Medical Sciences, University of Copenhagen, 2200 Copenhagen, Denmark

* Correspondence: pia.aehnlich@regionh.dk (P.A.); richard.morgan.powell@regionh.dk (R.M.P.); Per.Thor.Straten@regionh.dk (P.t.S.)

† Authors contributed equally to this work.

Simple Summary: TAM receptors are a family of receptor tyrosine kinases, comprising Tyro3, Axl and MerTK. Their primary role is in digestion of dying cells by macrophages without alarming the immune system. TAM receptors are also expressed by cancer cells in which signaling is oncogenic, and for this reason there is growing interest and research into TAM inhibition. This approach to cancer treatment may, however, come into conflict with beneficial and costimulatory TAM receptor signaling in T cells and natural killer (NK) cells. The aim of this review is to explore in detail the effects of TAM receptor inhibition on cancer cells and immune cells, and how the ramifications of this inhibition may affect cancer treatment in humans.

Abstract: Tyro3, Axl and MerTK (TAM) receptors are receptor tyrosine kinases which play important roles in efferocytosis and in the balancing of immune responses and inflammation. TAM receptor activation is induced upon binding of the ligands protein S (Pros1) or growth arrest-specific protein 6 (Gas6) which act as bridging molecules for binding of phosphatidyl serine (PtdSer) exposed on apoptotic cell membranes. Upon clearance of apoptotic cell material, TAM receptor activation on innate cells suppresses proinflammatory functions, thereby ensuring the immunologically silent removal of apoptotic material in the absence of deleterious immune responses. However, in T cells, MerTK signaling is costimulatory and promotes activation and functional output of the cell. MerTK and Axl are also aberrantly expressed in a range of both hematological and solid tumor malignancies, including breast, lung, melanoma and acute myeloid leukemia, where they have a role in oncogenic signaling. Consequently, TAM receptors are being investigated as therapeutic targets using small molecule inhibitors and have already demonstrated efficacy in mouse tumor models. Thus, inhibition of TAM signaling in cancer cells could have therapeutic value but given the opposing roles of TAM signaling in innate cells and T cells, TAM inhibition could also jeopardize anticancer immune responses. This conflict is discussed in this review, describing the effects of TAM inhibition on cancer cells as well as immune cells, while also examining the intricate interplay of cancer and immune cells in the tumor microenvironment.

Keywords: TAM receptors; Axl; MerTK; PD-1; small molecule inhibitors; cancer

Citation: Aehnlich, P.; Powell, R.M.; Peeters, M.J.W.; Rahbech, A.; thor Straten, P. TAM Receptor Inhibition–Implications for Cancer and the Immune System. *Cancers* **2021**, *13*, 1195. https://doi.org/10.3390/cancers13061195

Academic Editors: Michael Kershaw and Clare Slaney

Received: 20 February 2021
Accepted: 8 March 2021
Published: 10 March 2021

Publisher's Note: MDPI stays neutral with regard to jurisdictional claims in published maps and institutional affiliations.

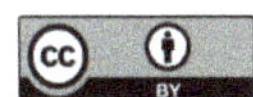

1. Introduction

The TAM receptors—Tyro3, Axl, MerTK—are a family of receptor tyrosine kinases that were discovered three decades ago, and are broadly expressed by a variety of cells and tissues in the body [1]. Ligands for the receptors are protein S (Pros1) and growth arrest-specific protein 6 (Gas6). Pros1 acts as ligand for Tyro3 and MerTK, whereas Gas6 is ligand for all three TAMs. Optimal signaling through the receptor is induced only when Pros1 and Gas6 act as bridging ligands for phosphatidyl serine (PtdSer), typically expressed on the outer membrane of apoptotic cells [2]. This leads to homodimerization and autophosphorylation of the TAM and downstream signaling; the outcome of which is highly cell-dependent but goes through pathways such as MEK/ERK, PI3K/AKT and JAK/STAT [3]. TAM receptors and ligands Pros1 and/or Gas6 are often co-expressed, and signaling is largely associated with efferocytosis, whereby TAM receptors expressed by macrophages, via Pros1/Gas6, bind PtdSer exposed by apoptotic cells or cell debris. The resultant signaling directs macrophages to an M2 phenotype, ensuring silent removal of dead cells and repair of tissues [4]. TAM receptors are also essential in regulation and control of inflammatory immune responses. Innate immune cells express pattern recognition receptors, e.g., toll-like receptors (TLR), which recognize microbial structures and upon ligand engagement induce an immune response [5]. To prevent a superfluous immune reaction, TAM signaling in dendritic cells (DC) functions as negative feedback to TLR signaling by induction of SOCS1/SOCS3 expression, thereby dampening the inflammatory response [6]. Axl signaling in murine natural killer (NK) cells limits the functional capacity of the cell [7], and activated T cells secrete Pros1, which works as an additional feedback mechanism to DCs and limits the immune response in a TAM-dependent manner [8]. As discussed in more detail later, we have shown that activated T cells express MerTK, which upon activation delivers a costimulatory signal to the T cell [9].

MerTK and Axl are expressed in a wide range of cancer types, including non-small cell lung cancer [10], breast cancer [11], colorectal cancer [12], ovarian cancer [13] and melanoma [14], with 50–70% of patient samples being positive. Not only solid cancers, but also leukemias express Axl and MerTK [15,16]. For a comprehensive list of MerTK and Axl expression in cancers, refer to Graham et al., 2014 [4]. Cancer cells express both TAM molecules and their ligands, and, despite not being apoptotic, they also expose PtdSer on the outer membrane. This phenomenon of apoptotic mimicry was first described in virally infected cells as a means to dampen antiviral immune responses in the host [17]. PtdSer expression of cancer cells similarly dampens immune responses by interacting with TAM on antigen-presenting cells [18]. Furthermore, the co-expression of TAM, ligand(s) and PtdSer on cancer cells allows for autocrine signaling through the receptors, i.e., typical oncogenic signaling pathways like MEK/ERK, PI3K/AKT and JAK/STAT. In cancer cells, additional oncogenic pathways are associated with TAM receptor signaling. Anti-apoptosis and survival are promoted through activation of the NF-κB pathway and signaling via BCL-2 and ACK1 [10,19,20]. In regards to metastasis, TAM signaling regulates migration and invasion through promotion of proteins such as RHO and FAK1 [21] as well as MMP9 [22]. Axl additionally upregulates Snail and Slug, which induces epithelial-to-mesenchymal transition (EMT) [23] (see Figure 1).

Expression of TAM is associated with a worse disease outcome in a range of cancer diagnoses, both solid and hematological (reviewed in [4]), which has prompted the development of strategies to block or inhibit TAM signaling in cancer cells [24]. While most aspects of Tyro3 are understudied, data are accumulating concerning the complex biology of MerTK and Axl in cells, tissues, the immune system and cancer. In this review, we highlight the key roles of MerTK and Axl as both oncogenes and immune system regulators. We discuss the current standing and future prospects of MerTK and Axl inhibition in the treatment of cancer and the balancing act that must be maintained to limit any potential detrimental effects on immune cells.

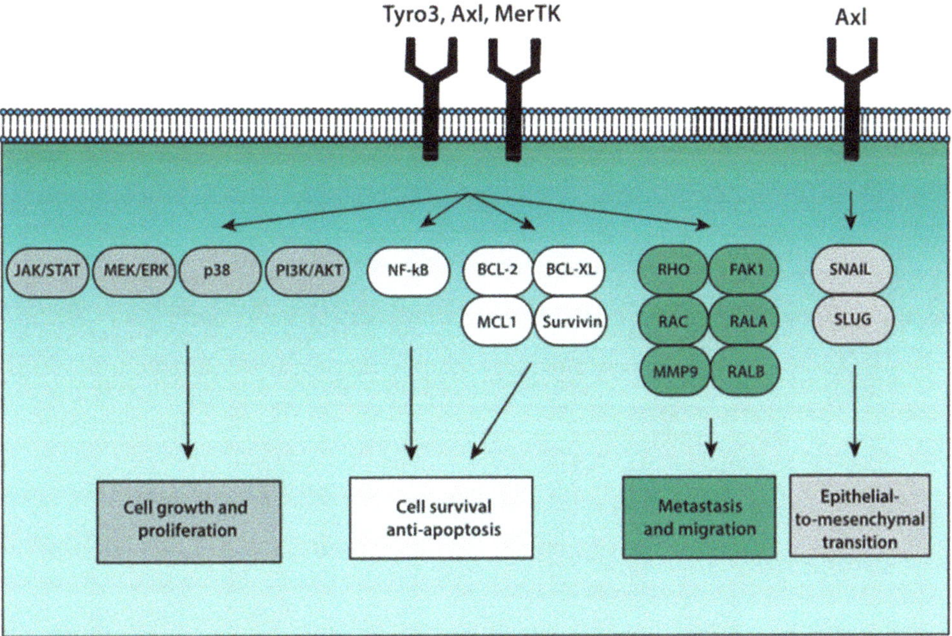

Figure 1. Activation of Tyro3, Axl and MerTK (TAM) receptors on cancer cells results in downstream oncogenic signaling. First, JAK/STAT, MEK/ERK, p38 and PI3K/AKT promote cell growth and proliferation in tumors. Second, cell survival and anti-apoptosis is induced through NF-κβ and BCL-2 pathways. Third, RHO and FAK1 signaling promote metastasis and migration. Lastly, epithelial-to-mesenchymal transition (EMT) is promoted through the SNAIL/SLUG signaling pathway.

2. MerTK

2.1. Targeting MerTK in Cancer

A wide range of cancers have been demonstrated to express high levels of MerTK, in both blood malignancies and solid cancers [24], resulting in gathering interest in the targeting of MerTK for cancer treatment. MerTK was first identified on a B lymphoblast library [25], and later characterization of acute myeloid leukemia (AML) and acute lymphocytic leukemia (ALL) showed expression in more than 80% of patient samples [15]. Importantly, numerous studies in various cancer diseases have been able to show that expression of MerTK is associated with a worse outcome [24]. Cancer cells that express high levels of TAM receptors, including MerTK, also express the ligands Gas6 and/or Pros1, as well as PtdSer on the outer membrane [26]. As a consequence, cancer cells express all the prerequisites to MerTK autosignaling, which has been demonstrated to assist in formation of metastases, chemoresistance and proliferation [4].

These findings have led to the development of MerTK-targeting therapies in the form of small molecule inhibitors as well as blocking antibodies. Preclinical studies have shown that MerTK inhibitors can be effective in certain MerTK-sensitive tumors. MerTK/FLT3-specific small molecule inhibitors UNC2025, MRX2843 and UNC1666 were shown to have significant effect on tumor growth of AML, ALL and melanoma in cell lines, murine models and primary patient tumor samples [27–30].

Apart from cancer-intrinsic features, MerTK signaling on tumor cells has been shown to also increase expression of PD-L1 [31], potentially limiting cytotoxic T cell antitumoral responses. Obviously, this phenomenon is associated with therapeutic implications, since the main breakthrough in cancer immunotherapy is treatment based on breach of the PD-L1/PD-1 axis between cancer cells and cytotoxic T cells. In addition, it has been demonstrated that MerTK signaling in APC promotes tolerogenic signaling and thus limits the ability of the APC to activate T cells [32]. Due to apoptotic mimicry, cancer cells seduce macrophages to silent phagocytosis via MerTK signaling instead of triggering an inflammatory response. Therefore, it is postulated that MerTK inhibition can be used to both control tumor growth directly and convert an immunosuppressive tumor microenvironment into an antitumoral microenvironment more prone to response to immunotherapy. To this end, Cook et al. demonstrated that MerTK knockout in a murine breast cancer model both reduced tumor growth and increased CD8 T cell infiltration [33]. Similarly, Tormoen et al. revealed that MerTK knockout in colorectal cancer and pancreatic ductal adenocarcinoma was responsible for control of tumor growth mediated by CD8 T cells and macrophages [34]. However, independent of any tumor model, Shao et al. showed that B cells in MerTK knockout mouse maintained normal activation, proliferation and antigen processing; however, their ability to activate T cells was decreased. The authors suggest this could be due to a reduced ability to effectively present antigen to CD4 T cells, illustrating that research on nontumoral effects of MerTK inhibition is required [35].

In recent years, the antitumor efficacy of small molecule inhibitors and MerTK-specific monoclonal antibodies (mAb) was demonstrated in a range of tumor models. In contrast to the previously mentioned studies that utilized MerTK knockout mouse models [33–35], MerTK inhibition alone was not always sufficient to impact on tumor outgrowth. It is, thus, highly important to point out that all the following studies required combination therapy involving αPD-1 treatment to facilitate antitumoral effects. Yokoyama et al. and Zhou et al. both studied PD-1 blockade and MerTK inhibition in the colorectal cancer mouse model, MC38. They demonstrated improved antitumor response, with increased Ki67+ CD8+ T cell infiltration and inflammatory cytokine profiles, when PD-1 blockade was used in conjunction with the MerTK small molecule inhibitor RDX106 or a MerTK monoclonal antibody [36,37]. In a lung xenograft carcinoma model, Caetano et al. showed that treatment involving αMerTK mAb and αPD-1 increased tumor infiltration of CD8 and NK cells. CD8+ CD103+ T cells were pointed out as a key phenotype that conveyed antitumoral effect [38]. A pan-TAM inhibitor, BMS 777607, was used by Kasikara et al. in a triple negative breast cancer model and it was revealed that this combination with PD-1 blockade again increased CD8 T cell infiltration, inflammatory cytokine profiles and, in this case, increased infiltration of Th1 type CD4 T cells [39]. The necessity of a combination therapy with anti-PD-1 is potentially due to the fact that PD-1 expression was increased on CD8+ T cells [36,37] and in the case of Kasikara et al., PD-L1 and PD-1 expression was increased in the tumor environment. It can therefore be posited that PD-1 blockade was required to unleash antitumor T cell response in these studies [39].

MerTK inhibition in murine tumor models has also revealed how macrophages and myeloid-derived suppressor cells (MDSCs) are affected in the context of an immune-driven antitumor response. A key mechanism is the ability of MerTK inhibition to switch M2 to M1 type macrophages and their relevant proinflammatory cytokine milieu [40]. Using MerTK inhibitor MRX2843, Lee-Sherrick et al. and Su et al. demonstrated in leukemia and glioblastoma models, respectively, that MerTK inhibition played a role in altering macrophage phenotype [41,42]. A switch from CD206+ M2-like macrophages to M1-like macrophages was reported with reduced PD-L1 expression, in conjunction with increased inflammatory cytokines and reduced regulatory T cell numbers. Holtzhausen et al. revealed that tumor-associated MDSCs express TAM receptors and that TAM inhibitor UNC4241, in conjunction with αPD-1, reduced tumor growth in melanoma models [43]. The MDSC's suppressive capacity was functionally reduced and infiltration of CD8 T cells was increased. Du et al. utilized a broad spectrum TAM inhibitor to demonstrate that in lung and breast cancer models, MDSCs and M2-like macrophages were reduced along with reduced anti-inflammatory Arg-1 and IL-4 in the tumor-microenvironment [44]. However, they did show that PD-L1 and PD-1 were increased and therefore combination therapy with αPD-1 was required to sufficiently reduce tumor growth.

2.2. The Function of MerTK on T Cells

The wealth of evidence from combination therapy involving MerTK inhibition in murine models suggests this route of treatment is beneficial for CD8 T cell-mediated antitumoral responses. This is somewhat controversial as recent papers have demonstrated that MERTK is expressed by activated T cells [45]. Initially, MerTK expression on mouse splenocytes or human T cells was found to be absent following two-day stimulation with PMA/PHA [46,47]. However, Cabezón et al. clarified that human CD4+ T cells expressed MerTK three days after activation when using αCD3/CD28 [32]. This was supported by a paper from Peeters et al., who moreover exposed MerTK expression on human CD8+ T cells to have a late costimulatory role [9]. Inhibition of MerTK signaling by the inhibitor UNC2025 or by siRNA resulted in decreased release of interferon (IFN)-γ and had a negative impact on proliferation of human CD8+ T cells. This costimulatory role was contrary to its previously described role as a negative regulator of the innate immune response [6] and APC activation [32]. Thus, MerTK signaling has shown ambivalent roles depending on cell subset, species origin and type of T cell stimulation, which further complicates the idea of therapeutic targeting.

As previously mentioned, an interplay between MerTK and PD-1 has been suggested, mainly based on murine studies using combination therapies with αPD-1 [36–39]. This was further confirmed by unpublished data from our group. Flow cytometric staining of activated human T cells indicated co-expression of MerTK and PD-1, as MerTK positive cells showed significantly higher levels of PD-1 expression compared to MerTK negative cells. Additionally, the expression kinetics of both molecules seem to go hand in hand over several days. PD-1 is known to be expressed by activated T cells and to be dependent on TCR signaling. PD-1 is furthermore used as a marker of tumor-reactive T cells among tumor-infiltrating lymphocytes (TIL) [48]. Based on our previously described costimulatory role of MerTK and this well-known role of PD-1, the MerTK and PD1+ double positive T cells seem to have a tumor-reactive phenotype. If PD-1 is decreased upon MerTK inhibition, as described by Lee-Sherick et al. [41], it might thus result in less activated, less tumor-reactive T cells. While this might not pose a problem in short-term assays, as we have seen in most mouse model studies, it should perhaps be considered in the more long-term clinical setting.

MerTK signaling seems to have a regulatory role in T cell memory responses. Observations from Peeters et al. showed a significantly higher level of MerTK expression on the T_{CM} CD8+ subset [9]. This was further supported by data indicating that expression kinetics of MerTK follow the fraction of the central memory T cell (T_{CM}) subset. Moreover, upon restimulation of the T cells, the percentage of MerTK-expressing cells increased significantly. Additional analysis of the T_{CM} subset upon restimulation revealed a higher fraction of T_{CM} within the MerTK-expressing cells (unpublished data). It, therefore, seems that MerTK signaling supports the formation of a central memory response. Thus, generation of long-term memory T cell responses could be jeopardized by MerTK inhibition. Importantly, it remains understudied if mouse T cells express MerTK upon activation. Surely, if this is not the case, this important role of MerTK in human T cells would not be illuminated in mouse tumor models.

2.3. MerTK in the Crossfire of Cancer Cells and T Cells

Due to the direct effect MerTK inhibitors have on their respective tumor targets, research into potential off-target effects on other cell types is scarce so far. Evidence suggests higher concentrations of inhibitors, i.e., >500 nM, impact colony formation of cord blood cells [27–29]. Since we know that T cells express MerTK and that it plays a role in costimulation and memory formation, further research needs to be undertaken to assess direct effects of new and potent MerTK-specific inhibitors. Two studies have briefly assessed the effect on CD8 T cells, suggesting no direct effect on CD8 T cell proliferation when their respective inhibitors were used [36,43]. However, the concentration tested was not stated or very low. Concentration is key in this respect, given that a balance needs to be struck between a direct tumor effect versus any detrimental effect on MerTK+ T cells. Since both cancer cells and immune cells express MerTK, it is important to investigate the role of MerTK signaling in the tumor context. It is firmly established that MERTK inhibition on cancer cells inhibits survival signaling pathways. Moreover, MerTK inhibition on APCs would block efferocytosis and render the cells more capable in priming T cell responses. On the other hand, blocking MERTK signaling on T cells would render the T cell less capable of cytokine production, proliferation and killing.

To answer this question of how MerTK inhibition may affect MerTK+ T cells in an antitumor cell response, we studied MerTK signaling in melanoma TILs by examining the impact of Pros1 [9]. Melanoma TILs are used for adoptive cell therapy (ACT) at our research center and TIL expansion represents a crucial step in the process since failure to grow cells obviously jeopardizes patient treatment. Clearance of Pros1 by an αPros1 antibody during TIL expansion resulted in a significant decrease in fold expansion rate. Similarly, we studied if addition of increasing Pros1 concentrations would impact the cytotoxicity of expanded TILs against an autologous melanoma cell line. These data indicated a trend, albeit non-significant, that higher Pros1 levels corresponded with enhanced killing activity of the T cells.

MerTK activation initiates a signaling cascade in cancer cells that classically promotes cancer cell survival, and in T cells provides a costimulatory signal. In the TME, this sets the stage for competition for Pros1 between cancer cells and T cells, and this balance may affect aspects of immune microenvironment resolution. In co-culture studies with the breast cancer cell line MDA-MB.231, which expresses high levels of MerTK, we could show that low concentrations of Pros1 resulted in an enhanced inhibition of T cell activation by the cancer cells. This competitive effect was abrogated when an excess amount of Pros1 was present in the co-culture media [9]. Cancer cell lines express a higher level of TAM receptors than activated T cells, which explains a higher Pros1 consumption by MDA-MB.231 cells compared to activated T cells. This shows how TAM expression by cancer cells, or any cell of the TME, could set the stage for ligand competition and Pros1 starving of T cells. One strategy to overcome this ligand competition could be to equip T cells with a constitutively active MerTK construct [49], thereby increasing MerTK signaling and rendering the T cell insensitive to Pros1 starvation.

3. Axl

3.1. Axl Drives Cancer Cell Survival, EMT and Chemoresistance

In recent years, Axl has been investigated to a great extent for its role as an oncogene and driver of cancer cell survival. It was this very role that led to the discovery of Axl in the first place; the gene was isolated from two patients with chronic myelogenous leukemia (CML) and shown to cause neoplastic transformation in NIH3T3 cells [50]. Following this discovery, a myriad of articles have been published to unravel Axl's involvement in cancer cell survival and metastasis in many cancer types (as reviewed in [51]). Downstream signaling of Axl resembles many other receptor tyrosine kinase signaling pathways and their specific activation seems to be dependent on cell and tissue type [51]. In general, Axl mediates both tumor-proliferating and anti-apoptotic functions, which synergize in promoting cancer cell survival. In addition, Axl signaling has more specialized features in cancer cells, two of which will be highlighted in the following.

First, Axl has repeatedly been shown to be involved in epithelial-to-mesenchymal transition (EMT), thus being a crucial player in enabling cancer cell metastasis [52]. Axl has been pointed out both as an upstream regulator [23] and a downstream effector [53] of EMT. Asiedu et al. showed that vector-based overexpression of Axl in human breast epithelial cells resulted in downregulation of the epithelial marker E-cadherin and a concurrent up-regulation of mesenchymal markers N-cadherin, Snail and Slug [23]. This EMT phenotype was suppressed when silencing Axl with shRNA or when blocking the NFκB pathway with proteasome inhibitor MG132. This elegantly demonstrated the role of Axl in inducing EMT, in part at least via activating NFκB. A recent study supported these results, as the ectopic expression of Axl in human gastric cancer cell lines also downregulated E-cadherin and upregulated the mesenchymal marker vimentin [54]. In both studies [23,54], inactivation of Axl in in vivo models slowed tumor outgrowth. As Axl is not only implicated as an inducer but also an effector of EMT, this strongly points towards a positive feedback loop to sustain the EMT phenotype of tumor cells. The induction of Axl by the EMT program has been observed in different tumor types, such as breast cancer [53,55], skin cancer [56], esophageal cancer [57] and ovarian cancer [58]. Axl signaling was shown to facilitate cancer cell invasion in esophageal cancer by increasing extracellular acidification by upregulation of lactate transporters. The increased extracellular pH, in turn, led to a peripheral distribution of lysosomes and enhanced lysosomal exocytosis and secretion of cathepsin B, a protease involved in extracellular matrix degradation. This paved the way for cancer cell migration from the primary site [57].

Second, expression of Axl plays a role in mediating chemoresistance, which is a major challenge in providing long-lasting treatment to cancer patients. Some cancers are more prone to chemoresistance than others and increased frequency of chemoresistance often goes hand in hand with a poorer prognosis. This, for instance, is the case for ovarian cancer, in which resistance to the first-line platinum-based chemotherapeutics is very common [13,59]. The chemoresistance against platins in ovarian cancer has been shown to be mediated by Axl by different mechanisms. Axl signaling was found to hamper intracellular accumulation of carboplatin in ovarian cancer cell line POV71-hTERT, thus keeping intracellular carboplatin concentrations at suboptimal levels [13]. Axl blockade in POV71-hTERT cells revealed an upregulation of multidrug resistance gene P-glycoprotein expression. P-glycoprotein is an ATP-dependent efflux pump, which could potentially export carboplatin from the cell. Therefore, this could indicate a pretarget resistance mechanism, as per classification of platinum resistance mechanisms by Galluzzi et al. [60]. Additionally, Axl has been implied in an off-target resistance mechanism against cisplatin: Axl seems to increase aerobic glycolysis of ovarian cancer cells, also known as the Warburg effect [59]. Specifically, Axl was shown to phosphorylate the pyruvate kinase isoform PKM2 at tyrosine 105, which favors ATP production by aerobic glycolysis over the Krebs cycle. This altered metabolism, with its increased energy production and biosynthesis, was suggested to compensate for the lethal cisplatin signaling. The diversity of chemoresistance mechanisms induced by Axl illustrates the key role that Axl plays in platinum resistance. Apart from ovarian cancer and platinum, Axl mediates chemoresistance in a range of other cancers and drugs. Just to name a few, Axl was shown to cause resistance of astrocytoma cell line A172 to carboplatin [61], resistance of FLT3-internal tandem duplication AML to quizartinib [62] or resistance of EGFR-mutated lung cancer to osimertinib [63].

Taken together, this shows that Axl signaling has a variety of beneficial effects on cancer cells that could be exploited therapeutically.

3.2. Targeting Axl on Cancer Cells and Its Implications

The strong oncogenic properties of Axl expression and signaling have led to the development of Axl inhibitors; one of the best known to date is bemcentinib (formerly BGB324 or R428). It has been shown to block proliferation and growth signaling [16] as well as tumor metastasis [52]. Furthermore, Axl inhibition enhances apoptosis mediated by chemotherapeutic drugs [64]. Due to the success of Axl inhibitors in preclinical models, some treatment prospects have been advanced into clinical testing. The lead candidate is bemcentinib, being tested in as much as ten clinical phase I/II studies registered on ClinicalTrials.gov (accessed on 28/10/2020). The clinical trials cover a wide range of tumor diagnoses, from brain cancer over triple-negative breast cancer to acute myeloid leukemia. Bemcentinib is being tested as a single-treatment agent as well as in combination with, e.g., chemotherapy, targeted therapy and immune checkpoint blockade. To date, only one study is registered as completed. TP-0903 is another candidate in clinical testing, comprising four registered in-patient trials. To our knowledge, only preliminary clinical data has been made available for these trials, showing some promising responses.

Besides merely being a treatment target, Axl has often been implied as a prognostic factor for cancer patients. High Axl expression is usually associated with a worse outcome [65]. These associations are mostly based on cancer gene signatures, allowing for determination of expression of Axl RNA. Axl RNA expression, however, has been shown to not directly correlate to Axl protein expression [66], which is necessary for functionality of the receptor. In their murine studies, Zagórska and colleagues demonstrated that Axl mRNA copy number is very similar in DCs and bone marrow-derived macrophages. Despite this, Axl protein expression is high on DCs, but low on bone marrow-derived macrophages, suggesting that post-transcriptional or post-translational mechanisms regulate Axl expression. Therefore, it should be considered that PCR-based evidence for high Axl expression on cancer cells does not necessarily translate into high expression of Axl protein.

Nevertheless, whether Axl is expressed on cancer cells or not, emerging evidence suggests that Axl inhibitors could affect cancer cells regardless of Axl expression. In a study by Chen et al., Axl inhibitor bemcentinib induced cancer cell apoptosis in cell lines, in which Axl was knocked down by a siRNA approach. They demonstrated that bemcentinib blocks Axl phosphorylation short-term and induced Axl upregulation, while still causing increased apoptosis—this increased apoptosis was observed even in Axl knockdown cell lines [67]. This was traced down to protonation of bemcentinib following accumulation in the lysosomes, which altered lysosomal pH. In turn, the altered pH disturbed lysosomal degradation leading to vacuolization, and eventually triggered cell death. This is underlined by R428′s molecular structure, which resembles other lysomotropic agents that induce vacuolization. An important consideration is that the entrapment of bemcentinib in lysosomes could explain the merely transient effect as an Axl inhibitor. Furthermore, Chen et al. showed that bemcentinib initiated autophagy, possibly as a feedback signal to compensate for the disrupted autophagic protein processing in the lysosomes, which, however, aggravates the problem. Increased autophagic flux was also observed upon treatment of renal cancer cells with bemcentinib [64]. These results, though, stand in contrast to a study by Lotsberg et al. [68], which showed that bemcentinib abrogates autophagy in non-small cell lung cancer (NSCLC) and thus induces immunogenic cell death. These differences could be related to different cancer cell lines studied, but also illustrate very well that the mechanism(s) of small molecule Axl inhibitors are not entirely clarified yet.

Upregulation of Axl caused by a small molecule Axl inhibitor as described by Chen et al. was later confirmed in another study with Axl TKI BMS777607 [69]. The authors found that Axl phosphorylation upon Gas6 stimulation is necessary for the protein to be ubiquitinylated, internalized and degraded by the lysosomal pathway. However, blocking receptor activation with a tyrosine kinase inhibitor also blocks this required phosphorylation, which leads to an accumulation of an inactive Axl receptor on the cell surface. Phosphorylation of this receptor can still take place, even after days, which causes severe consequences in the tumor microenvironment. In sections of tumors where the drug gradient might fall below inhibitory concentrations, accumulated Axl receptors may start to signal again, reversing any desired effect of treatment.

3.3. Axl Plays a Role in Immune Homeostasis

Axl can be expressed by various immune cells, which implies that targeting of Axl in cancer therapy may also have an impact on the immune system.

In DCs, Axl signaling plays a major role in terminating immune responses at the end of an infection [6]. TLR activation on DCs upregulates Axl expression via STAT1 signaling. Upon activation, Axl hijacks the IFNAR-STAT1 signaling cassette to induce SOCS1 and SOCS3. These molecules then suppress TLR signaling, terminating DC priming of T cells. Blocking this pathway could avoid the negative feedback mechanism, allowing continued immune responses.

Macrophages are another cell type in the myeloid compartment that expresses Axl. TAM receptor expression on macrophages is crucial in the process of efferocytosis, the immune-quiescent phagocytosis of apoptotic cells. While MerTK surely takes the lead role in this process [70], nuclear receptor signaling following efferocytosis is suggested to also upregulate Axl transcription in macrophages [71]. Blockade of Axl, or TAM receptors in general, can thus hinder efferocytosis [72]. Consequently, phagocytosis of (dying) tumor cells would trigger an inflammatory response, which could attract more immune cells to the crime scene. In the tumor context, Axl is also suggested to play a role in polarization of tumor-associated macrophages (as reviewed in [73]). There is conflicting evidence on Axl's involvement; while Axl inhibition with R428 decreased M2-associated factors (IL-10 and TGF-β) in mineral trioxide aggregate-treated THP-1 cells [74], blocking Axl with a monoclonal antibody in an MDA-MB231 xenograft model decreased M1-associated factors (IL-6, TNF-α, G-CSF) [75].

Furthermore, Axl signaling has been implied in optimal NK cell differentiation [76,77]. It should be considered that Axl inhibition could therefore hamper differentiation from immature NK cells into cytotoxic NK cells. Similar to DCs, Axl could possibly also be implicated in the negative regulation of NK cells [78]. Upon stimulation with interleukin-15, NK cells were shown to have reduced IFN-γ secretion if pretreated with type I interferons. This went hand in hand with an upregulation of Axl on NK cells, leading to the suggestion that Axl might be the mediator of diminished IFN-γ secretion. However, this mechanism remains to be fully investigated.

3.4. Axl Inhibition and the Effect on the Immune Response against Cancer

The previous sections have illustrated that Axl plays a role both in tumor biology and in the immune system. In an era during which the immune system's ability to control tumor growth is increasingly harnessed by immunotherapies, it is worth investigating which role Axl plays in this interaction between cancer and immune cells.

Besides its direct effects on cancer cell survival and invasion, blocking of Axl signaling has other antitumor effects, which render the tumor more susceptible to immune cell killing. Recently, Axl targeting was discovered to have a positive impact on the expression of ICAM-1 and ULBP-1 on lung carcinoma [79]. ICAM-1 is an adhesion molecule implicated in lymphocyte tissue migration and stabilization of cell–cell junctions, whereas ULBP-1 is a ligand for NKG2D, an activating NK receptor. By upregulation of these molecules, the lung carcinoma cell line clones displayed increased sensitivity to NK- and T cell-mediated killing. Likewise, Woo et al. found that R428 could enhance the effect of TRAIL-mediated killing [64]. TRAIL is a death receptor ligand, which is expressed by various immune cells. In their study, apoptosis induced by recombinant TRAIL was increased by R428 in a variety of cancer cell lines. They demonstrated that R428 induced upregulation of miR-708, which inhibits c-FLIP expression. Additionally, R428 triggered proteasomal degradation of survivin. Both c-FLIP and survivin are anti-apoptotic proteins, which explains why their downregulation allows increased apoptosis.

Apart from targeting tumor cells, Axl inhibition also has direct effects on the immune system, which could aid the immune cells in destructing the cancer cells. Specifically, the role of Axl in terminating immune responses should be discussed. Both in DCs and in NK cells, Axl has been implied in negative feedback loops and breaking these loops could restore essential immune responses in the tumor microenvironment. This concept is emphasized by a study by Guo et al., in which they could show that Axl inhibition (both by bemcentinib and SGI-7079) reprogrammed the tumor microenvironment in two different mouse tumor models [80]. They found that Axl inhibition caused a reduction of monocytes/macrophages and granulocytes in the tumor, but an accumulation of CD103+cDCs. These cDCs also expressed higher amounts of activation markers CD40 and CD86. Concomitantly, this led to increased infiltration of activated proliferating T cells (Ki67 and CD69 positive) to the tumor. This could suggest that the activated DCs induced a heightened T cell response, which was also underlined by higher Th1-associated gene expression in the tumor. However, this adaptive immune response was counteracted by PD-L1 upregulation on the tumor cells. This went hand in hand with an induction of PD-1 expression on the tumor-infiltrating T cells, which suggested a formation of an adaptive immune resistance.

PD-1 blockade could reverse this acquired resistance, to the degree that a third of mice treated with αPD-1 mAb and an Axl inhibitor were cured and resistant to rechallenge.

Similarly, in mice, TAM receptor signaling was suggested to attenuate NK cell responses via ubiquitin ligase Cbl-b. Hence, inhibition of TAM receptors, including Axl, could enhance NK cell function, shown by a decreased metastatic load in mice models [7,81]. Moreover, blockade of Axl ligand Gas6 signaling was also shown to activate NK cells, which further underlined this mechanism in murine tumors [82]. However, expression of Axl on mature human NK cells is debated: mRNA expression of Axl was shown to disappear on day 10 of NK cell differentiation from CD34+ human pluripotent stem cells [76]. On the contrary, a study on NK cells isolated from peripheral blood mononuclear cells found that a fraction of NK cells expressed Axl (approx. 1%) and that this expression was tripled by IFN-β stimulation [78]. Still, this raises questions about the functional relevance of Axl on human NK cells, and thus the effect of Axl inhibitors.

4. Conclusions

Thirty years after their characterization, TAM receptors are now recognized as important molecules in a range of normal physiological functions, e.g., efferocytosis, tissue repair, innate immune regulation and costimulation on T cells. TAM receptors also play important roles in cancer biology, which has prompted investigations on inhibition of mainly Axl and MerTK as a therapeutic strategy. To this end, various small molecule inhibitors have been developed, alongside a smaller number of blocking antibodies. In vitro inhibition of both MerTK and Axl has a negative impact on cancer cell survival, with enhanced apoptosis and diminished proliferation (see Figures 2 and 3 for MerTK and Axl inhibition, respectively). Blocking of Axl also impedes EMT and reverses chemoresistance. The favorable attributes of TAM inhibition could also be translated in vivo, since blocking TAM receptors prevented tumor outgrowth in several murine studies. In these studies, increased inflammatory tumor cell killing was observed when Axl or MerTK signaling was abrogated by small molecule inhibitors, blocking antibodies or gene knockout. The heightened immune response is mainly ascribed to an increased CD8 T cell infiltration. MerTK inhibition is also associated with M1 macrophage polarization and a reduced number of MDSCs (see Figure 2). Axl inhibition, in contrast, is suggested to block negative feedback loops in DCs and NK cells (see Figure 3). Despite inducing an inflammatory tumor microenvironment, TAM inhibition leads to an adaptive resistance to immune cell killing by upregulating molecules of the PD-1/PD-L1 axis. Therefore, combining TAM inhibition with anti-PD-1 blockade seems necessary and has proven efficacious in mouse models. Still, the desired effect of TAM inhibition, even as combination therapy, may come into conflict with undesirable effects on the immune system: Axl signaling plays a role in NK cell differentiation and MerTK signaling provides costimulation to T cells. Indeed, our research has demonstrated direct adverse effects of MerTK inhibition on T cells, including reduced proliferation and cytokine production (see Figure 2). Furthermore, MerTK-positive T cells that are restimulated generate a significantly increased central memory pool. Upon use of MerTK inhibitors, this mechanism may be disrupted, favoring short-lived effector T cell responses over generation of memory pools. While this may result in effective treatment in the short term, an insufficient adaptive T cell memory pool may fail to prevent relapse in the long term. Further study is required to fully interrogate the duality between beneficial and detrimental effects of MerTK and Axl inhibition in cancer treatment and its consequences for the immune system.

Clinical trials are ongoing to investigate the therapeutic potential of Axl and MerTK small molecule inhibitors in cancer and data from these trials will provide valuable insights into the precise mechanism of action. Preclinical data have shown that Axl small molecule inhibitors likely affect cellular degradation pathways, even independent of Axl expression. This illustrates the need for careful monitoring of early clinical data to harness merely the beneficial effects of TAM small molecule inhibitors. In the future, this will possibly prepare the platform for intelligent combination treatments with conventional therapies, including immunotherapy.

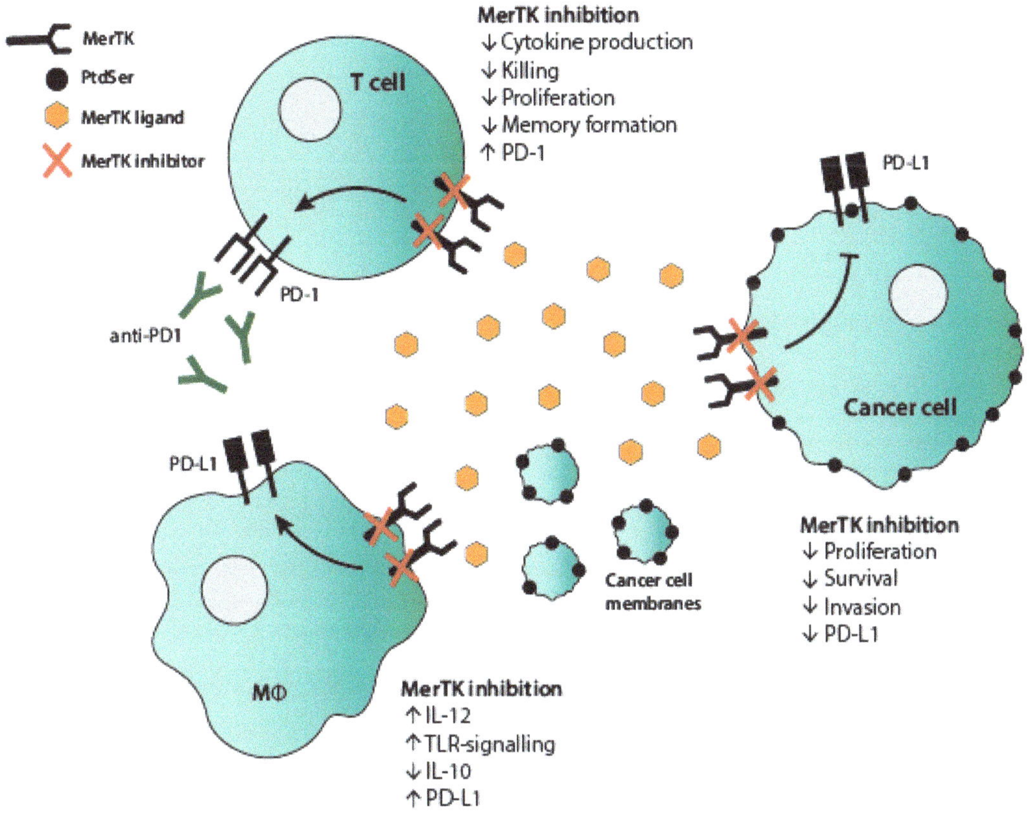

Figure 2. MerTK inhibition affects cancer cells, macrophages and T cells. In cancer cells, inhibition of MerTK signaling leads to reduced proliferation, survival and invasion. It also hampers upregulation of PD-L1 in cancer cells. In macrophages, MerTK inhibition increases IL-12 production, toll-like receptors (TLR) signaling and PD-L1 expression, while decreasing IL-10 production. MerTK blockade in T cells results in reduced cytokine production, cytotoxicity, proliferation and memory formation. It also induces expression of PD-1, thus, anti-PD-1 treatment should be considered in combination with MerTK inhibition.

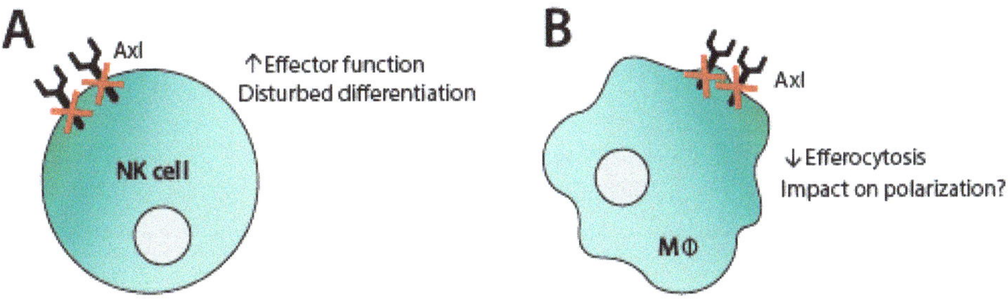

Figure 3. *Cont.*

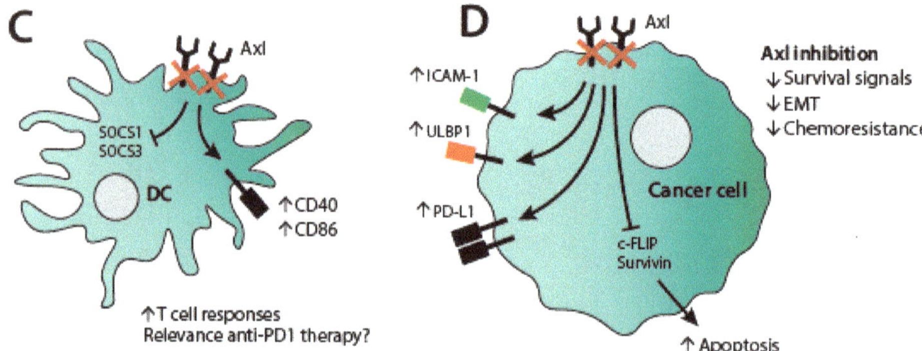

Figure 3. Axl inhibition influences both cancer and immune cells. (**A**) Blockade of Axl signaling in natural killer (NK) cells enhances effector function but has also been implied to disturb NK cell differentiation. (**B**) In macrophages, Axl inhibition leads to reduced efferocytosis and could also impact polarization. (**C**) Axl inhibition in dendritic cells (DCs) blocks SOCS1/3 signaling and upregulates CD40 and CD86. This results in increased T cell responses, which might need to be unleashed by PD-1 blockade. (**D**) Inhibition of Axl signaling in cancer cells diminishes survival signals, EMT as well as impedes chemoresistance. It also induces upregulation of ICAM-1, ULBP1 and PD-L1, while it downregulates c-FLIP and survivin and thus enhances apoptosis.

Author Contributions: P.A., R.M.P., A.R. and P.t.S. wrote the manuscript. M.J.W.P. designed the figures. All authors have read and agreed to the published version of the manuscript.

Funding: This study was supported by the Danish Council for Independent Research (Grant No. DFF-1331-00095B), Danish Cancer Society (Grant No. R72-A4396-13-S2), The Danielsen Foundation, Dagmar Marshalls Fond, Else og Mogens Wedell-Wedellsborg Fond, AP Møller Fonden, Den Bøhmske Fond, KV foundation, Familien Erichsens Mindefond, Axel Muusfeldts Fond and the Danish Health Authority under "Empowering cancer immunotherapy in Denmark". P.A. received a partial PhD stipend from the Clinical Academic Group in Translational Hematology, part of Greater Copenhagen Health Science Partners, and likewise a partial PhD stipend from Dept. of Immunology and Microbiology, University of Copenhagen.

Conflicts of Interest: The authors declare no conflict of interest.

References

1. Lai, C.; Lemke, G. An extended family of protein-tyrosine kinase genes differentially expressed in the vertebrate nervous system. *Neuron* **1991**, *6*, 691–704. [CrossRef]
2. Lew, E.D.; Oh, J.; Burrola, P.G.; Lax, I.; Zagórska, A.; Través, P.G.; Schlessinger, J.; Lemke, G. Differential TAM Receptor—Ligand—Phospholipid Interactions Delimit Differential TAM Bioactivities. *eLife* **2014**, *3*, e03385. [CrossRef]
3. Rothlin, C.V.; Carrera-Silva, E.A.; Bosurgi, L.; Ghosh, S. TAM Receptor Signaling in Immune Homeostasis. *Annu. Rev. Immunol.* **2015**, *33*, 355–391. [CrossRef]
4. Graham, D.K.; DeRyckere, D.; Davies, K.D.; Earp, H.S. The TAM family: Phosphatidylserine-sensing receptor tyrosine kinases gone awry in cancer. *Nat. Rev. Cancer* **2014**, *14*, 769–785. [CrossRef]
5. Creagh, E.M.; O'Neill, L.A.J. TLRs, NLRs and RLRs: A trinity of pathogen sensors that co-operate in innate immunity. *Trends Immunol.* **2006**, *27*, 352–357. [CrossRef]
6. Rothlin, C.V.; Ghosh, S.; Zuniga, E.I.; Oldstone, M.B.; Lemke, G. TAM Receptors Are Pleiotropic Inhibitors of the Innate Immune Response. *Cell* **2007**, *131*, 1124–1136. [CrossRef]
7. Paolino, M.; Choidas, A.; Wallner, S.; Pranjic, B.; Uribesalgo, I.; Loeser, S.; Jamieson, A.M.; Langdon, W.Y.; Ikeda, F.; Fededa, J.P.; et al. The E3 ligase Cbl-b and TAM receptors regulate cancer metastasis via natural killer cells. *Nature* **2014**, *507*, 508–512. [CrossRef]
8. Silva, E.A.C.; Chan, P.Y.; Joannas, L.; Errasti, A.E.; Gagliani, N.; Bosurgi, L.; Jabbour, M.; Perry, A.; Smith-Chakmakova, F.; Mucida, D.; et al. T Cell-Derived Protein S Engages TAM Receptor Signaling in Dendritic Cells to Control the Magnitude of the Immune Response. *Immunity* **2013**, *39*, 160–170. [CrossRef]
9. Peeters, M.J.; Dulkeviciute, D.; Draghi, A.; Ritter, C.; Rahbech, A.; Skadborg, S.K.; Seremet, T.; Simões, A.M.C.; Martinenaite, E.; Halldórsdóttir, H.R.; et al. MERTK Acts as a Costimulatory Receptor on Human CD8+ T Cells. *Cancer Immunol. Res.* **2019**, *7*, 1472–1484. [CrossRef]

10. Linger, R.M.A.; Cohen, R.A.; Cummings, C.T.; Sather, S.; Migdall-Wilson, J.; Middleton, D.H.G.; Lu, X.; Barón, A.E.; Franklin, W.A.; Merrick, D.T.; et al. Mer or Axl receptor tyrosine kinase inhibition promotes apoptosis, blocks growth and enhances chemosensitivity of human non-small cell lung cancer. *Oncogene* **2013**, *32*, 3420–3431. [CrossRef]

11. Png, K.J.; Halberg, N.; Yoshida, M.; Tavazoie, S.F. A microRNA regulon that mediates endothelial recruitment and metastasis by cancer cells. *Nature* **2012**, *481*, 190–196. [CrossRef] [PubMed]

12. Bosurgi, L.; Bernink, J.H.; Cuevas, V.D.; Gagliani, N.; Joannas, L.; Schmid, E.T.; Booth, C.J.; Ghosh, S.; Rothlin, C.V. Paradoxical role of the proto-oncogene Axl and Mer receptor tyrosine kinases in colon cancer. *Proc. Natl. Acad. Sci. USA* **2013**, *110*, 13091–13096. [CrossRef]

13. Quinn, J.M.; Greenwade, M.M.; Palisoul, M.L.; Opara, G.; Massad, K.; Guo, L.; Zhao, P.; Beck-Noia, H.; Hagemann, I.S.; Hagemann, A.R.; et al. Therapeutic inhibition of the receptor tyrosine kinase AXL improves sensitivity to platinum and taxane in ovarian cancer. *Mol. Cancer Ther.* **2019**, *18*, 389–398. [CrossRef] [PubMed]

14. Tworkoski, K.; Singhal, G.; Szpakowski, S.; Zito, C.I.; Bacchiocchi, A.; Muthusamy, V.; Bosenberg, M.; Krauthammer, M.; Halaban, R.; Stern, D.F. Phosphoproteomic screen identifies potential therapeutic targets in melanoma. *Mol. Cancer Res.* **2011**, *9*, 801–812. [CrossRef] [PubMed]

15. Lee-Sherick, A.B.; Eisenman, K.M.; Sather, S.; McGranahan, A.; Armistead, P.M.; McGary, C.S.; Hunsucker, S.A.; Schlegel, J.; Martinson, H.; Cannon, C.; et al. Aberrant Mer receptor tyrosine kinase expression contributes to leukemogenesis in acute myeloid leukemia. *Oncogene* **2013**, *32*, 5359–5368. [CrossRef] [PubMed]

16. Ben-Batalla, I.; Schultze, A.; Wroblewski, M.; Erdmann, R.; Heuser, M.; Waizenegger, J.S.; Riecken, K.; Binder, M.; Schewe, D.; Sawall, S.; et al. Axl, a prognostic and therapeutic target in acute myeloid leukemia mediates paracrine crosstalk of leukemia cells with bone marrow stroma. *Blood* **2013**, *122*, 2443–2452. [CrossRef] [PubMed]

17. Amara, A.; Mercer, J. Viral apoptotic mimicry. *Nat. Rev. Microbiol.* **2015**, *13*, 461–469. [CrossRef] [PubMed]

18. Lemke, G.; Rothlin, C.V. Immunobiology of the TAM receptors. *Nat. Rev. Immunol.* **2008**, *8*, 327–336. [CrossRef]

19. Georgescu, M.-M.; Kirsch, K.H.; Shishido, T.; Zong, C.; Hanafusa, H. Biological Effects of c-Mer Receptor Tyrosine Kinase in Hematopoietic Cells Depend on the Grb2 Binding Site in the Receptor and Activation of NF-κB. *Mol. Cell. Biol.* **1999**, *19*, 1171–1181. [CrossRef] [PubMed]

20. Mahajan, N.P.; Whang, Y.E.; Mohler, J.L.; Earp, H.S. Activated tyrosine kinase Ack1 promotes prostate tumorigenesis: Role of Ack1 in polyubiquitination of tumor suppressor Wwox. *Cancer Res.* **2005**, *65*, 10514–10523. [CrossRef]

21. Rogers, A.E.J.; Le, J.P.; Sather, S.; Pernu, B.M.; Graham, D.K.; Pierce, A.M.; Keating, A.K. Mer receptor tyrosine kinase inhibition impedes glioblastoma multiforme migration and alters cellular morphology. *Oncogene* **2012**, *31*, 4171–4181. [CrossRef] [PubMed]

22. Tai, K.-Y.; Shieh, Y.-S.; Lee, C.-S.; Shiah, S.-G.; Wu, C.-W. Axl promotes cell invasion by inducing MMP-9 activity through activation of NF-κB and Brg-1. *Oncogene* **2008**, *27*, 4044–4055. [CrossRef]

23. Asiedu, M.K.; Beauchamp-Perez, F.D.; Ingle, J.N.; Behrens, M.D.; Radisky, D.C.; Knutson, K.L. AXL induces epithelial-to-mesenchymal transition and regulates the function of breast cancer stem cells. *Oncogene* **2014**, *33*, 1316–1324. [CrossRef] [PubMed]

24. Huelse, J.M.; Fridlyand, D.M.; Earp, S.; DeRyckere, D.; Graham, D.K. MERTK in cancer therapy: Targeting the receptor tyrosine kinase in tumor cells and the immune system. *Pharmacol. Ther.* **2020**, *213*, 107577. [CrossRef] [PubMed]

25. Graham, D.K.; Dawson, T.L.; Mullaney, D.L.; Snodgrass, H.R.; Earp, H.S. Cloning and mRNA expression analysis of a novel human protooncogene, c-mer. *Cell Growth Differ.* **1994**, *5*, 647–657. [PubMed]

26. Segawa, K.; Suzuki, J.; Nagata, S. Constitutive exposure of phosphatidylserine on viable cells. *Proc. Natl. Acad. Sci. USA* **2011**, *108*, 19246–19251. [CrossRef] [PubMed]

27. Lee-Sherick, A.B.; Zhang, W.; Menachof, K.K.; Hill, A.A.; Rinella, S.; Kirkpatrick, G.; Page, L.S.; Stashko, M.A.; Jordan, C.T.; Wei, Q.; et al. Efficacy of a Mer and Flt3 tyrosine kinase small molecule inhibitor, UNC1666, in acute myeloid leukemia. *Oncotarget* **2015**, *6*, 6722–6736. [CrossRef] [PubMed]

28. Minson, K.A.; Smith, C.C.; DeRyckere, D.; Libbrecht, C.; Lee-Sherick, A.B.; Huey, M.G.; Lasater, E.A.; Kirkpatrick, G.D.; Stashko, M.A.; Zhang, W.; et al. The MERTK/FLT3 inhibitor MRX-2843 overcomes resistance-conferring FLT3 mutations in acute myeloid leukemia. *JCI Insight* **2016**, *1*, e85630. [CrossRef]

29. DeRyckere, D.; Lee-Sherick, A.B.; Huey, M.G.; Hill, A.A.; Tyner, J.W.; Jacobsen, K.M.; Page, L.S.; Kirkpatrick, G.G.; Eryildiz, F.; Montgomery, S.A.; et al. UNC2025, a MERTK Small-Molecule Inhibitor, Is Therapeutically Effective Alone and in Combination with Methotrexate in Leukemia Models. *Clin. Cancer Res.* **2017**, *23*, 1481–1492. [CrossRef]

30. Sinik, L.; Minson, K.A.; Tentler, J.J.; Carrico, J.; Bagby, S.M.; Robinson, W.A.; Kami, R.; Burstyn-Cohen, T.; Eckhardt, S.G.; Wang, X.; et al. Inhibition of MERTK Promotes Suppression of Tumor Growth in BRAF Mutant and BRAF Wild-Type Melanoma. *Mol. Cancer Ther.* **2019**, *18*, 278–288. [CrossRef]

31. Kasikara, C.; Kumar, S.; Kimani, S.; Tsou, W.I.; Geng, K.; Davra, V.; Sriram, G.; Devoe, C.; Nguyen, K.Q.N.; Antes, A.; et al. Phosphatidylserine sensing by TAM receptors regulates AKT-dependent chemoresistance and PD-L1 expression. *Mol. Cancer Res.* **2017**, *15*, 753–764. [CrossRef] [PubMed]

32. Cabezón, R.; Carrera-Silva, E.A.; Flórez-Grau, G.; Errasti, A.E.; Calderón-Gómez, E.; Lozano, J.J.; España, C.; Ricart, E.; Panés, J.; Rothlin, C.V.; et al. MERTK as negative regulator of human T cell activation. *J. Leukoc. Biol.* **2015**, *97*, 751–760. [CrossRef]

33. Cook, R.S.; Jacobsen, K.M.; Wofford, A.M.; DeRyckere, D.; Stanford, J.; Prieto, A.L.; Redente, E.; Sandahl, M.; Hunter, D.M.; Strunk, K.E.; et al. MerTK inhibition in tumor leukocytes decreases tumor growth and metastasis. *J. Clin. Investig.* **2013**, *123*, 3231–3242. [CrossRef] [PubMed]

34. Tormoen, G.W.; Blair, T.C.; Bambina, S.; Kramer, G.; Baird, J.; Rahmani, R.; Holland, J.M.; McCarty, O.J.T.; Baine, M.J.; Verma, V.; et al. Targeting MerTK Enhances Adaptive Immune Responses after Radiation Therapy. *Int. J. Radiat. Oncol.* **2020**, *108*, 93–103. [CrossRef] [PubMed]

35. Shao, W.H.; Zhen, Y.; Finkelman, F.D.; Cohen, P.L. The Mertk receptor tyrosine kinase promotes T-B interaction stimulated by IgD B-cell receptor cross-linking. *J. Autoimmun.* **2014**, *53*, 78–84. [CrossRef]

36. Yokoyama, Y.; Lew, E.D.; Seelige, R.; Tindall, E.A.; Walsh, C.; Fagan, P.C.; Lee, J.Y.; Nevarez, R.; Oh, J.; Tucker, K.D.; et al. Immuno-oncological Efficacy of RXDX-106, a Novel TAM (TYRO3, AXL, MER) Family Small-Molecule Kinase Inhibitor. *Cancer Res.* **2019**, *79*, 1996–2008. [CrossRef]

37. Zhou, Y.; Fei, M.; Zhang, G.; Liang, W.C.; Lin, W.Y.; Wu, Y.; Piskol, R.; Ridgway, J.; McNamara, E.; Huang, H.; et al. Blockade of the Phagocytic Receptor MerTK on Tumor-Associated Macrophages Enhances P2X7R-Dependent STING Activation by Tumor-Derived cGAMP. *Immunity* **2020**, *52*, 357–373. [CrossRef]

38. Caetano, M.S.; Younes, A.I.; Barsoumian, H.B.; Quigley, M.; Menon, H.; Gao, C.; Spires, T.; Reilly, T.P.; Cadena, A.P.; Cushman, T.R.; et al. Triple therapy with MeRTK and PD1 inhibition plus radiotherapy promotes abscopal antitumor immune responses. *Clin. Cancer Res.* **2019**, *25*, 7576–7584. [CrossRef] [PubMed]

39. Kasikara, C.; Davra, V.; Calianese, D.; Geng, K.; Spires, T.E.; Quigley, M.; Wichroski, M.; Sriram, G.; Suarez-Lopez, L.; Yaffe, M.B.; et al. Pan-TAM tyrosine kinase inhibitor BMS-777607 Enhances Anti-PD-1 mAb efficacy in a murine model of triple-negative breast cancer. *Cancer Res.* **2019**, *79*, 2669–2683. [CrossRef] [PubMed]

40. Takeda, S.; Andreu-Agullo, C.; Sridhar, S.; Halberg, N.; Lorenz, I.C.; Tavazoie, S.; Kurth, I.; Tavazoie, M. *Abstract LB-277: Characterization of the Anti-Cancer and Immunologic Activity of RGX-019, a Novel Pre-Clinical Stage Humanized Monoclonal Antibody Targeting the MERTK Receptor;* Cancer Research; American Association for Cancer Research (AACR): Philadelphia, PA, USA, 2019.

41. Lee-Sherick, A.B.; Jacobsen, K.M.; Henry, C.J.; Huey, M.G.; Parker, R.E.; Page, L.S.; Hill, A.A.; Wang, X.; Frye, S.V.; Earp, H.S.; et al. MERTK inhibition alters the PD-1 axis and promotes anti-leukemia immunity. *JCI Insight* **2018**, *3*, 1–17. [CrossRef]

42. Su, Y.-T.; Butler, M.; Zhang, M.; Zhang, W.; Song, H.; Hwang, L.; Tran, A.D.; Bash, R.E.; Schorzman, A.N.; Pang, Y.; et al. MerTK inhibition decreases immune suppressive glioblastoma-associated macrophages and neoangiogenesis in glioblastoma microenvironment. *Neuro Oncol. Adv.* **2020**, *2*, 1–13. [CrossRef] [PubMed]

43. Holtzhausen, A.; Harris, W.; Ubil, E.; Hunter, D.M.; Zhao, J.; Zhang, Y.; Zhang, D.; Liu, Q.; Wang, X.; Graham, D.K.; et al. TAM family receptor kinase inhibition reverses MDSC-mediated suppression and augments anti—PD-1 therapy in melanoma. *Cancer Immunol. Res.* **2019**, *7*, 1672–1686. [CrossRef] [PubMed]

44. Du, W.; Huang, H.; Sorrelle, N.; Brekken, R.A. Sitravatinib potentiates immune checkpoint blockade in refractory cancer models. *JCI Insight* **2018**, *3*, e12184. [CrossRef]

45. Peeters, M.J.W.; Rahbech, A.; Straten, P.T. TAM-ing T cells in the tumor microenvironment: Implications for TAM receptor targeting. *Cancer Immunol. Immunother.* **2020**, *69*, 237–244. [CrossRef]

46. Graham, D.K.; Salzberg, D.B.; Kurtzberg, J.; Sather, S.; Matsushima, G.K.; Keating, A.K.; Liang, X.; Lovell, M.A.; Williams, S.A.; Dawson, T.L.; et al. Ectopic expression of the proto-oncogene Mer in pediatric T-cell acute lymphoblastic leukemia. *Clin. Cancer Res.* **2006**, *12*, 2662–2669. [CrossRef]

47. Behrens, E.M.; Gadue, P.; Gong, S.Y.; Garrett, S.; Stein, P.L.; Cohen, P.L. The mer receptor tyrosine kinase: Expression and function suggest a role in innate immunity. *Eur. J. Immunol.* **2003**, *33*, 2160–2167. [CrossRef]

48. Simon, S.; Labarriere, N. PD-1 expression on tumor-specific T cells: Friend or foe for immunotherapy? *Oncoimmunology* **2018**, *7*, 1–7. [CrossRef] [PubMed]

49. Nguyen, K.Q.N.; Tsou, W.I.; Calarese, D.A.; Kimani, S.G.; Singh, S.; Hsieh, S.; Liu, Y.; Lu, B.; Wu, Y.; Garforth, S.J.; et al. Overexpression of MERTK receptor tyrosine kinase in epithelial cancer cells drives efferocytosis in a gain-of-function capacity. *J. Biol. Chem.* **2014**, *289*, 25737–25749. [CrossRef]

50. O'Bryan, J.P.; Frye, R.A.; Cogswell, P.C.; Neubauer, A.; Kitch, B.; Prokop, C.; Espinosa, R.; Le Beau, M.M.; Earp, H.S.; Liu, E.T. Axl, a transforming gene isolated from primary human myeloid leukemia cells, encodes a novel receptor tyrosine kinase. *Mol. Cell. Biol.* **1991**, *11*, 5016–5031. [CrossRef]

51. Axelrod, H.; Pienta, K.J. Axl as a mediator of cellular growth and survival. *Oncotarget* **2014**, *5*, 8818–8852. [CrossRef]

52. Holland, S.J.; Pan, A.; Franci, C.; Hu, Y.; Chang, B.; Li, W.; Duan, M.; Torneros, A.; Yu, J.; Heckrodt, T.J.; et al. R428, a selective small molecule inhibitor of Axl kinase, blocks tumor spread and prolongs survival in models of metastatic breast cancer. *Cancer Res.* **2010**, *70*, 1544–1554. [CrossRef]

53. Gjerdrum, C.; Tiron, C.; Hoiby, T.; Stefansson, I.; Haugen, H.; Sandal, T.; Collett, K.; Li, S.; McCormack, E.; Gjertsen, B.T.; et al. Axl is an essential epithelial-to-mesenchymal transition-induced regulator of breast cancer metastasis and patient survival. *Proc. Natl. Acad. Sci. USA* **2010**, *107*, 1124–1129. [CrossRef]

54. He, L.; Lei, Y.; Hou, J.; Wu, J.; Lv, G. Implications of the Receptor Tyrosine Kinase Axl in Gastric Cancer Progression. *OncoTargets Ther.* **2020**, *13*, 5901–5911. [CrossRef] [PubMed]

55. Vuoriluoto, K.; Haugen, H.; Kiviluoto, S.; Mpindi, J.-P.; Nevo, J.; Gjerdrum, C.; Tiron, C.; Lorens, J.B.; Ivaska, J. Vimentin regulates EMT induction by Slug and oncogenic H-Ras and migration by governing Axl expression in breast cancer. *Oncogene* **2011**, *30*, 1436–1448. [CrossRef] [PubMed]

56. Cichoń, M.A.; Szentpetery, Z.; Caley, M.P.; Papadakis, E.S.; Mackenzie, I.C.; Brennan, C.H.; O'Toole, E.A. The receptor tyrosine kinase Axl regulates cell—Cell adhesion and stemness in cutaneous squamous cell carcinoma. *Oncogene* **2014**, *33*, 4185–4192. [CrossRef]

57. Maacha, S.; Hong, J.; von Lersner, A.; Zijlstra, A.; Belkhiri, A. AXL Mediates Esophageal Adenocarcinoma Cell Invasion through Regulation of Extracellular Acidification and Lysosome Trafficking. *Neoplasia* **2018**, *20*, 1008–1022. [CrossRef] [PubMed]
58. Antony, J.; Tan, T.Z.; Kelly, Z.; Low, J.; Choolani, M.; Recchi, C.; Gabra, H.; Thiery, J.P.; Huang, R.Y.-J. The GAS6-AXL signaling network is a mesenchymal (Mes) molecular subtype-specific therapeutic target for ovarian cancer. *Sci. Signal.* **2016**, *9*, ra97. [CrossRef] [PubMed]
59. Tian, M.; Chen, X.; Li, L.; Wu, H.; Zeng, D.; Wang, X.; Zhang, Y.; Xiao, S.; Cheng, Y. Inhibition of AXL enhances chemosensitivity of human ovarian cancer cells to cisplatin via decreasing glycolysis. *Acta Pharmacol. Sin.* **2020**, 1–10. [CrossRef]
60. Galluzzi, L.; Senovilla, L.; Vitale, I.; Michels, J.; Martins, I.; Kepp, O.; Castedo, M.; Kroemer, G. Molecular mechanisms of cisplatin resistance. *Oncogene* **2012**, *31*, 1869–1883. [CrossRef]
61. Keating, A.K.; Kim, G.K.; Jones, A.E.; Donson, A.M.; Ware, K.; Mulcahy, J.M.; Salzberg, D.B.; Foreman, N.K.; Liang, X.; Thorburn, A.; et al. Inhibition of Mer and Axl Receptor Tyrosine Kinases in Astrocytoma Cells Leads to Increased Apoptosis and Improved Chemosensitivity. *Mol. Cancer Ther.* **2010**, *9*, 1298–1307. [CrossRef]
62. Dumas, P.Y.; Naudin, C.; Martin-Lannerée, S.; Izac, B.; Casetti, L.; Mansier, O.; Rousseau, B.; Artus, A.; Dufossée, M.; Giese, A.; et al. Hematopoietic niche drives FLT3-ITD acute myeloid leukemia resistance to quizartinib via STAT5- And hypoxia-dependent upregulation of AXL. *Haematologica* **2019**, *104*, 2017–2027. [CrossRef]
63. Taniguchi, H.; Yamada, T.; Wang, R.; Tanimura, K.; Adachi, Y.; Nishiyama, A.; Tanimoto, A.; Takeuchi, S.; Araujo, L.H.; Boroni, M.; et al. AXL confers intrinsic resistance to osimertinib and advances the emergence of tolerant cells. *Nat. Commun.* **2019**, *10*, 259. [CrossRef]
64. Woo, S.M.; Min, K.J.; Seo, S.U.; Kim, S.; Kubatka, P.; Park, J.W.; Kwon, T.K. Axl inhibitor R428 enhances TRAIL-mediated apoptosis through downregulation of c-FLIP and survivin expression in renal carcinoma. *Int. J. Mol. Sci.* **2019**, *20*. [CrossRef]
65. Zhang, S.; Xu, X.S.; Yang, J.X.; Guo, J.H.; Chao, T.F.; Tong, Y. The prognostic role of Gas6/Axl axis in solid malignancies: A meta-analysis and literature review. *OncoTargets Ther.* **2018**, *11*, 509–519. [CrossRef] [PubMed]
66. Zagórska, A.; Través, P.G.; Lew, E.D.; Dransfield, I.; Lemke, G. Diversification of TAM receptor tyrosine kinase function. *Nat. Immunol.* **2014**, *15*, 920–928. [CrossRef]
67. Chen, F.; Song, Q.; Yu, Q. Axl inhibitor R428 induces apoptosis of cancer cells by blocking lysosomal acidification and recycling independent of Axl inhibition. *Am. J. Cancer Res.* **2018**, *8*, 1466–1482. [PubMed]
68. Lotsberg, M.L.; Wnuk-Lipinska, K.; Terry, S.; Tan, T.Z.; Lu, N.; Trachsel-Moncho, L.; Røsland, G.V.; Siraji, M.I.; Hellesøy, M.; Rayford, A.; et al. AXL Targeting Abrogates Autophagic Flux and Induces Immunogenic Cell Death in Drug-Resistant Cancer Cells. *J. Thorac. Oncol.* **2020**, *15*, 973–999. [CrossRef] [PubMed]
69. Lauter, M.; Weber, A.; Torka, R. Targeting of the AXL receptor tyrosine kinase by small molecule inhibitor leads to AXL cell surface accumulation by impairing the ubiquitin-dependent receptor degradation. *Cell Commun. Signal.* **2019**, *17*, 59. [CrossRef]
70. Scott, R.S.; McMahon, E.J.; Pop, S.M.; Reap, E.A.; Caricchio, R.; Cohen, P.L.; Earp, H.S.; Matsushima, G.K. Phagocytosis and clearance of apoptotic cells is mediated by MER. *Nature* **2001**, *411*, 207–211. [CrossRef] [PubMed]
71. Majai, G.; Sarang, Z.; Csomós, K.; Zahuczky, G.; Fésüs, L. PPARγ-dependent regulation of human macrophages in phagocytosis of apoptotic cells. *Eur. J. Immunol.* **2007**, *37*, 1343–1354. [CrossRef]
72. Seitz, H.M.; Camenisch, T.D.; Lemke, G.; Earp, H.S.; Matsushima, G.K. Macrophages and Dendritic Cells Use Different Axl/Mertk/Tyro3 Receptors in Clearance of Apoptotic Cells. *J. Immunol.* **2007**, *178*, 5635–5642. [CrossRef]
73. Myers, K.V.; Amend, S.R.; Pienta, K.J. Targeting Tyro3, Axl and MerTK (TAM receptors): Implications for macrophages in the tumor microenvironment. *Mol. Cancer* **2019**, *18*, 94. [CrossRef]
74. Yeh, H.-W.; Chiang, C.-F.; Chen, P.-H.; Su, C.-C.; Wu, Y.-C.; Chou, L.; Huang, R.-Y.; Liu, S.-Y.; Shieh, Y.-S. Axl Involved in Mineral Trioxide Aggregate Induces Macrophage Polarization. *J. Endod.* **2018**, *44*, 1542–1548. [CrossRef]
75. Ye, X.; Li, Y.; Stawicki, S.; Couto, S.; Eastham-Anderson, J.; Kallop, D.; Weimer, R.; Wu, Y.; Pei, L. An anti-Axl monoclonal antibody attenuates xenograft tumor growth and enhances the effect of multiple anticancer therapies. *Oncogene* **2010**, *29*, 5254–5264. [CrossRef] [PubMed]
76. Park, I.-K.; Giovenzana, C.; Hughes, T.L.; Yu, J.; Trotta, R.; Caligiuri, M.A. The Axl/Gas6 pathway is required for optimal cytokine signaling during human natural killer cell development. *Blood* **2009**, *113*, 2470–2477. [CrossRef]
77. Caraux, A.; Lu, Q.; Fernandez, N.; Riou, S.; Di Santo, J.P.; Raulet, D.H.; Lemke, G.; Roth, C. Natural killer cell differentiation driven by Tyro3 receptor tyrosine kinases. *Nat. Immunol.* **2006**, *7*, 747–754. [CrossRef] [PubMed]
78. Lee, A.J.; Mian, F.; Poznanski, S.M.; Stackaruk, M.; Chan, T.; Chew, M.V.; Ashkar, A.A. Type I interferon receptor on NK cells negatively regulates interferon-γ production. *Front. Immunol.* **2019**, *10*, 1–11. [CrossRef]
79. Terry, S.; Abdou, A.; Engelsen, A.S.T.; Buart, S.; Dessen, P.; Corgnac, S.; Collares, D.; Meurice, G.; Gausdal, G.; Baud, V.; et al. AXL targeting overcomes human lung cancer cell resistance to NK- And CTL-mediated cytotoxicity. *Cancer Immunol. Res.* **2019**, *7*, 1789–1802. [CrossRef] [PubMed]
80. Guo, Z.; Li, Y.; Zhang, D.; Ma, J. Axl inhibition induces the antitumor immune response which can be further potentiated by PD-1 blockade in the mouse cancer models. *Oncotarget* **2017**, *8*, 89761–89774. [CrossRef]
81. Chirino, L.M.; Kumar, S.; Okumura, M.; Sterner, D.E.; Mattern, M.; Butt, T.R.; Kambayashi, T. TAM receptors attenuate murine NK-cell responses via E3 ubiquitin ligase Cbl-b. *Eur. J. Immunol.* **2020**, *50*, 48–55. [CrossRef]
82. Ireland, L.; Luckett, T.; Schmid, M.C.; Mielgo, A. Blockade of Stromal Gas6 Alters Cancer Cell Plasticity, Activates NK Cells, and Inhibits Pancreatic Cancer Metastasis. *Front. Immunol.* **2020**, *11*, 1–16. [CrossRef] [PubMed]

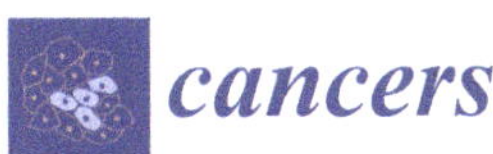

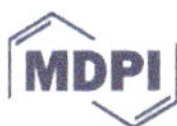

Review

Natural Killer Cells and Anti-Cancer Therapies: Reciprocal Effects on Immune Function and Therapeutic Response

Elisa C. Toffoli [1,†], Abdolkarim Sheikhi [1,2,†], Yannick D. Höppner [1], Pita de Kok [1], Mahsa Yazdanpanah-Samani [3], Jan Spanholtz [4], Henk M. W. Verheul [5], Hans J. van der Vliet [1,6] and Tanja D. de Gruijl [1,*]

[1]   Cancer Center Amsterdam, Department of Medical Oncology, Amsterdam UMC, Vrije Universiteit
        Amsterdam, De Boelelaan 1117, 1081 HV Amsterdam, The Netherlands; e.toffoli@amsterdamumc.nl (E.C.T.);
        sheikhi@queensu.ca (A.S.); yannick.hoeppner@bnitm.de (Y.D.H.); pitadk@outlook.com (P.d.K.);
        jj.vandervliet@amsterdamumc.nl (H.J.v.d.V.)
[2]   Department of Immunology, School of Medicine, Dezful University of Medical Sciences,
        Dezful 64616-43993, Iran
[3]   Department of Medical Biotechnology, School of Advanced Medical Sciences and Technologies, Shiraz
        University of Medical Sciences, Shiraz 71348-45794, Iran; myazdanpanah@sums.ac.ir
[4]   Glycostem, Kloosterstraat 9, 5349 AB Oss, The Netherlands; jan@glycostem.com
[5]   Department of Medical Oncology, Radboud Institute for Health Sciences, Radboud University Medical
        Center, Geert Grooteplein Zuid 10, 6525 GA Nijmegen, The Netherlands; Henk.Verheul@radboudumc.nl
[6]   Lava Therapeutics, Yalelaan 60, 3584 CM Utrecht, The Netherlands
*   Correspondence: td.degruijl@amsterdamumc.nl; Tel.: +31-20-4444063
†   These authors contributed equally to this paper.

Citation: Toffoli, E.C.; Sheikhi, A.; Höppner, Y.D.; de Kok, P.; Yazdanpanah-Samani, M.; Spanholtz, J.; Verheul, H.M.W.; van der Vliet, H.J.; de Gruijl, T.D. Natural Killer Cells and Anti-Cancer Therapies: Reciprocal Effects on Immune Function and Therapeutic Response. *Cancers* 2021, 13, 711. https://doi.org/10.3390/cancers 13040711

Academic Editor: Michael Kershaw
Received: 31 December 2020
Accepted: 6 February 2021
Published: 9 February 2021

Publisher's Note: MDPI stays neutral with regard to jurisdictional claims in published maps and institutional affiliations.

Simple Summary: Natural Killer (NK) cells are innate lymphocytes that play an important role in the immune response against cancer. Their activity is controlled by a balance of inhibitory and activating receptors, which in cancer can be skewed to favor their suppression in support of immune escape. It is therefore imperative to find ways to optimize their antitumor functionality. In this review, we explore and discuss how their activity influences, or even mediates, the efficacy of various anti-cancer therapies and, vice versa, how their activity can be affected by these therapies. Knowledge of the mechanisms underlying these observations could provide rationales for combining anti-cancer treatments with strategies enhancing NK cell function in order to improve their therapeutic efficacy.

Abstract: Natural Killer (NK) cells are innate immune cells with the unique ability to recognize and kill virus-infected and cancer cells without prior immune sensitization. Due to their expression of the Fc receptor CD16, effector NK cells can kill tumor cells through antibody-dependent cytotoxicity, making them relevant players in antibody-based cancer therapies. The role of NK cells in other approved and experimental anti-cancer therapies is more elusive. Here, we review the possible role of NK cells in the efficacy of various anti-tumor therapies, including radiotherapy, chemotherapy, and immunotherapy, as well as the impact of these therapies on NK cell function.

Keywords: NK cells; radiotherapy; local ablation therapies; checkpoint inhibitors; chemotherapy; protein kinase inhibitors; oncolytic virus; cancer; anti-cancer therapies

1. Introduction

Natural killer (NK) cells are large granular lymphocytes, part of the innate immune system, and are characterized by the expression of CD56, the absence of CD3 [1], and the ability to kill virus-infected and tumor cells without prior immune sensitization [2]. Classically, NK cells can be divided into two main subsets with distinct properties: the $CD56^{dim}$ effector NK cells with high cytotoxic capacity and the $CD56^{bright}$ NK cells, which exert mainly a regulatory function [3]. NK cell activity is controlled by a balance of inhibitory and activating receptors (Figure 1) [1]. Killer cell immunoglobulin-like receptors (KIR) and the natural killer receptor (NKG) 2A are examples of inhibitory receptors that are important to suppress non-specific cytotoxic activity and killing of healthy cells. They bind to multiple human leukocyte antigens (HLA), which can be downregulated by tumor and virus-infected cells to escape T cell recognition leading to increased NK cell recognition. In addition, NK cells can express other inhibitory receptors recognizing non-MHC molecules, such as the Lectin-like Transcript-1 (LLT-1), which binds to NKR-P1A. The activating receptors, such as natural killer group 2 member (NKG2)D/C/E, and natural cytotoxicity receptors (NCRs), such as NKp30, NKp46, and NKp44, recognize specific ligands, like MHC class I polypeptide–related sequence A/B (MICA/B), UL16 binding protein 1-6 (ULBP1-6), and heparan sulfate proteoglycan (HSPG), that are overexpressed by infected and malignant cells [1,2]. When the balance of these receptors is skewed towards activation, either due to a lack of inhibitory signals or the dominance of activating signals, NK cells are triggered to release cytotoxic granules and cytotoxic effector proteins like granzymes and perforin in order to kill the target cell [4,5]. NK cells can also induce apoptosis via Fas ligand and tumor necrosis factor (TNF)–related apoptosis-inducing ligand (TRAIL), which bind to the Fas receptor and the death receptor 5 (DR5) expressed on target cells [4]. Moreover, thanks to the expression of CD16 (Fc receptor: FcRγIII), NK cells can also kill through antibody-dependent cell-mediated cytotoxicity (ADCC) [6].

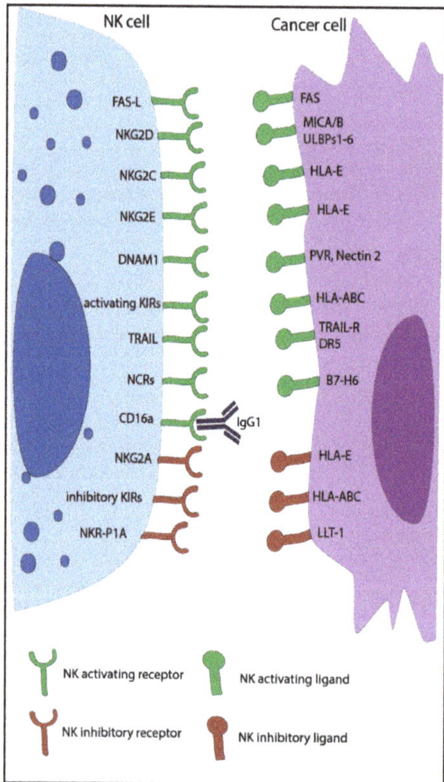

Figure 1. Overview of major natural killer (NK) cell activating and inhibitory receptors and their corresponding ligands expressed on tumor cells. KIR: killer cell immunoglobulin-like receptors; NKG: natural killer receptor; TRAIL: tumor necrosis factor-related apoptosis-inducing ligand; NCR: natural cytotoxicity receptors; HLA: human leukocyte antigen; MICA: MHC class I polypeptide–related sequence; PVR: poliovirus receptor; DR5: death receptor 5; DNAM1: DNAX Accessory Molecule-1, ULBP1-6: UL16 binding protein 1-6, LLT-1: lectin-like Transcript-1.

Cancer is a leading cause of death worldwide, and the number of new patients diagnosed with cancer is still rising globally [7]. In Europe, 20% of deaths are caused by cancer [8]. Although multiple therapeutic approaches are currently available, cancer remains a clinical challenge, and therefore new insights into this disease are necessary. NK cells are known to play a pivotal role in cancer. Patients with higher NK cell activity were found to have a better prognosis [9,10], and thanks to their ability to kill circulating cancer stem cells, which have high metastatic potential, NK cells play an essential role in the prevention of metastasis [11]. While the role of NK cells in monoclonal antibody-based therapies is well established [12], less is known on the function that NK cells have in other anti-cancer therapies. This review will focus on the effects that various anti-cancer therapies have on NK cells and the possible role that NK cells play in these therapies. An overview of clinical observations is presented in Supplementary Table S1.

2. Radiotherapy

Radiotherapy is an anti-cancer strategy based on the administration of ionizing radiation, which induces DNA damage and cell death, and that is currently included in more than 50% of all anti-cancer treatments [13,14]. Radiotherapy affects NK cells both directly and indirectly (Figure 2).

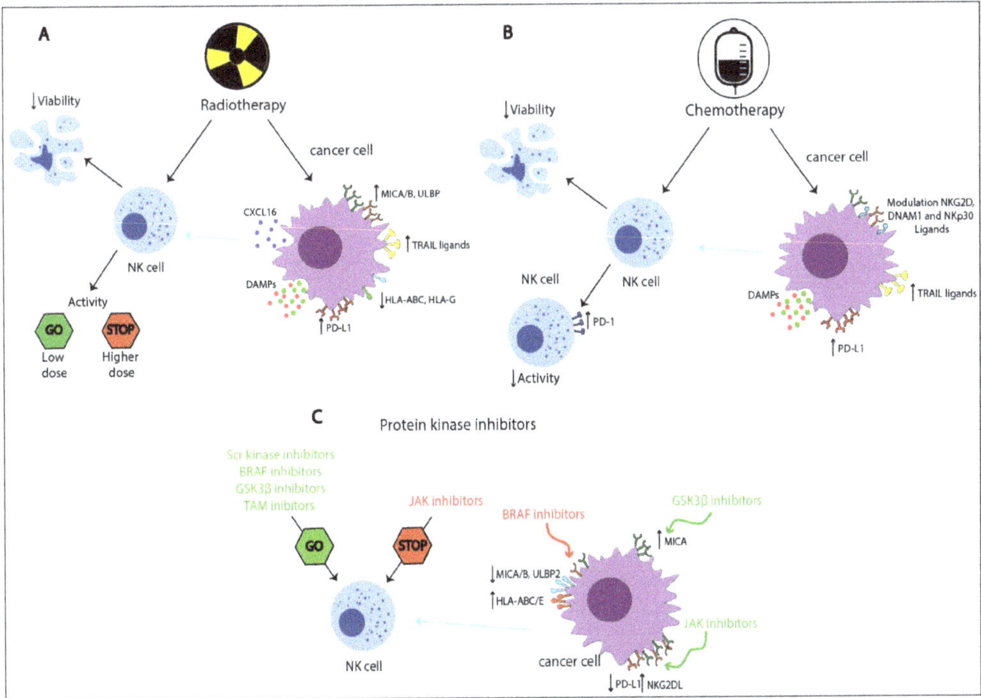

Figure 2. Direct and indirect effects of radiotherapy, chemotherapy, and protein kinase inhibitors on NK cell activity. Radiotherapy (**A**) and chemotherapy (**B**) cause cell damage, often leading to NK cell impairment, whereas protein kinase inhibitors (**C**) target specific signaling pathways resulting in either increased or decreased NK cell activity depending on the pathway involved. These treatments can also induce the modulation of various NK cell ligands on tumor cells and the release of damage-associated molecular patterns (DAMPs), indirectly affecting NK cell functions. Red arrows: inhibitory effects; green arrows: stimulatory effects; blue arrows: indirect effects, modulating the tumor cell's susceptibility to NK-mediated cytolysis. ULBP1-6: UL16 binding protein 1-6; MICA: MHC class I polypeptide–related sequence; TRAIL: tumor necrosis factor-related apoptosis-inducing ligand; HLA: human leukocyte antigen; PD-(L)1: programmed cell death protein (ligand) 1, NKG: natural killer receptor; NCR: natural cytotoxicity receptors; BRAF: B-rapidly accelerated fibrosarcoma; GSK-3β: Glycogen synthase kinase-3β; JAK: Janus kinase.

The viability of ex vivo irradiated NK cells from healthy donors was shown to be reduced, and this decrease was directly correlated with a higher single radiation dose and the length of the post-irradiation measurement interval [15–17]. For instance, the mean percentage of dead NK cells after the administration of 1 Gy ranged from 1.3% to 20.7% after 2 and 42 h, respectively, whereas at the same time points, a dose of 10 Gy induced the death of 2.7% to 67.5% NK cells [15]. At low radiation doses (<0.1 Gy), *ex vivo* irradiated NK cells from healthy donors actually demonstrated higher levels of cytotoxicity compared to non-irradiated NK cells. Moreover, higher expression of TNFα and interferon-γ (IFNγ) was observed. Interestingly, the addition of a specific P38 inhibitor hampered the positive effect of low dose radiation on NK cell cytotoxicity, suggesting that the p38-mitogen-activated protein kinase (MAPK) pathway might mediate this effect [18]. In another study, occasionally higher NK cell cytotoxicity was found when ex vivo NK cells from healthy donors were irradiated with a single dose between 1–10 Gy compared to non-irradiated cells [15]. In addition, the administration of a total dose of 10 Gy in two fractions was observed to enhance *ex vivo* healthy donor NK cell cytotoxicity compared to the non-fractionated dose [17]. In contrast, a reduction in cytotoxicity was reported when ex vivo isolated NK cells from healthy donors were treated with higher radiation doses (>20 Gy) [15,17].

Multiple studies focusing on patients with cancer undergoing radiotherapy also unveiled reductions in the absolute number of various peripheral blood (PB) lymphocyte subsets, including NK cells [19–25], and impaired NK cell activity compared to pre-treatment levels [26,27], suggesting that radiotherapy directly decreases both NK cell viability and function in a dose-dependent manner.

The indirect effects of radiotherapy on NK cells can be divided into three categories: the modulation of activating and inhibitory NK ligands, the release of damage-associated molecular patterns (DAMPs), and the enhancement of NK cell migration to the tumor. Upon radiotherapy, many cell types, including tumor cells, modulate the expression of NK cell ligands with a crucial impact on the sensitization to NK cell responses. Cancer cells from various solid tumor types were discovered to upregulate MICA/B and ULPB1–3 [28–31], whereas they downregulated the KIR2D ligands HLA-ABC and HLA-G [32–35], suggesting a higher sensitivity to NK cell-mediated cytotoxicity. Moreover, multiple irradiated cancer cell lines showed an increased expression of the intracellular adhesion molecule 1 (ICAM1), which was described to enhance NK cell-mediated killing by increasing cell-to-cell adhesion, and the Fas receptor, possibly indicating higher susceptibility to NK cell-mediated apoptosis [32,33,36]. Of note, also cancer stem cells (CSC), which represent a small radio-resistant population, were found not only to upregulate the Fas receptor in an irradiation dose-dependent manner but also to upregulate MICA/B, suggesting higher sensitization to NK cell killing [37]. On the other hand, other irradiated cancer cell lines demonstrated to be more resistant to NK cell cytotoxicity by the downregulation of MICA/B, ULPB 1–3, or the upregulation of HLA-ABC [33,38]. It is important to note that different tumor cell lines were used to analyze these effects and that the discrepancies in the responses could be due to cell line specific properties. Indeed, a study analyzing expression levels of various proteins related to NK cell sensitivity (e.g., of Fas, HLA-ABC) on human colon, lung, and prostate cancer cell lines upon irradiation found heterogeneous responses [33]. Moreover, variation in the expression of NKG2D ligands (NKG2D-L; e.g., MICA/B, ULBP1-3) might be due to the upregulation of matrix-bound metalloproteinases (MMPs) by cancer cells, which can shed NKG2D-L from the tumor cell surface leading to decreased membrane expression, consequently reducing NK cell recognition and activation [31].

Radiotherapy can also induce the release of DAMPs by tumor cells, such as heat shock proteins (Hsp), which are a family of stress-inducible factors with anti-apoptotic function regularly expressed by tumor cells [39]. Higher levels of Hsp70 are produced in response to cellular stress, which can be caused by radiotherapy [40,41]. In addition to the intracellular anti-apoptotic function, the release of Hps70, or its expression on the cell surface, can function as a DAMP triggering anti-tumor immune responses. In particular, membrane-bound Hsp70 (mHsp70) can elicit NK cell activation and tumor cell killing through binding to NKG2A/C/E and the co-receptor CD94 [42,43]. However, the expression of HLA-E by tumor cells can hinder this mechanism, significantly reducing Hsp70-dependent activation [44]. Radiotherapy and genotoxic stress can also induce the release of other DAMPs such as adenosine triphosphate (ATP), which can be bound and processed into adenosine (ADO) by multiple cells in the tumor microenvironment (TME) (e.g., tumor cells, regulatory T cells (Treg), and CD8[+] T cells) through their expression of CD39 and/or CD73. ADO is a highly immunosuppressive factor that impairs the function of multiple immune cells through the binding with its receptor, which is also expressed by NK cells [45,46].

Finally, radiotherapy enhanced NK cell migration to tumor cells in vitro. Multiple irradiated breast cancer cell lines were shown to increase their in vitro production of CXCL16, a CXCR6 ligand, leading to higher NK cell trans-well migration [47]. In conclusion, radiotherapy directly impaired NK cell viability and activity in a dose-dependent manner while modulating tumor cell sensitivity to NK cell-mediated cytotoxicity and the TME, potentially both promoting and impairing NK cell function, depending on dose and tumor heterogeneity, suggesting that combining radiotherapy with strategies to maintain NK cell viability and activity could be beneficial.

3. Local Ablation Therapies

Local ablation therapies are minimally invasive therapeutic approaches, whereby tumor cell death is caused by locally applied heat, cold, ultrasound, microwaves, irreversible electroporation, high-frequency electromagnetic currents, or chemicals. Here, we will focus on the effects of thermal ablation therapies on NK cells because, to our knowledge, the effects of other approaches on NK cells have not been investigated.

3.1. Radiofrequency Ablation

Radiofrequency ablation (RFA) is a technique based on alternating electromagnetic currents, which, by inducing ionic agitation, create local heat and, consequently, induce tumor necrosis [48,49]. RFA was found to positively affect NK cell frequency and activation. Multiple tumor-bearing animal models (i.e., mouse, rabbit, and rat) exhibited higher levels of peripheral blood (pb)NK cells after treatment with RFA [50,51]. Moreover, tumor-bearing rats treated with RFA had higher levels of intratumoral NK cells compared to untreated rats [52]. The effects of RFA on NK cell activation were studied in a rabbit model where higher *ex vivo* production of IFNγ and TNFα by NK cells was found after treatment as well as higher *ex vivo* cytotoxic activity compared to NK cells from non-treated rabbits, which was dependent on the expression of NKG2D [51].

In humans, no differences in pbNK cell percentages were measured after RFA compared to baseline in patients with renal cell carcinoma [53]. In contrast, patients with hepatocellular carcinoma (HCC) showed higher levels of pbNK cells after RFA treatment [54,55]. This increment was described to be mostly due to elevated levels of CD56[dim] pbNK cells, which were accompanied by increases in the expression of various NK cell-activating receptors (NKG2D, CD16, NKp30, and NKp46), a reduction in the expression of the inhibitory receptor NKG2A and higher in vitro NK cell cytotoxicity, ADCC, and IFNγ production compared to baseline, suggesting that RFA enhances NK cell activation. Interestingly, elevated levels of IFNγ release and NK cell cytotoxicity at 4 weeks after RFA were associated with longer disease-free survival [54]. However, in a cohort of 80 patients with HCC, a reduction in the percentage of NKp30[+] pbNK cells occurred one day after RFA treatment, which normalized after one month. In this study, higher frequency of NKp30[+] NK cells 1 day after RFA correlated to lower tumor recurrence, whereas a delayed increase of total NK cells and higher percentages of CD56[bright] NK cells at 1 month after RFA were associated with more tumor recurrence in patients with HCC [56], suggesting that NK cell dynamics play an important role in response to this therapy.

3.2. Microwave Ablation Therapy

Microwave ablation therapy (MWA) is a treatment whereby, similarly to RFA, electromagnetic energy is used to increase intratumoral temperature and, consequently, induce tumor necrosis. MWA is different as it uses frequencies $\geq$ 900 kHz, whereas this is lower for RFA treatments (400–500 kHz) [57]. The effects of MWA on NK cells have been studied in two mouse tumor models where higher levels of NK cells were found in PB as well as infiltrating in MWA-treated tumors. Moreover, MWA was shown to induce NK cell activation, which was dependent on intratumoral macrophage-derived interleukin(IL)-15. In the same study, NK cell depletion, but not $CD4^+$ or $CD8^+$ T cell depletion, significantly decreased overall survival and metastatic control, suggesting that NK cells played a pivotal role in response to MWA [58].

In humans, higher levels of tumor-infiltrating NK cells were described in patients with HCC treated with MWA. Interestingly, in this study, MWA also triggered (though to a lesser extent) NK cell infiltration in distant (non-MWA treated) lesions suggesting that the treatment could have induced an abscopal effect [59]. The frequency of pbNK cells has also been studied in patients with HCC, but no significant differences were shown before and after treatment [60]. In contrast, MWA-treated patients with early-stage breast cancer exhibited higher levels of pbNK cells compared to untreated controls [58]. NK cell activity has been studied in patients with prostate cancer (PC) treated with MWA, where higher levels of *ex vivo* NK cell cytotoxicity were described compared to baseline levels. Interestingly, MWA-treated patients with severely symptomatic benign prostatic hyperplasia exhibited no increases [61], suggesting that specifically tumor-related factors enhanced NK cell effector function. Finally, in patients with HCC or prostate cancer, higher *in vitro* NK cell cytotoxicity and intratumoral NK cell frequency after MWA treatment have both been correlated to therapeutic response [59,61], suggesting that in humans, NK cells also play an important role in response to this therapy.

3.3. High Intensity Focused Ultrasound Ablation

High intensity focused ultrasound ablation (HIFU) is a relatively new hyperthermia technique, whereby ultrasound waves induce the oscillation of water molecules to increase the intratumoral temperature ($\geq$60 °C) and consequently, induce cell damage [48]. HIFU therapy has been shown to be an effective treatment approach in multiple solid cancers (e.g., liver, breast, and pancreatic cancer) [62]. The frequency of pbNK cells after HIFU has been studied in patients with various solid malignancies and patients with uterine fibroids and exhibited no difference compared to pre-treatment levels [63,64]. However, higher levels of pbNK cells, assessed using an enzyme-linked immunosorbent assay, were observed after HIFU treatment in patients with primary liver cancer [65]. NK cell tumor infiltration after HIFU was studied in patients with breast cancer, where higher infiltration of $CD57^+$ cells was described after treatment [66]. However, CD57 can also be expressed by, e.g., senescent T cells, making this analysis non-specific for NK cells [67].

In conclusion, in animal models, both RFA and MWA seem to positively affect NK cell activity and frequency, both intratumorally and peripherally, whereas more discrepancies can be found in human studies, possibly due to differences in analyzed tumor types. The frequency of NK cells has also been studied after HIFU; however, the impact of this therapy on NK cells is less clear. Finally, NK cells seem to play a positive role in determining treatment response to both MWA and RFA. However, due to the small amount of available data, more studies are needed to further clarify and confirm these results.

4. Checkpoint Inhibitors

4.1. PD-1-PD-L1 Axis

Programmed cell death protein 1 (PD-1) and its ligand (PD-L1) are known for their role in controlling T cell activation, and multiple antibodies targeting this pathway are currently approved for clinical use [68]. Recent studies found that NK cells also play a pivotal part in determining the efficacy of these therapies in both a direct and indirect manner. PD-1$^+$ NK cells have been described in patients with multiple cancer types both in PB and, in higher percentages, in the TME [69–74]. Multiple studies using both mouse models and human NK cells showed that PD-1$^+$ NK cells became impaired upon binding to PD-L1 [70,71,73–75], whereas PD-1-PD-L1 blockade at least partially reversed this impairment [68,70,72,73] (Figure 3). Interestingly, it was found that PD-1-PD-L1 blockade could also indirectly influence NK cells by decreasing the expansion of PD-L1-induced Tregs, which could reduce both NK cell function and survival via the release of TGFβ and the seizing of IL-2 [73,76]. In multiple mouse models, NK cells played a key role in the efficacy of PD-1-PD-L1 blockade in both effector T cell-resistant (i.e., MHC-I^{lo}) tumors, where the effects of the therapies were NK cell-dependent, and T cell-sensitive tumors (MHC-I^{hi}), where the depletion of either CD8$^+$ T cells or NK cells led to similar increases in tumor growth suggesting that also in T cell sensitive tumors, NK cells play a role in the efficacy of PD-1-PD-L1 blockade [75]. In keeping with this notion, no response to PD-1 blockade was found after NK cell depletion in mice lacking T cells [72]. Enhanced *in vitro* NK cell-mediated ADCC was observed by applying the checkpoint inhibitor avelumab, an IgG1 monoclonal antibody (mAb) targeting PD-L1 [77,78]. NK cells also play an indirect role in the efficacy of PD-1-PD-L1 blockade. Via the production of chemokines (CCL5, XCL1) and the cytokine fms-related tyrosine kinase 3 ligand (FLT3-L), NK cells can enhance the migration and maintain the survival of type-1 conventional dendritic cells (DC), a rare CD141$^+$ DC population, which demonstrated to be particularly efficient in antigen cross-presentation and to be required for an effective anti-PD-1-response [79]. Moreover, high levels of IFNγ, produced also by activated NK cells, induced the expression of PD-L1 on tumor cells [73,76], which could sensitize PD-L1$^-$ tumor to PD-1-PD-L1 checkpoint inhibitor therapies.

Other anti-cancer therapies may be more effective when combined with PD-1-PD-L1 blockade, partially as a result of its activating effects on NK cells. For example, cetuximab-activated NK cells were found to express PD-1 and to induce the expression of PD-L1 on tumor cells upon IFNγ release [73]. Similarly, some chemotherapeutic agents induced PD-1 on NK cells, and higher expression levels of PD-L1 on tumor cells were described after exposure to both chemotherapy and radiotherapy, suggesting that combining these therapies with PD-1-PD-L1 blockade might enhance NK cell activity [38,80,81].

In conclusion, PD-1 is an important regulator of NK cell function, and its blockade was shown to enhance NK cell activity leading to increased tumor control. Moreover, NK cells were shown to play a role in response to PD-1-PD-L1 based therapies against tumors both sensitive and resistant to T cell-mediated cytotoxicity.

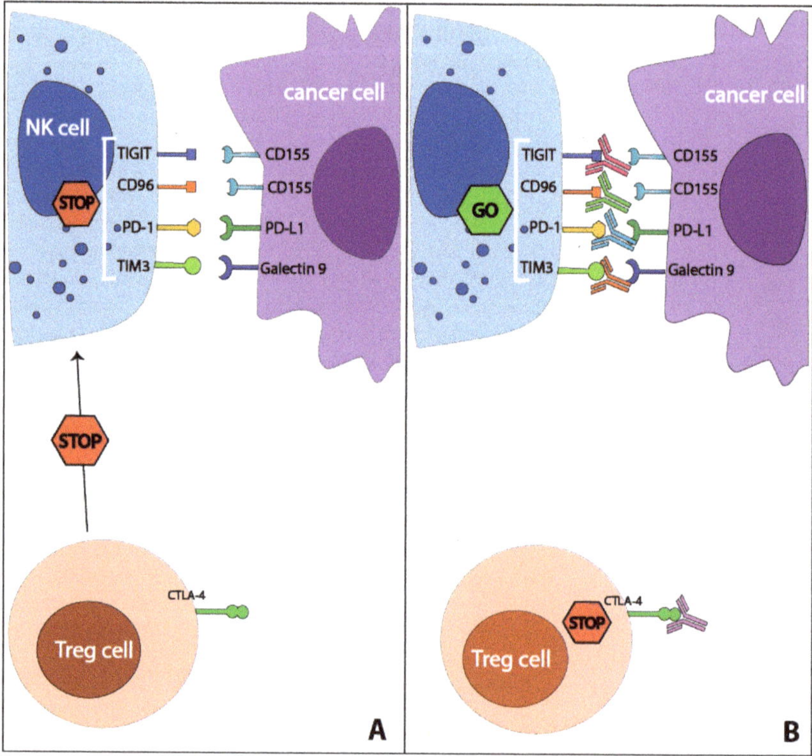

Figure 3. Effects of immune checkpoint inhibitor therapies on NK cells. NK cells can express various immune checkpoints such as PD-1, TIM3, TIGIT, CD96, which, upon binding to their ligands, impair NK cell function (**A**). Antibodies targeting these immune checkpoints were shown to restore NK cell activity (**B**). CTLA-4 is not expressed by human NK cells; however, anti-CTLA-4 therapy positively affects NK cell activity by reducing Treg-mediated suppression. A selection of immune checkpoint ligands is shown in the figure. TIGIT: T cell immunoglobulin and immunoreceptor tyrosine-based inhibitory motif domain; PD-(L)1: programmed cell death protein (ligand) 1; TIM3: T-cell immunoglobulin- and mucin-domain-containing molecule-3; CTLA-4: cytotoxic T-lymphocyte-associated protein 4.

4.2. CTLA-4

Cytotoxic T-lymphocyte-associated protein 4 (CTLA-4) is a T cell immune checkpoint receptor abundantly expressed by Tregs and, upon stimulation, by cytotoxic T cells. Antibodies targeting CTLA-4 are currently used as a therapy against multiple solid tumors [82–84]. Limited knowledge is available on the role of NK cells in CTLA-4-based therapies. Although it was shown that mouse NK cells could express membrane CTLA-4 upon stimulation with IL-2 [85], this has not been confirmed in humans [86]. In mice, anti-CTLA-4 was described to positively affect intratumoral NK cell frequency [87,88]. In humans, higher levels of intratumoral NK cells have been correlated with response to anti-CTLA-4 [89,90]. Moreover, in patients with malignant mesothelioma, a perturbation of the PB CD56bright/dim ratio was observed compared to healthy donors, which normalized in favor of the $CD56^{dim}$ effector NK cells after treatment with tremelimumab, an IgG2 anti-CTLA-4 mAb [91]. Interestingly, in patients with melanoma, lower levels of $CD56^{dim}$ NK cells were also found, which increased after treatment with ipilimumab, the first approved anti-CTLA-4 mAb [92]. These data suggest that CTLA-4 blockade influences NK cell dynamics. One factor that could play a role in these observations is the reduction of Tregs upon anti-CTLA-4 therapy, which can reduce Treg-mediated NK cell impairment and thereby increase NK cell activity [93] (Figure 3). A treatment-induced reduction of tumor load might also positively influence the frequency and function of NK cells. Finally, anti-CTLA-4 treatment could also stimulate NK cell ADCC. A recent study showed that in mice, anti-CTLA-4 antibodies can trigger NK cell activation and cytotoxicity against Tregs in an FcR-dependent matter [89]. However, ipilimumab, an IgG1 triggering CD16, induced ADCC against Tregs by monocytes and pro-inflammatory macrophages but not by intratumoral NK cells [93–95], whereas tremelimumab was shown to trigger ADCC by classical monocytes expressing CD32a, the main IgG2 receptor [96]. Nevertheless, it was shown that pbNK cells could induce a selective reduction of FOXp3[+] Treg when TILs, derived from patients with head and neck cancer, were co-cultured with isolated NK cells in the presence of ipilimumab [93]. Furthermore, ipilimumab induced ADCC by pbNK cells from healthy volunteers against CTLA-4[+] melanoma cells [97]. Of note, no NK cell-mediated ADCC was found against other CTLA-4[+] T cells [93,97], suggesting that other tumor-specific factors might play a role in the selectivity of this process. In conclusion, anti-CTLA-4 indirectly influenced NK cell activity, possibly through the (relative) reduction of Tregs and tumor load. Moreover, ipilimumab induced ADCC *in vitro* by pbNK but not by intratumoral NK cells, possibly due to differences in functionality.

4.3. TIM3

The immunoregulatory protein T-cell immunoglobulin- and mucin-domain-containing molecule-3 (TIM3) is an immune checkpoint receptor originally identified on T cells, which, upon binding with its cognate ligands (e.g., Galactin-9, phosphatidylserine,) inhibits T cell activity [68]. TIM3 has been described on pbNK cells both from healthy donors and, at higher levels, from patients with cancer and on intratumoral NK cells [74,98–101]. Purified TIM3[+] NK cells, both from HCC-bearing mice and patients with melanoma, were found to be functionally impaired against tumor cells expressing TIM3 ligands. In both cases, NK cell activity was restored with anti-TIM3 antibodies, which also led to enhanced NK cell proliferation [98,102] (Figure 3). These data were confirmed in two T-cell deficient murine models where anti-TIM3 antibody therapy led to prolonged overall survival and tumor control in an NK cell-dependent manner [102,103]. However, surprisingly, the production of IFNγ by TIM3[+] NK92 cells, a human NK cell line, was also found enhanced upon binding to its ligand galectin-9 [104]. Interestingly, NK cells exhibited TIM3 upregulation in response to different stimuli (e.g., various cytokines such as IL-2, IL-15, IL-12, IL-18, and antibody stimulation), but the *initial* priming factor responsible for the induction of TIM3 was described to primarily influence the function of TIM3[+] NK cells, possibly explaining some apparent discrepancies in the literature. For example, both IL-12/IL-18 and CD16-stimulation with IgG1 Fc multimers were shown to induce TIM3 expression on NK cells but solely the former led to enhanced IFNγ production [105]. In conclusion, TIM3 was able to regulate NK cell activity both positively and negatively, suggesting that other factors might differentially influence the functionality of NK cells through TIM3 induction. Clearly, detailed analysis is required to unravel these potentially opposing effects further.

4.4. TIGIT-CD96

TIGIT (T cell immunoglobulin and immunoreceptor tyrosine-based inhibitory motif domain) and CD96 are two inhibitory receptors that are expressed by NK cells and T cells and bind to the poliovirus receptor (PVR and CD155) and nectin (CD112), which are expressed by antigen-presenting cells and, upon cellular stress, by malignant and virus-infected cells [106,107]. These receptors are described in the same paragraph as they both bind the ligands of DNAX Accessory Molecule-1 (DNAM1), an NK cell activating receptor, thus potentially outcompeting its stimulatory effects. TIGIT[+] NK cells have been found in PBMC, both from healthy donors and patients with cancer [74,108,109] and in the TME [74,110]. It was shown *both in vitro* and *in vivo* that TIGIT could impair NK cell activity upon binding with its ligands and that NK cell function could be restored by blocking TIGIT [106,108,110,111] (Figure 3). The role of NK cells in TIGIT blockade-based therapies was analyzed in multiple mouse models where the efficacy of TIGIT blockade was dependent on both direct NK cell activation and on NK cell-dependent secondary T cell activation. Upon NK cell depletion, CD8$^+$ T cells expressed less CD107a, IFNγ, or TNFα, suggesting that NK cells support CD8$^+$ T cell function and/or prevent their exhaustion. Moreover, in NK cell-deficient mice, the therapeutic effect of TIGIT blockade was abolished even in the presence of TIGIT$^+$CD8$^+$ T cells, suggesting that, in this setting, NK cells support CD8$^+$ T cell function [110].

CD96$^+$ NK cells were found in PB of both healthy donors and patients with cancer and in the TME [109,112]. The effects of CD96 on NK cell activity were studied ex vivo using mouse NK cells wherein IFNγ production by NK cells was impaired in the presence of a stimulating CD155-Fc antibody construct, whereas the addition of an anti-CD96 mAb or the use of CD96$^{-/-}$ NK cells could reverse this effect (Figure 3). Moreover, CD96 had higher in vitro affinity for CD155 as compared to DNAM1/CD226, an NK cell activating receptor that recognizes the same ligands, suggesting that CD96 could hinder DNAM1-dependent NK cell activation [113]. The contribution of NK cells to the efficacy of CD96 blockade was studied in multiple mouse models, where an antagonistic anti-CD96 improved metastasis control in an NK cell and IFNγ dependent manner [107,112,114,115]. Interestingly, the effects of anti-CD96 were found to also be dependent on the presence of DNAM1, suggesting that CD96 is a critical regulator of DNAM1-dependent NK cell activation, likely through the aforementioned competition for binding to ligands [107,113,115]. Finally, in mice, the combination of anti-CD96 mAb with other immune checkpoint inhibitors (i.e., CTLA-4 and PD-1) or chemotherapy (e.g., doxorubicin and gemcitabine) demonstrated to be beneficial, suggesting a supportive role for CD96 blockade in combination with other anti-cancer therapies [107,114]. In line with the murine results, CD96$^+$ healthy donor NK cells showed lower levels of activation compared to CD96$^-$ NK cells. In the same study, CD96$^+$ NK cells were co-cultured with a CD155 expressing cell line, and higher levels of cytotoxicity were found in the presence of a CD96 blocking mAb [112], indicating that also in humans, CD96 could play an important role in the regulation of NK cell activity. In conclusion, both TIGIT and CD96 were demonstrated to negatively regulate NK cell activity, and preventing the binding of these receptors with their ligands could benefit NK cell-mediated anti-tumor functions.

4.5. LAG3

Lymphocyte activation gene-3 (LAG3) is an immune checkpoint receptor that has been described to be expressed on both activated T cells and NK cells [116]. However, yet little is known about its role on NK cells. In one human study, the presence of anti-LAG3 blocking mAbs or a recombinant soluble form of LAG3 did not influence LAG3$^+$ NK cell cytotoxicity against multiple tumor cell lines, suggesting that in humans, LAG3 may not have a major influence on NK cell activity [117].

In conclusion, multiple immune checkpoints contribute to the regulation of NK cell activity. PD-1, TIGIT, and CD96 can negatively affect NK cell function, and targeting these receptors with immune checkpoint inhibitors was found to enhance the anti-tumor response both in vitro and in vivo. In contrast, TIM3 was described to potentially both enhance and inhibit NK cell function, suggesting that other factors play a role in this pathway, urging the need for further studies. CTLA-4 blockade was observed to indirectly influence NK cells by reducing Treg and tumor-related immune suppression, but the potential ADCC effect by NK cells and its possible role in anti-CTLA-efficacy is still unclear. Finally, although LAG3 can be expressed by NK cells, its role on NK cell activity seems to be limited.

5. Chemotherapy

Experimental and clinical studies have shown that some chemotherapeutic agents may influence anti-cancer immune responses by directly modulating NK cell function [118–121]. Moreover, in response to cytotoxic agents, stressed or dying tumor cells up-regulate the expression of death receptors and different NK cell ligands on tumor cells and release DAMPs, which indirectly influence the immune response in the TME [118,119,122] Figure 2). Below different classes of chemotherapeutic agents, according to their mechanism of action, will be discussed in relation to their effects on NK cells and the possible involvement of NK cells in their efficacy.

5.1. Alkylating and Alkylating-Like Agents

Alkylating agents are chemotherapeutic drugs characterized by the ability to transfer alkyl-group to DNA bases leading to DNA damage and cell cycle arrest [123]. These compounds were shown to also directly affect NK cell function. In vitro, a reduction of NK cell cytotoxicity was reported upon exposure to chlorambucil [124]. Similarly, ifosfamide decreased in vitro NK cell activity in a dose-dependent manner through the reduction of intracellular glutathione [125–127]. Interestingly, cyclophosphamide indirectly enhanced ex vivo NK cell activity when administered in low doses in patients with end-stage cancer by inducing a selective depletion of Treg. However, this effect was lost when the dose of cyclophosphamide was increased, causing pan-lymphopenia [128].

Platinum drugs are chemotherapeutic agents that can form covalent bonds between the DNA and the platinum component, leading to DNA damage. These compounds are also known as alkylating-like agents due to the similarity in the mechanism of action [123]. Oxaliplatin and carboplatin had minimal impact on in vitro NK cell activity against the cell line K562 [124], whereas the exposure to single-dose oxaliplatin was observed to upregulate multiple NK cell-activating ligands (NKG2D, DNAM1, and TRAIL ligands) on ovarian cancer cells leading to increased NK cell-mediated lysis [129]. In contrast, no changes in the expression of NK cell ligands were found when multiple neuroblastoma and breast cancer cell lines were exposed to single-dose cisplatin [129,130]. It is noticeable that oxaliplatin, but not cisplatin, was shown to induce immunologic cell death, possibly explaining such apparent discrepancies [131]. Moreover, different responses to cisplatin have been described using other tumor cell lines, suggesting that the effects might also be dependent on the tumor cell type. For example, it was reported that single and repeated *in vitro* exposure of non-small cell lung cancer (NSCLC) cell lines to cisplatin lead to the upregulation of MICA/B through the regulation of ataxia-telangiectasia mutated (ATM), ataxia-telangiectasia, and Rad3-related (ATR) signaling pathways, as well as other NKG2D-L (ULBP1, ULBP2/5/6, ULBP3, and ULPB4), resulting in increased NK cell activity [132,133]. Similarly, HCC cell lines exhibited higher levels of ULBP2 upon exposure to low doses of cisplatin, which was also observed to enhance tumor control in HCC-bearing mice when combined with allogeneic NK cells [134]. In contrast, in patients with NSCLC, treated with more than two cycles of cisplatin-based chemotherapy followed by surgery, MICA/B and ULBP 2/3/4 were shown to be downregulated in 5/10 patients after treatment [133]. A possible explanation for this discrepancy is that the *in vivo* upregulation of these ligands by a subpopulation of tumor cells might have induced a selective NK cell response resulting in a general reduction in the expression. Cisplatin was also found to enhance the *in vitro* expression of B7-H6, a ligand of the activating NKp30 NK cell receptor, on tumor cells, making them more sensitive to NK cell lysis [135]. Finally, both alkylating and platinum agents were shown to induce the release of DAMPs, such as the high-mobility group box 1 protein (HMGB1), which can activate the innate immune system [131,136], and ATP, which, as mentioned, can be enzymatically converted to ADO leading to immune suppression [137].

5.2. Microtubule Targeting Agents

Microtubule targeting agents (MTAs) are a group of chemical compounds with the ability to interfere with the function of microtubules leading to cell death [138]. *In vitro*, multiple MTAs were described to substantially reduce NK cell cytotoxicity in a dose-dependent manner [124]. Similarly, patients with NSCLC treated with paclitaxel exhibited lower levels of *ex vivo* NK cell cytotoxicity [139]. These findings can be explained considering that NK cell activity was shown to be dependent on microtubule and microfilament integrity [140]. Moreover, a decrease in pbNK cells occurred in patients with various advanced cancers treated with docetaxel. Interestingly, this decrease was not shown in patients treated with paclitaxel alone [139,140] or in combination with carboplatin [141]. The reasons for this discrepancy are currently unclear and, as reductions in pbNK frequency were also observed following docetaxel treatment, this effect is probably not related to the chemotherapeutic class. MTAs were described to also influence NK cell activity indirectly. *In vitro*, cytochalasin D, nocodazole, and docetaxel induced the expression of several NKG2D and DNAM1 ligands on tumor cells leading to increased sensitivity to NK cell-mediated killing [142,143]. Interestingly, docetaxel enhanced NKG2D expression on NK cells in patients with breast cancer, suggesting a higher lytic ability [143].

5.3. Antimetabolites

Antimetabolites are small molecules related to nucleotide metabolites with the ability to interfere with DNA replication [123,144]. Multiple antimetabolite agents (e.g., methotrexate and fluorouracil) were described to have minimal or no effects on *in vitro* NK cell function except for the purine antagonist cladribine [124]. However, some antimetabolites indirectly affect NK cell function. Melphalan triggered the DNA damage response pathway of various multiple myeloma (MM) cell lines, which stimulated the *in vitro* up-regulation of MICA/B and PVR through the ATM-ATR pathway [145,146]. Also, 5- fluorouracil induced the *in vitro* expression of B7-H6 on tumor cells, making them more susceptible to NK cell killing [135].

5.4. Anthracyclines

Anthracyclines are a group of chemotherapeutic drugs extracted from Streptomyces species plural that function through multiple mechanisms of action, including interacting with the enzyme topoisomerase-II, interfering with DNA replication, and inducing the release of reactive oxygen species [147]. Daunorubicin, epirubicin, and doxorubicin were shown to have minimal effects on *in vitro* NK cell activity against K562 [124]. On the other hand, similarly to the antimetabolite melphalan, doxorubicin enhanced the *in vitro* expression of MICA/B and PVR on various MM cell lines through the ATM-ATR signaling [145,146]. In line with this, epirubicin induced higher levels of MICA/B, ULBP1/2, and Fas on breast cancer cell lines resulting in higher *in vitro* NK cell-mediated oncolysis [148]. In contrast, no changes in MICA/B were found on other tumor cell lines (renal cell carcinoma (RCC), melanoma, and bladder cancer) treated with doxorubicin. In this setting, higher levels of TRAIL and increased sensitivity to NK cell-mediated lysis were detected [149], suggesting differences in the NK cell response based on tumor type.

5.5. Other Anti-Cancer Agents

Histone deacetylases inhibitors (HDACi) are epigenetic regulators used for the treatment of hematological malignancies [150]. These agents demonstrated to inhibit NK cell activity. The *in vitro* exposure of NK cells to the HDACi valproic acid (VPA) and suberoylanilide hydroxamic acid decreased NK cell degranulation and cytotoxicity [151,152]. Moreover, in patients with cutaneous T-cell lymphoma treated with romidepsin, lower levels of K562-induced NK cell degranulation were observed compared to pretreatment levels [153]. HDACi were also found to modulate the expression of various ligands on the surface of tumor cells. In particular, HDACi upregulated NKG2D-L, such as MICA/B and ULBP1, on multiple tumor cell lines, both from hematological and solid tumors and on patient-derived acute myeloid leukemia (AML) cells, leading to increased sensitivity to NK cell-mediated cytotoxicity [154–157]. Similarly, VPA enhanced NK92-mediated tumor control in a pancreatic-mouse model by upregulating MICA/B [155]. HDACi were also shown to downregulate B7-H6 leading to the reduction of NK cell degranulation also against cell lines upregulating NKG2D-L in response to HDCAi, suggesting that this might limit NK cell response efficacy induced by HDACi [158]. Finally, various HDACi were described to induce the expression of TRAIL receptors on various malignant cell types [159–161].

Proteasome inhibitors are anti-cancer agents targeting the ubiquitin-proteasome pathway [162]. Bortezomib, a proteasome inhibitor approved for relapsed and refractory MM [162], was found to negatively impact NK cell activity *in vitro* in a dose-dependent manner [124]. Interestingly, at a low dose, bortezomib enhanced the expression of MICA/B on hepatocellular lines without negatively affecting NK cell activity [163]. Similar results were observed with MM cell lines and patient-derived malignant plasma cells in which higher levels of PVR and Nectin-2 upon *in vitro* exposure to low-dose bortezomib were found [145,164]. However, no changes in the expression of NKG2D-L have been described on other MM and various RCC cell lines cultured with low-dose bortezomib [165,166], suggesting differences in response to bortezomib. Finally, bortezomib enhanced the expression of DR5, a TRAIL ligand, on various tumor cells, increasing NK cell-mediated cytotoxicity [166–168].

5.6. Combination Therapies

Apart from single class effects, chemotherapeutic agents are often given in combination to maximize the anti-tumor effects. The effects of adjunctive chemotherapeutic treatments on pbNK cells frequency have been analyzed in various patient groups showing reductions in pbNK cell frequency after chemotherapy in patients with NSCLC (cisplatin/nedaplatin and pemetrexed), triple-negative breast cancer (epirubicin and cyclophosphamide), colorectal cancer (5-fluorouracil, oxaliplatin, and leucovorin) [169–171]. Combination therapies were also found to impact NK cell activity. Two studies analyzing the effects of chemotherapy (5-fluorouracil, cyclophosphamide combined with adriamycin or methotrexate) in patients with breast cancer reported a reduction in *ex vivo* NK cell-mediated cytotoxicity compared to pretreatment [172,173]. Similarly, a decline in NK cell activity was observed in patients with various stages of breast cancer treated with different chemotherapy regimens [174]. In contrast, a study analyzing patients with advanced ovarian cancer, treated with paclitaxel and carboplatin, found no change in NK cell activity after chemotherapy [141]. Interestingly, studies comparing different chemotherapy regimens in patients with cancer reported that the effects of the agents on NK cell frequency and activity differed based on both disease type and intensity of the therapy [174,175], possibly explaining the apparently conflicting reports on NK cell responses.

In conclusion, despite differences between the various chemotherapeutic agents, the exposure of NK cells to chemotherapy overall seems to reduce their activity while it increases the sensitivity of tumor cells to NK cell killing, suggesting that strategies to maintain NK cell activity during chemotherapy might be beneficial.

6. Protein Kinase Inhibitors

Protein kinase inhibitors are a group of agents that exert their function by blocking the activity of one or more protein kinases [176,177], enzymes that play a vital role in the regulation of important cellular pathways [178,179]. The dysregulation of protein kinases leads to multiple pathological conditions, including cancer [180–182]. Some protein kinase inhibitors have both a direct and indirect effect on NK cell activity (Figure 2).

6.1. Src-Kinase Inhibitors

Multiple protein tyrosine kinases of the Src-family were found to be involved in NK cell activity [183]. Dasatinib, a second-generation broad Src-kinase inhibitor used for the treatment of chronic myeloid leukemia (CML), reduced in vitro NK cell functions in a dose-dependent manner [184]. In contrast, NK cells isolated from patients with leukemia treated with dasatinib showed higher levels of ex vivo degranulation and cytotoxicity compared to either pretreatment measurement or untreated controls, suggesting differential effects of in vitro versus in vivo exposure [185,186]. Moreover, higher levels of ex vivo NK cytotoxicity were found in the patients with a complete cytogenetic response [186], which might be related to the eradication of the tumor and, consequently, of the tumor-related immune suppression. In contrast, findings on imatinib, another broad Src-kinase inhibitor approved for the treatment of various cancer types, are less clear. While one study described higher levels of *ex vivo* NK cell degranulation after 3 months of therapy [187], others found no changes in NK cell activity compared to either baseline or untreated controls both immediately after administration (2 h) and after long term therapy (median: 936 days; range: 28–2448) [185,186]. This discrepancy could, at least partially, be explained by the different time points at which NK cell activity was analyzed. Interestingly, in patients with CML treated for at least 3 years with imatinib and with a sustained molecular response, higher levels of effector NK cells at imatinib discontinuation correlated to better relapse-free survival, suggesting that NK cells have a role in tumor control after therapy discontinuation [188,189].

6.2. BRAF Inhibitors

As a part of the MAPK pathway, which regulates cell proliferation, survival, and metastasis [190], B-rapidly accelerated fibrosarcoma (BRAF)/MAPK has a significant role in cancer development [191]. Currently, there are three BRAF inhibitors (BRAFi) approved for clinical use in the treatment of advanced melanoma: vemurafenib, dabrafenib, and encorafenib [192,193]. The *in vitro* exposure to vemurafenib was shown to enhance ERK1/2 phosphorylation, CD69 expression and induce higher levels of IL-2 dependent IFNγ production in NK cells suggesting that BRAFi can directly enhance NK cell function. Moreover, in a mouse model, NK cells played a critical role in the antimetastatic function of vemurafenib in a perforin-dependent manner, which was enhanced by the combination with IL-2 [194]. In contrast, vemurafenib indirectly hampered NK cell activity by modulating the expression of various NK cell ligands on the surface of tumor cells. In particular, vemurafenib downregulated expression of the activating MICA and ULBP2 ligands while it upregulated expression of the inhibitory HLA-E and HLA-ABC receptors [195,196]. Interestingly, in melanoma cell lines, the downregulation of MICA and ULBP2/5/6 induced by vemurafenib was counterbalanced by the addition of HDACi, potent NKG2D ligand inducers, to the *in vitro* culture, leading to enhanced NK cell activity [196]. This suggests that the combination with HDACi could increase the efficacy of BRAFi in an NK cell-dependent manner. Finally, different melanoma cell lines with acquired resistance to vemurafenib and dabrafenib were described to modulate the expression of various NK cell ligands (e.g., MICA/B and HLA-ABC), resulting in higher sensitivity to NK cell lysis compared to the parental cell lines, suggesting patients gaining such resistance might benefit from strategies to enhance NK cell activity [197,198].

6.3. GSK-3β Inhibitors

Glycogen synthase kinase-3β (GSK-3β) is a Serine/Threonine kinase that plays a pivotal role in many cellular processes. Although multiple GSK-3β inhibitors are currently under preclinical and clinical evaluation, no compound has yet been approved for cancer treatment [199]. In NK cells, active GSK-3β has been associated with functional impairment and in line treatment with GSK-3β inhibitors increased in vitro cytotoxicity mediated by NK cells derived from both healthy donors and patients with cancer [200,201]. GSK-3β was shown to be inhibited via ERK or AKT signaling upon binding of NKG2D to its ligands, leading to activation of NK cells, confirming the negative regulatory role of GSK-3β in NK cell function [202]. Moreover, in MM cell lines treated with a GSK-3β inhibitor, higher expression levels of MICA were found, which was further augmented in combination with chemotherapeutics, and significantly improved NK cell cytotoxic activity through NKG2D recognition, suggesting that also indirect effects of GSK-3beta therapy can affect NK cell activity [203].

6.4. Other Protein Kinase Inhibitors

Sunitinib and sorafenib are two multi-target small-molecule tyrosine kinase inhibitors (TKI) used for the treatment of multiple cancers [192]. In vitro, exposure of NK cells to pharmacological levels of sorafenib, but not sunitinib, suppressed NK cell cytotoxicity and IFNγ production by reducing the levels of IL-2-induced ERK1/2 phosphorylation [204]. Interestingly, NK cell activity and ERK1/2 phosphorylation were enhanced when NK cells were exposed to a lower dose of sorafenib, indicating a dose-dependent effect [205]. Sunitinib and sorafenib indirectly enhanced *in vitro* NK cell activity against tumor cell lines by inducing the expression of NKG2D ligands on tumor cells through the noncanonical NF-κβ signaling pathway [206,207].

Janus kinase (JAK) and signal transducer and activator of transcription proteins (STATs) are part of a signaling pathway that mediates cellular response to cytokines and growth factors. This pathway was found to be critical for NK cell development and activation [208]. Ruxolitinib, the first JAK 1/2/(3) inhibitor approved for clinical use, was shown to directly inhibit NK cell function and maturation [209]. In contrast, other JAK inhibitors were found to indirectly enhance NK cell activity *in vitro* by impeding downregulation of NKG2D ligands and inducing upregulation of PD-L1 in NSCLC and PC cell lines, by IFNγ and IL-6 respectively, leading to enhanced NK cell-mediated killing [133,210]. It is currently unclear which of these contrasting effects prevails in vivo, thus determining the NK cell response.

Casitas B-lymphoma (Cbl)-b is an E3 protein ubiquitin-ligase expressed by all leukocytes that negatively regulate immune activation. Multiple drugs targeting one or more members of this family have currently been approved for clinical use for various cancer types (e.g., NSCLC, CML, and AML) [211]. On NK cells, Cbl-b was shown to target members of the TAM receptor family (Tyro3, Axl, and Mer), interfering with NK cell function [212]. In agreement with these findings, the administration of an experimental TAM inhibitor in multiple mouse tumor models led to the release of IFNγ and NK cell-dependent tumor control [213].

In conclusion, multiple protein kinases directly reduce NK cell activity, and the inhibition of these pathways through protein kinases inhibitors is mostly beneficial except for the JAK kinase inhibitors, which were shown to negatively impact NK cell functions. Moreover, several protein kinase inhibitors were observed to modulate the expression of various NK cell ligands on the surface of tumor cells, thus indirectly regulating NK cell activity.

7. Oncolytic Viruses

Oncolytic virus (OV) immunotherapy is a therapeutic approach that exploits native or genetically engineered viruses to selectively replicate in tumor cells leading to cell lysis and immune activation through the release of neoantigens, pathogen-associated molecular patterns, DAMPs, and various cytokines (e.g., type-I IFN, TNFα, IFNγ, and IL-12) [214,215]. Currently, multiple oncolytic viruses are under clinical evaluation. In 2005, the use of Oncorine, an engineered adenovirus, was approved in China for the treatment of nasopharyngeal carcinoma. Moreover, the FDA approved the use of Talimogene laherparepvec, an engineered oncolytic herpes simplex virus (oHSV), for the treatment of advanced melanoma [216]. Although to our knowledge, the role of NK cells in approved OV therapies has not been analyzed, in multiple experimental OV therapies, NK cells were described to play a dual role, both enhancing and limiting their therapeutic efficacy (Figure 4).

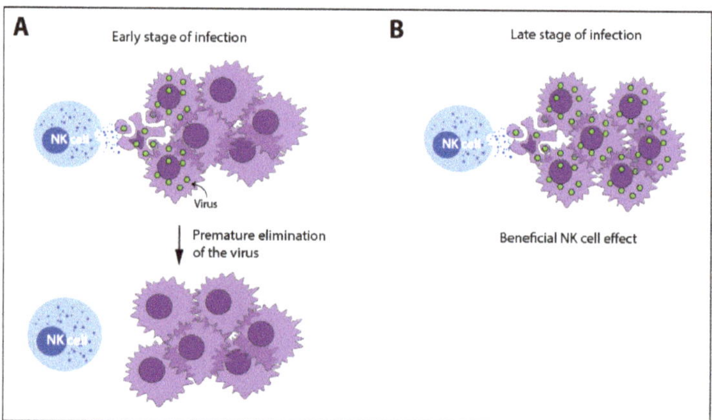

Figure 4. A dual role of NK cells in oncolytic virus therapies. Due to their ability to recognize and kill virus-infected cells, NK cells can cause a premature elimination of the virus, limiting its efficacy (**A**). However, thanks to this ability, NK cells can also enhance the clinical response by eliminating tumor cells in later stages of oncolytic virus (OV) therapy (**B**).

In support of the former, it was described that OVs enhance specific NK cell anti-tumor activity against various tumor cell lines. This increase was shown to be related to higher expression of NCR ligands or the downregulation of MHC-I [217–221]. In mice, multiple OVs induced mobilization, tumor recruitment, and activation of NK cells [222]. Moreover, in tumor bearing-mice, the treatment with an oHSV or an oncolytic Vesicular Stomatitis Virus (oVSV) was hampered when NK cells, or CD8[+] T cells, were depleted [223,224]. Interestingly, the preoperative administration of oncolytic parapoxvirus ovis could counteract surgery-induced suppression of NK cells, leading to higher metastatic control in tumor-bearing mice [225].

However, NK cells can also act as antagonists of OV therapy thanks to their ability to recognize virus-infected cells, which can often lead to the premature elimination of virus-infected tumor cell, thus interfering in the further viral spread and sequential waves of oncolysis, thus reducing the actual efficacy of this therapy [214]. In HCC-bearing rats treated with oVSV, NK cell depletion or strategies to hamper NK cell tumor-migration were found to increase OV efficacy [226]. Similarly, a novel oHSV, encoding E-cadherin, an adhesion molecule, and a ligand for killer cell lectin-like receptor G1, an inhibitory receptor expressed by NK and T cells, increased survival in glioblastoma-bearing mice by facilitating the cell-to-cell infection and preventing NK cell-mediated killing [227]. Moreover, in other glioblastoma-mouse models, it was shown that NK cell depletion or the combination with HDACi, which impaired NK cell anti-viral activity, enhanced the efficacy of oHSV [228,229]. In conclusion, NK cells exert both agonist and antagonistic effects in OV-based therapies. Interestingly, the ability of these therapies to enhance NK cell function might play a positive role when combined, with the appropriate timing, with other anti-cancer therapies that modulate NK cell activity and the TME. In line with this hypothesis, a study analyzing the optimal NK cell response dynamics during OV-bortezomib therapy showed that a temporary NK cell-depletion before virus therapy followed by NK cell adjuvant therapy administered after OV-bortezomib therapy might maximize the therapeutic benefits [230].

8. Conclusions

In this review, we have discussed how different anti-cancer therapies affect and are affected by NK cells. All considered treatments were found to impact NK cell function, while less is known on the contribution of NK cells to the efficacy of these treatments. Conventional anti-cancer therapies, such as radiotherapy and chemotherapy, which induce non-specific cell damage, were demonstrated to impact the viability and the function of both NK and tumor cells. The latter, upon genotoxic stress, was described to enhance the expression of NK cell ligands and to release DAMPs leading to both enhanced and impaired NK activity. Immune checkpoint and protein kinases inhibitors were mostly found to release NK cell activity by targeting specific receptors or pathways involved in dampening NK cell function. Moreover, protein kinase inhibitors also indirectly affected NK cells by modulating the expression of NK cell ligands on the surface of tumor cells. Results from animal studies suggest that NK cells contribute to the efficacy of some checkpoint inhibitors (i.e., PD-1-PD-L1, TIM3, TIGIT, and CD96) and protein kinase inhibitors (i.e., BRAFi). The findings on local ablation therapies are less clear due to the limited amount of available data and discrepancies in results. Therefore, no firm conclusions can be drawn. However, NK cell dynamics were correlated with efficacy in patients treated with MWA and RFA, suggesting that NK cells play a role in response to these treatments. Finally, NK cells were described to play a dual role in OV therapies, being activated by the therapy, on the one hand, thus contributing to tumor kill, but recognizing virus-infected cells, leading to the premature clearance of the OV, on the other hand. In mouse studies, NK cell depletion or strategies to hamper their function were both found to abolish and enhance the efficacy of OVs. In this setting, the timing of NK cell activation might be relevant in determining a more positive or negative effect. A better understanding of NK cell function in anti-cancer therapies could lead to a rationale for combining these treatments with strategies to modulate NK cell activity and thereby increase therapeutic efficacy. For example, bispecific antibodies or Fc-optimized mAb can represent useful strategies to enhance NK cell recognition and activation to specific targets [6]. Similarly, OVs might also induce specific NK cell effector function when combined, at the right time, with therapies that impair NK cell activity. NK cell allogeneic transfer could also represent a useful approach to increase NK cell numbers and tumor recognition, particularly in the setting of KIR or HLA mismatch [6]. The development of chimeric antigen receptor (CAR)-NK cells might further enhance the tumor specificity of allogeneic NK cells leading to promising future combination therapies. In conclusion, NK cells play a pivotal role against cancer and multiple anti-cancer therapies through various mechanisms have an impact on their function. The understanding of the underlying mechanisms opens opportunities to enhance NK cell activity and has the potential to increase the anti-cancer efficacy of these therapies.

Supplementary Materials: The following are available online at https://www.mdpi.com/2072-669 4/13/4/711/s1, Table S1: Clinical evaluations and studies included.

Author Contributions: Conceptualization and methodology: E.C.T., A.S., T.D.d.G., and H.J.v.d.V.; Investigation: E.C.T., A.S., Y.D.H., P.d.K., and M.Y.-S.; Writing—original draft preparation: E.C.T., A.S.; Writing—Review and Editing: E.C.T., A.S., T.D.d.G., H.J.v.d.V., J.S., and H.M.W.V.; Supervision: T.D.d.G., H.J.v.d.V., J.S., and H.M.W.V. All authors have read and agreed to the published version of the manuscript.

Funding: This work was supported by a research grant from Glycostem BV and a grant (DUMS-1397-3-19-1121) from the Dezful University of Medical Sciences.

Institutional Review Board Statement: Not applicable.

Informed Consent Statement: Not applicable.

Data Availability Statement: No new data were created or analyzed in this study. Data sharing is not applicable to this article.

Conflicts of Interest: J. Spanholtz is the chief scientific officer at Glycostem BV. H.J. van der Vliet is the chief scientific officer at Lava Therapeutics. We report no other conflict of interest.

References

1. Campbell, K.S.; Hasegawa, J. Natural killer cell biology: An update and future directions. *J. Allergy Clin. Immunol.* **2013**, *132*, 536–544. [CrossRef]

2. Vivier, E.; Tomasello, E.; Baratin, M.; Walzer, T.; Ugolini, S. Functions of natural killer cells. *Nat. Immunol.* **2008**, *9*, 503–510. [CrossRef]

3. Cooper, M.A.; Fehniger, T.A.; Caligiuri, M.A. The biology of human natural killer-cell subsets. *Trends Immunol.* **2001**, *22*, 633–640. [CrossRef]

4. Zamai, L.; Ahmad, M.; Bennett, I.M.; Azzoni, L.; Alnemri, E.S.; Perussia, B. Natural killer (NK) cell-mediated cytotoxicity: Differential use of TRAIL and Fas ligand by immature and mature primary human NK cells. *J. Exp. Med.* **1998**, *188*, 2375–2380. [CrossRef] [PubMed]

5. Lanier, L.L. Up on the tightrope: Natural killer cell activation and inhibition. *Nat. Immunol.* **2008**, *9*, 495–502. [CrossRef]

6. Veluchamy, J.P.; Kok, N.; van der Vliet, H.J.; Verheul, H.M.W.; de Gruijl, T.D.; Spanholtz, J. The rise of allogeneic Natural killer cells as a platform for cancer immunotherapy: Recent innovations and future developments. *Front. Immunol.* **2017**, *8*. [CrossRef] [PubMed]

7. WHO Key Statistics. Available online: https://www.who.int/cancer/resources/keyfacts/en/ (accessed on 30 October 2020).

8. WHO Europe Cancer. Available online: https://www.euro.who.int/en/health-topics/noncommunicable-diseases/cancer/cancer (accessed on 30 October 2020).

9. Takeuchi, H.; Maehara, Y.; Tokunaga, E.; Koga, T.; Kakeji, Y.; Sugimachi, K. Prognostic significance of natural killer cell activity in patients with gastric carcinoma: A multivariate analysis. *Am. J. Gastroenterol.* **2001**, *96*, 574–578. [CrossRef] [PubMed]

10. Tartter, P.I.; Steinberg, B.; Barron, D.M.; Martinelli, G. The Prognostic Significance of Natural Killer Cytotoxicity in Patients with Colorectal Cancer. *Arch. Surg.* **1987**, *122*, 1264–1268. [CrossRef]

11. Luna, J.I.; Grossenbacher, S.K.; Murphy, W.J.; Canter, R.J. Natural Killer Cell Immunotherapy Targeting Cancer Stem Cells. *Expert Opin. Biol. Ther.* **2018**, *17*, 313–324. [CrossRef]

12. Battella, S.; Cox, M.C.; Santoni, A.; Palmieri, G. Natural killer (NK) cells and anti-tumor therapeutic mAb: Unexplored interactions. *J. Leukoc. Biol.* **2016**, *99*, 87–96. [CrossRef]

13. Baskar, R.; Lee, K.A.; Yeo, R.; Yeoh, K.W. Cancer and radiation therapy: Current advances and future directions. *Int. J. Med. Sci.* **2012**, *9*, 193–199. [CrossRef] [PubMed]

14. Delaney, G.; Jacob, S.; Featherstone, C.; Barton, M. The role of Radiother in cancer treatment: Estimating optimal utilization from a review of evidence-based clinical guidelines. *Cancer* **2005**, *104*, 1129–1137. [CrossRef]

15. Hietanen, T.; Pitkänen, M.; Kapanen, M.; Kellokumpu-Lehtinen, P.L. Post-irradiation viability and cytotoxicity of natural killer cells isolated from human peripheral blood using different methods. *Int. J. Radiat. Biol.* **2016**, *92*, 71–79. [CrossRef] [PubMed]

16. Falcke, S.E.; Rühle, P.F.; Deloch, L.; Fietkau, R.; Frey, B.; Gaipl, U.S. Clinically relevant radiation exposure differentially impacts forms of cell death in human cells of the innate and adaptive immune system. *Int. J. Mol. Sci.* **2018**, *19*, 3574. [CrossRef]

17. Hietanen, T.; Pitkänen, M.; Kapanen, M.; Kellokumpu-Lehtinen, P.L. Effects of single and fractionated irradiation on natural killer cell populations: Radiobiological characteristics of viability and cytotoxicity in vitro. *Anticancer Res.* **2015**, *35*, 5193–5200.

18. Yang, G.; Kong, Q.; Wang, G.; Jin, H.; Zhou, L.; Yu, D.; Niu, C.; Han, W.; Li, W.; Cui, J. Low-dose ionizing radiation induces direct activation of natural killer cells and provides a novel approach for adoptive cellular immunotherapy. *Cancer Biother. Radiopharm.* **2014**, *29*. [CrossRef] [PubMed]

19. Eric, A.; Juranic, Z.; Tisma, N.; Plesinac, V.; Borojevic, N.; Jovanovic, D.; Milovanovic, Z.; Gavrilovic, D.; Ilic, B. Radiotherapy-induced changes of peripheral blood lymphocyte subpopulations in cervical cancer patients: Relationship to clinical response. *J. BUON* **2009**, *14*, 79–83. [PubMed]

20. Clave, E.; Socié, G.; Cosset, J.M.; Chaillet, M.P.; Tartour, E.; Girinsky, T.; Carosella, E.; Fridman, H.; Gluckman, E.; Mathiot, C. Multicolor flow cytometry analysis of blood cell subsets in patients given total body irradiation before bone marrow transplantation. *Int. J. Radiat. Oncol. Biol. Phys.* **1995**. [CrossRef]

21. Louagie, H.; van Eijkeren, M.; Philippe, J.; Thierens, H.; de Ridder, L. Changes in peripheral blood lymphocyte subsets in patients undergoing radiotherapy. *Int. J. Radiat. Biol.* **1999**, *75*, 767–771. [CrossRef]

22. Mozaffari, F.; Lindemalm, C.; Choudhury, A.; Granstam-Björneklett, H.; Helander, I.; Lekander, M.; Mikaelsson, E.; Nilsson, B.; Ojutkangas, M.L.; Österborg, A.; et al. NK-cell and T-cell functions in patients with breast cancer: Effects of surgery and adjuvant chemo- and radiotherapy. *Br. J. Cancer* **2007**, *97*, 105–111. [CrossRef] [PubMed]

23. Nakayama, Y.; Makino, S.; Fukuda, Y.; Ikemoto, T.; Shimizu, A. Varied Effects of Thoracic Irradiation on Peripheral Lymphocyte Subsets in Lung Cancer Patients. *Intern. Med.* **1995**. [CrossRef] [PubMed]

24. Belka, C.; Ottinger, H.; Kreuzfelder, E.; Weinmann, M.; Lindemann, M.; Lepple-Wienhues, A.; Budach, W.; Grosse-Wilde, H.; Bamberg, M. Impact of localized radiotherapy on blood immune cells counts and function in humans. *Radiother. Oncol.* **1999**. [CrossRef]

25. Domouchtsidou, A.; Barsegian, V.; Mueller, S.P.; Best, J.; Ertle, J.; Bedreli, S.; Horn, P.A.; Bockisch, A.; Lindemann, M. Impaired lymphocyte function in patients with hepatic malignancies after selective internal radiotherapy. *Cancer Immunol. Immunother.* **2018**. [CrossRef]

26. Yamaue, H.; Tanimura, H.; Aoki, Y.; Tsunoda, T.; Iwahashi, M.; Tani, M.; Tamai, M.; Noguchi, K.; Kashiwagi, H.; Sasaki, M.; et al. Clinical and immunological evaluation of intraoperative radiation therapy for patients with unresectable pancreatic cancer. *J. Surg. Oncol.* **1992**. [CrossRef]

27. Blomgren, H.; Baral, E.; Edsmyr, F.; Strender, L.E.; Petrini, B.; Wasserman, J. Natural killer activity in peripheral lymphocyte population following local radiation therapy. *Acta Radiol. Oncol. Radiat. Phys. Biol.* **1980**, *19*, 139–143. [CrossRef]

28. Kim, J.Y.; Son, Y.O.; Park, S.W.; Bae, J.H.; Joo, S.C.; Hyung, H.K.; Chung, B.S.; Kim, S.H.; Kang, C.D. Increase of NKG2D ligands and sensitivity to NK cell-mediated cytotoxicity of tumor cells by heat shock and ionizing radiation. *Exp. Mol. Med.* **2006**, *38*, 474–484. [CrossRef]
29. Fine, J.H.; Chen, P.; Mesci, A.; Allan, D.S.J.; Gasser, S.; Raulet, D.H.; Carlyle, J.R. Chemotherapy-induced genotoxic stress promotes sensitivity to natural killer cell cytotoxicity by enabling missing-self recognition. *Cancer Res.* **2010**, *70*, 7102–7113. [CrossRef]
30. Balaji, G.R.; Aguilar, O.A.; Tanaka, M.; Shingu-Vazquez, M.A.; Fu, Z.; Gully, B.S.; Lanier, L.L.; Carlyle, J.R.; Rossjohn, J.; Berry, R. Recognition of host Clr-b by the inhibitory NKR-P1B receptor provides a basis for missing-self recognition. *Nat. Commun.* **2018**, *9*. [CrossRef]
31. Heo, W.; Lee, Y.S.; Son, C.H.; Yang, K.; Park, Y.S.; Bae, J. Radiation-induced matrix metalloproteinases limit natural killer cell-mediated anticancer immunityin NCI-H23 lung cancer cells. *Mol. Med. Rep.* **2015**, 1800–1806. [CrossRef] [PubMed]
32. Kim, H.W.; Kim, J.E.; Hwang, M.H.; Jeon, Y.H.; Lee, S.W.; Lee, J.; Zeon, S.K.; Ahn, B.C. Enhancement of Natural Killer Cell Cytotoxicity by Sodium/Iodide Symporter Gene-Mediated Radioiodine Pretreatment in Breast Cancer Cells. *PLoS ONE* **2013**, *8*, e70194. [CrossRef] [PubMed]
33. Garnett, C.T.; Palena, C.; Chakarborty, M.; Tsang, K.Y.; Schlom, J.; Hodge, J.W. Sublethal irradiation of human tumor cells modulates phenotype resulting in enhanced killing by cytotoxic T lymphocytes. *Cancer Res.* **2004**, *64*, 7985–7994. [CrossRef]
34. Michelin, S.; Gallegos, C.E.; Dubner, D.; Favier, B.; Carosella, E.D. Ionizing radiation modulates the surface expression of human leukocyte antigen-G in a human melanoma cell line. *Hum. Immunol.* **2009**, *70*, 1010–1015. [CrossRef]
35. Urosevic, M.; Kempf, W.; Zagrodnik, B.; Panizzon, R.; Burg, G.; Dummer, R. HLA-G expression in basal cell carcinomas of the skin recurring after radiotherapy. *Clin. Exp. Derm.* **2005**, 422–425. [CrossRef]
36. Jeong, J.U.; Uong, T.N.T.; Chung, W.K.; Nam, T.K.; Ahn, S.J.; Song, J.Y.; Kim, S.K.; Shin, D.J.; Cho, E.; Kim, K.W.; et al. Effect of irradiation-induced intercellular adhesion molecule-1 expression on natural killer cell-mediated cytotoxicity toward human cancer cells. *Cytotherapy* **2018**, *20*, 715–727. [CrossRef] [PubMed]
37. Ames, E.; Canter, R.J.; Grossenbacher, S.K.; Mac, S.; Smith, R.C.; Monjazeb, A.M.; Chen, M.; Murphy, W.J. Enhanced targeting of stem-like solid tumor cells with radiation and natural killer cells. *OncoImmunology* **2015**, *4*, 1–11. [CrossRef] [PubMed]
38. Shen, M.J.; Xu, L.J.; Yang, L.; Tsai, Y.; Keng, P.C.; Chen, Y.; Lee, S.O.; Chen, Y. Radiation alters PD-L1/NKG2D ligand levels in lung cancer cells and leads to immune escape from NK cell cytotoxicity via IL-6- MEK/Erk signaling pathway. *Oncotarget* **2017**, *8*, 80506–80520. [CrossRef] [PubMed]
39. Multhoff, G.; Botzler, C.; Jennen, L.; Schmidt, J.; Ellwart, J.; Issels, R. Heat shock protein 72 on tumor cells: A recognition structure for natural killer cells. *J. Immunol.* **1997**, 4341–4350.
40. Multhoff, G.; Pockley, A.G.; Schmid, T.E.; Schilling, D. The role of heat shock protein 70 (Hsp70) in radiation-induced immunomodulation. *Cancer Lett.* **2015**, 179–184. [CrossRef]
41. Calini, V.; Urani, C.; Camatini, M. Overexpression of HSP70 is induced by ionizing radiation in C3H 10T1/2 cells and protects from DNA damage. *Toxicol. In Vitro* **2003**, *17*, 561–566. [CrossRef]
42. Gastpar, R.; Gross, C.; Rossbacher, L.; Ellwart, J.; Riegger, J.; Multhoff, G. The Cell Surface-Localized Heat Shock Protein 70 Epitope TKD Induces Migration and Cytolytic Activity Selectively in Human NK Cells. *J. Immunol.* **2004**. [CrossRef]
43. Multhoff, G.; Mizzen, L.; Winchester, C.C.; Milner, C.M.; Wenk, S.; Eissner, G.; Kampinga, H.H.; Laumbacher, B.; Johnson, J. Heat shock protein 70 (Hsp70) stimulates proliferation and cytolytic activity of natural killer cells. *Exp. Hematol.* **1999**, *27*, 1627–1636. [CrossRef]
44. Stangl, S.; Gross, C.; Pockley, A.G.; Asea, A.A.; Multhoff, G. Influence of Hsp70 and HLA-E on the killing of leukemic blasts by cytokine/Hsp70 peptide-activated human natural killer (NK) cells. *Cell Stress Chaperones* **2008**, *13*, 221–230. [CrossRef] [PubMed]
45. Vaupel, P.; Multhoff, G. Adenosine can thwart anti-tumor immune responses elicited by radiotherapy. *Strahlenther. Und Onkol.* **2016**, *192*, 279–287. [CrossRef]
46. Young, A.; Ngiow, S.F.; Gao, Y.; Patch, A.M.; Barkauskas, D.S.; Messaoudene, M.; Lin, G.; Coudert, J.D.; Stannard, K.A.; Zitvogel, L.; et al. A2AR adenosine signaling suppresses natural killer cell maturation in the tumor microenvironment. *Cancer Res.* **2018**, *78*, 1003–1016. [CrossRef]
47. Yoon, M.S.; Pham, C.T.; Phan, M.T.T.; Shin, D.J.; Jang, Y.Y.; Park, M.H.; Kim, S.K.; Kim, S.; Cho, D. Irradiation of breast cancer cells enhances CXCL16 ligand expression and induces the migration of natural killer cells expressing the CXCR6 receptor. *Cytotherapy* **2016**, *18*, 1532–1542. [CrossRef]
48. Thandassery, R.B.; Goenka, U.; Goenka, M.K. Role of Local Ablative Therapy for hepatocellular carcinoma. *J. Clin. Exp. Hepatol.* **2014**, *4*, S104–S111. [CrossRef] [PubMed]
49. Smith, S.L.; Jennings, P.E. Lung radiofrequency and microwave ablation: A review of indications, techniques and post-procedural imaging appearances. *Br. J. Radiol.* **2015**, *88*. [CrossRef]
50. Deng, Z.; Zhang, W.; Han, Y.; Zhang, S. Radiofrequency ablation inhibits lung metastasis ofbreast cancer in mice. *Zhonghua Zhong Liu Za Zhi* **2015**, *37*, 497–500. [PubMed]
51. Mo, Z.; Lu, H.; Mo, S.; Fu, X.; Chang, S.; Yue, J. Ultrasound-guided radiofrequency ablation enhances natural killer-mediated antitumor immunity against liver cancer. *Oncol. Lett.* **2018**, *15*, 7014–7020. [CrossRef]
52. Todorova, V.K.; Klimberg, V.S.; Hennings, L.; Kieber-Emmons, T.; Pashov, A. Immunomodulatory effects of radiofrequency ablation in a breast cancer model. *Immunol. Investig.* **2010**, *39*, 74–92. [CrossRef] [PubMed]

53. Matuszewski, M.; Michajłowski, J.; Michajłowski, I.; Ruckermann-Dizurdzińska, K.; Witkowski, J.M.; Biernat, W.; Krajka, K. Impact of radiofrequency ablation on PBMC subpopulation in patients with renal cell carcinoma. *Urol. Oncol. Semin. Orig. Investig.* **2011**, *29*, 724–730. [CrossRef] [PubMed]

54. Zerbini, A.; Pilli, M.; Laccabue, D.; Pelosi, G.; Molinari, A.; Negri, E.; Cerioni, S.; Fagnoni, F.; Soliani, P.; Ferrari, C.; et al. Radiofrequency Thermal Ablation for Hepatocellular Carcinoma Stimulates Autologous NK-Cell Response. *Gastroenterology* **2010**, *138*, 1931–1942.e2. [CrossRef] [PubMed]

55. Guan, H.T.; Wang, J.; Yang, M.; Song, L.; Tong, X.Q.; Zou, Y.H. Changes in immunological function after treatment with transarterial chemoembolization plus radiofrequency ablation in hepatocellular carcinoma patients. *Chin. Med. J.* **2013**, *126*, 3651–3655. [CrossRef]

56. Rochigneux, P.; Nault, J.C.; Mallet, F.; Chretien, A.S.; Barget, N.; Garcia, A.J.; del Pozo, L.; Bourcier, V.; Blaise, L.; Grando-Lemaire, V.; et al. Dynamic of systemic immunity and its impact on tumor recurrence after radiofrequency ablation of hepatocellular carcinoma. *OncoImmunology* **2019**, *8*, 1–11. [CrossRef]

57. Lencioni, R. Loco-regional treatment of hepatocellular carcinoma. *Hepatology* **2010**, *52*, 762–773. [CrossRef]

58. Yu, M.; Pan, H.; Che, N.; Li, L.; Wang, C.; Wang, Y.; Ma, G.; Qian, M.; Liu, J.; Zheng, M.; et al. Microwave ablation of primary breast cancer inhibits metastatic progression in model mice via activation of natural killer cells. *Cell. Mol. Immunol.* **2020**, 1–12. [CrossRef]

59. Dong, B.W.; Zhang, J.; Liang, P.; Yu, X.L.; Su, L.; Yu, D.J.; Ji, X.L.; Yu, G. Sequential pathological and immunologic analysis of percutaneous microwave coagulation therapy of hepatocellular carcinoma. *Int. J. Hyperth.* **2003**, *19*, 119–133. [CrossRef]

60. Zhang, H.; Hou, X.; Cai, H.; Zhuang, X. Effects of microwave ablation on T-cell subsets and cytokines of patients with hepatocellular carcinoma. *Minim. Invasive Allied Technol.* **2017**, *26*, 207–211. [CrossRef]

61. Szmigielski, S.; Sobczynski, J.; Sokolska, G.; Stawarz, B.; Zielinski, H.; Petrovich, Z. Effects of local prostatic hyperthermia on human NK and t cell function. *Int. J. Hyperth.* **1991**, *7*, 869–880. [CrossRef] [PubMed]

62. Zhang, L.; Wang, Z.B. High-intensity focused ultrasound tumor ablation: Review of ten years of clinical experience. *Front. Med. China* **2010**, *4*, 294–302. [CrossRef]

63. Wu, F.; Wang, Z.B.; Lu, P.; Xu, Z.L.; Chen, W.Z.; Zhu, H.; Jin, C.B. Activated anti-tumor immunity in cancer patients after high intensity focused ultrasound ablation. *Ultrasound Med. Biol.* **2004**, *30*, 1217–1222. [CrossRef] [PubMed]

64. Wang, X.; Qin, J.; Chen, J.; Wang, L.; Chen, W.; Tang, L. The effect of high-intensity focused ultrasound treatment on immune function in patients with uterine fibroids. *Int. J. Hyperth.* **2013**, *29*, 225–233. [CrossRef]

65. Ma, B.; Liu, X.; Yu, Z. The effect of high intensity focused ultrasound on the treatment of liver cancer and patients' immunity. *Cancer Biomark.* **2019**, *24*, 85–90. [CrossRef]

66. Lu, P.; Zhu, X.Q.; Xu, Z.L.; Zhou, Q.; Zhang, J.; Wu, F. Increased infiltration of activated tumor-infiltrating lymphocytes after high intensity focused ultrasound ablation of human breast cancer. *Surgery* **2009**, *145*, 286–293. [CrossRef] [PubMed]

67. Nielsen, C.M.; White, M.J.; Goodier, M.R.; Riley, E.M. Functional significance of CD57 expression on human NK cells and relevance to disease. *Front. Immunol.* **2013**, *4*, 422. [CrossRef]

68. Kim, N.; Kim, H.S. Targeting checkpoint receptors and molecules for therapeutic modulation of natural killer cells. *Front. Immunol.* **2018**, *9*, 2041. [CrossRef]

69. Niu, C.; Li, M.; Zhu, S.; Chen, Y.; Zhou, L.; Xu, D.; Xu, J.; Li, Z.; Li, W.; Cui, J. Pd-1-positive natural killer cells have a weaker antitumor function than that of pd-1-negative natural killer cells in lung cancer. *Int. J. Med. Sci.* **2020**, *17*, 1964–1973. [CrossRef]

70. Pesce, S.; Greppi, M.; Tabellini, G.; Rampinelli, F.; Parolini, S.; Olive, D.; Moretta, L.; Moretta, A.; Marcenaro, E. Identification of a subset of human natural killer cells expressing high levels of programmed death 1: A phenotypic and functional characterization. *J. Allergy Clin. Immunol.* **2017**, *139*, 335–346.e3. [CrossRef]

71. Tumino, N.; Martini, S.; Munari, E.; Scordamaglia, F.; Besi, F.; Mariotti, F.R.; Bogina, G.; Mingari, M.C.; Vacca, P.; Moretta, L. Presence of innate lymphoid cells in pleural effusions of primary and metastatic tumors: Functional analysis and expression of PD-1 receptor. *Int. J. Cancer* **2019**, *145*, 1660–1668. [CrossRef] [PubMed]

72. Liu, Y.; Cheng, Y.; Xu, Y.; Wang, Z.; Du, X.; Li, C.; Peng, J.; Gao, L.; Liang, X.; Ma, C. Increased expression of programmed cell death protein 1 on NK cells inhibits NK-cell-mediated anti-tumor function and indicates poor prognosis in digestive cancers. *Oncogene* **2017**, *36*, 6143–6153. [CrossRef]

73. Concha-Benavente, F.; Kansy, B.; Moskovitz, J.; Moy, J.; Chandran, U.; Ferris, R.L. PD-L1 Mediates Dysfunction in Activated PD-1+ NK Cells in Head and Neck Cancer Patients. *Cancer Immunol. Res.* **2018**, *6*, 1548–1560. [CrossRef]

74. Trefny, M.P.; Kaiser, M.; Stanczak, M.A.; Herzig, P.; Savic, S.; Wiese, M.; Lardinois, D.; Läubli, H.; Uhlenbrock, F.; Zippelius, A. PD-1+ natural killer cells in human non-small cell lung cancer can be activated by PD-1/PD-L1 blockade. *Cancer Immunol. Immunother.* **2020**, *69*, 1505–1517. [CrossRef]

75. Hsu, J.; Hodgins, J.J.; Marathe, M.; Nicolai, C.J.; Bourgeois-Daigneault, M.C.; Trevino, T.N.; Azimi, C.S.; Scheer, A.K.; Randolph, H.E.; Thompson, T.W.; et al. Contribution of NK cells to immunotherapy mediated by PD-1/PD-L1 blockade. *J. Clin. Investig.* **2018**, *128*, 4654–4668. [CrossRef] [PubMed]

76. Oyer, J.L.; Gitto, S.B.; Altomare, D.A.; Copik, A.J. PD-L1 blockade enhances anti-tumor efficacy of NK cells. *Oncoimmunology* **2018**, *7*. [CrossRef]

77. Juliá, E.P.; Amante, A.; Pampena, M.B.; Mordoh, J.; Levy, E.M. Avelumab, an IgG1 anti-PD-L1 immune checkpoint inhibitor, triggers NK cell-mediated cytotoxicity and cytokine production against triple negative breast cancer cells. *Front. Immunol.* **2018**, *9*. [CrossRef]

78. Boyerinas, B.; Jochems, C.; Fantini, M.; Heery, C.R.; Gulley, J.L.; Tsang, K.Y.; Schlom, J. Antibody-dependent cellular cytotoxicity activity of a Novel Anti-PD-L1 antibody avelumab (MSB0010718C) on human tumor cells. *Cancer Immunol. Res.* **2015**, *3*, 1148–1157. [CrossRef]

79. Barry, K.C.; Hsu, J.; Broz, M.L.; Cueto, F.J.; Binnewies, M.; Combes, A.J.; Nelson, A.E.; Loo, K.; Kumar, R.; Rosenblum, M.D.; et al. A natural killer–dendritic cell axis defines checkpoint therapy–responsive tumor microenvironments. *Nat. Med.* **2018**, *24*, 1178–1191. [CrossRef]

80. Deng, L.; Weichselbaum, R.R.; Fu, Y.; Deng, L.; Liang, H.; Burnette, B.; Beckett, M. Irradiation and anti—PD-L1 treatment synergistically promote antitumor immunity in mice Find the latest version: Irradiation and anti—PD-L1 treatment synergistically promote antitumor immunity in mice. *J. Clin. Investig.* **2014**, *124*, 687–695. [CrossRef]

81. Makowska, A.; Meier, S.; Shen, L.; Busson, P.; Baloche, V.; Kontny, U. Anti-PD-1 antibody increases NK cell cytotoxicity towards nasopharyngeal carcinoma cells in the context of chemotherapy-induced upregulation of PD-1 and PD-L1. *Cancer Immunol. Immunother.* **2020**. [CrossRef] [PubMed]

82. Cameron, F.; Whiteside, G.; Perry, C. Ipilimumab: First global approval. *Drugs* **2011**, *71*, 1093–1104. [CrossRef] [PubMed]

83. Patel, V.; Gandhi, H.; Upaganlawar, A. Ipilimumab: Melanoma and beyond. *J. Pharm. Bioallied Sci.* **2011**, *3*, 546.

84. Cabel, L.; Loir, E.; Gravis, G.; Lavaud, P.; Massard, C.; Albiges, L.; Baciarello, G.; Loriot, Y.; Fizazi, K. Long-term complete remission with Ipilimumab in metastatic castrate-resistant prostate cancer: Case report of two patients. *J. Immunother. Cancer* **2017**, *5*. [CrossRef]

85. Stojanovic, A.; Fiegler, N.; Brunner-Weinzierl, M.; Cerwenka, A. CTLA-4 Is Expressed by Activated Mouse NK Cells and Inhibits NK Cell IFN-γ Production in Response to Mature Dendritic Cells. *J. Immunol.* **2014**, *192*, 4184–4191. [CrossRef]

86. Lang, S.; Vujanovic, N.L.; Wollenberg, B.; Whiteside, T.L. Absence of B7.1-CD28/CTLA-4-mediated co-stimulation in human NK cells. *Eur. J. Immunol.* **1998**, *28*, 780–786. [CrossRef]

87. Hutmacher, C.; Nuñez, N.G.; Liuzzi, A.R.; Becher, B.; Neri, D. Targeted delivery of IL2 to the tumor stroma potentiates the action of immune checkpoint inhibitors by preferential activation of NK and CD8þ T cells. *Cancer Immunol. Res.* **2019**, *7*, 572–583. [CrossRef]

88. Kohlhapp, F.J.; Broucek, J.R.; Hughes, T.; Huelsmann, E.J.; Lusciks, J.; Zayas, J.P.; Dolubizno, H.; Fleetwood, V.A.; Grin, A.; Hill, G.E.; et al. NK cells and CD8+ T cells cooperate to improve therapeutic responses in melanoma treated with interleukin-2 (IL-2) and CTLA-4 blockade. *J. Immunother. Cancer* **2015**, *3*. [CrossRef]

89. Sanseviero, E.; Karras, J.R.; Shabaneh, T.B.; Arman, B.; Xu, W.; Zheng, C.; Yin, X.; Xu, X.; Karakousis, G.; Nam, B.T.; et al. Anti-CTLA4 activates intratumoral NK cells and combination with IL15/IL15Rα complexes enhances tumor control. *Cancer Immunol. Res.* **2020**, *7*, 1371–1380. [CrossRef]

90. Tallerico, R.; Cristiani, C.M.; Staaf, E.; Garofalo, C.; Sottile, R.; Capone, M.; de Coaña, Y.P.; Madonna, G.; Palella, E.; Wolodarski, M.; et al. IL-15, TIM-3 and NK cells subsets predict responsiveness to anti-CTLA-4 treatment in melanoma patients. *OncoImmunology* **2017**, *6*. [CrossRef]

91. Sottile, R.; Tannazi, M.; Johansson, M.H.; Cristiani, C.M.; Calabró, L.; Ventura, V.; Cutaia, O.; Chiarucci, C.; Covre, A.; Garofalo, C.; et al. NK- and T-cell subsets in malignant mesothelioma patients: Baseline pattern and changes in the context of anti-CTLA-4 therapy. *Int. J. Cancer* **2019**, *145*, 2238–2248. [CrossRef]

92. Tietze, J.K.; Angelova, D.; Heppt, M.V.; Ruzicka, T.; Berking, C. Low baseline levels of NK cells may predict a positive response to ipilimumab in melanoma therapy. *Exp. Derm.* **2017**, *26*, 622–629. [CrossRef] [PubMed]

93. Jie, H.B.; Schuler, P.J.; Lee, S.C.; Srivastava, R.M.; Argiris, A.; Ferrone, S.; Whiteside, T.L.; Ferris, R.L. CTLA-4+ regulatory t cells increased in cetuximab-treated head and neck cancer patients suppress nk cell cytotoxicity and correlate with poor prognosis. *Cancer Res.* **2015**, *75*, 2200–2210. [CrossRef] [PubMed]

94. Romano, E.; Kusio-Kobialka, M.; Foukas, P.G.; Baumgaertner, P.; Meyer, C.; Ballabeni, P.; Michielin, O.; Weide, B.; Romero, P.; Speiser, D.E. Ipilimumab-dependent cell-mediated cytotoxicity of regulatory T cells ex vivo by nonclassical monocytes in melanoma patients. *Proc. Natl. Acad. Sci. USA* **2015**. [CrossRef]

95. Simpson, T.R.; Li, F.; Montalvo-Ortiz, W.; Sepulveda, M.A.; Bergerhoff, K.; Arce, F.; Roddie, C.; Henry, J.Y.; Yagita, H.; Wolchok, J.D.; et al. Fc-dependent depletion of tumor-infiltrating regulatory t cells co-defines the efficacy of anti-CTLA-4 therapy against melanoma. *J. Exp. Med.* **2013**. [CrossRef]

96. Vargas, F.A.; Furness, A.J.S.; Litchfield, K.; Joshi, K.; Rosenthal, R.; Ghorani, E.; Solomon, I.; Lesko, M.H.; Ruef, N.; Roddie, C.; et al. Fc Effector Function Contributes to the Activity of Human Anti-CTLA-4 Antibodies. *Cancer Cell* **2018**, *33*, 649–663.e4. [CrossRef]

97. Laurent, S.; Queirolo, P.; Boero, S.; Salvi, S.; Piccioli, P.; Boccardo, S.; Minghelli, S.; Morabito, A.; Fontana, V.; Pietra, G.; et al. The engagement of CTLA-4 on primary melanoma cell lines induces antibody-dependent cellular cytotoxicity and TNF-α production. *J. Transl. Med.* **2013**, *11*, 1–13. [CrossRef]

98. Da Silva, I.P.; Gallois, A.; Jimenez-Baranda, S.; Khan, S.; Anderson, A.C.; Kuchroo, V.K.; Osman, I.; Bhardwaj, N. Reversal of NK-cell exhaustion in advanced melanoma by Tim-3 blockade. *Cancer Immunol. Res.* **2014**, *2*, 410–422. [CrossRef]

99. Komita, H.; Koido, S.; Hayashi, K.; Kan, S.; Ito, M.; Kamata, Y.; Suzuki, M.; Homma, S. Expression of immune checkpoint molecules of T cell immunoglobulin and mucin protein 3/galectin-9 for NK cell suppression in human gastrointestinal stromal tumors. *Oncol. Rep.* **2015**, *34*, 2099–2105. [CrossRef] [PubMed]

100. Xu, L.; Huang, Y.; Tan, L.; Yu, W.; Chen, D.; Lu, C.; He, J.; Wu, G.; Liu, X.; Zhang, Y. Increased Tim-3 expression in peripheral NK cells predicts a poorer prognosis and Tim-3 blockade improves NK cell-mediated cytotoxicity in human lung adenocarcinoma. *Int. Immunopharmacol.* **2015**, *29*, 635–641. [CrossRef]

101. Datar, I.; Sanmamed, M.F.; Wang, J.; Henick, B.S.; Choi, J.; Badri, T.; Dong, W.; Mani, N.; Toki, M.; Mejías, L.D.; et al. Expression analysis and significance of PD-1, LAG-3, and TIM-3 in human non-small cell lung cancer using spatially resolved and multiparametric single-cell analysis. *Clin. Cancer Res.* **2019**, *25*, 4663–4673. [CrossRef] [PubMed]

102. Tan, S.; Xu, Y.; Wang, Z.; Wang, T.; Du, X.; Song, X.; Guo, X.; Peng, J.; Zhang, J.; Liang, Y.; et al. Tim-3 hampers tumor surveillance of liver-resident and conventional NK cells by disrupting PI3K signaling. *Cancer Res.* **2020**, *80*, 1130–1142. [CrossRef]

103. Seo, H.; Kim, B.S.; Bae, E.A.; Min, B.S.; Han, Y.D.; Shin, S.J.; Kang, C.Y. IL21 therapy combined with PD-1 and Tim-3 blockade provides enhanced NK cell antitumor activity against MHC class I-deficient tumors. *Cancer Immunol. Res.* **2018**, *6*, 685–695. [CrossRef]

104. Gleason, M.K.; Lenvik, T.R.; McCullar, V.; Felices, M.; O'Brien, M.S.; Cooley, S.A.; Verneris, M.R.; Cichocki, F.; Holman, C.J.; Panoskaltsis-Mortari, A.; et al. Tim-3 is an inducible human natural killer cell receptor that enhances interferon gamma production in response to galectin-9. *Blood* **2012**, *119*, 3064–3072. [CrossRef] [PubMed]

105. So, E.C.; Khaladj-Ghom, A.; Ji, Y.; Amin, J.; Song, Y.; Burch, E.; Zhou, H.; Sun, H.; Chen, S.; Bentzen, S.; et al. NK cell expression of Tim-3: First impressions matter. *Immunobiology* **2019**, *224*, 362–370. [CrossRef] [PubMed]

106. Sarhan, D.; Cichocki, F.; Zhang, B.; Yingst, A.; Spellman, S.R.; Cooley, S.; Verneris, M.R.; Blazar, B.R.; Miller, J.S. Adaptive NK cells with low TIGIT expression are inherently resistant to myeloid-derived suppressor cells. *Cancer Res.* **2016**, *76*, 5696–5706. [CrossRef] [PubMed]

107. Blake, S.J.; Stannard, K.; Liu, J.; Allen, S.; Yong, M.C.R.; Mittal, D.; Aguilera, A.R.; Miles, J.J.; Lutzky, V.P.; de Andrade, L.F.; et al. Suppression of metastases using a new lymphocyte checkpoint target for cancer immunotherapy. *Cancer Discov.* **2016**, *6*, 446–459. [CrossRef]

108. Wang, F.; Hou, H.; Wu, S.; Tang, Q.; Liu, W.; Huang, M.; Yin, B.; Huang, J.; Mao, L.; Lu, Y.; et al. TIGIT expression levels on human NK cells correlate with functional heterogeneity among healthy individuals. *Eur. J. Immunol.* **2015**, *45*, 2886–2897. [CrossRef]

109. Peng, Y.P.; Xi, C.H.; Zhu, Y.; di Yin, L.; Wei, J.S.; Zhang, J.J.; Liu, X.C.; Guo, S.; Fu, Y.; Miao, Y. Altered expression of CD226 and CD96 on natural killer cells in patients with pancreatic cancer. *Oncotarget* **2016**, *7*, 66586–66594. [CrossRef]

110. Zhang, Q.; Bi, J.; Zheng, X.; Chen, Y.; Wang, H.; Wu, W.; Wang, Z.; Wu, Q.; Peng, H.; Wei, H.; et al. Blockade of the checkpoint receptor TIGIT prevents NK cell exhaustion and elicits potent anti-tumor immunity. *Nat. Immunol.* **2018**, *19*, 723–732. [CrossRef]

111. Stanietsky, N.; Simic, H.; Arapovic, J.; Toporik, A.; Levy, O.; Novik, A.; Levine, Z.; Beiman, M.; Dassa, L.; Achdout, H.; et al. The interaction of TIGIT with PVR and PVRL2 inhibits human NK cell cytotoxicity. *Proc. Natl. Acad. Sci. USA* **2009**, *106*, 17858–17863. [CrossRef]

112. Sun, H.; Huang, Q.; Huang, M.; Wen, H.; Lin, R.; Zheng, M.; Qu, K.; Li, K.; Wei, H.; Xiao, W.; et al. Human CD96 Correlates to Natural Killer Cell Exhaustion and Predicts the Prognosis of Human Hepatocellular Carcinoma. *Hepatology* **2019**, *70*. [CrossRef] [PubMed]

113. Chan, C.J.; Martinet, L.; Gilfillan, S.; Souza-Fonseca-Guimaraes, F.; Chow, M.T.; Town, L.; Ritchie, D.S.; Colonna, M.; Andrews, D.M.; Smyth, M.J. The receptors CD96 and CD226 oppose each other in the regulation of natural killer cell functions. *Nat. Immunol.* **2014**, *15*, 431–438. [CrossRef]

114. Brooks, J.; Fleischmann-Mundt, B.; Woller, N.; Niemann, J.; Ribback, S.; Peters, K.; Demir, I.E.; Armbrecht, N.; Ceyhan, G.O.; Manns, M.P.; et al. Perioperative, spatiotemporally coordinated activation of T and NK cells prevents recurrence of pancreatic cancer. *Cancer Res.* **2018**, *78*, 475–488. [CrossRef]

115. Roman Aguilera, A.; Lutzky, V.P.; Mittal, D.; Li, X.Y.; Stannard, K.; Takeda, K.; Bernhardt, G.; Teng, M.W.L.; Dougall, W.C.; Smyth, M.J. CD96 targeted antibodies need not block CD96-CD155 interactions to promote NK cell anti-metastatic activity. *OncoImmunology* **2018**, *7*. [CrossRef] [PubMed]

116. Baixeras, E.; Huard, B.; Miossec, C.; Jitsukawa, S.; Martin, M.; Hercend, T.; Auffray, C.; Triebel, F.; Piatier-Tonneau, D. Characterization of the Lymphocyte Activation Gene 3-Encoded Protein. A New Ligand for Human Leukocy Antigen Class H Antigens. *J. Exp. Med.* **1992**, *176*, 327–337. [CrossRef] [PubMed]

117. Huard, B.; Tournier, M.; Triebel, F. LAG-3 does not define a specific mode of natural killing in human. *Immunol. Lett.* **1998**, *61*, 109–112. [CrossRef]

118. Zingoni, A.; Fionda, C.; Borrelli, C.; Cippitelli, M.; Santoni, A.; Soriani, A. Natural Killer Cell Response to Chemotherapy-Stressed Cancer Cells: Role in Tumor Immunosurveillance. *Front. Immunol.* **2017**, *8*, 1194. [CrossRef] [PubMed]

119. Zitvogel, L.; Apetoh, L.; Ghiringhelli, F.; Kroemer, G. Immunological aspects of cancer chemotherapy. *Nat. Rev. Immunol.* **2008**, *8*, 59–73. [CrossRef] [PubMed]

120. Carson, W.E., 3rd; Shapiro, C.L.; Crespin, T.R.; Thornton, L.M.; Andersen, B.L. Cellular immunity in breast cancer patients completing taxane treatment. *Clin. Cancer Res.* **2004**, *10*, 3401–3409. [CrossRef] [PubMed]

121. Verma, C.; Kaewkangsadan, V.; Eremin, J.M.; Cowley, G.P.; Ilyas, M.; El-Sheemy, M.A.; Eremin, O. Natural killer (NK) cell profiles in blood and tumour in women with large and locally advanced breast cancer (LLABC) and their contribution to a

pathological complete response (PCR) in the tumour following neoadjuvant chemotherapy (NAC): Differential rest. *J. Transl. Med.* **2015**, *13*, 180. [CrossRef]

122. Krysko, D.V.; Garg, A.D.; Kaczmarek, A.; Krysko, O.; Agostinis, P.; Vandenabeele, P. Immunogenic cell death and DAMPs in cancer therapy. *Nat. Rev. Cancer* **2012**, *12*, 860–875. [CrossRef]

123. Swift, L.H.; Golsteyn, R.M. Genotoxic Anti-Cancer Agents and Their Relationship to DNA Damage, Mitosis, and Checkpoint Adaptation in Proliferating Cancer Cells. *Int. J. Mol. Sci.* **2014**, *15*, 3403–3431. [CrossRef]

124. Markasz, L.; Stuber, G.; Vanherberghen, B.; Flaberg, E.; Olah, E.; Carbone, E.; Eksborg, S.; Klein, E.; Skribek, H.; Szekely, L. Effect of frequently used chemotherapeutic drugs on the cytotoxic activity of human natural killer cells. *Mol. Cancer* **2007**, *6*, 644. [CrossRef]

125. Multhoff, G.; Meier, T.; Botzler, C.; Wiesnet, M.; Allenbacher, A.; Wilmanns, W.; Issels, R.D. Differential effects of ifosfamide on the capacity of cytotoxic T lymphocytes and natural killer cells to lyse their target cells correlate with intracellular glutathione levels. *Blood* **1995**, *85*, 2124–2131. [CrossRef]

126. Botzler, C.; Kis, K.; Issels, R.; Multhoff, G. A comparison of the effects of ifosfamide vs. mafosfamide treatment on intracellular glutathione levels and immunological functions of immunocompetent lymphocyte subsets. *Exp. Hematol.* **1997**, *25*, 338–344.

127. Kuppner, M.C.; Bleifuß, E.; Noessner, E.; Mocikat, R.; von Hesler, C.; Mayerhofer, C.; Issels, R.D. Differential effects of ifos-famide on dendritic cell-mediated stimulation of T cell interleukin-2 production, natural killer cell cytotoxicity and interferon-γ production. *Clin. Exp. Immunol.* **2008**, *153*, 429–438. [CrossRef]

128. Ghiringhelli, F.; Menard, C.; Puig, P.E.; Ladoire, S.; Roux, S.; Martin, F.; Solary, E.; le Cesne, A.; Zitvogel, L.; Chauffert, B. Metronomic cyclophosphamide regimen selectively depletes CD4+ CD25+ regulatory T cells and restores T and NK effector functions in end stage cancer patients. *Cancer Immunol. Immunother.* **2007**, *56*, 641–648. [CrossRef]

129. Siew, Y.Y.; Neo, S.Y.; Yew, H.C.; Lim, S.W.; Ng, Y.C.; Lew, S.M.; Seetoh, W.G.; Seow, S.V.; Koh, H.L. Oxaliplatin regulates expression of stress ligands in ovarian cancer cells and modulates their susceptibility to natural killer cell-mediated cytotoxicity. *Int. Immunol.* **2015**, *27*, 621–632. [CrossRef] [PubMed]

130. Veneziani, I.; Brandetti, E.; Ognibene, M.; Pezzolo, A.; Pistoia, V.; Cifaldi, L. Neuroblastoma cell lines are refractory to genotoxic drug-mediated induction of ligands for NK cell-activating receptors. *J. Immunol. Res.* **2018**, *2018*. [CrossRef] [PubMed]

131. Tesniere, A.; Schlemmer, F.; Boige, V.; Kepp, O.; Martins, I.; Ghiringhelli, F.; Aymeric, L.; Michaud, M.; Apetoh, L.; Barault, L.; et al. Immunogenic death of colon cancer cells treated with oxaliplatin. *Oncogene* **2010**, *29*, 482–491. [CrossRef] [PubMed]

132. Okita, R.; Yukawa, T.; Nojima, Y.; Maeda, A.; Saisho, S.; Shimizu, K.; Nakata, M. MHC class I chain-related molecule A and B expression is upregulated by cisplatin and associated with good prognosis in patients with non-small cell lung cancer. *Cancer Immunol. Immunother.* **2016**, *65*, 499–509. [CrossRef]

133. Okita, R.; Maeda, A.; Shimizu, K.; Nojima, Y.; Saisho, S.; Nakata, M. Effect of platinum-based chemotherapy on the expression of natural killer group 2 member D ligands, programmed cell death-1 ligand 1 and HLA class i in non-small cell lung cancer. *Oncol. Rep.* **2019**, *42*, 839–848. [CrossRef]

134. Shi, L.; Lin, H.; Li, G.; Sun, Y.; Shen, J.; Xu, J.; Lin, C.; Yeh, S.; Cai, X.; Chang, C. Cisplatin enhances NK cells immunotherapy efficacy to suppress HCC progression via altering the androgen receptor (AR)-ULBP2 signals. *Cancer Lett.* **2016**, *373*, 45–56. [CrossRef]

135. Cao, G.; Wang, J.; Zheng, X.; Wei, H.; Tian, Z.; Sun, R. Tumor Therapeutics Work as Stress Inducers to Enhance Tumor Sensitivity to Natural Killer (NK) Cell Cytolysis by Up-regulating NKp30 Ligand B7-H6. *J. Biol. Chem.* **2015**, *290*, 29964–29973. [CrossRef]

136. Guerriero, J.L.; Ditsworth, D.; Catanzaro, J.M.; Sabino, G.; Furie, M.B.; Kew, R.R.; Crawford, H.C.; Zong, W.-X. DNA Alkylating Therapy Induces Tumor Regression through an HMGB1-Mediated Activation of Innate Immunity. *J. Immunol.* **2011**, *186*, 3517–3526. [CrossRef] [PubMed]

137. Martins, I.; Tesniere, A.; Kepp, O.; Michaud, M.; Schlemmer, F.; Senovilla, L.; Séror, C.; Métivier, D.; Perfettini, J.-L.; Zitvogel, L.; et al. Chemotherapy induces ATP release from tumor cells. *Cell Cycle* **2009**, *8*, 3723–3728. [CrossRef] [PubMed]

138. Čermák, V.; Dostál, V.; Jelínek, M.; Libusová, L.; Kovář, J.; Rösel, D.; Brábek, J. Microtubule-targeting agents and their impact on cancer treatment. *Eur. J. Cell Biol.* **2020**, *99*, 151075. [CrossRef]

139. Sako, T.; Burioka, N.; Yasuda, K.; Tomita, K.; Miyata, M.; Kurai, J.; Chikumi, H.; Watanabe, M.; Suyama, H.; Fukuoka, Y.; et al. Cellular Immune Profile in Patients with Non-small Cell Lung Cancer after Weekly Paclitaxel Therapy. *Acta Oncol.* **2004**, *43*, 15–19. [CrossRef]

140. Tong, A.W.; Seamour, B.; Lawson, J.M.; Ordonez, G.; Vukelja, S.; Hyman, W.; Richards, D.; Stein, L.; Maples, P.B.; Nemunaitis, J. Cellular immune profile of patients with advanced cancer before and after taxane treatment. *Am. J. Clin. Oncol. Cancer Clin. Trials* **2000**, *23*, 463–472. [CrossRef]

141. Wu, X.; Feng, Q.M.; Wang, Y.; Shi, J.; Ge, H.I.; Di, W. The immunologic aspects in advanced ovarian cancer patients treated with paclitaxel and carboplatin chemotherapy. *Cancer Immunol. Immunother.* **2010**, *59*, 279–291. [CrossRef] [PubMed]

142. Acebes-Huerta, A.; Lorenzo-Herrero, S.; Folgueras, A.R.; Huergo-Zapico, L.; Lopez-Larrea, C.; López-Soto, A.; Gonzalez, S. Drug-induced hyperploidy stimulates an antitumor NK cell response mediated by NKG2D and DNAM-1 receptors. *OncoImmunology* **2016**, *5*. [CrossRef] [PubMed]

143. di Modica, M.; Sfondrini, L.; Regondi, V.; Varchetta, S.; Oliviero, B.; Mariani, G.; Bianchi, G.V.; Generali, D.; Balsari, A.; Triulzi, T.; et al. Taxanes enhance trastuzumab-mediated ADCC on tumor cells through NKG2D-mediated NK cell recognition. *Oncotarget* **2016**, *7*, 255–265. [CrossRef]

144. Luengo, A.; Gui, D.Y.; van der Heiden, M.G. Targeting Metabolism for Cancer Therapy. *Cell Chem. Biol.* **2017**, *24*, 1161–1180. [CrossRef]

145. Soriani, A.; Zingoni, A.; Cerboni, C.; Iannitto, M.L.; Ricciardi, M.R.; di Gialleonardo, V.; Cippitelli, M.; Fionda, C.; Petrucci, M.T.; Guarini, A.; et al. ATM-ATR–dependent up-regulation of DNAM-1 and NKG2D ligands on multiple myeloma cells by therapeutic agents results in enhanced NK-cell susceptibility and is associated with a senescent phenotype. *Blood* **2009**, *113*, 3503–3511. [CrossRef]

146. Soriani, A.; Iannitto, M.L.; Ricci, B.; Fionda, C.; Malgarini, G.; Morrone, S.; Peruzzi, G.; Ricciardi, M.R.; Petrucci, M.T.; Cippitelli, M.; et al. Reactive oxygen species–and DNA damage response–dependent NK cell activating ligand upregulation occurs at transcriptional levels and requires the transcriptional factor E2F1. *J. Immunol.* **2014**. [CrossRef] [PubMed]

147. Rayner, D.M.; Cutts, S.M. Anthracyclines. In *Side Effects of Drugs Annual*; Elsevier B.V.: Amsterdam, The Netherlands, 2014; Volume 36, pp. 683–694.

148. Feng, H.; Dong, Y.; Wu, J.; Qiao, Y.; Zhu, G.; Jin, H.; Cui, J.; Li, W.; Liu, Y.J.; Chen, J.; et al. Epirubicin pretreatment enhances NK cell-mediated cytotoxicity against breast cancer cells in vitro. *Am. J. Transl. Res.* **2016**, *8*, 473–484.

149. Wennerberg, E.; Sarhan, D.; Carlsten, M.; Kaminskyy, V.O.; D'Arcy, P.; Zhivotovsky, B.; Childs, R.; Lundqvist, A. Doxorubicin sensitizes human tumor cells to NK cell- and T-cell-mediated killing by augmented TRAIL receptor signaling. *Int. J. Cancer* **2013**, *133*, 1643–1652. [CrossRef] [PubMed]

150. Hull, E.E.; Montgomery, M.R.; Leyva, K.J. HDAC Inhibitors as Epigenetic Regulators of the Immune System: Impacts on Cancer Therapy and Inflammatory Diseases. *BioMed Res. Int.* **2016**, *2016*, 1–15. [CrossRef]

151. Ogbomo, H.; Michaelis, M.; Kreuter, J.; Doerr, H.W.; Cinatl, J. Histone deacetylase inhibitors suppress natural killer cell cytolytic activity. *Febs Lett.* **2007**, *581*, 1317–1322. [CrossRef]

152. Ni, L.; Wang, L.; Yao, C.; Ni, Z.; Liu, F.; Gong, C.; Zhu, X.; Yan, X.; Watowich, S.S.; Lee, D.A.; et al. The histone deacetylase inhibitor valproic acid inhibits NKG2D expression in natural killer cells through suppression of STAT3 and HDAC3. *Sci. Rep.* **2017**, *7*. [CrossRef] [PubMed]

153. Kelly-Sell, M.J.; Kim, Y.H.; Straus, S.; Benoit, B.; Harrison, C.; Sutherland, K.; Armstrong, R.; Weng, W.-K.; Showe, L.C.; Wysocka, M.; et al. The histone deacetylase inhibitor, romidepsin, suppresses cellular immune functions of cutaneous T-cell lymphoma patients. *Am. J. Hematol.* **2012**, *87*, 354–360. [CrossRef] [PubMed]

154. Armeanu, S.; Bitzer, M.; Lauer, U.M.; Venturelli, S.; Pathil, A.; Krusch, M.; Kaiser, S.; Jobst, J.; Smirnow, I.; Wagner, A.; et al. Natural killer cell-mediated lysis of hepatoma cells via specific induction of NKG2D ligands by the histone deacetylase inhibitor sodium valproate. *Cancer Res.* **2005**, *65*, 6321–6329. [CrossRef]

155. Shi, P.; Yin, T.; Zhou, F.; Cui, P.; Gou, S.; Wang, C. Valproic acid sensitizes pancreatic cancer cells to natural killer cell-mediated lysis by upregulating MICA and MICB via the PI3K/Akt signaling pathway. *BMC Cancer* **2014**, *14*. [CrossRef]

156. Diermayr, S.; Himmelreich, H.; Durovic, B.; Mathys-Schneeberger, A.; Siegler, U.; Langenkamp, U.; Hofsteenge, J.; Gratwohl, A.; Tichelli, A.; Paluszewska, M.; et al. NKG2D ligand expression in AML increases in response to HDAC inhibitor valproic acid and contributes to allorecognition by NK-cell lines with single KIR-HLA class I specificities. *Blood* **2008**, *111*, 1428–1436. [CrossRef] [PubMed]

157. Kato, N.; Tanaka, J.; Sugita, J.; Toubai, T.; Miura, Y.; Ibata, M.; Syono, Y.; Ota, S.; Kondo, T.; Asaka, M.; et al. Regulation of the expression of MHC class I-related chain A, B (MICA, MICB) via chromatin remodeling and its impact on the susceptibility of leukemic cells to the cytotoxicity of NKG2D-expressing cells. *Leukemia* **2007**, *21*, 2103–2108. [CrossRef]

158. Fiegler, N.; Textor, S.; Arnold, A.; Rölle, A.; Oehme, I.; Breuhahn, K.; Moldenhauer, G.; Witzens-Harig, M.; Cerwenka, A. Downregulation of the activating NKp30 ligand B7-H6 by HDAC inhibitors impairs tumor cell recognition by NK cells. *Blood* **2013**, *122*, 684–693. [CrossRef]

159. Nakata, S.; Yoshida, T.; Horinaka, M.; Shiraishi, T.; Wakada, M.; Sakai, T. Histone deacetylase inhibitors upregulate death receptor 5/TRAIL-R2 and sensitize apoptosis induced by TRAIL/APO2-L in human malignant tumor cells. *Oncogene* **2004**, *23*, 6261–6271. [CrossRef] [PubMed]

160. Kim, Y.-H. Sodium butyrate sensitizes TRAIL-mediated apoptosis by induction of transcription from the DR5 gene promoter through Sp1 sites in colon cancer cells. *Carcinogenesis* **2004**, *25*, 1813–1820. [CrossRef] [PubMed]

161. Insinga, A.; Monestiroli, S.; Ronzoni, S.; Gelmetti, V.; Marchesi, F.; Viale, A.; Altucci, L.; Nervi, C.; Minucci, S.; Pelicci, P.G. Inhibitors of histone deacetylases induce tumor-selective apoptosis through activation of the death receptor pathway. *Nat. Med.* **2005**, *11*, 71–76. [CrossRef] [PubMed]

162. Manasanch, E.E.; Orlowski, R.Z. Proteasome Inhibitors in Cancer Therapy HHS Public Access. *Nat. Rev. Clin. Oncol.* **2017**, *14*, 417–433. [CrossRef]

163. Armeanu, S.; Krusch, M.; Baltz, K.M.; Weiss, T.S.; Smirnow, I.; Steinle, A.; Lauer, U.M.; Bitzer, M.; Salih, H.R. Direct and natural killer cell-mediated antitumor effects of low-dose bortezomib in hepatocellular carcinoma. *Clin. Cancer Res.* **2008**, *14*, 3520–3528. [CrossRef]

164. Niu, C.; Jin, H.; Li, M.; Zhu, S.; Zhou, L.; Jin, F.; Zhou, Y.; Xu, D.; Xu, J.; Zhao, L.; et al. Low-dose bortezomib increases the expression of NKG2D and DNAM-1 ligands and enhances induced NK and γδ T cellmediated lysis in multiple myeloma. *Oncotarget* **2017**, *8*, 5954–5964. [CrossRef]

165. Shi, J.; Tricot, G.J.; Garg, T.K.; Malaviarachchi, P.A.; Szmania, S.M.; Kellum, R.E.; Storrie, B.; Mulder, A.; Shaughnessy, J.D.; Barlogie, B.; et al. Bortezomib down-regulates the cell-surface expression of HLA class I and enhances natural killer cell-mediated lysis of myeloma. *Blood* **2008**, *111*, 1309–1317. [CrossRef]

166. Lundqvist, A.; Abrams, S.I.; Schrump, D.S.; Alvarez, G.; Suffredini, D.; Berg, M.; Childs, R. Bortezomib and depsipeptide sensitize tumors to tumor necrosis factor-related apoptosis-inducing ligand: A novel method to potentiate natural killer cell tumor cytotoxicity. *Cancer Res.* **2006**, *66*, 7317–7325. [CrossRef]

167. Kabore, A.F.; Sun, J.; Hu, X.; McCrea, K.; Johnston, J.B.; Gibson, S.B. The TRAIL apoptotic pathway mediates proteasome inhibitor induced apoptosis in primary chronic lymphocytic leukemia cells. *Apoptosis* **2006**, *11*, 1175–1193. [CrossRef]

168. Liu, X.; Yue, P.; Chen, S.; Hu, L.; Lonial, S.; Khuri, F.R.; Sun, S.Y. The proteasome inhibitor PS-341 (bortezomib) up-regulates DR5 expression leading to induction of apoptosis and enhancement of TRAIL-induced apoptosis despite up-regulation of c-FLIP and survivin expression in human NSCLC cells. *Cancer Res.* **2007**, *67*, 4981–4988. [CrossRef] [PubMed]

169. Massa, C.; Karn, T.; Denkert, C.; Schneeweiss, A.; Hanusch, C.; Blohmer, J.U.; Zahm, D.M.; Jackisch, C.; van Mackelenbergh, M.; Thomalla, J.; et al. Differential effect on different immune subsets of neoadjuvant chemotherapy in patients with TNBC. *J. Immunother. Cancer* **2020**, *8*. [CrossRef] [PubMed]

170. Aldarouish, M.; Su, X.; Qiao, J.; Gao, C.; Chen, Y.; Dai, A.; Zhang, T.; Shu, Y.; Wang, C. Immunomodulatory effects of chemotherapy on blood lymphocytes and survival of patients with advanced non-small cell lung cancer. *Int. J. Immunopathol. Pharmacol.* **2019**, *33*, 2058738419839592. [CrossRef] [PubMed]

171. Shinko, D.; McGuire, H.M.; Diakos, C.I.; Pavlakis, N.; Clarke, S.J.; Byrne, S.N.; Charles, K.A. Mass Cytometry Reveals a Sustained Reduction in CD16+ Natural Killer Cells Following Chemotherapy in Colorectal Cancer Patients. *Front. Immunol.* **2019**, *10*. [CrossRef]

172. Beitsch, P.; Lotzová, E.; Hortobagyi, G.; Pollock, R. Natural immunity in breast cancer patients during neoadjuvant chemotherapy and after surgery. *Surg. Oncol.* **1994**, *3*, 211–219. [CrossRef]

173. Sewell, H.F.; Halbert, C.F.; Robins, R.A.; Galvin, A.; Chan, S.; Blamey, R.W. Chemotherapy-induced differential changes in lymphocyte subsets and natural-killer-cell function in patients with advanced breast cancer. *Int. J. Cancer* **1993**, *55*, 735–738. [CrossRef]

174. Brenner, B.G.; Margolese, R.G. The relationship of chemotherapeutic and endocrine intervention on natural killer cell activity in human breast cancer. *Cancer* **1991**, *68*, 482–488. [CrossRef]

175. Ogura, M.; Ishida, T.; Tsukasaki, K.; Takahashi, T.; Utsunomiya, A. Effects of first-line chemotherapy on natural killer cells in adult T-cell leukemia–lymphoma and peripheral T-cell lymphoma. *Cancer Chemother. Pharm.* **2016**, *78*, 199–207. [CrossRef] [PubMed]

176. Wullschleger, S.; Loewith, R.; Hall, M.N. TOR Signaling in Growth and Metabolism. *Cell* **2006**, *124*, 471–484. [CrossRef] [PubMed]

177. Bhullar, K.S.; Lagarón, N.O.; McGowan, E.M.; Parmar, I.; Jha, A.; Hubbard, B.P.; Rupasinghe, H.P.V. Kinase-targeted cancer therapies: Progress, challenges and future directions. *Mol. Cancer* **2018**, *17*, 48. [CrossRef]

178. Adams, J.A. Kinetic and catalytic mechanisms of protein kinases. *Chem. Rev.* **2001**, *101*, 2271–2290. [CrossRef]

179. Johnson, L.N.; Lewis, R.J. Structural basis for control by phosphorylation. *Chem. Rev.* **2001**, *101*, 2209–2242. [CrossRef] [PubMed]

180. DiDonato, J.A.; Mercurio, F.; Karin, M. NF-κB and the link between inflammation and cancer. *Immunol. Rev.* **2012**, *246*, 379–400. [CrossRef]

181. Sun, C.; Bernards, R. Feedback and redundancy in receptor tyrosine kinase signaling: Relevance to cancer therapies. *Trends Biochem. Sci.* **2014**, *39*, 465–474. [CrossRef] [PubMed]

182. Huang, M.; Shen, A.; Ding, J.; Geng, M. Molecularly targeted cancer therapy: Some lessons from the past decade. *Trends Pharm. Sci.* **2014**, *35*, 41–50. [CrossRef]

183. Kreutzman, A.; Porkka, K.; Mustjoki, S. Immunomodulatory effects of tyrosine kinase inhibitors. *Int. Trends Immun.* **2013**, *1*, 17–28.

184. Blake, S.J.; Lyons, A.B.; Fraser, C.K.; Hayball, J.D.; Hughes, T.P. Dasatinib suppresses in vitro natural killer cell cytotoxicity. *Blood* **2008**, *111*, 4415–4416. [CrossRef]

185. Mustjoki, S.; Auvinen, K.; Kreutzman, A.; Rousselot, P.; Hernesniemi, S.; Melo, T.; Lahesmaa-Korpinen, A.-M.; Hautaniemi, S.; Bouchet, S.; Molimard, M.; et al. Rapid mobilization of cytotoxic lymphocytes induced by dasatinib therapy. *Leukemia* **2013**, *27*, 914–924. [CrossRef]

186. Hayashi, Y.; Nakamae, H.; Katayama, T.; Nakane, T.; Koh, H.; Nakamae, M.; Hirose, A.; Hagihara, K.; Terada, Y.; Nakao, Y.; et al. Different immunoprofiles in patients with chronic myeloid leukemia treated with imatinib, nilotinib or dasatinib. *Leuk. Lymphoma* **2012**, *53*, 1084–1089. [CrossRef]

187. Kreutzman, A.; Yadav, B.; Brummendorf, T.H.; Gjertsen, B.T.; Lee, M.H.; Janssen, J.; Kasanen, T.; Koskenvesa, P.; Lotfi, K.; Markevärn, B.; et al. Immunological monitoring of newly diagnosed CML patients treated with bosutinib or imatinib first-line. *Oncoimmunology* **2019**, *8*. [CrossRef] [PubMed]

188. Ilander, M.; Olsson-Strömberg, U.; Schlums, H.; Guilhot, J.; Brück, O.; Lähteenmäki, H.; Kasanen, T.; Koskenvesa, P.; Söderlund, S.; Höglund, M.; et al. Increased proportion of mature NK cells is associated with successful imatinib discontinuation in chronic myeloid leukemia. *Leukemia* **2017**, *31*, 1108–1116. [CrossRef]

189. Rea, D.; Henry, G.; Khaznadar, Z.; Etienne, G.; Guilhot, F.; Nicolini, F.; Guilhot, J.; Rousselot, P.; Huguet, F.; Legros, L.; et al. Natural killer-cell counts are associated with molecular relapse-free survival after imatinib discontinuation in chronic myeloid leukemia: The IMMUNOSTIM study. *Haematologica* **2017**, *102*, 1368–1377. [CrossRef] [PubMed]

190. Roberts, P.J.; Der, C.J. Targeting the Raf-MEK-ERK mitogen-activated protein kinase cascade for the treatment of cancer. *Oncogene* **2007**, *26*, 3291–3310. [CrossRef]
191. Subbiah, V.; Baik, C.; Kirkwood, J.M. Clinical Development of BRAF plus MEK Inhibitor Combinations. *Trends Cancer* **2020**, *6*, 797–810. [CrossRef]
192. Kannaiyan, R.; Mahadevan, D. A comprehensive review of protein kinase inhibitors for cancer therapy HHS Public Access. *Expert Rev. Anticancer* **2018**, *18*, 1249–1270. [CrossRef] [PubMed]
193. Shirley, M. Encorafenib and Binimetinib: First Global Approvals. *Drugs* **2018**, *78*, 1277–1284. [CrossRef] [PubMed]
194. De Andrade, L.F.; Ngiow, S.F.; Stannard, K.; Rusakiewicz, S.; Kalimutho, M.; Khanna, K.K.; Tey, S.K.; Takeda, K.; Zitvogel, L.; Martinet, L.; et al. Natural killer cells are essential for the ability of BRAF inhibitors to control BRAFV600E-mutant metastatic melanoma. *Cancer Res.* **2014**, *74*, 7298–7308. [CrossRef]
195. Frazao, A.; Colombo, M.; Fourmentraux-Neves, E.; Messaoudene, M.; Rusakiewicz, S.; Zitvogel, L.; Vivier, E.; Vély, F.; Faure, F.; Dréno, B.; et al. Shifting the Balance of Activating and Inhibitory Natural Killer Receptor Ligands on BRAF(V600E) Melanoma Lines with Vemurafenib. *Cancer Immunol. Res.* **2017**, *5*, 582–593. [CrossRef] [PubMed]
196. López-Cobo, S.; Pieper, N.; Campos-Silva, C.; García-Cuesta, E.M.; Reyburn, H.T.; Paschen, A.; Valés-Gómez, M. Impaired NK cell recognition of vemurafenib-treated melanoma cells is overcome by simultaneous application of histone deacetylase inhibitors. *OncoImmunology* **2018**, *7*. [CrossRef]
197. Frazao, A.; Rethacker, L.; Jeudy, G.; Colombo, M.; Pasmant, E.; Avril, M.-F.; Toubert, A.; Moins-Teisserenc, H.; Roelens, M.; Dalac, S.; et al. BRAF inhibitor resistance of melanoma cells triggers increased susceptibility to natural killer cell-mediated lysis. *J. Immunother. Cancer* **2020**, *8*, e000275. [CrossRef]
198. Sottile, R.; Pangigadde, P.N.; Tan, T.; Anichini, A.; Sabbatino, F.; Trecroci, F.; Favoino, E.; Orgiano, L.; Roberts, J.; Ferrone, S.; et al. HLA class I downregulation is associated with enhanced NK-cell killing of melanoma cells with acquired drug resistance to BRAF inhibitors. *Eur. J. Immunol.* **2016**, *46*, 409–419. [CrossRef] [PubMed]
199. Augello, G.; Emma, M.R.; Cusimano, A.; Azzolina, A.; Montalto, G.; McCubrey, J.A.; Cervello, M. The Role of GSK-3 in Cancer Immunotherapy: GSK-3 Inhibitors as a New Frontier in Cancer Treatment. *Cells* **2020**, *9*, 1427. [CrossRef]
200. Parameswaran, R.; Ramakrishnan, P.; Moreton, S.A.; Xia, Z.; Hou, Y.; Lee, D.A.; Gupta, K.; Delima, M.; Beck, R.C.; Wald, D.N. Repression of GSK3 restores NK cell cytotoxicity in AML patients. *Nat. Commun.* **2016**, *7*. [CrossRef] [PubMed]
201. Cichocki, F.; Valamehr, B.; Bjordahl, R.; Zhang, B.; Rezner, B.; Rogers, P.; Gaidarova, S.; Moreno, S.; Tuininga, K.; Dougherty, P.; et al. GSK3 inhibition drives maturation of NK cells and enhances their antitumor activity. *Cancer Res.* **2017**, *77*, 5664–5675. [CrossRef]
202. Cosman, D.; Müllberg, J.; Sutherland, C.L.; Chin, W.; Armitage, R.; Fanslow, W.; Kubin, M.; Chalupny, N.J. ULBPs, novel MHC class I-related molecules, bind to CMV glycoprotein UL16 and stimulate NK cytotoxicity through the NKG2D receptor. *Immunity* **2001**, *14*, 123–133. [CrossRef]
203. Fionda, C.; Malgarini, G.; Soriani, A.; Zingoni, A.; Cecere, F.; Iannitto, M.L.; Ricciardi, M.R.; Federico, V.; Petrucci, M.T.; Santoni, A.; et al. Inhibition of glycogen synthase kinase-3 increases NKG2D ligand MICA expression and sensitivity to NK cell-mediated cytotoxicity in multiple myeloma cells: Role of STAT3. *J. Immunol.* **2013**, *190*, 6662–6672. [CrossRef]
204. Krusch, M.; Salih, J.; Schlicke, M.; Baessler, T.; Kampa, K.M.; Mayer, F.; Salih, H.R. The Kinase Inhibitors Sunitinib and Sorafenib Differentially Affect NK Cell Antitumor Reactivity In Vitro. *J. Immunol.* **2009**, *183*, 8286–8294. [CrossRef]
205. Lohmeyer, J.; Nerreter, T.; Dotterweich, J.; Einsele, H.; Seggewiss-Bernhardt, R. Sorafenib paradoxically activates the RAS/RAF/ERK pathway in polyclonal human NK cells during expansion and thereby enhances effector functions in a dose- and time-dependent manner. *Clin. Exp. Immunol.* **2018**, *193*, 64–72. [CrossRef]
206. Huang, Y.X.; Chen, X.T.; Guo, K.Y.; Li, Y.H.; Wu, B.Y.; Song, C.Y.; He, Y.J. Sunitinib induces NK-κB-dependent NKG2D ligand expression in nasopharyngeal carcinoma and hepatoma cells. *J. Immunother.* **2017**, *40*, 164–174. [CrossRef]
207. Huang, Y.; Wang, Y.; Li, Y.; Guo, K.; He, Y. Role of sorafenib and sunitinib in the induction of expressions of NKG2D ligands in nasopharyngeal carcinoma with high expression of ABCG2. *J. Cancer Res. Clin. Oncol.* **2011**, *137*, 829–837. [CrossRef]
208. Harrison, D.A. The JAK/STAT pathway. *Cold Spring Harb. Perspect. Biol.* **2012**, *4*. [CrossRef]
209. Schönberg, K.; Rudolph, J.; Wolf, D. NK cell modulation by JAK inhibition. *Oncoscience* **2015**, *2*, 677. [CrossRef]
210. Xu, L.J.; Chen, X.D.; Shen, M.J.; Yang, D.R.; Fang, L.; Weng, G.; Tsai, Y.; Keng, P.C.; Chen, Y.; Lee, S.O. Inhibition of IL-6-JAK/Stat3 signaling in castration-resistant prostate cancer cells enhances the NK cell-mediated cytotoxicity via alteration of PD-L1/NKG2D ligand levels. *Mol. Oncol.* **2018**, *12*, 269–286. [CrossRef] [PubMed]
211. Zhu, C.; Wei, Y.; Wei, X. AXL receptor tyrosine kinase as a promising anti-cancer approach: Functions, molecular mechanisms and clinical applications. *Mol. Cancer* **2019**, *18*. [CrossRef] [PubMed]
212. Lutz-Nicoladoni, C.; Wolf, D.; Sopper, S.; Sharabi, A.; Palmer, D. Modulation of immune cell functions by the E3 ligase Cbl-b. *Front. Oncol.* **2015**, *5*. [CrossRef] [PubMed]
213. Paolino, M.; Choidas, A.; Wallner, S.; Pranjic, B.; Uribesalgo, I.; Loeser, S.; Jamieson, A.M.; Langdon, W.Y.; Ikeda, F.; Fededa, J.P.; et al. The E3 ligase Cbl-b and TAM receptors regulate cancer metastasis via natural killer cells. *Nature* **2014**, *507*, 508–512. [CrossRef]
214. Kaufman, H.L.; Kohlhapp, F.J.; Zloza, A. Oncolytic viruses: A new class of immunotherapy drugs. *Nat. Rev. Drug Discov.* **2015**, *14*, 642–662. [CrossRef] [PubMed]

215. Fukuhara, H.; Ino, Y.; Todo, T. Oncolytic virus therapy: A new era of cancer treatment at dawn. *Cancer Sci.* **2016**, *107*, 1373–1379. [CrossRef] [PubMed]
216. Hamid, O.; Ismail, R.; Puzanov, I. Intratumoral Immunotherapy—Update 2019. *Oncologist* **2020**, *25*. [CrossRef]
217. Samudio, I.; Hofs, E.; Cho, B.; Li, M.; Bolduc, K.; Bu, L.; Liu, G.; Lam, V.; Rennie, P.; Jia, W.; et al. UV Light-inactivated HSV-1 Stimulates Natural Killer Cell-induced Killing of Prostate Cancer Cells. *J. Immunother.* **2019**, *42*, 162–174. [CrossRef] [PubMed]
218. Bhat, R.; Rommelaere, J. NK-cell-dependent killing of colon carcinoma cells is mediated by natural cytotoxicity receptors (NCRs) and stimulated by parvovirus infection of target cells. *BMC Cancer* **2013**, *13*. [CrossRef] [PubMed]
219. Ogbomo, H.; Michaelis, M.; Geiler, J.; van Rikxoort, M.; Muster, T.; Egorov, A.; Doerr, H.W.; Cinatl, J. Tumor cells infected with oncolytic influenza a virus prime natural killer cells for lysis of resistant tumor cells. *Med. Microbiol. Immunol.* **2010**, *199*, 93–101. [CrossRef] [PubMed]
220. Jarahian, M.; Watzl, C.; Fournier, P.; Arnold, A.; Djandji, D.; Zahedi, S.; Cerwenka, A.; Paschen, A.; Schirrmacher, V.; Momburg, F. Activation of Natural Killer Cells by Newcastle Disease Virus Hemagglutinin-Neuraminidase. *J. Virol.* **2009**, *83*, 8108–8121. [CrossRef] [PubMed]
221. Ogbomo, H.; Zemp, F.J.; Lun, X.; Zhang, J.; Stack, D.; Rahman, M.M.; Mcfadden, G.; Mody, C.H.; Forsyth, P.A. Myxoma Virus Infection Promotes NK Lysis of Malignant Gliomas In Vitro and In Vivo. *PLoS ONE* **2013**, *8*. [CrossRef]
222. Bhat, R.; Rommelaere, J. Emerging role of Natural killer cells in oncolytic virotherapy. *Immuno Targets Ther.* **2015**, *4*, 65–77. [CrossRef]
223. Diaz, R.M.; Galivo, F.; Kottke, T.; Wongthida, P.; Qiao, J.; Thompson, J.; Valdes, M.; Barber, G.; Vile, R.G. Oncolytic immunovirotherapy for melanoma using vesicular stomatitis virus. *Cancer Res.* **2007**, *67*, 2840–2848. [CrossRef]
224. Miller, C.G.; Fraser, N.W. Requirement of an integrated immune response for successful neuroattenuated HSV-1 therapy in an intracranial metastatic melanoma model. *Mol. Ther.* **2003**, *7*, 741–747. [CrossRef]
225. Tai, L.H.; de Souza, C.T.; Bélanger, S.; Ly, L.; Alkayyal, A.A.; Zhang, J.; Rintoul, J.L.; Ananth, A.A.; Lam, T.; Breitbach, C.J.; et al. Preventing postoperative metastatic disease by inhibiting surgery-induced dysfunction in natural killer cells. *Cancer Res.* **2013**, *73*, 97–107. [CrossRef]
226. Altomonte, J.; Wu, L.; Chen, L.; Meseck, M.; Ebert, O.; García-Sastre, A.; Fallon, J.; Woo, S.L. Exponential enhancement of oncolytic vesicular stomatitis virus potency by vector-mediated suppression of inflammatory responses in vivo. *Mol. Ther.* **2008**, *16*, 146–153. [CrossRef] [PubMed]
227. Xu, B.; Ma, R.; Russell, L.; Yoo, J.Y.; Han, J.; Cui, H.; Yi, P.; Zhang, J.; Nakashima, H.; Dai, H.; et al. An oncolytic herpesvirus expressing E-cadherin improves survival in mouse models of glioblastoma. *Nat. Biotechnol.* **2019**, *37*, 45–54. [CrossRef] [PubMed]
228. Alvarez-Breckenridge, C.A.; Yu, J.; Price, R.; Wojton, J.; Pradarelli, J.; Mao, H.; Wei, M.; Wang, Y.; He, S.; Hardcastle, J.; et al. NK cells impede glioblastoma virotherapy through NKp30 and NKp46 natural cytotoxicity receptors. *Nat. Med.* **2012**, *18*, 1827–1834. [CrossRef] [PubMed]
229. Alvarez-Breckenridge, C.A.; Yu, J.; Price, R.; Wei, M.; Wang, Y.; Nowicki, M.O.; Ha, Y.P.; Bergin, S.; Hwang, C.; Fernandez, S.A.; et al. The Histone Deacetylase Inhibitor Valproic Acid Lessens NK Cell Action against Oncolytic Virus-Infected Glioblastoma Cells by Inhibition of STAT5/T-BET Signaling and Generation of Gamma Interferon. *J. Virol.* **2012**, *86*, 4566–4577. [CrossRef] [PubMed]
230. Kim, Y.; Yoo, J.Y.; Lee, T.J.; Liu, J.; Yu, J.; Caligiuri, M.A.; Kaur, B.; Friedman, A. Complex role of NK cells in regulation of oncolytic virus–bortezomib therapy. *Proc. Natl. Acad. Sci. USA* **2018**, *115*, 4927–4932. [CrossRef]

Review

Harnessing Tumor Necrosis Factor Alpha to Achieve Effective Cancer Immunotherapy

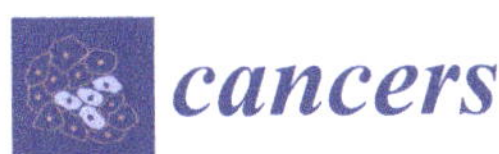

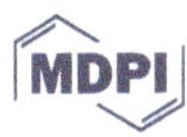

María Florencia Mercogliano [1], Sofía Bruni [2], Florencia Mauro [2], Patricia Virginia Elizalde [2] and Roxana Schillaci [2,*]

[1] Laboratorio de Biofisicoquímica de Proteínas, Instituto de Química Biológica de la Facultad de Ciencias Exactas y Naturales-Consejo Nacional de Investigaciones Científicas y Técnicas (IQUIBICEN-CONICET), Buenos Aires 1428, Argentina; florenciamercogliano@qb.fcen.uba.ar

[2] Laboratory of Molecular Mechanisms of Carcinogenesis, Instituto de Biología y Medicina Experimental (IBYME-CONICET), Buenos Aires 1428, Argentina; sbruni@dna.uba.ar (S.B.); fmauro@dna.uba.ar (F.M.); patriciaelizalde@ibyme.conicet.gov.ar (P.V.E.)

* Correspondence: rschillaci@ibyme.conicet.gov.ar; Tel.: +54-11-4783-2869; Fax: +54-11-4786-2564

Simple Summary: Inflammation has been acknowledged as one of the causes of increased cancer risk. Among the pro-inflammatory mediators, tumor necrosis factor alpha (TNFα) has been identified as an important player in cancer progression and metastasis. On the other hand, TNFα has a central role in promoting innate and adaptive immune responses. These apparently controversial effects are now starting to be uncovered through different studies on TNFα isoforms and distinct mechanisms of action of TNFα receptors. The use of immunotherapies for cancer treatment such as monoclonal antibodies against cancer cells or immune checkpoints and adoptive cell therapy, are beginning to broaden our understanding of TNFα's actions and its potential therapeutic role. This work describes TNFα participation as a source of treatment resistance and its implication in side effects to immunotherapy, as well as its participation in different cancer types, where TNFα can be a suitable target to improve therapy outcome.

Abstract: Tumor necrosis factor alpha (TNFα) is a pleiotropic cytokine known to have contradictory roles in oncoimmunology. Indeed, TNFα has a central role in the onset of the immune response, inducing both activation and the effector function of macrophages, dendritic cells, natural killer (NK) cells, and B and T lymphocytes. Within the tumor microenvironment, however, TNFα is one of the main mediators of cancer-related inflammation. It is involved in the recruitment and differentiation of immune suppressor cells, leading to evasion of tumor immune surveillance. These characteristics turn TNFα into an attractive target to overcome therapy resistance and tackle cancer. This review focuses on the diverse molecular mechanisms that place TNFα as a source of resistance to immunotherapy such as monoclonal antibodies against cancer cells or immune checkpoints and adoptive cell therapy. We also expose the benefits of TNFα blocking strategies in combination with immunotherapy to improve the antitumor effect and prevent or treat adverse immune-related effects.

Keywords: TNFα; immunotherapy; adoptive cell therapy; monoclonal antibody; immune checkpoint inhibitor; cancer

Citation: Mercogliano, M.F.; Bruni, S.; Mauro, F.; Elizalde, P.V.; Schillaci, R. Harnessing Tumor Necrosis Factor Alpha to Achieve Effective Cancer Immunotherapy. *Cancers* **2021**, *13*, 564. https://doi.org/10.3390/cancers13030564

Academic Editors: Michael Kershaw and George Mosialos
Received: 7 December 2020
Accepted: 22 January 2021
Published: 2 February 2021

Publisher's Note: MDPI stays neutral with regard to jurisdictional claims in published maps and institutional affiliations.

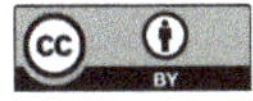

1. Introduction

It is well known that tumor necrosis factor alpha (TNFα) participates as a proinflammatory cytokine, increasing the risk of several cancers, such as colorectal, esophageal, pancreatic, liver, and breast cancer [1]. However, another layer of complexity in TNFα functions was added with the emergence of immunotherapy. In this review we highlight recent data pointing out TNFα participation in the effectiveness of monoclonal antibodies (mAbs) targeting cancer cells, immune checkpoint inhibitors, and adoptive cell therapy (ACT), as well as its involvement in the adverse immune effects of immunotherapy.

2. TNFα Overview

TNFα was identified in 1975 as a molecule capable of causing tumor necrosis at high concentration [2–4]. Many studies on TNFα showed that it is a pleiotropic proinflammatory cytokine involved in a wide variety of cellular processes and, moreover, has contradictory effects ranging from cell proliferation to cell death. First, it was described that TNFα was involved in immune system regulation and was mainly secreted by cells such as monocytes, macrophages, natural killer (NK) cells, T lymphocytes, mast cells, and neutrophils, but later several works showed that it is also produced by non-immune cells like endothelial cells, adipocytes, neurons, fibroblasts, and smooth muscle, among others [5–9].

The human TNFα gene consists of a single copy located in chromosome 6 near the major histocompatibility complex genes [10]. It comprises four exons and three introns. The first exon contains the leader peptide sequence and the last ones the information for the protein. TNFα transcription is stimulated by NF-κB [11], AP-1, c-Jun, and Nuclear Factor of Activated T-cells (NFAT) [6]. TNFα is present in either of two forms: transmembrane (tmTNFα) or soluble TNFα (sTNFα). tmTNFα is classified as a type II membrane protein, like many of the TNF-related ligands; it has a molecular weight of 26 kDa and forms a homotrimer that can also act as a receptor. TNFα can regulate several pathological and physiological processes beyond the immune system. The duality of many members of the TNF superfamily, as ligand and receptor, gives rise to the particular phenomenon of reverse signaling [12]: when acting as a receptor, tmTNFα can signal outside-to-inside back to the tmTNFα expressing cell. This mechanism has been mostly described in the regulation of the immune system but has not yet been completely characterized. On the other hand, sTNFα of 17 kDa is generated through proteolytic cleavage of tmTNFα by the TNFα Converting Enzyme (TACE/ADAM17) [13]. The active mature sTNFα also forms a homotrimer of 52 kDa that exerts a powerful autocrine, paracrine, and endocrine effect [14].

There are two membrane receptors for TNFα, also classified as type I membrane proteins, TNFα receptor 1 (TNFR1/CD120a, 55 kDa) and 2 (TNFR2/CD120b, 75 kDa) [15], and tm- and sTNFα can bind to them. Both isoforms of TNFα trigger receptor trimerization and subsequent recruitment of scaffold proteins to the cytoplasmic domain to induce different signaling pathways depending on the receptor involved, the type of TNFα that activated the receptor, the cell type, and the cellular context [16]. Pleiotropic effects of TNFα can be due not only to its two forms but also to the low homology of the ligand binding domain and no homology in the intracellular domain of the receptors, which have no enzymatic activity and therefore have to recruit scaffold proteins to unleash the signaling cascade [16]. Another particularity of the TNFα pathway, which explains its contradictory and varied effects, is that both TNFR1 and TNFR2 have soluble forms that are cleaved by TACE/ADAM17. The function of soluble receptors is to regulate TNFα availability and protect this cytokine from degradation to accomplish a sustained signal [17,18]. Most nucleated cells of the body express TNFR1, which can be activated by both forms of TNFα [19]. On the contrary, TNFR2 is expressed mainly in immune cells and in limited cell types like neurons, oligodendrocytes, astrocytes, and endothelial cells, among others, and can only be fully activated by tmTNFα [20,21].

Regarding the signaling of each receptor, TNFR1 has a cytoplasmic death domain, which can recruit TNFR1-Associated Death Domain (TRADD) protein and TNF Receptor-Associated Factor 2 (TRAF2), which can form two complexes: complex I, which stimulates cell survival and proliferation through JNK, NF-κB, AP-1, and MAPK pathways [22], and complex II, which, on the contrary, recruits Fas-Associated protein with Dead Domain (FADD) and pro-caspases that constitute a death-inducing signaling complex [23], which ends in apoptosis [24]. Which of these pathways prevails is determined by the signaling molecules of the scaffold, signal strength, and crosstalk with other pathways [25]. TNFR2, instead, lacks the death domain and mainly regulates cell activation, migration, and proliferation [26]. Nonetheless, TNFR2 can also bind TRAF2 through TRAF1, concluding in the activation of both the canonical and non-canonical NF-κB pathway like TNFR1, but activation is slower and more sustained [27,28]. It has also been reported that TNFR2 can activate the abovementioned TNFR1 pathways through recruitment of Receptor Interacting Protein 1 (RIP-1) and TRADD via TRAF2, resulting in apoptosis.

Briefly, the convoluted pathway of TNFα involves a transmembrane and a soluble form, as well as two distinct receptors, which also exist in a soluble form. The combination of these elements activates distinct and unique signaling pathways that account for the pleiotropic effects of this cytokine. To add to the complexity, the pathways stimulated by each receptor can converge depending on different factors such as the adaptor proteins, TNFα concentration, cell type, and cellular context.

3. TNFα and the Immune System

Regulation of the innate immune system is the main role of TNFα, and it has been reviewed extensively throughout time. In particular, it is a major protagonist in immunity against intracellular organisms [29–32], has been intensively studied in *Mycobacterium* infection [33], and is responsible for the proliferation of thymocytes [34]. TNFα is also the main player in the initiation of inflammatory reactions characterizing the onset of the immune response.

Neither the TNFα nor TNFRs knockout model is lethal, but lymphoid organs and the immune response are affected. TNFα and its receptors are essential for the regulation of pro- and anti-inflammatory processes [30], the formation of Peyer's patches [35], and the adaptive B cell immune response [36], since it is involved in the generation of B cell follicles and germinal centers, and consequently, they affect the humoral immune response, among others.

TNFα also has contradictory effects in the immune system, since it can act as an immunosuppressor or an immunostimulant [2,37]. TNFα activates macrophages that produce more TNFα, generating a feed-forward loop, and is essential in guiding proliferation and proper effector function of several cell populations of the immune system, such as T, B, NK, and dendritic cells (DC). TNFα immunosuppressor effects encompass the regulation of suppressor cell populations like regulatory T and B cells (Tregs and Bregs, respectively) [38–40] and myeloid-derived suppressor cells (MDSCs) [41,42].

The central role of TNFα as an immunostimulant is to initiate the inflammatory response of the innate immune system and stimulate the Th1 profile. When a pathogen enters the organism, TNFα expression is induced. The elevated level of TNFα induces a chemokine/cytokine signaling cascade which, at the site of injury, induces certain adhesion molecule expression on the endothelial cells and immune cells, which allow neutrophil extravasation and the recruitment of macrophages and lymphocytes. It is noteworthy that TNFα generates a positive autocrine feedback loop that activates NF-κB, which increases GM-CSF, IL-8, and TNFα itself [43].

As stated before, TNFR2 is mainly expressed in immune cells, and when TNFα binds to it, TRAF1, 2, and 3 are recruited together with cIAP1/2 to activate canonical and non-canonical NF-κB and PI3K-Akt pathways, which consequently guides cell proliferation and survival. TNFR2 expression is higher in Tregs with respect to the rest of the T cell population, and in humans, this set of Tregs also expresses higher levels of cytotoxic T lymphocyte antigen 4 (CTLA-4), a well-known immunomodulator. TNFR2 has also been found to be involved in the suppressive activity of Tregs, but the mechanisms behind this process remain to be elucidated. Tregs also produce TNFα in certain inflammatory pathologies, and their function depends on the context, indicating that TNFα could be an attractive target to treat these inflammatory diseases. This proves once again the pleiotropic activity of TNFα, since it can promote the inhibition of Treg function in co-culture conditions with effector T lymphocytes but can also stimulate their immunosuppressive role, promoting Treg proliferation and survival, depending on the context [44–46]. Unstimulated CD4+ T lymphocytes increase MDSC accumulation [47] through tmTNFα via TNFR2 [48] and through 17-β-estradiol [49], and enhance their immunosuppressive activity through Nos2 [42].

4. TNFα in Cancer

TNFα has a plethora of functions and implications, and this also applies to cancer cells. TNFα has been described as having contradictory effects on almost every type of cancer. In high concentrations, TNFα is able to eliminate methylcolanthrene (MCA)-induced sarcomas, as first described by Carswell [2], and approximately 28% of cancers are sensitive to sTNFα [50]. TNFα antitumor mechanisms are varied and include the following: mediating cellular apoptosis extensively reviewed by Rath et al. [51]; directing tumor-associated macrophages (TAMs) to the M1 profile (antitumoral phenotype) [52]; guiding neutrophils and monocytes to tumor sites [53,54], activating macrophages and inhibiting monocyte differentiation to immunosuppressive phenotypes [55]; and inducing disruption of tumor vasculature [56,57]. Despite the above, TNFα expression at low levels can be pro-tumorigenic, an effect broadly reviewed by Balkwill [37,58].

There has been a large amount of evidence linking pro-inflammatory cytokines to cancer and the association with poor prognosis (reviewed by Mantovani) [59]. TNFα is one of the major pro-inflammatory cytokines of the immune system and has been found in several human cancers, such as breast [60], gastric [61], pancreatic [62], ovarian [63,64], endometrial [65], prostate [45], bladder [66], colorectal [67], oral [68], and liver [69]. It has also been detected in leukemias and lymphomas. Even so, there has been disagreement in considering TNFα expression as a biomarker, since the cytokine is increased in numerous other pathologies as well.

The distinct and opposing effects of TNFα in cancer depend on cytokine concentration and s- TNFα or tm- TNFα isoforms, distinct caspase activation, varied expression of adaptor proteins, different expression levels of members of the Bcl-2 family, among others [70]. TNFα acts as a pro-tumoral cytokine involved in different processes, such as cell proliferation, tumor progression, migration, epithelial-to-mesenchymal transition (EMT), angiogenesis and metastasis in several cancer types. The pro- and anti-tumorigenic/tumoral effects of TNFα are shown in Table 1 for different types of cancers.

Concerning breast cancer, our group has extensively reviewed TNFα impact/role on the different subtypes [71]. Regarding TNFα involvement in resistance to therapy, we have described TNFα involvement in trastuzumab resistance in HER2+ breast and gastric cancer. In the case of gastric cancer, the HER2 expressing gastric cancer cell line sensitive to trastuzumab NCI-N87 becomes refractory to the antibody after TNFα exposure [72]. In pancreatic cancer, blocking TNFα strategies proved to be effective in animal models [62] and in patients [73].

In melanoma, TNFα induces cell invasion [74] and aggressiveness [75], extravascular migration of cancer cells [76] and impairs CD8 T lymphocytes accumulation in the TME [77], moreover blocking TNFα prevents metastasis formation in the lungs in pre-clinical models [78]. TNFα is also overexpressed in oral squamous cell carcinoma (OSCC) [79], promotes the sphere-forming abilities of its cells maintaining a cancer stem cell-like phenotype [80], and increases proliferation in leukemia stem cells [81]. Interestingly, TNFα at low doses increases CD20 expression in B chronic lymphocytic leukemia, which can take advantage of the proven anti-CD20 therapy [82].

There are reports pointing to TNFα having no effect in endometrial cancer [83,84]. On the other hand, elevated pre-diagnostic concentrations of TNFα and its soluble receptors and the activation of TNFα-related pathways have been related to higher risk and poorer survival in endometrial cancer [85], prostate cancer [86] where could induce a shift to an untreatable phenotype [87]. In OSCC correlates with progression [88,89] and with relapse in children with B-lineage acute lymphoblastic leukemia (ALL) [90], but not with response to treatment [91] and in patients with non-Hodgkin's lymphoma [92] and diffuse large B cell lymphoma, TNFα is useful to differentiate risk groups [93]. In the latter TNFR1 expression in the tumor is also a good biomarker for prognosis [94].

Regarding TNFα as a potential biomarker, it was shown that TNFα polymorphisms in the gene promoter or coding region are associated with a risk of progression in patients with gastric lesions [95,96], with worse prognosis in prostate cancer patients [97], with tumor stage in bladder cancer [98], with risk of recurrence in hepatocellular carcinoma [99] and with higher risk in non-Hodgkin's lymphoma [100], T cell lymphoma [101], and gastric B cell lymphoma [102]. In ovarian cancer, TNFα gene polymorphisms are associated with pathogenesis but remains to be validated [103].

Table 1. Dual role of tumor necrosis factor alpha (TNFα) in cancer.

Cancer Type	Pro-Tumorigenic	References	Anti-Tumorigenic	References
Breast	Promotes proliferation, progression, and metastasis	[70]	Apoptosis and inhibition of proliferation	[70]
Gastric	Proliferation, progression and metastasis	[104–108]	Apoptosis acting together with TGFβ	[109]
Pancreatic	Promotes tumor progression Generates a immune evasive microenvironment	[110,111] [115]	Apoptosis -	[112–114] -
Ovarian	Tumor promotion through TNFR1 and IL-17 Generates a immunosuppresor microenvironment Contributes to the EMT process through the NF-κB pathway Tumor proliferation, progression, and invasion.	[116] [117] [64] [118–120]	- - - -	- - - -
Prostate	Survival and proliferation, progression, angiogenesis and metastasis	[121–126]	Apoptosis	[127,128]
Bladder	Migration and invasion through the p38 MAPK pathway	[129–131]	Apoptosis	[132,133]
Colorectal	Together with Th17-cytokines promotes immune escape, proliferation, survival, progression, and metastasis	[134–136]	-	-
Oral	Promotes immune evasion Promotes cell viability Promotes angiogenesis, invasion and metastasis	[137] [138] [139,140]	-	- - -
Liver	Induces PTTG1, which in turn upregulates c-myc Promotes proliferation and metastasis in HCC through p38 MAPK, Erk1/2 and β-catenin Promotes resistance to the adaptive immune response through PD-L1 and PD-L2	[141] [143–145] [146]	In combination with IFN-γ showed reduction of liver tumors - -	[142] - -
Melanoma	Induces cell invasion and metastasis Increases aggressiveness	[74,76] [75]	Reduces tumor growth Apoptosis	[147,148] [149]
Hematological	Cell survival Promotes progression through the NF-κB pathway and proliferation thorugh GM-CSF Promotes cell survival in Burkitt's lymphoma through reverse signaling - - - -	[150–152] [81,155,156] [157] - - - -	Apoptosis thorugh TNFR1, iNOS and PKC Increases efficacy of anti-CD20 therapy Induces maturation of AML generating specific cytotoxic CD8+ lymphocytes targeting leukemic disease Activate B cells to fight again lymphoma cells Combined with IL-1 and IFN-γ has an antiproliferative effect Participates in the crosstalk between DC and NK cells Promotes cell death in Burkitt's lymphoma through forward signaling	[153,154] [82] [158] [159] [160] [161] [157]

TGFβ: Transforming Growth Factor beta; EMT: epithelial-to-mesenchymal transition; p38MAPK: p38 Mitogen-Activated Protein Kinase; PTTG1: Pituitary Tumor Transforming Gene 1; IFN-γ: Interferon gamma; HCC: hepatocellular carcinoma; PD-L1: Programmed Death Ligand 1; PD-L2: Programmed Death Ligand 2; iNOS: Inducible Nitric Oxide Synthase; PKC: Protein Kinase C; GM-CSF: Granulocyte-Macrophage Colony-Stimulating Factor; AML: Acute Myeloid Leukemia; DC: dendritic cells; NK: natural killer cells.

Comprehensively, the data presented in this section point to the central role of TNFα in cancer initiation, progression, and metastasis, despite its potential to activate cell death when present in high concentrations. A plethora of accumulated evidence highlights TNFα as a pro-tumoral cytokine, which stresses its appeal as a potential target to treat different cancers.

5. Immunotherapy Overview

The concept of using immune response specificity to target cancer cells has been investigated for a long time and has given rise to different strategies. So-called passive immunotherapy is based on the administration of antibodies or adoptive cell therapy, including chimeric antigen receptor (CAR)-T cells. Active immunotherapy, on the other hand, relies on several approaches, including the use of cancer vaccines, which can, for example, enhance antigen uptake and presentation, and the administration of antibodies that release the brakes of the immune response, known as immune checkpoint inhibitors. TNFα participation in these immunotherapies, either by hampering their success or mediating side effects, is discussed below and summarized in Table 2. For cancer vaccines, we refer to several recent reviews [162–164].

Table 2. Impact of anti-TNFα drugs in cancer immunotherapies.

IT	Target/Cell Type	Drug Name	Anti-TNFa	Effect on Cancer	Side Effects of IT	Ref.
Monoclonal antibodies	HER2	Trastuzumab	Etanercept	Overcomes trastuzumab resistance in HER2+ breast cancer	NT	[72]
			INB03	Overcomes trastuzumab resistance in HER2+ breast cancer	-	[165]
	CD20	Rituximab	Etanercept	Improves disease-related symptoms and increases OS in chronic lymphocytic leukemia patients	NT	[166,167]
	PD-1	anti-PD-1	Anti-TNFR1 or anti-TNFa	Prevents T lymphocytes exhaustion and death by anti PD-1 treatment in melanoma	Prevents immune-related adverse effect	[168]
		Pembrolizumab	Infliximab	NT	Treatement of immune-related adverse effects	[169–171]
	PD-1+ CTLA-4	anti-PD-1 + anti CTL-4	Etanercept	Improves antitumor effect of anti PD-1+ anti CTL-4 antibodies in colon cancer	Prevents immune-related adverse effect	[172]
	CTLA-4	Ipilimumab	Infliximab	NT	Treatement of immune-related adverse effects	[169,170, 173,174]
	PD-L1	Atezolizumab, duvalumab and avelumab	Infliximab	NT	Treatement of immune-related adverse effects	[170]
CAR-T cells	CD19	-	Etanercept	NT	Treatment of systemic inflammatory response syndrome	[175]

IT: immunotherapy; OS: overall survival; NT: not tested; TNFα: Tumor necrosis factor alpha; TNFR1: TNFα receptor 1; PD-1: programmed cell death protein 1; PD-L1: PD-ligand 1; CTLA-4: cytotoxic T-lymphocyte-associated protein 4; CAR-T cells: chimeric antigen receptor T cell.

5.1. Monoclonal Antibodies

The mAbs, widely used to treat cancer and inflammatory diseases, are either chimeric, humanized, or fully human mAbs [176–178]. In this section, we outline the different cancer therapies based on mAbs targeting cancer cells and, in the following section, the mAbs directed to immune checkpoints, highlighting the implications of combining them with TNFα blocking agents.

Anti-TNFα Drugs

The first attempts to target TNFα were made decades ago, with the understanding that this cytokine was the major mediator of inflammation and its deregulation was implicated in a variety of autoimmune diseases, such as rheumatoid arthritis (RA), multiple sclerosis, psoriasis, Crohn's disease, scleroderma, systemic lupus erythematosus, ankylosing spondylitis, and diabetes. The pro-inflammatory effects of TNFα are mediated mainly by the activation of the NF-κB pathway, which, in turn, promotes the transcription of inflammatory proteins, generating a positive feedback loop.

In several models of experimental metastasis in mice, both endogenous and exogenous administration of TNFα increased the development and number of metastatic lesions [179–181]. Additionally, TNFα is known to be a major inducer of chemokines [182] such as CCL2 and IL-6 in the TME, thus increasing monocyte and macrophage infiltration [183] as well as tumor growth and angiogenesis [184], respectively. On the other hand, increasing evidence has been accumulating about the positive impact of TNFα-blocking strategies in cancer treatment. Balkwill and collaborators demonstrated that neutralization of TNFα during early stages of skin carcinogenesis is sufficient to inhibit tumor formation and set the basis of the rationale of anti-TNFα therapy for cancer treatment [185]. Given the mentioned effects of TNFα, several blocking agents have been developed against it for use in the clinical setting. In this review, we will address the well-known etanercept, infliximab, and adalimumab and the new blocking agent, INB03.

Etanercept is a fusion protein that consists of two extracellular portions of human TNFR2 linked to the Fc portion of human immunoglobulin 1 (IgG1) [19] and exerts its anti-inflammatory properties by competitively binding sTNFα and tmTNFα, preventing their interaction with their receptors and therefore inhibiting the activation of important inflammatory pathways. Its use in cancer is limited and certainly poorly explored. Kai Sha and collaborators proved that a TNFα–CCL2 paracrine loop is induced in response to androgen deprivation therapy with enzalutamide in prostate cancer patients and might account for some forms of prostate cancer therapy resistance. Moreover, they showed that TNFα inhibition with etanercept in castration-resistant prostate cancer cells blocked enzalutamide-induced CCL2 protein secretion and mRNA expression. These data suggest that TNFα blockade would be a suitable therapy combined with androgen deprivation therapy in prostate cancer patients with primary tumors prior to the onset of castration-resistant prostate cancer and metastasis [186]. Almost two decades ago, etanercept was evaluated in a phase II clinical trial on patients with advanced metastatic breast cancer [187] who had shown incomplete or partial response, and a decrease in TNFα and CCL2 concentration in plasma samples was shown. A phase I trial assessing the clinical benefit of infliximab in patients with advanced cancer also reported no objective responses (either complete or partial). However, several patients achieved disease stabilization, which correlated with undetectable TNFα, CCL2, and IL-6 plasma levels [188]. These trials highlighted the need to further explore the use of TNFα-blocking agents in combination with radiotherapy and chemotherapy for advanced cancer treatment, yet scarce progress has been made in this direction.

Another TNFα blocking agent is the chimeric human-murine mAb infliximab, initially approved by the FDA in 1999 to treat patients with Crohn's disease who failed to respond to conventional therapy. Its structure consists of human constant regions and murine variable regions that specifically bind to human TNFα [189]. Like etanercept, this mAb binds both sTNFα and tmTNFα molecules and interferes with their activity. Moreover, the drug lyses cells bearing tmTNFα. However, infliximab contains 25% murine sequences in its structure, leading to the secretion of human anti-infliximab antibodies, which generates adverse reactions or a gradually increasing lack of efficacy [190].

The beneficial use of mAbs against TNFα has also been demonstrated in ovarian cancer xenografts; treatment of tumor-bearing mice with infliximab twice a week for 4 weeks resulted in reduced tumor burden, a significantly decreased proportion of infiltrating macrophages, and a marked reduction of IL-6 in the TME [191]. The authors suggested that targeting predominant cytokines like TNFα in the TME would be more useful in combination with conventional chemotherapy regimens or treatments that target malignant cells directly, and better tolerated as well, than simply addressing tumor cells with targeted therapy.

Another way in which this pro-inflammatory cytokine can orchestrate the TME in ovarian cancer was described by Charles and collaborators, who demonstrated that TNFα is able to bind to TNFR1 and maintain the production of IL-17 in CD4+ leukocytes [116]. This sustained TNFR1-dependent IL-17 production and secretion leads to recruitment of the myeloid cell population to the TME and increased tumor growth [116]. These data were confirmed after blocking TNFα with infliximab in a mouse model of ovarian cancer and were also consistent with clinical results; patients with advanced ovarian cancer treated with infliximab exhibited substantially reduced plasma and ascitic levels of IL-17. Additionally, the authors found an association between high activation of TNFα signaling and expression of genes related to Th17 cell activation and expansion [116]. Unfortunately, some tumor types showed no benefit from the combination regime of the gold standard with TNFα blocking agents. Such is the case with advanced renal cell carcinoma (RCC), where phase I and II clinical trials demonstrated that the combined administration of sorafenib and infliximab, whose acceptable safety and tolerability were duly reported, was not more efficient than sorafenib alone [192]. In line with these data, recent results indicate that TNFα pathway activation would play a crucial role in resistance to tyrosine kinase inhibitors (TKIs) in patients with clear RCC [193]. Moreover, the authors suggest that TNFR1 could be a predictive biomarker for patient responsiveness to TKI treatment since it is augmented in TKI-resistant RCC tumors. In addition, the potential antitumor activity of infliximab has been reported in advanced RCC patients who progressed on cytokine therapy [194,195]. Therefore, a combination using infliximab or other TNFα inhibitors still holds promise as a therapeutic strategy for patients with RCC.

Adalimumab is a fully human recombinant mAb that binds and neutralizes both TNFα isoforms. Moreover, this mAb also induces apoptosis in immune cells bearing TNFα receptors. It was first approved by the FDA in 2008 for psoriasis treatment, but it is currently used in many other inflammatory diseases, such as RA, ankylosing spondylitis, Crohn's disease, ulcerative colitis and certain types of uveitis [196]. Its role in clinical oncology is not certain, but there is evidence that proves its efficacy in inhibiting TNFα tumor-promoting properties. In colorectal cancer cells, treatment with adalimumab hindered the induction of the Metastasis-Associated in Colon Cancer 1 (MACC1), a crucial oncogene that promotes cell proliferation, motility, and survival, increasing metastasis in preclinical models [197]. The authors proved that the expression of MACC1 in inflamed tissues from ulcerative colitis and Crohn's disease patients is upregulated by TNFα through NF-κB signaling pathway, via TNFR1, which lead to an increase in cell migration. These effects were abolished using anti-TNFR1 antibodies or adalimumab, suggesting a potential role of this mAb in MACC1 driven colorectal tumors. Moreover, adalimumab has demonstrated a high efficacy to delay the acquisition of the senescence associated secretory phenotype (SASP) in endothelial cells, which is strictly related to inflammation and cancer progression [198]. Treatment of HUVEC cells with adalimumab generated a decrease in the release of the SASP marker IL-6, together with an upregulation of eNOS, indicating an enhanced endothelial function. Interestingly, TNFα inhibition by adalimumab in senescent endothelial cells diminished the tumor-promoting and pro-metastatic properties of their conditioned medium since the authors observed a decreased migration rate and mammospheres formation of MCF-7 breast cancer cells in the presence of such senescent secretome. These data highlight the potential role of adalimumab in restraining the SASP and delaying the consequent age-related diseases onset and progression in patients with a chronic inflammation background.

Etanercept, infliximab and adalimumab are based on the structure and function of mAbs, but there are other approaches to neutralize this cytokine. An example is INB03, a dominant-negative TNFα biologic that selectively neutralizes sTNFα without affecting the tmTNFα variant [199]. INB03 consists of a sTNFα mutant that forms inactive heterotrimers with the native cytokine. This differential blockade of TNFα isoforms is critical for activating the immune system in cancer patients, since it is known that the tmTNFα–TNFR2 interaction is necessary for the crosstalk between DC and NK cells, which does not depend on the sTNFα-TNFR1 axis [200–202]. This crosstalk acts as an immunomodulatory mechanism inducing an increase in Th1-type cytokines and promotes antitumor response [203]. There is evidence, including results from our own team, that confirms the pivotal role of sTNFα in the recruitment and expansion of MDSCs in the tumor bed, generating immunosuppression and favoring tumor progression [71,165,200]. Sobo-Vujanovic and collaborators proved that selectively blocking sTNFα with INB03 reduced tumor incidence and growth rate in mice with chemically induced carcinogenesis, compared to MCA-injected mice treated with etanercept or with vehicle [200]. Moreover, the authors demonstrated that wild-type mice and TNFR2 knockout mice treated with MCA exhibited significantly higher tumor incidence and poorer survival than TNFR1 knockout mice. These results suggest that sTNFα is the one that drives tumor progression and is critical for MCA-induced carcinogenesis, while tmTNFα is dispensable for tumor growth but has a pivotal role in immune system activation and promotion of its antitumor activity. In addition, they propose that tmTNFα could have a protective role in cancer and should therefore not be inhibited during treatment regimens [200]. These data place INB03 as the most appealing treatment option to block TNFα and avoid compromising the immune system in order to mount an antitumor response.

5.2. Monoclonal Antibodies Targeting Cancer Cells

5.2.1. HER2

HER2 tyrosine kinase receptor is overexpressed in 13–20% of human breast cancer cases and in 60% of metastases to bone and is associated with poor outcome. Additionally, it is amplified in 80% and 12% of urinary bladder and ovarian tumors, respectively, as well as in pancreatic adenocarcinoma and gastric cancer [204,205]. Moreover, when small-cell lung cancer (SCLC) cells acquire chemoresistance, HER2 is frequently upregulated and acts as a biomarker of poor prognosis in advanced cases [206–208]. As it constitutes an interesting target for directed therapy, several mAbs have been developed against it.

Trastuzumab is a humanized mAb that recognizes the fourth domain of the extracellular region of HER2 [177] and was approved in 1998 by the FDA as the first mAb for solid tumors, particularly for breast cancer treatment. We have also demonstrated that blockade of tmTNFα and sTNFα with etanercept downregulates the membrane glycoprotein mucin 4 (MUC4) expression and overcomes trastuzumab de novo or acquired resistance in HER2+MUC4+ breast cancer cells and xenografts. Moreover, we disclosed that it is sTNFα and not tmTNFα that drives MUC4 expression; we observed that HER2+MUC4+ breast cancer cells and tumors were also sensitized to trastuzumab in combination with INB03 [165]. TNFα blockade overcomes trastuzumab resistance in HER2+ breast cancer tumors not only by downregulating MUC4 expression, but also by transforming the TME to a less immunosuppressive state, characterized by increased NK cell activation and degranulation, a higher M1/M2 ratio, and decreased MDSC infiltration [71]. Tumor heterogeneity poses an immense challenge, which is why current therapeutic research is intended to develop several strategies to tackle HER2. sTNFα is certainly an interesting target for HER2+ breast cancer, and its combination with HER2 blocking agents should be further investigated to offer better treatment for patients.

T-DM1 is an antibody–drug conjugate (ADC) that combines trastuzumab with maytansine, a cytotoxic agent that inhibits microtubule polymerizationT-DM1 has also shown efficacy in women with progressive disease as second-line HER2-targeted therapy for metastatic breast cancer [209]. Results from our team demonstrate that TNFα expression and secretion by tumor cells is implicated in the resistance of HER2+ breast cancer cells to T-DM1 therapy by the upregulation of MUC4 [72].

5.2.2. EGFR/HER1

It is common knowledge that chemokines play a substantial role in cancer progression and metastasis, as they regulate cell migration in and out of the TME, among other cellular processes that promote metastasis formation [210,211]. TNFα has been implicated in the transactivation of EGFR signaling to promote survival of colon epithelial cells [212]. It has been demonstrated that TNFα signaling, through its receptors, stimulates EGFR phosphorylation and promotes cellular proliferation, migration, and survival [213,214], and both TNFα and EGF can induce expression and secretion of cyclooxygenase 2 (COX-2), a prostaglandin synthase implicated in several biologic responses through prostaglandins [215,216]. Chronically elevated COX-2 levels correlate with increased risk for colorectal adenocarcinomas, and the use of chronic nonsteroidal anti-inflammatory drugs and administration of TNFα blocking antibodies have been associated with a decreased risk of developing colorectal cancer [217,218]. In this respect, it has been demonstrated that the induction of COX-2 expression by TNFα in gastrointestinal epithelial cells is dependent on TNFα-induced EGFR transactivation, promoting cell survival and proliferation. Furthermore, it has been elucidated that COX-2 expression is driven by the TNFR1 signaling pathway and not by TNFR2, by means of an EGFR-, Src-, and MAPK-dependent mechanism. These results add to accumulating evidence in favor of a critical role of sTNFα in colorectal cancer, which should be addressed by TNFα-blocking agents [191].

Interestingly, it has recently been demonstrated that in several ovarian cancer cell lines, cytokines like CCL20, CXCL1-3, and CXCL8 are the primary cytokines induced by EGFR activation or TNFα, through the NF-κB and PI3K-Akt signaling pathways [219], indicating that TNFα could be a suitable target in ovarian cancer. We speculate that it would be beneficial for patients with EGFR+ ovarian tumors that secrete TNFα to consider a combination regime of anti-EGFR mAb, like cetuximab, and TNFα blocking agents. Considering all the above, it seems that TNFα is the driving force of the increased expression of pro-inflammatory cytokines in several cancer types and that it promotes this increase by transactivating the EGFR molecule and the consequent autocrine and paracrine loop with its ligands, EGF and TGFα. These data suggest the potential use of TNFα blocking agents in combination with anti-EGFR therapies to overcome resistance and target the pro-inflammatory and tumor promoting TME for better outcomes for said patients.

5.2.3. CD20

It is known that TNFα inhibits CLL cell death by upregulating Bcl-2, among other antiapoptotic proteins, while it increases the proliferation of malignant cells [220]. In addition, TNFα is one of the main cytokines released as part of the toxicity in CLL patients receiving weekly treatment with rituximab [221,222].

Several clinical trials have been carried out to test the potential improvement of the anti-CD20 mAb rituximab treatment in combination with TNFα blocking agents, such as etanercept. Administration of etanercept has been shown to be safe in patients with CLL and other hematologic malignancies, whose disease-related symptoms also improved [166]. Particularly, in a phase I/II clinical trial, Woyach and collaborators showed that 75% of patients treated with rituximab in combination with etanercept exhibited a response, either complete or partial (29%), or had stable disease (56%) and did not require further treatment for 12 months after trial completion [167]. Moreover, the combination of rituximab and etanercept showed increased OS in responder patients, suggesting an improved outcome when compared to historical cytotoxic agent-based therapies. Furthermore, the addition of anti-TNFα mAb mitigated the toxicity of rituximab treatment [167]. The authors claimed that this combination regime would benefit fludarabine-refractory patients and people who are not eligible for more aggressive therapy, such as chemoimmunotherapy or rituximab alone, due to their high infusion toxicity.

Another fact that favors the study of TNFα in hematologic malignancies is that TNFα concentration is higher in the serum of patients with progressive CLL compared to healthy donors or patients with indolent disease [223]. Furthermore, it has been identified that TNFα overproduction in progressive CLL patients and CLL mouse models induces a decrease of plasmacytoid dendritic cells (pDCs), an immune cell population crucial for antiviral immunity and antitumor responses. The reduction in number and functionality of pDCs causes impaired INFα production due to the decreased expression of FMS-like tyrosine kinase 3 receptor (Flt3) and Toll-like receptor 9 (TLR9). This effect was reverted when splenocytes from progressing CLL mice were treated with anti-TNFα mAbs, upon which increased pDC numbers and restored Flt3 expression were observed [223]. Similar results, along with reduced splenic tumor burden and increased splenic pDCs, were obtained by injection of anti-TNFα mAbs in mice with progressive CLL compared to control mice. In addition, anti-TNFα therapy promoted an increase in serum IFNα production and augmented CD8+ T lymphocytes [223]. Blocking TNFα may be a potential strategy for immune reactivation in CLL patients. These results confirm the role of TNFα in CLL and the importance of addressing this pro-inflammatory cytokine as a therapeutic target in combination regimes with targeted therapies such as rituximab or standard cytotoxic agents like chemotherapy.

5.3. Monoclonal Antibodies against Immune Checkpoints

One of the shutdown mechanisms that are triggered after T lymphocyte activation operates through checkpoint inhibitors. The most well-known checkpoints in the context of cancer immunotherapy are CTLA-4 and programmed cell death protein 1 (PD-1, CD279), which are transmembrane molecules expressed by T lymphocytes after their activation. CTLA-4 binds to CD80 (B7-1) and CD86 (B7-2) expressed in DC, and PD-1 interacts with PD-ligand 1 (PD-L1, CD274) present in T lymphocytes, B lymphocytes, APCs, and tissues with immunological tolerance such as placenta and pancreatic islets, and with PD-L2 (CD273), expressed in APCs, thus mediating T lymphocytesinhibition [224–228]. Both immune checkpoints are hijacked by cancer cells, which promote CTLA-4 induction in T lymphocytes and induce PD-L1 expression in tumor cells as a mechanism of immune evasion. Thus, the interest in preventing CTLA-4/CD80/86 and PD-1/PD-L1 interactions derived in the development of antibodies against them as T cell-targeted immunomodulators [229,230] whose action is based on reinvigoration of the antitumor immune response. The impressive clinical benefit of this strategy, obtained first in melanoma patients [231], triggered a large number of clinical trials for the treatment of almost all types of cancer (Table S1).

There is plenty of evidence that TNFα upregulates PD-L1 expression in several cancer types. In prostate cancer cell lines HCT116 and LNCaP, TNFα increase PD-L1 mRNA and protein expression. In the case of LNCaP cells [232], the pathways involved in PD-L1 upregulation, dependent on ERK1/2 activation in HCT116 and in Akt and NF-κB. In ovarian cancer cell lines HO8910 and SKOV3, it was demonstrated that TAMs or cytokines released from them, like IFN-γ, TNFα, IL-10, and IL-6, are responsible for the upregulation of PD-L1 expression in the surface of these cells, but no modification in its mRNA was observed. The increase in PD-L1 levels produced by IFN-γ and TNFα was due to the activation of PI-3K and ERK1/2 pathways, respectively. In a preclinical model, treatment with anti-PD-1 or anti-PD-L1 was able to inhibit SKOV3 tumor growth [233] and was associated with decreased PD-1+ CD8+ T lymphocytes infiltration. A study demonstrated a progressive increase in PD-L1 levels ranging from immature bone marrow monocytes in tumor to circulating monocytes and to tumor tissue macrophages, the latter exhibiting the highest expression.

TNFα has been identified as the cytokine present in tumor-conditioned medium from B16 melanoma cells and 4T1 breast cancer cells that causes upregulation of PD-L1 in monocytes. In addition, tumor cells secrete versican, which stimulates TNFα production by monocytes via activation of TLR2 [234]. The role of adipocytes in PD-L1 expression was also addressed. Using an obese mouse model, it was demonstrated that B16-F10 melanomas and Hep-G2 hepatomas grew faster in the treated mice than in control animals, which was correlated with PD-L1 expression in cancer cells. Conditioned medium of adipocytes was able to increase PD-L1 levels due to the presence of TNFα and IL-6, both regulating the NF-κB and STAT3 pathways (Figure 1) [235].

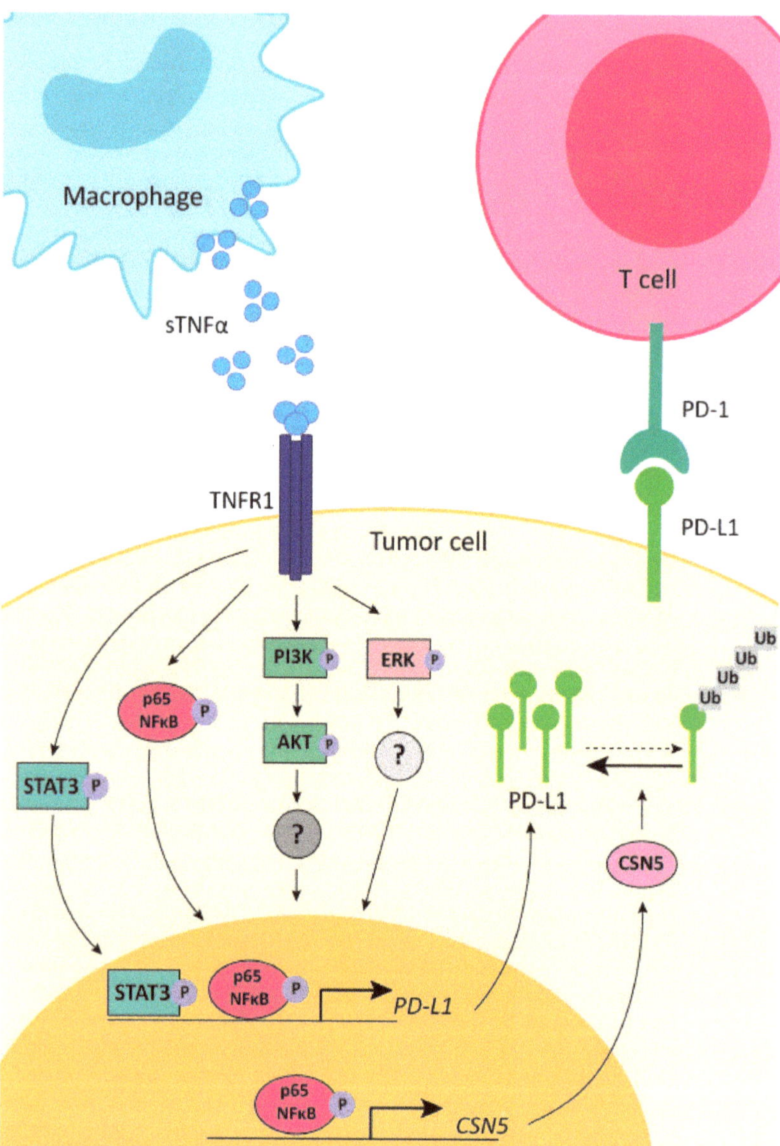

Figure 1. Tumor necrosis factor alpha (TNFα) modulates programmed death ligand 1 (PD-L1) expression transcriptionally and post-transcriptionally. TNFα, acting through TNFα receptor 1 (TNFR1), activates extracellular signal-regulated kinase (ERK) and phosphatidylinositol-3-kinase (PI-3K/AKT) pathways and nuclear factor kappa B (NF-κB) and signal transducer and activator of transcription 3 (STAT3) transcription factors that promote PD-L1 gene transcription. In addition, NF-κB also induces transcription of the deubiquitinase COP9 signalosome 5 (CSN5), which promotes PD-L1 protein stability. Ub: ubiquitin, sTNFα: soluble TNFα.

In addition, PD-L1 expression induced by TNFα was also proved in gastric cancer, where mast cell infiltration was directly related to its progression and reduced overall survival. A direct correlation was demonstrated between PD-L1+ mast cells and TNFα in gastric cancer specimens. TNFα secreted from gastric cancer cells induces PD-L1 expression in mast cells via activation of the NF-κB signaling pathway [236]. It was recently demonstrated that PD-L1 expression in gastric cancer was dependent on TNFα and IL-6 produced by infiltrating macrophages. These cytokines promote PD-L1 expression through the activation of NF-κB and STAT3 signaling [237]. Similar findings were observed in pancreatic cancer, where TNFα was the macrophage-secreted cytokine responsible for upregulation of PD-L1 in pancreatic ductal adenocarcinoma cells. In pancreatic cancer specimens, PD-L1 expression in tumor cells directly correlated with macrophage infiltration and poor survival [115].

PD-L1 expression can also be regulated at the posttranscriptional level. Seminal work by Hung's lab demonstrated that TNFα can increase PD-L1 expression in breast cancer cells by posttranscriptional regulation. TNFα stabilizes PD-L1 protein by inducing the expression of the deubiquitinating enzyme COP9 signalosome 5 (CSN5) via NF-κB activation. This PD-L1 stabilization by TNFα also affects dendritic and T lymphocytes, inducing an immunosuppressive response (Figure 1) [238].

5.4. TNFα in Resistance to Anti-PD-1/PD-L1 and Anti-CTLA-4 Therapies

Several antibodies were designed to interfere with the PD-1/PD-L1 interaction and have been approved by the FDA for the treatment of different types of cancer at different stages (Table S1). These are the anti-PD-1 antibodies nivolumab, pembrolizumab, cemiplimab, and sintinimab and the anti-PD-L1 antibodies atezolizumab, durvalumab, and avelumab. In addition, CTLA-4 was effectively targeted by ipilimumab. Nivolumab, cemiplimab, sintinimab, avelumab, and ipilimumab are human monoclonal antibodies, while pembrolizumab, atezolizumab, and durvalumab are humanized monoclonal antibodies. The impressive clinical impact of these antibodies in the oncology arena was recognized by the 2018 Nobel Prize in Physiology or Medicine awarded to Dr. James Allison (MD Anderson Cancer Center at the University of Texas, Houston, TX, USA) and Dr. Tasuku Honjo (Kyoto University, Kyoto, Japan), for their contributions to the research on CTLA-4 and PD-1, respectively [239]. However, some patients exhibit resistance to anti-immune checkpoint treatment, depending on their cancer type and stage. Here, we highlight TNFα involvement in treatment failure based on immune checkpoint blockade.

In a preclinical melanoma model, TNFα, acting through TNFR1, impaired the infiltration of CD8+T lymphocytes into the TME and promoted their activation-induced cell death, facilitating tumor growth [77]. In addition, TNFR1 blockade improved the efficacy of anti-PD-1 treatment. Preventing TNFα upregulation of PD-L1 and TIM-3 expression by CD8+ tumor infiltrating lymphocytes (TILs) causes reinvigoration of the antitumor immune response, consequently overcoming anti-PD-1 resistance (Figure 2). These findings were validated using TCGA melanoma data, where a direct correlation was observed between TNFα and an immune escape signature, particularly with genes encoding PD-L1, PD-L2, and TIM-3 [168].

In an experimental melanoma, it was determined that anti-CTLA-4 treatment increased the production of TNFα associated with T lymphocytes infiltration, which in turn upregulated Ezh2, silencing tumor cell immunogenicity and antigen presentation. The inhibition of Ezh2 improved the effectiveness of anti-CTLA-4 and IL-2 immunotherapy [240].

The metabolic status of the tumor also conditions the efficacy of PD-L1 antibodies. In NSCLC, it was found that TNFα-induced aerobic glycolysis of TAMs was associated with tumor hypoxia in preclinical and clinical settings. TAM depletion facilitates the upregulation of PD-L1 in tumor cells, which can then be effectively targeted by anti-PD-L1 antibodies [241]. In addition, NSCLC patients with increased IFN-γ, TNFα, IL-1β, IL-2, IL-4, IL-5, IL-6, IL-8, IL-10, and IL-12 serum levels at diagnosis and at 3 months post initiation of anti-PD-1 treatment exhibited longer OS [242]. Determination of these cytokines was proposed as a biomarker of patient selection for anti-PD-1 treatment.

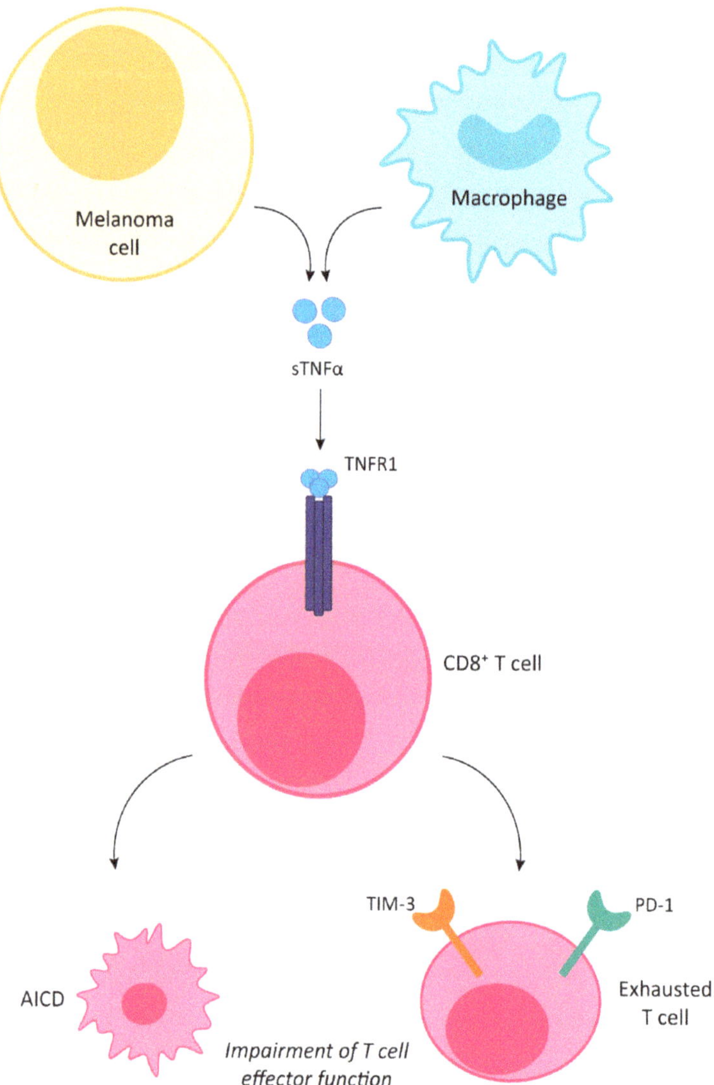

Figure 2. TNFα induces anti-immune checkpoint therapy resistance acting on CD8+ T lymphocytes. TNFα, produced by either tumor cells or macrophages from the tumor microenvironment, induces activation-induced cell death (AICD) and exhaustion of CD8+ T lymphocytes, impairing the effectiveness of anti-immune checkpoint therapy. TIM3: T-cell immunoglobulin and mucin-domain containing-3.

5.5. TNFα Involvement in the Adverse Effects of Immune Checkpoint Inhibitors

Releasing the brakes of the immune system through immune checkpoint blockade can trigger nonspecific immunologic activation that resembles autoimmune disease. These secondary effects, known as immune-related adverse effects (irAEs), can compromise the liver and skin (rash, pruritus, and vitiligo) and the endocrine (hypophysitis, hypothyroidism, and thyroiditis) and gastrointestinal (diarrhea and colitis) systems, among others [243]. About 50% of patients treated with anti-immune checkpoint therapy experienced some form of irAE and 20% suffered grade 3 or 4 toxicity, limiting the implementation of this treatment [244–246]. irAEs sometimes lead to discontinuation of treatment or administration of corticosteroids or other immunosuppressive agents or TNFα antagonists [169–171,173,174]. The combination of anti-CTLA-4 and anti-PD-1 or PD-L1 antibodies is now more frequently used because of its increased clinical benefit compared to monotherapy regimens [247], but it also increases the severity of irAEs.

While in several cancers, such as lung and bladder cancer, there is an association between clinical benefit and irAEs, in melanoma the results are contradictory. In melanoma, the presence of irAEs does not guarantee tumor response, whereas the absence of side effects can be accompanied by clinical benefit [248,249]. In this respect, Perez-Ruiz et al., using melanoma and colon carcinoma models, demonstrated that the combined administration of anti-CTLA-4 and anti-PD-1 antibodies with anti-TNFα or etanercept reduced colitis and hepatitis in mice [172]. Importantly, they also showed that TNFα blockade enhanced the antitumor effect of immune checkpoint inhibitor treatment in melanoma and colon cancer, revealing that TNFα mediates irAEs [172]. This is an important piece of evidence indicating that preventing irAEs with TNF blocking agents allows the antitumor effect of immune checkpoint blockade.

Another work analyzed the effect of anti-TNFα treatment concomitant with or after anti-CTL-4 administration on irAEs and the antitumor effect. Results showed that although the antitumor effect on breast and colon cancer models of anti-CD40 decreased, the most suitable combination was simultaneous rather than delayed treatment with anti-TNFα administration. In this way, irAEs were prevented [250]. In the clinical setting, a recent report on patients from the Dutch Melanoma Treatment Registry showed that those treated with ipilimumab and anti-PD1 with severe irAEs had longer survival. However, treatment with infliximab blunted this clinical benefit [251]. Using large cohorts of 225,090 and 188,420 patients with Crohn's disease or ulcerative colitis, respectively, it was demonstrated that those treated with anti-TNFα agents were less likely to develop colorectal cancer. Further studies in different cancer types are needed to define the clinical benefit of TNFα blockade in terms of dose and administration in patients undergoing anti-immune checkpoint treatment [252].

5.6. Adoptive Cell Therapies

The development of ACTs has increased greatly in the last four years. Hundreds of new cell therapies have been added since 2017, quadrupling in 2020. Even in the current year, despite the COVID-19 pandemic, the number of cellular therapies has outgrown that of all existing types of immunotherapy [253].

In recent years, many advances have been made in immunotherapy for ALL [254]. ACTs have been developed with CAR-T cells, which consist of genetically modified T lymphocytes obtained from patients themselves, resulting in cells that combine an extracellular antigen-binding domain with one or more intracellular T lymphocytes signaling domains, leading to the activation of T lymphocytes and finally the elimination of lymphoblasts. In other words, these modified T lymphocytes are redirected to target specific antigens on the surface of lymphoblasts [255–257]. The CD19 antigen is a transmembrane protein expressed in all cells of the B lineage and is thus an attractive target for CAR-T cell therapy toward ALL B lymphoblasts [258,259]. Indeed, in 2017 the FDA approved an anti-CD19 CAR-T called CTL019 for the treatment of B cell ALL that is refractory to treatment or for second or later relapse of patients up to 25 years of age. The future of ACTs with CAR-T cells for B cell ALL is promising. Currently, various groups are working on addressing different targets such as CD22 for patients with CD19 negative relapses, optimizing the dose of CAR-T cells, and standardizing the management of neurological toxicity and systemic inflammatory response syndrome (SIRS) [254].

SIRS is the most common toxicity associated with CAR-T cell therapies. SIRS is generated due to the release of proinflammatory cytokines such as IL-6, IL-10, and IFN-γ (and possibly TNF-α and IL-1α) after the activation of CAR-T cells. SIRS causes symptoms that range from myalgia, fever, and flu-like symptoms to capillary leak, vascular collapse, pulmonary edema, coagulopathy, and multiple organ failure [260]. Another highly unwanted possible adverse effect of CAR-T cell infusion is anaphylactic shock [261]. Treatment of

SIRS still remains challenging, and management is not well established. Corticosteroids have been used to treat severe SIRS with some success, but such treatment may interfere with the efficacy of CAR-T cell therapy itself [262]. Other anti-inflammatory agents have also been proposed, such as the IL-1 receptor antagonist anakinra or etanercept [175].

A barrier to ACTs in solid tumors is the formation of abnormal blood vessels, which hinders tumor infiltration of T lymphocytes [263]. Hypoxia can lead to the formation of new, tortuous, and leaky vessels, thus generating irregular blood flow and increased interstitial tumor pressure. Furthermore, endothelial cells fail to express leukocyte adhesion molecules correctly, an event known as endothelial anergy [264]. Therefore, crossing the abnormal endothelial barrier and interstitium in solid tumors is a major obstacle for cells of the immune system and CAR-T cell therapy [265]. This may also explain the resistance of some solid tumors to immune checkpoint inhibitors [266,267]. It has been shown that minimizing the amount of TNFα targeting the vascular endothelium with Cys-Asn-Gly-Arg-Cys-Gly-TNFα (NGR-TNF), a fusion protein targeting the tumor vasculature [147], can activate the endothelial cells and enhance tumor infiltration by cytotoxic T lymphocytes [268]. This approach has also been shown to enhance ACT with TCR redirected T lymphocytes [269]. Based on this, Elia et al. proposed using low doses of TNFα directed toward the tumor vasculature in association with ACT, which may represent a novel strategy to improve the infiltration of T cells in solid tumors and overcome the resistance to CAR-T cells and anti-immune checkpoint inhibitor therapy [263].

Anti-cancer ACT with tumor-specific cytotoxic T lymphocytes has been well documented in animal models, where infusion of modified T lymphocytes into mice resulted in tumor eradication [270–272]. The results of Ye et al. show that cytotoxic T lymphocytes transfected with adenovirus genetically modified to express TNFα, cytotoxicity, and survival of lymphocytes were improved [273]. Furthermore, ACT induces long-term antitumor immunity by generating memory T lymphocytes after ACT. Therefore, cytotoxic T lymphocytes designed to secrete TNFα may be useful when designing strategies for ACT in solid tumors [273].

Induction of antitumor immunity by DC vaccines correlates with their maturation stage. TNFα appears to have profound effects on DC function, as it contributes to activation [274], maturation [275], subsequent migration and accumulation in lymph nodes [276], and significantly reduces inhibition of these processes mediated by IL-10 [277]. Based on this, and the previously mentioned characteristics of TNFα as an antitumor cytokine, Liu et al. proposed the use of combination immunotherapy [278]. Gene therapy with adenoviruses expressing TNFα and DC vaccines genetically modified to overexpress TNFα were used to treat well-established tumors in animal models. The modified DCs stimulated cytotoxic T lymphocytes in vitro and in vivo and produced more efficient antitumor immune responses than wild-type DCs [278].

Lymphodepletion is a preconditioning strategy carried out by high-dose chemotherapy and is commonly used to increase the clinical efficacy of adoptive T cell therapy. Suppression of the host's immune system ensures that the transferred immune cells will be capable of surviving and proliferating, since they would otherwise be suppressed or deprived of key cytokines for their functioning [279]. However, as might be expected, this type of treatment can become highly toxic to patients, causing severe cytopenias [280,281]. In contrast, oncolytic adenoviruses are safer and, when engineered to express IL-2 and TNFα, can achieve lymphodepletion-like antitumor immunomodulatory effects [282]. When produced from these adenoviruses, IL-2 and TNFα can recruit NK and T lymphocytes into the tumor bed [283]. Studies in patients and mice revealed that toxicity was minimal. These findings demonstrate that ACT can be facilitated by adenoviruses that encode cytokines, thus avoiding lymphodepletion and its consequences [282].

In the case of melanoma, ACT with cytotoxic T lymphocytes that target melanocytic antigens can achieve remission in patients with metastatic melanomas, but tumors often relapse [284,285]. Landsberg et al. demonstrated that melanoma cells can resist ACT through a reversible dedifferentiation process in response to the inflammatory microenvironment induced by T lymphocytes [286]. TNFα secreted by macrophages induces dedifferentiation of human melanoma cells, leading to impaired recognition by cytotoxic T lymphocytes specific for melanocytic antigens. These results demonstrate that an inflammatory microenvironment is responsible for the phenotypic plasticity of melanoma cells, contributing to tumor relapse after initially successful T lymphocyte immunotherapy [286]. This inflammation-induced dedifferentiation mechanism from tumor cells to precursor cells was also shown in a case report of a 60-year-old male patient with metastatic melanoma who received specific ACT against the melanocytic antigen MART-1 and developed resistance to therapy in association with a dedifferentiated tumor phenotype lacking conventional melanocytic antigens [287]. In vitro assays showed that TNFα treatment led to dedifferentiation of tumor cells. The dedifferentiation process was proved to be reversible upon removal of inflammatory media from cultures. The RNA of different melanoma cell lines treated with TNFα was also sequenced, and it was seen that the pathways of dedifferentiation induced by inflammation may overlap with those of innate resistance to anti-PD-1 gene signature [288], which includes genes related to EMT transition, hypoxia, and angiogenesis, and suggests that dedifferentiation may reflect a more invasive phenotype. The data exposed here highlight the need to deepen studies of the underlying mechanisms of ACT resistance in humans [287].

6. Clinical Implications

The administration of anti-TNFα drugs was originally limited to inflammatory and autoimmune pathologies, where they proved to be beneficial for patients [289]. Nevertheless, about 40% of patients did not respond to anti-TNFα treatment [290]. The different anti-TNFα biologics show no differences in the treatment of inflammatory pathologies such as RA and spondyloarthritis [291]. Regarding treatment effectiveness, it has been shown that polymorphisms in the TNFα promoter or the gene region can predict response to TNFα inhibition therapy. Meta-analyses showed that TNFα -308 G and -238 G alleles predicted good response to anti-TNFα therapy, and this prediction was more powerful for etanercept than for infliximab in patients with spondyloarthritis [292] or refractory sarcoidosis. Regarding patients with psoriatic arthritis, another study found that the polymorphism in +489 A exhibited a trend of association with better response to etanercept [293].

One of the main concerns of anti-TNFα treatment is the increased risk of infection upon therapy administration, a matter extensively studied in patients with inflammatory diseases. In these patients, TNFα-blocking therapies are administered alone or in combination with disease-modifying anti-rheumatic drugs (DMARDs) [294–296]. Concerning opportunistic intracellular bacterial infections, tuberculosis (TB) is one of the most studied, since TNFα is responsible for the recruitment and effector function of neutrophils and lymphocytes to battle the infection [297,298]. It was shown that TNFα or TNFR1 knockout mice, as well as those treated with TNFα inhibitors, cannot fight TB infection [299]. There are controversial studies about the adverse effects of TNFα inhibitor administration [300]. While several works show no correlation between adverse effects and TNFα inhibitor treatment [301–303], a substantial number show the opposite [304–307]. These works underline the importance of appropriate TB screening before TNFα inhibitor administration. Similar results were found for L. monocytogenes infection [304]. Something similar also occurs in viral and fungal infections. While there are reports that show no correlation between herpes zoster infection and TNFα blockage [308], others show the opposite [304,309,310]. Other detrimental effects of TNFα inhibitors were described regarding the nervous system, with headache as the most common event. Other serious neurological events [311,312] were also reported: multiple sclerosis [313], central and peripheral demyelinating events, vasculitis, and transverse myelitis, among others [314–316]. Regarding cardiac disease, it was demonstrated that anti-TNFα therapy is injurious [317]. Surprisingly, TNFα inhibition can cause de novo disease or reactivation of inflammatory disease, such as psoriasis, arthritis, colitis, uveitis, etc. [318].

Given the mentioned pivotal role of TNFα in the immune system, another important concern regarding its blockade is related to cancer development. Numerous studies have addressed this issue in patients with inflammatory diseases. At present, there is increasing evidence that TNFα inhibition does not correlate with an augmented incidence of cancer [319–321], but there are a few reports that show the opposite [322], including two reports that indicate an elevated risk of hematological malignancies and nonmelanoma skin cancers in patients with RA [298,323]. It is noteworthy that these studies also claim that an increased risk of lymphoma is associated with RA regardless of the anti-TNFα therapy, which inhibits any conclusion regarding the treatment. Instead, more recent studies show that, plausibly, the underlying inflammation caused by the pathology is more likely to promote the development of malignancy than the therapy itself [321,324]. Moreover, they claim the treatment can have positive implications in preventing cancer. There is a study on inflammatory bowel disease in patients with a prior history of cancer showing that TNFα inhibition poses a mild risk of acquiring cancer. This report poses a conundrum, since it is an established fact that former cancer patients have a higher probability of developing new cancers, once again highlighting that the results cannot be ascribed to the anti-TNFα therapy. These data indicate that TNFα-blocking treatments should not be administered to patients with cancer in their clinical history [325].

There are limited reports in the field of cancer and TNFα inhibitors. Only one phase II clinical trial studied the effect of etanercept in breast cancer patients, and the results showed that there was no objective response to treatment, which could, however, be due to the advanced tumor stage of the cohort [187]. Polymorphisms in the TNFα gene have also been studied related to cancer incidence. In breast cancer, it was reported that the TNFα -308 G>A allele is associated with higher expression of TNFα, but no predisposition for any breast cancer subtype was found, although this polymorphism is associated with an increased risk of metastasis in triple-negative breast cancer [326]. Another study showed that the same polymorphism was correlated with vascular invasion in breast cancer [327], while another group found a possible association between the -308 G>A polymorphism and lower OS in cancer patients [328]. However, these polymorphisms could be meaningful regarding responsiveness to anti-TNFα therapy. The matter remains to be explored in cohorts of patients with malignancies receiving anti-TNFα treatment.

Various reports have acknowledged the pro-tumorigenic role of TNFR1, which indicates that hindering sTNFα action could be a potential new strategy to tackle cancer [37,329]. In this regard, it has been shown that targeting sTNFα prevents skin carcinogenesis [203] and overcomes trastuzumab resistance in HER2+ breast cancer [72].

Besides targeting TNFα, another interesting approach is the development of therapies directed to TNFRs. One of the strategies is based on the fact that soluble TNFRs (sTNFR) are immunosuppressive because they impede TNF-α activity. Therefore, a selective apheresis to remove sTNFRs from systemic circulation can release TNFα and reactivate an effective antitumor immune response. In the beginnings, the apheresis column contained anti-TNFR and antiIL-2R antibodies and the treatment was effective in reducing patient's tumor burden [330]. Now an improvement was achieved using single-chain TNFα as bait [331] and this strategy has shown to be effective in the treatment of canine cancers [332]. On the other hand, TNFR2 is expressed in Tregs and particularly in a subset that present the most immunosuppressive characteristics [333]. Tregs in general have been a potential target for cancer therapy [334], but delivery to the TME has been challenging [335]. TNFR2 induces activation of NF-κB and PI3K/Akt pathways, which finalizes in cell proliferation, augmenting the number of Tregs [336], positioning TNFR2 as an attractive target. In addition, MDSCs also express TNFR2 in mice, and their inhibition diminished metastasis in a liver cancer model [337]. Furthermore, TNFR2 expression has been proved in different cancers, such as RCC [338], colorectal cancer [339], Hodgkin's lymphoma [340], multiple myeloma [341], and ovarian cancer [342]. Interestingly, several studies show that tumors can escape immune checkpoint inhibitor therapy by upregulating TNFR2 expression in Tregs [343]. Moreover, TNFα/TNFR2 axis supports angiogenesis promoting VEGF secretion and neovascularization via endothelial colony forming cells [344]. Recently, it has been demonstrated that endothelial progenitor cells secrete immunosuppressive cytokines in a TNFR2-dependent manner and inhibit T lymphocytes proliferation [345]. All this evidence points to the need to develop TNFR2-targeted therapy to diminish tumor-infiltrating Tregs, to impair MDSCs differentiation and endothelial cell neovascularization and to directly attack TNFR2-expressing tumor cells. In this respect, Vanamee et al. postulated that TNFR2 inhibitors could be safer than immune checkpoint inhibitors for cancer treatment, given the restricted expression of the receptor [346]. TNFR2 antagonistic antibodies were successfully tested in the OVCAR3 preclinical model and proved to be effective in killing Tregs from ascites and ovarian cells [347]. Finally, an IgG2 antibody targeting TNFR2 proved to be effective in killing cancer cells in direct correlation to their TNFR2 expression density. It was also shown that this antibody modified the TME eliminating Tregs while preserving viability of effector T cells [348]. Therefore, a new horizon of specific treatment targeting immunosuppressive cells is open with anti-TNFR2 strategies.

7. Conclusions

The clinical relevance of TNFα to either fostering or hindering the success of immunotherapy has not yet been fully elucidated. In practice, however, the clinical application of anti-TNFα drugs to prevent irAEs produced by immune checkpoint inhibitors and ACTs has provided interesting results, showing that neutralizing this cytokine has potential antitumor benefit. In addition, several clinical trials have demonstrated the importance of TNFα blockade in prostate and renal cancer and in hematologic malignancies, as it promotes higher OS. Furthermore, there is plenty of preclinical evidence showing that TNFα is able to induce immunotherapy resistance. For example, TNFα can induce PD-L1 overexpression in a large variety of tumors, rendering an immunosuppressive TME, impairing inhibition of immune checkpoints, and inducing resistance to targeted therapies [72,165–168,172,232–238]. All of the above therefore suggest that the use of TNFα inhibitors should be considered as a novel strategy in cancer treatment, particularly in combination with the gold standard therapy for each particular cancer.

On the other hand, due to its potent antitumor activity, the production of TNFα by DC and cytotoxic T lymphocytes is important in ACT. In addition, the administration of a fusion protein of TNFα targeting tumor vessels can rescue their normal permeability and promote tumor infiltration by cytotoxic T lymphocytes, enhancing the effectiveness of immune checkpoint inhibitors.

In conclusion, the administration of TNFα-blocking agents emerges as a promising option in the oncology arena, but their combination with other therapies in specific tumor types needs to be further studied to attain optimal clinical results.

Supplementary Materials: The following are available online at https://www.mdpi.com/2072-6694/13/3/564/s1, Table S1: FDA approved drugs targeting PD-1, PD-L1 and CTLA-4 (current as November 2020).

Author Contributions: M.F.M. and P.V.E. wrote and edited the manuscript, S.B. wrote, revised the manuscript and prepared the figures, F.M. wrote, revised the manuscript and prepared the table, R.S. conceptualized, wrote, and edited the manuscript. All authors have read and agreed to the published version of the manuscript.

Funding: This work was supported by grants from National Cancer Institute (Argentina) 2018, IDB/PICT 2017-1517 and 2018-2086 from the National Agency of Scientific Promotion of Argentina (ANPCyT), Florencio Fiorini Foundation and Alberto J. Roemmers Foundation awarded to RS; a grant from Oncomed-Reno, CONICET 1819/03, awarded to PVE and RS; grants from National Cancer Institute (Argentina) 2018, IDB/PICT 2015-1587, IDB/PICT 2017-1587, from ANPCyT, PID 2012-066 from Consejo Nacional de InvestigacionesCientíficas y Técnicas and from the National Institute of Cancer from Argentina (Argentina) 2018-2019, all of them awarded to PVE. We are grateful to Fundación René Baron and Fundación Williams for their institutional support to IBYME-CONICET.

Conflicts of Interest: The authors declare no conflict of interest.

References

1. Coussens, L.M.L.M.; Werb, Z. Inflammation and Cancer. *Nature* **2002**, *420*, 860–867. [CrossRef]
2. Carswell, E.A.; Old, L.J.; Kassel, R.L.; Green, S.; Fiore, N.; Williamson, B. An Endotoxin-Induced Serum Factor That Causes Necrosis of Tumors. *Proc. Natl. Acad. Sci. USA* **1975**, *72*, 3666–3670. [CrossRef]
3. Green, S.; Dobrjansky, A.; Carswell, E.A.; Kassel, R.L.; Old, L.J.; Fiore, N.; Schwartz, M.K. Partial Purification of a Serum Factor That Causes Necrosis of Tumors. *Proc. Natl. Acad. Sci. USA* **1976**, *73*, 381–385. [CrossRef] [PubMed]
4. Pennica, D.; Nedwin, G.E.; Hayflick, J.S.; Seeburg, P.H.; Derynck, R.; Palladino, M.A.; Kohr, W.J.; Aggarwal, B.B.; Goeddel, D.V. Human Tumour Necrosis Factor: Precursor Structure, Expression and Homology to Lymphotoxin. *Nature* **1984**, *312*, 724–729. [CrossRef] [PubMed]
5. Falvo, J.V.; Tsytsykova, A.V.; Goldfeld, A.E. Transcriptional Control of the TNF Gene. *Curr. Dir. Autoimmun.* **2010**, *11*, 27–60. [CrossRef] [PubMed]
6. Tsai, E.Y.; Yie, J.; Thanos, D.; Goldfeld, A.E. Cell-Type-Specific Regulation of the Human Tumor Necrosis Factor Alpha Gene in B Cells and T Cells by NFATp and ATF-2/JUN. *Mol. Cell. Biol.* **1996**, *16*, 5232–5244. [CrossRef] [PubMed]
7. Gahring, L.C.; Carlson, N.G.; Kulmar, R.A.; Rogers, S.W. Neuronal Expression of Tumor Necrosis Factor Alpha in the Murine Brain. *Neuroimmunomodulation* **1996**, *3*, 289–303. [CrossRef]
8. Ranta, V.; Orpana, A.; Carpén, O.; Turpeinen, U.; Ylikorkala, O.; Viinikka, L. Human Vascular Endothelial Cells Produce Tumor Necrosis Factor-Alpha in Response to Proinflammatory Cytokine Stimulation. *Crit. Care Med.* **1999**, *27*, 2184–2187. [CrossRef]
9. Rydén, M.; Arner, P. Tumour Necrosis Factor-Alpha in Human Adipose Tissue-from Signalling Mechanisms to Clinical Implications. *J. Intern. Med.* **2007**, *262*, 431–438. [CrossRef]
10. Spriggs, D.R.; Deutsch, S.; Kufe, D.W. Genomic Structure, Induction, and Production of TNF-Alpha. *Immunol. Ser.* **1992**, *56*, 3–34.
11. Shakhov, A.N.; Collart, M.A.; Vassalli, P.; Nedospasov, S.A.; Jongeneel, C.V. Kappa B-Type Enhancers Are Involved in Lipopolysaccharide-Mediated Transcriptional Activation of the Tumor Necrosis Factor Alpha Gene in Primary Macrophages. *J. Exp. Med.* **1990**, *171*, 35–47. [CrossRef] [PubMed]
12. Qu, Y.; Zhao, G.; Li, H. Forward and Reverse Signaling Mediated by Transmembrane Tumor Necrosis Factor-Alpha and TNF Receptor 2: Potential Roles in an Immunosuppressive Tumor Microenvironment. *Front. Immunol.* **2017**, *8*. [CrossRef] [PubMed]
13. Kriegler, M.; Perez, C.; DeFay, K.; Albert, I.; Lu, S.D. A Novel Form of TNF/Cachectin Is a Cell Surface Cytotoxic Transmembrane Protein: Ramifications for the Complex Physiology of TNF. *Cell* **2018**, *53*, 45–53. [CrossRef]
14. Perez, C.; Albert, I.; DeFay, K.; Zachariades, N.; Gooding, L.; Kriegler, M. A Nonsecretable Cell Surface Mutant of Tumor Necrosis Factor (TNF) Kills by Cell-to-Cell Contact. *Cell* **1990**, *63*, 251–258. [CrossRef]
15. Tartaglia, L.A.; Weber, R.F.; Figari, I.S.; Reynolds, C.; Palladino, M.A., Jr.; Goeddel, D.V. The Two Different Receptors for Tumor Necrosis Factor Mediate Distinct Cellular Responses. *Proc. Natl. Acad. Sci. USA* **1991**, *88*, 9292–9296. [CrossRef]
16. Ledgerwood, E.C.; Pober, J.S.; Bradley, J.R. Recent Advances in the Molecular Basis of TNF Signal Transduction. *Lab. Invest.* **1999**, *79*, 1041–1050.
17. Aderka, D.; Engelmann, H.; Maor, Y.; Brakebusch, C.; Wallach, D. Stabilization of the Bioactivity of Tumor Necrosis Factor by Its Soluble Receptors. *J. Exp. Med.* **1992**, *175*, 323–329. [CrossRef]
18. Watts, A.D.; Hunt, N.H.; Madigan, M.C.; Chaudhri, G. Soluble TNF-Alpha Receptors Bind and Neutralize over-Expressed Transmembrane TNF-Alpha on Macrophages, but Do Not Inhibit Its Processing. *J. Leukoc. Biol.* **1999**, *66*, 1005–1013. [CrossRef]
19. Tracey, D.; Klareskog, L.; Sasso, E.H.; Salfeld, J.G.; Tak, P.P. Tumor Necrosis Factor Antagonist Mechanisms of Action: A Comprehensive Review. *Pharmacol. Ther.* **2008**, *117*, 244–279. [CrossRef]
20. Choi, S.J.; Lee, K.H.; Park, H.S.; Kim, S.K.; Koh, C.M.; Park, J.Y. Differential Expression, Shedding, Cytokine Regulation and Function of TNFR1 and TNFR2 in Human Fetal Astrocytes. *Yonsei Med. J.* **2005**, *46*, 818–826. [CrossRef]
21. Faustman, D.; Davis, M. TNF Receptor 2 Pathway: Drug Target for Autoimmune Diseases. *Nat. Rev. Drug Discov.* **2010**, *9*, 482. [CrossRef] [PubMed]
22. Liu, Z.G.; Hsu, H.; Goeddel, D.V.; Karin, M. Dissection of TNF Receptor 1 Effector Functions: JNK Activation Is Not Linked to Apoptosis While NF-KappaB Activation Prevents Cell Death. *Cell* **1996**, *87*, 565–576. [CrossRef]
23. Chinnaiyan, A.M.; Tepper, C.G.; Seldin, M.F.; O'Rourke, K.; Kischkel, F.C.; Hellbardt, S.; Krammer, P.H.; Peter, M.E.; Dixit, V.M. FADD/MORT1 Is a Common Mediator of CD95 (Fas/APO-1) and Tumor Necrosis Factor Receptor-Induced Apoptosis. *J. Biol. Chem.* **1996**, *271*, 4961–4965. [CrossRef]
24. Kischkel, F.C.; Hellbardt, S.; Behrmann, I.; Germer, M.; Pawlita, M.; Krammer, P.H.; Peter, M.E. Cytotoxicity-Dependent APO-1 (Fas/CD95)-Associated Proteins Form a Death-Inducing Signaling Complex (DISC) with the Receptor. *Embo J.* **1995**, *14*, 5579–5588. [CrossRef] [PubMed]
25. Ihnatko, R.; Kubes, M. TNF Signaling: Early Events and Phosphorylation. *Gen. Physiol. Biophys.* **2007**, *26*, 159–167. [PubMed]
26. Bradley, J.R. TNF-Mediated Inflammatory Disease. *J. Pathol.* **2008**, *214*, 149–160. [CrossRef]
27. Rothe, M.; Wong, S.C.; Henzel, W.J.; Goeddel, D.V. A Novel Family of Putative Signal Transducers Associated with the Cytoplasmic Domain of the 75 KDa Tumor Necrosis Factor Receptor. *Cell* **1994**, *78*, 681–692. [CrossRef]
28. Naudé, P.J.W.; den Boer, J.A.; Luiten, P.G.M.; Eisel, U.L.M. Tumor Necrosis Factor Receptor Cross-Talk. *FEBS J.* **2011**, *278*, 888–898. [CrossRef]
29. Nunes-Alves, C.; Booty, M.G.; Carpenter, S.M.; Jayaraman, P.; Rothchild, A.C.; Behar, S.M. In Search of a New Paradigm for Protective Immunity to TB. *Nat. Rev. Microbiol.* **2014**, *12*, 289–299. [CrossRef]

30. Marino, M.W.; Dunn, A.; Grail, D.; Inglese, M.; Noguchi, Y.; Richards, E.; Jungbluth, A.; Wada, H.; Moore, M.; Williamson, B.; et al. Characterization of Tumor Necrosis Factor-Deficient Mice. *Proc. Natl. Acad. Sci. USA* **1997**, *94*, 8093–8098. [CrossRef]
31. Lin, P.L.; Myers, A.; Smith, L.; Bigbee, C.; Bigbee, M.; Fuhrman, C.; Grieser, H.; Chiosea, I.; Voitenek, N.N.; Capuano, S.V.; et al. Tumor Necrosis Factor Neutralization Results in Disseminated Disease in Acute and Latent Mycobacterium Tuberculosis Infection with Normal Granuloma Structure in a Cynomolgus Macaque Model. *Arthritis Rheum.* **2010**, *62*, 340–350. [CrossRef] [PubMed]
32. Bruns, H.; Meinken, C.; Schauenberg, P.; Härter, G.; Kern, P.; Modlin, R.L.; Antoni, C.; Stenger, S. Anti-TNF Immunotherapy Reduces CD8+ T Cell-Mediated Antimicrobial Activity against Mycobacterium Tuberculosis in Humans. *J. Clin. Investig.* **2009**, *119*, 1167–1177. [CrossRef] [PubMed]
33. Matucci, A.; Maggi, E.; Vultaggio, A. Cellular and Humoral Immune Responses during Tuberculosis Infection: Useful Knowledge in the Era of Biological Agents. *J. Rheumatol. Suppl.* **2014**, *91*, 17–23. [CrossRef] [PubMed]
34. Baseta, J.G.; Stutman, O. TNF Regulates Thymocyte Production by Apoptosis and Proliferation of the Triple Negative (CD3-CD4-CD8-) Subset. *J. Immunol.* **2000**, *165*, 5621–5630. [CrossRef] [PubMed]
35. Neumann, B.; Luz, A.; Pfeffer, K.; Holzmann, B. Defective Peyer's Patch Organogenesis in Mice Lacking the 55-KD Receptor for Tumor Necrosis Factor. *J. Exp. Med.* **1996**, *184*, 259–264. [CrossRef]
36. Pasparakis, M.; Alexopoulou, L.; Episkopou, V.; Kollias, G. Immune and Inflammatory Responses in TNF Alpha-Deficient Mice: A Critical Requirement for TNF Alpha in the Formation of Primary B Cell Follicles, Follicular Dendritic Cell Networks and Germinal Centers, and in the Maturation of the Humoral Immune Respons. *J. Exp. Med.* **1996**, *184*, 1397–1411. [CrossRef]
37. Balkwill, F. Tumour Necrosis Factor and Cancer. *Nat. Rev. Cancer* **2009**, *9*, 361–371. [CrossRef]
38. Jung, M.K.; Lee, J.S.; Kwak, J.E.; Shin, E.C. Tumor Necrosis Factor and Regulatory T Cells. *Yonsei Med. J.* **2019**, *60*, 126–131. [CrossRef]
39. Schioppa, T.; Moore, R.; Thompson, R.G.; Rosser, E.C.; Kulbe, H.; Nedospasov, S.; Mauri, C.; Coussens, L.M.; Balkwill, F.R. B Regulatory Cells and the Tumor-Promoting Actions of TNF-α during Squamous Carcinogenesis. *Proc. Natl. Acad. Sci. USA* **2011**, *108*, 10662–10667. [CrossRef]
40. Mauri, C.; Menon, M. Human Regulatory B Cells in Health and Disease: Therapeutic Potential. *J. Clin. Investig.* **2017**, *127*, 772–779. [CrossRef]
41. Zhao, X.X.; Rong, L.; Zhao, X.X.; Li, X.; Liu, X.; Deng, J.; Wu, H.; Xu, X.; Erben, U.; Wu, P.; et al. TNF Signaling Drives Myeloid-Derived Suppressor Cell Accumulation. *J. Clin. Investig.* **2012**, *122*, 4094–4104. [CrossRef] [PubMed]
42. Schröder, M.; Krötschel, M.; Conrad, L.; Naumann, S.K.; Bachran, C.; Rolfe, A.; Umansky, V.; Helming, L.; Swee, L.K. Genetic Screen in Myeloid Cells Identifies TNF-α Autocrine Secretion as a Factor Increasing MDSC Suppressive Activity via Nos2 up-Regulation. *Sci. Rep.* **2018**, *8*, 13399. [CrossRef] [PubMed]
43. Xue, Q.; Lu, Y.; Eisele, M.R.; Sulistijo, E.S.; Khan, N.; Fan, R.; Miller-Jensen, K. Analysis of Single-Cell Cytokine Secretion Reveals a Role for Paracrine Signaling in Coordinating Macrophage Responses to TLR4 Stimulation. *Sci. Signal.* **2015**, *8*, ra59. [CrossRef] [PubMed]
44. Nagar, M.; Jacob-Hirsch, J.; Vernitsky, H.; Berkun, Y.; Ben-Horin, S.; Amariglio, N.; Bank, I.; Kloog, Y.; Rechavi, G.; Goldstein, I. TNF Activates a NF-KappaB-Regulated Cellular Program in Human CD45RA-Regulatory T Cells That Modulates Their Suppressive Function. *J. Immunol.* **2010**, *184*, 3570–3581. [CrossRef]
45. Balkwill, F.; Mantovani, A. Inflammation and Cancer: Back to Virchow? *Lancet* **2018**, *357*, 539–545. [CrossRef]
46. Waters, J.P.; Pober, J.S.; Bradley, J.R. Tumour Necrosis Factor and Cancer. *J. Pathol.* **2013**, *230*, 241–248. [CrossRef]
47. Bauswein, M.; Singh, A.; Ralhan, A.; Neri, D.; Fuchs, K.; Blanz, K.D.; Schäfer, I.; Hector, A.; Handgretinger, R.; Hartl, D.; et al. Human T Cells Modulate Myeloid-Derived Suppressor Cells through a TNF-α-Mediated Mechanism. *Immunol. Lett.* **2018**, *202*, 31–37. [CrossRef]
48. Hu, X.; Li, B.; Li, X.; Zhao, X.; Wan, L.; Lin, G.; Yu, M.; Wang, J.; Jiang, X.; Feng, W.; et al. Transmembrane TNF-α Promotes Suppressive Activities of Myeloid-Derived Suppressor Cells via TNFR2. *J. Immunol.* **2014**, *192*, 1320–1331. [CrossRef]
49. Dong, G.; You, M.; Fan, H.; Ji, J.; Ding, L.; Li, P.; Hou, Y. 17β-Estradiol Contributes to the Accumulation of Myeloid-Derived Suppressor Cells in Blood by Promoting TNF-α Secretion. *Acta Biochim. Biophys. Sin.* **2015**, *47*, 620–629. [CrossRef]
50. Greish, K.; Taurin, S.; Morsy, M.A. The Effect of Adjuvant Therapy with TNF-α on Animal Model of Triple-Negative Breast Cancer. *Ther. Deliv.* **2018**, *9*, 333–342. [CrossRef]
51. Rath, P.C.; Aggarwal, B.B. TNF-Induced Signaling in Apoptosis. *J. Clin. Immunol.* **1999**, *19*, 350–364. [CrossRef] [PubMed]
52. Benoit, M.; Desnues, B.; Mege, J.-L. Macrophage Polarization in Bacterial Infections. *J. Immunol.* **2008**, *181*, 3733–3739. [CrossRef] [PubMed]
53. Lejeune, F.J.; Liénard, D.; Matter, M.; Rüegg, C. Efficiency of Recombinant Human TNF in Human Cancer Therapy. *Cancer Immun.* **2006**, *6*, 6. [PubMed]
54. Qiao, Y.; Huang, X.; Nimmagadda, S.; Bai, R.; Staedtke, V.; Foss, C.A.; Cheong, I.; Holdhoff, M.; Kato, Y.; Pomper, M.G.; et al. A Robust Approach to Enhance Tumor-Selective Accumulation of Nanoparticles. *Oncotarget* **2011**, *2*, 59–68. [CrossRef]
55. Kratochvill, F.; Neale, G.; Haverkamp, J.M.; Van de Velde, L.-A.; Smith, A.M.; Kawauchi, D.; McEvoy, J.; Roussel, M.F.; Dyer, M.A.; Qualls, J.E.; et al. TNF Counterbalances the Emergence of M2 Tumor Macrophages. *Cell Rep.* **2015**, *12*, 1902–1914. [CrossRef]
56. Hoving, S.; Seynhaeve, A.L.B.; van Tiel, S.T.; Aan de Wiel-Ambagtsheer, G.; de Bruijn, E.A.; Eggermont, A.M.M.; ten Hagen, T.L.M. Early Destruction of Tumor Vasculature in Tumor Necrosis Factor-Alpha-Based Isolated Limb Perfusion Is Responsible for Tumor Response. *Anticancer Drugs* **2006**, *17*, 949–959. [CrossRef]
57. Mackay, F.; Loetscher, H.; Stueber, D.; Gehr, G.; Lesslauer, W. Tumor Necrosis Factor Alpha (TNF-Alpha)-Induced Cell Adhesion to Human Endothelial Cells Is under Dominant Control of One TNF Receptor Type, TNF-R55. *J. Exp. Med.* **1993**, *177*, 1277–1286. [CrossRef]
58. Balkwill, F. TNF-Alpha in Promotion and Progression of Cancer. *Cancer Metastasis Rev.* **2006**, *25*, 409–416. [CrossRef]
59. Mantovani, A.; Allavena, P.; Sica, A.; Balkwill, F. Cancer-Related Inflammation. *Nature* **2008**, *454*, 436–444. [CrossRef]

60. Cruceriu, D.; Baldasici, O.; Balacescu, O. The Dual Role of Tumor Necrosis Factor-Alpha (TNF- α) in Breast Cancer: Molecular Insights and Therapeutic Approaches. *Cell. Oncol.* **2020**, 1–18. [CrossRef]
61. Zhao, C.; Lu, X.; Bu, X.; Zhang, N.; Wang, W. Involvement of Tumor Necrosis Factor-Alpha in the Upregulation of CXCR4 Expression in Gastric Cancer Induced by Helicobacter Pylori. *BMC Cancer* **2010**, *10*, 419. [CrossRef] [PubMed]
62. Egberts, J.-H.; Cloosters, V.; Noack, A.; Schniewind, B.; Thon, L.; Klose, S.; Kettler, B.; von Forstner, C.; Kneitz, C.; Tepel, J.; et al. Anti-Tumor Necrosis Factor Therapy Inhibits Pancreatic Tumor Growth and Metastasis. *Cancer Res.* **2008**, *68*, 1443–1450. [CrossRef] [PubMed]
63. Gupta, M.; Babic, A.; Beck, A.H.; Terry, K. TNF-α Expression, Risk Factors, and Inflammatory Exposures in Ovarian Cancer: Evidence for an Inflammatory Pathway of Ovarian Carcinogenesis? *Hum. Pathol.* **2016**, *54*, 82–91. [CrossRef] [PubMed]
64. Naylor, M.S.; Malik, S.T.; Stamp, G.W.; Jobling, T.; Balkwill, F.R. In Situ Detection of Tumour Necrosis Factor in Human Ovarian Cancer Specimens. *Eur. J. Cancer* **1990**, *26*, 1027–1030. [CrossRef]
65. Morgado, M.; Sutton, M.N.; Simmons, M.; Warren, C.R.; Lu, Z.; Constantinou, P.E.; Liu, J.; Francis, L.L.W.; Steven Conlan, R.; Bast, R.C.; et al. Tumor Necrosis Factor-α and Interferon-γ Stimulate MUC16 (CA125) Expression in Breast, Endometrial and Ovarian Cancers through NFκB. *Oncotarget* **2016**, *7*, 14871–14884. [CrossRef]
66. Sethi, G.; Shanmugam, M.K.; Ramachandran, L.; Kumar, A.P.; Tergaonkar, V. Multifaceted Link between Cancer and Inflammation. *Biosci. Rep.* **2012**, *32*, 1–15. [CrossRef]
67. Li, X.; Wang, S.; Ren, H.J.; Ma, J.; Sun, X.; Li, N.; Liu, C.; Huang, K.; Xu, M.; Ming, L. Molecular Correlates and Prognostic Value of TmTNF-α Expression in Colorectal Cancer of 5-Fluorouracil-Based Adjuvant Therapy. *Cancer Biol. Ther.* **2016**, *17*, 684–692. [CrossRef]
68. Tang, D.; Tao, D.; Fang, Y.; Deng, C.; Xu, Q.; Zhou, J. TNF-Alpha Promotes Invasion and Metastasis via NF-Kappa B Pathway in Oral Squamous Cell Carcinoma. *Med. Sci. Monit. Basic Res.* **2017**, *23*, 141–149. [CrossRef]
69. Roberts, R.A.; Kimber, I. Cytokines in Non-Genotoxic Hepatocarcinogenesis. *Carcinogenesis* **1999**, *20*, 1397–1401. [CrossRef]
70. Burow, M.E.; Weldon, C.B.; Tang, Y.; Navar, G.L.; Krajewski, S.; Reed, J.C.; Hammond, T.G.; Clejan, S.; Beckman, B.S. Differences in Susceptibility to Tumor Necrosis Factor α-Induced Apoptosis among MCF-7 Breast Cancer Cell Variants. *Cancer Res.* **1998**, *58*, 4940–4946.
71. Mercogliano, M.F.; Bruni, S.; Elizalde, P.V.; Schillaci, R. Tumor Necrosis Factor α Blockade: An Opportunity to Tackle Breast Cancer. *Front. Oncol.* **2020**, *10*. [CrossRef] [PubMed]
72. Mercogliano, M.F.; De Martino, M.; Venturutti, L.; Rivas, M.A.; Proietti, C.J.; Inurrigarro, G.; Frahm, I.; Allemand, D.H.; Deza, E.G.; Ares, S.; et al. TNFα-Induced Mucin 4 Expression Elicits Trastuzumab Resistance in HER2-Positive Breast Cancer. *Clin. Cancer Res.* **2017**, *23*, 636–648. [CrossRef] [PubMed]
73. Wu, C.; Fernandez, S.A.; Criswell, T.; Chidiac, T.A.; Guttridge, D.; Villalona-Calero, M.; Bekaii-Saab, T.S. Disrupting Cytokine Signaling in Pancreatic Cancer: A Phase I/II Study of Etanercept in Combination with Gemcitabine in Patients with Advanced Disease. *Pancreas* **2013**, *42*, 813–818. [CrossRef]
74. Katerinaki, E.; Evans, G.S.; Lorigan, P.C.; MacNeil, S. TNF-Alpha Increases Human Melanoma Cell Invasion and Migration in Vitro: The Role of Proteolytic Enzymes. *Br. J. Cancer* **2003**, *89*, 1123–1129. [CrossRef] [PubMed]
75. Rossi, S.; Cordella, M.; Tabolacci, C.; Nassa, G.; D'Arcangelo, D.; Senatore, C.; Pagnotto, P.; Magliozzi, R.; Salvati, A.; Weisz, A.; et al. TNF-Alpha and Metalloproteases as Key Players in Melanoma Cells Aggressiveness. *J. Exp. Clin. Cancer Res.* **2018**, *37*, 326. [CrossRef]
76. Bald, T.; Quast, T.; Landsberg, J.; Rogava, M.; Glodde, N.; Lopez-Ramos, D.; Kohlmeyer, J.; Riesenberg, S.; van den Boorn-Konijnenberg, D.; Hömig-Hölzel, C.; et al. Ultraviolet-Radiation-Induced Inflammation Promotes Angiotropism and Metastasis in Melanoma. *Nature* **2014**, *507*, 109–113. [CrossRef]
77. Bertrand, F.; Rochotte, J.; Colacios, C.; Montfort, A.; Tilkin-Mariamé, A.-F.; Touriol, C.; Rochaix, P.; Lajoie-Mazenc, I.; Andrieu-Abadie, N.; Levade, T.; et al. Blocking Tumor Necrosis Factor α Enhances CD8 T-Cell-Dependent Immunity in Experimental Melanoma. *Cancer Res.* **2015**, *75*, 2619–2628. [CrossRef]
78. Waterston, A.M.; Salway, F.; Andreakos, E.; Butler, D.M.; Feldmann, M.; Coombes, R.C. TNF Autovaccination Induces Self Anti-TNF Antibodies and Inhibits Metastasis in a Murine Melanoma Model. *Br. J. Cancer* **2004**, *90*, 1279–1284. [CrossRef]
79. St John, M.A.R.; Li, Y.; Zhou, X.; Denny, P.; Ho, C.-M.; Montemagno, C.; Shi, W.; Qi, F.; Wu, B.; Sinha, U.; et al. Interleukin 6 and Interleukin 8 as Potential Biomarkers for Oral Cavity and Oropharyngeal Squamous Cell Carcinoma. *Arch. Otolaryngol. Head Neck Surg.* **2004**, *130*, 929–935. [CrossRef]
80. Lee, S.H.; Hong, H.S.; Liu, Z.X.; Kim, R.H.; Kang, M.K.; Park, N.-H.; Shin, K.-H. TNFα Enhances Cancer Stem Cell-like Phenotype via Notch-Hes1 Activation in Oral Squamous Cell Carcinoma Cells. *Biochem. Biophys. Res. Commun.* **2012**, *424*, 58–64. [CrossRef]
81. Zhou, X.; Zhou, S.; Li, B.; Li, Q.; Gao, L.; Li, D.; Gong, Q.; Zhu, L.; Wang, J.; Wang, N.; et al. Transmembrane TNF-α Preferentially Expressed by Leukemia Stem Cells and Blasts Is a Potent Target for Antibody Therapy. *Blood* **2015**, *126*, 1433–1442. [CrossRef] [PubMed]
82. Sivaraman, S.; Deshpande, C.G.; Ranganathan, R.; Huang, X.; Jajeh, A.; O'Brien, T.; Huang, R.W.; Gregory, S.A.; Venugopal, P.; Preisler, H.D. Tumor Necrosis Factor Modulates CD 20 Expression on Cells from Chronic Lymphocytic Leukemia: A New Role for TNF Alpha? *Microsc. Res. Tech.* **2000**, *50*, 251–257. [CrossRef]
83. Chopra, V.; Dinh, T.V.; Hannigan, E.V. Serum Levels of Interleukins, Growth Factors and Angiogenin in Patients with Endometrial Cancer. *J. Cancer Res. Clin. Oncol.* **1997**, *123*, 167–172. [CrossRef] [PubMed]
84. Ellis, P.E.; Barron, G.A.; Bermano, G. Adipocytokines and Their Relationship to Endometrial Cancer Risk: A Systematic Review and Meta-Analysis. *Gynecol. Oncol.* **2020**, *158*, 507–516. [CrossRef] [PubMed]

85. Dossus, L.; Becker, S.; Rinaldi, S.; Lukanova, A.; Tjønneland, A.; Olsen, A.; Overvad, K.; Chabbert-Buffet, N.; Boutron-Ruault, M.-C.; Clavel-Chapelon, F.; et al. Tumor Necrosis Factor (TNF)-α, Soluble TNF Receptors and Endometrial Cancer Risk: The EPIC Study. *Int. J. Cancer* **2011**, *129*, 2032–2037. [CrossRef] [PubMed]
86. Sharma, J.; Gray, K.P.; Harshman, L.C.; Evan, C.; Nakabayashi, M.; Fichorova, R.; Rider, J.; Mucci, L.; Kantoff, P.W.; Sweeney, C.J. Elevated IL-8, TNF-α, and MCP-1 in Men with Metastatic Prostate Cancer Starting Androgen-Deprivation Therapy (ADT) Are Associated with Shorter Time to Castration-Resistance and Overall Survival. *Prostate* **2014**, *74*, 820–828. [CrossRef]
87. Banzola, I.; Mengus, C.; Wyler, S.; Hudolin, T.; Manzella, G.; Chiarugi, A.; Boldorini, R.; Sais, G.; Schmidli, T.S.; Chiffi, G.; et al. Expression of Indoleamine 2,3-Dioxygenase Induced by IFN-γ and TNF-α as Potential Biomarker of Prostate Cancer Progression. *Front. Immunol.* **2018**, *9*, 1051. [CrossRef]
88. Sahibzada, H.A.; Khurshid, Z.; Khan, R.S.; Naseem, M.; Siddique, K.M.; Mali, M.; Zafar, M.S. Salivary IL-8, IL-6 and TNF-α as Potential Diagnostic Biomarkers for Oral Cancer. *Diagnostics* **2017**, *7*, 21. [CrossRef]
89. Dantas, T.S.; de Barros Silva, P.G.; Lima Verde, M.E.Q.; de Ribeiro Junior, A.L.; do Cunha, M.P.S.S.; Mota, M.R.L.; Alves, A.P.N.N.; de Leitão, R.F.C.; Sousa, F.B. Role of Inflammatory Markers in Prognosis of Oral Squamous Cell Carcinoma. *Asian Pac. J. Cancer Prev.* **2019**, *20*, 3635–3642. [CrossRef]
90. Jaime-Pérez, J.C.; Gamboa-Alonso, C.M.; Jiménez-Castillo, R.A.; López-Silva, L.J.; Pinzón-Uresti, M.A.; Gómez-De León, A.; Gómez-Almaguer, D. TNF-α Increases in the CSF of Children with Acute Lymphoblastic Leukemia before CNS Relapse. *Blood Cells Mol. Dis.* **2017**, *63*, 27–31. [CrossRef]
91. Potapnev, M.P.; Petyovka, N.V.; Belevtsev, M.V.; Savitskiy, V.P.; Migal, N.V. Plasma Level of Tumor Necrosis Factor-Alpha (TNF-Alpha) Correlates with Leukocytosis and Biological Features of Leukemic Cells, but Not Treatment Response of Children with Acute Lymphoblastic Leukemia. *Leuk. Lymphoma* **2003**, 1077–1079. [CrossRef] [PubMed]
92. Macia, J.; Gomez, X.; Esquerda, A.; Perez, B.; Callao, V.; Marzo, C. Value of the Determination of TNF-Alpha in the Plasma of Patients with Non-Hodgkins Lymphoma. *Leuk. Lymphoma* **1996**, *20*, 481–486. [CrossRef] [PubMed]
93. Lech-Maranda, E.; Bienvenu, J.; Broussais-Guillaumot, F.; Warzocha, K.; Michallet, A.-S.; Robak, T.; Coiffier, B.; Salles, G. Plasma TNF-Alpha and IL-10 Level-Based Prognostic Model Predicts Outcome of Patients with Diffuse Large B-Cell Lymphoma in Different Risk Groups Defined by the International Prognostic Index. *Arch. Immunol. Exp.* **2010**, *58*, 131–141. [CrossRef]
94. Nakayama, S.; Yokote, T.; Tsuji, M.; Akioka, T.; Miyoshi, T.; Hirata, Y.; Hiraoka, N.; Iwaki, K.; Takayama, A.; Nishiwaki, U.; et al. TNF-α Receptor 1 Expression Predicts Poor Prognosis of Diffuse Large B-Cell Lymphoma, Not Otherwise Specified. *Am. J. Surg. Pathol.* **2014**, *38*, 1138–1146. [CrossRef] [PubMed]
95. Dantas, R.N.; de Souza, A.M.; Herrero, S.S.T.; Kassab, P.; Malheiros, C.A.; Lima, E.M. Association between PSCA, TNF-α, PARP1 and TP53 Gene Polymorphisms and Gastric Cancer Susceptibility in the Brazilian Population. *Asian Pac. J. Cancer Prev.* **2020**, *21*, 43–48. [CrossRef]
96. Du, L.C.; Gao, R. Role of TNF-α -308G/A Gene Polymorphism in Gastric Cancer Risk: A Case Control Study and Meta-Analysis. *J. Turk. Soc. Gastroenterol.* **2017**, *28*, 272–282. [CrossRef]
97. Pardo, T.; Salcedo, P.; Quintero, J.M.; Borjas, L.; Fernández-Mestre, M.; Sánchez, Y.; Carrillo, Z.; Rivera, S. Study of the association between the polymorphism of the TNF-α gene and prostate cáncer. *Rev. Alerg. Mex.* **2019**, *66*, 154–162. [CrossRef]
98. Shi, H.-Z.; Ren, P.; Lu, Q.-J.; Niedrgethmnn, M.; Wu, G.-Y. Association between EGF, TGF-B1 and TNF-α Gene Polymorphisms and Hepatocellular Carcinoma. *Asian Pac. J. Cancer Prev.* **2012**, *13*, 6217–6220. [CrossRef]
99. Verma, H.K.; Merchant, N.; Bhaskar, L.V.K.S. Tumor Necrosis Factor-Alpha Gene Promoter (TNF-α G-308A) Polymorphisms Increase the Risk of Hepatocellular Carcinoma in Asians: A Meta-Analysis. *Crit. Rev. Oncog.* **2020**, *25*, 11–20. [CrossRef]
100. He, Y.-Q.; Zhu, J.-H.; Huang, S.-Y.; Cui, Z.; He, J.; Jia, W.-H. The Association between the Polymorphisms of TNF-α and Non-Hodgkin Lymphoma: A Meta-Analysis. *Tumour Biol. J. Int. Soc. Oncodevelopmental Biol. Med.* **2014**, *35*, 12509–12517. [CrossRef]
101. Liu, J.; Liu, J.; Song, B.; Wang, T.; Liu, Y.; Hao, J.; Yu, J. Genetic Variations in CTLA-4, TNF-α, and LTA and Susceptibility to T-Cell Lymphoma in a Chinese Population. *Cancer Epidemiol.* **2013**, *37*, 930–934. [CrossRef] [PubMed]
102. Hellmig, S.; Fischbach, W.; Goebeler-Kolve, M.-E.; Fölsch, U.R.; Hampe, J.; Schreiber, S. A Functional Promotor Polymorphism of TNF-Alpha Is Associated with Primary Gastric B-Cell Lymphoma. *Am. J. Gastroenterol.* **2005**, *100*, 2644–2649. [CrossRef] [PubMed]
103. Ahmed, A.B.; Zidi, S.; Sghaier, I.; Ghazouani, E.; Mezlini, A.; Almawi, W.; Loueslati, B.Y. Common Variants in IL-1RN, IL-1β and TNF-α and the Risk of Ovarian Cancer: A Case Control Study. *Cent. J. Immunol.* **2017**, *42*, 150–155. [CrossRef] [PubMed]
104. Kanda, K.; Komekado, H.; Sawabu, T.; Ishizu, S.; Nakanishi, Y.; Nakatsuji, M.; Akitake-Kawano, R.; Ohno, M.; Hiraoka, Y.; Kawada, M.; et al. Nardilysin and ADAM Proteases Promote Gastric Cancer Cell Growth by Activating Intrinsic Cytokine Signalling via Enhanced Ectodomain Shedding of TNF-α. *Embo Mol. Med.* **2012**, *4*, 396–411. [CrossRef]
105. Mochizuki, Y.; Nakanishi, H.; Kodera, Y.; Ito, S.; Yamamura, Y.; Kato, T.; Hibi, K.; Akiyama, S.; Nakao, A.; Tatematsu, M. TNF-Alpha Promotes Progression of Peritoneal Metastasis as Demonstrated Using a Green Fluorescence Protein (GFP)-Tagged Human Gastric Cancer Cell Line. *Clin. Exp. Metastasis* **2004**, *21*, 39–47. [CrossRef]
106. Cui, X.; Zhang, H.; Cao, A.; Cao, L.; Hu, X. Cytokine TNF-α Promotes Invasion and Metastasis of Gastric Cancer by down-Regulating Pentraxin3. *J. Cancer* **2020**, *11*, 1800–1807. [CrossRef]
107. Zhou, Q.; Wu, X.; Wang, X.; Yu, Z.; Pan, T.; Li, Z.; Chang, X.; Jin, Z.; Li, J.; Zhu, Z.; et al. The Reciprocal Interaction between Tumor Cells and Activated Fibroblasts Mediated by TNF-α/IL-33/ST2L Signaling Promotes Gastric Cancer Metastasis. *Oncogene* **2020**, *39*, 1414–1428. [CrossRef]

108. Kim, S.; Choi, M.G.; Lee, H.S.; Lee, S.K.; Kim, S.H.; Kim, W.W.; Hur, S.M.; Kim, J.-H.; Choe, J.-H.; Nam, S.J.; et al. Silibinin Suppresses TNF-Alpha-Induced MMP-9 Expression in Gastric Cancer Cells through Inhibition of the MAPK Pathway. *Molecules* **2009**, *14*, 4300–4311. [CrossRef]

109. Ha Thi, H.T.; Lim, H.-S.; Kim, J.; Kim, Y.-M.; Kim, H.-Y.; Hong, S. Transcriptional and Post-Translational Regulation of Bim Is Essential for TGF-β and TNF-α-Induced Apoptosis of Gastric Cancer Cell. *Biochim. Biophys. Acta* **2013**, *1830*, 3584–3592. [CrossRef]

110. Alam, M.S.; Gaida, M.M.; Bergmann, F.; Lasitschka, F.; Giese, T.; Giese, N.A.; Hackert, T.; Hinz, U.; Hussain, S.P.; Kozlov, S.V.; et al. Selective Inhibition of the P38 Alternative Activation Pathway in Infiltrating T Cells Inhibits Pancreatic Cancer Progression. *Nat. Med.* **2015**, *21*, 1337–1343. [CrossRef]

111. Aida, K.; Miyakawa, R.; Suzuki, K.; Narumi, K.; Udagawa, T.; Yamamoto, Y.; Chikaraishi, T.; Yoshida, T.; Aoki, K. Suppression of Tregs by Anti-Glucocorticoid Induced TNF Receptor Antibody Enhances the Antitumor Immunity of Interferon-α Gene Therapy for Pancreatic Cancer. *Cancer Sci.* **2014**, *105*, 159–167. [CrossRef] [PubMed]

112. Bharadwaj, U.; Marin-Muller, C.; Li, M.; Chen, C.; Yao, Q. Mesothelin Confers Pancreatic Cancer Cell Resistance to TNF-α-Induced Apoptosis through Akt/PI3K/NF-KB Activation and IL-6/Mcl-1 Overexpression. *Mol. Cancer* **2011**, *10*, 106. [CrossRef] [PubMed]

113. Guo, X.; Li, T.; Wang, Y.; Shao, L.; Zhang, Y.; Ma, D.; Han, W. CMTM5 Induces Apoptosis of Pancreatic Cancer Cells and Has Synergistic Effects with TNF-Alpha. *Biochem. Biophys. Res. Commun.* **2009**, *387*, 139–142. [CrossRef] [PubMed]

114. Murugesan, S.R.; King, C.R.; Osborn, R.; Fairweather, W.R.; O'Reilly, E.M.; Thornton, M.O.; Wei, L.L. Combination of Human Tumor Necrosis Factor-Alpha (HTNF-Alpha) Gene Delivery with Gemcitabine Is Effective in Models of Pancreatic Cancer. *Cancer Gene Ther.* **2009**, *16*, 841–847. [CrossRef] [PubMed]

115. Tsukamoto, M.; Imai, K.; Ishimoto, T.; Komohara, Y.; Yamashita, Y.-I.; Nakagawa, S.; Umezaki, N.; Yamao, T.; Kitano, Y.; Miyata, T.; et al. PD-L1 Expression Enhancement by Infiltrating Macrophage-Derived Tumor Necrosis Factor-α Leads to Poor Pancreatic Cancer Prognosis. *Cancer Sci.* **2019**, *110*, 310–320. [CrossRef]

116. Charles, K.A.; Kulbe, H.; Soper, R.; Escorcio-Correia, M.; Lawrence, T.; Schultheis, A.; Chakravarty, P.; Thompson, R.G.; Kollias, G.; Smyth, J.F.; et al. The Tumor-Promoting Actions of TNF-Alpha Involve TNFR1 and IL-17 in Ovarian Cancer in Mice and Humans. *J. Clin. Investig.* **2009**, *119*, 3011–3023. [CrossRef] [PubMed]

117. Hassan, M.I.; Kassim, S.K.; Saeda, L.; Laban, M.; Khalifa, A. Ovarian Cancer-Induced Immunosuppression: Relationship to Tumor Necrosis Factor-Alpha (TNF-Alpha) Release from Ovarian Tissue. *Anticancer Res.* **1999**, *19*, 5657–5662.

118. Wu, S.; Rodabaugh, K.; Martinez-Maza, O.; Watson, J.M.; Silberstein, D.S.; Boyer, C.M.; Peters, W.P.; Weinberg, J.B.; Berek, J.S.; Bast, R.C.J. Stimulation of Ovarian Tumor Cell Proliferation with Monocyte Products Including Interleukin-1, Interleukin-6, and Tumor Necrosis Factor-Alpha. *Am. J. Obstet. Gynecol.* **1992**, *166*, 997–1007. [CrossRef]

119. Li, H.; Chen, A.; Yuan, Q.; Chen, W.; Zhong, H.; Teng, M.; Xu, C.; Qiu, Y.; Cao, J. NF-KB/Twist Axis Is Involved in Chysin Inhibition of Ovarian Cancer Stem Cell Features Induced by Co-Treatment of TNF-α and TGF-β. *Int. J. Clin. Exp. Pathol.* **2019**, *12*, 101–112.

120. Kim, D.S.; Jang, Y.-J.; Jeon, O.-H.; Kim, D.-S. Saxatilin, a Snake Venom Disintegrin, Suppresses TNF-Alpha-Induced Ovarian Cancer Cell Invasion. *J. Biochem. Mol. Biol.* **2007**, *40*, 290–294. [CrossRef]

121. Schröder, S.K.; Asimakopoulou, A.; Tillmann, S.; Koschmieder, S.; Weiskirchen, R. TNF-α Controls Lipocalin-2 Expression in PC-3 Prostate Cancer Cells. *Cytokine* **2020**, *135*, 155214. [CrossRef] [PubMed]

122. Safari, H.; Zabihi, E.; Pouramir, M.; Morakabati, P.; Abedian, Z.; Karkhah, A.; Nouri, H.R. Decrease of Intracellular ROS by Arbutin Is Associated with Apoptosis Induction and Downregulation of IL-1β and TNF-α in LNCaP.; Prostate Cancer. *J. Food Biochem.* **2020**, e13360. [CrossRef] [PubMed]

123. Mu, H.Q.; He, Y.H.; Wang, S.B.; Yang, S.; Wang, Y.J.; Nan, C.J.; Bao, Y.F.; Xie, Q.P.; Chen, Y.H. MiR-130b/TNF-α/NF-KB/VEGFA Loop Inhibits Prostate Cancer Angiogenesis. *Clin. Transl. Oncol.* **2020**, *22*, 111–121. [CrossRef] [PubMed]

124. Lv, L.; Yuan, J.; Huang, T.; Zhang, C.; Zhu, Z.; Wang, L.; Jiang, G.; Zeng, F. Stabilization of Snail by HIF-1α and TNF-α Is Required for Hypoxia-Induced Invasion in Prostate Cancer PC3 Cells. *Mol. Biol. Rep.* **2014**, *41*, 4573–4582. [CrossRef]

125. Maolake, A.; Izumi, K.; Natsagdorj, A.; Iwamoto, H.; Kadomoto, S.; Makino, T.; Naito, R.; Shigehara, K.; Kadono, Y.; Hiratsuka, K.; et al. Tumor Necrosis Factor-α Induces Prostate Cancer Cell Migration in Lymphatic Metastasis through CCR7 Upregulation. *Cancer Sci.* **2018**, *109*, 1524–1531. [CrossRef]

126. Wang, H.; Fang, R.; Wang, X.-F.; Zhang, F.; Chen, D.-Y.; Zhou, B.; Wang, H.-S.; Cai, S.-H.; Du, J. Stabilization of Snail through AKT/GSK-3β Signaling Pathway Is Required for TNF-α-Induced Epithelial-Mesenchymal Transition in Prostate Cancer PC3 Cells. *Eur. J. Pharm.* **2013**, *714*, 48–55. [CrossRef]

127. Pilling, A.B.; Hwang, O.; Boudreault, A.; Laurent, A.; Hwang, C. IAP Antagonists Enhance Apoptotic Response to Enzalutamide in Castration-Resistant Prostate Cancer Cells via Autocrine TNF-α Signaling. *Prostate* **2017**, *77*, 866–877. [CrossRef]

128. Shi, J.; Chen, J.; Serradji, N.; Xu, X.; Zhou, H.; Ma, Y.; Sun, Z.; Jiang, P.; Du, Y.; Yang, J.; et al. PMS1077 Sensitizes TNF-α Induced Apoptosis in Human Prostate Cancer Cells by Blocking NF-KB Signaling Pathway. *PLoS ONE* **2013**, *8*, e61132. [CrossRef]

129. Lee, E.-J.; Kim, W.-J.; Moon, S.-K. Cordycepin Suppresses TNF-Alpha-Induced Invasion, Migration and Matrix Metalloproteinase-9 Expression in Human Bladder Cancer Cells. *Phytother. Res.* **2010**, *24*, 1755–1761. [CrossRef]

130. Lee, S.-J.; Park, S.-S.; Lee, U.-S.; Kim, W.-J.; Moon, S.-K. Signaling Pathway for TNF-Alpha-Induced MMP-9 Expression: Mediation through P38 MAP Kinase, and Inhibition by Anti-Cancer Molecule Magnolol in Human Urinary Bladder Cancer 5637 Cells. *Int. Immunopharmacol.* **2008**, *8*, 1821–1826. [CrossRef]

131. Lee, S.-J.; Park, S.-S.; Cho, Y.-H.; Park, K.; Kim, E.-J.; Jung, K.-H.; Kim, S.-K.; Kim, W.-J.; Moon, S.-K. Activation of Matrix Metalloproteinase-9 by TNF-Alpha in Human Urinary Bladder Cancer HT1376 Cells: The Role of MAP Kinase Signaling Pathways. *Oncol. Rep.* **2008**, *19*, 1007–1013. [PubMed]

132. Yang, T.; Shi, R.; Chang, L.; Tang, K.; Chen, K.; Yu, G.; Tian, Y.; Guo, Y.; He, W.; Song, X.; et al. Huachansu Suppresses Human Bladder Cancer Cell Growth through the Fas/Fasl and TNF- Alpha/TNFR1 Pathway in Vitro and in Vivo. *J. Exp. Clin. Cancer Res.* **2015**, *34*, 21. [CrossRef] [PubMed]

133. Wang, Z.; Cheng, Y.; Zheng, R.; Qin, D.; Liu, G. Effect of TNF-Alpha and IFN-Alpha on the Proliferation and Cytotoxicity of Lymphokine-Activated Killer Cells in Patients with Bladder Cancer. *Chin. Med. J.* **1997**, *110*, 180–183. [PubMed]

134. Grimm, M.; Lazariotou, M.; Kircher, S.; Höfelmayr, A.; Germer, C.T.; von Rahden, B.H.A.; Waaga-Gasser, A.M.; Gasser, M. Tumor Necrosis Factor-α Is Associated with Positive Lymph Node Status in Patients with Recurrence of Colorectal Cancer–Indications for Anti-TNF-α Agents in Cancer Treatment. *Anal. Cell. Pathol.* **2010**, *33*, 151–163. [CrossRef]

135. Shen, Z.; Zhou, R.; Liu, C.; Wang, Y.; Zhan, W.; Shao, Z.; Liu, J.; Zhang, F.; Xu, L.; Zhou, X.; et al. MicroRNA-105 Is Involved in TNF-α-Related Tumor Microenvironment Enhanced Colorectal Cancer Progression. *Cell Death Dis.* **2017**, *8*, 3213. [CrossRef]

136. Møller, T.; James, J.P.; Holmstrøm, K.; Sørensen, F.B.; Lindebjerg, J.; Nielsen, B.S. Co-Detection of MiR-21 and TNF-α MRNA in Budding Cancer Cells in Colorectal Cancer. *Int. J. Mol. Sci.* **2019**, *20*, 1907. [CrossRef]

137. Kassouf, N.; Thornhill, M.H. Oral Cancer Cell Lines Can Use Multiple Ligands, Including Fas-L, TRAIL and TNF-Alpha, to Induce Apoptosis in Jurkat T Cells: Possible Mechanisms for Immune Escape by Head and Neck Cancers. *Oral Oncol.* **2008**, *44*, 672–682. [CrossRef]

138. Iulia Irimie, A.; Braicu, C.; Zanoaga, O.; Pileczki, V.; Soritau, O.; Berindan-Neagoe, I.; Septimiu Campian, R. Inhibition of Tumor Necrosis Factor Alpha Using RNA Interference in Oral Squamous Cell Carcinoma. *J. Buon.* **2015**, *20*, 1107–1114.

139. Lai, K.-C.; Liu, C.-J.; Lin, T.-J.; Mar, A.-C.; Wang, H.-H.; Chen, C.-W.; Hong, Z.-X.; Lee, T.-C. Blocking TNF-α Inhibits Angiogenesis and Growth of IFIT2-Depleted Metastatic Oral Squamous Cell Carcinoma Cells. *Cancer Lett.* **2016**, *370*, 207–215. [CrossRef]

140. Hsing, E.-W.; Shiah, S.-G.; Peng, H.-Y.; Chen, Y.-W.; Chuu, C.-P.; Hsiao, J.-R.; Lyu, P.-C.; Chang, J.-Y. TNF-α-Induced MiR-450a Mediates TMEM182 Expression to Promote Oral Squamous Cell Carcinoma Motility. *PLoS ONE* **2019**, *14*, e0213463. [CrossRef]

141. Lin, X.; Yang, Y.; Guo, Y.; Liu, H.; Jiang, J.; Zheng, F.; Wu, B. PTTG1 Is Involved in TNF-α-Related Hepatocellular Carcinoma via the Induction of c-Myc. *Cancer Med.* **2019**, *8*, 5702–5715. [CrossRef] [PubMed]

142. Yang, R.; Liu, Q.; Rescorla, F.J.; Grosfeld, J.L. Experimental Liver Cancer: Improved Response after Hepatic Artery Ligation and Infusion of Tumor Necrosis Factor-Alpha and Interferon-Gamma. *Surgery* **1995**, *118*, 764–768. [CrossRef]

143. Zhang, Y.H.; Yan, H.Q.; Wang, F.; Wang, Y.Y.; Jiang, Y.N.; Wang, Y.N.; Gao, F.G. TIPE2 Inhibits TNF-α-Induced Hepatocellular Carcinoma Cell Metastasis via Erk1/2 Downregulation and NF-KB Activation. *Int. J. Oncol.* **2015**, *46*, 254–264. [CrossRef] [PubMed]

144. Zhang, G.-P.; Yue, X.; Li, S.-Q. Cathepsin C Interacts with TNF-α/P38 MAPK Signaling Pathway to Promote Proliferation and Metastasis in Hepatocellular Carcinoma. *Cancer Res. Treat.* **2020**, *52*, 10–23. [CrossRef] [PubMed]

145. Chen, Y.; Wen, H.; Zhou, C.; Su, Q.; Lin, Y.; Xie, Y.; Huang, Y.; Qiu, Q.; Lin, J.; Huang, X.; et al. TNF-α Derived from M2 Tumor-Associated Macrophages Promotes Epithelial-Mesenchymal Transition and Cancer Stemness through the Wnt/β-Catenin Pathway in SMMC-7721 Hepatocellular Carcinoma Cells. *Exp. Cell Res.* **2019**, *378*, 41–50. [CrossRef]

146. Li, N.; Wang, J.; Zhang, N.; Zhuang, M.; Zong, Z.; Zou, J.; Li, G.; Wang, X.; Zhou, H.; Zhang, L.; et al. Cross-Talk between TNF-α and IFN-γ Signaling in Induction of B7-H1 Expression in Hepatocellular Carcinoma Cells. *Cancer Immunol. Immunother.* **2018**, *67*, 271–283. [CrossRef]

147. Curnis, F.; Sacchi, A.; Borgna, L.; Magni, F.; Gasparri, A.; Corti, A. Enhancement of Tumor Necrosis Factor Alpha Antitumor Immunotherapeutic Properties by Targeted Delivery to Aminopeptidase N (CD13). *Nat. Biotechnol.* **2000**, *18*, 1185–1190. [CrossRef]

148. Cervera-Carrascon, V.; Siurala, M.; Santos, J.M.; Havunen, R.; Tähtinen, S.; Karell, P.; Sorsa, S.; Kanerva, A.; Hemminki, A. TNFa and IL-2 Armed Adenoviruses Enable Complete Responses by Anti-PD-1 Checkpoint Blockade. *Oncoimmunology* **2018**, *7*, e1412902. [CrossRef]

149. Broussard, L.; Howland, A.; Ryu, S.; Song, K.; Norris, D.; Armstrong, C.A.; Song, P.I. Melanoma Cell Death Mechanisms. *Chonnam Med. J.* **2018**, *54*, 135–142. [CrossRef]

150. Warzocha, K.; Robak, T. Antileukemic Effects of Recombinant Human Tumor Necrosis Factor Alpha (Rh-TNF Alpha) with Cyclophosphamide or Methotrexate on Leukemia L1210 and Leukemia P388 in Mice. *Acta Haematol. Pol.* **1992**, *23*, 55–62.

151. Kitajima, I.; Nakajima, T.; Imamura, T.; Takasaki, I.; Kawahara, K.; Okano, T.; Tokioka, T.; Soejima, Y.; Abeyama, K.; Maruyama, I. Induction of Apoptosis in Murine Clonal Osteoblasts Expressed by Human T-Cell Leukemia Virus Type I Tax by NF-Kappa B and TNF-Alpha. *J. Bone Miner. Res.* **1996**, *11*, 200–210. [CrossRef]

152. Gautam, S.C.; Pindolia, K.R.; Xu, Y.X.; Janakiraman, N.; Chapman, R.A.; Freytag, S.O. Antileukemic Activity of TNF-Alpha Gene Therapy with Myeloid Progenitor Cells against Minimal Leukemia. *J. Hematother.* **1998**, *7*, 115–125. [CrossRef] [PubMed]

153. Qin, Y.; Auh, S.; Blokh, L.; Long, C.; Gagnon, I.; Hamann, K.J. TNF-Alpha Induces Transient Resistance to Fas-Induced Apoptosis in Eosinophilic Acute Myeloid Leukemia Cells. *Cell. Mol. Immunol.* **2007**, *4*, 43–52.

154. D'Alessandro, N.; Flugy, A.; Tolomeo, M.; Dusonchet, L. The Apoptotic Signaling of TNF-Alpha in Multidrug Resistant Friend Leukemia Cells. *Anticancer Res.* **1998**, *18*, 3065–3072. [PubMed]

155. Kagoya, Y.; Yoshimi, A.; Kataoka, K.; Nakagawa, M.; Kumano, K.; Arai, S.; Kobayashi, H.; Saito, T.; Iwakura, Y.; Kurokawa, M. Positive Feedback between NF-KB and TNF-α Promotes Leukemia-Initiating Cell Capacity. *J. Clin. Investig.* **2014**, *124*, 528–542. [CrossRef] [PubMed]

156. Brailly, H.; Pebusque, M.J.; Tabilio, A.; Mannoni, P. TNF Alpha Acts in Synergy with GM-CSF to Induce Proliferation of Acute Myeloid Leukemia Cells by up-Regulating the GM-CSF Receptor and GM-CSF Gene Expression. *Leukemia* **1993**, *7*, 1557–1563.

157. Zhang, H.; Yan, D.; Shi, X.; Liang, H.; Pang, Y.; Qin, N.; Chen, H.; Wang, J.; Yin, B.; Jiang, X.; et al. Transmembrane TNF-Alpha Mediates "Forward" and "Reverse" Signaling, Inducing Cell Death or Survival via the NF-KappaB Pathway in Raji Burkitt Lymphoma Cells. *J. Leukoc. Biol.* **2008**, *84*, 789–797. [CrossRef] [PubMed]

158. Saudemont, A.; Corm, S.; Wickham, T.; Hetuin, D.; Quesnel, B. Induction of Leukemia-Specific CD8+ Cytotoxic T Cells with Autologous Myeloid Leukemic Cells Matured with a Fiber-Modified Adenovirus Encoding TNF-Alpha. *Mol. Ther.* **2005**, *11*, 950–959. [CrossRef] [PubMed]

159. Heilig, B.; Mapara, M.; Bargou, R.; Fiehn, C.; Dörken, B. TNF Alpha Therapy Activates Human B-Lymphoma Cells in Vivo and May Protect Myelopoiesis. *Leuk. Res.* **1992**, *16*, 769–773. [CrossRef]

160. Di Pietro, R.; Robuffo, I.; Pucci, A.M.; Bosco, D.; Santavenere, E. Effects of TNF-Alpha/Colchicine Combined Treatment on Burkitt Lymphoma Cells: Molecular and Ultrastructural Changes. *Cytokine* **1999**, *11*, 144–150. [CrossRef]

161. Gupta, U.; Hira, S.K.; Singh, R.; Paladhi, A.; Srivastava, P.; Pratim Manna, P. Essential Role of TNF-α in Gamma c Cytokine Aided Crosstalk between Dendritic Cells and Natural Killer Cells in Experimental Murine Lymphoma. *Int. Immunopharmacol.* **2020**, *78*, 106031. [CrossRef] [PubMed]

162. Perez, C.R.; De Palma, M. Engineering Dendritic Cell Vaccines to Improve Cancer Immunotherapy. *Nat. Commun.* **2019**, *10*, 5408. [CrossRef] [PubMed]

163. Bowen, W.S.; Svrivastava, A.K.; Batra, L.; Barsoumian, H.; Shirwan, H. Current Challenges for Cancer Vaccine Adjuvant Development. *Expert Rev. Vaccines* **2018**, *17*, 207–215. [CrossRef] [PubMed]

164. Aurisicchio, L.; Pallocca, M.; Ciliberto, G.; Palombo, F. The Perfect Personalized Cancer Therapy: Cancer Vaccines against Neoantigens. *J. Exp. Clin. Cancer Res.* **2018**, *37*, 86. [CrossRef] [PubMed]

165. Schillaci, R.; Bruni, S.; De Martino, M.; Mercogliano, M.F.; Inurrigarro, G.; Frahm, I.; Proietti, C.J.; Elizalde, P.V. Abstract P6-20-14: Neutralizing Soluble Tumor Necrosis Factor Alpha Overcomes Trastuzumab-Resistant Breast Cancer Immune Evasion by Down-regulating Mucin 4, Improving NK Cell Function and Decreasing Myeloid-Derived Suppressor Cells in Tumor Microenvironmen. *Cancer Res.* **2019**, *79* (Suppl. S4), P6-20-14. [CrossRef]

166. Tsimberidou, A.-M.; Thomas, D.; O'Brien, S.; Andreeff, M.; Kurzrock, R.; Keating, M.; Albitar, M.; Kantarjian, H.; Giles, F. Recombinant Human Soluble Tumor Necrosis Factor (TNF) Receptor (P75) Fusion Protein Enbrel in Patients with Refractory Hematologic Malignancies. *Cancer Chemother. Pharm.* **2002**, *50*, 237–242. [CrossRef]

167. Woyach, J.A.; Lin, T.S.; Lucas, M.S.; Heerema, N.; Moran, M.E.; Cheney, C.; Lucas, D.M.; Wei, L.; Caligiuri, M.A.; Byrd, J.C. A Phase I/II Study of Rituximab and Etanercept in Patients with Chronic Lymphocytic Leukemia and Small Lymphocytic Lymphoma. *Leukemia* **2009**, *23*, 912–918. [CrossRef]

168. Bertrand, F.; Montfort, A.; Marcheteau, E.; Imbert, C.; Gilhodes, J.; Filleron, T.; Rochaix, P.; Andrieu-Abadie, N.; Levade, T.; Meyer, N.; et al. TNFα Blockade Overcomes Resistance to Anti-PD-1 in Experimental Melanoma. *Nat. Commun.* **2017**, *8*. [CrossRef]

169. Stucci, S.; Palmirotta, R.; Passarelli, A.; Silvestris, E.; Argentiero, A.; Lanotte, L.; Acquafredda, S.; Todisco, A.; Silvestris, F. Immune-Related Adverse Events during Anticancer Immunotherapy: Pathogenesis and Management. *Oncol. Lett.* **2017**, *14*, 5671–5680. [CrossRef]

170. Puzanov, I.; Diab, A.; Abdallah, K.; Bingham III, C.O.; Brogdon, C.; Dadu, R.; Hamad, L.; Kim, S.; Lacouture, M.E.; LeBoeuf, N.R.; et al. Managing Toxicities Associated with Immune Checkpoint Inhibitors: Consensus Recommendations from the Society for Immunotherapy of Cancer (SITC) Toxicity Management Working Group. *J. Immunother. Cancer* **2017**, *5*, 95. [CrossRef]

171. Badran, Y.R.; Cohen, J.V.; Brastianos, P.K.; Parikh, A.R.; Hong, T.S.; Dougan, M. Concurrent Therapy with Immune Checkpoint Inhibitors and TNFα Blockade in Patients with Gastrointestinal Immune-Related Adverse Events. *J. Immunother. Cancer* **2019**, *7*, 226. [CrossRef] [PubMed]

172. Perez-Ruiz, E.; Minute, L.; Otano, I.; Alvarez, M.; Ochoa, M.C.; Belsue, V.; de Andrea, C.; Rodriguez-Ruiz, M.E.; Perez-Gracia, J.L.; Marquez-Rodas, I.; et al. Prophylactic TNF Blockade Uncouples Efficacy and Toxicity in Dual CTLA-4 and PD-1 Immunotherapy. *Nature* **2019**, *569*, 428–432. [CrossRef] [PubMed]

173. Arriola, E.; Wheater, M.; Karydis, I.; Thomas, G.; Ottensmeier, C. Infliximab for IPILIMUMAB-Related Colitis-Letter. *Clin. Cancer Res.* **2015**, *21*, 5642–5643. [CrossRef] [PubMed]

174. Horvat, T.Z.; Adel, N.G.; Dang, T.-O.; Momtaz, P.; Postow, M.A.; Callahan, M.K.; Carvajal, R.D.; Dickson, M.A.; D'Angelo, S.P.; Woo, K.M.; et al. Immune-Related Adverse Events, Need for Systemic Immunosuppression, and Effects on Survival and Time to Treatment Failure in Patients With Melanoma Treated With Ipilimumab at Memorial Sloan Kettering Cancer Center. *J. Clin. Oncol.* **2015**, *33*, 3193–3198. [CrossRef]

175. Figueroa, J.A.; Reidy, A.; Mirandola, L.; Trotter, K.; Suvorava, N.; Figueroa, A.; Konala, V.; Aulakh, A.; Littlefield, L.; Grizzi, F.; et al. Chimeric Antigen Receptor Engineering: A Right Step in the Evolution of Adoptive Cellular Immunotherapy. *Int. Rev. Immunol.* **2015**, *34*, 154–187. [CrossRef]

176. von Mehren, M.; Adams, G.P.; Weiner, L.M. Monoclonal Antibody Therapy for Cancer. *Annu. Rev. Med.* **2003**, *54*, 343–369. [CrossRef]

177. Adams, G.P.; Weiner, L.M. Monoclonal Antibody Therapy of Cancer. *Nat. Biotechnol.* **2005**, *23*, 1147–1157. [CrossRef]

178. Harding, F.A.; Stickler, M.M.; Razo, J.; DuBridge, R.B. The Immunogenicity of Humanized and Fully Human Antibodies: Residual Immunogenicity Resides in the CDR Regions. *MAbs* **2010**, *2*, 256–265. [CrossRef]

179. Luo, J.-L.; Maeda, S.; Hsu, L.-C.; Yagita, H.; Karin, M. Inhibition of NF-KappaB in Cancer Cells Converts Inflammation- Induced Tumor Growth Mediated by TNFalpha to TRAIL-Mediated Tumor Regression. *Cancer Cell* **2004**, *6*, 297–305. [CrossRef]

180. Orosz, P.; Echtenacher, B.; Falk, W.; Rüschoff, J.; Weber, D.; Männel, D.N. Enhancement of Experimental Metastasis by Tumor Necrosis Factor. *J. Exp. Med.* **1993**, *177*, 1391–1398. [CrossRef]

181. Kitakata, H.; Nemoto-Sasaki, Y.; Takahashi, Y.; Kondo, T.; Mai, M.; Mukaida, N. Essential Roles of Tumor Necrosis Factor Receptor P55 in Liver Metastasis of Intrasplenic Administration of Colon 26 Cells. *Cancer Res.* **2002**, *62*, 6682–6687. [PubMed]

182. Wilson, J.; Balkwill, F. The Role of Cytokines in the Epithelial Cancer Microenvironment. *Semin. Cancer Biol.* **2002**, *12*, 113–120. [CrossRef] [PubMed]

183. Ueno, T.; Toi, M.; Saji, H.; Muta, M.; Bando, H.; Kuroi, K.; Koike, M.; Inadera, H.; Matsushima, K. Significance of Macrophage Chemoattractant Protein-1 in Macrophage Recruitment, Angiogenesis, and Survival in Human Breast Cancer. *Clin. Cancer Res.* **2000**, *6*, 3282–3289. [PubMed]

184. Kishimoto, T.; Akira, S.; Narazaki, M.; Taga, T. Interleukin-6 Family of Cytokines and Gp130. *Blood* **1995**, *86*, 1243–1254. [CrossRef] [PubMed]

185. Scott, K.A.; Moore, R.J.; Arnott, C.H.; East, N.; Thompson, R.G.; Scallon, B.J.; Shealy, D.J.; Balkwill, F.R. An Anti-Tumor Necrosis Factor-Alpha Antibody Inhibits the Development of Experimental Skin Tumors. *Mol. Cancer Ther.* **2003**, *2*, 445–451.

186. Sha, K.; Yeh, S.; Chang, C.; Nastiuk, K.L.; Krolewski, J.J. TNF Signaling Mediates an Enzalutamide-Induced Metastatic Phenotype of Prostate Cancer and Microenvironment Cell Co-Cultures. *Oncotarget* **2015**, *6*, 25726–25740. [CrossRef]

187. Madhusudan, S.; Foster, M.; Muthuramalingam, S.R.; Braybrooke, J.P.; Wilner, S.; Kaur, K.; Han, C.; Hoare, S.; Balkwill, F.; Talbot, D.C.; et al. A Phase II Study of Etanercept (Enbrel), a Tumor Necrosis Factor α Inhibitor in Patients with Metastatic Breast Cancer. *Clin. Cancer Res.* **2004**, *10*, 6528–6534. [CrossRef] [PubMed]

188. Brown, E.R.; Charles, K.A.; Hoare, S.A.; Rye, R.L.; Jodrell, D.I.; Aird, R.E.; Vora, R.; Prabhakar, U.; Nakada, M.; Corringham, R.E.; et al. A Clinical Study Assessing the Tolerability and Biological Effects of Infliximab, a TNF-Alpha Inhibitor, in Patients with Advanced Cancer. *Ann. Oncol.* **2008**, *19*, 1340–1346. [CrossRef]

189. Rutgeerts, P.; Van Assche, G.; Vermeire, S. Optimizing Anti-TNF Treatment in Inflammatory Bowel Disease. *Gastroenterology* **2004**, *126*, 1593–1610. [CrossRef]

190. Atzeni, F.; Sarzi-Puttini, P. *Autoimmunity and the Newer Biopharmaceuticals*; Chapter 92; Shoenfeld, Y., Meroni, P.L., Gershwin, M.E.B.T.-A., Third, E., Eds.; Elsevier: San Diego, CA, USA, 2014; pp. 795–802. [CrossRef]

191. Kulbe, H.; Chakravarty, P.; Leinster, D.A.; Charles, K.A.; Kwong, J.; Thompson, R.G.; Coward, J.I.; Schioppa, T.; Robinson, S.C.; Gallagher, W.M.; et al. A Dynamic Inflammatory Cytokine Network in the Human Ovarian Cancer Microenvironment. *Cancer Res.* **2012**, *72*, 66–75. [CrossRef]

192. Larkin, J.M.G.; Ferguson, T.R.; Pickering, L.M.; Edmonds, K.; James, M.G.; Thomas, K.; Banerji, U.; Berns, B.; de Boer, C.; Gore, M.E. A Phase I/II Trial of Sorafenib and Infliximab in Advanced Renal Cell Carcinoma. *Br. J. Cancer* **2010**, *103*, 1149–1153. [CrossRef] [PubMed]

193. Hwang, H.S.; Park, Y.Y.; Shin, S.J.; Go, H.; Park, J.M.; Yoon, S.Y.; Lee, J.L.; Cho, Y.M. Involvement of the TNF-α Pathway in TKI Resistance and Suggestion of TNFR1 as a Predictive Biomarker for TKI Responsiveness in Clear Cell Renal Cell Carcinoma. *J. Korean Med. Sci.* **2020**, *35*, e31. [CrossRef] [PubMed]

194. Harrison, M.L.; Obermueller, E.; Maisey, N.R.; Hoare, S.; Edmonds, K.; Li, N.F.; Chao, D.; Hall, K.; Lee, C.; Timotheadou, E.; et al. Tumor Necrosis Factor Alpha as a New Target for Renal Cell Carcinoma: Two Sequential Phase II Trials of Infliximab at Standard and High Dose. *J. Clin. Oncol.* **2007**, *25*, 4542–4549. [CrossRef]

195. Maisey, N. Antitumor Necrosis Factor (TNF-a) Antibodies in the Treatment of Renal Cell Cancer. *Cancer Invest.* **2007**, *25*, 589–593. [CrossRef]

196. Navarro-Sarabia, F.; Ariza-Ariza, R.; Hernández-Cruz, B.; Villanueva, I. Adalimumab for Treating Rheumatoid Arthritis. *J. Rheumatol.* **2006**, *33*, 1075–1081. [CrossRef]

197. Kobelt, D.; Zhang, C.; Clayton-Lucey, I.A.; Glauben, R.; Voss, C.; Siegmund, B.; Stein, U. Pro-Inflammatory TNF-α and IFN-γ Promote Tumor Growth and Metastasis via Induction of MACC1. *Front. Immunol.* **2020**, *11*, 980. [CrossRef]

198. Prattichizzo, F.; Giuliani, A.; Recchioni, R.; Bonafè, M.; Marcheselli, F.; De Carolis, S.; Campanati, A.; Giuliodori, K.; Rippo, M.R.; Brugè, F.; et al. Anti-TNF-α Treatment Modulates SASP and SASP-Related MicroRNAs in Endothelial Cells and in Circulating Angiogenic Cells. *Oncotarget* **2016**, *7*, 11945–11958. [CrossRef]

199. Steed, P.M.; Tansey, M.G.; Zalevsky, J.; Zhukovsky, E.A.; Desjarlais, J.R.; Szymkowski, D.E.; Abbott, C.; Carmichael, D.; Chan, C.; Cherry, L.; et al. Inactivation of TNF Signaling by Rationally Designed Dominant-Negative TNF Variants. *Science* **2003**, *301*, 1895–1898. [CrossRef]

200. Xu, J.; Chakrabarti, A.K.; Tan, J.L.; Ge, L.; Gambotto, A.; Vujanovic, N.L. Essential Role of the TNF-TNFR2 Cognate Interaction in Mouse Dendritic Cell-Natural Killer Cell Crosstalk. *Blood* **2007**, *109*, 3333–3341. [CrossRef]

201. Vujanovic, L.; Szymkowski, D.E.; Alber, S.; Watkins, S.C.; Vujanovic, N.L.; Butterfield, L.H. Virally Infected and Matured Human Dendritic Cells Activate Natural Killer Cells via Cooperative Activity of Plasma Membrane-Bound TNF and IL-15. *Blood* **2010**, *116*, 575–583. [CrossRef]

202. Vujanovic, N.L. Role of TNF Superfamily Ligands in Innate Immunity. *Immunol. Res.* **2011**, *50*, 159–174. [CrossRef] [PubMed]

203. Andrea, S.V.; Lazar, V.; Albert, B.D.L.; Fernando, C.B.; Robert, L.F.; Yan, L.; Nikola, L.V. Inhibition of Soluble Tumor Necrosis Factor Prevents Chemically Induced Carcinogenesis in Mice. *Cancer Immunol. Res.* **2016**, *4*, 441–451. [CrossRef]

204. Slamon, D.J.; Godolphin, W.; Jones, L.A.; Holt, J.A.; Wong, S.G.; Keith, D.E.; Levin, W.J.; Stuart, S.G.; Udove, J.; Ullrich, A. Studies of the HER-2/Neu Proto-Oncogene in Human Breast and Ovarian Cancer. *Science* **1989**, *244*, 707–712. [CrossRef] [PubMed]

205. Braun, S.; Schlimok, G.; Heumos, I.; Schaller, G.; Riethdorf, L.; Riethmüller, G.; Pantel, K. ErbB2 Overexpression on Occult Metastatic Cells in Bone Marrow Predicts Poor Clinical Outcome of Stage I-III Breast Cancer Patients. *Cancer Res.* **2001**, *61*, 1890–1895. [PubMed]

206. Potti, A.; Willardson, J.; Forseen, C.; Kishor Ganti, A.; Koch, M.; Hebert, B.; Levitt, R.; Mehdi, S.A. Predictive Role of HER-2/Neu Overexpression and Clinical Features at Initial Presentation in Patients with Extensive Stage Small Cell Lung Carcinoma. *Lung Cancer* **2002**, *36*, 257–261. [CrossRef]

207. Canoz, O.; Ozkan, M.; Arsav, V.; Er, O.; Coskun, H.S.; Soyuer, S.; Altinbas, M. The Role of C-ErbB-2 Expression on the Survival of Patients with Small-Cell Lung Cancer. *Lung* **2006**, *184*, 267–272. [CrossRef] [PubMed]

208. Minami, T.; Kijima, T.; Kohmo, S.; Arase, H.; Otani, Y.; Nagatomo, I.; Takahashi, R.; Miyake, K.; Higashiguchi, M.; Morimura, O.; et al. Overcoming Chemoresistance of Small-Cell Lung Cancer through Stepwise HER2-Targeted Antibody-Dependent Cell-Mediated Cytotoxicity and VEGF-Targeted Antiangiogenesis. *Sci. Rep.* **2013**, *3*, 2669. [CrossRef] [PubMed]

209. Krop, I.E.; Kim, S.-B.; González-Martín, A.; LoRusso, P.M.; Ferrero, J.-M.; Smitt, M.; Yu, R.; Leung, A.C.F.; Wildiers, H. Trastuzumab Emtansine versus Treatment of Physician's Choice for Pretreated HER2-Positive Advanced Breast Cancer (TH3RESA): A Randomised, Open-Label, Phase 3 Trial. *Lancet Oncol.* **2014**, *15*, 689–699. [CrossRef]

210. Singh, R.; Lillard, J.W.J.; Singh, S. Chemokines: Key Players in Cancer Progression and Metastasis. *Front. Biosci.* **2011**, *3*, 1569–1582. [CrossRef]

211. Balkwill, F.R. The Chemokine System and Cancer. *J. Pathol.* **2012**, *226*, 148–157. [CrossRef]

212. Hobbs, S.S.; Goettel, J.A.; Liang, D.; Yan, F.; Edelblum, K.L.; Frey, M.R.; Mullane, M.T.; Polk, D.B. TNF Transactivation of EGFR Stimulates Cytoprotective COX-2 Expression in Gastrointestinal Epithelial Cells. *Am. J. Physiol. Gastrointest. Liver Physiol.* **2011**, *301*, G220–G229. [CrossRef] [PubMed]

213. Argast, G.M.; Campbell, J.S.; Brooling, J.T.; Fausto, N. Epidermal Growth Factor Receptor Transactivation Mediates Tumor Necrosis Factor-Induced Hepatocyte Replication. *J. Biol. Chem.* **2004**, *279*, 34530–34536. [CrossRef] [PubMed]

214. Ueno, Y.; Sakurai, H.; Matsuo, M.; Choo, M.K.; Koizumi, K.; Saiki, I. Selective Inhibition of TNF-Alpha-Induced Activation of Mitogen-Activated Protein Kinases and Metastatic Activities by Gefitinib. *Br. J. Cancer* **2005**, *92*, 1690–1695. [CrossRef] [PubMed]

215. Tsatsanis, C.; Androulidaki, A.; Venihaki, M.; Margioris, A.N. Signalling Networks Regulating Cyclooxygenase-2. *Int. J. Biochem. Cell Biol.* **2006**, *38*, 1654–1661. [CrossRef]

216. Chun, K.-S.; Surh, Y.-J. Signal Transduction Pathways Regulating Cyclooxygenase-2 Expression: Potential Molecular Targets for Chemoprevention. *Biochem. Pharmacol.* **2004**, *68*, 1089–1100. [CrossRef]

217. Giovannucci, E.; Rimm, E.B.; Stampfer, M.J.; Colditz, G.A.; Ascherio, A.; Willett, W.C. Aspirin Use and the Risk for Colorectal Cancer and Adenoma in Male Health Professionals. *Ann. Intern. Med.* **1994**, *121*, 241–246. [CrossRef]

218. Greenberg, E.R.; Baron, J.A.; Freeman, D.H.J.; Mandel, J.S.; Haile, R. Reduced Risk of Large-Bowel Adenomas among Aspirin Users. The Polyp Prevention Study Group. *J. Natl. Cancer Inst.* **1993**, *85*, 912–916. [CrossRef]

219. Son, D.-S.; Kabir, S.M.; Dong, Y.; Lee, E.; Adunyah, S.E. Characteristics of Chemokine Signatures Elicited by EGF and TNF in Ovarian Cancer Cells. *J. Inflamm.* **2013**, *10*, 25. [CrossRef]

220. Freedman, M.H.; Cohen, A.; Grunberger, T.; Bunin, N.; Luddy, R.E.; Saunders, E.F.; Shahidi, N.; Lau, A.; Estrov, Z. Central Role of Tumour Necrosis Factor, GM-CSF, and Interleukin 1 in the Pathogenesis of Juvenile Chronic Myelogenous Leukaemia. *Br. J. Haematol.* **1992**, *80*, 40–48. [CrossRef]

221. Shan, D.; Ledbetter, J.A.; Press, O.W. Signaling Events Involved in Anti-CD20-Induced Apoptosis of Malignant Human B Cells. *Cancer Immunol. Immunother.* **2000**, *48*, 673–683. [CrossRef]

222. Adami, F.; Guarini, A.; Pini, M.; Siviero, F.; Sancetta, R.; Massaia, M.; Trentin, L.; Foà, R.; Semenzato, G. Serum Levels of Tumour Necrosis Factor-Alpha in Patients with B-Cell Chronic Lymphocytic Leukaemia. *Eur. J. Cancer* **1994**, *30A*, 1259–1263. [CrossRef]

223. Saulep-Easton, D.; Vincent, F.B.; Le Page, M.; Wei, A.; Ting, S.B.; Croce, C.M.; Tam, C.; Mackay, F. Cytokine-Driven Loss of Plasmacytoid Dendritic Cell Function in Chronic Lymphocytic Leukemia. *Leukemia* **2014**, *28*, 2005–2015. [CrossRef] [PubMed]

224. Francisco, L.M.; Sage, P.T.; Sharpe, A.H. The PD-1 Pathway in Tolerance and Autoimmunity. *Immunol. Rev.* **2010**, *236*, 219–242. [CrossRef] [PubMed]

225. Guleria, I.; Khosroshahi, A.; Ansari, M.J.; Habicht, A.; Azuma, M.; Yagita, H.; Noelle, R.J.; Coyle, A.; Mellor, A.L.; Khoury, S.J.; et al. A Critical Role for the Programmed Death Ligand 1 in Fetomaternal Tolerance. *J. Exp. Med.* **2005**, *202*, 231–237. [CrossRef] [PubMed]

226. Butte, M.J.; Keir, M.E.; Phamduy, T.B.; Sharpe, A.H.; Freeman, G.J. Programmed Death-1 Ligand 1 Interacts Specifically with the B7-1 Costimulatory Molecule to Inhibit T Cell Responses. *Immunity* **2007**, *27*, 111–122. [CrossRef]

227. Curiel, T.J.; Wei, S.; Dong, H.; Alvarez, X.; Cheng, P.; Mottram, P.; Krzysiek, R.; Knutson, K.L.; Daniel, B.; Zimmermann, M.C.; et al. Blockade of B7-H1 Improves Myeloid Dendritic Cell-Mediated Antitumor Immunity. *Nat. Med.* **2003**, *9*, 562–567. [CrossRef]

228. Latchman, Y.E.; Liang, S.C.; Wu, Y.; Chernova, T.; Sobel, R.A.; Klemm, M.; Kuchroo, V.K.; Freeman, G.J.; Sharpe, A.H. PD-L1-Deficient Mice Show That PD-L1 on T Cells, Antigen-Presenting Cells, and Host Tissues Negatively Regulates T Cells. *Proc. Natl. Acad. Sci. USA* **2004**, *101*, 10691–10696. [CrossRef]

229. Freeman, G.J.; Long, A.J.; Iwai, Y.; Bourque, K.; Chernova, T.; Nishimura, H.; Fitz, L.J.; Malenkovich, N.; Okazaki, T.; Byrne, M.C.; et al. Engagement of the PD-1 Immunoinhibitory Receptor by a Novel B7 Family Member Leads to Negative Regulation of Lymphocyte Activation. *J. Exp. Med.* **2000**, *192*, 1027–1034. [CrossRef]

230. Leach, D.R.; Krummel, M.F.; Allison, J.P. Enhancement of Antitumor Immunity by CTLA-4 Blockade. *Science* **1996**, *271*, 1734–1736. [CrossRef]

231. Hodi, F.S.; O'Day, S.J.; McDermott, D.F.; Weber, R.W.; Sosman, J.A.; Haanen, J.B.; Gonzalez, R.; Robert, C.; Schadendorf, D.; Hassel, J.C.; et al. Improved Survival with Ipilimumab in Patients with Metastatic Melanoma. *N. Engl. J. Med.* **2010**, *363*, 711–723. [CrossRef]

232. Wang, X.; Yang, L.; Huang, F.; Zhang, Q.; Liu, S.; Ma, L.; You, Z. Inflammatory Cytokines IL-17 and TNF-α up-Regulate PD-L1 Expression in Human Prostate and Colon Cancer Cells. *Immunol. Lett.* **2017**, *184*, 7–14. [CrossRef] [PubMed]

233. Qu, Q.-X.; Xie, F.; Huang, Q.; Zhang, X.-G. Membranous and Cytoplasmic Expression of PD-L1 in Ovarian Cancer Cells. *Cell. Physiol. Biochem. Int. J. Exp. Cell. Physiol. Biochem. Pharm.* **2017**, *43*, 1893–1906. [CrossRef] [PubMed]

234. Hartley, G.; Regan, D.; Guth, A.; Dow, S. Regulation of PD-L1 Expression on Murine Tumor-Associated Monocytes and Macrophages by Locally Produced TNF-α. *Cancer Immunol. Immunother.* **2017**, *66*, 523–535. [CrossRef] [PubMed]

235. Li, Z.; Zhang, C.; Du, J.-X.; Zhao, J.; Shi, M.-T.; Jin, M.-W.; Liu, H. Adipocytes Promote Tumor Progression and Induce PD-L1 Expression via TNF-α/IL-6 Signaling. *Cancer Cell Int.* **2020**, *20*, 179. [CrossRef]

236. Lv, Y.; Zhao, Y.; Wang, X.; Chen, N.; Mao, F.; Teng, Y.; Wang, T.; Peng, L.; Zhang, J.; Cheng, P.; et al. Increased Intratumoral Mast Cells Foster Immune Suppression and Gastric Cancer Progression through TNF-α-PD-L1 Pathway. *J. Immunother. Cancer* **2019**, *7*, 54. [CrossRef]

237. Ju, X.; Zhang, H.; Zhou, Z.; Chen, M.; Wang, Q. Tumor-Associated Macrophages Induce PD-L1 Expression in Gastric Cancer Cells through IL-6 and TNF-α Signaling. *Exp. Cell Res.* **2020**, *396*, 112315. [CrossRef]

238. Lim, S.-O.; Li, C.-W.; Xia, W.; Cha, J.-H.; Chan, L.-C.; Wu, Y.; Chang, S.-S.; Lin, W.-C.; Hsu, J.-M.; Hsu, Y.-H.; et al. Deubiquitination and Stabilization of PD-L1 by CSN5. *Cancer Cell* **2016**, *30*, 925–939. [CrossRef]

239. Rotte, A.; D'Orazi, G.; Bhandaru, M. Nobel Committee Honors Tumor Immunologists. *J. Exp. Clin. Cancer Res.* **2018**, *37*, 262. [CrossRef]

240. Zingg, D.; Arenas-Ramirez, N.; Sahin, D.; Rosalia, R.A.; Antunes, A.T.; Haeusel, J.; Sommer, L.; Boyman, O. The Histone Methyltransferase Ezh2 Controls Mechanisms of Adaptive Resistance to Tumor Immunotherapy. *Cell Rep.* **2017**, *20*, 854–867. [CrossRef]

241. Jeong, H.; Kim, S.; Hong, B.-J.; Lee, C.-J.; Kim, Y.-E.; Bok, S.; Oh, J.-M.; Gwak, S.-H.; Yoo, M.Y.; Lee, M.S.; et al. Tumor-Associated Macrophages Enhance Tumor Hypoxia and Aerobic Glycolysis. *Cancer Res.* **2019**, *79*, 795–806. [CrossRef]

242. Boutsikou, E.; Domvri, K.; Hardavella, G.; Tsiouda, D.; Zarogoulidis, K.; Kontakiotis, T. Tumour Necrosis Factor, Interferon-Gamma and Interleukins as Predictive Markers of Antiprogrammed Cell-Death Protein-1 Treatment in Advanced Non-Small Cell Lung Cancer: A Pragmatic Approach in Clinical Practice. *Ther. Adv. Med. Oncol.* **2018**, *10*. [CrossRef] [PubMed]

243. Blidner, A.G.; Choi, J.; Cooksley, T.; Dougan, M.; Glezerman, I.; Ginex, P.; Girotra, M.; Gupta, D.; Johnson, D.; Shannon, V.R.; et al. Cancer Immunotherapy-Related Adverse Events: Causes and Challenges. *Support. Care Cancer Off. J. Multinatl. Assoc. Support. Care Cancer* **2020**, *28*, 6111–6117. [CrossRef] [PubMed]

244. Flaherty, K.T.; Infante, J.R.; Daud, A.; Gonzalez, R.; Kefford, R.F.; Sosman, J.; Hamid, O.; Schuchter, L.; Cebon, J.; Ibrahim, N.; et al. Combined BRAF and MEK Inhibition in Melanoma with BRAF V600 Mutations. *N. Engl. J. Med.* **2012**, *367*, 1694–1703. [CrossRef] [PubMed]

245. Wang, D.Y.; Salem, J.-E.; Cohen, J.V.; Chandra, S.; Menzer, C.; Ye, F.; Zhao, S.; Das, S.; Beckermann, K.E.; Ha, L.; et al. Fatal Toxic Effects Associated With Immune Checkpoint Inhibitors: A Systematic Review and Meta-Analysis. *JAMA Oncol.* **2018**, *4*, 1721–1728. [CrossRef]

246. Boutros, C.; Tarhini, A.; Routier, E.; Lambotte, O.; Ladurie, F.L.; Carbonnel, F.; Izzeddine, H.; Marabelle, A.; Champiat, S.; Berdelou, A.; et al. Safety Profiles of Anti-CTLA-4 and Anti-PD-1 Antibodies Alone and in Combination. *Nat. Rev. Clin. Oncol.* **2016**, *13*, 473–486. [CrossRef]

247. Larkin, J.; Chiarion-Sileni, V.; Gonzalez, R.; Grob, J.J.; Cowey, C.L.; Lao, C.D.; Schadendorf, D.; Dummer, R.; Smylie, M.; Rutkowski, P.; et al. Combined Nivolumab and Ipilimumab or Monotherapy in Untreated Melanoma. *N. Engl. J. Med.* **2015**, *373*, 23–34. [CrossRef]

248. Naidoo, J.; Page, D.B.; Li, B.T.; Connell, L.C.; Schindler, K.; Lacouture, M.E.; Postow, M.A.; Wolchok, J.D. Toxicities of the Anti-PD-1 and Anti-PD-L1 Immune Checkpoint Antibodies. *Ann. Oncol.* **2015**, *26*, 2375–2391. [CrossRef]

249. Ribas, A.; Wolchok, J.D. Cancer Immunotherapy Using Checkpoint Blockade. *Science* **2018**, *359*, 1350–1355. [CrossRef]

250. Jacoberger-Foissac, C.; Blake, S.J.; Liu, J.; McDonald, E.; Triscott, H.; Nakamura, K.; Smyth, M.J.; Teng, M.W. Concomitant or Delayed Anti-TNF Differentially Impact on Immune-Related Adverse Events and Antitumor Efficacy after Anti-CD40 Therapy. *J. Immunother. Cancer* **2020**, *8*. [CrossRef]

251. Verheijden, R.J.; May, A.M.; Blank, C.U.; Aarts, M.J.B.; van den Berkmortel, F.W.P.J.; van den Eertwegh, A.J.M.; de Groot, J.W.B.; Boers-Sonderen, M.J.; van der Hoeven, J.J.M.; Hospers, G.A.; et al. Association of Anti-TNF with Decreased Survival in Steroid Refractory Ipilimumab and Anti-PD1-Treated Patients in the Dutch Melanoma Treatment Registry. *Clin. Cancer Res.* **2020**, *26*, 2268–2274. [CrossRef]

252. Montfort, A.; Dufau, C.; Colacios, C.; Andrieu-Abadie, N.; Levade, T.; Filleron, T.; Delord, J.-P.; Ayyoub, M.; Meyer, N.; Ségui, B. Anti-TNF, a Magic Bullet in Cancer Immunotherapy? *J. Immunother. Cancer* **2019**, *7*, 303. [CrossRef] [PubMed]

253. Upadhaya, S.; Hubbard-Lucey, V.M.; Yu, J.X. Immuno-Oncology Drug Development Forges on despite COVID-19. *Nat. Rev. Drug Discov.* **2020**, 751–752. [CrossRef] [PubMed]

254. Phelan, K.W.; Advani, A.S. Novel Therapies in Acute Lymphoblastic Leukemia. *Curr. Hematol. Malig. Rep.* **2018**, *13*, 289–299. [CrossRef] [PubMed]

255. Dai, H.; Wang, Y.; Lu, X.; Han, W. Chimeric Antigen Receptors Modified T-Cells for Cancer Therapy. *J. Natl. Cancer Inst.* **2016**, *108*. [CrossRef] [PubMed]

256. Frey, N. The What, When and How of CAR T Cell Therapy for ALL. *Best Pr. Res. Clin. Haematol.* **2017**, *30*, 275–281. [CrossRef]

257. Grupp, S.A.; Kalos, M.; Barrett, D.; Aplenc, R.; Porter, D.L.; Rheingold, S.R.; Teachey, D.T.; Chew, A.; Hauck, B.; Wright, J.F.; et al. Chimeric Antigen Receptor-Modified T Cells for Acute Lymphoid Leukemia. *N. Engl. J. Med.* **2013**, *368*, 1509–1518. [CrossRef]

258. Raponi, S.; De Propris, M.S.; Intoppa, S.; Milani, M.L.; Vitale, A.; Elia, L.; Perbellini, O.; Pizzolo, G.; Foá, R.; Guarini, A. Flow Cytometric Study of Potential Target Antigens (CD19, CD20, CD22, CD33) for Antibody-Based Immunotherapy in Acute Lymphoblastic Leukemia: Analysis of 552 Cases. *Leuk. Lymphoma* **2011**, *52*, 1098–1107. [CrossRef]
259. Scheuermann, R.H.; Racila, E. CD19 Antigen in Leukemia and Lymphoma Diagnosis and Immunotherapy. *Leuk. Lymphoma* **1995**, *18*, 385–397. [CrossRef]
260. Maude, S.L.; Barrett, D.; Teachey, D.T.; Grupp, S.A. Managing Cytokine Release Syndrome Associated with Novel T Cell-Engaging Therapies. *Cancer J.* **2014**, *20*, 119–122. [CrossRef]
261. Maus, M.V.; Haas, A.R.; Beatty, G.L.; Albelda, S.M.; Levine, B.L.; Liu, X.; Zhao, Y.; Kalos, M.; June, C.H. T Cells Expressing Chimeric Antigen Receptors Can Cause Anaphylaxis in Humans. *Cancer Immunol. Res.* **2013**, *1*, 26–31. [CrossRef]
262. Brentjens, R.J.; Davila, M.L.; Riviere, I.; Park, J.; Wang, X.; Cowell, L.G.; Bartido, S.; Stefanski, J.; Taylor, C.; Olszewska, M.; et al. CD19-Targeted T Cells Rapidly Induce Molecular Remissions in Adults with Chemotherapy-Refractory Acute Lymphoblastic Leukemia. *Sci. Transl. Med.* **2013**, *5*, 177ra38. [CrossRef] [PubMed]
263. Elia, A.R.; Grioni, M.; Basso, V.; Curnis, F.; Freschi, M.; Corti, A.; Mondino, A.; Bellone, M. Targeting Tumor Vasculature with TNF Leads Effector T Cells to the Tumor and Enhances Therapeutic Efficacy of Immune Checkpoint Blockers in Combination with Adoptive Cell Therapy. *Clin. Cancer Res.* **2018**, *24*, 2171–2181. [CrossRef] [PubMed]
264. Piali, L.; Fichtel, A.; Terpe, H.J.; Imhof, B.A.; Gisler, R.H. Endothelial Vascular Cell Adhesion Molecule 1 Expression Is Suppressed by Melanoma and Carcinoma. *J. Exp. Med.* **1995**, *181*, 811–816. [CrossRef] [PubMed]
265. Bellone, M.; Calcinotto, A. Ways to Enhance Lymphocyte Trafficking into Tumors and Fitness of Tumor Infiltrating Lymphocytes. *Front. Oncol.* **2013**, *3*, 231. [CrossRef] [PubMed]
266. Sharma, P.; Hu-Lieskovan, S.; Wargo, J.A.; Ribas, A. Primary, Adaptive, and Acquired Resistance to Cancer Immunotherapy. *Cell* **2017**, *168*, 707–723. [CrossRef]
267. Bellone, M.; Elia, A.R. Constitutive and Acquired Mechanisms of Resistance to Immune Checkpoint Blockade in Human Cancer. *Cytokine Growth Factor Rev.* **2017**, *36*, 17–24. [CrossRef]
268. Calcinotto, A.; Grioni, M.; Jachetti, E.; Curnis, F.; Mondino, A.; Parmiani, G.; Corti, A.; Bellone, M. Targeting TNF-α to Neoangiogenic Vessels Enhances Lymphocyte Infiltration in Tumors and Increases the Therapeutic Potential of Immunotherapy. *J. Immunol.* **2012**, *188*, 2687–2694. [CrossRef]
269. Manzo, T.; Sturmheit, T.; Basso, V.; Petrozziello, E.; Hess Michelini, R.; Riba, M.; Freschi, M.; Elia, A.R.; Grioni, M.; Curnis, F.; et al. T Cells Redirected to a Minor Histocompatibility Antigen Instruct Intratumoral TNFα Expression and Empower Adoptive Cell Therapy for Solid Tumors. *Cancer Res.* **2017**, *77*, 658–671. [CrossRef]
270. Plautz, G.E.; Touhalisky, J.E.; Shu, S. Treatment of Murine Gliomas by Adoptive Transfer of Ex Vivo Activated Tumor-Draining Lymph Node Cells. *Cell. Immunol.* **1997**, *178*, 101–107. [CrossRef]
271. Peng, L.; Shu, S.; Krauss, J.C. Treatment of Subcutaneous Tumor with Adoptively Transferred T Cells. *Cell. Immunol.* **1997**, *178*, 24–32. [CrossRef]
272. Tanaka, H.; Yoshizawa, H.; Yamaguchi, Y.; Ito, K.; Kagamu, H.; Suzuki, E.; Gejyo, F.; Hamada, H.; Arakawa, M. Successful Adoptive Immunotherapy of Murine Poorly Immunogenic Tumor with Specific Effector Cells Generated from Gene-Modified Tumor-Primed Lymph Node Cells. *J. Immunol.* **1999**, *162*, 3574–3582. [PubMed]
273. Ye, Z.; Shi, M.; Chan, T.; Sas, S.; Xu, S.; Xiang, J. Engineered CD8+ Cytotoxic T Cells with Fiber-Modified Adenovirus-Mediated TNF-Alpha Gene Transfection Counteract Immunosuppressive Interleukin-10-Secreting Lung Metastasis and Solid Tumors. *Cancer Gene* **2007**, *14*, 661–675. [CrossRef] [PubMed]
274. Pedersen, A.E.; Thorn, M.; Gad, M.; Walter, M.R.; Johnsen, H.E.; Gaarsdal, E.; Nikolajsen, K.; Buus, S.; Claesson, M.H.; Svane, I.M. Phenotypic and Functional Characterization of Clinical Grade Dendritic Cells Generated from Patients with Advanced Breast Cancer for Therapeutic Vaccination. *Scand. J. Immunol.* **2005**, 147–156. [CrossRef] [PubMed]
275. Brunner, C.; Seiderer, J.; Schlamp, A.; Bidlingmaier, M.; Eigler, A.; Haimerl, W.; Lehr, H.A.; Krieg, A.M.; Hartmann, G.; Endres, S. Enhanced Dendritic Cell Maturation by TNF-Alpha or Cytidine-Phosphate-Guanosine DNA Drives T Cell Activation in Vitro and Therapeutic Anti-Tumor Immune Responses in Vivo. *J. Immunol.* **2000**, *165*, 6278–6286. [CrossRef] [PubMed]
276. Cumberbatch, M.; Kimber, I. Tumour Necrosis Factor-Alpha Is Required for Accumulation of Dendritic Cells in Draining Lymph Nodes and for Optimal Contact Sensitization. *Immunology* **1995**, *84*, 31–35.
277. Hogquist, K.A.; Jameson, S.C.; Heath, W.R.; Howard, J.L.; Bevan, M.J.; Carbone, F.R. T Cell Receptor Antagonist Peptides Induce Positive Selection. *Cell* **1994**, *76*, 17–27. [CrossRef]
278. Liu, Y.; Saxena, A.; Zheng, C.; Carlsen, S.; Xiang, J. Combined Alpha Tumor Necrosis Factor Gene Therapy and Engineered Dendritic Cell Vaccine in Combating Well-Established Tumors. *J. Gene Med.* **2004**, *6*, 857–868. [CrossRef]
279. Klebanoff, C.A.; Khong, H.T.; Antony, P.A.; Palmer, D.C.; Restifo, N.P. Sinks, Suppressors and Antigen Presenters: How Lymphodepletion Enhances T Cell-Mediated Tumor Immunotherapy. *Trends Immunol.* **2005**, *26*, 111–117. [CrossRef]
280. Dudley, M.E.; Wunderlich, J.R.; Yang, J.C.; Sherry, R.M.; Topalian, S.L.; Restifo, N.P.; Royal, R.E.; Kammula, U.; White, D.E.; Mavroukakis, S.A.; et al. Adoptive Cell Transfer Therapy Following Non-Myeloablative but Lymphodepleting Chemotherapy for the Treatment of Patients with Refractory Metastatic Melanoma. *J. Clin. Oncol.* **2005**, *23*, 2346–2357. [CrossRef]
281. Dudley, M.E.; Gross, C.A.; Langhan, M.M.; Garcia, M.R.; Sherry, R.M.; Yang, J.C.; Phan, G.Q.; Kammula, U.S.; Hughes, M.S.; Citrin, D.E.; et al. CD8+ Enriched "Young" Tumor Infiltrating Lymphocytes Can Mediate Regression of Metastatic Melanoma. *Clin. Cancer Res.* **2010**, *16*, 6122–6131. [CrossRef]

282. Santos, J.M.; Cervera-carrascon, V.; Havunen, R.; Zafar, S.; Siurala, M.; Sorsa, S.; Anttila, M.; Kanerva, A.; Hemminki, A. Adenovirus Coding for Interleukin-2 and Tumor Necrosis Factor Alpha Replaces Lymphodepleting Chemotherapy in Adoptive T Cell Therapy. *Mol. Ther.* **2018**, *26*, 2243–2254. [CrossRef] [PubMed]
283. Siurala, M.; Havunen, R.; Saha, D.; Lumen, D.; Airaksinen, A.J.; Tähtinen, S.; Cervera-Carrascon, V.; Bramante, S.; Parviainen, S.; Vähä-Koskela, M.; et al. Adenoviral Delivery of Tumor Necrosis Factor-α and Interleukin-2 Enables Successful Adoptive Cell Therapy of Immunosuppressive Melanoma. *Mol. Ther.* **2016**, *24*, 1435–1443. [CrossRef] [PubMed]
284. Restifo, N.P.; Dudley, M.E.; Rosenberg, S.A. Adoptive Immunotherapy for Cancer: Harnessing the T Cell Response. *Nat. Rev. Immunol.* **2012**, *12*, 269–281. [CrossRef] [PubMed]
285. Rosenberg, S.A.; Yang, J.C.; Sherry, R.M.; Kammula, U.S.; Hughes, M.S.; Phan, G.Q.; Citrin, D.E.; Restifo, N.P.; Robbins, P.F.; Wunderlich, J.R.; et al. Durable Complete Responses in Heavily Pretreated Patients with Metastatic Melanoma Using T-Cell Transfer Immunotherapy. *Clin. Cancer Res.* **2011**, *17*, 4550–4557. [CrossRef]
286. Landsberg, J.; Kohlmeyer, J.; Renn, M.; Bald, T.; Rogava, M.; Cron, M.; Fatho, M.; Lennerz, V.; Wölfel, T.; Hölzel, M.; et al. Melanomas Resist T-Cell Therapy through Inflammation-Induced Reversible Dedifferentiation. *Nature* **2012**, *490*, 412–416. [CrossRef] [PubMed]
287. Mehta, A.; Kim, Y.J.; Robert, L.; Tsoi, J.; Comin-Anduix, B.; Berent-Maoz, B.; Cochran, A.J.; Economou, J.S.; Tumeh, P.C.; Puig-Saus, C.; et al. Immunotherapy Resistance by Inflammation-Induced Dedifferentiation. *Cancer Discov.* **2018**, *8*, 935–943. [CrossRef]
288. Hugo, W.; Zaretsky, J.M.; Sun, L.; Song, C.; Moreno, B.H.; Hu-Lieskovan, S.; Berent-Maoz, B.; Pang, J.; Chmielowski, B.; Cherry, G.; et al. Genomic and Transcriptomic Features of Response to Anti-PD-1 Therapy in Metastatic Melanoma. *Cell* **2017**, *168*, 542. [CrossRef]
289. Willrich, M.A.V.; Murray, D.L.; Snyder, M.R. Tumor Necrosis Factor Inhibitors: Clinical Utility in Autoimmune Diseases. *Transl. Res.* **2015**, *165*, 270–282. [CrossRef]
290. Roda, G.; Jharap, B.; Neeraj, N.; Colombel, J.-F. Loss of Response to Anti-TNFs: Definition, Epidemiology, and Management. *Clin. Transl. Gastroenterol.* **2016**, *7*, e135. [CrossRef]
291. Rubbert-Roth, A.; Atzeni, F.; Masala, I.F.; Caporali, R.; Montecucco, C.; Sarzi-Puttini, P. TNF Inhibitors in Rheumatoid Arthritis and Spondyloarthritis: Are They the Same? *Autoimmun. Rev.* **2018**, *17*, 24–28. [CrossRef]
292. Liu, J.; Dong, Z.; Zhu, Q.; He, D.; Ma, Y.; Du, A.; He, F.; Zhao, D.; Xu, X.; Zhang, H.; et al. TNF-α Promoter Polymorphisms Predict the Response to Etanercept More Powerfully than That to Infliximab/Adalimumab in Spondyloarthritis. *Sci. Rep.* **2016**, *6*, 1–9. [CrossRef] [PubMed]
293. Murdaca, G.; Gulli, R.; Spanò, F.; Lantieri, F.; Burlando, M.; Parodi, A.; Mandich, P.; Puppo, F. TNF-α Gene Polymorphisms: Association with Disease Susceptibility and Response to Anti-TNF-α Treatment in Psoriatic Arthritis. *J. Invest. Derm.* **2014**, *134*, 2503–2509. [CrossRef] [PubMed]
294. Hochberg, M.C.; Lebwohl, M.G.; Plevy, S.E.; Hobbs, K.F.; Yocum, D.E. The Benefit/Risk Profile of TNF-Blocking Agents: Findings of a Consensus Panel. *Semin. Arthritis Rheum.* **2005**, *34*, 819–836. [CrossRef] [PubMed]
295. Taylor, P.C. Antibody Therapy for Rheumatoid Arthritis. *Curr. Opin. Pharm.* **2003**, *3*, 323–328. [CrossRef]
296. Chang, J.; Girgis, L. Clinical Use of Anti-TNF-Alpha Biological Agents—A Guide for GPs. *Aust. Fam. Physician* **2007**, *36*, 1035–1038.
297. Roach, D.R.; Bean, A.G.D.; Demangel, C.; France, M.P.; Briscoe, H.; Britton, W.J. TNF Regulates Chemokine Induction Essential for Cell Recruitment, Granuloma Formation, and Clearance of Mycobacterial Infection. *J. Immunol.* **2002**, *168*, 4620–4627. [CrossRef]
298. Antoni, C.; Braun, J. Side Effects of Anti-TNF Therapy: Current Knowledge. *Clin. Exp. Rheumatol.* **2002**, *20* (Suppl. S28), S152–S157.
299. Bean, A.G.; Roach, D.R.; Briscoe, H.; France, M.P.; Korner, H.; Sedgwick, J.D.; Britton, W.J. Structural Deficiencies in Granuloma Formation in TNF Gene-Targeted Mice Underlie the Heightened Susceptibility to Aerosol Mycobacterium Tuberculosis Infection, Which Is Not Compensated for by Lymphotoxin. *J. Immunol.* **1999**, *162*, 3504–3511.
300. Her, M.; Kavanaugh, A. Alterations in Immune Function with Biologic Therapies for Autoimmune Disease. *J. Allergy Clin. Immunol.* **2016**, *137*, 19–27. [CrossRef]
301. Leombruno, J.P.; Einarson, T.R.; Keystone, E.C. The Safety of Anti-Tumour Necrosis Factor Treatments in Rheumatoid Arthritis: Meta and Exposure-Adjusted Pooled Analyses of Serious Adverse Events. *Ann. Rheum. Dis.* **2009**, *68*, 1136–1145. [CrossRef]
302. Thompson, A.E.; Rieder, S.W.; Pope, J.E. Tumor Necrosis Factor Therapy and the Risk of Serious Infection and Malignancy in Patients with Early Rheumatoid Arthritis: A Meta-Analysis of Randomized Controlled Trials. *Arthritis Rheum.* **2011**, *63*, 1479–1485. [CrossRef] [PubMed]
303. Grijalva, C.G.; Chen, L.; Delzell, E.; Baddley, J.W.; Beukelman, T.; Winthrop, K.L.; Griffin, M.R.; Herrinton, L.J.; Liu, L.; Ouellet-Hellstrom, R.; et al. Initiation of Tumor Necrosis Factor-α Antagonists and the Risk of Hospitalization for Infection in Patients with Autoimmune Diseases. *JAMA* **2011**, *306*, 2331–2339. [CrossRef] [PubMed]
304. Murdaca, G.; Negrini, S.; Pellecchio, M.; Greco, M.; Schiavi, C.; Giusti, F.; Puppo, F. Update upon the Infection Risk in Patients Receiving TNF Alpha Inhibitors. *Expert Opin. Drug Saf.* **2019**, *18*, 219–229. [CrossRef] [PubMed]
305. Zhang, Z.; Fan, W.; Yang, G.; Xu, Z.; Wang, J.; Cheng, Q.; Yu, M. Risk of Tuberculosis in Patients Treated with TNF-α Antagonists: A Systematic Review and Meta-Analysis of Randomised Controlled Trials. *BMJ Open* **2017**, *7*, 1–8. [CrossRef]
306. Ramiro, S.; Sepriano, A.; Chatzidionysiou, K.; Nam, J.L.; Smolen, J.S.; van der Heijde, D.; Dougados, M.; van Vollenhoven, R.; Bijlsma, J.W.; Burmester, G.R.; et al. Safety of Synthetic and Biological DMARDs: A Systematic Literature Review Informing the 2016 Update of the EULAR Recommendations for Management of Rheumatoid Arthritis. *Ann. Rheum. Dis.* **2017**, *76*, 1101–1136. [CrossRef]

307. Cao, B.L.; Qasem, A.; Sharp, R.C.; Abdelli, L.S.; Naser, S.A. Systematic Review and Meta-Analysis on the Association of Tuberculosis in Crohn's Disease Patients Treated with Tumor Necrosis Factor-α Inhibitors (Anti-TNFα). *World J. Gastroenterol.* **2018**, *24*, 2764–2775. [CrossRef]

308. McDonald, J.R.; Zeringue, A.L.; Caplan, L.; Ranganathan, P.; Xian, H.; Burroughs, T.E.; Fraser, V.J.; Cunningham, F.; Eisen, S.A. Herpes Zoster Risk Factors in a National Cohort of Veterans with Rheumatoid Arthritis. *Clin. Infect. Dis.* **2009**, *48*, 1364–1371. [CrossRef]

309. Che, H.; Lukas, C.; Morel, J.; Combe, B. Risk of Herpes/Herpes Zoster during Anti-Tumor Necrosis Factor Therapy in Patients with Rheumatoid Arthritis. Systematic Review and Meta-Analysis. *Jt. Bone Spine* **2014**, *81*, 215–221. [CrossRef]

310. Winthrop, K.L.; Baddley, J.W.; Chen, L.; Liu, L.; Grijalva, C.G.; Delzell, E.; Beukelman, T.; Patkar, N.M.; Xie, F.; Saag, K.G.; et al. Association between the Initiation of Anti-Tumor Necrosis Factor Therapy and the Risk of Herpes Zoster. *JAMA* **2013**, *309*, 887–895. [CrossRef]

311. Deepak, P.; Stobaugh, D.J.; Sherid, M.; Sifuentes, H.; Ehrenpreis, E.D. Neurological Events with Tumour Necrosis Factor Alpha Inhibitors Reported to the Food and Drug Administration Adverse Event Reporting System. *Aliment. Pharm.* **2013**, *38*, 388–396. [CrossRef]

312. Kaltsonoudis, E.; Zikou, A.K.; Voulgari, P.V.; Konitsiotis, S.; Argyropoulou, M.I.; Drosos, A.A. Neurological Adverse Events in Patients Receiving Anti-TNF Therapy: A Prospective Imaging and Electrophysiological Study. *Arthritis Res.* **2014**, *16*, R125. [CrossRef] [PubMed]

313. Robinson, W.H.; Genovese, M.C.; Moreland, L.W. Demyelinating and Neurologic Events Reported in Association with Tumor Necrosis Factor Alpha Antagonism: By What Mechanisms Could Tumor Necrosis Factor Alpha Antagonists Improve Rheumatoid Arthritis but Exacerbate Multiple Sclerosis? *Arthritis Rheum.* **2001**, *44*, 1977–1983. [CrossRef]

314. Solomon, A.J.; Spain, R.I.; Kruer, M.C.; Bourdette, D. Inflammatory Neurological Disease in Patients Treated with Tumor Necrosis Factor Alpha Inhibitors. *Mult. Scler.* **2011**, *17*, 1472–1487. [CrossRef] [PubMed]

315. Saffra, N.; Astafurov, K. Visual Loss Induced by Adalimumab Used for Plaque Psoriasis. *Case Rep. Dermatol.* **2017**, 60–64. [CrossRef] [PubMed]

316. Tanno, M.; Nakamura, I.; Kobayashi, S.; Kurihara, K.; Ito, K. New-Onset Demyelination Induced by Infliximab Therapy in Two Rheumatoid Arthritis Patients. *Clin. Rheumatol.* **2006**, *25*, 929–933. [CrossRef] [PubMed]

317. Balakumar, P.; Singh, M. Anti-Tumour Necrosis Factor-Alpha Therapy in Heart Failure: Future Directions. *Basic Clin. Pharm. Toxicol.* **2006**, *99*, 391–397. [CrossRef]

318. Bucalo, A.; Rega, F.; Zangrilli, A.; Silvestri, V.; Valentini, V.; Scafetta, G.; Marraffa, F.; Grassi, S.; Rogante, E.; Piccolo, A.; et al. Paradoxical Psoriasis Induced by Anti-TNFα Treatment: Evaluation of Disease-Specific Clinical and Genetic Markers. *Int. J. Mol. Sci.* **2020**, *21*, 7873. [CrossRef]

319. Bonovas, S.; Minozzi, S.; Lytras, T.; González-Lorenzo, M.; Pecoraro, V.; Colombo, S.; Polloni, I.; Moja, L.; Cinquini, M.; Marino, V.; et al. Risk of Malignancies Using Anti-TNF Agents in Rheumatoid Arthritis, Psoriatic Arthritis, and Ankylosing Spondylitis: A Systematic Review and Meta-Analysis. *Expert Opin. Drug Saf.* **2016**, *15*, 35–54. [CrossRef]

320. Chen, Y.; Sun, J.; Yang, Y.; Huang, Y.; Liu, G. Malignancy Risk of Anti-Tumor Necrosis Factor Alpha Blockers: An Overview of Systematic Reviews and Meta-Analyses. *Clin. Rheumatol.* **2016**, *35*, 1–18. [CrossRef]

321. Shelton, E.; Laharie, D.; Scott, F.I.; Mamtani, R.; Lewis, J.D.; Colombel, J.-F.; Ananthakrishnan, A.N. Cancer Recurrence Following Immune-Suppressive Therapies in Patients With Immune-Mediated Diseases: A Systematic Review and Meta-Analysis. *Gastroenterology* **2016**, *151*, 97–109.e4. [CrossRef]

322. Bongartz, T.; Sutton, A.J.; Sweeting, M.J.; Buchan, I.; Matteson, E.L.; Montori, V. Anti-TNF Antibody Therapy in Rheumatoid Arthritis and the Risk of Serious Infections and Malignancies: Systematic Review and Meta-Analysis of Rare Harmful Effects in Randomized Controlled Trials. *JAMA* **2006**, *295*, 2275–2285. [CrossRef] [PubMed]

323. Askling, J.; Fored, C.M.; Baecklund, E.; Brandt, L.; Backlin, C.; Ekbom, A.; Sundström, C.; Bertilsson, L.; Cöster, L.; Geborek, P.; et al. Haematopoietic Malignancies in Rheumatoid Arthritis: Lymphoma Risk and Characteristics after Exposure to Tumour Necrosis Factor Antagonists. *Ann. Rheum. Dis.* **2005**, *64*, 1414–1420. [CrossRef] [PubMed]

324. Minozzi, S.; Bonovas, S.; Lytras, T.; Pecoraro, V.; González-Lorenzo, M.; Bastiampillai, A.J.; Gabrielli, E.M.; Lonati, A.C.; Moja, L.; Cinquini, M.; et al. Risk of Infections Using Anti-TNF Agents in Rheumatoid Arthritis, Psoriatic Arthritis, and Ankylosing Spondylitis: A Systematic Review and Meta-Analysis. *Expert Opin. Drug Saf.* **2016**, *15* (Suppl. S1), 11–34. [CrossRef] [PubMed]

325. Dignass, A.; Van Assche, G.; Lindsay, J.O.; Lémann, M.; Söderholm, J.; Colombel, J.F.; Danese, S.; D'Hoore, A.; Gassull, M.; Gomollón, F.; et al. The Second European Evidence-Based Consensus on the Diagnosis and Management of Crohn's Disease: Current Management. *J. Crohns. Colitis* **2010**, *4*, 28–62. [CrossRef] [PubMed]

326. Li, H.H.; Zhu, H.; Liu, L.S.; Huang, Y.; Guo, J.; Li, J.; Sun, X.P.; Chang, C.X.; Wang, Z.H.; Zhai, K. Tumour Necrosis Factor-α Gene Polymorphism Is Associated with Metastasis in Patients with Triple Negative Breast Cancer. *Sci. Rep.* **2015**, *5*, 10244. [CrossRef]

327. Azmy, I.A.F.; Balasubramanian, S.P.; Wilson, A.G.; Stephenson, T.J.; Cox, A.; Brown, N.J.; Reed, M.W.R. Role of Tumour Necrosis Factor Gene Polymorphisms (-308 and -238) in Breast Cancer Susceptibility and Severity. *Breast Cancer Res.* **2004**, *6*, 395–400. [CrossRef]

328. Yi, F.; Shi, X.; Pei, X.; Wu, X. Tumor Necrosis Factor-Alpha-308 Gene Promoter Polymorphism Associates with Survival of Cancer Patients: A Meta-Analysis. *Medicine (Baltimore)* **2018**, *97*, e13160. [CrossRef]

329. Balkwill, F. Mantovani, a. Cancer and Inflammation: Implications for Pharmacology and Therapeutics. *Clin. Pharm.* **2010**, *87*, 401–406. [CrossRef]

330. Lentz, M.; Kumar, K. Reduction of Plasma Levels of Soluble Tumor Necrosis Factor and Interleukin-2 Receptors by Means of a Novel Immunoadsorption Column. *Ther. Apher. Dial.* **2008**, *12*, 491–499. [CrossRef]

331. Krippner-Heidenreich, A.; Grunwald, I.; Zimmermann, G.; Kühnle, M.; Gerspach, J.; Sterns, T.; Shnyder, S.D.; Gill, J.H.; Männel, D.N.; Pfizenmaier, K.; et al. Single-Chain TNF, a TNF Derivative with Enhanced Stability and Antitumoral Activity. *J. Immunol.* **2008**, *180*, 8176–8183. [CrossRef]
332. Josephs, S.F.; Ichim, T.E.; Prince, S.M.; Kesari, S.; Marincola, F.M.; Escobedo, A.R.; Jafri, A. Unleashing Endogenous TNF-Alpha as a Cancer Immunotherapeutic. *J. Transl. Med.* **2018**, *16*, 1–8. [CrossRef] [PubMed]
333. Chen, X.; Subleski, J.J.; Kopf, H.; Howard, O.M.Z.; Männel, D.N.; Oppenheim, J.J. Cutting Edge: Expression of TNFR2 Defines a Maximally Suppressive Subset of Mouse CD4+CD25+FoxP3+ T Regulatory Cells: Applicability to Tumor-Infiltrating T Regulatory Cells. *J. Immunol.* **2008**, *180*, 6467–6471. [CrossRef] [PubMed]
334. Facciabene, A.; Motz, G.T.; Coukos, G. T-Regulatory Cells: Key Players in Tumor Immune Escape and Angiogenesis. *Cancer Res.* **2012**, *72*, 2162–2171. [CrossRef]
335. Smyth, M.J.; Ngiow, S.F.; Teng, M.W.L. Targeting Regulatory T Cells in Tumor Immunotherapy. *Immunol. Cell Biol.* **2014**, *92*, 473–474. [CrossRef]
336. Okubo, Y.; Mera, T.; Wang, L.; Faustman, D.L. Homogeneous Expansion of Human T-Regulatory Cells via Tumor Necrosis Factor Receptor 2. *Sci. Rep.* **2013**, *3*, 3153. [CrossRef]
337. Ham, B.; Wang, N.; D'Costa, Z.; Fernandez, M.C.; Bourdeau, F.; Auguste, P.; Illemann, M.; Eefsen, R.L.; Høyer-Hansen, G.; Vainer, B.; et al. TNF Receptor-2 Facilitates an Immunosuppressive Microenvironment in the Liver to Promote the Colonization and Growth of Hepatic Metastases. *Cancer Res.* **2015**, *75*, 5235–5247. [CrossRef] [PubMed]
338. Wang, J.; Al-Lamki, R.S. Tumor Necrosis Factor Receptor 2: Its Contribution to Acute Cellular Rejection and Clear Cell Renal Carcinoma. *Biomed Res. Int.* **2013**, *2013*, 821310. [CrossRef] [PubMed]
339. Hamilton, K.E.; Simmons, J.G.; Ding, S.; Van Landeghem, L.; Lund, P.K. Cytokine Induction of Tumor Necrosis Factor Receptor 2 Is Mediated by STAT3 in Colon Cancer Cells. *Mol. Cancer Res.* **2011**, *9*, 1718–1731. [CrossRef]
340. Nakayama, S.; Yokote, T.; Tsuji, M.; Akioka, T.; Miyoshi, T.; Hirata, Y.; Hiraoka, N.; Iwaki, K.; Takayama, A.; Nishiwaki, U.; et al. Expression of Tumour Necrosis Factor-α and Its Receptors in Hodgkin Lymphoma. *Br. J. Haematol.* **2014**, 574–577. [CrossRef]
341. Rauert, H.; Stühmer, T.; Bargou, R.; Wajant, H.; Siegmund, D. TNFR1 and TNFR2 Regulate the Extrinsic Apoptotic Pathway in Myeloma Cells by Multiple Mechanisms. *Cell Death Dis.* **2011**, *2*, e194. [CrossRef]
342. Uhlén, M.; Björling, E.; Agaton, C.; Szigyarto, C.A.-K.; Amini, B.; Andersen, E.; Andersson, A.-C.; Angelidou, P.; Asplund, A.; Asplund, C.; et al. A Human Protein Atlas for Normal and Cancer Tissues Based on Antibody Proteomics. *Mol. Cell. Proteom.* **2005**, *4*, 1920–1932. [CrossRef] [PubMed]
343. Williams, G.S.; Mistry, B.; Guillard, S.; Ulrichsen, J.C.; Sandercock, A.M.; Wang, J.; González-Muñoz, A.; Parmentier, J.; Black, C.; Soden, J.; et al. Phenotypic Screening Reveals TNFR2 as a Promising Target for Cancer Immunotherapy. *Oncotarget* **2016**, *7*, 68278–68291. [CrossRef] [PubMed]
344. Goukassian, D.A.; Qin, G.; Dolan, C.; Murayama, T.; Silver, M.; Curry, C.; Eaton, E.; Luedemann, C.; Ma, H.; Asahara, T.; et al. Tumor Necrosis Factor-Alpha Receptor P75 Is Required in Ischemia-Induced Neovascularization. *Circulation* **2007**, *115*, 752–762. [CrossRef] [PubMed]
345. Naserian, S.; Abdelgawad, M.E.; Afshar Bakshloo, M.; Ha, G.; Arouche, N.; Cohen, J.L.; Salomon, B.L.; Uzan, G. The TNF/TNFR2 Signaling Pathway Is a Key Regulatory Factor in Endothelial Progenitor Cell Immunosuppressive Effect. *Cell Commun. Signal.* **2020**, *18*, 94. [CrossRef] [PubMed]
346. Vanamee, É.S.; Faustman, D.L. TNFR2: A Novel Target for Cancer Immunotherapy. *Trends Mol. Med.* **2017**, *23*, 1037–1046. [CrossRef]
347. Torrey, H.; Butterworth, J.; Mera, T.; Okubo, Y.; Wang, L.; Baum, D.; Defusco, A.; Plager, S.; Warden, S.; Huang, D.; et al. Targeting TNFR2 with Antagonistic Antibodies Inhibits Proliferation of Ovarian Cancer Cells and Tumor-Associated Tregs. *Sci. Signal.* **2017**, *10*, eaaf8608. [CrossRef] [PubMed]
348. Yang, M.; Tran, L.; Torrey, H.; Song, Y.; Perkins, H.; Case, K.; Zheng, H.; Takahashi, H.; Kuhtreiber, W.M.; Faustman, D.L. Optimizing TNFR2 Antagonism for Immunotherapy with Tumor Microenvironment Specificity. *J. Leukoc. Biol.* **2020**, *107*, 971–980. [CrossRef]

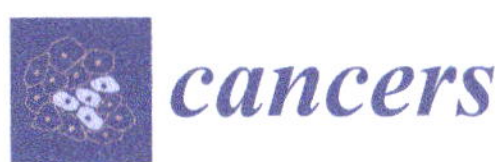

MDPI

Review

Chimeric Antigen Receptor beyond CAR-T Cells

Vicky Mengfei Qin [1,2], Criselle D'Souza [1,3], Paul J. Neeson [1,3,*] and Joe Jiang Zhu [1,3,*]

1   Cancer Immunology Program, Peter MacCallum Cancer Centre, Melbourne, VIC 3000, Australia; Vicky.Qin@petermac.org (V.M.Q.); Criselle.DSouza@petermac.org (C.D.)
2   Department of Clinical Pathology, University of Melbourne, Melbourne, VIC 3010, Australia
3   Sir Peter MacCallum Department of Oncology, University of Melbourne, Melbourne, VIC 3010, Australia
*   Correspondence: Paul.Neeson@petermac.org (P.J.N.); Joe.Zhu@petermac.org (J.J.Z.)

Simple Summary: Chimeric antigen receptors (CAR) are engineered molecules expressed on the cell surface that can recognise specific proteins and deliver an activation signal to the cells. Human T lymphocytes equipped with CAR, also called CAR-T cells, can target and kill tumour cells. This technology has been successfully used in treating some of the blood cancers in the last decade. Although the majority of research interest in CAR technology has been focused on CAR-T cells to date, the CAR design has also been used in other types of immune cells to fight against cancers. In this review, we discuss recent advances in CAR design beyond that used in conventional CAR-T cells and their novel indications to develop more potent CAR-based therapy for cancers.

Abstract: Chimeric antigen receptors (CAR) are genetically engineered receptors that can recognise specific antigens and subsequently activate downstream signalling. Human T cells engineered to express a CAR, also known as CAR-T cells, can target a specific tumour antigen on the cell surface to mediate a cytotoxic response against the tumour. CAR-T cell therapy has achieved remarkable success in treating hematologic malignancies, but not in solid tumours. Currently, extensive research is being carried out to make CAR-T cells a therapy for solid tumours. To date, most of the research interest in the field has focused on cytotoxic T lymphocytes as the carrier of CAR products. However, in addition to T cells, the CAR design can be introduced in other immune cells, such as natural killer (NK)/NKT cells, γδ T cells, mucosal-associated invariant T (MAIT) cells, dendritic cells (DC), macrophages, regulatory T cells (Treg), B cells, etc. Some of the CAR-engineered immune cells, such as CAR- γδ T and CAR-NK/NK-T cells, are directly involved in the anti-tumour response, demonstrated in preclinical studies and/or clinical trials. CAR-Tregs showed promising therapeutic potential in treating autoimmune diseases. In particular, B cells engineered with chimeric receptors can be used as a platform for long-term delivery of therapeutic proteins, such as recombinant antibodies or protein replacement, in an antigen-specific manner. CAR technology is one of the most powerful engineering platforms in immunotherapy, especially for the treatment of cancers. In this review, we will discuss the recent application of the CAR design in non-CAR-T cells and future opportunities in immunotherapy.

Keywords: chimeric antigen receptor; immune cell; endodomain; combination therapy

Citation: Qin, V.M.; D'Souza, C.; Neeson, P.J.; Zhu, J.J. Chimeric Antigen Receptor beyond CAR-T Cells. *Cancers* **2021**, *13*, 404. https://doi.org/10.3390/cancers13030404

Received: 18 December 2020
Accepted: 20 January 2021
Published: 22 January 2021

Publisher's Note: MDPI stays neutral with regard to jurisdictional claims in published maps and institutional affiliations.

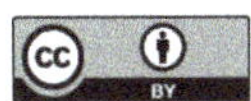

1. Introduction

Adoptive cell transfer was first introduced by Steven Rosenberg in 1986 to treat cancer patients with their own immune cells [1]. In 1992, Michel Sadelain began to genetically engineer primary T cells against cancer [2]. In the following year, the first-generation chimeric antigen receptor T (CAR-T) cells were developed by Zelig Eshhar [3], although they did not persist in vivo and were not effective against cancer cells. Chimeric antigen receptors are synthetic receptors that ligate to a surface antigen and transduce the target recognition into a signalling cascade. The molecular architecture of this chimeric fusion protein comprises (1) a single-chain variable fragment (scFv) extracellular domain targeting a protein, lipid or glycan, (2) a hinge region and transmembrane domain as a membrane anchor, and (3) intracellular signalling domains [4,5].

In 2002, the second-generation of CAR-T cells was developed and proved to be effective in vitro [6] and in 2003, Dr Sadelain demonstrated that the CD19-targeted CAR-T cells could kill leukemia cells in a mouse model [7], which had an enormous impact in the future development of CAR-T therapy. Since then, CAR technology has been developed for several generations, and many innovative constructs have been introduced to improve clinical efficacy. To date, the most commonly used design in the clinic is the second-generation CAR, with either a CD28 or 4-1BB endodomain, displaying significant anti-tumour efficacy, whilst more toxicity was observed with the third generation CAR that contains both endodomains [8]. Nonetheless, this may not happen with other CAR-based cellular therapies. By converting the antigen engagement into an antibody-based binding, CARs overcome potential immune escape associated with major histocompatibility complex (MHC)-downregulation and loss of co-stimulation. This endows CAR-T cells with intrinsic anti-tumour advantages over the endogenous T cells.

To date, CAR-T therapy has shown unprecedented success in B cell malignancies, and most patients have long-lasting complete remission [9,10]. However, antigen loss and treatment-related toxicity—cytokine release syndrome (CRS) and immune effector cell-associated neurotoxicity (ICANS)—are issues that need to be resolved [11,12]. In addition to B cell malignancies, extensive research has been done to explore the application of CAR-T therapy in solid tumours. However, to date, the anti-tumour efficacy is poor. To increase efficacy in treating solid tumours, CAR-T cells need to tackle several unique obstacles: impaired homing and trafficking, low persistence, immunosuppressive tumour microenvironment (TME) and antigen heterogeneity. To address these issues, innovative T cell engineering strategies have been developed; these have been extensively reviewed elsewhere [13–15]. Alternatively, promising proof-of-concept studies in conventional T cells raise the prospect of developing CAR-based approaches in non-conventional T cells, and other immune cell types to combat cancer or autoimmune diseases. In this review, we discuss recent advances in CAR design beyond that used in conventional T cells and their novel indications to develop more potent CAR-based cellular platforms in the clinic.

2. $\gamma\delta$ T Cells

T cells that express heterodimeric T-cell receptors (TCRs) comprised of γ and δ chains are characterised as 'unconventional' T cells [16]. These cells display features of innate and adaptive immune systems. As the major circulating $\gamma\delta$ T population, Vδ2/Vγ9 T cells recognise phosphoantigens. Indeed, aminobiphosphonates (e.g., zoledronate) are broadly used for their ex vivo expansion [17]. Other $\gamma\delta$ T cell subsets account for rarer populations, among which Vδ1 subsets confer residency in mucosal epithelia [18]. $\gamma\delta$ T cells are crucial players in tumour defence and distinguish stress-induced self-antigens in transformed cells. Upon ligation with TCR and/or NK cell receptors, $\gamma\delta$ T cells target tumour cells through Th1-biased cytokines, antibody-dependent cellular cytotoxicity (ADCC), antigen presentation, and cytotoxic activity via perforin-granzyme axis [19,20]. In contrast with $\alpha\beta$ T cells, their antigen sensing does not rely on MHC molecules; therefore, allogeneic $\gamma\delta$ T cells could be more readily used for adoptive transfer without unwanted side effects, especially graft-versus-host disease (GvHD).

In preclinical studies, $\gamma\delta$ T cells were engineered with CAR to generate CAR-$\gamma\delta$ T cells, which showed anti-tumour efficacy in leukemia models. Transduction of polyclonal $\gamma\delta$ T cells with a CD19-targeted CAR resulted in enriched IFN-γ and TNF-α responses and systemically reduced leukemic burden in vivo [21]. A direct comparison with conventional CD19-CAR-T cells demonstrated comparable killing in aggressive leukemia xenograft but also superior cytotoxicity against leukemia cells with loss of CD19 [22]. These results illustrate that the CAR can efficiently boost anti-tumour capacity in $\gamma\delta$ T cells, while retaining their innate cytotoxicity, providing great potential to counter antigen loss in haematological cancers. In the context of solid tumours, GD2-targeting CAR $\gamma\delta$ T cells had equivalent lysis of neuroblastoma cells as conventional CAR-T cells, and cross-presented antigens to activate $\alpha\beta$ T cells in vitro [23]. CAR-$\gamma\delta$ T cells might act as professional antigen-presentation cells to induce endogenous immunity, therefore coping with antigen heterogeneity in solid tumours. However, in vivo efficacy has not yet been evaluated in neuroblastoma or other solid tumour models, and thus requires further investigation.

CAR has also been explored in $\gamma\delta$ T cells to minimise on-target/off-tumour toxicity. One powerful approach is combinatorial antigen sensing which controls the CAR-T cell response via a logic gate, commonly termed 'AND-NOT' gates. This gate provides exquisite tuning of the T cell response and is dependent on the expression of two antigens on the tumour cell surface. For example, $\gamma\delta$ T cells recognised cognate antigen through $\gamma\delta$ TCR and ganglioside GD-2 through DAP10-CAR, which mimics NKG2D co-stimulation. CAR-$\gamma\delta$ T cells induced full activation only in the presence of dual antigens, resulting in equivalent killing as CD28-CD3ζ-CAR T cells against neuroblastoma and Ewings sarcoma cells [24]. This precise discrimination provides a safeguard for solid tumours that lack tumour-specific antigens. Additionally, separating co-stimulatory signals can abrogate tonic signalling, mirrored by potent effector functions and lower exhaustion marker expression [25]. This feature may prolong the in vivo persistence of the gene-modified T cells. Notwithstanding, antigen loss could compromise their cytotoxicity and consequently hinder long-term immunosurveillance. Alternatively, non-integrating transient expression of CAR in $\gamma\delta$ T cells through mRNA electroporation has been reported to alleviate long-term toxicity while maintaining comparable potency as CAR-T cells [26]. Moreover, CAR without signalling domains can be used as a non-activating anchor to drive $\gamma\delta$ T cell residence in proximity with malignant cells and elicit an anti-tumour response through intrinsic cytotoxicity [27]. Collectively, these examples are encouraging by leveraging temporal and spatial control on CAR-$\gamma\delta$ T cells to develop a safe platform and retain effective anti-tumour activity.

Preclinical results have not yet demonstrated superior therapeutic efficacy, but more residual disease was observed than CAR-$\alpha\beta$ T cells in the long-term [22]. Poor in vivo expansion and proliferation, at least in part, can be attributable to this, and are concerns that must be considered in future clinical trials. Nonetheless, CAR-$\gamma\delta$ T cells retained TCR function and innate cytotoxicity, indicating promising effector function. It is not known what percentage of transduced $\gamma\delta$ T cells can conserve these functional capacities after expansion in the GMP product, and this needs to be further characterised. Moreover, it also remains unclear how CAR-$\gamma\delta$ T cells will be applied in the allogeneic setting for 'off-the-shelf' product. Hence, CAR-$\gamma\delta$ T cells may not be sufficient as a stand-alone therapy. They may be used in combination with CAR-$\alpha\beta$ T cells to alleviate immune escape.

3. Regulatory T Cells

Regulatory T cells (Treg), a subset of conventional CD4+ T cells, harbour immunoregulatory properties and can be divided into two types: thymus-derived and peripheral-induced Tregs [28]. Tregs can modulate effector T cells or antigen-presenting cells through soluble anti-inflammatory mediators or cell-cell interactions [29,30]. In cancer, Treg cells behave as negative regulators in the TME, and they are central players in inducing immune tolerance to avoid tissue damage and autoimmune responses.

Synthetic biology and cell engineering has accelerated the application of CAR technology to Tregs. In preclinical studies, Tregs transduced with second-generation CARs showed antigen-specific immunosuppression of T cell responses in GvHD, solid organ transplantation, type 1 diabetes and colitis [31–33]. Interestingly, another study showed that CAR-Tregs elicited bystander suppression of T cells with diverse specificities [34]. This may provide widespread protection against auto-/alloreactive responses in the local environment. In other studies, CAR-Tregs were capable of inhibiting autoimmune antibody response and B cell activities [34,35]. Taken together, CAR-Tregs maintain natural immunoregulatory properties and induce peripheral tolerance. Potential cross-talk with other immune cells as indirect suppressive mechanisms might also be beneficial in highly inflammatory conditions, and thus merit further studies.

Although CAR-Tregs convey potent immunosuppression, some studies demonstrated pro-inflammatory cytokines and antigen-specific cytotoxicity [35,36]. This may be a cause for concern about safety and stability of CAR-Tregs to generate long-term suppression. Optimising CAR-construct might be one strategy. Most studies report that the CD28 endodomain imparts superior suppressive functions in Tregs and promotes longer persistence than the 4-1BB signalling domain [37,38]. Additionally, it is not clear whether CAR-Tregs are sufficient as a single regimen to generate a durable response. In addition, their effect under established immunosuppressive therapies should be considered in different disease models.

4. Mucosal Associated Invariant T Cells

Mucosal-associated invariant T cells (MAIT) are a subset of T cells that recognise vitamin B2 metabolites (5-(2-oxoethylideneamino)-6-D-ribitylaminouracil (5-OP-RU) and structural analogues) as antigens presented on non-classical molecule MR-1 [39]. These cells are highly abundant in human tissues such as the liver and can be up to 10% of $CD8^+$ T cells in the peripheral blood [40]. MAIT cell responses have been studied against bacterial, fungal, and certain viral infections, as previously reviewed [41]. A few studies have demonstrated that MAIT cells play a role in cancer, either protective or pathogenic [41].

MAIT cells have great potential as CAR-T cells because they are MR1-restricted and also have a restricted TCR usage. MR1 is a highly conserved non-classical MHC Class 1B molecule [42]. This suggests that MAIT cells are unlikely to induce GvHD. Hence, CAR-MAIT cells could be used as universal CAR-T cells and an 'off-the-shelf' therapy.

However, current strategies of isolating, expanding, and transferring MAIT cells back into patients is challenging using current CAR-T GMP production approaches. MAIT cells can be expanded ex vivo using the ligand 5-OP-RU in the presence of MR-1 expressing APCs or TLR stimulation [43,44]. As MAIT cell numbers vary in individuals (5–10% of T cells) in peripheral blood, the CAR-MAIT numbers obtained after expansion will also be limited as compared to the ex vivo expansion of all T cells. PD-1 upregulation and exhaustion phenotypes have been observed on MAIT cells in chronic viral hepatitis [45], and this may also be the case with cancers. Therefore, a combination approach with anti-PD1 may possibly overcome this hurdle.

5. Tissue-Resident Memory T Cells

Tissue-resident memory T cells (TRM) are long-lived non-circulating memory T cells that persist in peripheral tissue at sites of previous antigen counter such as in infections or cancer [46]. TRM cells provide long-term immune protection through enhanced effector function against a known pathogen and recruitment of circulating T cells [46]. Due to these properties, TRM cells are an attractive option as CAR- TRM cells. CAR-TRMs could be generated against known cancer antigens. However, TRM differentiation is formed from circulating precursor cells under the influence of tissue factors, including TGF-β [47]. Therefore, the CAR-T cell product would need to have these TRM precursor cells [48]. An alternate strategy is to generate CAR-T cells with an inducible system, where once the CAR recognises the target antigen, this would in turn switch on or off genes that can convert these cells to tissue-resident CAR-T cells. Some of the genes known to drive TRM differentiation and maintenance include CD69, expression of transcription factors Blimp1, Hobit, and Runx3, and downregulation of KLF2, as reviewed elsewhere [49].

6. Natural Killer Cells

Natural killer cells (NK) are professional killer cells from the innate lymphoid family and have critical roles in cancer immunosurveillance. Unlike T cells, NK cells require joint signals from different activating and inhibitory receptors to target tumours [50]. They can induce rapid cytotoxicity predominantly via perforin and granzyme or through death-receptor pathways (FasL or TNF-related apoptosis-inducing ligand TRAIL-mediated) [51–53]. Non-MHC-restricted NK cells confer limited alloreactivity and no GvHD in adoptive transfer [54].

Despite the limited number of clinical trials, CAR-NK cells consistently show a favourable safety profile while maintaining potent reactivity. A phase I/II trial of cord blood (CB)-derived HLA-mismatched CD19-CAR-NK cells with an escalating dose was conducted in relapsed or refractory chronic lymphocytic leukemia (CLL) or non-Hodgkin's lymphoma patients (NCT03056339) [55]. None of the patients had any side-effects, such as CRS, neurotoxicity, or GvHD, and the maximum tolerated dose was not reached. Seven out of 11 patients had complete remission, and six patients tested negative for minimal residual disease, revealing that CAR-NK cells are an effective treatment strategy against CLL. This is in line with another phase I trial for metastatic colorectal cancer with local delivery of autologous or allogeneic NKG2D-DAP12 CAR-NK cells (NCT03415100), in which all three patients significantly reduced their tumour burden with transient grade I CRS [56]. This study demonstrates the successful protection of CAR-induced killing mediated by NK cells in the context of solid tumours. Moreover, NK-92-derived CD33-CAR-NK cells were well-tolerated in a phase I trial of 3 patients with acute myeloid leukemia (AML) (NCT02944162). In contrast with CAR-T cells, repeated infusion with high-dose third-generation CAR-NK cells only caused mild elevation of CRS-related cytokines [57]. Together, these data highlight that CAR-NK cells are a safer strategy for cancer patients with a minimised risk of undesirable side effects. Additionally, different non-autologous sources were employed, including NK-92, CB-derived and allogeneic NK cells, underpinning the great therapeutic potential for NK cells coupled with CARs to provide 'off-the-shelf' product.

Post-infusion NK cell behaviour is vital for CAR-mediated surveillance and durable remission in patients. For example, a significantly lower early expansion of CB-derived CAR-NK cells was found in non-responding patients [55], suggesting the correlation between in vivo proliferation of CAR-NK cells with treatment responsiveness. In addition, the persistence of the CAR-NK products is still not clear, as most patients went on post-treatment due to the sign of disease progression or relapse. To prolong persistence, deleting cytokine-inducible SH2-containing protein (CIS) (a negative regulator of interleukin (IL)-15) was shown to achieve synergism with IL-15 signalling in CAR-NK cells, leading to doubled persistence and tumour eradication in lymphoma xenografts [58]. Alternatively, coupling Myd88/CD40 with ectopic expression of IL-15 in CAR-NK cells, in an attempt to mimic the Toll-like receptor (TLR) signalling, resulted in the robust proliferation and prolonged persistence in vivo [59]. As these examples illustrate, extended persistence holds promise as a means of augmenting CAR-NK cell function. However, caution is still warranted given the short-lived nature of mature NK cells and in vivo expansion, and persistence would be a major concern that impairs the anti-tumour efficacy when reaching the clinic.

Of note, CAR-NK cells exhibited efficient homing to the disease site with rapid cytotoxicity against tumours in patients. This brings about opportunities to use CAR-NK cells as a bridging therapy prior to CAR-T therapy to fulfil the demand of patients with advanced disease. With the early onset of anti-tumour activity of CAR-NK cells to lyse tumour targets, CAR-T cells may perform better with less suppression from the tumour, followed by sustained memory CAR-T repertoire to eliminate residual disease and retain immune surveillance.

7. Natural Killer T Cells

Natural killer T cells (NKT) are $\alpha\beta$T cells restricted by CD1d, which is an HLA-like molecule presenting lipid antigen. NKT cells can be divided into invariant NKT cells (iNKT) recognising α-galactosylceramide (α-GalCer), and diverse NKT cells express more variant TCRs. While most studies suggest that diverse NKT cells inhibit anti-tumour immunity, iNKT cells contribute to natural tumour surveillance with immediate cytokine secretion (IFN-γ, TNF, IL-13, IL-17, IL-4, IL21, IL-22) and FasL/TRAIL pathways [60,61]. Furthermore, iNKT are clinically feasible in the allogeneic setting without GvHD; thus, universal CAR-NKT cells can be obtained from healthy donors to circumvent production and quality issues from autologous cells. Together with their effector properties, iNKT cells are an attractive platform for CAR-based therapy.

Different CAR constructs have been explored to impart iNKT cells with efficient anti-tumour properties. iNKT cells engineered with a third-generation CAR specific for ganglioside GD2 fostered expansion and persistence accompanied by superior efficacy than the second-generation counterpart in metastatic neuroblastoma xenografts without CAR-related toxicity [62]. Clinically, iNKT cells might be an optimal carrier for third-generation CAR by surmounting the unwanted side effects in CAR-T cells, and this underpins the importance of selecting co-stimulatory domains in different immune subsets. Notably, CAR-iNKT cells recapitulated the polarised T helper 1 (Th1) cytokine profile with a high IFN-γ/IL-4 ratio and increased granzyme B regardless of different endodomains [63,64]. iNKT cells naturally harbour both Th1 and Th2 cytokine profile; therefore, CAR-iNKT cells can tilt the balance towards Th1 pro-inflammatory cytokines with enhanced cytotoxic potential. These properties are favourable in attacking the tumour and could maximise their anti-tumour capacity.

To counter the lack of deep remission with conventional CARs, armoured CAR-iNKT cells have been developed and achieved marked success. Secretion of IL-15 by anti-GD2 CAR-iNKT cells improved disease-free survival with long-term persistence in bone metastasised sites and decreased the expression of exhaustion markers such as PD-1 in neuroblastoma xenograft [65]. Thus, IL-15 provides a favourable phenotype for transfer and promotes persistence, leading to greater anti-tumour potential. Based on encouraging proof-of-concept studies, a phase I trial for children with neuroblastoma is currently underway and has obtained promising safety data from initial results (NCT03294954) [66]. Alternatively, CAR iNKT cells maintained CD62L expression, acting as central memory-like cells, which enhanced their proliferative capacity and resulted in a substantial reduction in tumour burden in mice xenografted with lymphoma [67]. IL-21 in iNKT cell ex vivo expansion cultures altered the iNKT cells enhancing cytotoxicity and persistence of CD62L+ CAR-iNKT with better tumour protection [63]. Changing phenotypic composition in CAR-iNKT cells might also play a role in therapeutic efficacy as a means of prolonging persistence; nevertheless, whether this less-differentiated phenotype can be maintained over time, and help them resist T cell exhaustion, is currently unknown. Together, these data suggest superior in vivo survival, and prolonged persistence is of importance for CAR iNKT cells to harbour effective killing, but the duration of their persistence remains to be fully determined.

Building on intrinsic properties, iNKT with CARs reveals several advantages over CAR-T therapy. Rotolo et al. demonstrated that CAR-iNKT cells preserved endogenous TCR-activation in the presence of CAR-stimulation, mirrored by an improved capacity for tumour clearance in lymphoma xenografts as compared to CAR-T cells [64]. Dual targeting by CD1d and CAR as cooperative killing resulted in synergistic cytotoxicity, therefore mitigating the risk of immune escape. Different preclinical models have shown that CAR-iNKT express a higher level of chemokine receptors and exhibit augmented infiltration at the tumour lesion than CAR-T cells [62,64]. This illustrates that CAR-iNKT cells retain their physiological capacity of chemotaxis to localise to the tumour as compared to effector conventional T cells leading to better tumour control. Notably, CAR iNKT cells have shown a protective role against GvHD while their invariant TCR was intact in neuroblastoma and lymphoma xenograft [62–65]. Due to the non-polymorphic nature of CD1d, CAR-iNKT cells limit off-target reactivity, serving as a safe platform for allogeneic use. However, there are limiting aspects of iNKT cells, in that iNKT cells only account for 0.01 to 0.1% of T cells in humans and harvesting sufficient iNKT cells from an apheresis product is not feasible. Additionally, lacking a highly purified initial product would also dampen the therapeutic efficacy. Therefore, robust production of CAR-iNKT cells in the clinic still requires further investigation.

8. Macrophages

Macrophages as innate myeloid cells are professional phagocytes capable of orchestrating homeostasis of the adaptive immune system. Given their high abundance in many solid tumours, tumour-associated macrophages (TAM) occupy a special niche in TME, and many mediators can tailor their phenotype [68]. Immunosuppressive TAMs (M2) can dampen T cell response and facilitate tumour progression [69,70]. In contrast, M1 polarisation encompasses pro-inflammatory phenotype and harbours anti-tumour activity [71,72], thereby leading to great interest in engineering macrophages in cancer to assist immune surveillance.

CAR endows macrophages with the specificity of response against tumour-associated antigens (TAAs) in parallel with enhanced effector functions against the tumour. For example, macrophages can be engineered with CD19-CAR incorporating cytosolic domains of Megf10 or FcRγ to mimic phagocytic signalling. Consequently, this triggered antigen-specific phagocytosis and trogocytosis of lymphoma cells in an in vitro model [73]. In another study, CD3ζ-CAR macrophage also demonstrated active phagocytosis equivalent to FcRγ-CAR [74]. As such, redirected antigen-specific phagocytosis bestows spatial control and precision on eliminating cancer cells and ultimately contributes to the therapeutic effect. Furthermore, macrophages transduced with conventional CAR via adenoviral vectors polarised towards pro-inflammatory M1 phenotype and stimulated T cell responses, leading to marked tumour regression and prolonged survival in mouse models with ovarian cancer [74]. This suggests potential epitope spreading and a broader anti-tumour response propagated by CAR-macrophages within TME. Besides directly targeting tumour cells, macrophages can be transduced with CAR incorporating CD147 endodomain to express matrix metalloproteinase (MMP). This improved capacity to remodel the extracellular matrix (ECM) subsequently promoted T cell infiltration to inhibit tumour growth in breast cancer xenografts [75]. This would be beneficial for stroma-enriched solid tumours by removing physical barriers for killer cells to access tumour cells and exert cytotoxicity. CAR engineering recapitulates immune functional programs built on canonical signalling network of macrophages and therefore provides new opportunities using innate immune cells as effective CAR-carriers to treat patients with solid tumours.

As observed in the studies discussed above, CAR-macrophages have the potential to address some challenges of CAR-T cells in TME: immune cell penetration and immunosuppressive milieu. Additionally, there was evidence of cross-talk mediated by CAR-macrophages to re-educate the M2 phenotype into the M1 phenotype, facilitate maturation of dendritic cells, and cross-present antigens to activate T cells [74]. CAR-macrophages may convert the TME into an inflammatory environment and thus potentially can be used as a supportive regimen for CAR-T cells or other immunotherapies. Conversely, in vivo phenotype plasticity of macrophage should not be underestimated. There is still limited understanding as to whether CAR-macrophages can resist the suppression from regulatory cells in TME: Tregs and myeloid-derived suppressive cells (MDSC). Concerning the safety profile, there are two remaining issues. Firstly, peripheral blood-derived monocytes are highly heterogenous and manufactured CAR-macrophages could potentially develop biodistribution bias to healthy tissues with systemic administration. Secondly, macrophages have been considered as key mediators of CRS [76], thus necessitating closer attention.

9. Dendritic Cells

Dendritic cells (DC), a heterogeneous subset, are professional antigen-presenting cells that prime naïve T cells and reactivate memory responses. In cancer, DCs sense environmental cues in lymphoid organs or the TME and sensing of danger signals induces DC maturation leading to either immune tolerance or a tumour-specific response [77,78]. Importantly, cytotoxic CD8+ T cells can be activated by DCs through cross-presentation of TAAs or neoantigens to promote a stronger anti-tumour response [79]. These have key implications for cancer immunotherapy, and CAR becomes an emerging strategy to manipulate DCs for an effective response against the tumour.

Intra-tumoural DCs are considered paramount in modulating T cell functions in TME. DC engineered with CAR have been documented in a preclinical AML model to support CAR-T cells by providing immunomodulatory cytokines (activation signal 3). DC expressing a CAR containing the 4-1BB-signalling domain facilitated differentiation into the intra-tumoural DC subset, resulting in augmented cytotoxicity of infused CD33-CAR T cells with higher cytokine production and better survival in AML mice xenograft than CAR-T alone [80]. This underpins active interactions between CAR-DCs with CAR-T cells to orchestrate anti-tumour response and a synergistic therapeutic efficacy. Enhancing DC functionality may further break tolerance to tumours with the activation of bystander immune cells. On the other hand, DCs may be exploited by tumour cells or immunosuppressive mediators to subdue their function; yet evidence of CAR-DC behaviour in the TME has not been elucidated in immunocompetent models. Another topic of interest is how heterogeneous subsets of human DCs may induce different effects with CAR-T cells and their optimal ratio for patients. Notwithstanding, their clinical safety needs to be further explored, since the high level of secreted IL-12 may induce systemic toxicity [81].

10. B Cells

B cells and long-lived plasma cells are classically known to modulate humoral response by producing antibodies, and coordinate T cell response. They have been uncovered as active participants in tumour-draining lymph nodes, tumour-associated tertiary lymphoid structures and TME to prompt anti-tumour response, although specific subsets are polarised with pro-tumoural effects [82–84]. Their prevailing natures convey several advantages, making B cells attractive as a therapeutic cellular platform such as antigen-specific activation, in vivo persistence, memory pool formation and the potential to secrete proteins in large quantities.

While ex vivo manipulation of primary B cells has been limited by technical challenges, one clinical study has reported a case of CAR-transduced leukemic B cell [85]. Recently, clustered regularly interspaced short palindromic repeats (CRISPR) and CRISPR-associated protein 9 (Cas9) induced homolog-directed repair was successfully used to introduce CAR-expression cassettes into B cells. CARs equipped with the CD79β signalling domain, which is a component of B cell receptor (BCR) complex for activation, can be engineered in primary murine B cells to induce robust surface expression and antigen-recognition independent of endogenous BCR [86]. B cells could be feasible carriers for CAR-based therapy by exploiting endogenous BCR signalling, although human B cells' functionality (e.g., proliferative capacity and antibody secretion) should be evaluated in future studies.

Considering the clinical translation, directly engineering primary human B cells and plasma cells to effectively secrete immunoglobulin and therapeutic proteins have been shown in preclinical studies to address infectious disease and protein deficiency, respectively [87,88]. In line with this concept, CAR-B cells can be used to drive the local delivery of monoclonal antibodies at the tumour site by targeting a particular TAA. This introduces the possibility of CAR-B cells as safe and controllable vehicles for releasing efficacious therapeutic antibodies that convey severe toxicity in systemic administration. Alternatively, CAR-B cells can be a novel platform for autoimmune disease and prophylactic vaccines.

11. The Design of CAR Constructs

The CAR construct used in conventional CAR-T cells is designed to initiate the cytotoxic killing upon antigen recognition. The application of the CAR construct in other immune subsets relies on the conserved activation pathways and/or the canonical signalling molecules in the engineered cells. Thus, the anti-tumour activities may vary in a cell type-specific manner. An optimised approach is to change the components in the CAR construct based on the activating signalling chains and inherent biological properties of engineered cells. For instance, DAP12 demonstrated superior cytotoxicity than CD3ζ in CAR-NK cells in a colorectal cancer xenograft model [56]. Distinct cellular functions beyond the cytolysis can also be induced by altering the endodomains, such as antibody production in CAR-B cells and matrix metalloproteinase secretion in CAR-macrophages. Furthermore, the extracellular domain can be derived from receptors (e.g., NKG2D) or scFv targeting non-tumour cells, such as stromal components (e.g., MDSC). The optimisation of the transmembrane domain and hinge regions may also enhance the surface expression of CAR and its functionality; however, this remains an area of ongoing investigations.

12. Challenges and Opportunities in Solid Tumours

To date, conventional CAR-T efficacy in solid tumours has been poor. Barriers to CAR-T cell success in solid tumours include the immunosuppressive and immune exclusive tumour microenvironment, tumour antigen heterogeneity and poor T cell trafficking. Given the distinct characteristics of the CAR immune cells described above, they may provide promising improvements in treating solid tumours in combination of conventional CAR-T cells. CAR-$\gamma\delta$ T cells can act as professional antigen-presentation cells to cross-present antigens to conventional $\alpha\beta$ CAR-T and endogenous T cells. These features provide great potential for CAR-$\gamma\delta$ T cells to cope with the issue of the tumour heterogeneity. Similarly to CAR-$\gamma\delta$ T cells, CAR-NK/NK-T cells can be used in combination with conventional CAR-T cells or as bridging therapy prior to CAR-T therapy. The superior anti-tumour efficacy and efficient trafficking capability of CAR-NK cells facilitate the early onset of anti-tumour cytotoxicity and induce the recruitment of CAR-T cells to the tumour site. CAR-DC may synergize the anti-tumour activity of the CAR-T cells, and it may also engage and activate the bystander T cells in the tumour microenvironment. Similarly, CAR-macrophage (M1) can also crosstalk with CAR-T or bystander T cells in the tumour through cytokines and chemokines, facilitating the antigen presentation and immune cell recruitment. In addition, CAR-macrophages can remodel the extracellular matrix through the production of MMP, enabling the T cell penetration into the stroma-rich solid tumours. In summary, a combination of CAR-immune cells may support the conventional CAR-T cells to overcome the current challenges in solid tumour.

13. Manufacture of Clinical Product

Successful ex vivo generation of CAR-immune cell products is essential for clinical application. Leukapheresis can be used for most cases. Immune subsets can be enriched by clinical grade purification through positive (e.g., NKT and $\gamma\delta$ T cells) or negative selection (NK cells), although they represent a minority of peripheral blood lymphocytes [55,66]. These cells can be further sorted for a defined phenotype, which may have an impact on the functional activity of the final product [67]. Current expansion protocols typically incorporate engineered feeder cells and cytokine exposure (IL-2, IL-7, IL-15 and IL-21) [63,66]. Nonetheless, methodologies heavily rely on the cell type, and some expansion protocols require synthetic ligands (e.g., zoledronate, α-GalCer) [64]. Similarly, peripheral blood monocytes can be purified and induced into macrophages or dendritic cells. For example, dendritic cells in autologous cancer vaccine Sipuleucel-T can be cultured and expanded ex vivo to a high cell number (10^7–10^9 cells) [89,90]. In addition, induced pluripotent stem cells (iPSCs) can potentially provide an unlimited supply for CAR-immune cells, such as CAR-NK cells or CAR-macrophages [91,92]. Attractively, CAR-NK cells can also be generated from cord blood, as shown in a Phase I clinical trial [55]. Although the productivity of ex vivo generation of CAR-immune cells may be limited compared with that of conventional CAR-T cells, it is still feasible for the clinical application. As discussed in the above sections, most of the CAR-immune cells will be used in combination with conventional CAR-T cells, and the required dose will be much less than that of conventional CAR-T cells currently used in the clinic. Thus, not only the manufacturing time but also the cost of the production will be significantly reduced, which can further promote the combination immunotherapy for cancers.

14. Conclusions and Prospects

In the last twenty years, CAR technology has been developed for several generations; however, the conventional T lymphocytes still remain the major target for CAR engineering. Until recently, the CAR had been introduced into γδ T cells, NK/NK-T cells, DCs, macrophages and B cells, showing the great potential of CAR application in non-conventional T cells and other immune cell subsets.

The CAR technology enables host cells to specifically recognise cells expressing the target antigens on the cell surface, and subsequently trigger the downstream intracellular signalling. As the CAR design adopts the scFv from antibodies, any antigen that can be recognised by an antibody, including proteins and polysaccharides, can be used as the target for CARs. The choices of intracellular signalling are also diverse, including T-cell co-stimulatory signalling for cytotoxicity, MMP signalling for extracellular matrix remodelling, apoptosis signalling for suicide, and transcription signalling for producing specific protein, etc. (Table 1). These flexibilities facilitate distinctive approaches to target cancer cells and the tumour microenvironment by different immune cells equipped with various CARs.

Table 1. The CAR designs are different in non-conventional T cells and other immune cell subsets.

Immune Cell Type	Extracellular scFv (Anti-)	Intracellular Domain	CAR Generation	Targeted Disease	Clinical Trials	Reference
γδ T	CD19	CD28-CD3ζ	2nd	B-ALL	-	[21,22]
	GD2	CD28-CD3ζ	2nd	Neuroblastoma	-	[23]
	MCSP	CD28-CD3ζ	2nd	Melanoma	-	[26]
	GD2	DAP10	1st	Neuroblastoma	-	[24,25]
	CD5	Non-signalling CAR	-	T-ALL	-	[27]
NKT	GD2	CD3ζ 4-1BB-CD3ζ CD28-CD3ζ CD28-4-1BB-CD3ζ	2nd and 3rd	Neuroblastoma	-	[62]
	CD19	CD28-CD3ζ CD28-OX40-CD3ζ	2nd and 3rd	B cell lymphoma	-	[64]
	CD19	4-1BB-CD3ζ	2nd	B cell lymphoma	-	[63,67]
	GD2	CD28-CD3ζ 4-1BB-CD3ζ Armoured with IL-15	2nd	Neuroblastoma	NCT03294954	[65,66]
NK	CD19	CD28-CD3ζ Armoured with IL-15	2nd	CLL, NHL	NCT03056339	[55,58]
	CD33	CD28-4-1BB-CD3ζ	3rd	AML	NCT02944162	[57]
	NKG2D	DAP12	1st	Colorectal cancer	NCT03415100	[56]
	BCMA	CD3ζ Armoured with IL15, MyD88-CD40	1st	Multiple myeloma	-	[59]

Table 1. *Cont.*

Immune Cell Type	Extracellular scFv (Anti-)	Intracellular Domain	CAR Generation	Targeted Disease	Clinical Trials	Reference
Macrophage	CD19	Megf10 FcRγ FcRγ-CD19	1st	B cell malignancies	-	[73]
	Her2	CD147	1st	Breast cancer	-	[75]
	Her2	CD3ζ	1st	Ovarian cancer	-	[74]
DC	CD33	4-1BB-CD3ζ	2nd	AML	-	[80]
B cell	Hen Egg Lysozyme	CD79β	-	-	-	[86]
Treg	CD19	4-1BB-CD3ζ	2nd	Tissue-specific immune suppression	-	[38]
	CD19	CD28-CD3ζ	2nd	Autoantibody-mediated autoimmune disease	-	[35,38]
	Factor VIII	CD28-CD3ζ	2nd	Hemophilia A	-	[34]
	HLA-A2	CD28-CD3ζ	2nd	GvHD	-	[36]

MCSP: melanoma-associated chondroitin sulfate proteoglycan; BCMA: B cell maturation antigen; B-ALL: B cell acute lymphoblastic leukemia; T-ALL: T cell acute lymphoblastic leukemia; CLL: chronic lymphocytic leukemia; NHL: non-Hodgkin's lymphoma; AML: acute myeloid leukemia.

The current issues for conventional CAR-T cell therapy, especially in solid tumours, include tumour heterogeneity, trafficking, and infiltration into the tumour, in vivo activation/persistence of CAR-T cells and tumour microenvironment. Using various CAR-engineered immune cells may help to address these complex issues. One rationale for the CAR combination could be utilising conventional CAR-T cells in combination with CAR-NK cells, CAR-γδ T cells, CAR-DC, CAR-macrophages, and possibly CAR-B cells (Figure 1).

Unlike the conventional CAR-T cells, most of the intracellular signalling domains in non-conventional CAR-immune cells vary greatly depending on the host cells; for example, DAP12 for CAR-NK cells, and Megf10 for CAR-macrophages. Thus, selecting the appropriate intracellular signalling for non-conventional CAR-immune cells will be the key for the therapeutic efficacy. It should also be noted that unlike T lymphocytes, some immune cell populations are difficult or expensive to expand ex vivo, due to the low ex vivo proliferation or limited source from human peripheral blood. One possible solution is to use an alternative source to produce these CAR-engineered immune cells, for example, using induced pluripotent stem cell (iPSC) to generate CAR-NK cells or CAR-macrophages derived from iPSC or monocytes. Until now, except for CAR-NK/NK-T cells, most of the CAR-engineered immune cells are still at the preclinical stage, and some of them are even at the early proof-of-concept phase, such as CAR-MAIT and CAR-TRM cells. Further studies will be needed to explore the anti-tumour efficacy, as well as safety, of these CAR-engineered immune cells.

CAR technology is a powerful and versatile tool for immunotherapy. However, in the last few years, further modifications of the CAR itself on T cells did not achieve significant clinical improvement in solid tumours. By reviewing the pros and cons of the non-conventional CAR-immune cells, it appears promising that the combination treatment with non-conventional CAR-immune cells may overcome the major hurdles in solid cancers. Future development of the non-conventional CAR-immune cells may involve (i) customisation of appropriate intracellular signalling domain for each host cell, (ii) evaluation of the anti-tumour efficacy and safety, and (iii) optimisation of the ex vivo expansion of the non-conventional CAR-immune cells in a clinically and commercially adequate manner.

Once solved, the combination CAR-immune cell therapy may become an efficient, safe, and affordable therapy for cancer treatment, and as well as other immune-related diseases.

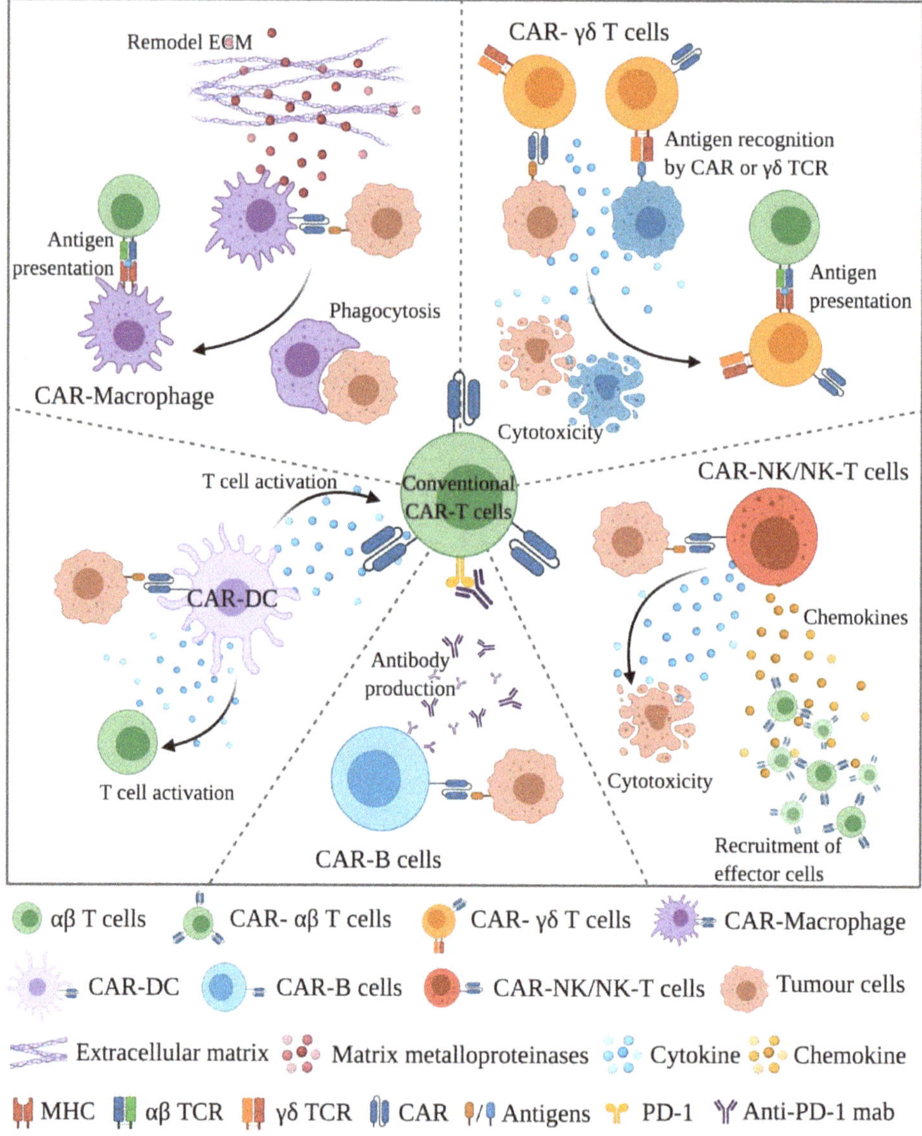

Figure 1. A schematic diagram demonstrating the concept of using conventional CAR-T cells in the combination of CAR-immune cells. In the combination, CAR-γδ T cells and CAR-macrophages can directly kill tumour cells and facilitate antigen presentation to cope with the tumour heterogeneity issue. CAR-macrophages can also remodel the extracellular matrix through the production of MMP. CAR-NK/NK-T cells can induce the early onset of anti-tumour activity, followed by the recruitment of CAR-T cells through chemokines. CAR-DC can support the full activation signals to CAR-T and the bystander T cells. CAR-B cells can be used as an ideal platform to deliver therapeutic antibodies, such as anti-PD1 antibody. (The figure is created with BioRender.com).

Author Contributions: Writing—original draft preparation, V.M.Q., C.D., J.J.Z.; Writing—review and editing, P.J.N., J.J.Z.; Supervision, P.J.N. All authors have read and agreed to the published version of the manuscript.

Funding: This research received no external funding.

Institutional Review Board Statement: Not applicable.

Informed Consent Statement: Not applicable.

Data Availability Statement: No new data were created or analyzed in this study. Data sharing is not applicable to this article.

Conflicts of Interest: The authors declare no conflict of interest.

References

1. Rosenberg, S.A.; Spiess, P.; Lafreniere, R. A new approach to the adoptive immunotherapy of cancer with tumor-infiltrating lymphocytes. *Science* **1986**, *233*, 1318–1321. [CrossRef]
2. Sadelain, M.; Riviere, I.; Riddell, S. Therapeutic T cell engineering. *Nature* **2017**, *545*, 423–431. [CrossRef]
3. Eshhar, Z.; Waks, T.; Gross, G.; Schindler, D.G. Specific activation and targeting of cytotoxic lymphocytes through chimeric single chains consisting of antibody-binding domains and the gamma or zeta subunits of the immunoglobulin and T-cell receptors. *Proc. Natl. Acad. Sci. USA* **1993**, *90*, 720–724. [CrossRef]
4. Fesnak, A.D.; June, C.H.; Levine, B.L. Engineered T cells: The promise and challenges of cancer immunotherapy. *Nat. Rev. Cancer* **2016**, *16*, 566–581. [CrossRef]
5. Sadelain, M.; Brentjens, R.; Riviere, I. The basic principles of chimeric antigen receptor design. *Cancer Discov.* **2013**, *3*, 388–398. [CrossRef]
6. Maher, J.; Brentjens, R.J.; Gunset, G.; Riviere, I.; Sadelain, M. Human T-lymphocyte cytotoxicity and proliferation directed by a single chimeric TCRzeta/CD28 receptor. *Nat. Biotechnol.* **2002**, *20*, 70–75. [CrossRef]
7. Brentjens, R.J.; Latouche, J.B.; Santos, E.; Marti, F.; Gong, M.C.; Lyddane, C.; King, P.D.; Larson, S.; Weiss, M.; Riviere, I.; et al. Eradication of systemic B-cell tumors by genetically targeted human T lymphocytes co-stimulated by CD80 and interleukin-15. *Nat. Med.* **2003**, *9*, 279–286. [CrossRef]
8. Morgan, R.A.; Yang, J.C.; Kitano, M.; Dudley, M.E.; Laurencot, C.M.; Rosenberg, S.A. Case report of a serious adverse event following the administration of T cells transduced with a chimeric antigen receptor recognizing ERBB2. *Mol. Ther.* **2010**, *18*, 843–851. [CrossRef]
9. Srour, S.A.; Singh, H.; McCarty, J.; de Groot, E.; Huls, H.; Rondon, G.; Qazilbash, M.; Ciurea, S.; Bardelli, G.; Buck, J.; et al. Long-term outcomes of Sleeping Beauty-generated CD19-specific CAR T-cell therapy for relapsed-refractory B-cell lymphomas. *Blood* **2020**, *135*, 862–865. [CrossRef]
10. Park, J.H.; Riviere, I.; Gonen, M.; Wang, X.; Senechal, B.; Curran, K.J.; Sauter, C.; Wang, Y.; Santomasso, B.; Mead, E.; et al. Long-Term Follow-up of CD19 CAR Therapy in Acute Lymphoblastic Leukemia. *N. Engl. J. Med.* **2018**, *378*, 449–459. [CrossRef]
11. Wang, M.; Munoz, J.; Goy, A.; Locke, F.L.; Jacobson, C.A.; Hill, B.T.; Timmerman, J.M.; Holmes, H.; Jaglowski, S.; Flinn, I.W.; et al. KTE-X19 CAR T-Cell Therapy in Relapsed or Refractory Mantle-Cell Lymphoma. *N. Engl. J. Med.* **2020**, *382*, 1331–1342. [CrossRef]
12. Fry, T.J.; Shah, N.N.; Orentas, R.J.; Stetler-Stevenson, M.; Yuan, C.M.; Ramakrishna, S.; Wolters, P.; Martin, S.; Delbrook, C.; Yates, B.; et al. CD22-targeted CAR T cells induce remission in B-ALL that is naive or resistant to CD19-targeted CAR immunotherapy. *Nat. Med.* **2018**, *24*, 20–28. [CrossRef]
13. Mardiana, S.; Solomon, B.J.; Darcy, P.K.; Beavis, P.A. Supercharging adoptive T cell therapy to overcome solid tumor-induced immunosuppression. *Sci. Transl. Med.* **2019**, *11*, eaaw2293. [CrossRef]
14. Rafiq, S.; Hackett, C.S.; Brentjens, R.J. Engineering strategies to overcome the current roadblocks in CAR T cell therapy. *Nat. Rev. Clin. Oncol.* **2020**, *17*, 147–167. [CrossRef]
15. Hong, M.; Clubb, J.D.; Chen, Y.Y. Engineering CAR-T Cells for Next-Generation Cancer Therapy. *Cancer Cell* **2020**, *38*, 473–488. [CrossRef]
16. Godfrey, D.I.; Uldrich, A.P.; McCluskey, J.; Rossjohn, J.; Moody, D.B. The burgeoning family of unconventional T cells. *Nat. Immunol.* **2015**, *16*, 1114–1123. [CrossRef]
17. Kakimi, K.; Matsushita, H.; Masuzawa, K.; Karasaki, T.; Kobayashi, Y.; Nagaoka, K.; Hosoi, A.; Ikemura, S.; Kitano, K.; Kawada, I.; et al. Adoptive transfer of zoledronate-expanded autologous Vgamma9Vdelta2 T-cells in patients with treatment-refractory non-small-cell lung cancer: A multicenter, open-label, single-arm, phase 2 study. *J. Immunother. Cancer* **2020**, *8*, e001185. [CrossRef]
18. Mikulak, J.; Oriolo, F.; Bruni, E.; Roberto, A.; Colombo, F.S.; Villa, A.; Bosticardo, M.; Bortolomai, I.; Lo Presti, E.; Meraviglia, S.; et al. NKp46-expressing human gut-resident intraepithelial Vdelta1 T cell subpopulation exhibits high antitumor activity against colorectal cancer. *JCI Insight* **2019**, *4*, e125884. [CrossRef]
19. Sebestyen, Z.; Prinz, I.; Dechanet-Merville, J.; Silva-Santos, B.; Kuball, J. Translating gammadelta (gammadelta) T cells and their receptors into cancer cell therapies. *Nat. Rev. Drug Discov.* **2020**, *19*, 169–184. [CrossRef]

20. Silva-Santos, B.; Mensurado, S.; Coffelt, S.B. γδ T cells: Pleiotropic immune effectors with therapeutic potential in cancer. *Nat. Rev. Cancer* **2019**, *19*, 392–404. [CrossRef]
21. Deniger, D.C.; Switzer, K.; Mi, T.; Maiti, S.; Hurton, L.; Singh, H.; Huls, H.; Olivares, S.; Lee, D.A.; Champlin, R.E.; et al. Bispecific T-cells expressing polyclonal repertoire of endogenous gammadelta T-cell receptors and introduced CD19-specific chimeric antigen receptor. *Mol. Ther.* **2013**, *21*, 638–647. [CrossRef] [PubMed]
22. Rozenbaum, M.; Meir, A.; Aharony, Y.; Itzhaki, O.; Schachter, J.; Bank, I.; Jacoby, E.; Besser, M.J. Gamma-Delta CAR-T Cells Show CAR-Directed and Independent Activity Against Leukemia. *Front. Immunol.* **2020**, *11*, 1347. [CrossRef] [PubMed]
23. Capsomidis, A.; Benthall, G.; Van Acker, H.H.; Fisher, J.; Kramer, A.M.; Abeln, Z.; Majani, Y.; Gileadi, T.; Wallace, R.; Gustafsson, K.; et al. Chimeric Antigen Receptor-Engineered Human Gamma Delta T Cells: Enhanced Cytotoxicity with Retention of Cross Presentation. *Mol. Ther.* **2018**, *26*, 354–365. [CrossRef] [PubMed]
24. Fisher, J.; Abramowski, P.; Wisidagamage Don, N.D.; Flutter, B.; Capsomidis, A.; Cheung, G.W.; Gustafsson, K.; Anderson, J. Avoidance of On-Target Off-Tumor Activation Using a Co-stimulation-Only Chimeric Antigen Receptor. *Mol. Ther.* **2017**, *25*, 1234–1247. [CrossRef]
25. Fisher, J.; Sharma, R.; Don, D.W.; Barisa, M.; Hurtado, M.O.; Abramowski, P.; Porter, L.; Day, W.; Borea, R.; Inglott, S.; et al. Engineering gammadelta T cells limits tonic signaling associated with chimeric antigen receptors. *Sci. Signal.* **2019**, *12*. [CrossRef]
26. Harrer, D.C.; Simon, B.; Fujii, S.I.; Shimizu, K.; Uslu, U.; Schuler, G.; Gerer, K.F.; Hoyer, S.; Dorrie, J.; Schaft, N. RNA-transfection of gamma/delta T cells with a chimeric antigen receptor or an alpha/beta T-cell receptor: A safer alternative to genetically engineered alpha/beta T cells for the immunotherapy of melanoma. *BMC Cancer* **2017**, *17*, 551. [CrossRef]
27. Fleischer, L.C.; Becker, S.A.; Ryan, R.E.; Fedanov, A.; Doering, C.B.; Spencer, H.T. Non-signaling Chimeric Antigen Receptors Enhance Antigen-Directed Killing by gammadelta T Cells in Contrast to alphabeta T Cells. *Mol. Ther. Oncolytics* **2020**, *18*, 149–160. [CrossRef]
28. Plitas, G.; Rudensky, A.Y. Regulatory T Cells: Differentiation and Function. *Cancer Immunol. Res.* **2016**, *4*, 721–725. [CrossRef]
29. Sharabi, A.; Tsokos, M.G.; Ding, Y.; Malek, T.R.; Klatzmann, D.; Tsokos, G.C. Regulatory T cells in the treatment of disease. *Nat. Rev. Drug Discov.* **2018**, *17*, 823–844. [CrossRef]
30. Lucca, L.E.; Dominguez-Villar, M. Modulation of regulatory T cell function and stability by co-inhibitory receptors. *Nat. Rev. Immunol.* **2020**, *20*, 680–693. [CrossRef]
31. Tenspolde, M.; Zimmermann, K.; Weber, L.C.; Hapke, M.; Lieber, M.; Dywicki, J.; Frenzel, A.; Hust, M.; Galla, M.; Buitrago-Molina, L.E.; et al. Regulatory T cells engineered with a novel insulin-specific chimeric antigen receptor as a candidate immunotherapy for type 1 diabetes. *J. Autoimmun.* **2019**, *103*, 102289. [CrossRef] [PubMed]
32. Blat, D.; Zigmond, E.; Alteber, Z.; Waks, T.; Eshhar, Z. Suppression of murine colitis and its associated cancer by carcinoembryonic antigen-specific regulatory T cells. *Mol. Ther.* **2014**, *22*, 1018–1028. [CrossRef] [PubMed]
33. Pierini, A.; Iliopoulou, B.P.; Peiris, H.; Perez-Cruz, M.; Baker, J.; Hsu, K.; Gu, X.; Zheng, P.P.; Erkers, T.; Tang, S.W.; et al. T cells expressing chimeric antigen receptor promote immune tolerance. *JCI Insight* **2017**, *2*, e92865. [CrossRef]
34. Yoon, J.; Schmidt, A.; Zhang, A.H.; Konigs, C.; Kim, Y.C.; Scott, D.W. FVIII-specific human chimeric antigen receptor T-regulatory cells suppress T- and B-cell responses to FVIII. *Blood* **2017**, *129*, 238–245. [CrossRef]
35. Imura, Y.; Ando, M.; Kondo, T.; Ito, M.; Yoshimura, A. CD19-targeted CAR regulatory T cells suppress B cell pathology without GvHD. *JCI Insight* **2020**, *5*, e136185. [CrossRef]
36. MacDonald, K.G.; Hoeppli, R.E.; Huang, Q.; Gillies, J.; Luciani, D.S.; Orban, P.C.; Broady, R.; Levings, M.K. Alloantigen-specific regulatory T cells generated with a chimeric antigen receptor. *J. Clin. Investig.* **2016**, *126*, 1413–1424. [CrossRef]
37. Dawson, N.A.J.; Rosado-Sanchez, I.; Novakovsky, G.E.; Fung, V.C.W.; Huang, Q.; McIver, E.; Sun, G.; Gillies, J.; Speck, M.; Orban, P.C.; et al. Functional effects of chimeric antigen receptor co-receptor signaling domains in human regulatory T cells. *Sci. Transl. Med.* **2020**, *12*, eaaz3866. [CrossRef]
38. Boroughs, A.C.; Larson, R.C.; Choi, B.D.; Bouffard, A.A.; Riley, L.S.; Schiferle, E.; Kulkarni, A.S.; Cetrulo, C.L.; Ting, D.; Blazar, B.R.; et al. Chimeric antigen receptor costimulation domains modulate human regulatory T cell function. *JCI Insight* **2019**, *4*, e126194. [CrossRef]
39. Corbett, A.J.; Eckle, S.B.; Birkinshaw, R.W.; Liu, L.; Patel, O.; Mahony, J.; Chen, Z.; Reantragoon, R.; Meehan, B.; Cao, H.; et al. T-cell activation by transitory neo-antigens derived from distinct microbial pathways. *Nature* **2014**, *509*, 361–365. [CrossRef]
40. Gherardin, N.A.; Keller, A.N.; Woolley, R.E.; Le Nours, J.; Ritchie, D.S.; Neeson, P.J.; Birkinshaw, R.W.; Eckle, S.B.G.; Waddington, J.N.; Liu, L.; et al. Diversity of T Cells Restricted by the MHC Class I-Related Molecule MR1 Facilitates Differential Antigen Recognition. *Immunity* **2016**, *44*, 32–45. [CrossRef]
41. D'Souza, C.; Chen, Z.; Corbett, A.J. Revealing the protective and pathogenic potential of MAIT cells. *Mol. Immunol.* **2018**, *103*, 46–54. [CrossRef] [PubMed]
42. Riegert, P.; Wanner, V.; Bahram, S. Genomics, isoforms, expression, and phylogeny of the MHC class I-related MR1 gene. *J. Immunol.* **1998**, *161*, 4066–4077. [PubMed]
43. Chen, Z.; Wang, H.; D'Souza, C.; Sun, S.; Kostenko, L.; Eckle, S.B.; Meehan, B.S.; Jackson, D.C.; Strugnell, R.A.; Cao, H.; et al. Mucosal-associated invariant T-cell activation and accumulation after in vivo infection depends on microbial riboflavin synthesis and co-stimulatory signals. *Mucosal Immunol.* **2017**, *10*, 58–68. [CrossRef] [PubMed]

44. Koay, H.F.; Gherardin, N.A.; Enders, A.; Loh, L.; Mackay, L.K.; Almeida, C.F.; Russ, B.E.; Nold-Petry, C.A.; Nold, M.F.; Bedoui, S.; et al. A three-stage intrathymic development pathway for the mucosal-associated invariant T cell lineage. *Nat. Immunol.* **2016**, *17*, 1300–1311. [CrossRef]

45. Yong, Y.K.; Saeidi, A.; Tan, H.Y.; Rosmawati, M.; Enstrom, P.F.; Batran, R.A.; Vasuki, V.; Chattopadhyay, I.; Murugesan, A.; Vignesh, R.; et al. Hyper-Expression of PD-1 Is Associated with the Levels of Exhausted and Dysfunctional Phenotypes of Circulating CD161++TCR iValpha7.2+ Mucosal-Associated Invariant T Cells in Chronic Hepatitis B Virus Infection. *Front. Immunol.* **2018**, *9*, 472. [CrossRef]

46. Schenkel, J.M.; Masopust, D. Tissue-resident memory T cells. *Immunity* **2014**, *41*, 886–897. [CrossRef] [PubMed]

47. Mackay, L.K.; Wynne-Jones, E.; Freestone, D.; Pellicci, D.G.; Mielke, L.A.; Newman, D.M.; Braun, A.; Masson, F.; Kallies, A.; Belz, G.T.; et al. T-box Transcription Factors Combine with the Cytokines TGF-beta and IL-15 to Control Tissue-Resident Memory T Cell Fate. *Immunity* **2015**, *43*, 1101–1111. [CrossRef] [PubMed]

48. Kok, L.; Dijkgraaf, F.E.; Urbanus, J.; Bresser, K.; Vredevoogd, D.W.; Cardoso, R.F.; Perie, L.; Beltman, J.B.; Schumacher, T.N. A committed tissue-resident memory T cell precursor within the circulating CD8+ effector T cell pool. *J. Exp. Med.* **2020**, *217*, e20191711. [CrossRef] [PubMed]

49. Steinbach, K.; Vincenti, I.; Merkler, D. Resident-Memory T Cells in Tissue-Restricted Immune Responses: For Better or Worse? *Front. Immunol.* **2018**, *9*, 2827. [CrossRef] [PubMed]

50. Bald, T.; Krummel, M.F.; Smyth, M.J.; Barry, K.C. The NK cell-cancer cycle: Advances and new challenges in NK cell-based immunotherapies. *Nat. Immunol.* **2020**, *21*, 835–847. [CrossRef]

51. Lelaidier, M.; Diaz-Rodriguez, Y.; Cordeau, M.; Cordeiro, P.; Haddad, E.; Herblot, S.; Duval, M. TRAIL-mediated killing of acute lymphoblastic leukemia by plasmacytoid dendritic cell-activated natural killer cells. *Oncotarget* **2015**, *6*, 29440–29455. [CrossRef]

52. Prager, I.; Liesche, C.; van Ooijen, H.; Urlaub, D.; Verron, Q.; Sandstrom, N.; Fasbender, F.; Claus, M.; Eils, R.; Beaudouin, J.; et al. NK cells switch from granzyme B to death receptor-mediated cytotoxicity during serial killing. *J. Exp. Med.* **2019**, *216*, 2113–2127. [CrossRef]

53. Shimasaki, N.; Jain, A.; Campana, D. NK cells for cancer immunotherapy. *Nat. Rev. Drug Discov.* **2020**, *19*, 200–218. [CrossRef]

54. Miller, J.S.; Soignier, Y.; Panoskaltsis-Mortari, A.; McNearney, S.A.; Yun, G.H.; Fautsch, S.K.; McKenna, D.; Le, C.; Defor, T.E.; Burns, L.J.; et al. Successful adoptive transfer and in vivo expansion of human haploidentical NK cells in patients with cancer. *Blood* **2005**, *105*, 3051–3057. [CrossRef] [PubMed]

55. Liu, E.; Marin, D.; Banerjee, P.; Macapinlac, H.A.; Thompson, P.; Basar, R.; Nassif Kerbauy, L.; Overman, B.; Thall, P.; Kaplan, M.; et al. Use of CAR-Transduced Natural Killer Cells in CD19-Positive Lymphoid Tumors. *N. Engl. J. Med.* **2020**, *382*, 545–553. [CrossRef]

56. Xiao, L.; Cen, D.; Gan, H.; Sun, Y.; Huang, N.; Xiong, H.; Jin, Q.; Su, L.; Liu, X.; Wang, K.; et al. Adoptive Transfer of NKG2D CAR mRNA-Engineered Natural Killer Cells in Colorectal Cancer Patients. *Mol. Ther.* **2019**, *27*, 1114–1125. [CrossRef]

57. Tang, X.; Yang, L.; Li, Z.; Nalin, A.P.; Dai, H.; Xu, T.; Yin, J.; You, F.; Zhu, M.; Shen, W.; et al. First-in-man clinical trial of CAR NK-92 cells: Safety test of CD33-CAR NK-92 cells in patients with relapsed and refractory acute myeloid leukemia. *Am. J. Cancer Res.* **2018**, *8*, 1083–1089.

58. Daher, M.; Basar, R.; Gokdemir, E.; Baran, N.; Uprety, N.; Nunez Cortes, A.K.; Mendt, M.; Kerbauy, L.N.; Banerjee, P.P.; Hernandez Sanabria, M.; et al. Targeting a cytokine checkpoint enhances the fitness of armored cord blood CAR-NK cells. *Blood* **2020**. [CrossRef] [PubMed]

59. Wang, X.; Jasinski, D.L.; Medina, J.L.; Spencer, D.M.; Foster, A.E.; Bayle, J.H. Inducible MyD88/CD40 synergizes with IL-15 to enhance antitumor efficacy of CAR-NK cells. *Blood Adv.* **2020**, *4*, 1950–1964. [CrossRef] [PubMed]

60. Godfrey, D.I.; Le Nours, J.; Andrews, D.M.; Uldrich, A.P.; Rossjohn, J. Unconventional T Cell Targets for Cancer Immunotherapy. *Immunity* **2018**, *48*, 453–473. [CrossRef]

61. McEwen-Smith, R.M.; Salio, M.; Cerundolo, V. The regulatory role of invariant NKT cells in tumor immunity. *Cancer Immunol. Res.* **2015**, *3*, 425–435. [CrossRef] [PubMed]

62. Heczey, A.; Liu, D.; Tian, G.; Courtney, A.N.; Wei, J.; Marinova, E.; Gao, X.; Guo, L.; Yvon, E.; Hicks, J.; et al. Invariant NKT cells with chimeric antigen receptor provide a novel platform for safe and effective cancer immunotherapy. *Blood* **2014**, *124*, 2824–2833. [CrossRef] [PubMed]

63. Ngai, H.; Tian, G.; Courtney, A.N.; Ravari, S.B.; Guo, L.; Liu, B.; Jin, J.; Shen, E.T.; Di Pierro, E.J.; Metelitsa, L.S. IL-21 Selectively Protects CD62L+ NKT Cells and Enhances Their Effector Functions for Adoptive Immunotherapy. *J. Immunol.* **2018**, *201*, 2141–2153. [CrossRef] [PubMed]

64. Rotolo, A.; Caputo, V.S.; Holubova, M.; Baxan, N.; Dubois, O.; Chaudhry, M.S.; Xiao, X.; Goudevenou, K.; Pitcher, D.S.; Petevi, K.; et al. Enhanced Anti-lymphoma Activity of CAR19-iNKT Cells Underpinned by Dual CD19 and CD1d Targeting. *Cancer Cell* **2018**, *34*, 596–610. [CrossRef] [PubMed]

65. Xu, X.; Huang, W.; Heczey, A.; Liu, D.; Guo, L.; Wood, M.; Jin, J.; Courtney, A.N.; Liu, B.; Di Pierro, E.J.; et al. NKT Cells Coexpressing a GD2-Specific Chimeric Antigen Receptor and IL15 Show Enhanced In Vivo Persistence and Antitumor Activity against Neuroblastoma. *Clin. Cancer Res.* **2019**, *25*, 7126–7138. [CrossRef] [PubMed]

66. Heczey, A.; Courtney, A.N.; Montalbano, A.; Robinson, S.; Liu, K.; Li, M.; Ghatwai, N.; Dakhova, O.; Liu, B.; Raveh-Sadka, T.; et al. Anti-GD2 CAR-NKT cells in patients with relapsed or refractory neuroblastoma: An interim analysis. *Nat. Med.* **2020**, *26*, 1686–1690. [CrossRef] [PubMed]

67. Tian, G.; Courtney, A.N.; Jena, B.; Heczey, A.; Liu, D.; Marinova, E.; Guo, L.; Xu, X.; Torikai, H.; Mo, Q.; et al. CD62L⁺ NKT cells have prolonged persistence and antitumor activity in vivo. *J. Clin. Investig.* **2016**, *126*, 2341–2355. [CrossRef]
68. Malfitano, A.M.; Pisanti, S.; Napolitano, F.; Di Somma, S.; Martinelli, R.; Portella, G. Tumor-Associated Macrophage Status in Cancer Treatment. *Cancers* **2020**, *12*, 1987. [CrossRef]
69. Kaneda, M.M.; Messer, K.S.; Ralainirina, N.; Li, H.; Leem, C.J.; Gorjestani, S.; Woo, G.; Nguyen, A.V.; Figueiredo, C.C.; Foubert, P.; et al. PI3Kgamma is a molecular switch that controls immune suppression. *Nature* **2016**, *539*, 437–442. [CrossRef]
70. Nielsen, S.R.; Quaranta, V.; Linford, A.; Emeagi, P.; Rainer, C.; Santos, A.; Ireland, L.; Sakai, T.; Sakai, K.; Kim, Y.S.; et al. Macrophage-secreted granulin supports pancreatic cancer metastasis by inducing liver fibrosis. *Nat. Cell Biol.* **2016**, *18*, 549–560. [CrossRef]
71. Di Mitri, D.; Mirenda, M.; Vasilevska, J.; Calcinotto, A.; Delaleu, N.; Revandkar, A.; Gil, V.; Boysen, G.; Losa, M.; Mosole, S.; et al. Re-education of Tumor-Associated Macrophages by CXCR2 Blockade Drives Senescence and Tumor Inhibition in Advanced Prostate Cancer. *Cell Rep.* **2019**, *28*, 2156–2168. [CrossRef] [PubMed]
72. Guerriero, J.L.; Sotayo, A.; Ponichtera, H.E.; Castrillon, J.A.; Pourzia, A.L.; Schad, S.; Johnson, S.F.; Carrasco, R.D.; Lazo, S.; Bronson, R.T.; et al. Class IIa HDAC inhibition reduces breast tumours and metastases through anti-tumour macrophages. *Nature* **2017**, *543*, 428–432. [CrossRef] [PubMed]
73. Morrissey, M.A.; Williamson, A.P.; Steinbach, A.M.; Roberts, E.W.; Kern, N.; Headley, M.B.; Vale, R.D. Chimeric antigen receptors that trigger phagocytosis. *Elife* **2018**, *7*, e36688. [CrossRef] [PubMed]
74. Klichinsky, M.; Ruella, M.; Shestova, O.; Lu, X.M.; Best, A.; Zeeman, M.; Schmierer, M.; Gabrusiewicz, K.; Anderson, N.R.; Petty, N.E.; et al. Human chimeric antigen receptor macrophages for cancer immunotherapy. *Nat. Biotechnol.* **2020**, *38*, 947–953. [CrossRef]
75. Zhang, W.; Liu, L.; Su, H.; Liu, Q.; Shen, J.; Dai, H.; Zheng, W.; Lu, Y.; Zhang, W.; Bei, Y.; et al. Chimeric antigen receptor macrophage therapy for breast tumours mediated by targeting the tumour extracellular matrix. *Br. J. Cancer* **2019**, *121*, 837–845. [CrossRef]
76. Giavridis, T.; van der Stegen, S.J.C.; Eyquem, J.; Hamieh, M.; Piersigilli, A.; Sadelain, M. CAR T cell-induced cytokine release syndrome is mediated by macrophages and abated by IL-1 blockade. *Nat. Med.* **2018**, *24*, 731–738. [CrossRef]
77. Williford, J.M.; Ishihara, J.; Ishihara, A.; Mansurov, A.; Hosseinchi, P.; Marchell, T.M.; Potin, L.; Swartz, M.A.; Hubbell, J.A. Recruitment of CD103⁺ dendritic cells via tumor-targeted chemokine delivery enhances efficacy of checkpoint inhibitor immunotherapy. *Sci. Adv.* **2019**, *5*, eaay1357. [CrossRef]
78. Maier, B.; Leader, A.M.; Chen, S.T.; Tung, N.; Chang, C.; LeBerichel, J.; Chudnovskiy, A.; Maskey, S.; Walker, L.; Finnigan, J.P.; et al. A conserved dendritic-cell regulatory program limits antitumour immunity. *Nature* **2020**, *580*, 257–262. [CrossRef]
79. Hildner, K.; Edelson, B.T.; Purtha, W.E.; Diamond, M.; Matsushita, H.; Kohyama, M.; Calderon, B.; Schraml, B.U.; Unanue, E.R.; Diamond, M.S.; et al. Batf3 deficiency reveals a critical role for CD8alpha+ dendritic cells in cytotoxic T cell immunity. *Science* **2008**, *322*, 1097–1100. [CrossRef]
80. Suh, H.C.; Pohl, K.A.; Termini, C.; Kan, J.; Timmerman, J.M.; Slamon, D.J.; Chute, J.P. Bioengineered Autologous Dendritic Cells Enhance CAR T Cell Cytotoxicity By Providing Cytokine Stimulation and Intratumoral Dendritic Cells. *Blood* **2018**, *132*, 3693. [CrossRef]
81. Zhang, L.; Morgan, R.A.; Beane, J.D.; Zheng, Z.; Dudley, M.E.; Kassim, S.H.; Nahvi, A.V.; Ngo, L.T.; Sherry, R.M.; Phan, G.Q.; et al. Tumor-infiltrating lymphocytes genetically engineered with an inducible gene encoding interleukin-12 for the immunotherapy of metastatic melanoma. *Clin. Cancer Res.* **2015**, *21*, 2278–2288. [CrossRef] [PubMed]
82. Shalapour, S.; Font-Burgada, J.; Di Caro, G.; Zhong, Z.; Sanchez-Lopez, E.; Dhar, D.; Willimsky, G.; Ammirante, M.; Strasner, A.; Hansel, D.E.; et al. Immunosuppressive plasma cells impede T-cell-dependent immunogenic chemotherapy. *Nature* **2015**, *521*, 94–98. [CrossRef]
83. Helmink, B.A.; Reddy, S.M.; Gao, J.; Zhang, S.; Basar, R.; Thakur, R.; Yizhak, K.; Sade-Feldman, M.; Blando, J.; Han, G.; et al. B cells and tertiary lymphoid structures promote immunotherapy response. *Nature* **2020**, *577*, 549–555. [CrossRef] [PubMed]
84. McDaniel, J.R.; Pero, S.C.; Voss, W.N.; Shukla, G.S.; Sun, Y.; Schaetzle, S.; Lee, C.H.; Horton, A.P.; Harlow, S.; Gollihar, J.; et al. Identification of tumor-reactive B cells and systemic IgG in breast cancer based on clonal frequency in the sentinel lymph node. *Cancer Immunol. Immunother.* **2018**, *67*, 729–738. [CrossRef] [PubMed]
85. Ruella, M.; Xu, J.; Barrett, D.M.; Fraietta, J.A.; Reich, T.J.; Ambrose, D.E.; Klichinsky, M.; Shestova, O.; Patel, P.R.; Kulikovskaya, I.; et al. Induction of resistance to chimeric antigen receptor T cell therapy by transduction of a single leukemic B cell. *Nat. Med.* **2018**, *24*, 1499–1503. [CrossRef]
86. Pesch, T.; Bonati, L.; Kelton, W.; Parola, C.; Ehling, R.A.; Csepregi, L.; Kitamura, D.; Reddy, S.T. Molecular Design, Optimization, and Genomic Integration of Chimeric B Cell Receptors in Murine B Cells. *Front. Immunol.* **2019**, *10*, 2630. [CrossRef]
87. Hung, K.L.; Meitlis, I.; Hale, M.; Chen, C.Y.; Singh, S.; Jackson, S.W.; Miao, C.H.; Khan, I.F.; Rawlings, D.J.; James, R.G. Engineering Protein-Secreting Plasma Cells by Homology-Directed Repair in Primary Human B Cells. *Mol. Ther.* **2018**, *26*, 456–467. [CrossRef]
88. Moffett, H.F.; Harms, C.K.; Fitzpatrick, K.S.; Tooley, M.R.; Boonyaratanakornkit, J.; Taylor, J.J. B cells engineered to express pathogen-specific antibodies protect against infection. *Sci. Immunol.* **2019**, *4*, eaax0644. [CrossRef]
89. Kantoff, P.W.; Higano, C.S.; Shore, N.D.; Berger, E.R.; Small, E.J.; Penson, D.F.; Redfern, C.H.; Ferrari, A.C.; Dreicer, R.; Sims, R.B.; et al. Sipuleucel-T immunotherapy for castration-resistant prostate cancer. *N. Engl. J. Med.* **2010**, *363*, 411–422. [CrossRef]

90. Small, E.J.; Schellhammer, P.F.; Higano, C.S.; Redfern, C.H.; Nemunaitis, J.J.; Valone, F.H.; Verjee, S.S.; Jones, L.A.; Hershberg, R.M. Placebo-controlled phase III trial of immunologic therapy with sipuleucel-T (APC8015) in patients with metastatic, asymptomatic hormone refractory prostate cancer. *J. Clin. Oncol.* **2006**, *24*, 3089–3094. [CrossRef]
91. Li, Y.; Hermanson, D.L.; Moriarity, B.S.; Kaufman, D.S. Human iPSC-Derived Natural Killer Cells Engineered with Chimeric Antigen Receptors Enhance Anti-tumor Activity. *Cell Stem Cell* **2018**, *23*, 181–192. [CrossRef] [PubMed]
92. Zhang, L.; Tian, L.; Dai, X.; Yu, H.; Wang, J.; Lei, A.; Zhu, M.; Xu, J.; Zhao, W.; Zhu, Y.; et al. Pluripotent stem cell-derived CAR-macrophage cells with antigen-dependent anti-cancer cell functions. *J. Hematol. Oncol.* **2020**, *13*, 153. [CrossRef] [PubMed]

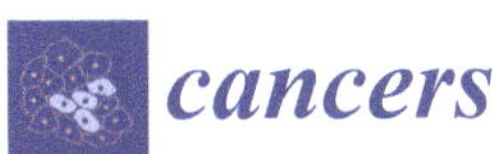

Review

Overcoming Challenges for CD3-Bispecific Antibody Therapy in Solid Tumors

Jim Middelburg [1], Kristel Kemper [2], Patrick Engelberts [2], Aran F. Labrijn [2], Janine Schuurman [2] and Thorbald van Hall [1,*]

[1] Department of Medical Oncology, Oncode Institute, Leiden University Medical Center, 2333 ZA Leiden, The Netherlands; j.middelburg@lumc.nl
[2] Genmab, 3584 CT Utrecht, The Netherlands; kke@genmab.com (K.K.); pen@genmab.com (P.E.); ala@genmab.com (A.F.L.); jsc@genmab.com (J.S.)
* Correspondence: T.van_Hall@lumc.nl; Tel.: +31-71-5266945

Simple Summary: CD3-bispecific antibody therapy is a form of immunotherapy that enables soldier cells of the immune system to recognize and kill tumor cells. This type of therapy is currently successfully used in the clinic to treat tumors in the blood and is under investigation for tumors in our organs. The treatment of these solid tumors faces more pronounced hurdles, which affect the safety and efficacy of CD3-bispecific antibody therapy. In this review, we provide a brief status update of this field and identify intrinsic hurdles for solid cancers. Furthermore, we describe potential solutions and combinatorial approaches to overcome these challenges in order to generate safer and more effective therapies.

Abstract: Immunotherapy of cancer with CD3-bispecific antibodies is an approved therapeutic option for some hematological malignancies and is under clinical investigation for solid cancers. However, the treatment of solid tumors faces more pronounced hurdles, such as increased on-target off-tumor toxicities, sparse T-cell infiltration and impaired T-cell quality due to the presence of an immunosuppressive tumor microenvironment, which affect the safety and limit efficacy of CD3-bispecific antibody therapy. In this review, we provide a brief status update of the CD3-bispecific antibody therapy field and identify intrinsic hurdles in solid cancers. Furthermore, we describe potential combinatorial approaches to overcome these challenges in order to generate selective and more effective responses.

Keywords: antibody therapy; immuno-oncology; CD3-bispecific antibody; T-cell engager; solid tumors; on-target off-tumor toxicity; T-cell co-stimulation; tumor-associated antigens

Citation: Middelburg, J.; Kemper, K.; Engelberts, P.; Labrijn, A.F.; Schuurman, J.; van Hall, T. Overcoming Challenges for CD3-Bispecific Antibody Therapy in Solid Tumors. *Cancers* **2021**, *13*, 287. https://doi.org/10.3390/cancers13020287

Received: 14 December 2020
Accepted: 10 January 2021
Published: 14 January 2021

Publisher's Note: MDPI stays neutral with regard to jurisdictional clai-ms in published maps and institutio-nal affiliations.

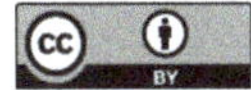

1. Introduction

CD3-bispecific antibodies (CD3-BsAbs) are an emerging treatment modality in the field of cancer immunotherapy. BsAbs can recognize distinct antigens with each of their antigen-binding domains, in contrast to conventional Abs that recognize the same antigen with both Fab arms. The exception is IgG4, which has been reported to naturally exchange arms to attain bispecificity [1]. CD3-BsAbs act by simultaneous binding to a tumor-associated antigen (TAA) expressed on tumor cells and to CD3 on a T cell (CD3xTAA) [2]. Crosslinking of these two cell types by CD3-BsAbs allows the formation of an immunological synapse, similar to that of a natural T-cell receptor (TCR)/peptide–major histocompatibility complex (MHC) complex [3]. This synapse results in T-cell activation and thereby the secretion of inflammatory cytokines and cytolytic molecules that are able to kill the tumor cells in the process. The strength of CD3-BsAbs lies in the fact that any T cell could serve as an effector cell, regardless of TCR specificity, as for these BsAbs, TCR signaling does not require engagement of the antigen-binding domain of the TCR, but is initiated via CD3 [4].

Therefore, CD3-BsAbs can employ all available T cells and are not limited to tumor-specific T cells, contrary to the key requirement for effective immune checkpoint therapy [5].

CD3-BsAb therapy is a passive form of immunotherapy and shows striking kinship with the adoptive cell transfer of T cells expressing chimeric antigen receptor (CAR) transgenes [6]. CARs consist of TAA binding domains from antibodies directly linked to the intracellular CD3ζ chain and domains from costimulatory receptors (e.g., 4-1BB) and thereby activate T cells upon antigen recognition. CD3-BsAbs and CAR T cells are similar in many ways: both target a surface TAA, both exploit T-cell effector functions and both are successfully used in the clinic for hematological malignancies and show a similar type of toxicity profile [7,8]. Some disadvantages of currently clinically approved CAR T cells compared to CD3-BsAbs are: (1) patients are required to be lymphodepleted prior to infusion of CAR T cells, (2) CAR T cells have to be individually produced for each patient, whereas CD3-BsAbs can serve as off-the-shelf therapeutics, (3) CAR T cells remain in the patients after the tumor is cleared, resulting in continuous B-cell depletion in the case of CD19-targeting CAR T cells, whereas CD3-BsAbs are cleared from the blood over time and (4) unlike CD3-BsAbs, dosing cannot be adjusted to minimize adverse events [7,9]. Nevertheless, it will be important to learn from the CAR T cell field to potentially extrapolate new findings to the CD3-BsAb field.

Over the last few years, new insights in BsAb biology and enabling technologies resulted in the generation of many different formats of CD3-BsAbs, which was elaborately reviewed by Labrijn et al. [10]. As of December 2020, over 100 different CD3-BsAb formats are known, ranging from very small fragments containing two different variable domains without an Fc tail, conventional antibody structures (two Fab arms linked to an Fc tail) and larger structures with additional variable domains linked to the conventional antibody structure. These different formats determine important features, such as antibody half-life via neonatal Fc receptor (FcRn)-mediated recycling, immunogenicity, type of effector response via altered immune synapse formation and ability to penetrate in solid tumors [11]. The presence and functionality of the Fc tail determines whether the BsAb is able to bind to and activate Fc receptor (FcR)-expressing immune cells, which could lead to stronger inflammatory responses, but also allows activation of immune cells in the absence of TAA, potentially resulting in more severe adverse events (AEs) [12].

Currently, CD3-BsAbs show great potential for hematological cancers, with the FDA-approved blinatumomab (CD3xCD19) being successfully used in the clinic to treat some B-cell malignancies. Many other CD3-BsAbs are being tested in (pre)clinical studies for both hematological and solid tumors. However, contrary to the success of CD3-BsAbs in hematological malignancies, the effect of these antibodies in solid tumors is still rather limited [13]. This review will focus on essential hurdles for CD3-BsAbs for solid tumors, such as critical on-target off-tumor binding, sparse T-cell infiltration and quality of tumor-infiltrating lymphocyte (TIL) effector cells due to the presence of an immunosuppressive tumor microenvironment (TME). Lastly, we will discuss potential combination strategies to overcome these hurdles.

2. Main Text

2.1. CD3-BsAbs in Hematological Malignancies

CD3-BsAbs received a lot of attention due to their success in hematological cancers. Blinatumomab (a CD3xCD19 BsAb without an Fc tail) was FDA approved in 2014 and is now successfully used in the clinic to treat patients suffering from relapsed or refractory B-cell precursor acute lymphoblastic leukemia (ALL) [14]. Over 40% of adult patients treated with blinatumomab show a complete or partial response and median overall survival is improved by several months compared to standard of care chemotherapy [15–17]. Unfortunately, most patients still relapse eventually after primary response to blinatumomab therapy. These relapses are currently being extensively investigated and the data have thus far indicated that relapses are frequently found at immune-privileged extramedullary locations and some relapses have lost CD19 antigen expression, but more research is required to further elucidate these resistance mechanisms [18,19].

Apart from blinatumomab, many other CD3-BsAbs are currently in clinical trials targeting well-established B-cell markers, like CD19, CD20, CD38 and B-cell maturation antigen (BCMA) and myeloid markers, like CD33 and CD123. For instance, in a phase I/II study, patients suffering from acute myeloid leukemia (AML) were treated with flotetuzumab (CD3xCD123 BsAb) and showed promising overall response rates (complete response with full, partial or incomplete recovery of blood cells) of 30% [20]. In another phase I/II study for patients suffering from diffuse large B-cell lymphoma (DLBCL), high-grade B-cell lymphoma (HGBCL) or follicular lymphoma (FL), epcoritamab (CD3xCD20 BsAb) therapy generated impressive responses: 44% complete response (CR) and 11% partial response (PR) for patients with DLBCL or HGBCL and 100% PR for patients with FL [21]. Comparable results were obtained with other CD3xCD20 bispecifics [22,23]. In NOD/SCID-gamma null (NSG) mice, REGN1979 (CD3xCD20) delayed tumor outgrowth better than rituximab, thereby further indicating the strength of CD3-BsAbs [24]. Interestingly, some of these trials target the same B-cell or myeloid antigens, however, with different CD3-BsAb formats. Therefore, these clinical studies could potentially inform on the role of different antibody formats' treatment safety and efficacy.

Clinical trials with blinatumomab revealed that cytokine release syndrome (CRS) is one of the major safety-related AEs [25]. The availability of CD19$^+$ tumor cells and healthy B- and T cells in the same compartment allows acute and synchronic CD3-BsAb-mediated T-cell activation, followed by excessive release of inflammatory cytokines, such as IFN-γ, IL-6 and TNF-α, resulting in symptoms ranging from mild fever to multi-organ system failure [26]. However, CRS is not a specific problem for blinatumomab, but is observed for all CD3-BsAbs and CAR T-cell therapies in both hematological and solid cancer indications with CRS severities dependent on the type of therapy and target [27,28]. Preclinical research using a humanized mouse model showed that the primary mediator of CD3-BsAb-induced CRS was TNF-α produced by activated T cells, leading to massive secretion of inflammatory cytokines by monocytes [29]. The blockade of upstream TNF-α and downstream IL-1β or IL-6 can mitigate CRS [29–31]. Others have reported that step-up dosing, or subcutaneous administration of CD3-BsAbs, decreased the extent of CRS [32,33]. Furthermore, several preclinical studies in mouse and cynomolgus monkey models showed that reducing CD3 affinity could reduce treatment-induced cytokine levels [34–37].

2.2. Historical Perspective and Current Status of CD3-BsAbs in Solid Cancers

Despite the fact that CD3-BsAbs are mostly known for their use in hematological malignancies, the first European medicines agency (EMA)-approved CD3 bispecific antibody was catumaxomab, a CD3xEpCAM BsAb for the intraperitoneal treatment of epithelial cell adhesion molecule (EpCAM)-positive malignant ascites [38]. This antibody was actually trifunctional, as its Fc was able to bind FcR-expressing cells and induced strong immunological responses [39]. Severe liver toxicity was also observed due to the activation of Kupffer cells when administered intravenously [12]. Catumaxomab was eventually withdrawn for commercial reasons in 2017, but taught the field an important lesson about the potential dangers of the presence of an active Fc in CD3-BsAbs. All current full length CD3-BsAbs in development contain Fc-silent backbones with mutations impairing the binding of FcγR and C1q [10]. Moreover, preclinical studies showed that Fc-silenced full length CD3-BsAbs improved T-cell trafficking towards the tumor and induced better anti-tumor responses. Wang et al. showed that CD3-BsAbs with an active Fc backbone failed to drive T cells to the tumor, but instead induced either T-cell depletion or the accumulation of T cells in the lungs [40]. This observed effect was attributed to the capacity of the Fc backbone to be bound by FcγR-expressing myeloid cells. Fc-silenced CD3-BsAbs did not lead to sequestration of T cells in the lungs, but they arrived in the tumor. More importantly, therapeutic efficacy was greatly improved in Fc-silenced CD3-BsAb-treated mice. A similar trend was also observed in a syngeneic mouse model, where CD3xTrp1 (tyrosinase-related protein 1) was used to treat Trp1-positive B16F10 tumor cells [41].

As of December 2020, no CD3-BsAbs are approved for the treatment of solid tumors in the clinic. However, many different targets are being explored in clinical studies, of which most are focusing on classical TAAs, such as carcinoembryonic antigen (CEA), epidermal growth factor receptor (EGFR), EpCAM, HER2 and prostate-specific membrane antigen (PSMA). Other TAAs are also being explored (see Table 1 for an elaborate list). Most of these studies simply inject CD3-BsAbs, however, in some studies, these Abs piggyback with infused T cells as "bispecific-armed T cells". Furthermore, this table also includes CD3-BsAb formats based on affinity-enhanced TCR-like domains that recognize peptide–human leukocyte antigen (HLA) complexes (immune mobilizing monoclonal T-cell receptors against cancer (ImmTACs)) [42]. Multiple other TAAs are currently pursued in preclinical studies hoping to make their way to the clinic, including B7-H4, CD133, CD155, claudin 6 (CLDN6), cellular mesenchymal to epithelial transcription factor (C-MET), ephrin receptor A10 (EphA10), folate receptor 1 (FOLR1), HLA-A*24:survivin $2B_{80\text{-}88}$, integrin $\beta4$ (ITGB4), P-cadherin, prolactin receptor (PRLR), receptor tyrosine kinase-like orphan receptor 1 (ROR1), TNF-related apoptosis-inducing ligand receptor (TRAIL-R2), transferrin receptor (TfR) and tumor-associated calcium signal transducer 2 (Trop-2) [43–69].

Table 1. Overview of clinical studies involving CD3-BsAbs targeting solid tumors.

TAA	Disease	Phase
Completed Clinical Trials		
CEA	CEA-positive tumors	Phase I (NCT02324257, completed)
CEA	Gastrointestinal adenocarcinomas	Phase I NCT01284231, completed)
CEA	Advanced CEA-positive solid tumors	Phase I (NCT02291614, completed)
CEA	Advanced CEA-positive solid tumors	Phase I (NCT02650713, completed)
EGFR	Brain and central nervous system tumors	Phase I (NCT00005813, completed)
EpCAM	Solid tumors	Phase I (NCT00635596, completed)
EpCAM	Ascites, ovarian cancer, fallopian tube cancer, peritoneal cancer	Phase II (NCT00326885, completed)
EpCAM	Ovarian cancer, fallopian tube cancer, peritoneal cancer	Phase II (NCT00377429, completed)
EpCAM	Recurrent ovarian cancer, fallopian tube cancer, peritoneal carcinomatosis	Phase II (NCT01815528, completed)
EpCAM	Ovarian cancer, fallopian tube cancer, peritoneal cancer	Phase II (NCT01246440, completed)
EpCAM	Ovarian cancer	Phase II (NCT00563836, completed)
EpCAM	Ascites, carcinoma, epithelial cancer	Phase II (NCT01065246, completed)
EpCAM	Ovarian cancer, gastric cancer, pancreatic cancer, malignant ascites	Phase II (2005-001700-39, completed)
EpCAM	Gastric cancer and gastric adenocarcinoma	Phase II (NCT00352833, completed)
EpCAM	Peritoneal carcinomatosis and gastric adenocarcinoma	Phase II (NCT01504256, completed)
EpCAM	Ovarian cancer, fallopian tube cancer, peritoneal cancer	Phase II (NCT00189345, completed)
EpCAM	Gastric cancer and gastric adenocarcinoma	Phase II (NCT00464893, completed)
EpCAM	Malignant ascites and EpCAM-positive tumors	Phase II/III, (NCT00836654, completed)
EpCAM	EpCAM-positive solid cancers	Phase III (NCT00822809, completed)
GD2	Neuroblastoma	Phase I (NCT00877110, completed)
gpA33	Colorectal carcinoma	Phase I (NCT02248805, completed)
GPC3	Solid tumors	Phase I (NCT02748837, completed)
HER2	Breast cancer, metastatic breast cancer	Phase I (NCT00027807, completed)
HLA-A*02:01:gp100	Melanoma, advanced melanoma	Phase I (NCT01209676, completed)
HLA-A*02:01:gp100	Malignant melanoma	Phase I (NCT01211262, completed)
PSMA	Prostate cancer	Phase I (NCT02262910, completed)
PSMA	Prostatic neoplasms	Phase I (NCT01723475, completed)

Table 1. *Cont.*

TAA	Disease	Phase
Active clinical trials *		
5T4	Malignant solid tumors	Phase I/II (NCT04424641, recruiting)
B7-H3	Advanced solid tumors, metastatic solid tumors	Phase I (NCT03406949, active not recruiting)
CEA	Colorectal cancers	Phase I (NCT03866239, recruiting)
CEA	NSCLC	Phase I/II (NCT03337698, recruiting)
CEA, EGFR, GPC3, HER2, MUC1	Malignant solid tumors	Phase I (NCT04076137, recruiting)
CEA, EpCAM, GPC3, MUC1	Advanced liver cancer	Phase II (NCT03146637, recruiting)
CLDN18.2	Gastric and gastroesophageal junction adenocarcinoma	Phase I (NCT04260191, recruiting)
DLL3	Small cell lung carcinoma	Phase I (NCT03319940, recruiting)
DLL3	Small cell lung cancer, advanced cancers	Phase I/II (NCT04471727, not yet recruiting)
EGFR	Multiple solid gastrointestinal tumors	Phase I (NCT01420874, active not recruiting)
EGFR	Glioblastoma multiforme, gliosarcoma	Phase I (NCT03344250, recruiting)
EGFR	Pancreatic cancer	Phase I (NCT04137536, recruiting)
EGFR	Advanced pancreatic cancer	Phase Ib/II (NCT02620865, active not recruiting)
EGFR	Advanced and metastatic pancreatic adenocarcinoma	Phase Ib/II (NCT03269526, recruiting)
EGFRv3	Glioblastoma multiforme, malignant glioma	Phase I (NCT03296696, active not recruiting)
EpCAM	Large bowel (colon) cancer, colorectal cancer	Phase U (ChiCTR-ROC-16008620, not yet recruiting)
EpCAM	Malignant ascites, advanced solid tumors	Phase I (CTR20181212, recruiting)
EpCAM	Ascites, advanced solid tumors	Phase I (ChiCTR1900024144, recruiting)
EpCAM	Malignant ascites	Phase I (NCT04501744, recruiting)
EpCAM	Gastric adenocarcinoma, peritoneal carcinomatosis, colorectal adenocarcinoma	Phase II (2010-022810-26, recruiting)
EpCAM	Advanced gastric cancer, stomach cancer, gastric cancer	Phase III (NCT04222114, recruiting)
GD2	Neuroblastoma	Phase I (NCT02650648, active not recruiting)
GD2	Neuroblastoma, osteosarcoma, other solid tumors	Phase I/II (NCT03860207, recruiting)
GD2	Neuroblastoma, osteosarcoma	Phase I/II (NCT02173093, recruiting)
gpA33	Metastatic colorectal cancer	Phase I/II (NCT03531632, active not recruiting)
GPC3	Advanced solid tumors, recurrent solid tumors	Phase I (JapicCTI-194805, recruiting)
GUCY2C	Gastrointestinal malignancies, esophageal cancer	Phase I (NCT04171141, recruiting)
HER2	Breast cancer	Phase U (ChiCTR-ROC-16008650, not yet recruiting)
HER2	HER2-positive solid tumors	Phase I (NCT04501770, recruiting)
HER2	Breast cancer and leptomeningeal metastases	Phase I (NCT03661424, recruiting)
HER2	Esophageal, gastric, pancreatic, liver, gallbladder and bowel cancer	Phase I (NCT02662348, unknown status)
HER2	Advanced solid tumors	Phase I (NCT03448042, recruiting)
HER2	Advanced solid tumors	Phase I (CTR20171194, recruiting)
HER2	Solid tumors, advanced solid tumors	Phase I (ChiCTR1900024128, recruiting)
HER2	Breast cancer	Phase I/II (NCT03983395, recruiting)
HER2	Metastatic breast cancer	Phase I/II NCT03272334, recruiting)
HER2	Metastatic castration resistant prostate cancer	Phase II (NCT03406858, status unknown)
HER2	Breast cancer	Phase II (NCT01147016, status unknown)
HER2	Breast cancer	Phase II (NCT01022138, status unknown)
HLA-A*02:01:gp100	Uveal melanoma	Phase I/II (NCT02570308, active not recruiting)
HLA-A*02:01:gp100	Melanoma	Phase I/II (NCT02535078, active not recruiting)

Table 1. *Cont.*

TAA	Disease	Phase
HLA-A*02:01:gp100	Uveal melanoma, metastatic uveal melanoma, advanced uveal melanoma	Phase II (NCT03070392, active not recruiting)
HLA-A*02:MAGE-A4	Advanced solid tumors, metastatic solid tumors	Phase I/II (NCT03973333, recruiting)
MSLN	Mesotheliomas, ovarian cancers, pancreatic cancers	Phase I/II (NCT03872206, recruiting)
MUC16	Ovarian cancer fallopian tube cancer, peritoneal cancer	Phase I/II (NCT04590326, not yet recruiting)
MUC16	Ovarian cancer fallopian tube cancer, peritoneal cancer	Phase I/II, (NCT03564340, recruiting)
MUC17	Gastric and gastroesophageal junction cancer	Phase I (NCT04117958, recruiting)
NY-ESO1	NY-ESO1-positive tumors	Phase I/II (NCT03515551, recruiting)
PRAME	Advanced solid tumors, cancer indications	Phase I/II (NCT04262466, recruiting)
PSCA	NSCLC, breast cancer, pancreatic cancer, urogenital cancer	Phase I NCT(03927573, recruiting)
PSMA	Prostate cancer	Phase I (NCT04077021, recruiting)
PSMA	Prostate cancers, advanced solid tumors, neoplasms, renal cancers, small cell lung cancer	Phase I (NCT03926013, recruiting)
PSMA	Castration-resistant prostate carcinoma	Phase I (NCT04104607, recruiting)
PSMA	Metastatic castration-resistant prostate cancer	Phase I (NCT03792841, recruiting)
PSMA	Squamous cell lung carcinoma	Phase I/II NCT04496674, not yet recruiting)
PSMA	Prostate cancer	Phase I/II (NCT03577028, recruiting)
SSTR2	Neuroendocrine tumors and gastrointestinal neoplasms	Phase I (NCT03411915, recruiting)
SSTR2	Merkel cell carcinoma and small cell lung cancer	Phase I/II (NCT04590781, not yet recruiting)
STEAP1	Metastatic castration-resistant prostate cancer	Phase I (NCT04221542, recruiting)

* Data as of 13 November 2020. Clinical studies are ordered based on the targeted tumor-associated antigen (TAA). CEA, carcinoembryonic antigen; CLDN18.2, claudin18 isoform 2; DLL3, delta-like ligand 3; EGFR, epidermal growth factor receptor, EpCAM, epithelial cell adhesion molecule; GD2, disialoganglioside; gp100, glycoprotein 100; gpA33, glycoprotein A33; GPC3, glypican 3; GUCY2C, guanylyl cyclase C; HER2, human epidermal growth factor receptor 2; HLA, human leukocyte antigen; MAGE-A4, melanoma-associated antigen 4; MSLN, mesothelin, MUC16, mucin 16; NSCLC, non-small cell lung cancer; NY-ESO1, New York esophageal squamous cell carcinoma 1; PRAME, preferentially expressed antigen in melanoma; PSCA, prostate stem cell antigen; PSMA, prostate-specific membrane antigen; SSTR2, somostatin receptor 2; STEAP1, six-transmembrane epithelial antigen of the prostate 1.

Most of these studies are currently still enrolling patients and we are only starting to get a view on CD3-BsAb therapy safety and efficacy in solid cancers. First, in three different studies, patients were treated with an i.p. infusion of catumaxomab, which resulted in frequent but manageable toxicities and increased time between paracentesis in all studies and even a significant improvement in overall survival (OS) in one study [38,70,71]. Other clinical trials in solid tumors reported dose-limiting toxicities (DLTs) for CD3-BsAbs targeting CEA, EpCAM and HLA-A*02:01:gp100 [70–73]. These toxicities consisted of abnormal liver parameters, colitis, CRS, diarrhea, dyspnea, hypotension, hypoxia, respiratory failure and tachycardia. Some of these toxicities were caused by tumor lesion inflammation, however, most were reversible upon treatment discontinuation. Responses to CD3-BsAbs varied from only 1.5% partial response (PR) [70], up to 15% PR and 46% stable disease (SD) [73] and everything in between [73–75]. Pasotuxizumab, a CD3-BsAb targeting PSMA, obtained the most impressive results with two long-term responders, of which one had marked regression of soft tissue and bone metastases [74]. Overall, some evidence for efficacy induced by CD3-BsAbs in solid tumors has been found, however, with only a handful of long-term survivors, some partial responses and the occurrence of multiple DLTs, the development of CD3-BsAbs in solid tumors lags behind that in hematological malignancies.

2.3. Hurdles in Solid Tumors

The observation that CD3-BsAbs seem more efficacious in hematological malignancies than in solid tumors can be attributed to several challenges that are specific to solid tumors. The first hurdle is on-target off-tumor toxicities, as these seem less forgiving for TAAs selected for solid tumor targeting, when compared to hematologic TAAs [76]. In the case of hematological cancers, the temporary depletion of B cells or myeloid subsets is reversible, as long as hematopoietic stem cells are not targeted, allowing replenishment of the blood pool. However, solid tumor TAAs are often also expressed on tissues of healthy organs, which can lead to immune pathology and organ failure with potential fatality, as shown in a preclinical mouse study using a CD3-BsAb targeting EGFR [75]. Critical selection of a tumor-specific TAA is thus crucial.

The second hurdle is the availability of effector cells in the TME. For hematological malignancies, cancer cells in the blood are surrounded by T cells, allowing the CD3-BsAb to draw from an endless pool of effector cells, whereas solid tumors require T-cell infiltration for therapeutic efficacy. In this context, three immune landscapes have been described: (1) "inflamed" tumors, which are infiltrated by immune cells and frequently respond to immune checkpoint therapy [77], (2) "immune desert" tumors, which have a reduced or absent immunogenicity, resulting in very few primed tumor-specific T cells that home to the tumor [78] and (3) "immune-excluded" tumors, which display T-cell infiltration in the stroma, but not the tumor nests [79,80]. For these immune-excluded tumors, the deposition of extracellular matrix (ECM) components in the stroma results in a physical barrier surrounding the tumor parenchyma. Apart from this physical barrier, the secretion of soluble factors such as transforming growth factor beta (TGF-β) and C-X-C motif chemokine ligand 12 (CXCL12) further frustrates T-cell infiltration. Since T-cell trafficking to solid tumors can be scarce in immune desert or immune-excluded tumors, CD3-BsAbs might have only a few T cells available in the TME (see Scheme 1 for T-cell development and trafficking). The requirement of T-cell infiltrate for effective CD3-BsAb therapy was described by Ströhlein et al. in a clinical study with catumaxomab [81].

T cells originate in bone marrow and progenitor stem cells are educated in the thymus, where they mature and undergo positive and negative selection, to largely exclude "self-reactivity" and release non-self-specific T cells [82]. After this education, the newly formed naïve T cells remain in the peripheral blood and lymph system via the expression of chemokine receptor type 7 (CCR7) and lymph node-produced cognate C-C chemokine ligand 19 (CCL19)/CCL21, in addition to the sphingosine-1-phosphate (S1P) system [83,84]. After activation by dendritic cells (DCs), T cells differentiate into effector cells and different types of memory cells. T cells lose CCR7 expression after this priming event, while they gain expression of other chemokine receptors, such as C-X-C chemokine receptor type 3 (CXCR3) [85]. This enables them to follow chemokine gradients of C-X-C motif chemokines like CXCL9 and CXCL10 towards inflamed tissues, which they enter via selectin/integrin-mediated intravasation [86]. T cells are retained in tissues to clear pathogens and tumors by the expression of retention integrins such as CD103 [87]. Central memory T cells regain CCR7 and recirculate in blood and lymph nodes, whereas effector memory T cells and tissue-resident memory T cells are still able to enter and reside in tissues [88].

Scheme 1. Explanation about T cell development and trafficking [82–88].

The third and final hurdle concerns the quality of infiltrating T cells. TILs can be dysfunctional, with impaired ability to proliferate and produce cytolytic molecules, including granzymes and perforins [89]. Immunosuppressive cells in the TME, including cancer-associated fibroblasts (CAFs), myeloid-derived suppressor cells (MDSCs) and regulatory T cells (T_{regs}) produce factors such as TGF-β, IL-10, indoleamine 2,3-dioxygenase (IDO) and arginase, which hamper T-cell metabolism and activation [90]. Additionally, effector T cells were shown to exhibit an "exhausted" profile due to chronic antigen stimulation, as witnessed by the expression of inhibitory immune checkpoints, such as programmed cell death protein 1 (PD-1) and cytotoxic T-lymphocyte antigen 4 (CTLA-4) [91]. Furthermore, it has been reported that CD3-BsAbs might induce TIL apoptosis via activation-induced cell death, which hampers a strong anti-tumor response [48]. Some of the discovered TME obstacles have only been described in resistance upon immune checkpoint therapy, however, we expect these hurdles to also play a role in CD3-BsAb therapy. An overview of these hurdles is shown in Figure 1.

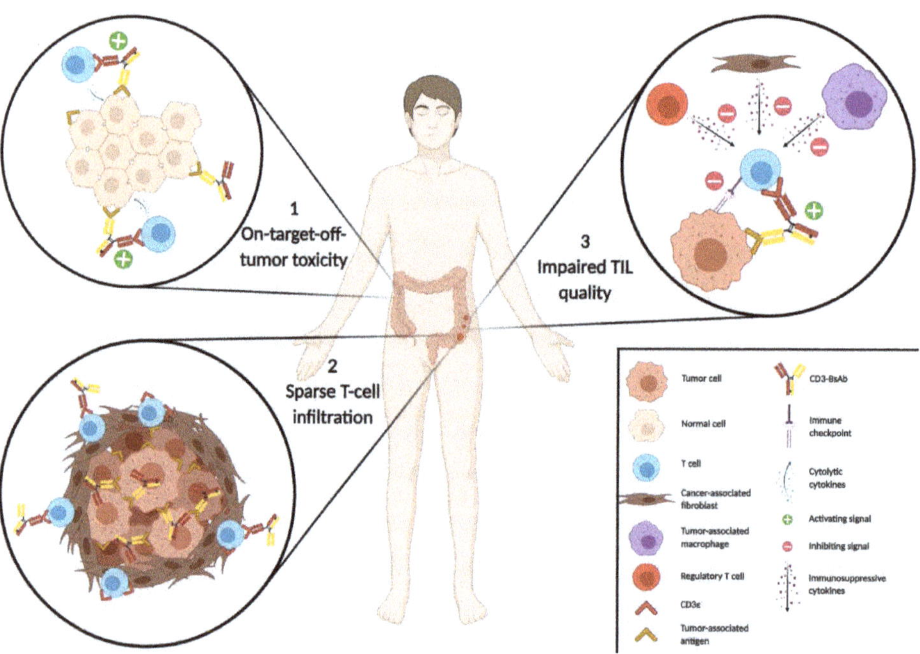

Figure 1. Three main hurdles for CD3-BsAb therapy in solid tumors. (**1**) CD3-BsAbs can generate on-target off-tumor toxicities by binding with the TAA arm to the same antigen on healthy cells, thereby redirecting T cells towards normal tissues, resulting in permanent tissue destruction. (**2**) Certain types of solid tumors ("immune desert" and "immune-excluded") have sparse or even no T-cell infiltration, thereby preventing CD3-BsAb from cross-linking T cells to tumor cells, resulting in limited treatment efficacy. (**3**) The tumor microenvironment (TME) of solid tumors contains multiple immunosuppressive cell types, including cancer-associated fibroblasts, regulatory T cells and tumor-associated macrophages, thereby hampering the quality of effector T cells. Furthermore, immune checkpoints further decrease tumor-infiltrating lymphocyte (TIL) effector functions.

2.4. Solutions and Opportunities

2.4.1. Mitigating of On-Target Off-Tumor Toxicities

Most alterations in cells during the process of oncogenesis affect intracellular circuits involved in the cell cycle, survival and invasive growth [92]. As such, the surface proteome is relatively conserved between cancer cells and their healthy counterparts, with the exception of tyrosine kinase growth receptors, e.g., EGFR family members, which are overexpressed and sometimes truncated in extracellular domains [93]. The search for suitable TAAs for targeting by CD3-BsAbs is therefore complicated, as these targets should be surface proteins that are exclusively expressed by tumor cells and absent in healthy cells. HLA molecules can present small neo-antigenic peptides derived from mutated proteins or peptides from tumor virus proteins and these peptide/HLA complexes can serve as highly cancer-specific TAAs [94]. Their disadvantage is that most identified neoantigens are patient specific and viral antigens are observed in only a subset of cancers [95,96]. A lot of research is currently being performed to identify new and more common neoantigens, which may result in promising future TAAs for CD3-BsAb therapy [97]. The next best targets are overexpressed proteins on tumor cells compared to healthy cells, which is the case for most of the clinically targeted TAAs, such as CEA, EGFR, EpCAM and HER2 [98,99]. Targeting these TAAs offers some selectivity of tumor cells over healthy cells dependent on the extent of overexpression, however, healthy tissues can still be affected.

Some of the most differentially expressed genes in cancer are actually intracellular proteins, which cannot be reached by conventional antibodies [100]. This intracellular proteome is only approachable via HLA class I molecules, which present them to the outer world. These surface peptide/HLA complexes can be targeted with peptide-specific antibody formats or by TCR molecules, such as ImmTACs or T-cell engaging receptor (TCER) molecules [101,102]. The TCR arms of ImmTACs and TCERs are affinity enhanced to low nM ranges to obtain sufficient TAA binding strength to the cancer cell in order to successfully engage effector T cells with the CD3-binding arm. However, major disadvantages of TCR-like CD3-BsAbs are HLA restrictions and vulnerability towards HLA downregulation in the tumor. ESK1, an ImmTAC recognizing intracellular Wilms' tumor 1 (WT1) antigen presented in HLA-A*02:01, was able to lyse WT1-positive tumor cells in vitro and reduce tumor outgrowth of AML, ALL and mesothelioma tumors in NSG mice [103]. A clinical trial with the ImmTAC tebentafusp targeting gp100 presented on HLA-A2*02:01 has successfully been completed and response rates of 15% PR and 46% SD were reported. Unfortunately, DLTs in the form of hypotension were observed in four patients receiving the highest dose [73]. These intracellular targets are both overexpressed TAAs and still seem to generate on-target off-tumor toxicity (as described for tebentafusp). The development of ImmTACs targeting more specific TAAs, such as neoantigens derived from highly conserved Ras mutations in various cancers, E6 and E7 peptides from human papilloma virus (HPV)-induced cancers or T-cell epitopes associated with impaired peptide processing (TEIPP) antigens for cancers with defects in transport associated with antigen processing (TAP) function, could be promising [104–106].

To improve tumor selectivity and specificity and mitigate on-target off-tumor toxicities, the TAA avidity could be increased, for instance, by generating so-called 2:1 CD3-BsAbs. These 2:1 CD3-BsAbs contain a second TAA binding fragment, resulting in a CD3xTAAxTAA bispecific antibody [107]. Slaga et al. showed that specificity for high-expressing HER2 cells was significantly increased when using a 2:1 HER2-targeting CD3-BsAb in vitro [108]. More importantly, tumor growth of high HER2-expressing tumors in NSG mice was efficiently delayed by the 2:1 CD3-BsAb, whereas no anti-tumor efficacy was observed in low HER2-expressing tumors. In contrast, the 1:1 CD3-BsAb was able to effectively delay tumor growth in both high and low HER2-expressing tumors (used here as a model for healthy tissue). In cynomolgus monkeys, i.v. infusion of the 2:1 CD3-BsAB did not result in an increase in C-reactive protein (CRP), T-cell activation or alanine or aspartate aminotransferase (ALT and AST) levels in blood upon exposure to the endogenous expression of HER2 on healthy cells. However, a direct comparison between these two formats was not feasible, as similar cynomolgus monkey data were not generated for the 1:1 CD3-BsAb. A similar improved selectivity was observed for a 2:1 CEA-targeting CD3-BsAb [109]. This CD3-BsAb was tested in patients with advanced CEA-positive carcinomas and displayed signs of anti-tumor effects (5% PR, 11% SD) with a manageable toxicity profile, which was most likely associated with tumor lesion inflammation [72]. In this 2:1 format, TAA affinity plays a very important role: when the TAA affinity is too high, there is no increased specificity, as the BsAb can still bind to low levels of the TAA expressed on healthy cells. On the other hand, if the TAA affinity is too low, the potency of the CD3-BsAb will be compromised. Therefore, modulating TAA affinity could be seen as a tight balance between specificity and efficacy [110]. In a similar fashion, specificity could also be improved for 1:1 CD3-BsAbs by lowering TAA affinity, however, due to the lower avidity compared to 2:1 BsAbs, it is expected to be harder to achieve the optimal balance [111].

A conceptual novelty in this area is the generation of CD3-BsAbs as prodrugs that are activated in the TME. Differences in physiological features, such as hypoxia-related low pH, excessive production of ECM and increased proteolysis, distinguish solid tumors from healthy tissues [112,113]. These differences warranted the development of CD3-BsAbs with binding regions that are masked with protease-cleavable linkers. Boustany et al. developed a masked CD3xEGFR BsAb, which blocked both CD3 and EGFR binding [114]. The binding of this BsAb to CD3 and EGFR was strongly reduced in vitro in the absence of proteases, whereas in vivo anti-tumor efficacy was retained. In cynomolgus monkeys, the maximum tolerated dose (MTD) for masked CD3xEGFR was 60-fold higher than the unmasked variant. Additionally, the masked variant greatly prolonged plasma concentrations at higher dosing concentrations. Very recently, Panchal et al. described the development of conditional bispecific-redirected activation (COBRA) T-cell engagers [115]. This format separates the α-CD3 V_H and V_L via a matrix metallopeptidase 9 (MMP9)-degradable linker, thereby only allowing CD3 binding after linker cleavage, while constantly allowing EGFR and serum albumin binding (to increase half-life). In co-cultures of T cells with tumor cell lines, a dependency on the presence of MMP9 was demonstrated for T-cell-mediated cytotoxicity. In vivo, COBRA BsAb could completely eradicate established HT-29 colorectal tumors in NSG mice, whereas their non-cleavable BsAb counterpart displayed no anti-tumor activity. Furthermore, Geiger et al. described a folate receptor 1 (FOLR1)-targeting CD3-BsAb (Prot-FOLR1-TCB) that linked a protease-cleavable anti-idiotypic anti-CD3 mask to the CD3 arm [116]. This masked the CD3-binding domain of the BsAb and was cleaved by proteases produced in the TME, resulting in selective T-cell activation after the addition of protease in vitro. In humanized mice, Prot-FOLR1-TCB was able to delay tumor outgrowth to a similar extent to the non-masked BsAb. Other approaches that have split the anti-CD3 modality into two separate components, which only functionally recombine at the tumor surface when both bind to separate TAAs, are also being explored [117,118].

Another way to mitigate on-target off-tumor toxicities is to alter CD3-BsAb distribution, for example, by the modification of CD3 affinity. In a preclinical mouse study, the distribution of radiolabeled CD3xHER2 BsAbs with different CD3 affinities was followed by single-photon emission computed tomographic (SPECT) imaging. This study showed that CD3-BsAbs with a high affinity CD3 arm accumulated in T-cell-rich tissues, such as the spleen and lymph nodes, whereas CD3-low affinity BsAbs accumulated mainly in the HER2$^+$ tumor, thereby affecting the biodistribution and treatment outcome [119]. Instead of the systemic administration of (conditionally active) CD3-BsAb, another option to alter distribution could be to administer CD3-BsAbs intratumorally. Although this would not completely prevent systemic spreading, as some CD3-BsAb will probably enter the blood by diffusion, local administration can strongly reduce on-target off-tumor toxicity [120]. Although local administration is possible under ultrasound guidance for non-superficial tumors, this method is still complicated because multiple injections are required. Alternatively, delivery systems can be exploited that would selectively release or produce CD3-BsAb in the tumor. One such method is the use of transduced (tumor-specific) T cells, that are engineered to express CD3-BsAbs upon T-cell activation, also called the secretion of T-bsAbs by engineered (STAb)-T cells [121]. Iwahori et al. generated STAb-T cells recognizing the erythropoietin-producing hepatocellular carcinoma A2 (EphA2) antigen that produced CD3xEphA2 BsAb upon T-cell activation [122]. They showed effective anti-tumor activity in U373 glioma and A549 lung tumors in NSG mice, while systemic exposure to the CD3-BsAb seemed to be minimal, as indicated by the absence of human cytokines in peripheral blood. Alternatively, BsAb constructs can be expressed in producer lines or non-specific T cells, however, this approach is not well developed at the moment [123,124]. Oncolytic virus (OV) was also used as a delivery vehicle as it selectively replicates in transformed cancerous cells over healthy cells [125]. Fajardo et al. described an oncolytic adenovirus encoding CD3xEGFR BsAb and observed a modest but significant delay in tumor outgrowth when used either by intratumoral or i.v. administration in NSG mice [126]. In a different study, oncolytic measles virus encoding CD3xCEA BsAb was developed and used to treat patient-derived colorectal cancer xenografts in NSG mice [127]. Tumor outgrowth was moderately delayed in mice treated intratumorally, without detectable BsAb in serum. However, when mice were treated i.v., only low BsAb levels were detected in the tumor in contrast to high BsAb concentrations in peripheral blood. Other groups also used OVs encoding CD3-BsAbs targeting EpCAM, Eph-A2 and CD44v6 and observed anti-tumor activities against several tumor models [128–130]. However, in all of these studies, OV encoding CD3-BsAb was administered locally and toxicity evaluation was not reported. An overview of mitigation strategies to overcome off-tumor on-target toxicities is depicted in Figure 2.

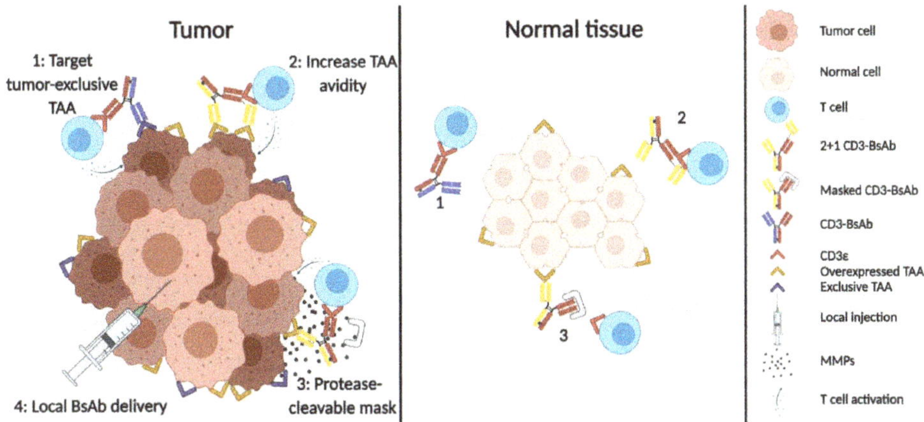

Figure 2. Solutions to mitigate hurdle 1: on-target off-tumor toxicities. (**1**) Target TAAs that are exclusively expressed by tumor cells, such as human leukocyte antigen (HLA)-presented neo-antigens, or surface antigens from virally induced cancers. (**2**) The avidity for TAAs can be increased with formats that include multiple TAA binding arms. This results in increased selectivity for tumor targeting over healthy tissues. (**3**) Binding arms of CD3-BsAbs can be masked using a protease-cleavable linker, making the BsAb only active inside the tumor. In healthy tissues, a minimal presence of proteases limits unmasking of the CD3 arm, whereas the abundance of matrix metallopeptidases (MMPs) in the TME allows the CD3-BsAb to redirect T cells towards the tumor. (**4**) Ensure local delivery of CD3-BsAbs to decrease systemic exposure by either local injection, or using delivery systems that locally produce these BsAbs, such as oncolytic viruses (OVs) and STAb-T cells.

2.4.2. Increasing the Number of Intratumoral T cells

Tumors can be classified in three categories regarding T-cell infiltration: immune desert, immune-excluded and inflamed [79]. Immune desert tumors barely contain T cells at all, not in the tumor nests nor surrounding the rims, thereby potentially limiting CD3-BsAb therapy efficacy. Interestingly, intratumoral OV administration can ignite T-cell influx in immune desert tumors. The replication of oncolytic virus can generate an interferon response in the TME and induce an innate and adaptive antiviral immune response [131–133]. We used this concept to pre-treat immune desert murine tumors (B16F10 melanoma and (LSL-Kras^{G12D}, LSL-Trp53^{R172H}, Pdx-1-Cre) KPC pancreatic carcinoma) with OV, which induced sensitization and generated major T-cell influx peaking around day 7, allowing strong tumor regression upon CD3-BsAb treatment [134]. In the absence of OV sensitization, CD3-BsAb did not even delay tumor growth, underlining the importance of an inflammatory TME. Of note, we found that the simultaneous administration of CD3-BsAb and OV did not provide survival benefit, indicating that the timing of OV and CD3-BsAb is an important aspect.

Immune-excluded tumors have T cells surrounding the tumor, but penetration into tumor beds is hindered by physical barriers or soluble factors. Efforts to improve therapy efficacy in these types of tumors should therefore focus on removing these obstructions. The physical barrier is mainly formed by ECM structures, which forces T cells to move along areas of increased stiffness instead of following the chemokine gradient in a process called haptotaxis [135]. This barrier consists of proteoglycans and fibrous proteins such as collagen, elastin and laminin, which are mainly produced by CAFs, but also by tumor cells and stellate cells [135,136]. The ECM could be targeted by the direct destruction of ECM components, such as collagen and hyaluronic acid (HA), a process which is also studied in the context of chemotherapeutic drug delivery to the tumor [137–139]. Guan et al. used hyaluronidase to break down HA, which increased the infiltration of tumor-specific T cells and greatly improved treatment efficacy in a B16.OVA melanoma mouse model [140]. Not only ECM components, but also their cellular producers could be targeted. CAFs are the major producers of ECM products and highly express fibroblast activation protein (FAP), which constitutes an attractive target for immunotherapy. In several mouse tumor models, T-cell infiltration was increased upon CAF targeting using DNA vaccines or fibrosis inhibitors [141–143]. OV encoding a CD3-BsAb targeting FAP was elegantly used in several studies to kill CAFs and simultaneously enhance T-cell infiltration [144–146].

Apart from creating a physical barrier, CAFs can also influence T-cell infiltration by various secreted molecules [147]. CAFs are the major source of the chemokine CXCL12, which has been implicated to mediate T-cell exclusion in solid tumors [148]. The inhibition of CXCL12 or its receptor CXCR4 resulted in increased T-cell infiltration and rendered tumors vulnerable towards checkpoint inhibition therapy in mouse models for pancreatic and colorectal cancer [148,149]. Furthermore, TGF-β has been implicated in hampering T-cell infiltration. This immunosuppressive cytokine is produced by CAFs, but also many other cells, including T_{regs} and M2 macrophages [147]. Similar to CXCL12 signaling inhibition, blocking TGF-β signaling resulted in more T-cell infiltration and increased sensitivity to checkpoint inhibition therapy in multiple mouse models for breast cancer and colorectal cancer [150–152]. Post-translational modifications of secreted factors in the TME can also affect T-cell attraction, as was reported for CCL2 [153]. Nitrification of CCL2 by reactive nitrogen species (RNS) in the TME resulted in T cells being stuck in the stroma surrounding the tumor cells. The inhibition of RNS production greatly improved T-cell infiltration in several mouse tumor models and thereby improved survival as a monotherapy or in combination with adoptive cell transfer. An overview of solutions to overcome sparse T-cell infiltration is shown in Figure 3.

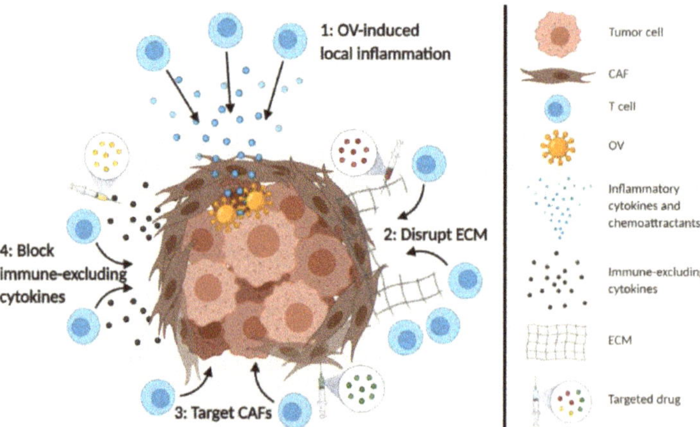

Figure 3. Solutions for hurdle 2: sparse T-cell infiltration. (**1**) Pre-treatment with OV generates a strong interferon response in the tumor, resulting in local innate and adaptive immune responses and strong T-cell infiltration. (**2**) Disruption of the physical extracellular matrix (ECM) barrier prevents T cells from getting stuck in the ECM and allows infiltration into the tumor nests. (**3**) Targeting cancer-associated fibroblasts (CAFs) removes the major producers of ECM components and immune-excluding cytokines, thereby improving T-cell infiltration. (**4**) Blockade of immune-excluding cytokines reduces limiting factors for T-cell infiltration, resulting in better infiltrated tumors.

2.4.3. Improving the Quality of T-cell Responses

When the CD3-BsAb and sufficient T cells have finally reached the tumor, they are faced with another challenge: a hostile and immunosuppressive TME. Firstly, immune checkpoint ligands are known to be expressed in the TME, such as programmed death ligand 1 (PD-L1) and HLA-E [154,155]. PD-L1 is upregulated on tumor, stromal and immune cells upon local interferon release by immune cells [156–158]. Most intratumoral T cells already express PD-1 and the CD3-BsAb-mediated activation of T cells further stimulates the expression of this inhibitory co-receptor, thereby hampering effector functions and treatment efficacy [159,160]. Combination therapies of CD3-BsAbs and checkpoint blockade have been widely investigated in multiple in vitro studies and mouse models and resulted in improved tumor control [44,161,162]. Interestingly, Osada et al. reported that PD-1/PD-L1 blockade could not improve T-cell functioning in an in vitro setting if blockade is applied after T cells have engaged tumor cells [163]. Exhausted cells could no longer be rescued when blockade was applied too late, thereby emphasizing the importance of timing. The combination of CD3-BsAbs with checkpoint blockade is also being explored in several clinical studies (NCT03319940, NCT03531632, NCT03406858, NCT03272334, NCT03564340, NCT03792841, NCT04590781 and NCT02324257). The NCT02324257 study (CD3xCEA in combination with atezolizumab (anti-PD-L1) for patients with advanced CEA-positive tumors) has been completed and seemed to be in line with previous preclinical results: the combination of CD3-BsAbs with checkpoint blockade showed better anti-tumor responses when compared to CD3-BsAb monotherapy and they found no evidence of increased toxicities [72]. Therefore, this combination holds great promise.

Unfortunately, not only immune checkpoints have the capability to dampen T-cell function. Due to their rapid glycolysis-dependent proliferation, tumor cells generate a hypoxic and low-glucose TME [164]. In these hypoxic conditions, hypoxia-induced factors (HIFs) initiate the expression of CD39 and CD73 by multiple cell types in the TME; CD39 and CD73 convert free ATP in the TME into adenosine [165]. Adenosine has been reported to counteract TCR activation by binding to adenosine A_{2A} receptors via protein kinase A and cyclic Amp signaling, which suppresses the effector functions of T cells [161,162]. Furthermore, low glucose concentrations have been reported to dampen the anti-tumoral cytokine production and survival of effector T cells, as they rely heavily on glucose for their functioning [166,167]. Apart from these tumor-mediated factors, stromal cells, infiltrating T_{regs} and MDSCs secrete other immunosuppressive factors, such as IDO, TGF-β, IL-10 and arginase. IDO has been reported to degrade the amino acid tryptophan into kynurenine, resulting in decreased effector function via downregulation of the CD3 ζ-chain, and induce apoptosis in T cells [164,168]. TGF-β is able to suppress T-cell effector function and inhibit the differentiation of CD4$^+$ cells into effector cells, while promoting T_{reg} differentiation [169–171]. IL-10 has been described to induce T-cell anergy and prevent the development of new effector T cells by decreasing antigen presentation and costimulation on antigen-presenting cells (APCs) [172,173]. Arginase breaks down the amino acid arginine and, similar to IDO, results in the downregulation of the CD3 ζ-chain and thereby decreased cytotoxic and proliferative capacity of T cells [174,175].

Most of these immunosuppressive factors do not only act on T cells but also on other cells in the TME to generate a negative feedback loop and dampen the inflammatory response. The inhibitory effect on T cells could be overcome by decreasing the amount of immunosuppressive signals, which could be accomplished by blocking receptor–ligand interactions for these molecules. Several studies have been published reporting improved T-cell effector function after blocking adenosine, arginase, IDO, IL-10 and TGF-β [176–181]. CD3-BsAb therapy has thus far only been combined preclinically with IDO blockade. Hong et al. showed improved in vitro killing and in vivo tumor control of EpCAM- and IDO-positive murine breast cancer cells using a combination of an EpCAMxCD3 BsAb with IDO blockade [182]. The cells producing these immunosuppressive factors can also be targeted, which is already being extensively studied for CAFs, as described above. MDSCs are popular targets as well, with therapies being developed to deplete them and prevent migration into the TME, resulting in improved anti-tumor activity in combination with several different types of immunotherapy [183–190]. Currently, no combinations of CD3-BsAbs and MDSC targeting have been reported for solid tumors. However, several studies in hematological malignancies showed that CD3xCD33 BsAbs mediated both AML and MDSC killing, yielding promising treatment outcomes [191,192]. Finally, depleting T_{regs} in combination with CD3-BsAb treatment could be favorable in two ways: (1) T_{regs} secrete immunosuppressive cytokines such as IL-4, IL-10 and TGF-β and, more importantly, (2) T_{regs} are suggested to be activated by CD3-BsAbs, resulting in a dampened treatment effect [193,194]. Forkhead box protein P3 (FoxP3)-positive T_{regs} highly express OX40, CTLA-4 and CD25 and can be depleted to achieve stronger anti-tumor effects in combinatorial strategies [195–199]. One study investigated the effect of combining CD3xEGFR-armed T cells with T_{reg}-depleting ipilimumab (anti-CTLA-4) on T-cell activation and proliferation when co-cultured with tumor cell lines or primary tumor cells and found enhanced T-cell-mediated cytotoxicity and increased T-cell proliferation [200]. Thus far, there are some promising preclinical results for combining CD3-BsAbs with IDO blockade, MDSC depletion and T_{reg} depletion, warranting further exploitation of these combinations.

Instead of decreasing T-cell inhibitory signals, another approach would be to trigger stimulatory receptors on T cells, which could be induced by administering agonistic antibodies for these receptors on T cells, such as CD28 and 4-1BB. This approach parallels the addition of a costimulatory intracellular signaling domain to improve efficacy for second generation CAR T cells [201]. The combination of CD3-BsAbs with costimulatory antibodies has been successfully used in many different tumor models in mice [202,203]. Chiu et al. showed in a humanized mouse model that combination of a CD3xPSMA BsAb with a costimulatory agonistic 4-1BB Ab greatly enhanced anti-tumor efficacy [204]. The combination successfully improved the survival of mice bearing large tumors in contrast to CD3-BsAb monotherapy and, more importantly, generated a memory response that protected surviving mice from a second tumor challenge. However, weight loss was reported in the mice receiving the combination treatment, which is in line with reported toxicities for the administration of bivalent agonistic 4-1BB costimulatory Abs [205,206]. Conditional costimulation only in the tumor TME can be generated by CD28xTAA BsAbs [207]. Using this localized costimulation, Skokos et al. observed no toxicities in in vitro assays as well as in cynomolgus monkey toxicity studies, while these combinations still displayed impressive enhancements in anti-tumor activity in various mouse models [207]. Therefore, the combination of CD3-BsAbs with TME-targeted costimulatory BsAbs seems promising. Furthermore, additional costimulation has been reported to protect T cells from Fas-mediated apoptosis after activation by CD3-BsAb [208]. Currently, a clinical trial is investigating the combination of CD3xMUC1 with CD28xMUC1 and we are looking forward to seeing if the promising preclinical results will translate to clinical efficacy (NCT04590326). Finally, T-cell-sustaining cytokines can be coinjected, or engineered onto CD3-BsAbs. Rossi et al. reported that IFN-α enhanced T-cell activation and delayed tumor outgrowth in two mouse models [209]. Schmol et al. linked IL-15 to a bispecific natural killer (NK) cell engager and showed enhanced NK cell proliferation, activation and survival in vitro. This finding could potentially be translated to CD3-BsAbs as well, since IL-15 also promotes T-cell survival [210]. An overview of the solutions to improve T-cell quality is depicted in Figure 4.

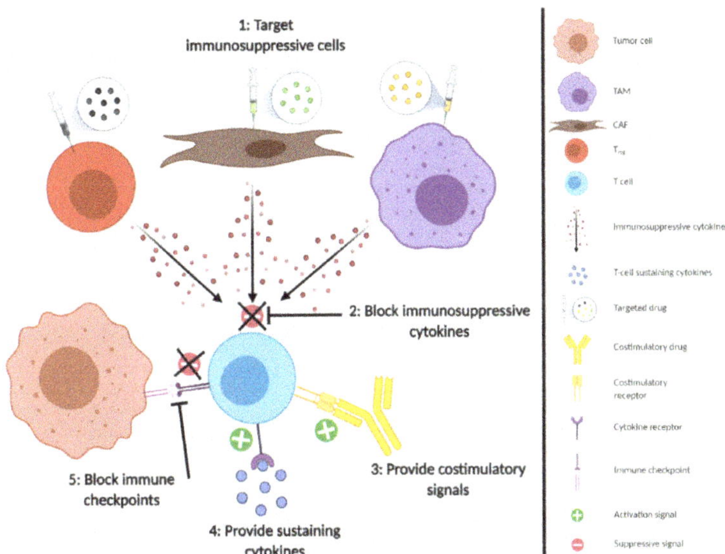

Figure 4. Solutions for hurdle 3: impaired TIL quality. (**1**) Targeting immunosuppressive cells such as CAFs, T_{regs} and tumor-associated macrophages (TAMs) depletes producers of immuno-suppressive cytokines, thereby decreasing suppressive signals for T cells, improving their effector functions. (**2**) Direct blockade of immunosuppressive cytokines, instead of targeting their cellular producers, is able to achieve the same. (**3**) Addition of costimulation provides positive signals for T-cell effector functions and survival. (**4**) Providing sustaining cytokines can also improve T-cell functioning. (**5**) Blockade of immune checkpoints can prevent T-cell dysfunction and allow stronger anti-tumor responses.

3. Future Perspectives

CD3-BsAbs are an emerging and promising class of immunotherapy due to their impressive treatment outcomes in hematological malignancies, however, prominent anti-tumor efficacy in solid tumors still needs to be delivered clinically. Particularly, a whole array of hurdles arises in solid cancers, ranging from on-target off-tumor toxicities and the absence of T-cell infiltration in the TME, to hampered T-cell function attributable to a hostile and immunosuppressive microenvironment. Due to continuous research efforts, more tumor-specific TAAs become available every year for use in CD3-BsAb formats. Combined with constantly evolving technologies allowing conditional masking of BsAbs, on-target off-tumor effects should be manageable in the near future. Some interesting pre-clinical concepts have been published to enhance T-cell infiltration in the tumor, such as pre-treatment with OV to facilitate massive T-cell infiltration and create an inflammatory TME. OV treatment seems most promising, as the inflamed TME also contributes to the quality of the TILs. Many options are available in terms of improving TIL quality, however, apart from checkpoint blockade or costimulation, only very few of them have been tested in combination with CD3-BsAbs. Nevertheless, based on elegant preclinical studies, we are convinced that a combination CD3-BsAbs with (tumor-targeted) costimulation is able to overcome many of the hurdles set by the TME of solid tumors.

We anticipate a future where the immune landscape of the tumor from a biopsy guides the selection of the best treatment combination. However, since many of these combinations have only just started to emerge, it will be intriguing to follow the results of new pre-clinical studies and see how those results translate to the clinic. Ultimately, based on these novel approaches, we foresee a bright future for CD3-BsAb-based therapy in solid tumors and are interested to see if comparable anti-tumor efficacy can be observed in solid cancer as seen in hematological cancers.

Author Contributions: Original draft preparation: J.M. and T.v.H.; review and draft editing: K.K., P.E. and A.F.L.; supervision: J.S. All authors have read and agreed to the published version of the manuscript.

Funding: J.M. works on a grant provided by Genmab to T.v.H., K.K., P.E., A.F.L. and J.S. have ownership interests (including stocks, warrants, patents, etc.) in Genmab.

Institutional Review Board Statement: Not applicable.

Informed Consent Statement: Not applicable.

Data Availability Statement: No new data were created or analyzed in this study. Data sharing is not applicable to this article.

Acknowledgments: The authors thank Gijs Zom, Katy Lloyd, Lars Guelen and Judith Klimovsky for critically reading the manuscript. All figures were created with BioRender software (BioRender.com).

Conflicts of Interest: K.K., P.E., A.F.L. and J.S. are all Genmab employees and own stock and/or warrants in the company. Furthermore, K.K., P.E., A.F.L. and J.S. are listed as inventors on patents relating to CD3-BsAb or the DuoBody BsAb technology platform.

References

1. van der Neut Kolfschoten, M.; Schuurman, J.; Losen, M.; Bleeker, W.K.; Martinez-Martinez, P.; Vermeulen, E.; den Bleker, T.H.; Wiegman, L.; Vink, T.; Aarden, L.A.; et al. Anti-inflammatory activity of human IgG4 antibodies by dynamic Fab arm exchange. *Science* **2007**, *317*, 1554–1557. [CrossRef] [PubMed]
2. Dahlen, E.; Veitonmaki, N.; Norlen, P. Bispecific antibodies in cancer immunotherapy. *Ther. Adv. Vaccines Immunother.* **2018**, *6*, 3–17. [CrossRef] [PubMed]
3. Xu, H.; Cheng, M.; Guo, H.; Chen, Y.; Huse, M.; Cheung, N.K. Retargeting T cells to GD2 pentasaccharide on human tumors using Bispecific humanized antibody. *Cancer Immunol. Res.* **2015**, *3*, 266–277. [CrossRef] [PubMed]
4. Wu, Z.; Cheung, N.V. T cell engaging bispecific antibody (T-BsAb): From technology to therapeutics. *Pharmacol. Ther.* **2018**, *182*, 161–175. [CrossRef] [PubMed]
5. Fife, B.T.; Guleria, I.; Gubbels Bupp, M.; Eagar, T.N.; Tang, Q.; Bour-Jordan, H.; Yagita, H.; Azuma, M.; Sayegh, M.H.; Bluestone, J.A. Insulin-induced remission in new-onset NOD mice is maintained by the PD-1-PD-L1 pathway. *J. Exp. Med.* **2006**, *203*, 2737–2747. [CrossRef]
6. Miliotou, A.N.; Papadopoulou, L.C. CAR T-cell Therapy: A New Era in Cancer Immunotherapy. *Curr. Pharm. Biotechnol.* **2018**, *19*, 5–18. [CrossRef]
7. Slaney, C.Y.; Wang, P.; Darcy, P.K.; Kershaw, M.H. CARs versus BiTEs: A Comparison between T Cell-Redirection Strategies for Cancer Treatment. *Cancer Discov.* **2018**, *8*, 924–934. [CrossRef]
8. Sadelain, M. CD19 CAR T Cells. *Cell* **2017**, *171*, 1471. [CrossRef]
9. Scholler, J.; Brady, T.L.; Binder-Scholl, G.; Hwang, W.T.; Plesa, G.; Hege, K.M.; Vogel, A.N.; Kalos, M.; Riley, J.L.; Deeks, S.G.; et al. Decade-long safety and function of retroviral-modified chimeric antigen receptor T cells. *Sci. Transl. Med.* **2012**, *4*, 132ra153. [CrossRef]
10. Labrijn, A.F.; Janmaat, M.L.; Reichert, J.M.; Parren, P. Bispecific antibodies: A mechanistic review of the pipeline. *Nat. Rev. Drug Discov.* **2019**, *18*, 585–608. [CrossRef]
11. Suurs, F.V.; Lub-de Hooge, M.N.; de Vries, E.G.E.; de Groot, D.J.A. A review of bispecific antibodies and antibody constructs in oncology and clinical challenges. *Pharmacol. Ther.* **2019**, *201*, 103–119. [CrossRef] [PubMed]
12. Borlak, J.; Langer, F.; Spanel, R.; Schondorfer, G.; Dittrich, C. Immune-mediated liver injury of the cancer therapeutic antibody catumaxomab targeting EpCAM, CD3 and Fcgamma receptors. *Oncotarget* **2016**, *7*, 28059–28074. [CrossRef] [PubMed]
13. Clynes, R.A.; Desjarlais, J.R. Redirected T Cell Cytotoxicity in Cancer Therapy. *Annu. Rev. Med.* **2019**, *70*, 437–450. [CrossRef] [PubMed]
14. Przepiorka, D.; Ko, C.W.; Deisseroth, A.; Yancey, C.L.; Candau-Chacon, R.; Chiu, H.J.; Gehrke, B.J.; Gomez-Broughton, C.; Kane, R.C.; Kirshner, S.; et al. FDA Approval: Blinatumomab. *Clin. Cancer Res.* **2015**, *21*, 4035–4039. [CrossRef] [PubMed]
15. Martinelli, G.; Dombret, H.; Chevallier, P.; Ottmann, O.G.; Goekbuget, N.; Topp, M.S.; Fielding, A.K.; Sterling, L.R.; Benjamin, J.; Stein, A.S. Complete Molecular and Hematologic Response in Adult Patients with Relapsed/Refractory (R/R) Philadelphia Chromosome-Positive B-Precursor Acute Lymphoblastic Leukemia (ALL) Following Treatment with Blinatumomab: Results from a Phase 2 Single-Arm, Multicenter Study (ALCANTARA). *Blood* **2015**, *126*, 679. [CrossRef]
16. Kantarjian, H.; Stein, A.; Gokbuget, N.; Fielding, A.K.; Schuh, A.C.; Ribera, J.M.; Wei, A.; Dombret, H.; Foa, R.; Bassan, R.; et al. Blinatumomab versus Chemotherapy for Advanced Acute Lymphoblastic Leukemia. *N. Engl. J. Med.* **2017**, *376*, 836–847. [CrossRef] [PubMed]

17. Franquiz, M.J.; Short, N.J. Blinatumomab for the Treatment of Adult B-Cell Acute Lymphoblastic Leukemia: Toward a New Era of Targeted Immunotherapy. *Biologics* **2020**, *14*, 23–34. [CrossRef] [PubMed]
18. Lau, K.M.; Saunders, I.M.; Goodman, A.M. Characterization of relapse patterns in patients with acute lymphoblastic leukemia treated with blinatumomab. *J. Oncol. Pharm. Pract.* **2020**. [CrossRef]
19. Zhao, Y.; Aldoss, I.; Qu, C.; Crawford, J.C.; Gu, Z.; Allen, E.K.; Zamora, A.E.; Alexander, T.B.; Wang, J.; Goto, H.; et al. Tumor intrinsic and extrinsic determinants of response to blinatumomab in adults with B-ALL. *Blood* **2020**. [CrossRef]
20. Uy, G.L.; Aldoss, I.; Foster, M.C.; Sayre, P.H.; Wieduwilt, M.J.; Advani, A.S.; Godwin, J.E.; Arellano, M.L.; Sweet, K.; Emadi, A.; et al. Flotetuzumab as Salvage Immunotherapy for Refractory Acute Myeloid Leukemia. *Blood* **2020**. [CrossRef]
21. Hutchings, M.; Lugtenburg, P.; Mous, R.; Clausen, M.R.; Chamuleau, M.; Linton, K.; Rule, S.; Lopez, J.S.; Oliveri, R.S.; DeMarco, D.; et al. Epcoritamab (GEN3013; DuoBody-CD3×CD20) to induce complete response in patients with relapsed/refractory B-cell non-Hodgkin lymphoma (B-NHL): Complete dose escalation data and efficacy results from a phase I/II trial. *J. Clin. Oncol.* **2020**, *38*, 8009. [CrossRef]
22. Bannerji, R.; Allan, J.N.; Arnason, J.E.; Brown, J.R.; Advani, R.H.; Barnes, J.A.; Ansell, S.M.; O'Brien, S.M.; Chavez, J.; Duell, J.; et al. Clinical Activity of REGN1979, a Bispecific Human, Anti-CD20 x Anti-CD3 Antibody, in Patients with Relapsed/Refractory (R/R) B-Cell Non-Hodgkin Lymphoma (B-NHL). *Blood* **2019**, *134*, 762. [CrossRef]
23. Schuster, S.J.; Bartlett, N.L.; Assouline, S.; Yoon, S.-S.; Bosch, F.; Sehn, L.H.; Cheah, C.Y.; Shadman, M.; Gregory, G.P.; Ku, M.; et al. Mosunetuzumab Induces Complete Remissions in Poor Prognosis Non-Hodgkin Lymphoma Patients, Including Those Who Are Resistant to or Relapsing After Chimeric Antigen Receptor T-Cell (CAR-T) Therapies, and Is Active in Treatment through Multiple Lines. *Blood* **2019**, *134*, 6. [CrossRef]
24. Varghese, B.; Menon, J.; Rodriguez, L.; Haber, L.; Olson, K.; Duramad, P.; Oyejide, A.; Smith, E.; Thurston, G.; Kirshner, J. A Novel CD20xCD3 Bispecific Fully Human Antibody Induces Potent Anti-Tumor Effects Against B Cell Lymphoma in Mice. *Blood* **2014**, *124*, 4501. [CrossRef]
25. Teachey, D.T.; Rheingold, S.R.; Maude, S.L.; Zugmaier, G.; Barrett, D.M.; Seif, A.E.; Nichols, K.E.; Suppa, E.K.; Kalos, M.; Berg, R.A.; et al. Cytokine release syndrome after blinatumomab treatment related to abnormal macrophage activation and ameliorated with cytokine-directed therapy. *Blood* **2013**, *121*, 5154–5157. [CrossRef]
26. Shimabukuro-Vornhagen, A.; Godel, P.; Subklewe, M.; Stemmler, H.J.; Schlosser, H.A.; Schlaak, M.; Kochanek, M.; Boll, B.; von Bergwelt-Baildon, M.S. Cytokine release syndrome. *J. Immunother. Cancer* **2018**, *6*, 56. [CrossRef]
27. Maude, S.L.; Teachey, D.T.; Porter, D.L.; Grupp, S.A. CD19-targeted chimeric antigen receptor T-cell therapy for acute lymphoblastic leukemia. *Blood* **2015**, *125*, 4017–4023. [CrossRef]
28. Strohl, W.R.; Naso, M. Bispecific T-Cell Redirection versus Chimeric Antigen Receptor (CAR)-T Cells as Approaches to Kill Cancer Cells. *Antibodies* **2019**, *8*, 41. [CrossRef]
29. Li, J.; Piskol, R.; Ybarra, R.; Chen, Y.J.; Li, J.; Slaga, D.; Hristopoulos, M.; Clark, R.; Modrusan, Z.; Totpal, K.; et al. CD3 bispecific antibody-induced cytokine release is dispensable for cytotoxic T cell activity. *Sci. Transl. Med.* **2019**, *11*. [CrossRef]
30. Giavridis, T.; van der Stegen, S.J.C.; Eyquem, J.; Hamieh, M.; Piersigilli, A.; Sadelain, M. CAR T cell-induced cytokine release syndrome is mediated by macrophages and abated by IL-1 blockade. *Nat. Med.* **2018**, *24*, 731–738. [CrossRef]
31. Norelli, M.; Camisa, B.; Barbiera, G.; Falcone, L.; Purevdorj, A.; Genua, M.; Sanvito, F.; Ponzoni, M.; Doglioni, C.; Cristofori, P.; et al. Monocyte-derived IL-1 and IL-6 are differentially required for cytokine-release syndrome and neurotoxicity due to CAR T cells. *Nat. Med.* **2018**, *24*, 739–748. [CrossRef] [PubMed]
32. Iwata, Y.; Sasaki, M.; Harada, A.; Taketo, J.; Hara, T.; Akai, S.; Ishiguro, T.; Narita, A.; Kaneko, A.; Mishima, M. Daily ascending dosing in cynomolgus monkeys to mitigate cytokine release syndrome induced by ERY22, surrogate for T-cell redirecting bispecific antibody ERY974 for cancer immunotherapy. *Toxicol. Appl. Pharmacol.* **2019**, *379*, 114657. [CrossRef] [PubMed]
33. Deppisch, N.; Ruf, P.; Eissler, N.; Neff, F.; Buhmann, R.; Lindhofer, H.; Mocikat, R. Efficacy and Tolerability of a GD2-Directed Trifunctional Bispecific Antibody in a Preclinical Model: Subcutaneous Administration Is Superior to Intravenous Delivery. *Mol. Cancer Ther.* **2015**, *14*, 1877–1883. [CrossRef]
34. Trinklein, N.D.; Pham, D.; Schellenberger, U.; Buelow, B.; Boudreau, A.; Choudhry, P.; Clarke, S.C.; Dang, K.; Harris, K.E.; Iyer, S.; et al. Efficient tumor killing and minimal cytokine release with novel T-cell agonist bispecific antibodies. *MAbs* **2019**, *11*, 639–652. [CrossRef] [PubMed]
35. Leong, S.R.; Sukumaran, S.; Hristopoulos, M.; Totpal, K.; Stainton, S.; Lu, E.; Wong, A.; Tam, L.; Newman, R.; Vuillemenot, B.R.; et al. An anti-CD3/anti-CLL-1 bispecific antibody for the treatment of acute myeloid leukemia. *Blood* **2017**, *129*, 609–618. [CrossRef]
36. Staflin, K.; Zuch de Zafra, C.L.; Schutt, L.K.; Clark, V.; Zhong, F.; Hristopoulos, M.; Clark, R.; Li, J.; Mathieu, M.; Chen, X.; et al. Target arm affinities determine preclinical efficacy and safety of anti-HER2/CD3 bispecific antibody. *JCI Insight* **2020**, *5*. [CrossRef]
37. Vafa, O.; Trinklein, N.D. Perspective: Designing T-Cell Engagers With Better Therapeutic Windows. *Front. Oncol.* **2020**, *10*, 446. [CrossRef]
38. Heiss, M.M.; Murawa, P.; Koralewski, P.; Kutarska, E.; Kolesnik, O.O.; Ivanchenko, V.V.; Dudnichenko, A.S.; Aleknaviciene, B.; Razbadauskas, A.; Gore, M.; et al. The trifunctional antibody catumaxomab for the treatment of malignant ascites due to epithelial cancer: Results of a prospective randomized phase II/III trial. *Int. J. Cancer* **2010**, *127*, 2209–2221. [CrossRef]

39. Riesenberg, R.; Buchner, A.; Pohla, H.; Lindhofer, H. Lysis of prostate carcinoma cells by trifunctional bispecific antibodies (alpha EpCAM x alpha CD3). *J. Histochem. Cytochem.* **2001**, *49*, 911–917. [CrossRef]

40. Wang, L.; Hoseini, S.S.; Xu, H.; Ponomarev, V.; Cheung, N.K. Silencing Fc Domains in T cell-Engaging Bispecific Antibodies Improves T-cell Trafficking and Antitumor Potency. *Cancer Immunol. Res.* **2019**, *7*, 2013–2024. [CrossRef]

41. Labrijn, A.F.; Meesters, J.I.; Bunce, M.; Armstrong, A.A.; Somani, S.; Nesspor, T.C.; Chiu, M.L.; Altintas, I.; Verploegen, S.; Schuurman, J.; et al. Efficient Generation of Bispecific Murine Antibodies for Pre-Clinical Investigations in Syngeneic Rodent Models. *Sci. Rep.* **2017**, *7*, 2476. [CrossRef]

42. Oates, J.; Hassan, N.J.; Jakobsen, B.K. ImmTACs for targeted cancer therapy: Why, what, how, and which. *Mol. Immunol.* **2015**, *67*, 67–74. [CrossRef] [PubMed]

43. Chen, C.; Wang, Y.; Zhong, K.; Jiang, C.; Wang, L.; Yuan, Z.; Nie, C.; Xu, J.; Guo, G.; Zhou, L.; et al. Frequent B7-H3 overexpression in craniopharyngioma. *Biochem. Biophys. Res. Commun.* **2019**, *514*, 379–385. [CrossRef]

44. Crawford, A.; Haber, L.; Kelly, M.P.; Vazzana, K.; Canova, L.; Ram, P.; Pawashe, A.; Finney, J.; Jalal, S.; Chiu, D.; et al. A Mucin 16 bispecific T cell-engaging antibody for the treatment of ovarian cancer. *Sci. Transl. Med.* **2019**, *11*. [CrossRef] [PubMed]

45. Fisher, T.S.; Hooper, A.T.; Lucas, J.; Clark, T.H.; Rohner, A.K.; Peano, B.; Elliott, M.W.; Tsaparikos, K.; Wang, H.; Golas, J.; et al. A CD3-bispecific molecule targeting P-cadherin demonstrates T cell-mediated regression of established solid tumors in mice. *Cancer Immunol. Immunother.* **2018**, *67*, 247–259. [CrossRef] [PubMed]

46. Fu, M.; He, Q.; Guo, Z.; Zhou, X.; Li, H.; Zhao, L.; Tang, H.; Zhou, X.; Zhu, H.; Shen, G.; et al. Therapeutic Bispecific T-Cell Engager Antibody Targeting the Transferrin Receptor. *Front. Immunol.* **2019**, *10*, 1396. [CrossRef] [PubMed]

47. Fu, M.P.; Guo, Z.L.; Tang, H.L.; Zhu, H.F.; Shen, G.X.; He, Y.; Lei, P. Selection for Anti-transferrin Receptor Bispecific T-cell Engager in Different Molecular Formats. *Curr. Med. Sci.* **2020**, *40*, 28–34. [CrossRef]

48. Hettich, M.; Lahoti, J.; Prasad, S.; Niedermann, G. Checkpoint Antibodies but not T Cell-Recruiting Diabodies Effectively Synergize with TIL-Inducing gamma-Irradiation. *Cancer Res.* **2016**, *76*, 4673–4683. [CrossRef]

49. Huang, L.; Xie, K.; Li, H.; Wang, R.; Xu, X.; Chen, K.; Gu, H.; Fang, J. Suppression of c-Met-Overexpressing Tumors by a Novel c-Met/CD3 Bispecific Antibody. *Drug Des. Dev. Ther.* **2020**, *14*, 3201–3214. [CrossRef]

50. Iizuka, A.; Nonomura, C.; Ashizawa, T.; Kondou, R.; Ohshima, K.; Sugino, T.; Mitsuya, K.; Hayashi, N.; Nakasu, Y.; Maruyama, K.; et al. A T-cell-engaging B7-H4/CD3-bispecific Fab-scFv Antibody Targets Human Breast Cancer. *Clin. Cancer Res.* **2019**, *25*, 2925–2934. [CrossRef]

51. Kamada, H.; Taki, S.; Nagano, K.; Inoue, M.; Ando, D.; Mukai, Y.; Higashisaka, K.; Yoshioka, Y.; Tsutsumi, Y.; Tsunoda, S. Generation and characterization of a bispecific diabody targeting both EPH receptor A10 and CD3. *Biochem. Biophys. Res. Commun.* **2015**, *456*, 908–912. [CrossRef] [PubMed]

52. Kurosawa, N.; Wakata, Y.; Ida, K.; Midorikawa, A.; Isobe, M. High throughput development of TCR-mimic antibody that targets survivin-2B80-88/HLA-A*A24 and its application in a bispecific T-cell engager. *Sci. Rep.* **2019**, *9*, 9827. [CrossRef] [PubMed]

53. Li, H.; Huang, C.; Zhang, Z.; Feng, Y.; Wang, Z.; Tang, X.; Zhong, K.; Hu, Y.; Guo, G.; Zhou, L.; et al. MEK Inhibitor Augments Antitumor Activity of B7-H3-Redirected Bispecific Antibody. *Front. Oncol.* **2020**, *10*, 1527. [CrossRef] [PubMed]

54. Ma, J.; Shang, T.; Ma, P.; Sun, X.; Zhao, J.; Sun, X.; Zhang, M. Bispecific anti-CD3 x anti-B7-H3 antibody mediates T cell cytotoxic ability to human melanoma in vitro and in vivo. *Investig. New Drugs* **2019**, *37*, 1036–1043. [CrossRef] [PubMed]

55. Ma, W.; Ma, J.; Lei, T.; Zhao, M.; Zhang, M. Targeting immunotherapy for bladder cancer by using anti-CD3x CD155 bispecific antibody. *J. Cancer* **2019**, *10*, 5153–5161. [CrossRef] [PubMed]

56. Ma, W.; Ma, J.; Ma, P.; Lei, T.; Zhao, M.; Zhang, M. Targeting immunotherapy for bladder cancer using anti-CD3x B7-H3 bispecific antibody. *Cancer Med.* **2018**, *7*, 5167–5177. [CrossRef]

57. Martini, S.; Figini, M.; Croce, A.; Frigerio, B.; Pennati, M.; Gianni, A.M.; De Marco, C.; Daidone, M.G.; Argueta, C.; Landesman, Y.; et al. Selinexor Sensitizes TRAIL-R2-Positive TNBC Cells to the Activity of TRAIL-R2xCD3 Bispecific Antibody. *Cells* **2020**, *9*, 2231. [CrossRef]

58. Mathur, D.; Root, A.R.; Bugaj-Gaweda, B.; Bisulco, S.; Tan, X.; Fang, W.; Kearney, J.C.; Lucas, J.; Guffroy, M.; Golas, J.; et al. A Novel GUCY2C-CD3 T-Cell Engaging Bispecific Construct (PF-07062119) for the Treatment of Gastrointestinal Cancers. *Clin. Cancer Res.* **2020**, *26*, 2188–2202. [CrossRef]

59. Qi, J.; Hymel, D.; Nelson, C.G.; Burke, T.R., Jr.; Rader, C. Conventional and Chemically Programmed Asymmetric Bispecific Antibodies Targeting Folate Receptor 1. *Front. Immunol.* **2019**, *10*, 1994. [CrossRef]

60. Qi, J.; Li, X.; Peng, H.; Cook, E.M.; Dadashian, E.L.; Wiestner, A.; Park, H.; Rader, C. Potent and selective antitumor activity of a T cell-engaging bispecific antibody targeting a membrane-proximal epitope of ROR1. *Proc. Natl. Acad. Sci. USA* **2018**, *115*, E5467–E5476. [CrossRef]

61. Root, A.R.; Cao, W.; Li, B.; LaPan, P.; Meade, C.; Sanford, J.; Jin, M.; O'Sullivan, C.; Cummins, E.; Lambert, M.; et al. Development of PF-06671008, a Highly Potent Anti-P-cadherin/Anti-CD3 Bispecific DART Molecule with Extended Half-Life for the Treatment of Cancer. *Antibodies* **2016**, *5*, 6. [CrossRef]

62. Ruan, S.; Lin, M.; Zhu, Y.; Lum, L.; Thakur, A.; Jin, R.; Shao, W.; Zhang, Y.; Hu, Y.; Huang, S.; et al. Integrin beta4-Targeted Cancer Immunotherapies Inhibit Tumor Growth and Decrease Metastasis. *Cancer Res.* **2020**, *80*, 771–783. [CrossRef]

63. Satta, A.; Grazia, G.; Caroli, F.; Frigerio, B.; Di Nicola, M.; Raspagliesi, F.; Mezzanzanica, D.; Zaffaroni, N.; Gianni, A.M.; Anichini, A.; et al. A Bispecific Antibody to Link a TRAIL-Based Antitumor Approach to Immunotherapy. *Front. Immunol.* **2019**, *10*, 2514. [CrossRef]

64. Satta, A.; Mezzanzanica, D.; Caroli, F.; Frigerio, B.; Di Nicola, M.; Kontermann, R.E.; Iacovelli, F.; Desideri, A.; Anichini, A.; Canevari, S.; et al. Design, selection and optimization of an anti-TRAIL-R2/anti-CD3 bispecific antibody able to educate T cells to recognize and destroy cancer cells. *MAbs* **2018**, *10*, 1084–1097. [CrossRef] [PubMed]

65. Stadler, C.R.; Bahr-Mahmud, H.; Plum, L.M.; Schmoldt, K.; Kolsch, A.C.; Tureci, O.; Sahin, U. Characterization of the first-in-class T-cell-engaging bispecific single-chain antibody for targeted immunotherapy of solid tumors expressing the oncofetal protein claudin 6. *Oncoimmunology* **2016**, *5*, e1091555. [CrossRef] [PubMed]

66. Taki, S.; Kamada, H.; Inoue, M.; Nagano, K.; Mukai, Y.; Higashisaka, K.; Yoshioka, Y.; Tsutsumi, Y.; Tsunoda, S. A Novel Bispecific Antibody against Human CD3 and Ephrin Receptor A10 for Breast Cancer Therapy. *PLoS ONE* **2015**, *10*, e0144712. [CrossRef] [PubMed]

67. Zhao, H.; Ma, J.; Lei, T.; Ma, W.; Zhang, M. The bispecific anti-CD3 x anti-CD155 antibody mediates T cell immunotherapy for human prostate cancer. *Investig. New Drugs* **2019**, *37*, 810–817. [CrossRef]

68. Zhao, L.; Yang, Y.; Zhou, P.; Ma, H.; Zhao, X.; He, X.; Wang, T.; Zhang, J.; Liu, Y.; Zhang, T. Targeting CD133high Colorectal Cancer Cells In Vitro and In Vivo with an Asymmetric Bispecific Antibody. *J. Immunother.* **2015**, *38*, 217–228. [CrossRef]

69. Zhou, Y.; Zong, H.; Han, L.; Xie, Y.; Jiang, H.; Gilly, J.; Zhang, B.; Lu, H.; Chen, J.; Sun, R.; et al. A novel bispecific antibody targeting CD3 and prolactin receptor (PRLR) against PRLR-expression breast cancer. *J. Exp. Clin. Cancer Res.* **2020**, *39*, 87. [CrossRef]

70. Kebenko, M.; Goebeler, M.E.; Wolf, M.; Hasenburg, A.; Seggewiss-Bernhardt, R.; Ritter, B.; Rautenberg, B.; Atanackovic, D.; Kratzer, A.; Rottman, J.B.; et al. A multicenter phase 1 study of solitomab (MT110, AMG 110), a bispecific EpCAM/CD3 T-cell engager (BiTE(R)) antibody construct, in patients with refractory solid tumors. *Oncoimmunology* **2018**, *7*, e1450710. [CrossRef]

71. Pishvaian, M.; Morse, M.A.; McDevitt, J.; Norton, J.D.; Ren, S.; Robbie, G.J.; Ryan, P.C.; Soukharev, S.; Bao, H.; Denlinger, C.S. Phase 1 Dose Escalation Study of MEDI-565, a Bispecific T-Cell Engager that Targets Human Carcinoembryonic Antigen, in Patients With Advanced Gastrointestinal Adenocarcinomas. *Clin. Colorectal. Cancer* **2016**, *15*, 345–351. [CrossRef] [PubMed]

72. Tabernero, J.; Melero, I.; Ros, W.; Argiles, G.; Marabelle, A.; Rodriguez-Ruiz, M.E.; Albanell, J.; Calvo, E.; Moreno, V.; Cleary, J.M.; et al. Phase Ia and Ib studies of the novel carcinoembryonic antigen (CEA) T-cell bispecific (CEA CD3 TCB) antibody as a single agent and in combination with atezolizumab: Preliminary efficacy and safety in patients with metastatic colorectal cancer (mCRC). *J. Clin. Oncol.* **2017**, *35*, 3002. [CrossRef]

73. Middleton, M.R.; McAlpine, C.; Woodcock, V.K.; Corrie, P.; Infante, J.R.; Steven, N.M.; Evans, T.R.J.; Anthoney, A.; Shoushtari, A.N.; Hamid, O.; et al. Tebentafusp, A TCR/Anti-CD3 Bispecific Fusion Protein Targeting gp100, Potently Activated Antitumor Immune Responses in Patients with Metastatic Melanoma. *Clin. Cancer Res.* **2020**. [CrossRef] [PubMed]

74. Hummel, H.-D.; Kufer, P.; Grüllich, C.; Deschler-Baier, B.; Chatterjee, M.; Goebeler, M.-E.; Miller, K.; Santis, M.D.; Loidl, W.C.; Buck, A.; et al. Phase 1 study of pasotuxizumab (BAY 2010112), a PSMA-targeting Bispecific T cell Engager (BiTE) immunotherapy for metastatic castration-resistant prostate cancer (mCRPC). *J. Clin. Oncol.* **2019**, *37*, 5034. [CrossRef]

75. Lutterbuese, R.; Raum, T.; Kischel, R.; Hoffmann, P.; Mangold, S.; Rattel, B.; Friedrich, M.; Thomas, O.; Lorenczewski, G.; Rau, D.; et al. T cell-engaging BiTE antibodies specific for EGFR potently eliminate KRAS- and BRAF-mutated colorectal cancer cells. *Proc. Natl. Acad. Sci. USA* **2010**, *107*, 12605–12610. [CrossRef] [PubMed]

76. Ellerman, D. Bispecific T-cell engagers: Towards understanding variables influencing the in vitro potency and tumor selectivity and their modulation to enhance their efficacy and safety. *Methods* **2019**, *154*, 102–117. [CrossRef]

77. Chen, D.S.; Mellman, I. Elements of cancer immunity and the cancer-immune set point. *Nature* **2017**, *541*, 321–330. [CrossRef]

78. Lanitis, E.; Dangaj, D.; Irving, M.; Coukos, G. Mechanisms regulating T-cell infiltration and activity in solid tumors. *Ann. Oncol.* **2017**, *28*, xii18–xii32. [CrossRef]

79. Groeneveldt, C.; van Hall, T.; van der Burg, S.H.; Ten Dijke, P.; van Montfoort, N. Immunotherapeutic Potential of TGF-beta Inhibition and Oncolytic Viruses. *Trends Immunol.* **2020**, *41*, 406–420. [CrossRef]

80. Kuczek, D.E.; Larsen, A.M.H.; Thorseth, M.L.; Carretta, M.; Kalvisa, A.; Siersbaek, M.S.; Simoes, A.M.C.; Roslind, A.; Engelholm, L.H.; Noessner, E.; et al. Collagen density regulates the activity of tumor-infiltrating T cells. *J. Immunother. Cancer* **2019**, *7*, 68. [CrossRef]

81. Strohlein, M.A.; Lefering, R.; Bulian, D.R.; Heiss, M.M. Relative lymphocyte count is a prognostic parameter in cancer patients with catumaxomab immunotherapy. *Med. Hypotheses* **2014**, *82*, 295–299. [CrossRef] [PubMed]

82. Kumar, B.V.; Connors, T.J.; Farber, D.L. Human T Cell Development, Localization, and Function throughout Life. *Immunity* **2018**, *48*, 202–213. [CrossRef] [PubMed]

83. Halin, C.; Scimone, M.L.; Bonasio, R.; Gauguet, J.M.; Mempel, T.R.; Quackenbush, E.; Proia, R.L.; Mandala, S.; von Andrian, U.H. The S1P-analog FTY720 differentially modulates T-cell homing via HEV: T-cell-expressed S1P1 amplifies integrin activation in peripheral lymph nodes but not in Peyer patches. *Blood* **2005**, *106*, 1314–1322. [CrossRef] [PubMed]

84. Yan, Y.; Chen, R.; Wang, X.; Hu, K.; Huang, L.; Lu, M.; Hu, Q. CCL19 and CCR7 Expression, Signaling Pathways, and Adjuvant Functions in Viral Infection and Prevention. *Front. Cell Dev. Biol.* **2019**, *7*, 212. [CrossRef] [PubMed]

85. Groom, J.R.; Luster, A.D. CXCR3 in T cell function. *Exp. Cell Res.* **2011**, *317*, 620–631. [CrossRef]

86. Chow, M.T.; Luster, A.D. Chemokines in cancer. *Cancer Immunol. Res.* **2014**, *2*, 1125–1131. [CrossRef]

87. Iijima, N.; Iwasaki, A. Tissue instruction for migration and retention of TRM cells. *Trends Immunol.* **2015**, *36*, 556–564. [CrossRef]

88. Amsen, D.; van Gisbergen, K.; Hombrink, P.; van Lier, R.A.W. Tissue-resident memory T cells at the center of immunity to solid tumors. *Nat. Immunol.* **2018**, *19*, 538–546. [CrossRef] [PubMed]

89. Thommen, D.S.; Schumacher, T.N. T Cell Dysfunction in Cancer. *Cancer Cell* **2018**, *33*, 547–562. [CrossRef]
90. Tormoen, G.W.; Crittenden, M.R.; Gough, M.J. Role of the immunosuppressive microenvironment in immunotherapy. *Adv. Radiat. Oncol.* **2018**, *3*, 520–526. [CrossRef]
91. Grywalska, E.; Pasiarski, M.; Gozdz, S.; Rolinski, J. Immune-checkpoint inhibitors for combating T-cell dysfunction in cancer. *Onco Targets Ther.* **2018**, *11*, 6505–6524. [CrossRef] [PubMed]
92. Hanahan, D.; Weinberg, R.A. Hallmarks of cancer: The next generation. *Cell* **2011**, *144*, 646–674. [CrossRef] [PubMed]
93. Wee, P.; Wang, Z. Epidermal Growth Factor Receptor Cell Proliferation Signaling Pathways. *Cancers* **2017**, *9*, 52. [CrossRef]
94. Vigneron, N. Human Tumor Antigens and Cancer Immunotherapy. *Biomed. Res. Int.* **2015**, *2015*, 948501. [CrossRef] [PubMed]
95. Bansal, A.; Singh, M.P.; Rai, B. Human papillomavirus-associated cancers: A growing global problem. *Int. J. Appl. Basic Med. Res.* **2016**, *6*, 84–89. [CrossRef] [PubMed]
96. Wu, J.; Zhao, W.; Zhou, B.; Su, Z.; Gu, X.; Zhou, Z.; Chen, S. TSNAdb: A Database for Tumor-specific Neoantigens from Immunogenomics Data Analysis. *Genomics Proteomics Bioinform.* **2018**, *16*, 276–282. [CrossRef] [PubMed]
97. Koster, J.; Plasterk, R.H.A. A library of Neo Open Reading Frame peptides (NOPs) as a sustainable resource of common neoantigens in up to 50% of cancer patients. *Sci. Rep.* **2019**, *9*, 6577. [CrossRef]
98. Kraus, M.H.; Popescu, N.C.; Amsbaugh, S.C.; King, C.R. Overexpression of the EGF receptor-related proto-oncogene erbB-2 in human mammary tumor cell lines by different molecular mechanisms. *EMBO J.* **1987**, *6*, 605–610. [CrossRef]
99. Imrich, S.; Hachmeister, M.; Gires, O. EpCAM and its potential role in tumor-initiating cells. *Cell Adh. Migr.* **2012**, *6*, 30–38. [CrossRef]
100. Trenevska, I.; Li, D.; Banham, A.H. Therapeutic Antibodies against Intracellular Tumor Antigens. *Front. Immunol.* **2017**, *8*, 1001. [CrossRef]
101. Bunk, S.; Hofmann, M.; Unverdorben, F.; Hutt, M.; Pszolla, G.; Schwöbel, F.; Wagner, C.; Yousef, S.; Schuster, H.; Missel, S.; et al. Effective Targeting of PRAME-Positive Tumors with Bispecific T Cell-Engaging Receptor (TCER®) Molecules. *Blood* **2019**, *134*, 3368. [CrossRef]
102. Maruta, M.; Ochi, T.; Tanimoto, K.; Asai, H.; Saitou, T.; Fujiwara, H.; Imamura, T.; Takenaka, K.; Yasukawa, M. Direct comparison of target-reactivity and cross-reactivity induced by CAR- and BiTE-redirected T cells for the development of antibody-based T-cell therapy. *Sci. Rep.* **2019**, *9*, 13293. [CrossRef] [PubMed]
103. Dao, T.; Pankov, D.; Scott, A.; Korontsvit, T.; Zakhaleva, V.; Xu, Y.; Xiang, J.; Yan, S.; de Morais Guerreiro, M.D.; Veomett, N.; et al. Therapeutic bispecific T-cell engager antibody targeting the intracellular oncoprotein WT1. *Nat. Biotechnol.* **2015**, *33*, 1079–1086. [CrossRef] [PubMed]
104. Marijt, K.A.; Doorduijn, E.M.; van Hall, T. TEIPP antigens for T-cell based immunotherapy of immune-edited HLA class I(low) cancers. *Mol. Immunol.* **2019**, *113*, 43–49. [CrossRef] [PubMed]
105. Prior, I.A.; Lewis, P.D.; Mattos, C. A comprehensive survey of Ras mutations in cancer. *Cancer Res.* **2012**, *72*, 2457–2467. [CrossRef] [PubMed]
106. Ressing, M.E.; de Jong, J.H.; Brandt, R.M.; Drijfhout, J.W.; Benckhuijsen, W.E.; Schreuder, G.M.; Offringa, R.; Kast, W.M.; Melief, C.J. Differential binding of viral peptides to HLA-A2 alleles. Implications for human papillomavirus type 16 E7 peptide-based vaccination against cervical carcinoma. *Eur. J. Immunol.* **1999**, *29*, 1292–1303. [CrossRef]
107. Bacac, M.; Klein, C.; Umana, P. CEA TCB: A novel head-to-tail 2:1 T cell bispecific antibody for treatment of CEA-positive solid tumors. *Oncoimmunology* **2016**, *5*, e1203498. [CrossRef]
108. Slaga, D.; Ellerman, D.; Lombana, T.N.; Vij, R.; Li, J.; Hristopoulos, M.; Clark, R.; Johnston, J.; Shelton, A.; Mai, E.; et al. Avidity-based binding to HER2 results in selective killing of HER2-overexpressing cells by anti-HER2/CD3. *Sci. Transl. Med.* **2018**, *10*. [CrossRef]
109. Bacac, M.; Fauti, T.; Sam, J.; Colombetti, S.; Weinzierl, T.; Ouaret, D.; Bodmer, W.; Lehmann, S.; Hofer, T.; Hosse, R.J.; et al. A Novel Carcinoembryonic Antigen T-Cell Bispecific Antibody (CEA TCB) for the Treatment of Solid Tumors. *Clin. Cancer Res.* **2016**, *22*, 3286–3297. [CrossRef]
110. Panowski, S.H.; Kuo, T.C.; Zhang, Y.; Chen, A.; Geng, T.; Aschenbrenner, L.; Kamperschroer, C.; Pascua, E.; Chen, W.; Delaria, K.; et al. Preclinical Efficacy and Safety Comparison of CD3 Bispecific and ADC Modalities Targeting BCMA for the Treatment of Multiple Myeloma. *Mol. Cancer Ther.* **2019**, *18*, 2008–2020. [CrossRef]
111. Mazor, Y.; Sachsenmeier, K.F.; Yang, C.; Hansen, A.; Filderman, J.; Mulgrew, K.; Wu, H.; Dall'Acqua, W.F. Enhanced tumor-targeting selectivity by modulating bispecific antibody binding affinity and format valence. *Sci. Rep.* **2017**, *7*, 40098. [CrossRef] [PubMed]
112. DeClerck, Y.A.; Mercurio, A.M.; Stack, M.S.; Chapman, H.A.; Zutter, M.M.; Muschel, R.J.; Raz, A.; Matrisian, L.M.; Sloane, B.F.; Noel, A.; et al. Proteases, extracellular matrix, and cancer: A workshop of the path B study section. *Am. J. Pathol.* **2004**, *164*, 1131–1139. [CrossRef]
113. Stubbs, M.; McSheehy, P.M.; Griffiths, J.R.; Bashford, C.L. Causes and consequences of tumour acidity and implications for treatment. *Mol. Med. Today* **2000**, *6*, 15–19. [CrossRef]
114. Boustany, L.M.; Wong, L.; White, C.W.; Diep, L.; Huang, Y.; Liu, S.; Richardson, J.H.; Kavanaugh, W.M.; Irving, B.A. Abstract A164: EGFR-CD3 bispecific Probody™ therapeutic induces tumor regressions and increases maximum tolerated dose >60-fold in preclinical studies. *Mol. Cancer Ther.* **2018**, *17*, A164. [CrossRef]

115. Panchal, A.; Seto, P.; Wall, R.; Hillier, B.J.; Zhu, Y.; Krakow, J.; Datt, A.; Pongo, E.; Bagheri, A.; Chen, T.T.; et al. COBRA: A highly potent conditionally active T cell engager engineered for the treatment of solid tumors. *MAbs* **2020**, *12*, 1792130. [CrossRef]

116. Geiger, M.; Stubenrauch, K.-G.; Sam, J.; Richter, W.F.; Jordan, G.; Eckmann, J.; Hage, C.; Nicolini, V.; Freimoser-Grundschober, A.; Ritter, M.; et al. Protease-activation using anti-idiotypic masks enables tumor specificity of a folate receptor 1-T cell bispecific antibody. *Nat. Commun.* **2020**, *11*. [CrossRef]

117. Banaszek, A.; Bumm, T.G.P.; Nowotny, B.; Geis, M.; Jacob, K.; Wolfl, M.; Trebing, J.; Kucka, K.; Kouhestani, D.; Gogishvili, T.; et al. On-target restoration of a split T cell-engaging antibody for precision immunotherapy. *Nat. Commun.* **2019**, *10*, 5387. [CrossRef]

118. Minogue, E.; Millar, D.; Chuan, Y.; Zhang, S.; Grauwet, K.; Guo, M.; Langenbucher, A.; Benes, C.H.; Heather, J.; Minshull, J.; et al. Redirecting T-Cells Against AML in a Multidimensional Targeting Space Using T-Cell Engaging Antibody Circuits (TEAC). *Blood* **2019**, *134*, 2653. [CrossRef]

119. Mandikian, D.; Takahashi, N.; Lo, A.A.; Li, J.; Eastham-Anderson, J.; Slaga, D.; Ho, J.; Hristopoulos, M.; Clark, R.; Totpal, K.; et al. Relative Target Affinities of T-Cell-Dependent Bispecific Antibodies Determine Biodistribution in a Solid Tumor Mouse Model. *Mol. Cancer Ther.* **2018**, *17*, 776–785. [CrossRef]

120. Kroesen, B.J.; ter Haar, A.; Spakman, H.; Willemse, P.; Sleijfer, D.T.; de Vries, E.G.; Mulder, N.H.; Berendsen, H.H.; Limburg, P.C.; The, T.H.; et al. Local antitumour treatment in carcinoma patients with bispecific-monoclonal-antibody-redirected T cells. *Cancer Immunol. Immunother.* **1993**, *37*, 400–407. [CrossRef]

121. Blanco, B.; Ramirez-Fernandez, A.; Alvarez-Vallina, L. Engineering Immune Cells for in vivo Secretion of Tumor-Specific T Cell-Redirecting Bispecific Antibodies. *Front. Immunol.* **2020**, *11*, 1792. [CrossRef] [PubMed]

122. Iwahori, K.; Kakarla, S.; Velasquez, M.P.; Yu, F.; Yi, Z.; Gerken, C.; Song, X.T.; Gottschalk, S. Engager T cells: A new class of antigen-specific T cells that redirect bystander T cells. *Mol. Ther.* **2015**, *23*, 171–178. [CrossRef] [PubMed]

123. Blanco, B.; Holliger, P.; Vile, R.G.; Alvarez-Vallina, L. Induction of human T lymphocyte cytotoxicity and inhibition of tumor growth by tumor-specific diabody-based molecules secreted from gene-modified bystander cells. *J. Immunol.* **2003**, *171*, 1070–1077. [CrossRef]

124. Compte, M.; Blanco, B.; Serrano, F.; Cuesta, A.M.; Sanz, L.; Bernad, A.; Holliger, P.; Alvarez-Vallina, L. Inhibition of tumor growth in vivo by in situ secretion of bispecific anti-CEA x anti-CD3 diabodies from lentivirally transduced human lymphocytes. *Cancer Gene Ther.* **2007**, *14*, 380–388. [CrossRef] [PubMed]

125. Everts, B.; van der Poel, H.G. Replication-selective oncolytic viruses in the treatment of cancer. *Cancer Gene Ther.* **2005**, *12*, 141–161. [CrossRef]

126. Fajardo, C.A.; Guedan, S.; Rojas, L.A.; Moreno, R.; Arias-Badia, M.; de Sostoa, J.; June, C.H.; Alemany, R. Oncolytic Adenoviral Delivery of an EGFR-Targeting T-cell Engager Improves Antitumor Efficacy. *Cancer Res.* **2017**, *77*, 2052–2063. [CrossRef]

127. Speck, T.; Heidbuechel, J.P.W.; Veinalde, R.; Jaeger, D.; von Kalle, C.; Ball, C.R.; Ungerechts, G.; Engeland, C.E. Targeted BiTE Expression by an Oncolytic Vector Augments Therapeutic Efficacy Against Solid Tumors. *Clin. Cancer Res.* **2018**, *24*, 2128–2137. [CrossRef]

128. Freedman, J.D.; Hagel, J.; Scott, E.M.; Psallidas, I.; Gupta, A.; Spiers, L.; Miller, P.; Kanellakis, N.; Ashfield, R.; Fisher, K.D.; et al. Oncolytic adenovirus expressing bispecific antibody targets T-cell cytotoxicity in cancer biopsies. *EMBO Mol. Med.* **2017**, *9*, 1067–1087. [CrossRef]

129. Porter, C.E.; Rosewell Shaw, A.; Jung, Y.; Yip, T.; Castro, P.D.; Sandulache, V.C.; Sikora, A.; Gottschalk, S.; Ittman, M.M.; Brenner, M.K.; et al. Oncolytic Adenovirus Armed with BiTE, Cytokine, and Checkpoint Inhibitor Enables CAR T Cells to Control the Growth of Heterogeneous Tumors. *Mol. Ther.* **2020**, *28*, 1251–1262. [CrossRef]

130. Yu, F.; Wang, X.; Guo, Z.S.; Bartlett, D.L.; Gottschalk, S.M.; Song, X.T. T-cell engager-armed oncolytic vaccinia virus significantly enhances antitumor therapy. *Mol. Ther.* **2014**, *22*, 102–111. [CrossRef]

131. Gujar, S.; Pol, J.G.; Kroemer, G. Heating it up: Oncolytic viruses make tumors 'hot' and suitable for checkpoint blockade immunotherapies. *Oncoimmunology* **2018**, *7*, e1442169. [CrossRef] [PubMed]

132. Marchini, A.; Daeffler, L.; Pozdeev, V.I.; Angelova, A.; Rommelaere, J. Immune Conversion of Tumor Microenvironment by Oncolytic Viruses: The Protoparvovirus H-1PV Case Study. *Front. Immunol.* **2019**, *10*, 1848. [CrossRef]

133. Russell, L.; Peng, K.W.; Russell, S.J.; Diaz, R.M. Oncolytic Viruses: Priming Time for Cancer Immunotherapy. *BioDrugs* **2019**, *33*, 485–501. [CrossRef] [PubMed]

134. Groeneveldt, C.; Kinderman, P.; van den Wollenberg, D.J.M.; van den Oever, R.L.; Middelburg, J.; Mustafa, D.A.M.; Hoeben, R.C.; van der Burg, S.H.; van Hall, T.; van Montfoort, N. Preconditioning of the tumor microenvironment with oncolytic reovirus converts CD3-bispecific antibody treatment into effective immunotherapy. *J. Immunother. Cancer* **2020**, *8*. [CrossRef]

135. Henke, E.; Nandigama, R.; Ergun, S. Extracellular Matrix in the Tumor Microenvironment and Its Impact on Cancer Therapy. *Front. Mol. Biosci.* **2019**, *6*, 160. [CrossRef] [PubMed]

136. Coulouarn, C.; Clement, B. Stellate cells and the development of liver cancer: Therapeutic potential of targeting the stroma. *J. Hepatol.* **2014**, *60*, 1306–1309. [CrossRef] [PubMed]

137. Wang, X.; Luo, J.; He, L.; Cheng, X.; Yan, G.; Wang, J.; Tang, R. Hybrid pH-sensitive nanogels surface-functionalized with collagenase for enhanced tumor penetration. *J. Colloid Interface Sci.* **2018**, *525*, 269–281. [CrossRef]

138. Yoshida, E.; Kudo, D.; Nagase, H.; Suto, A.; Shimoda, H.; Suto, S.; Kakizaki, I.; Endo, M.; Hakamada, K. 4-Methylumbelliferone Decreases the Hyaluronan-rich Extracellular Matrix and Increases the Effectiveness of 5-Fluorouracil. *Anticancer Res.* **2018**, *38*, 5799–5804. [CrossRef]

139. Eikenes, L.; Tari, M.; Tufto, I.; Bruland, O.S.; de Lange Davies, C. Hyaluronidase induces a transcapillary pressure gradient and improves the distribution and uptake of liposomal doxorubicin (Caelyx) in human osteosarcoma xenografts. *Br. J. Cancer* **2005**, *93*, 81–88. [CrossRef]

140. Guan, X.; Chen, J.; Hu, Y.; Lin, L.; Sun, P.; Tian, H.; Chen, X. Highly enhanced cancer immunotherapy by combining nanovaccine with hyaluronidase. *Biomaterials* **2018**, *171*, 198–206. [CrossRef]

141. Wen, Y.; Wang, C.T.; Ma, T.T.; Li, Z.Y.; Zhou, L.N.; Mu, B.; Leng, F.; Shi, H.S.; Li, Y.O.; Wei, Y.Q. Immunotherapy targeting fibroblast activation protein inhibits tumor growth and increases survival in a murine colon cancer model. *Cancer Sci.* **2010**, *101*, 2325–2332. [CrossRef] [PubMed]

142. Kraman, M.; Bambrough, P.J.; Arnold, J.N.; Roberts, E.W.; Magiera, L.; Jones, J.O.; Gopinathan, A.; Tuveson, D.A.; Fearon, D.T. Suppression of antitumor immunity by stromal cells expressing fibroblast activation protein-alpha. *Science* **2010**, *330*, 827–830. [CrossRef] [PubMed]

143. Ohshio, Y.; Teramoto, K.; Hanaoka, J.; Tezuka, N.; Itoh, Y.; Asai, T.; Daigo, Y.; Ogasawara, K. Cancer-associated fibroblast-targeted strategy enhances antitumor immune responses in dendritic cell-based vaccine. *Cancer Sci.* **2015**, *106*, 134–142. [CrossRef] [PubMed]

144. Freedman, J.D.; Duffy, M.R.; Lei-Rossmann, J.; Muntzer, A.; Scott, E.M.; Hagel, J.; Campo, L.; Bryant, R.J.; Verrill, C.; Lambert, A.; et al. An Oncolytic Virus Expressing a T-cell Engager Simultaneously Targets Cancer and Immunosuppressive Stromal Cells. *Cancer Res.* **2018**, *78*, 6852–6865. [CrossRef] [PubMed]

145. de Sostoa, J.; Fajardo, C.A.; Moreno, R.; Ramos, M.D.; Farrera-Sal, M.; Alemany, R. Targeting the tumor stroma with an oncolytic adenovirus secreting a fibroblast activation protein-targeted bispecific T-cell engager. *J. Immunother. Cancer* **2019**, *7*, 19. [CrossRef] [PubMed]

146. Yu, F.; Hong, B.; Song, X.-T. A T-cell engager-armed oncolytic vaccinia virus to target the tumor stroma. *Cancer Transl. Med.* **2017**, *3*, 122–132. [CrossRef]

147. Harryvan, T.J.; Verdegaal, E.M.E.; Hardwick, J.C.H.; Hawinkels, L.; van der Burg, S.H. Targeting of the Cancer-Associated Fibroblast-T-Cell Axis in Solid Malignancies. *J. Clin. Med.* **2019**, *8*, 1989. [CrossRef]

148. Feig, C.; Jones, J.O.; Kraman, M.; Wells, R.J.; Deonarine, A.; Chan, D.S.; Connell, C.M.; Roberts, E.W.; Zhao, Q.; Caballero, O.L.; et al. Targeting CXCL12 from FAP-expressing carcinoma-associated fibroblasts synergizes with anti-PD-L1 immunotherapy in pancreatic cancer. *Proc. Natl. Acad. Sci. USA* **2013**, *110*, 20212–20217. [CrossRef]

149. Zboralski, D.; Hoehlig, K.; Eulberg, D.; Fromming, A.; Vater, A. Increasing Tumor-Infiltrating T Cells through Inhibition of CXCL12 with NOX-A12 Synergizes with PD-1 Blockade. *Cancer Immunol. Res.* **2017**, *5*, 950–956. [CrossRef]

150. Mariathasan, S.; Turley, S.J.; Nickles, D.; Castiglioni, A.; Yuen, K.; Wang, Y.; Kadel, E.E., III; Koeppen, H.; Astarita, J.L.; Cubas, R.; et al. TGFbeta attenuates tumour response to PD-L1 blockade by contributing to exclusion of T cells. *Nature* **2018**, *554*, 544–548. [CrossRef]

151. Tauriello, D.V.F.; Palomo-Ponce, S.; Stork, D.; Berenguer-Llergo, A.; Badia-Ramentol, J.; Iglesias, M.; Sevillano, M.; Ibiza, S.; Canellas, A.; Hernando-Momblona, X.; et al. TGFbeta drives immune evasion in genetically reconstituted colon cancer metastasis. *Nature* **2018**, *554*, 538–543. [CrossRef] [PubMed]

152. Holmgaard, R.B.; Schaer, D.A.; Li, Y.; Castaneda, S.P.; Murphy, M.Y.; Xu, X.; Inigo, I.; Dobkin, J.; Manro, J.R.; Iversen, P.W.; et al. Targeting the TGFbeta pathway with galunisertib, a TGFbetaRI small molecule inhibitor, promotes anti-tumor immunity leading to durable, complete responses, as monotherapy and in combination with checkpoint blockade. *J. Immunother. Cancer* **2018**, *6*, 47. [CrossRef] [PubMed]

153. Molon, B.; Ugel, S.; Del Pozzo, F.; Soldani, C.; Zilio, S.; Avella, D.; De Palma, A.; Mauri, P.; Monegal, A.; Rescigno, M.; et al. Chemokine nitration prevents intratumoral infiltration of antigen-specific T cells. *J. Exp. Med.* **2011**, *208*, 1949–1962. [CrossRef] [PubMed]

154. Rotte, A.; Jin, J.Y.; Lemaire, V. Mechanistic overview of immune checkpoints to support the rational design of their combinations in cancer immunotherapy. *Ann. Oncol.* **2018**, *29*, 71–83. [CrossRef] [PubMed]

155. Borst, L.; van der Burg, S.H.; van Hall, T. The NKG2A-HLA-E Axis as a Novel Checkpoint in the Tumor Microenvironment. *Clin. Cancer Res.* **2020**, *26*, 5549–5556. [CrossRef]

156. Jiang, X.; Wang, J.; Deng, X.; Xiong, F.; Ge, J.; Xiang, B.; Wu, X.; Ma, J.; Zhou, M.; Li, X.; et al. Role of the tumor microenvironment in PD-L1/PD-1-mediated tumor immune escape. *Mol. Cancer* **2019**, *18*, 10. [CrossRef]

157. Chen, S.; Crabill, G.A.; Pritchard, T.S.; McMiller, T.L.; Wei, P.; Pardoll, D.M.; Pan, F.; Topalian, S.L. Mechanisms regulating PD-L1 expression on tumor and immune cells. *J. Immunother. Cancer* **2019**, *7*, 305. [CrossRef]

158. Chikuma, S.; Terawaki, S.; Hayashi, T.; Nabeshima, R.; Yoshida, T.; Shibayama, S.; Okazaki, T.; Honjo, T. PD-1-mediated suppression of IL-2 production induces CD8+ T cell anergy in vivo. *J. Immunol.* **2009**, *182*, 6682–6689. [CrossRef]

159. Kobold, S.; Pantelyushin, S.; Rataj, F.; Vom Berg, J. Rationale for Combining Bispecific T Cell Activating Antibodies With Checkpoint Blockade for Cancer Therapy. *Front. Oncol.* **2018**, *8*, 285. [CrossRef]

160. Schreiner, J.; Thommen, D.S.; Herzig, P.; Bacac, M.; Klein, C.; Roller, A.; Belousov, A.; Levitsky, V.; Savic, S.; Moersig, W.; et al. Expression of inhibitory receptors on intratumoral T cells modulates the activity of a T cell-bispecific antibody targeting folate receptor. *Oncoimmunology* **2016**, *5*, e1062969. [CrossRef]

161. Huang, S.; Apasov, S.; Koshiba, M.; Sitkovsky, M. Role of A2a extracellular adenosine receptor-mediated signaling in adenosine-mediated inhibition of T-cell activation and expansion. *Blood* **1997**, *90*, 1600–1610. [CrossRef] [PubMed]

162. Linden, J.; Cekic, C. Regulation of lymphocyte function by adenosine. *Arterioscler. Thromb. Vasc. Biol.* **2012**, *32*, 2097–2103. [CrossRef] [PubMed]
163. Osada, T.; Patel, S.P.; Hammond, S.A.; Osada, K.; Morse, M.A.; Lyerly, H.K. CEA/CD3-bispecific T cell-engaging (BiTE) antibody-mediated T lymphocyte cytotoxicity maximized by inhibition of both PD1 and PD-L1. *Cancer Immunol. Immunother.* **2015**, *64*, 677–688. [CrossRef] [PubMed]
164. Singer, K.; Gottfried, E.; Kreutz, M.; Mackensen, A. Suppression of T-cell responses by tumor metabolites. *Cancer Immunol. Immunother.* **2011**, *60*, 425–431. [CrossRef] [PubMed]
165. Young, A.; Mittal, D.; Stagg, J.; Smyth, M.J. Targeting cancer-derived adenosine: New therapeutic approaches. *Cancer Discov.* **2014**, *4*, 879–888. [CrossRef]
166. Yin, Z.; Bai, L.; Li, W.; Zeng, T.; Tian, H.; Cui, J. Targeting T cell metabolism in the tumor microenvironment: An anti-cancer therapeutic strategy. *J. Exp. Clin. Cancer Res.* **2019**, *38*, 403. [CrossRef]
167. Zhao, E.; Maj, T.; Kryczek, I.; Li, W.; Wu, K.; Zhao, L.; Wei, S.; Crespo, J.; Wan, S.; Vatan, L.; et al. Cancer mediates effector T cell dysfunction by targeting microRNAs and EZH2 via glycolysis restriction. *Nat. Immunol.* **2016**, *17*, 95–103. [CrossRef]
168. Lee, G.K.; Park, H.J.; Macleod, M.; Chandler, P.; Munn, D.H.; Mellor, A.L. Tryptophan deprivation sensitizes activated T cells to apoptosis prior to cell division. *Immunology* **2002**, *107*, 452–460. [CrossRef]
169. Chen, W.; Jin, W.; Hardegen, N.; Lei, K.J.; Li, L.; Marinos, N.; McGrady, G.; Wahl, S.M. Conversion of peripheral CD4+CD25- naive T cells to CD4+CD25+ regulatory T cells by TGF-beta induction of transcription factor Foxp3. *J. Exp. Med.* **2003**, *198*, 1875–1886. [CrossRef]
170. Gorelik, L.; Constant, S.; Flavell, R.A. Mechanism of transforming growth factor beta-induced inhibition of T helper type 1 differentiation. *J. Exp. Med.* **2002**, *195*, 1499–1505. [CrossRef]
171. Yoon, J.H.; Jung, S.M.; Park, S.H.; Kato, M.; Yamashita, T.; Lee, I.K.; Sudo, K.; Nakae, S.; Han, J.S.; Kim, O.H.; et al. Activin receptor-like kinase5 inhibition suppresses mouse melanoma by ubiquitin degradation of Smad4, thereby derepressing eomesodermin in cytotoxic T lymphocytes. *EMBO Mol. Med.* **2013**, *5*, 1720–1739. [CrossRef] [PubMed]
172. Mittal, S.K.; Cho, K.J.; Ishido, S.; Roche, P.A. Interleukin 10 (IL-10)-mediated Immunosuppression: March-i induction regulates antigen presentation by macrophages but not Dendritic cells. *J. Biol. Chem.* **2015**, *290*, 27158–27167. [CrossRef] [PubMed]
173. Steinbrink, K.; Graulich, E.; Kubsch, S.; Knop, J.; Enk, A.H. CD4(+) and CD8(+) anergic T cells induced by interleukin-10-treated human dendritic cells display antigen-specific suppressor activity. *Blood* **2002**, *99*, 2468–2476. [CrossRef] [PubMed]
174. Rodriguez, P.C.; Zea, A.H.; DeSalvo, J.; Culotta, K.S.; Zabaleta, J.; Quiceno, D.G.; Ochoa, J.B.; Ochoa, A.C. L-arginine consumption by macrophages modulates the expression of CD3 zeta chain in T lymphocytes. *J. Immunol.* **2003**, *171*, 1232–1239. [CrossRef] [PubMed]
175. Taheri, F.; Ochoa, J.B.; Faghiri, Z.; Culotta, K.; Park, H.J.; Lan, M.S.; Zea, A.H.; Ochoa, A.C. L-Arginine regulates the expression of the T-cell receptor zeta chain (CD3zeta) in Jurkat cells. *Clin. Cancer Res.* **2001**, *7*, 958s–965s. [PubMed]
176. Steggerda, S.M.; Bennett, M.K.; Chen, J.; Emberley, E.; Huang, T.; Janes, J.R.; Li, W.; MacKinnon, A.L.; Makkouk, A.; Marguier, G.; et al. Inhibition of arginase by CB-1158 blocks myeloid cell-mediated immune suppression in the tumor microenvironment. *J. Immunother. Cancer* **2017**, *5*, 101. [CrossRef] [PubMed]
177. Ni, G.; Wang, T.; Walton, S.; Zhu, B.; Chen, S.; Wu, X.; Wang, Y.; Wei, M.Q.; Liu, X. Manipulating IL-10 signalling blockade for better immunotherapy. *Cell Immunol.* **2015**, *293*, 126–129. [CrossRef]
178. Hausler, S.F.; Del Barrio, I.M.; Diessner, J.; Stein, R.G.; Strohschein, J.; Honig, A.; Dietl, J.; Wischhusen, J. Anti-CD39 and anti-CD73 antibodies A1 and 7G2 improve targeted therapy in ovarian cancer by blocking adenosine-dependent immune evasion. *Am. J. Transl. Res.* **2014**, *6*, 129–139.
179. Stagg, J.; Divisekera, U.; McLaughlin, N.; Sharkey, J.; Pommey, S.; Denoyer, D.; Dwyer, K.M.; Smyth, M.J. Anti-CD73 antibody therapy inhibits breast tumor growth and metastasis. *Proc. Natl. Acad. Sci. USA* **2010**, *107*, 1547–1552. [CrossRef]
180. Holmgaard, R.B.; Zamarin, D.; Munn, D.H.; Wolchok, J.D.; Allison, J.P. Indoleamine 2,3-dioxygenase is a critical resistance mechanism in antitumor T cell immunotherapy targeting CTLA-4. *J. Exp. Med.* **2013**, *210*, 1389–1402. [CrossRef]
181. Spranger, S.; Koblish, H.K.; Horton, B.; Scherle, P.A.; Newton, R.; Gajewski, T.F. Mechanism of tumor rejection with doublets of CTLA-4, PD-1/PD-L1, or IDO blockade involves restored IL-2 production and proliferation of CD8(+) T cells directly within the tumor microenvironment. *J. Immunother. Cancer* **2014**, *2*, 3. [CrossRef] [PubMed]
182. Hong, R.; Zhou, Y.; Tian, X.; Wang, L.; Wu, X. Selective inhibition of IDO1, D-1-methyl-tryptophan (D-1MT), effectively increased EpCAM/CD3-bispecific BiTE antibody MT110 efficacy against IDO1(hi)breast cancer via enhancing immune cells activity. *Int. Immunopharmacol.* **2018**, *54*, 118–124. [CrossRef] [PubMed]
183. Suzuki, E.; Kapoor, V.; Jassar, A.S.; Kaiser, L.R.; Albelda, S.M. Gemcitabine selectively eliminates splenic Gr-1+/CD11b+ myeloid suppressor cells in tumor-bearing animals and enhances antitumor immune activity. *Clin. Cancer Res.* **2005**, *11*, 6713–6721. [CrossRef] [PubMed]
184. Sevko, A.; Michels, T.; Vrohlings, M.; Umansky, L.; Beckhove, P.; Kato, M.; Shurin, G.V.; Shurin, M.R.; Umansky, V. Antitumor effect of paclitaxel is mediated by inhibition of myeloid-derived suppressor cells and chronic inflammation in the spontaneous melanoma model. *J. Immunol.* **2013**, *190*, 2464–2471. [CrossRef]
185. Vincent, J.; Mignot, G.; Chalmin, F.; Ladoire, S.; Bruchard, M.; Chevriaux, A.; Martin, F.; Apetoh, L.; Rebe, C.; Ghiringhelli, F. 5-Fluorouracil selectively kills tumor-associated myeloid-derived suppressor cells resulting in enhanced T cell-dependent antitumor immunity. *Cancer Res.* **2010**, *70*, 3052–3061. [CrossRef] [PubMed]

186. Eriksson, E.; Wenthe, J.; Irenaeus, S.; Loskog, A.; Ullenhag, G. Gemcitabine reduces MDSCs, tregs and TGFbeta-1 while restoring the teff/treg ratio in patients with pancreatic cancer. *J. Transl. Med.* **2016**, *14*, 282. [CrossRef]
187. Highfill, S.L.; Cui, Y.; Giles, A.J.; Smith, J.P.; Zhang, H.; Morse, E.; Kaplan, R.N.; Mackall, C.L. Disruption of CXCR2-mediated MDSC tumor trafficking enhances anti-PD1 efficacy. *Sci. Transl. Med.* **2014**, *6*, 237ra267. [CrossRef]
188. Sun, L.; Clavijo, P.E.; Robbins, Y.; Patel, P.; Friedman, J.; Greene, S.; Das, R.; Silvin, C.; Van Waes, C.; Horn, L.A.; et al. Inhibiting myeloid-derived suppressor cell trafficking enhances T cell immunotherapy. *J. CI Insight* **2019**, *4*. [CrossRef]
189. Qin, H.; Lerman, B.; Sakamaki, I.; Wei, G.; Cha, S.C.; Rao, S.S.; Qian, J.; Hailemichael, Y.; Nurieva, R.; Dwyer, K.C.; et al. Generation of a new therapeutic peptide that depletes myeloid-derived suppressor cells in tumor-bearing mice. *Nat. Med.* **2014**, *20*, 676–681. [CrossRef]
190. Scott, E.M.; Jacobus, E.J.; Lyons, B.; Frost, S.; Freedman, J.D.; Dyer, A.; Khalique, H.; Taverner, W.K.; Carr, A.; Champion, B.R.; et al. Bi- and tri-valent T cell engagers deplete tumour-associated macrophages in cancer patient samples. *J. Immunother. Cancer* **2019**, *7*, 320. [CrossRef]
191. Cheng, P.; Eksioglu, E.; Chen, X.; Wei, M.; Guenot, J.; Fox, J.; List, A.F.; Wei, S. Immunodepletion of MDSC By AMV564, a Novel Tetravalent Bispecific CD33/CD3 T Cell Engager Restores Immune Homeostasis in MDS in Vitro. *Blood* **2017**, *130*, 51. [CrossRef]
192. Jitschin, R.; Saul, D.; Braun, M.; Tohumeken, S.; Volkl, S.; Kischel, R.; Lutteropp, M.; Dos Santos, C.; Mackensen, A.; Mougiakakos, D. CD33/CD3-bispecific T-cell engaging (BiTE(R)) antibody construct targets monocytic AML myeloid-derived suppressor cells. *J. Immunother. Cancer* **2018**, *6*, 116. [CrossRef] [PubMed]
193. Koristka, S.; Cartellieri, M.; Arndt, C.; Feldmann, A.; Seliger, B.; Ehninger, G.; Bachmann, M.P. Tregs activated by bispecific antibodies: Killers or suppressors? *Oncoimmunology* **2015**, *4*, e994441. [CrossRef]
194. Koristka, S.; Cartellieri, M.; Theil, A.; Feldmann, A.; Arndt, C.; Stamova, S.; Michalk, I.; Topfer, K.; Temme, A.; Kretschmer, K.; et al. Retargeting of human regulatory T cells by single-chain bispecific antibodies. *J. Immunol.* **2012**, *188*, 1551–1558. [CrossRef] [PubMed]
195. Kvarnhammar, A.M.; Veitonmaki, N.; Hagerbrand, K.; Dahlman, A.; Smith, K.E.; Fritzell, S.; von Schantz, L.; Thagesson, M.; Werchau, D.; Smedenfors, K.; et al. The CTLA-4 x OX40 bispecific antibody ATOR-1015 induces anti-tumor effects through tumor-directed immune activation. *J. Immunother. Cancer* **2019**, *7*, 103. [CrossRef]
196. Dao, T.; Mun, S.S.; Scott, A.C.; Jarvis, C.A.; Korontsvit, T.; Yang, Z.; Liu, L.; Klatt, M.G.; Guerreiro, M.; Selvakumar, A.; et al. Depleting T regulatory cells by targeting intracellular Foxp3 with a TCR mimic antibody. *Oncoimmunology* **2019**, *8*, 1570778. [CrossRef]
197. Morse, M.A.; Hobeika, A.C.; Osada, T.; Serra, D.; Niedzwiecki, D.; Lyerly, H.K.; Clay, T.M. Depletion of human regulatory T cells specifically enhances antigen-specific immune responses to cancer vaccines. *Blood* **2008**, *112*, 610–618. [CrossRef]
198. Onda, M.; Kobayashi, K.; Pastan, I. Depletion of regulatory T cells in tumors with an anti-CD25 immunotoxin induces CD8 T cell-mediated systemic antitumor immunity. *Proc. Natl. Acad. Sci. USA* **2019**, *116*, 4575–4582. [CrossRef]
199. Jarnicki, A.G.; Lysaght, J.; Todryk, S.; Mills, K.H. Suppression of antitumor immunity by IL-10 and TGF-beta-producing T cells infiltrating the growing tumor: Influence of tumor environment on the induction of CD4+ and CD8+ regulatory T cells. *J. Immunol.* **2006**, *177*, 896–904. [CrossRef]
200. Yano, H.; Thakur, A.; Tomaszewski, E.N.; Choi, M.; Deol, A.; Lum, L.G. Ipilimumab augments antitumor activity of bispecific antibody-armed T cells. *J. Transl. Med.* **2014**, *12*, 191. [CrossRef]
201. Tian, Y.; Li, Y.; Shao, Y.; Zhang, Y. Gene modification strategies for next-generation CAR T cells against solid cancers. *J. Hematol. Oncol.* **2020**, *13*, 54. [CrossRef] [PubMed]
202. Correnti, C.E.; Laszlo, G.S.; de van der Schueren, W.J.; Godwin, C.D.; Bandaranayake, A.; Busch, M.A.; Gudgeon, C.J.; Bates, O.M.; Olson, J.M.; Mehlin, C.; et al. Simultaneous multiple interaction T-cell engaging (SMITE) bispecific antibodies overcome bispecific T-cell engager (BiTE) resistance via CD28 co-stimulation. *Leukemia* **2018**, *32*, 1239–1243. [CrossRef] [PubMed]
203. Liu, R.; Jiang, W.; Yang, M.; Guo, H.; Zhang, Y.; Wang, J.; Zhu, H.; Shi, R.; Fan, D.; Yang, C.; et al. Efficient inhibition of human B-cell lymphoma in SCID mice by synergistic antitumor effect of human 4-1BB ligand/anti-CD20 fusion proteins and anti-CD3/anti-CD20 diabodies. *J. Immunother.* **2010**, *33*, 500–509. [CrossRef] [PubMed]
204. Chiu, D.; Tavare, R.; Haber, L.; Aina, O.H.; Vazzana, K.; Ram, P.; Danton, M.; Finney, J.; Jalal, S.; Krueger, P.; et al. A PSMA-Targeting CD3 Bispecific Antibody Induces Antitumor Responses that Are Enhanced by 4-1BB Costimulation. *Cancer Immunol. Res.* **2020**, *8*, 596–608. [CrossRef] [PubMed]
205. Dubrot, J.; Milheiro, F.; Alfaro, C.; Palazon, A.; Martinez-Forero, I.; Perez-Gracia, J.L.; Morales-Kastresana, A.; Romero-Trevejo, J.L.; Ochoa, M.C.; Hervas-Stubbs, S.; et al. Treatment with anti-CD137 mAbs causes intense accumulations of liver T cells without selective antitumor immunotherapeutic effects in this organ. *Cancer Immunol. Immunother.* **2010**, *59*, 1223–1233. [CrossRef] [PubMed]
206. Niu, L.; Strahotin, S.; Hewes, B.; Zhang, B.; Zhang, Y.; Archer, D.; Spencer, T.; Dillehay, D.; Kwon, B.; Chen, L.; et al. Cytokine-mediated disruption of lymphocyte trafficking, hemopoiesis, and induction of lymphopenia, anemia, and thrombocytopenia in anti-CD137-treated mice. *J. Immunol.* **2007**, *178*, 4194–4213. [CrossRef]
207. Skokos, D.; Waite, J.C.; Haber, L.; Crawford, A.; Hermann, A.; Ullman, E.; Slim, R.; Godin, S.; Ajithdoss, D.; Ye, X.; et al. A class of costimulatory CD28-bispecific antibodies that enhance the antitumor activity of CD3-bispecific antibodies. *Sci. Transl. Med.* **2020**, *12*. [CrossRef]

208. Daniel, P.T.; Kroidl, A.; Kopp, J.; Sturm, I.; Moldenhauer, G.; Dorken, B.; Pezzutto, A. Immunotherapy of B-cell lymphoma with CD3x19 bispecific antibodies: Costimulation via CD28 prevents "veto" apoptosis of antibody-targeted cytotoxic T cells. *Blood* **1998**, *92*, 4750–4757. [CrossRef]
209. Rossi, E.A.; Rossi, D.L.; Cardillo, T.M.; Chang, C.H.; Goldenberg, D.M. Redirected T-cell killing of solid cancers targeted with an anti-CD3/Trop-2-bispecific antibody is enhanced in combination with interferon-alpha. *Mol. Cancer Ther.* **2014**, *13*, 2341–2351. [CrossRef]
210. Schmohl, J.U.; Felices, M.; Taras, E.; Miller, J.S.; Vallera, D.A. Enhanced ADCC and NK Cell Activation of an Anticarcinoma Bispecific Antibody by Genetic Insertion of a Modified IL-15 Cross-linker. *Mol. Ther.* **2016**, *24*, 1312–1322. [CrossRef]

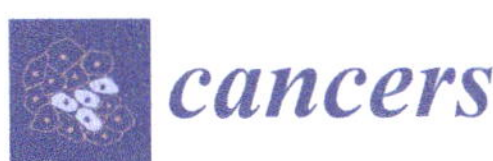

Review

IL-12 Family Cytokines in Cancer and Immunotherapy

Bhalchandra Mirlekar [1] and Yuliya Pylayeva-Gupta [1,2,*]

1 Lineberger Comprehensive Cancer Center, The University of North Carolina at Chapel Hill School of Medicine, Chapel Hill, NC 27599, USA; rmirlekar@med.unc.edu
2 Department of Genetics, The University of North Carolina at Chapel Hill School of Medicine, Chapel Hill, NC 27599, USA
* Correspondence: yuliyap1@email.unc.edu

Simple Summary: The IL-12 family cytokines play an important role in regulating the tumor immune contexture. Recent efforts geared towards the development of better immune therapeutic approaches have identified the need to overcome immune suppression and improve the quantity and quality of anti-tumor effector immune cells within the tumor milieu. In this review, we summarize the recent findings on IL-12 family cytokines in regulating anti-tumor immunity as well as the effectiveness and benefits of enhancing anti-tumor immunity in pre-clinical and clinical settings by targeting IL-12 family cytokines.

Abstract: The IL-12 family cytokines are a group of unique heterodimeric cytokines that include IL-12, IL-23, IL-27, IL-35 and, most recently, IL-39. Recent studies have solidified the importance of IL-12 cytokines in shaping innate and adaptive immune responses in cancer and identified multipronged roles for distinct IL-12 family members, ranging from effector to regulatory immune functions. These cytokines could serve as promising candidates for the development of immunomodulatory therapeutic approaches. Overall, IL-12 can be considered an effector cytokine and has been found to engage anti-tumor immunity by activating the effector Th1 response, which is required for the activation of cytotoxic T and NK cells and tumor clearance. IL-23 and IL-27 play dual roles in tumor immunity, as they can both activate effector immune responses and promote tumor growth by favoring immune suppression. IL-35 is a potent regulatory cytokine and plays a largely pro-tumorigenic role by inhibiting effector T cells. In this review, we summarize the recent findings on IL-12 family cytokines in the control of tumor growth with an emphasis primarily on immune regulation. We underscore the clinical implications for the use of these cytokines either in the setting of monotherapy or in combination with other conventional therapies for the more effective treatment of malignancies.

Keywords: IL-12 family cytokines; tumor microenvironment; cancer immunotherapy; anti-tumor immunity; STAT; B cell; T cell

Citation: Mirlekar, B.; Pylayeva-Gupta, Y. IL-12 Family Cytokines in Cancer and Immunotherapy. *Cancers* **2021**, *13*, 167. https://doi.org/10.3390/cancers13020167

Received: 1 December 2020
Accepted: 29 December 2020
Published: 6 January 2021

Publisher's Note: MDPI stays neutral with regard to jurisdictional clai-ms in published maps and institutio-nal affiliations.

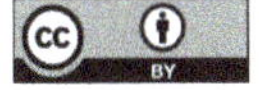

1. Introduction. IL-12 Family Cytokines: Composition, Signaling and Mechanism of Action

The IL-12 family cytokines are known to play essential roles in regulating innate and adaptive immune responses [1]. The functions of the IL-12 family cytokines have been widely studied in the settings of infection and auto-inflammatory diseases. The ability of these cytokines to modulate immune responses in cancer has been of significant interest. IL-12 family cytokines are typically secreted by innate immune cells but can also be secreted by adaptive immune cells depending on the disease and immune contexture. The members of this cytokine family are well known for shaping adaptive immune responses [2,3]. Due to their broad-spectrum roles in regulating immune responses, the IL-12 family cytokines are recognized as promising candidates for the modulation of anti-tumor immunity.

1.1. IL-12

IL-12 is a heterodimeric cytokine composed of p40 and p35 subunits and is considered a largely pro-inflammatory cytokine (Figure 1). It is produced by antigen-presenting cells, such as dendritic cells and macrophages, and is crucial for the recruitment and effector functions of CD8[+] T and NK cells [4]. Therefore, IL-12 is a major contributor to effective anti-tumor immune responses [5]. IL-12 signals through IL-12Rβ1 and IL-12Rβ2 receptors expressed on target cells, which allow downstream Jak2 and Tyk2 to promote the phosphorylation of and homo-dimerization of STAT4. The homodimer of pSTAT4 binds to its target genes and regulates gene expression [1]. In CD4[+] T cells, STAT4 activation by IL-12 is required for the transcription of T-bet, a positive regulator of Th1 cell differentiation. T-bet enhances the expression of Th1-specific cytokines, chemokines, and Th1's associated receptors. T-bet alone can positively regulate the expression of IFN-γ, while in combination with STAT4, it enhances transcription of CXCR3, IL-12Rβ1, CCL3 and CCL4 [6–8]. CCL3 and CCL4 are required for the intra-tumoral recruitment of cytotoxic NK cells and CD8[+] T cells [9–11]. In the presence of IL-12, NK cells are activated, express CD69 and CD25, and can further proliferate in the tumor niche [12,13]. Activated Th1 and NK cells proliferate and infiltrate into the tumor, where Th1 cells support the effector functions of tumor-specific cytotoxic T cells [4,12,13]. The IFN-γ, granzyme, and perforin secreted by cytotoxic NK and CD8[+] T cells can induce the apoptosis of cancer cells and control tumor growth. Moreover, IL-12 facilitates antigen presentation by upregulating MHCI on tumor cells, favoring polarization to M1 macrophages and attracting effector immune cells by enhancing the production of the chemokines CXCL9, CXCL10 and CXCL11 [5,14–16]. Additionally, T-bet and STAT4 act as negative regulators for RORγt and Foxp3, transcription factors responsible for Th17 and Treg generation, respectively, and limit their proliferation in the tumor microenvironment (TME) [17–20]. IL-12 can also neutralize signaling by negative regulatory receptors on CD8[+] T cells. For example, IL-12 downregulates PD-1 and IFNγR2 expression on CD8[+] T cells, protecting tumor infiltrating CD8[+] T cells from IFN-γ-induced cell death [21]. The activation of anti-tumor immunity by anti-PD1 requires IL-12-mediated crosstalk between T cells and dendritic cells that enables CD8[+] T cell-mediated tumor cell killing [22].

Besides its function in effector immune cells, IL-12 alters the plasticity of terminally differentiated Treg cells by converting Foxp3[+] Treg cells to IFN-γ-producing Foxp3[+] T cells. Treatment with IL-12 diminishes the level of IL-2, which is required for Treg cell survival and expansion [23]. IL-12 was shown to stimulate the IFN-γ-mediated inhibition of mouse Treg cell expansion. Mechanistically, IL-12-induced IFN-γ signaling causes cell cycle arrest in Treg cells and inhibits tumor-induced Treg cell proliferation. [23,24]. These studies demonstrate that IL-12 is not only required for the activation of effector anti-tumor immune responses but can also directly inhibit immune suppression. Thus, the use of IL-12 as a cancer immunotherapy could be beneficial in controlling tumor growth by activating anti-tumor cytotoxic immune responses. Overall, IL-12 targets and modulates T cells, NK cells and antigen-presenting cells (APCs) that regulate the fate of the anti-tumor immune response against the cancer cells.

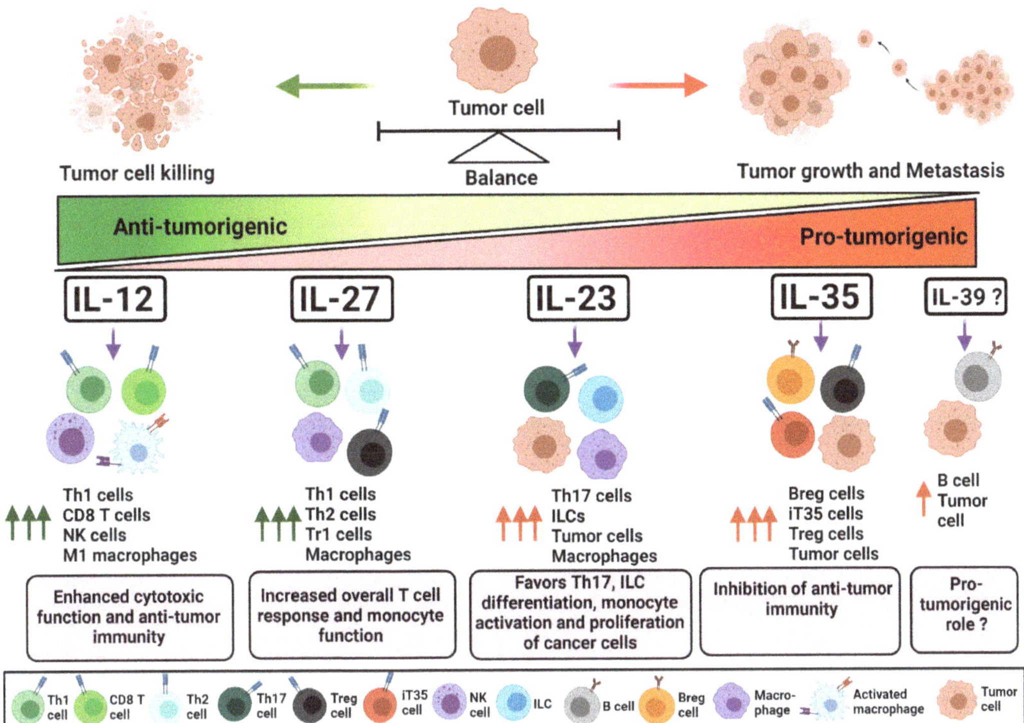

Figure 1. Role of IL-12 family cytokines in maintaining a balance between effector and regulatory immune responses in tumorigenesis. IL-12 activates an effector immune response against tumor cells by promoting both M1 macrophage polarization and IFN-γ- production by Th1 cells, which in turn, stimulate anti-tumor cytotoxic CD8[+] and NK cells. IL-27 and IL-23 have dual effects on immune cells in cancer. IL-27 and IL-23 can induce an overall T cell-mediated immune response and also modulate immune suppressive macrophages. Furthermore, IL-23 can stimulate the proliferation and growth of tumor cells. Conversely, IL-35 is a strong immune suppressive cytokine; it induces regulatory B and T cell activation and proliferation that subverts anti-tumor immunity and stimulates tumor growth and metastasis. IL-39 was recently shown to be secreted by B cells and may increase cancer cell proliferation. ↑ Arrow indicates increase in respective cell type activity; Tr1—T regulatory type 1; ILC—innate lymphoid cell; Breg—regulatory B cell; Treg—regulatory T cell; iT35—IL35-inducible regulatory T cell.

1.2. IL-12 in Cancer Immunotherapy

Cytokine-based immunotherapy can be effective in the treatment of numerous malignancies. IL-12 can be considered a strong candidate for immunotherapy-based interventions, as it potentiates tumor-specific cytotoxic NK and CD8[+] T cells that are largely responsible for tumor cell killing. However, the systemic administration of IL-12 is quite toxic; therefore, alternative methods of IL-12 delivery and/or the activation of T cells by IL-12 are needed [25,26]. To that extent, a recent report by Nguyen et al. provided comprehensive updates on the development and application of a localized delivery strategy for IL-12-based immunotherapy [27]. Wang et al. reported that systemic delivery via an oncolytic adenovirus encoding IL-12 lacking the signaling peptide reduced the toxic side effects and enhanced survival in mouse models of pancreatic cancer [26]. The nanoparticle-mediated delivery of IL-12 has also enhanced the cytotoxic activity against human hepatocellular carcinoma cells [28]. The in vitro nanoparticle-mediated delivery of IL-12 specifically into naïve CD8[+] T cells favored their expansion and the activation of the effector phenotype [28]. Several studies have shown that IL-12 favors the survival and differentiation of naïve CD8+ T cells towards the effector phenotype. IL-12 acts as an anti-apoptotic factor for CD8+ T cells by the impediment of the activation-induced cell death of CD8+CD62L^{hi} naïve CD8+ T cells, increased T cell homing, and has shown sustainable anti-tumor activity against mouse models of melanoma [29]. These findings suggest that the priming of naïve CD8+ T cells with IL-12 prior to adoptive cell therapy could increase their effectiveness and anti-tumor activity. Similar preclinical studies have reported the synergistic use of IL-12 with adoptive T-cell-based immunotherapies. In a syngeneic mouse model, the administration of anti–VEGFR-2 chimeric antigen receptor (CAR) and IL-12–co-transduced T cells directly into the tumor site modified the immune suppressive environment by ablating systemic and intra-tumoral VEGFR-2+ myeloid-derived suppressor cells (MDSCs) [30]. Moreover, genetically engineered T cells, which expressed high levels of IL-12, were therapeutically effective against established murine B16 melanoma tumors, even in the absence of a tumor vaccine and IL-2 [31]. Although the survival of IL-12 engineered cells was low compared to endogenous T cells, they demonstrated improved functionality, were detected at a higher frequency in the melanoma, and maintained the activity of endogenous NK and CD8+ T cells. In clinical trials, IL-12 was shown to have anti-cancer activity against human glioma [32]. In this case, 31 high-grade glioma patients were treated with human IL-12 vector (Ad-RTS-hIL-12) in a multicenter phase 1 dose-escalation trial (NCT02026271), and showed evidence of increased IFN-γ and PD-1+ tumor-infiltrating lymphocytes [32]. These findings suggest that increases in the concentration of intra-tumoral IL-12 improve the efficacy of adoptive T cell therapies.

Another recent advance in potentiating T cell-based anti-tumor activity has been increasing the load of IL-12 in CAR T cells. In a recent pre-clinical mouse study, Kueberuwa et al. used CAR T cells expressing IL-12 and showed that modified CAR T cells were able to cure B cell lymphoma and improve the long-term survival rate [33]. In this setting, IL-12-engineered CAR T cells recruited host immune cells to elicit an anti-tumor immune response. In addition, IL-12-producing CAR T cells directed against ovarian cancer cells showed robust proliferation and secretion of IFN-γ, which resulted in increased survival in a mouse model [34]. Similar preclinical studies in a hepatocellular carcinoma model indicated that IL-12-expressing CAR T cells produced high levels of effector cytokines, accompanied by attenuated Treg cell infiltration and induced tumor cell lysis [35]. In summary, these observations reveal that the inducible expression of IL-12 improves the anti-tumor functions of CAR T cells and might provide a promising treatment strategy for cancer patients (Figure 2). Nevertheless, CAR T or TCR T cells expressing IL-12 resulted in severe, edema-like toxicity and increased serum levels of IFN-γ and TNF-α in mice with melanoma [36]. Additionally, IL-12 overexpressing CAR T cells can lead to cytokine release syndrome (CRS) and cause systemic inflammatory responses in patients treated with CAR T cells [37,38]. These severe reactions should be considered before the use of genetically engineered T cells, particularly IL-12-producing CAR T cells.

While conventional immune checkpoint blockade, such as anti-PD-L1, is commonly used for the treatment of many cancers, its efficacy is not universal, and combination therapies that augment T cell responses are needed. Hewitt et al. demonstrated that intra-tumoral IL-12 mRNA (MEDI1191) therapy was able to stimulate IL-12 production within the tumor milieu without toxic effects [39]. MEDI1191 is currently being assessed in a phase I trial in patients with solid tumors (NCT03946800). The combination of this approach with anti-PD-L1 enhanced anti-tumor immunity by promoting IFN-γ+ Th1 cell differentiation. Fallon et al. engineered the fusion of two molecules of murine IL-12 (NHS-muIL12) with a longer half-life than recombinant murine IL-12 [40]. The combination of NHS-muIL12 and anti-PD-L1 boosted T cell activation and effector function within the TME and augmented tumor regression in murine tumor models. Other immunotherapy combinations could also be used. For example, combined immune therapy with IL-12 and tumor necrosis factor-related apoptosis-inducing ligand (TRAIL) in humanized mouse models of hepatocellular carcinoma increased the infiltration of IFN-γ-producing NK cells and promoted the apoptosis of cancer cells. Additionally, in the presence of IL-12,

TRAIL enhanced MHCI expression on antigen-presenting cells and downregulated the expression of intra-tumoral vascular endothelial growth factor (VEGF) and CD31 [41]. Another study showed that a combination of the immune-modulating protein aggregate magnesium–ammonium phospholinoleate–palmitoleate anhydride (P-MAPA) and human rIL-12 significantly reduced the migratory potential and invasion capacity by inducing the apoptosis of ovarian cancer cells [42]. These findings reveal that the use of IL-12 could substantially increase the effectiveness of cancer immunotherapy.

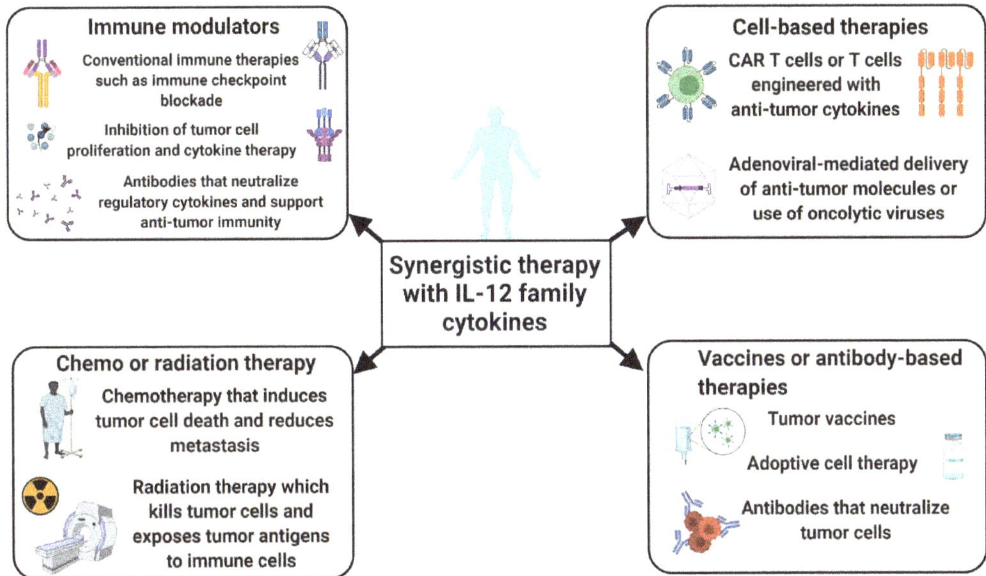

Figure 2. The therapeutic modulation of IL-12 family cytokines may enhance the efficacy of conventional therapy. Recent studies indicate that the therapies targeting (either upregulating or downregulating) the IL-12 family cytokines in combination with other standard therapies may increase treatment effectiveness. Context-dependent functions of IL-12 cytokines in cancer could drive the development of inhibitor or augmentative therapy axes, respectively. Drugs or antibodies targeting IL-12 family cytokines may help to restrain immune suppression within the tumor microenvironment (TME) and allow for the infiltration and proliferation of anti-tumor immune cells. Additionally, the targeted delivery of these cytokines with the help of adenovirus or chimeric antigen receptor (CAR) T cells may enhance cytotoxicity and tumor cell clearance. Such approaches could make tumor cells more sensitive to radiation, chemotherapy and immune checkpoint blockade therapy.

IL-12 may also have a beneficial role in synergizing with chemotherapy treatments. In patients with metastatic HER2$^+$ cancers, a synergistic treatment of IL-12 with chemotherapy, such as trastuzumab, stimulated NK cell activity [43]. Similar synergistic approaches could be used with radiation therapy. Deplanque et al. showed that radiation-induced immune suppression in well-established tumors could be overcome by increases in IL-12-dependent Th1 responses in mouse models of colon cancer [44]. Recent reports showed that radiation therapy in combination with IL-12 induced clonal epitope-specific T cell expansion and infiltration, blocked tumor growth and the improved survival of animals with human rhabdomyosarcoma xenografts [45]. Human recombinant IL-12 was also shown to have a protective role in cancer patients treated with radiation therapy. In this setting, it diminished the complications that can arise from radiation therapy, such as severe myelosuppression or pancytopenia [46]. In murine pancreatic cancer, immunotherapy using IL-12$^+$ microspheres in combination with stereotactic body radiation therapy induced intra-tumoral IFN-γ production, repolarized myeloid suppressors, promoted robust T cell activation and efficiently eliminated established liver metastases [47]. Overall, these observations reveal the importance of IL-12-based therapies in the initiation and stimulation of anti-tumor immune responses.

1.3. IL-23

IL-23 is a heterodimeric cytokine made up of p40 and p19 subunits. In cancer, IL-23 has been shown to have both pro- and anti-tumorigenic roles (Figure 1). Here, we discuss the dual role of IL-23 in modulating effector and/or regulatory immune responses in cancer.

1.3.1. IL-23 as a Suppressor of Anti-Tumor Immunity

The pro-tumorigenic role of IL-23 was first reported by Langowski et al., where it was observed that the genetic deletion or blockade of IL-23 in mice led to an increased infiltration of cytotoxic T cells with protective effects against cancer [48]. IL-23 can be secreted by dendritic cells, monocytes, neutrophils and innate lymphoid cells (ILCs) [49–52]. Upon stimulation, macrophages, dendritic cells and neutrophils have been shown to secrete IL-23 [53]. For example, IL-6, VEGF, CCL22 and/or PGE2 produced by tumor cells recruited tumor-associated macrophages, which in turn produced IL-23 and maintained suppressive Treg activity in the TME [54–58]. IL-23 produced by tumor-educated neutrophils activated downstream AKT and p38 pathways in mesenchymal stem cells and transformed those mesenchymal stem cells into cancer-associated fibroblasts [59]. CXCL5 could also induce the expression of IL-23 in neutrophils to enable the enhanced migration and invasion of gastric cancer cells [60]. Microbial products could also activate intra-tumoral myeloid cells, which in turn produced IL-23 and promoted colorectal neoplasms in mice [61]. Similar studies by Jin et al. reported that microbiota stimulated myeloid cells to induce IL-23 production in mouse models of lung cancer [62].

The role of IL-23 in regulating Th17 cell differentiation is widely studied and has been shown to play a critical role in Th17 cell expansion and the maintenance of the Th17 phenotype. IL-23 is required for the stabilization of RORγt, a transcription factor for Th17 cell generation, and facilitates the secretion of the effector cytokines IL-17 and IL-21 by Th17 cells [63,64]. IL-23 also stimulates IL-17 production from γδ T cells, which can support tumor growth [62,65–67]. IL-23 signals through IL-12Rβ1 and IL-23R in target cells and activates Jak2 and Tyk2, resulting in the phosphorylation of STAT3 and STAT4 [1]. IL-23R signaling in CD4$^+$ T cells activates STAT3, which in turn stabilizes RORγt expression and enhances IL-17 gene transcription [63,64]. IL-23 or IL-23-induced IL-17 signaling also activates NFkB, which regulates genes responsible for the recruitment of tumor-associated macrophages (TAMs) and MDSCs in the TME [68–70].

Thus, IL-23 is recognized as mediator of the Th17 response and plays an important role in shaping immune responses towards cancer. For example, CCL20 produced by tumor cells cooperated with stromal IL-23 to recruit IL-17-producing Th17 cells in the TME [71–74]. IL-17, in turn, promoted tumor angiogenesis by inducing angiogenic factors, such as VEGF and PGE2, and activated oncogenic STAT3 signaling, which was essential for the expression of pro-survival and pro-angiogenic genes [72–74].

IL-23 can also enhance inflammation in the TME and promote tumorigenesis independently of IL-17. The elevated expression of IL-23R on tumor cells enhanced tumor-associated inflammation and promoted the development and metastasis of cancer [75,76]. As one example, IL-23 induced the activation of STAT3 in lung cancer cells expressing IL-23R and stimulated their proliferation [77]. The expression of IL-12Rβ2 and IL-23R on laryngeal tumor cells mediated crosstalk between the cancer cells and tumor-infiltrating lymphocytes and affected the prognosis of laryngeal cancer patients [78]. Furthermore, the expression of IL-23R on B-acute lymphoblastic leukemia (B-ALL) cells in B-ALL patients was increased compared to normal B-lymphocytes and acted to upregulate miR15a and downregulate the pro-survival factor BCL2 [79]. These results indicate that, apart from regulating the Th17 response, IL-23 can also potentially alter the fate and function of cancer cells.

1.3.2. IL-23 as an Activator of Anti-Tumor Immunity

IL-23 is known to activate and maintain the expression of Th17-specific transcription factors, and these transcription factors can negatively regulate the immune-suppressive Treg cell response. IL-23 signaling can repress Treg differentiation and maintain the active transcription of IL-17, IL-21, IL-22 and IL-23R [63,64]. IL-23 can also regulate the function of diverse subsets of immune cells in the TME. For example, IL-23 upregulated the expression of IL-23R on type 3 innate lymphoid cells (ILC3), granulocytes and NK cells, which in turn induced their pro-inflammatory cytokine production and cytotoxic function [80–82]. In the presence of IL-23, intraepithelial cells secreted IL-22, which augmented their barrier function and maintained the CD4$^+$ T cells' effector phenotype [83–85]. On the other hand, activated fibroblasts secreted CCL5 and MCP-1, which recruited IL-23-producing macrophages [86,87]. IL-23$^+$ macrophages expanded anti-tumorigenic Th17 cells that had a distinct phenotype known as Th1-like Th17 cells and promoted tumor-specific immune responses by secreting IFN-γ, CXCL9 and CXCL10 [86,87]. Thus, IL-23 and IL-17 have been shown to play multipronged roles in tumorigenesis by activating or inhibiting effector anti-tumor immunity. These findings demonstrate that IL-23 could modulate pro- as well as anti-tumor immune responses (Figure 1).

Overall, IL-23 uses different downstream signaling pathways in tumor and immune cells that regulate pro-inflammatory and anti-inflammatory pathways. Overall, context-dependent functions of IL-23 in cancer could drive the development of inhibitor or augmentative therapy axes, respectively.

1.4. IL-23 in Cancer Immunotherapy

IL-23 is an important player in inflammatory responses, and IL-23-producing and responding cells are highly abundant in the tumor milieu [88,89]. In fact, the abundance of IL-23 in tumors is a general feature of cancer [85,88,90]. The levels of IL-23 and IL-23R were found to be significantly higher in breast cancer tissues and positively correlated with the patient's tumor size, TNM stage and metastasis [90]. In colorectal cancer, the levels of IL-23 in patients' serum samples were found to gradually increase with tumor stage progression [91,92]. IL-23 could activate Th17, ILC3, granulocytes, NK cells and intra-epithelial lymphocytes, which exaggerated gut inflammation and promoted the growth of colon cancer [93]. In multiple myeloma patients, IL-23 induced IL-17 and RORC in the bone marrow microenvironment [94]. Similar studies reported that IL-23 could promote IL-17-mediated tumorigenesis by converting type 1 innate lymphoid cells (ILC1) into ILC3, resulting in poor prognosis for patients with lung carcinoma [95]. Moreover, the overexpression of IL-23 mRNA was observed in serum samples of breast cancer patients, where IL-23 played a pro-tumorigenic role by upregulating the expression of regulatory cytokines [96]. Liu et al. observed elevated levels of serum IL-23 from hepatocellular carcinoma patients, and this was associated with poor clinical outcomes [97]. They demonstrated that ILC3 cells were the main source of IL-23 in hepatocellular carcinoma, and these cells directly suppressed the CD8$^+$ T cell response by enhancing apoptosis and preventing the proliferation of CD8$^+$ T cells [97].

Prostate cancer patients can exhibit resistance to androgen-deprivation therapy, a condition known as castration-resistant prostate cancer (CRPC). Increased levels of IL-23 were also observed in blood and tumor samples of patients with CRPC [98]. The major source of IL-23 was shown to be MDSCs. In a mouse model of CRPC, the blockade of IL-23 improved sensitivity to androgen deprivation and synergized with conventional therapies to boost anti-tumor immunity [98]. Another study showed that elevated IL-23 was associated with poor survival in renal cell carcinoma patients [99]. Mechanistically, intra-tumoral IL-23$^+$ macrophages augmented both Treg cell proliferation and IL-10/TGF-β secretion and suppressed the cytotoxic functionality of CD8$^+$ T cells. The blockade of IL-23 promoted CD8$^+$ T cell cytotoxicity and improved the overall survival of mice. Moreover, the blockade of IL-23 together with immune checkpoint blockade augmented therapeutic benefits [99]. Therefore, blockade of IL-23 in combination with immune checkpoint inhibitors can be a potential therapeutic approach in several cancer types (Figure 2). Conversely, reports from pancreatic cancer patients found that the levels of IL-23 decreased with tumor progression, and long-term survivors had increased IL-23 expression [100,101]. Similarly, IL-23 was shown to play a dual role in premalignant oral lesions to cancer in mice, where IL-23 was pro-inflammatory in premalignant oral lesions and inhibitory as the lesions progressed to cancer [102]. Thus, IL-23 may have distinct effects on anti-tumor immunity [103,104].

Sheng et al. showed that IL-23 can also enhance metastasis through the upregulation of anti-apoptotic factors in cancer cells [90]. In this case, the neutralization of IL-23p19 reduced cell proliferation and induced cell apoptosis by reducing the expression of BCL2 in breast cancer cell lines [90]. Besides its effects on the survival of tumor cells, IL-23 induced the expression of the proliferative marker Ki67 and endothelial marker CD31, promoting tumor cell proliferation, mammary tumor growth and pulmonary metastasis in mouse models of breast cancer [105]. Apart from the role of IL-23 in modulating the tumor cell cycle and growth, IL-23 exerts its effects on immune cells within the TME. IL-23 signaling stimulates the expression of regulatory genes, such as *IL-10, TGF-β* and *VEGF*, and increases the infiltration of immunosuppressive M2 macrophages and neutrophils that reduce the ability of effector CD4$^+$ and CD8$^+$ T cells to infiltrate tumors [105,106]. Zhang et al. showed that IL-23 is involved in the formation of immune-tolerant and pro-angiogenic TME through the induction of IL-17; this promoted the development of invasive prostate adenocarcinomas in mice [107]. These studies revealed the effects of IL-23 on the modulation of both immune cells and cancer cells. Thus, neutralizing IL-23 may augment tumor-specific immune responses and may control tumor cell proliferation and metastasis in certain cancer types.

Some preclinical studies have shown that IL-23 depletion combined with CAR T cells promotes tumor suppression, and neutralizing IL-23 can be effective particularly in combination with CAR T cell therapy [108]. The monoclonal antibody (mAB)-mediated depletion of IL-23 in mouse models of prostate cancer reinstated sensitivity to androgen deprivation therapy [98]. In one preclinical study, depleting IL-23mAB therapy in combination with CAR T cell therapy showed promising effects in the treatment of prostate cancer. The CAR T cells were generated by dual targeting using an IL-23-specific antibody and prostate-specific membrane antigen (PSMA)-specific mAB. IL-23mAB/PSMA CAR T cells had greater effectiveness than PSMA CAR only in the suppression of prostate cancer growth. Mechanistically, treatment with IL-23mAB/PSMA-CAR significantly enhanced CD45RO$^+$CD8$^+$ and CD127$^+$CD4$^+$ CAR T cells and indicated a potential role for IL-23 in the efficacy of CAR T cell therapy against prostate cancer [108,109]. By contrast, IL-23-expressing CARs were also shown to have anti-tumorigenic properties in preclinical studies. Ma et al. engineered the expression of the p40 subunit of IL-23 in T cells (p40-Td cells), and this enhanced the proliferation of activated T cells via autocrine signaling [110]. They also demonstrated in xenograft and syngeneic mouse models that p40-Td CAR T cells had enhanced anti-tumor capacity, with increases in granzyme B and decreases in PD-1 expression. Using neuroblastoma and pancreatic cancer models, they observed that p40-Td CAR T cells had greater efficacy in comparison to unmodified CAR T cells and exhibited diminished side effects in comparison to IL-18- or IL-15-producing CAR T cells [110]. Thus, the immune therapeutic strategies that target IL-23 may have use in the treatment of cancer.

1.5. IL-27

IL-27 is a heterodimeric cytokine consisting of EBi3 and p28 subunits [1]. IL-27 is generally involved in the differentiation and activation of different CD4$^+$ T cell subsets (Figure 1). Antigen-presenting cells stimulated by tumor antigens and CD40 can secrete IL-27, which has a dual function in regulating immune responses against cancer [111].

1.5.1. IL-27 as a Suppressor of Anti-Tumor Immunity

IL-27 has been shown to have anti-inflammatory properties. For example, IL-27 activated STAT3 and stabilized Foxp3 expression and IL-10 transcription in T cells, leading to sustained immune suppression [112]. Such IL-10-producing T cells are known as Tr1 cells [112,113]. Tr1 cells are immunosuppressive and downregulate the cytotoxic activity of CD8$^+$ T cells and NK cells, as well as preventing the production of TNF-α and IL-6 by monocytes, which are important for anti-tumor immunity [113,114]. Mechanistically, IL-27 signaling through STAT1 and STAT3 could activate the transcription factor c-Maf and induce the generation of Tr1 cells and IL-10 production by T cells [115–118]. IL-27 has also been shown to act as an anti-inflammatory cytokine by inhibiting Th2 and Th17 cell-specific immune responses and promoting the activation and proliferation of Treg cells [112,119,120]. Additionally, the activation of STAT1 and STAT3 by IL-27 can induce the expression of IL-1β, TNF-α and IL-18, which are important for the polarization of the immunosuppressive M2 phenotype [119,120]. In advanced non-small cell lung cancer (NSCLC) patients, IL-27 has also been shown to play a pro-tumorigenic role, where IL-27 induced tolerogenic dendritic cells that helped cancer cells to escape from immune surveillance [121].

1.5.2. IL-27 as an Activator of Anti-Tumor Immunity

On the other hand, IL-27 produced by dendritic cells, monocytes and macrophages following TLR activation may positively regulate Th1 differentiation through STAT1 dimerization. This subsequently leads to T-bet activation and Th1-specific gene expression [122–124]. IL-27 can also enhance the surface expression of MHCI and MHCII in monocytes as well as co-stimulatory CD80, CD86, and adhesion molecule CD54, overall promoting the pro-inflammatory activity of T cells [125]. IL-27 signals through IL-27R (WSX-1) and gp130 receptors on target cells [1]. IL-27R and gp130 receptors recruit Jak1 and Jak2, which in turn activate STAT1 and STAT3 [1]. IL-27 plays a critical role in the development of Th1 and IL-10-producing T cells. Th1 cells express T-bet and the effector cytokine IFN-γ through STAT1 dimerization induced by downstream IL-27 signaling [124,126]. In certain scenarios, the IL-27 receptor can also activate STAT4 and STAT5. For example, IL-27 signals through STAT1 and STAT4 to induce T-bet expression in CD4$^+$ T cells, which results in the upregulation of intracellular IFN-γ [124]. At the same time, the activation of STAT5 enhances the proliferation of Th1 cells in the TME [122,127]. For example, signaling through WSX-1 and gp130 on CD8$^+$ T cells activated STAT1 and STAT4 and resulted in the increased expression of granzyme, perforin and IFN-γ in a T-bet-dependent manner [128,129]. In NK cells, the activation of STAT1/STAT4 by IL-27 stimulated T-bet-dependent IFN-γ production and IL-27R expression [130,131]. These overall pro-inflammatory effects of IL-27 can stimulate anti-tumor immunity and contribute to tumor cell clearance [130–132]. Additionally, IL-27 may antagonize the production of IL-2, which is required for T cell activation, and regulated the intensity and duration of the effector CD4$^+$ T cell response [133,134].

IL-27 signaling in innate and adaptive immune cells as well as in cancer cells regulates the expression of distinct key molecules important for the activation of immune responses in the tumor milieu. To this end, IL-27 was reported to enhance the expression of DNAM-1, NKG2D and CD69 on NK cells [131]. NK cells also secreted high amounts of perforin and granzyme B and showed enhanced cytotoxic activity against cancer cells [131]. Moreover, the synergistic action of IL-27 with IL-18 activated and increased NK cell proliferation, cytotoxicity and IFN-γ production [131]. Another important aspect of IL-27 in regulating the NK cell response against uterine endometrial cancer cell (UECC) was recently reported by Zhou et al. In this study, the production of IL-27 by uterine endometrial cancer cells in the presence of rapamycin upregulated the expression of WSX-1 and gp130 on NK cells and increased their cytotoxic activity against cancer cells in a xenograft mouse model [135]. IL-27 also reduced the proliferation of human ovarian cancer cells by activating STAT3 and inhibiting Akt signaling pathways [136]. In mouse models of colon carcinoma, IL-27 induced NK cell-mediated cytotoxicity and anti-tumor immunity by activating STAT3 and triggering the expression of perforins [137].

IL-27 can also potentiate anti-tumor immunity by supporting the differentiation and expansion of myeloid progenitor cells into anti-tumorigenic M1 macrophages. For example,

IL-27 was shown to act on Sca-1$^+$c-Kit$^+$ cells in bone marrow and promoted their differentiation into M1 macrophages in preclinical mouse studies of B16F10 melanoma and MC38 colon adenocarcinoma [138]. IL-27 also enhanced the expression of inducible nitric oxide synthase, which sustained the anti-tumor activity of macrophages within the TME [138]. Similar studies in pancreatic cancer using co-cultures of human pancreatic cell lines and TAMs reported the role of IL-27 in restricting the differentiation of TAMs into immune suppressive M2 macrophages, which enhanced the effectiveness of gemcitabine [139]. Besides the role of IL-27 in regulating the differentiation of macrophages, IL-27 can also regulate several key surface molecules on cancer cells. Carbotti et al. showed that IL-27 triggered STAT1/STAT3 phosphorylation and upregulated the expression of surface MHC class I antigen on human small cell lung cancer cells, boosting the CD8$^+$ T cell response [140]. In non-small cell lung cancer patients, IL-27 promoted the anti-tumor function of myeloid cells and suppressed epithelial-to-mesenchymal transition (EMT) in cancer cells [141]. In human prostate cancer cells, IL-27 upregulated TLR3 expression and enhanced TLR-mediated cell death [142]. A relationship between IL-27 genetic polymorphisms and cancer risk has been identified. The IL-27 2905T/G genotype is linked with a decreased susceptibility to and development of cervical cancer in patients [143]. IL-27 also hindered NSCLC and squamous cell carcinoma (SCC) growth in cooperation with granulocyte and macrophage-driven necrosis, CXCL3 production, and diminished EMT-related gene expression [141]. These results indicate that IL-27 has great potential and can be utilized in the development of novel immune-therapeutic approaches.

1.6. IL-27 in Cancer Immunotherapy

Given the ability of IL-27 to regulate both pro-tumorigenic and anti-tumorigenic responses, the choice of the augmentation or blockade of IL-27 should be carefully evaluated given the tumor type and the immune contexture. Recent efforts have made therapeutic use of recombinant IL-27, either alone or in combination with other therapies. Majumder et al. demonstrated that treatment with rIL-27 ameliorated angiogenesis and immunosuppression in mouse models of benzo(a)pyrene (BaP)-induced lung carcinogenesis [144]. Zhu et al. also used an IL-27-expressing recombinant adeno-associated virus (AAV-IL-27) for the treatment of mouse models of lung cancer [145]. Such treatment significantly reduced tumor growth and enhanced the T cell response by downregulating the Treg cell frequency in the peripheral blood and in the TME [145]. These approaches could supplement current methods of Treg depletion, as attempts for total Treg cell depletion in cancer can result in autoimmunity. Furthermore, AAV-IL-27 drastically increased the efficacy of immune checkpoint blockade and Granulocyte Macrophage Colony Stimulating Factor (GM-CSF) vaccine treatment with no significant adverse effects [145]. Similar studies showed the recombinant adeno-associated virus (rAAV)-mediated delivery of IL-27 reduced Treg frequency and increased the effectiveness of immunotherapeutic agents in different mouse tumor models [146]. In this case, the intra-tumoral injection of AAV-IL-27 robustly increased anti-tumor immunity against plasmacytoma J558 and B16F10 mouse tumors by inducing the expression of CXCR3 in T cells and increasing responsiveness to anti-PD-1 or T cell adoptive transfer therapy [146]. These observations indicate that the intra-tumoral administration of IL-27 in combination with immune checkpoint blockade or adoptive T cell therapy could be a suitable approach for cancer treatment.

With regards to tackling the potential pro-tumor activity of IL-27, several studies have shown that IL-27 can regulate the immunosuppression and exhaustion of T cells. For example, IL-27 could also induce indoleamine 2,3-dioxygenase (IDO) and PD-L1 expression on monocytes and tumor-associated macrophages and on human prostate, breast and lung cancer cells [147–150]. Moreover, IL-27 signaling in human ovarian cancer cells activated STAT1/STAT3 and induced the constitutive expression of IDO [149]. These alterations on monocytes and tumor cells potentiate escape from immune attack. Similar studies in human lymphoma cell lines showed that the enhancement of IL-27 expression by tumor cells triggered the surface expression of PD-L1 on tumor-associated macrophages [151]. Moreover, IL-27 signaling on tumor cells activated STAT1; upregulated the expression of PD-L1 and production of IL-10, TGF-β and IDO; and downregulated MHCI expression [111,152]. Finally, IL-27 signaling in NK and CD8$^+$ T cells upregulated the cell surface expression of negative regulators, such as LAG3 and Tim3, contributing to the exhaustion of the effector phenotype [153,154]. In mouse models of melanoma, the inhibitory receptor Tim-3 was a crucial regulator of T cell dysfunction in tumorigenesis. IL-27 was shown to induce the expression of nuclear factor interleukin 3 regulated (NFIL3), which in association with T-bet, induced the expression of Tim-3 and the immunosuppressive cytokine IL-10 [153]. In this case, the blockade of IL-27 signaling resulted in reduced NFIL3 and Tim-3 expression, and decreased T cell exhaustion [153]. Similar studies reported pro-tumorigenic action of IL-27 favoring the expansion of Treg cells, where IL-27R$^{-/-}$ Treg cells were unable to suppress anti-tumor immunity in mouse models of melanoma [155]. Furthermore, IL-27 secreted by tumor-infiltrated neutrophils upregulated CD39 expression and enhanced the immune suppressive capacity of CD163$^+$ macrophages [156]. Here, the depletion of IL-27 attenuated the expression of PD-L1 and IL-10 in macrophages isolated from ovarian cancer patients [156]. These studies indicate that the IL-27/STAT3 axis can be a potential target for immunotherapy.

1.7. IL-35

IL-35 is a recent addition to the IL-12 family of cytokines and is composed of the p35 and EBi3 subunits [1,3]. IL-35 is a potent immune suppressive cytokine produced mostly by regulatory B (Breg) cells, iT35 cells and Treg cells and can play an important role in the suppression of effector immune responses [157]. IL-35 has also recently been detected in macrophages, dendritic cells and tumor cells [158–160]. The role of IL-35 in tumor growth is becoming more prominent due to its ability to inhibit effector immune responses (Figure 1). IL-35 regulates the differentiation of CD4$^+$ T cells and strongly favors regulatory T cell fate [161]. IL-35 is also thought to regulate the Th1 and Th17 lineage-specific transcription factors T-bet and RORγt as well as cytokines IFN-γ and IL-17 [162–164]. For example, IL-35 suppressed the effector functions of CD4$^+$ cells and favored tumor growth by facilitating the exhaustion of CD8$^+$ T cells [165,166]. Additionally, IL-35 restricted CD8$^+$ T cell activation by suppressing the expression of the costimulatory surface molecule CD28, and Th1 cytokine production, and reduced cytolytic functions by repressing the expression of perforins [167,168]. Furthermore, IL-35 converted effector T cells into IL-35-producing T cells known as iT35 cells and activated IL-35 production and the proliferation of Treg cells [163,169,170]. A subset of mouse and human regulatory B cells can be a major source of IL-35 in certain malignant tumor types [167,171,172]. Additionally, IL-35 can enhance its own expression in B cells through IL-12Rβ2 and IL-27Rα and the activation of STAT1 and STAT3, resulting in the augmented formation of Breg cells [173,174]. Mechanistically, the loss of IL-35 hindered pancreatic tumor growth via increases in effector CD4$^+$ T cells and CD8$^+$ T cells within the TME [165]. A specialized subset of B cells marked by CD21^{hi}CD1d^{hi}CD5$^+$ was identified as the main source of IL-35 in pancreatic cancer. The B cell-specific production of IL-35 promoted the expansion of Treg cells and blocked the anti-tumor activity of effector CD4$^+$ T cells [169]. Furthermore, IL-35 directly acted on CD8$^+$ T cells and suppressed their infiltration and effector function by downregulating the expression of IFN-γ and CXCR3 in a STAT3-dependent manner [169]. IL-35-producing B cells were also elevated in the peripheral blood of gastric cancer (GC) patients and were responsible for the accumulation of immune suppressive Treg cells, MDSCs, IL-10-producing B cells and CD14$^+$ monocytes [170].

IL-35 signals through IL-12Rβ2 and gp130 receptors in T cells, which triggers Jak1 and Jak2 to activate STAT1 and STAT4 [157]. IL-35-mediated signaling via STAT1/STAT4 in conventional T cells can polarize them to IL-35-producing iT35 cells [171]. The expression of IL-35 by Foxp3$^+$ Treg cells can reduce the proliferation of effector T cells and can lead to T cell exhaustion [171,172]. In this regard, Turnis at al. also demonstrated that IL-35$^+$ Treg cells could enhance the surface expression of the negative regulators Tim-

1, PD-1 and LAG3 on anti-tumor T cells [166]. A clinical study also showed that IL-35 produced by Treg cells promoted the growth of acute myeloid leukemia (AML) blasts in adult AML patients by limiting the activity of CD4$^+$CD25$^-$ T effector cells and increasing cancer cell proliferation [175]. IL-35 was reported to limit anti-tumor immunity in NSCLC patients by suppressing Th1 and Th17 responses and cytotoxic genes in CD8$^+$ T cells [176]. Apart from T cells, IL-35$^+$ macrophages were able to upregulate IL-12Rβ2 expression on cancer cells and make them more responsive to IL-35, facilitating the activation of JAK2–STAT6 and GATA3, and increased metastasis in mouse models of breast and lung cancer [159]. Moreover, Zou et al. showed that IL-35 facilitated the polarization of neutrophils, leading to increases in tumor growth in mouse models of melanoma and hepatocellular carcinoma [177]. Furthermore, IL-35 promoted immune suppression by favoring M2 macrophage polarization [178,179]. IL-35 also impeded DC maturation by reducing the cell surface expression of MHCI and MHCII and co-stimulatory molecules CD80/CD86 [180–182]. Overall, these observations indicate that IL-35 has a strong immune suppressive effect in the TME and could play a major role in controlling anti-tumor immunity; therefore, targeting IL-35 in cancer may hold substantial therapeutic potential for the treatment of patients with cancer.

1.8. IL-35 in Cancer Immunotherapy

A detailed understanding of IL-35 in cancer is essential. This information may lead to the development of new immunotherapeutic agents for the treatment of cancer patients, and it can be used as a potential biomarker for disease progression. As an example, elevated levels of IL-35 have been associated with poor prognosis in many solid cancer types [183–186].

1.8.1. IL-35 in Inhibiting Tumor Growth

Although IL-35 plays a pro-tumorigenic role in several cancer models, such as melanoma, pancreatic cancer, NSCLCC, breast cancer, lymphoma and gastric cancer, among others, Zhang et al. reported that IL-35 inhibited the cell migration, proliferation, colony formation and invasion of human colon cancer cells by suppressing β-catenin [187]. In this instance, IL-35 suppressed cancer growth in vivo and sensitized colon cancer cells to chemotherapy. Thus, IL-35 in combination with chemotherapy could be a useful treatment for colon cancer. Similar studies showed that IL-35 plays an inhibitory role in human NSCLC and colon cancer cells by suppressing cell migration and colony formation [188,189]. In hepatocellular carcinoma (HCC) patients, IL-35 expression was significantly reduced in patients with advanced cancer as compared to early stages. The HCC patients with reduced IL-35 had increased tumor size, distant metastases and positive microvascular invasion. Furthermore, the overexpression of IL-35 upregulated MHCI and CD95 in HepG2 cancer cells and reduced cell migration, colony formation and invasion. These data indicate that IL-35 plays an anti-tumorigenic role in HCC by enhancing MHCI-specific anti-tumor immunity and by reducing cancer cell migration. [190].

1.8.2. IL-35 in Promoting Tumor Growth

However, most research studies have reported that increased levels of IL-35 can be correlated with the pathogenicity and progression of cancer. The levels of IL-35 in the serum samples of prostate cancer patients were highly elevated compared with healthy controls and correlated with disease progression [184,191]. Similar studies reported elevated levels of circulating IL-35 in breast cancer patients, which positively correlated with the expression of Ki67, p53 and EGFR on breast cancer cells [192]. Furthermore, high levels of IL-35 were shown to be associated with the poor survival of diffuse-large B-cell lymphoma (DLBCL) patients treated with chemotherapy [193]. Additionally, increased levels of IL-35 were observed in the bone marrow of acute myeloid leukemia (AML) patients and correlated positively with clinical stages [194]. IL-35 can also be secreted by cancer cells and was shown to have a pro-tumorigenic effect particularly in pancreatic cancer. To this end, IL-35 was associated with poor prognosis in pancreatic cancer patients and is also thought to promote the growth of pancreatic cancer cells by enabling metastasis and extravasation [195]. In this case, IL-35 signaling in cancer cells activated STAT1 via the gp130 receptor, triggered the expression of ICAM1, and increased endothelial adhesion and metastasis. The human pancreatic cancer cell production of IL-35 also favored the proliferation of tumor cells by promoting the expression of cyclin B, cyclin D, Cdk2 and Cdk4, and it inhibited apoptosis by increasing levels of Bcl2 and decreasing levels of TRAILR1 [196]. Jin et al. showed that elevated levels of IL-35 in pancreatic cancer patients correlated with increases in tumor size, TNM staging and lymph node metastasis [197]. Furthermore, IL-35 produced by human nasopharyngeal carcinoma, B cell lymphoma and melanoma tumor cells enhanced the infiltration of CD11b$^+$Gr1$^+$ myeloid cells and promoted angiogenesis [160]. These findings indicate that IL-35 may have a distinct role in cancer when produced by immune cells or cancer cells.

Accumulating evidence suggests that IL-35 blockade could synergize with immunotherapy to ameliorate tumor growth. Turnis et al. showed that anti-PD-1 therapy combined with the depletion of IL-35 and/or deletion of Treg cell-specific IL-35 expression significantly limited murine melanoma and colon cancer growth by promoting cytotoxic T cell proliferation, effector function and long-term memory formation [166]. Similarly, the loss of B cell-specific IL-35 expression or antibody-based IL-35 blockade synergized with anti-PD1 treatment in a CD8$^+$ T cell-dependent manner to inhibit pancreatic cancer growth in preclinical models [169]. A similar approach of combining IL-35 blockade with the immune checkpoint inhibition of PD1 or PD-L1 was effective in NSCLC [185]. In this case, the neutralization of IL-35 hindered immunosuppressive macrophages and Treg cells while enhancing anti-tumor immunity. These findings identify the potential behind targeting IL-35-mediated immune suppression in the TME and highlight the importance of IL-35 as a therapeutic target in synergistic approaches with immune checkpoint therapy for the treatment of multiple cancer types.

1.9. IL-39

IL-39 is a newly proposed member of the IL-12 family. It is a heterodimeric cytokine consisting of the subunits p19 and EBi3 [198]. Most studies to date have only focused on cancer cell lines, and no concrete reports in animal models or human subjects are available yet. Thus, it is premature to designate IL-39 as an inflammatory or regulatory cytokine at this point in time. Wang et al. demonstrated that IL-39 could be secreted by LPS-stimulated B cells and could induce inflammation by activating STAT1/STAT3 in mouse models of lupus [198]. IL-39-producing B cells increased in mice with lupus, and the silencing of IL-39 led to reduced disease severity [199]. In this study, IL-39 induced the differentiation and expansion of CD11b$^+$Gr1$^+$ neutrophils in vivo. Furthermore, activated neutrophils could further potentiate the expression of B cell activation factor (BAFF) in GL7$^+$ B cells, creating a positive feedback loop that results in the increased production of IL-39 [199]. IL-39 was also shown to have a pro-tumorigenic function in pancreatic cancer, where in the presence of IL-39, colonies of human pancreatic cancer cells significantly increased their proliferation rate [200]. This was accompanied by the reduced expression of *p21* and *TRAILR1*. IL-39 is thought to signal via IL-23R and gp130 in target cells and to activate downstream STAT1 and STAT3 signaling [201,202]. Floss et al. engineered shuffled IL-12 family cytokine receptors, which are responsive to IL-39. The authors found that IL-39 may use two additional receptor combinations, IL-23R/IL-12Rβ2 and gp130/IL12Rβ1, in Ba/F3 cells [203]. These findings may highlight the flexibility of receptor usage by IL-39. More work needs to be done in order to understand the potential of targeting IL-39 in cancer immunotherapy.

2. Conclusions and Future Perspectives

IL-12 family cytokines play a critical role in the regulation of innate and adaptive immune responses. Their functions in the modulation of immune responses are well reported in autoimmunity and infectious diseases. These cytokines also play key roles in cancer initiation and progression. Tumor growth and spread have a direct relationship with host immune responses, and it is clear that IL-12 family cytokines can regulate tumor growth (Figure 1). Therefore, targeting or modifying the immune response against the tumor by harnessing the biological functionality of IL-12 family cytokines has recently gained lots of attention. The silent feature of various tumors is that they escape the host immune attack by favoring immune suppression within the TME. Cancer cells can secrete immune suppressive cytokines and chemokines and, in conjunction with regulatory immune cells, hinder the activity and proliferation of tumor-specific cytotoxic cells. Due to the "cold" nature of many cancers, therapies such as immune checkpoint blockade, adoptive T cell therapy, tumor vaccines, conventional chemotherapy and/or radiotherapy are frequently unable to manifest effective responses. Thus, strategies aiming to boost immune infiltration and functionality would be highly beneficial.

In this review, we summarized recent studies and advancements in the IL-12 field, namely, the roles and potential for the targeting of IL-12, IL-23, IL-27, IL-35 and IL-39 in tumorigenesis. The overarching objective is to make a tumor more susceptible to immune attack and become more responsive to conventional therapies. Targeting these cytokines may alter the tumor phenotype from immunologically "cold" to immunologically "hot". As discussed above, these cytokines are secreted not only by immune cells but also by tumor cells. Therefore, therapies focusing on IL-12 family cytokines can block the tumor cell cycle, induce apoptosis and prevent tumor cell proliferation, together with facilitating effector immune responses against cancer cells. Synergistic therapies that focus on IL-12 family cytokines and immune checkpoint blockade, such as anti-PD1, neutralizing antibodies, adoptive T cell therapy and CAR T cell therapy have shown promising effects in preclinical models. Localized IL-12 delivery and synergistic therapy consisting of IL-12 with immune checkpoint inhibitors and adoptive cell transfer is under investigation in clinical trials [27]. Hu et al. demonstrated that the combination of IL-12 and doxorubicin could enhance the infiltration of cytotoxic T cells into large solid tumors in different human xenograft models [204]. The local expression of IL-12 was achieved by injecting IL-12 DNA and conducting in vivo electroporation. This treatment hampered Treg cell infiltration and increased the effector functions of tumor-infiltrated T cells [204,205]. This strategy is under investigation in clinical trials (NCT01579318, NCT00323206, NCT01502293 and NCT02345330) and also in combination with pembrolizumab (NCT02493361 and NCT03132675) [205]. Although IL-12 is an effector cytokine and recruits a variety of effector immune cells at the tumoral site, it is possible that it can induce inflammatory effects. Therefore, future studies, particularly studies involving clinical trials, should consider the inflammatory effects associated with IL-12 family cytokines while using them as immunotherapy for cancer patients.

Future studies should place more emphasis on developing appropriate targeting reagents suitable for use in human clinical trials. More preclinical studies need to be performed, especially on IL-39. Given the role of IL-12 family cytokines in modulating the immune cell as well as cancer cell phenotype and receptor expression pattern, downstream signaling pathways need to be studied in detail, as they may dictate downstream therapeutic strategies. Preclinical studies using genetic mouse models need to include head-to-head comparisons across the distinct subunits that comprise IL-12 cytokines in order to establish which particular IL-12 family cytokine(s) play a role in a specific cancer type. Although IL-12 family cytokines seem to be promising candidates for the treatment of different malignancies, their associated side-effects and roles in regulating the local versus systemic immune system still need to be elaborated in detail.

Funding: This work was supported in part by National Institutes of Health R37 CA230786 (Y.P.-G.), University Cancer Research Fund at the University of North Carolina at Chapel Hill, and a Concern Foundation Conquer Cancer Now Award (Y.P.-G.).

Acknowledgments: We thank W.J. Bell for help with editing the manuscript. Figures created using BioRender.com.

Conflicts of Interest: The authors declare no conflict of interest.

References

1. Wojno, E.D.T.; Hunter, C.A.; Stumhofer, J.S. The immunobiology of the interleukin-12 family: Room for discovery. *Immunity* **2019**, *50*, 851–870. [CrossRef] [PubMed]
2. Mal, X.; Trinchieri, G. Regulation of interleukin-12 production in antigen-presenting cells. *Dev. Funct. Myeloid Subsets* **2001**, *79*, 55–92.
3. Vignali, D.A.; Kuchroo, V.K. Il-12 family cytokines: Immunological playmakers. *Nat. Immunol.* **2012**, *13*, 722–728.
4. Zundler, S.; Neurath, M.F. Interleukin-12: Functional activities and implications for disease. *Cytokine Growth Factor Rev.* **2015**, *26*, 559–568. [CrossRef]
5. Tugues, S.; Burkhard, S.; Ohs, I.; Vrohlings, M.; Nussbaum, K.; Berg, J.V.; Kulig, P.; Becher, B. New insights into il-12-mediated tumor suppression. *Cell Death Differ.* **2015**, *22*, 237–246. [CrossRef] [PubMed]
6. Thieu, V.T.; Yu, Q.; Chang, H.-C.; Yeh, N.; Nguyen, E.T.; Sehra, S.; Kaplan, M.H. Stat4 is required for t-bet to promote il-12-dependent th1 fate determination. *Immunity* **2008**, *29*, 679–690. [CrossRef] [PubMed]
7. Williams, C.L.; Schilling, M.M.; Cho, S.H.; Lee, K.; Wei, M.; Boothby, M. Stat4 and t-bet are required for the plasticity of ifn-γ expression across th2 ontogeny and influence changes in ifng promoter DNA methylation. *J. Immunol.* **2013**, *191*, 678–687. [CrossRef]
8. Jenner, R.G.; Townsend, M.J.; Jackson, I.; Sun, K.; Bouwman, R.D.; Young, R.A.; Glimcher, L.H.; Lord, G.M. The transcription factors t-bet and gata-3 control alternative pathways of T-cell differentiation through a shared set of target genes. *Proc. Natl. Acad. Sci. USA* **2009**, *106*, 17876–17881.
9. Vilgelm, A.E.; Richmond, A. Chemokines modulate immune surveillance in tumorigenesis, metastasis, and response to immunotherapy. *Front. Immunol.* **2019**, *10*, 333. [CrossRef]
10. Allen, F.; Bobanga, I.D.; Rauhe, P.; Barkauskas, D.; Teich, N.; Tong, C.; Myers, J.; Huang, A.Y. Ccl3 augments tumor rejection and enhances cd8$^+$ T cell infiltration through nk and cd103$^+$ dendritic cell recruitment via ifnγ. *Oncoimmunology* **2018**, *7*, e1393598. [CrossRef]
11. Allen, F.; Rauhe, P.; Askew, D.; Tong, A.A.; Nthale, J.; Eid, S.; Myers, J.T.; Tong, C.; Huang, A.Y. Ccl3 enhances antitumor immune priming in the lymph node via ifnγ with dependency on natural killer cells. *Front. Immunol.* **2017**, *8*, 1390. [CrossRef] [PubMed]
12. Zwirner, N.W.; Ziblat, A. Regulation of nk cell activation and effector functions by the il-12 family of cytokines: The case of il-27. *Front. Immunol.* **2017**, *8*, 25. [CrossRef] [PubMed]
13. Oka, N.; Markova, T.; Tsuzuki, K.; Li, W.; El-Darawish, Y.; Pencheva-Demireva, M.; Yamanishi, K.; Yamanishi, H.; Sakagami, M.; Tanaka, Y. Il-12 regulates the expansion, phenotype, and function of murine nk cells activated by il-15 and il-18. *Cancer Immunol. Immunother.* **2020**, *69*, 1699–1712. [CrossRef] [PubMed]
14. Yu, X.; Wu, B.; Ma, T.; Lin, Y.; Cheng, F.; Xiong, H.; Xie, C.; Liu, C.; Wang, Q.; Li, Z. Overexpression of il-12 reverses the phenotype and function of m2 macrophages to m1 macrophages. *Int. J. Clin. Exp. Pathol.* **2016**, *9*, 8963–8972.
15. Suzuki, S.; Umezu, Y.; Saijo, Y.; Satoh, G.; Abe, Y.; Satoh, K.; Nukiwa, T. Exogenous recombinant human il-12 augments mhc class i antigen expression on human cancer cells in vitro. *Tohoku J. Exp. Med.* **1998**, *185*, 223–226. [CrossRef]
16. Kerkar, S.P.; Goldszmid, R.S.; Muranski, P.; Chinnasamy, D.; Yu, Z.; Reger, R.N.; Leonardi, A.J.; Morgan, R.A.; Wang, E.; Marincola, F.M. Il-12 triggers a programmatic change in dysfunctional myeloid-derived cells within mouse tumors. *J. Clin. Investig.* **2011**, *121*, 4746–4757. [PubMed]
17. Lazarevic, V.; Chen, X.; Shim, J.; Hwang, E.; Jang, E.; Bolm, A.; Oukka, M.; Kuchroo, V.; Glimcher, L. Transcription factor t-bet represses th17 differentiation by preventing runx1-mediated activation of the ror7t gene. *Nat. Immunol.* **2011**, *12*, 96–104. [CrossRef]
18. Lin, Z.-W.; Wu, L.-X.; Xie, Y.; Ou, X.; Tian, P.-K.; Liu, X.-P.; Min, J.; Wang, J.; Chen, R.-F.; Chen, Y.-J. The expression levels of transcription factors t-bet, gata-3, rorγt and foxp3 in peripheral blood lymphocyte (pbl) of patients with liver cancer and their significance. *Int. J. Med Sci.* **2015**, *12*, 7–16. [CrossRef]
19. Li, C.; Jiang, P.; Wei, S.; Xu, X.; Wang, J. Regulatory t cells in tumor microenvironment: New mechanisms, potential therapeutic strategies and future prospects. *Mol. Cancer* **2020**, *19*, 1–23.
20. O'Malley, J.T.; Sehra, S.; Thieu, V.T.; Yu, Q.; Chang, H.C.; Stritesky, G.L.; Nguyen, E.T.; Mathur, A.N.; Levy, D.E.; Kaplan, M.H. Signal transducer and activator of transcription 4 limits the development of adaptive regulatory T cells. *Immunology* **2009**, *127*, 587–595.
21. Lin, L.; Rayman, P.; Pavicic, P.G.; Tannenbaum, C.; Hamilton, T.; Montero, A.; Ko, J.; Gastman, B.; Finke, J.; Ernstoff, M. Ex vivo conditioning with il-12 protects tumor-infiltrating cd8+ T cells from negative regulation by local ifn-γ. *Cancer Immunol. Immunother.* **2019**, *68*, 395–405. [CrossRef] [PubMed]
22. Garris, C.S.; Arlauckas, S.P.; Kohler, R.H.; Trefny, M.P.; Garren, S.; Piot, C.; Engblom, C.; Pfirschke, C.; Siwicki, M.; Gungabeesoon, J. Successful anti-pd-1 cancer immunotherapy requires T cell-dendritic cell crosstalk involving the cytokines ifn-γ and il-12. *Immunity* **2018**, *49*, 1148–1161.e7. [CrossRef] [PubMed]

23. Cao, X.; Leonard, K.; Collins, L.I.; Cai, S.F.; Mayer, J.C.; Payton, J.E.; Walter, M.J.; Piwnica-Worms, D.; Schreiber, R.D.; Ley, T.J. Interleukin 12 stimulates ifn-γ–mediated inhibition of tumor-induced regulatory T-cell proliferation and enhances tumor clearance. *Cancer Res.* **2009**, *69*, 8700–8709. [CrossRef] [PubMed]

24. Zhao, J.; Zhao, J.; Perlman, S. Differential effects of il-12 on tregs and non-treg T cells: Roles of ifn-γ, il-2 and il-2r. *PLoS ONE* **2012**, *7*, e46241. [CrossRef] [PubMed]

25. Leonard, J.P.; Sherman, M.L.; Fisher, G.L.; Buchanan, L.J.; Larsen, G.; Atkins, M.B.; Sosman, J.A.; Dutcher, J.P.; Vogelzang, N.J.; Ryan, J.L. Effects of single-dose interleukin-12 exposure on interleukin-12–associated toxicity and interferon-γ production. *Blood J. Am. Soc. Hematol.* **1997**, *90*, 2541–2548.

26. Wang, P.; Li, X.; Wang, J.; Gao, D.; Li, Y.; Li, H.; Chu, Y.; Zhang, Z.; Liu, H.; Jiang, G. Re-designing interleukin-12 to enhance its safety and potential as an anti-tumor immunotherapeutic agent. *Nat. Commun.* **2017**, *8*, 1–15.

27. Nguyen, K.G.; Vrabel, M.R.; Mantooth, S.M.; Hopkins, J.J.; Wagner, E.S.; Gabaldon, T.A.; Zaharoff, D.A. Localized interleukin-12 for cancer immunotherapy. *Front. Immunol.* **2020**, *11*, 575597. [CrossRef]

28. Li, J.; Lin, W.; Chen, H.; Xu, Z.; Ye, Y.; Chen, M. Dual-target il-12-containing nanoparticles enhance t cell functions for cancer immunotherapy. *Cell. Immunol.* **2020**, *349*, 104042. [CrossRef]

29. Díaz-Montero, C.M.; el Naggar, S.; al Khami, A.; el Naggar, R.; Montero, A.J.; Cole, D.J.; Salem, M.L. Priming of naive cd8+ T cells in the presence of il-12 selectively enhances the survival of cd8+ cd62l hi cells and results in superior anti-tumor activity in a tolerogenic murine model. *Cancer Immunol. Immunother.* **2008**, *57*, 563–572. [CrossRef]

30. Chinnasamy, D.; Yu, Z.; Kerkar, S.P.; Zhang, L.; Morgan, R.A.; Restifo, N.P.; Rosenberg, S.A. Local delivery of lnterleukin-12 using T cells targeting vegf receptor-2 eradicates multiple vascularized tumors in mice. *Clin. Cancer Res.* **2012**, *18*, 1672–1683. [CrossRef]

31. Kerkar, S.P.; Muranski, P.; Kaiser, A.; Boni, A.; Sanchez-Perez, L.; Yu, Z.; Palmer, D.C.; Reger, R.N.; Borman, Z.A.; Zhang, L. Tumor-specific cd8+ t cells expressing interleukin-12 eradicate established cancers in lymphodepleted hosts. *Cancer Res.* **2010**, *70*, 6725–6734. [CrossRef]

32. Chiocca, E.A.; John, S.Y.; Lukas, R.V.; Solomon, I.H.; Ligon, K.L.; Nakashima, H.; Triggs, D.A.; Reardon, D.A.; Wen, P.; Stopa, B.M. Regulatable interleukin-12 gene therapy in patients with recurrent high-grade glioma: Results of a phase 1 trial. *Sci. Transl. Med.* **2019**, *11*, eaaw5680. [CrossRef] [PubMed]

33. Kueberuwa, G.; Kalaitsidou, M.; Cheadle, E.; Hawkins, R.E.; Gilham, D.E. Cd19 car T cells expressing il-12 eradicate lymphoma in fully lymphoreplete mice through induction of host immunity. *Mol. Ther.-Oncolytics* **2018**, *8*, 41–51. [CrossRef]

34. Koneru, M.; Purdon, T.J.; Spriggs, D.; Koneru, S.; Brentjens, R.J. Il-12 secreting tumor-targeted chimeric antigen receptor T cells eradicate ovarian tumors in vivo. *Oncoimmunology* **2015**, *4*, e994446. [PubMed]

35. Liu, Y.; Di, S.; Shi, B.; Zhang, H.; Wang, Y.; Wu, X.; Luo, H.; Wang, H.; Li, Z.; Jiang, H. Armored inducible expression of il-12 enhances antitumor activity of glypican-3–targeted chimeric antigen receptor–engineered T cells in hepatocellular carcinoma. *J. Immunol.* **2019**, *203*, 198–207. [CrossRef]

36. Kunert, A.; Chmielewski, M.; Wijers, R.; Berrevoets, C.; Abken, H.; Debets, R. Intra-tumoral production of il18, but not il12, by tcr-engineered T cells is non-toxic and counteracts immune evasion of solid tumors. *Oncoimmunology* **2018**, *7*, e1378842. [CrossRef] [PubMed]

37. Brudno, J.N.; Kochenderfer, J.N. Toxicities of chimeric antigen receptor T cells: Recognition and management. *Blood* **2016**, *127*, 3321–3330. [CrossRef] [PubMed]

38. Bonifant, C.L.; Jackson, H.J.; Brentjens, R.J.; Curran, K.J. Toxicity and management in car T-cell therapy. *Mol. Ther.-Oncolytics* **2016**, *3*, 16011. [CrossRef] [PubMed]

39. Hewitt, S.L.; Bailey, D.; Zielinski, J.; Apte, A.; Musenge, F.; Karp, R.; Burke, S.; Garcon, F.; Mishra, A.; Gurumurthy, S. Intratumoral interleukin-12 mrna therapy promotes th1 transformation of the tumor microenvironment. *Clin. Cancer Res.* **2020**, *26*, 6284–6298. [CrossRef]

40. Fallon, J.K.; Vandeveer, A.J.; Schlom, J.; Greiner, J.W. Enhanced antitumor effects by combining an il-12/anti-DNA fusion protein with avelumab, an anti-pd-l1 antibody. *Oncotarget* **2017**, *8*, 20558–20571. [CrossRef]

41. El-Shemi, A.G.; Ashshi, A.M.; Na, Y.; Li, Y.; Basalamah, M.; Al-Allaf, F.A.; Oh, E.; Jung, B.-K.; Chae-Ok, Y. Combined therapy with oncolytic adenoviruses encoding trail and il-12 genes markedly suppressed human hepatocellular carcinoma both in vitro and in an orthotopic transplanted mouse model. *J. Exp. Clin. Cancer Res.* **2016**, *35*, 1–16. [CrossRef] [PubMed]

42. Lupi, L.A.; Delella, F.K.; Cucielo, M.S.; Romagnoli, G.G.; Kaneno, R.; Nunes, I.d.S.; Domeniconi, R.F.; Martinez, M.; Martinez, F.E.; Fávaro, W.J. P-mapa and interleukin-12 reduce cell migration/invasion and attenuate the toll-like receptor-mediated inflammatory response in ovarian cancer skov-3 cells: A preliminary study. *Molecules* **2020**, *25*, 5. [CrossRef] [PubMed]

43. Bekaii-Saab, T.S.; Roda, J.M.; Guenterberg, K.D.; Ramaswamy, B.; Young, D.C.; Ferketich, A.K.; Lamb, T.A.; Grever, M.R.; Shapiro, C.L.; Carson, W.E. A phase i trial of paclitaxel and trastuzumab in combination with interleukin-12 in patients with her2/neu-expressing malignancies. *Mol. Cancer Ther.* **2009**, *8*, 2983–2991. [CrossRef] [PubMed]

44. Deplanque, G.; Shabafrouz, K.; Obeid, M. Can local radiotherapy and il-12 synergise to overcome the immunosuppressive tumor microenvironment and allow "in situ tumor vaccination"? *Cancer Immunol. Immunother.* **2017**, *66*, 833–840. [CrossRef]

45. Eckert, F.; Jelas, I.; Oehme, M.; Huber, S.M.; Sonntag, K.; Welker, C.; Gillies, S.D.; Strittmatter, W.; Zips, D.; Handgretinger, R. Tumor-targeted il-12 combined with local irradiation leads to systemic tumor control via abscopal effects in vivo. *Oncoimmunology* **2017**, *6*, e1323161. [CrossRef]

46. Guo, N.; Wang, W.-Q.; Gong, X.-J.; Gao, L.; Yang, L.-R.; Yu, W.-N.; Shen, H.-Y.; Wan, L.-Q.; Jia, X.-F.; Wang, Y.-S. Study of recombinant human interleukin-12 for treatment of complications after radiotherapy for tumor patients. *World J. Clin. Oncol.* **2017**, *8*, 158–167. [CrossRef]

47. Mills, B.N.; Connolly, K.A.; Ye, J.; Murphy, J.D.; Uccello, T.P.; Han, B.J.; Zhao, T.; Drage, M.G.; Murthy, A.; Qiu, H. Stereotactic body radiation and interleukin-12 combination therapy eradicates pancreatic tumors by repolarizing the immune microenvironment. *Cell Rep.* **2019**, *29*, 406–421.e5. [CrossRef]

48. Langowski, J.L.; Zhang, X.; Wu, L.; Mattson, J.D.; Chen, T.; Smith, K.; Basham, B.; McClanahan, T.; Kastelein, R.A.; Oft, M. Il-23 promotes tumour incidence and growth. *Nature* **2006**, *442*, 461–465. [CrossRef]

49. Kastelein, R.A.; Hunter, C.A.; Cua, D.J. Discovery and biology of il-23 and il-27: Related but functionally distinct regulators of inflammation. *Annu. Rev. Immunol.* **2007**, *25*, 221–242. [CrossRef]

50. Ignacio, A.; Breda, C.N.S.; Camara, N.O.S. Innate lymphoid cells in tissue homeostasis and diseases. *World J. Hepatol.* **2017**, *9*, 979–989. [CrossRef]

51. Tian, Z.; van Velkinburgh, J.C.; Wu, Y.; Ni, B. Innate lymphoid cells involve in tumorigenesis. *Int. J. Cancer* **2016**, *138*, 22–29. [CrossRef] [PubMed]

52. Tamassia, N.; Arruda-Silva, F.; Wright, H.L.; Moots, R.J.; Gardiman, E.; Bianchetto-Aguilera, F.; Gasperini, S.; Capone, M.; Maggi, L.; Annunziato, F. Human neutrophils activated via tlr8 promote th17 polarization through il-23. *J. Leukoc. Biol.* **2019**, *105*, 1155–1165. [CrossRef] [PubMed]

53. Cauli, A.; Piga, M.; Floris, A.; Mathieu, A. Current Perspective on the Role of the Interleukin-23/Interleukin-17 Axis in Inflammation and Disease (Chronic Arthritis and Psoriasis). *ImmunoTargets Ther.* **2015**, *4*, 185–190. Available online: https://www.dovepress.com/front_end/cr_data/cache/pdf/download_1606621601_5fc319a1519b0/ITT-62870-current-perspectives-on-the-role-of-the-interleukin-23-inter_100115.pdf (accessed on 30 November 2020). [CrossRef] [PubMed]

54. Wang, K.; Karin, M. The il-23 to il-17 cascade inflammation-related cancers. *Clin. Exp. Rheumatol.* **2015**, *33*, S87–S90.

55. Qian, X.; Gu, L.; Ning, H.; Zhang, Y.; Hsueh, E.C.; Fu, M.; Hu, X.; Wei, L.; Hoft, D.F.; Liu, J. Increased th17 cells in the tumor microenvironment is mediated by il-23 via tumor-secreted prostaglandin e2. *J. Immunol.* **2013**, *190*, 5894–5902. [CrossRef] [PubMed]

56. Li, X.; Li, D.; Shi, Q.; Huang, X.; Ju, X. Umbilical cord blood-derived helios-positive regulatory t cells promote angiogenesis in acute lymphoblastic leukemia in mice via ccl22 and the vegfa-vegfr2 pathway. *Mol. Med. Rep.* **2019**, *19*, 4195–4204. [CrossRef]

57. Martinenaite, E.; Ahmad, S.M.; Hansen, M.; Met, Ö.; Westergaard, M.W.; Larsen, S.K.; Klausen, T.W.; Donia, M.; Svane, I.M.; Andersen, M.H. Ccl22-specific T cells: Modulating the immunosuppressive tumor microenvironment. *Oncoimmunology* **2016**, *5*, e1238541. [CrossRef]

58. Wiedemann, G.M.; Röhrle, N.; Makeschin, M.-C.; Fesseler, J.; Endres, S.; Mayr, D.; Anz, D. Peritumoural ccl1 and ccl22 expressing cells in hepatocellular carcinomas shape the tumour immune infiltrate. *Pathology* **2019**, *51*, 586–592. [CrossRef]

59. Zhang, J.; Ji, C.; Li, W.; Mao, Z.; Shi, Y.; Shi, H.; Ji, R.; Qian, H.; Xu, W.; Zhang, X. Tumor-educated neutrophils activate mesenchymal stem cells to promote gastric cancer growth and metastasis. *Front. Cell Dev. Biol.* **2020**, *8*, 788. [CrossRef]

60. Mao, Z.; Zhang, J.; Shi, Y.; Li, W.; Shi, H.; Ji, R.; Mao, F.; Qian, H.; Xu, W.; Zhang, X. Cxcl5 promotes gastric cancer metastasis by inducing epithelial-mesenchymal transition and activating neutrophils. *Oncogenesis* **2020**, *9*, 1–14.

61. Grivennikov, S.I.; Wang, K.; Mucida, D.; Stewart, C.A.; Schnabl, B.; Jauch, D.; Taniguchi, K.; Yu, G.-Y.; Österreicher, C.H.; Hung, K.E. Adenoma-linked barrier defects and microbial products drive il-23/il-17-mediated tumour growth. *Nature* **2012**, *491*, 254–258. [CrossRef] [PubMed]

62. Jin, C.; Lagoudas, G.K.; Zhao, C.; Bullman, S.; Bhutkar, A.; Hu, B.; Ameh, S.; Sandel, D.; Liang, X.S.; Mazzilli, S. Commensal microbiota promote lung cancer development via γδ T cells. *Cell* **2019**, *176*, 998–1013.e16. [CrossRef] [PubMed]

63. Gaffen, S.L.; Jain, R.; Garg, A.V.; Cua, D.J. The il-23–il-17 immune axis: From mechanisms to therapeutic testing. *Nat. Rev. Immunol.* **2014**, *14*, 585–600. [CrossRef] [PubMed]

64. Iwakura, Y.; Ishigame, H. The il-23/il-17 axis in inflammation. *J. Clin. Investig.* **2006**, *116*, 1218–1222. [CrossRef]

65. Ma, S.; Cheng, Q.; Cai, Y.; Gong, H.; Wu, Y.; Yu, X.; Shi, L.; Wu, D.; Dong, C.; Liu, H. Il-17a produced by γδ T cells promotes tumor growth in hepatocellular carcinoma. *Cancer Res.* **2014**, *74*, 1969–1982. [CrossRef]

66. Lee, J.S.; Tato, C.M.; Joyce-Shaikh, B.; Gulen, M.F.; Cayatte, C.; Chen, Y.; Blumenschein, W.M.; Judo, M.; Ayanoglu, G.; McClanahan, T.K. Interleukin-23-independent il-17 production regulates intestinal epithelial permeability. *Immunity* **2015**, *43*, 727–738. [CrossRef]

67. Kimura, Y.; Nagai, N.; Tsunekawa, N.; Sato-Matsushita, M.; Yoshimoto, T.; Cua, D.J.; Iwakura, Y.; Yagita, H.; Okada, F.; Tahara, H. Il-17a-producing cd 30+ vδ1 T cells drive inflammation-induced cancer progression. *Cancer Sci.* **2016**, *107*, 1206–1214. [CrossRef]

68. Pastor-Fernández, G.; Mariblanca, I.R.; Navarro, M.N. Decoding il-23 signaling cascade for new therapeutic opportunities. *Cells* **2020**, *9*, 2044. [CrossRef]

69. Tang, L.; Wang, K. Chronic inflammation in skin malignancies. *J. Mol. Signal.* **2016**, *11*, 2.

70. Wang, K.; Kim, M.K.; di Caro, G.; Wong, J.; Shalapour, S.; Wan, J.; Zhang, W.; Zhong, Z.; Sanchez-Lopez, E.; Wu, L.-W. Interleukin-17 receptor a signaling in transformed enterocytes promotes early colorectal tumorigenesis. *Immunity* **2014**, *41*, 1052–1063. [CrossRef]

71. Kirshberg, S.; Izhar, U.; Amir, G.; Demma, J.; Vernea, F.; Beider, K.; Shlomai, Z.; Wald, H.; Zamir, G.; Shapira, O.M. Involvement of ccr6/ccl20/il-17 axis in nsclc disease progression. *PLoS ONE* **2011**, *6*, e24856. [CrossRef] [PubMed]

72. Wu, X.; Yang, T.; Liu, X.; Guo, J.n.; Xie, T.; Ding, Y.; Lin, M.; Yang, H. Il-17 promotes tumor angiogenesis through stat3 pathway mediated upregulation of vegf in gastric cancer. *Tumor Biol.* **2016**, *37*, 5493–5501. [CrossRef] [PubMed]

73. Pan, B.; Shen, J.; Cao, J.; Zhou, Y.; Shang, L.; Jin, S.; Cao, S.; Che, D.; Liu, F.; Yu, Y. Interleukin-17 promotes angiogenesis by stimulating vegf production of cancer cells via the stat3/giv signaling pathway in non-small-cell lung cancer. *Sci. Rep.* **2015**, *5*, 16053. [CrossRef] [PubMed]

74. Wang, L.; Yi, T.; Kortylewski, M.; Pardoll, D.M.; Zeng, D.; Yu, H. Il-17 can promote tumor growth through an il-6–stat3 signaling pathway. *J. Exp. Med.* **2009**, *206*, 1457–1464. [PubMed]

75. Liu, J.; Wang, L.; Wang, T.; Wang, J. Expression of il-23r and il-17 and the pathology and prognosis of urinary bladder carcinoma. *Oncol. Lett.* **2018**, *16*, 4325–4330. [CrossRef] [PubMed]

76. Yan, J.; Smyth, M.J.; Teng, M.W. Interleukin (il)-12 and il-23 and their conflicting roles in cancer. *Cold Spring Harb. Perspect. Biol.* **2018**, *10*, a028530. [CrossRef]

77. Li, J.; Zhang, L.; Zhang, J.; Wei, Y.; Li, K.; Huang, L.; Zhang, S.; Gao, B.; Wang, X.; Lin, P. Interleukin 23 regulates proliferation of lung cancer cells in a concentration-dependent way in association with the interleukin-23 receptor. *Carcinogenesis* **2013**, *34*, 658–666.

78. Tao, Y.; Tao, T.; Gross, N.; Peng, X.; Li, Y.; Huang, Z.; Liu, L.; Li, G.; Chen, X.; Yang, J. Combined effect of il-12rβ2 and il-23r expression on prognosis of patients with laryngeal cancer. *Cell. Physiol. Biochem.* **2018**, *50*, 1041–1054. [CrossRef]

79. Cocco, C.; Canale, S.; Frasson, C.; di Carlo, E.; Ognio, E.; Ribatti, D.; Prigione, I.; Basso, G.; Airoldi, I. Interleukin-23 acts as antitumor agent on childhood b-acute lymphoblastic leukemia cells. *Blood J. Am. Soc. Hematol.* **2010**, *116*, 3887–3898. [CrossRef]

80. Chen, F.; Cao, A.; Yao, S.; Evans-Marin, H.L.; Liu, H.; Wu, W.; Carlsen, E.D.; Dann, S.M.; Soong, L.; Sun, J. Mtor mediates il-23 induction of neutrophil il-17 and il-22 production. *J. Immunol.* **2016**, *196*, 4390–4399.

81. Lee, P.W.; Smith, A.J.; Yang, Y.; Selhorst, A.J.; Liu, Y.; Racke, M.K.; Lovett-Racke, A.E. Il-23r–activated stat3/stat4 is essential for th1/th17-mediated cns autoimmunity. *JCI Insight* **2017**, *2*, e91663. [CrossRef] [PubMed]

82. Sun, R.; Hedl, M.; Abraham, C. Il23 group> il23r recycling and amplifies innate receptor-induced signalling and cytokines in human macrophages, and the ibd-protective il23r r381q variant modulates these outcomes. *Gut* **2020**, *69*, 264–273. [CrossRef] [PubMed]

83. McCuaig, S.; Barras, D.; Mann, E.; Friedrich, M.; Bullers, S.J.; Janney, A.; Garner, L.C.; Domingo, E.; Koelzer, V.H.; Delorenzi, M. The interleukin 22 pathway interacts with mutant kras to promote poor prognosis in colon cancer. *Clin. Cancer Res.* **2020**, *26*, 4313–4325. [CrossRef] [PubMed]

84. Aden, K.; Rehman, A.; Falk-Paulsen, M.; Secher, T.; Kuiper, J.; Tran, F.; Pfeuffer, S.; Sheibani-Tezerji, R.; Breuer, A.; Luzius, A. Epithelial il-23r signaling licenses protective il-22 responses in intestinal inflammation. *Cell Rep.* **2016**, *16*, 2208–2218. [CrossRef]

85. Markota, A.; Endres, S.; Kobold, S. Targeting interleukin-22 for cancer therapy. *Hum. Vaccines Immunother.* **2018**, *14*, 2012–2015.

86. Guéry, L.; Hugues, S. Th17 cell plasticity and functions in cancer immunity. *BioMed Res. Int.* **2015**, *2015*, 1–11.

87. Bailey, S.R.; Nelson, M.H.; Himes, R.A.; Li, Z.; Mehrotra, S.; Paulos, C.M. Th17 cells in cancer: The ultimate identity crisis. *Front. Immunol.* **2014**, *5*, 276.

88. Li, J.; Lau, G.; Chen, L.; Yuan, Y.-F.; Huang, J.; Luk, J.M.; Xie, D.; Guan, X.-Y. Interleukin 23 promotes hepatocellular carcinoma metastasis via nf-kappa b induced matrix metalloproteinase 9 expression. *PLoS ONE* **2012**, *7*, e46264. [CrossRef]

89. Chang, H.-H.; Young, S.H.; Sinnett-Smith, J.; Chou, C.E.N.; Moro, A.; Hertzer, K.M.; Hines, O.J.; Rozengurt, E.; Eibl, G. Prostaglandin e2 activates the mtorc1 pathway through an ep4/camp/pka-and ep1/ca2+-mediated mechanism in the human pancreatic carcinoma cell line panc-1. *Am. J. Physiol.-Cell Physiol.* **2015**, *309*, C639–C649. [CrossRef]

90. Sheng, S.; Zhang, J.; Ai, J.; Hao, X.; Luan, R. Aberrant expression of il-23/il-23r in patients with breast cancer and its clinical significance. *Mol. Med. Rep.* **2018**, *17*, 4639–4644.

91. Elessawi, D.F.; Alkady, M.M.; Ibrahim, I.M. Diagnostic and prognostic value of serum il-23 in colorectal cancer. *Arab J. Gastroenterol.* **2019**, *20*, 65–68. [CrossRef] [PubMed]

92. Stanilov, N.; Miteva, L.; Jovchev, J.; Cirovski, G.; Stanilova, S. The prognostic value of preoperative serum levels of il-12p40 and il-23 for survival of patients with colorectal cancer. *Apmis* **2014**, *122*, 1223–1229. [CrossRef] [PubMed]

93. Neurath, M.F. Il-23 in inflammatory bowel diseases and colon cancer. *Cytokine Growth Factor Rev.* **2019**, *45*, 1–8. [CrossRef] [PubMed]

94. Hmid, A.B.; Selmi, O.; Rekik, R.; Lamari, H.; Zamali, I.; Ladeb, S.; Safra, I.; Othman, T.B.; Romdhane, N.B.; Ahmed, M.B. Rorc overexpression as a sign of th17 lymphocytes accumulation in multiple myeloma bone marrow. *Cytokine* **2020**, *134*, 155210. [CrossRef]

95. Koh, J.; Kim, H.Y.; Lee, Y.; Park, I.K.; Kang, C.H.; Kim, Y.T.; Kim, J.-E.; Choi, M.; Lee, W.-W.; Jeon, Y.K. Il23-producing human lung cancer cells promote tumor growth via conversion of innate lymphoid cell 1 (ilc1) into ilc3. *Clin. Cancer Res.* **2019**, *25*, 4026–4037. [CrossRef]

96. Khodadadi, A.; Razmkhah, M.; Eskandari, A.-R.; Hosseini, A.; Habibagahi, M.; Ghaderi, A.; Jaberipour, M. Il-23/il-27 ratio in peripheral blood of patients with breast cancer. *Iran. J. Med. Sci.* **2014**, *39*, 350–356.

97. Liu, Y.; Song, Y.; Lin, D.; Lei, L.; Mei, Y.; Jin, Z.; Gong, H.; Zhu, Y.; Hu, B.; Zhang, Y. Ncr−group 3 innate lymphoid cells orchestrate il-23/il-17 axis to promote hepatocellular carcinoma development. *EBioMedicine* **2019**, *41*, 333–344. [CrossRef]

98. Calcinotto, A.; Spataro, C.; Zagato, E.; di Mitri, D.; Gil, V.; Crespo, M.; de Bernardis, G.; Losa, M.; Mirenda, M.; Pasquini, E. Il-23 secreted by myeloid cells drives castration-resistant prostate cancer. *Nature* **2018**, *559*, 363–369.

99. Fu, Q.; Xu, L.; Wang, Y.; Jiang, Q.; Liu, Z.; Zhang, J.; Zhou, Q.; Zeng, H.; Tong, S.; Wang, T. Tumor-associated macrophage-derived interleukin-23 interlinks kidney cancer glutamine addiction with immune evasion. *Eur. Urol.* **2019**, *75*, 752–763.

100. Błogowski, W.; Deskur, A.; Budkowska, M.; Sałata, D.; Madej-Michniewicz, A.; Dąbkowski, K.; Dołęgowska, B.; Starzyńska, T. Selected cytokines in patients with pancreatic cancer: A preliminary report. *PLoS ONE* **2014**, *9*, e97613. [CrossRef]

101. Hussain, S.M.; Reed, L.F.; Krasnick, B.A.; Miranda-Carboni, G.; Fields, R.C.; Bi, Y.; Elahi, A.; Ajidahun, A.; Dickson, P.V.; Deneve, J.L. Il23 and tgf-ss diminish macrophage associated metastasis in pancreatic carcinoma. *Sci. Rep.* **2018**, *8*, 1–9. [CrossRef] [PubMed]

102. Caughron, B.; Yang, Y.; Young, M.R.I. Role of il-23 signaling in the progression of premalignant oral lesions to cancer. *PLoS ONE* **2018**, *13*, e0196034. [CrossRef] [PubMed]

103. Baird, A.-M.; Leonard, J.; Naicker, K.M.; Kilmartin, L.; O'Byrne, K.J.; Gray, S.G. Il-23 is pro-proliferative, epigenetically regulated and modulated by chemotherapy in non-small cell lung cancer. *Lung Cancer* **2013**, *79*, 83–90. [CrossRef] [PubMed]

104. Fukuda, M.; Ehara, M.; Suzuki, S.; Ohmori, Y.; Sakashita, H. Il-23 promotes growth and proliferation in human squamous cell carcinoma of the oral cavity. *Int. J. Oncol.* **2010**, *36*, 1355–1365. [CrossRef] [PubMed]

105. Nie, W.; Yu, T.; Sang, Y.; Gao, X. Tumor-promoting effect of il-23 in mammary cancer mediated by infiltration of m2 macrophages and neutrophils in tumor microenvironment. *Biochem. Biophys. Res. Commun.* **2017**, *482*, 1400–1406. [CrossRef] [PubMed]

106. Kortlever, R.M.; Sodir, N.M.; Wilson, C.H.; Burkhart, D.L.; Pellegrinet, L.; Swigart, L.B.; Littlewood, T.D.; Evan, G.I. Myc cooperates with ras by programming inflammation and immune suppression. *Cell* **2017**, *171*, 1301–1315.e14. [CrossRef]

107. Zhang, Q.; Liu, S.; Zhang, Q.; Xiong, Z.; Wang, A.R.; Myers, L.; Melamed, J.; Tang, W.W.; You, Z. Interleukin-17 promotes development of castration-resistant prostate cancer potentially through creating an immunotolerant and pro-angiogenic tumor microenvironment. *Prostate* **2014**, *74*, 869–879. [CrossRef]

108. Wang, D.; Shao, Y.; Zhang, X.; Lu, G.; Liu, B. Il-23 and psma-targeted duo-car t cells in prostate cancer eradication in a preclinical model. *J. Transl. Med.* **2020**, *18*, 1–10. [CrossRef]

109. Testa, U.; Castelli, G.; Pelosi, E. Cellular and molecular mechanisms underlying prostate cancer development: Therapeutic implications. *Medicines* **2019**, *6*, 82. [CrossRef]

110. Ma, X.; Shou, P.; Smith, C.; Chen, Y.; Du, H.; Sun, C.; Kren, N.P.; Michaud, D.; Ahn, S.; Vincent, B. Interleukin-23 engineering improves car t cell function in solid tumors. *Nat. Biotechnol.* **2020**, *38*, 448–459. [CrossRef]

111. Fabbi, M.; Carbotti, G.; Ferrini, S. Dual roles of il-27 in cancer biology and immunotherapy. *Mediat. Inflamm.* **2017**, *2017*. [CrossRef] [PubMed]

112. Pot, C.; Apetoh, L.; Awasthi, A.; Kuchroo, V.K. Induction of regulatory tr1 cells and inhibition of th17 cells by il-27. *Semin. Immunol.* **2011**, *23*, 438–445. [CrossRef]

113. Pot, C.; Apetoh, L.; Awasthi, A.; Kuchroo, V.K. Molecular pathways in the induction of interleukin-27-driven regulatory type 1 cells. *J. Interf. Cytokine Res.* **2010**, *30*, 381–388. [CrossRef] [PubMed]

114. Murugaiyan, G.; Saha, B. Il-27 in tumor immunity and immunotherapy. *Trends Mol. Med.* **2013**, *19*, 108–116. [CrossRef] [PubMed]

115. Murugaiyan, G.; Mittal, A.; Lopez-Diego, R.; Maier, L.M.; Anderson, D.E.; Weiner, H.L. Il-27 is a key regulator of il-10 and il-17 production by human cd4+ T cells. *J. Immunol.* **2009**, *183*, 2435–2443. [CrossRef] [PubMed]

116. Qi, J.; Zhang, Z.; Tang, X.; Li, W.; Chen, W.; Yao, G. Il-27 regulated cd4+ il-10+ T cells in experimental sjögren syndrome. *Front. Immunol.* **2020**, *11*, 1699. [CrossRef]

117. Pot, C.; Jin, H.; Awasthi, A.; Liu, S.M.; Lai, C.-Y.; Madan, R.; Sharpe, A.H.; Karp, C.L.; Miaw, S.-C.; Ho, I.-C. Cutting edge: Il-27 induces the transcription factor c-maf, cytokine il-21, and the costimulatory receptor icos that coordinately act together to promote differentiation of il-10-producing tr1 cells. *J. Immunol.* **2009**, *183*, 797–801. [CrossRef]

118. Chang, K.-K.; Liu, L.-B.; Jin, L.-P.; Zhang, B.; Mei, J.; Li, H.; Wei, C.-Y.; Zhou, W.-J.; Zhu, X.-Y.; Shao, J. Il-27 triggers il-10 production in th17 cells via a c-maf/ror γ t/blimp-1 signal to promote the progression of endometriosis. *Cell Death Dis.* **2017**, *8*, e2666. [CrossRef]

119. Guzzo, C.; Mat, N.F.C.; Gee, K. Interleukin-27 induces a stat1/3-and nf-κb-dependent proinflammatory cytokine profile in human monocytes. *J. Biol. Chem.* **2010**, *285*, 24404–24411. [CrossRef]

120. Wang, N.; Liang, H.; Zen, K. Molecular mechanisms that influence the macrophage m1–m2 polarization balance. *Front. Immunol.* **2014**, *5*, 614. [CrossRef]

121. Lu, Y.; Xu, W.; Gu, Y.; Chang, X.; Wei, G.; Rong, Z.; Qin, L.; Chen, X.; Zhou, F. Non-small cell lung cancer cells modulate the development of human cd1c+ conventional dendritic cell subsets mediated by cd103 and cd205. *Front. Immunol.* **2019**, *10*, 2829. [CrossRef] [PubMed]

122. Iwasaki, Y.; Fujio, K.; Okamura, T.; Yamamoto, K. Interleukin-27 in t cell immunity. *Int. J. Mol. Sci.* **2015**, *16*, 2851–2863. [CrossRef] [PubMed]

123. Owaki, T.; Asakawa, M.; Morishima, N.; Hata, K.; Fukai, F.; Matsui, M.; Mizuguchi, J.; Yoshimoto, T. A role for il-27 in early regulation of th1 differentiation. *J. Immunol.* **2005**, *175*, 2191–2200. [CrossRef] [PubMed]

124. Kamiya, S.; Owaki, T.; Morishima, N.; Fukai, F.; Mizuguchi, J.; Yoshimoto, T. An indispensable role for stat1 in il-27-induced t-bet expression but not proliferation of naive cd4+ T cells. *J. Immunol.* **2004**, *173*, 3871–3877. [CrossRef]

125. Feng, X.M.; Liu, N.; Yang, S.G.; Hu, L.Y.; Chen, X.L.; Fang, Z.H.; Ren, Q.; Lu, S.H.; Liu, B.; Han, Z.C. Regulation of the class ii and class i mhc pathways in human thp-1 monocytic cells by interleukin-27. *Biochem. Biophys. Res. Commun.* **2008**, *367*, 553–559. [CrossRef]

126. Torrado, E.; Fountain, J.; Pearl, J.; Cooper, A. Il-27 sustains t-bet expression and promotes the development of terminally differentiated cd4 T cells during tuberculosis (59.5). *Am. Assoc. Immnol.* **2012**, *188* (Suppl. 1), 59.5.

127. Hirahara, K.; Onodera, A.; Villarino, A.V.; Bonelli, M.; Sciumè, G.; Laurence, A.; Sun, H.-W.; Brooks, S.R.; Vahedi, G.; Shih, H.-Y. Asymmetric action of stat transcription factors drives transcriptional outputs and cytokine specificity. *Immunity* **2015**, *42*, 877–889. [CrossRef]

128. Schneider, R.; Yaneva, T.; Beauseigle, D.; El-Khoury, L.; Arbour, N. Il-27 increases the proliferation and effector functions of human naive cd8+ t lymphocytes and promotes their development into tc1 cells. *Eur. J. Immunol.* **2011**, *41*, 47–59. [CrossRef]

129. Morishima, N.; Mizoguchi, I.; Okumura, M.; Chiba, Y.; Xu, M.; Shimizu, M.; Matsui, M.; Mizuguchi, J.; Yoshimoto, T. A pivotal role for interleukin-27 in cd8+ T cell functions and generation of cytotoxic t lymphocytes. *J. Biomed. Biotechnol.* **2010**, *2010*, 1–10. [CrossRef]

130. Gotthardt, D.; Trifinopoulos, J.; Sexl, V.; Putz, E.M. Jak/stat cytokine signaling at the crossroad of nk cell development and maturation. *Front. Immunol.* **2019**, *10*, 2590. [CrossRef]

131. Choi, Y.H.; Lim, E.J.; Kim, S.W.; Moon, Y.W.; Park, K.S.; An, H.-J. Il-27 enhances il-15/il-18-mediated activation of human natural killer cells. *J. Immunother. Cancer* **2019**, *7*, 168. [CrossRef] [PubMed]

132. Hisada, M.; Kamiya, S.; Fujita, K.; Belladonna, M.L.; Aoki, T.; Koyanagi, Y.; Mizuguchi, J.; Yoshimoto, T. Potent antitumor activity of interleukin-27. *Cancer Res.* **2004**, *64*, 1152–1156. [CrossRef] [PubMed]

133. Villarino, A.V.; Stumhofer, J.S.; Saris, C.J.; Kastelein, R.A.; de Sauvage, F.J.; Hunter, C.A. Il-27 limits il-2 production during th1 differentiation. *J. Immunol.* **2006**, *176*, 237–247. [CrossRef] [PubMed]

134. Owaki, T.; Asakawa, M.; Kamiya, S.; Takeda, K.; Fukai, F.; Mizuguchi, J.; Yoshimoto, T. Il-27 suppresses cd28-medicated il-2 production through suppressor of cytokine signaling 3. *J. Immunol.* **2006**, *176*, 2773–2780. [CrossRef]

135. Zhou, W.-J.; Chang, K.-K.; Wu, K.; Yang, H.-L.; Mei, J.; Xie, F.; Li, D.-J.; Li, M.-Q. Rapamycin synergizes with cisplatin in antiendometrial cancer activation by improving il-27–stimulated cytotoxicity of nk cells. *Neoplasia* **2018**, *20*, 69–79. [CrossRef] [PubMed]

136. Zhang, Z.; Zhou, B.; Zhang, K.; Song, Y.; Zhang, L.; Xi, M. Il-27 suppresses skov3 cells proliferation by enhancing stat3 and inhibiting the akt signal pathway. *Mol. Immunol.* **2016**, *78*, 155–163. [CrossRef] [PubMed]

137. Li, Q.; Sato, A.; Shimozato, O.; Shingyoji, M.; Tada, Y.; Tatsumi, K.; Shimada, H.; Hiroshima, K.; Tagawa, M. Administration of DNA encoding the interleukin-27 gene augments antitumour responses through non-adaptive immunity. *Scand. J. Immunol.* **2015**, *82*, 320–327. [CrossRef] [PubMed]

138. Chiba, Y.; Mizoguchi, I.; Furusawa, J.; Hasegawa, H.; Ohashi, M.; Xu, M.; Owaki, T.; Yoshimoto, T. Interleukin-27 exerts its antitumor effects by promoting differentiation of hematopoietic stem cells to m1 macrophages. *Cancer Res.* **2018**, *78*, 182–194. [CrossRef] [PubMed]

139. Yao, L.; Wang, M.; Niu, Z.; Liu, Q.; Gao, X.; Zhou, L.; Liao, Q.; Zhao, Y. Interleukin-27 inhibits malignant behaviors of pancreatic cancer cells by targeting m2 polarized tumor associated macrophages. *Cytokine* **2017**, *89*, 194–200. [CrossRef] [PubMed]

140. Carbotti, G.; Nikpoor, A.R.; Vacca, P.; Gangemi, R.; Giordano, C.; Campelli, F.; Ferrini, S.; Fabbi, M. Il-27 mediates hla class i up-regulation, which can be inhibited by the il-6 pathway, in hla-deficient small cell lung cancer cells. *J. Exp. Clin. Cancer Res.* **2017**, *36*, 140. [CrossRef]

141. Airoldi, I.; Tupone, M.G.; Esposito, S.; Russo, M.V.; Barbarito, G.; Cipollone, G.; di Carlo, E. Interleukin-27 re-educates intratumoral myeloid cells and down-regulates stemness genes in non-small cell lung cancer. *Oncotarget* **2015**, *6*, 3694–3708. [CrossRef] [PubMed]

142. Kourko, O.; Smyth, R.; Cino, D.; Seaver, K.; Petes, C.; Eo, S.Y.; Basta, S.; Gee, K. Poly (i: C)-mediated death of human prostate cancer cell lines is induced by interleukin-27 treatment. *J. Interf. Cytokine Res.* **2019**, *39*, 483–494. [CrossRef] [PubMed]

143. Wang, G.-Q.; Zhao, W.-H.; Zhao, X.-X.; Zhang, J.; Nan, K.-J. Association between il-27 2905t/g genotypes and the risk and survival of cervical cancer: A case-control study. *Biomarkers* **2016**, *21*, 272–275. [CrossRef] [PubMed]

144. Majumder, D.; Debnath, R.; Maiti, D. Il-27 along with il-28b ameliorates the pulmonary redox impairment, inflammation and immunosuppression in benzo (a) pyrene induced lung cancer bearing mice. *Life Sci.* **2020**, *260*, 118384. [CrossRef] [PubMed]

145. Zhu, J.; Liu, J.-Q.; Shi, M.; Cheng, X.; Ding, M.; Zhang, J.C.; Davis, J.P.; Varikuti, S.; Satoskar, A.R.; Lu, L. Il-27 gene therapy induces depletion of tregs and enhances the efficacy of cancer immunotherapy. *JCI Insight* **2018**, *3*. [CrossRef]

146. Hu, A.; Ding, M.; Zhu, J.; Liu, J.-Q.; Pan, X.; Ghoshal, K.; Bai, X.-F. Intra-tumoral delivery of il-27 using adeno-associated virus stimulates anti-tumor immunity and enhances the efficacy of immunotherapy. *Front. Cell Dev. Biol.* **2020**, *8*, 210. [CrossRef]

147. Yan, H.; Viswanadhapalli, S.; Chupp, D.; Fernandez, M.; Wu, S.; Wang, J.; Moroney, J.; Taylor, J.; Im, J.; Rivera, C. B cell-produced il-27 up-regulates pd-l1 expression in the tumor microenvironment to promote breast cancer development. *AACR* **2019**. [CrossRef]

148. Chen, S.; Crabill, G.A.; Pritchard, T.S.; McMiller, T.L.; Wei, P.; Pardoll, D.M.; Pan, F.; Topalian, S.L. Mechanisms regulating pd-l1 expression on tumor and immune cells. *J. Immunother. Cancer* **2019**, *7*, 1–12. [CrossRef]

149. Carbotti, G.; Barisione, G.; Airoldi, I.; Mezzanzanica, D.; Bagnoli, M.; Ferrero, S.; Petretto, A.; Fabbi, M.; Ferrini, S. Il-27 induces the expression of ido and pd-l1 in human cancer cells. *Oncotarget* **2015**, *6*, 43267–43280. [CrossRef]

150. Rolvering, C.; Zimmer, A.D.; Ginolhac, A.; Margue, C.; Kirchmeyer, M.; Servais, F.; Hermanns, H.M.; Hergovits, S.; Nazarov, P.V.; Nicot, N. The pd-l1-and il6-mediated dampening of the il27/stat1 anticancer responses are prevented by α-pd-l1 or α-il6 antibodies. *J. Leukoc. Biol.* **2018**, *104*, 969–985. [CrossRef]

151. Horlad, H.; Ma, C.; Yano, H.; Pan, C.; Ohnishi, K.; Fujiwara, Y.; Endo, S.; Kikukawa, Y.; Okuno, Y.; Matsuoka, M. An il-27/stat3 axis induces expression of programmed cell death 1 ligands (pd-l1/2) on infiltrating macrophages in lymphoma. *Cancer Sci.* **2016**, *107*, 1696–1704. [CrossRef] [PubMed]

152. Meissl, K.; Macho-Maschler, S.; Müller, M.; Strobl, B. The good and the bad faces of stat1 in solid tumours. *Cytokine* **2017**, *89*, 12–20. [CrossRef] [PubMed]

153. Zhu, C.; Sakuishi, K.; Xiao, S.; Sun, Z.; Zaghouani, S.; Gu, G.; Wang, C.; Tan, D.J.; Wu, C.; Rangachari, M. An il-27/nfil3 signalling axis drives tim-3 and il-10 expression and t-cell dysfunction. *Nat. Commun.* **2015**, *6*, 1–12.

154. Anderson, A.C.; Joller, N.; Kuchroo, V.K. Lag-3, tim-3, and tigit: Co-inhibitory receptors with specialized functions in immune regulation. *Immunity* **2016**, *44*, 989–1004. [CrossRef]

155. Park, Y.-J.; Ryu, H.; Choi, G.; Kim, B.-S.; Hwang, E.S.; Kim, H.S.; Chung, Y. Il-27 confers a protumorigenic activity of regulatory t cells via cd39. *Proc. Natl. Acad. Sci. USA* **2019**, *116*, 3106–3111. [CrossRef]

156. d'Almeida, S.M.; Kauffenstein, G.; Roy, C.; Basset, L.; Papargyris, L.; Henrion, D.; Catros, V.; Ifrah, N.; Descamps, P.; Croue, A. The ecto-atpdase cd39 is involved in the acquisition of the immunoregulatory phenotype by m-csf-macrophages and ovarian cancer tumor-associated macrophages: Regulatory role of il-27. *Oncoimmunology* **2016**, *5*, e1178025. [CrossRef]

157. Pylayeva-Gupta, Y. Molecular pathways: Interleukin-35 in autoimmunity and cancer. *Clin. Cancer Res.* **2016**, *22*, 4973–4978. [CrossRef]

158. Hao, S.; Chen, X.; Wang, F.; Shao, Q.; Liu, J.; Zhao, H.; Yuan, C.; Ren, H.; Mao, H. Breast cancer cell–derived il-35 promotes tumor progression via induction of il-35-producing induced regulatory T cells. *Carcinogenesis* **2018**, *39*, 1488–1496. [CrossRef]

159. Lee, C.-C.; Lin, J.-C.; Hwang, W.-L.; Kuo, Y.-J.; Chen, H.-K.; Tai, S.-K.; Lin, C.-C.; Yang, M.-H. Macrophage-secreted interleukin-35 regulates cancer cell plasticity to facilitate metastatic colonization. *Nat. Commun.* **2018**, *9*, 1–18.

160. Wang, Z.; Liu, J.-Q.; Liu, Z.; Shen, R.; Zhang, G.; Xu, J.; Basu, S.; Feng, Y.; Bai, X.-F. Tumor-derived il-35 promotes tumor growth by enhancing myeloid cell accumulation and angiogenesis. *J. Immunol.* **2013**, *190*, 2415–2423. [CrossRef]

161. Collison, L.W.; Workman, C.J.; Kuo, T.T.; Boyd, K.; Wang, Y.; Vignali, K.M.; Cross, R.; Sehy, D.; Blumberg, R.S.; Vignali, D.A. The inhibitory cytokine il-35 contributes to regulatory T-cell function. *Nature* **2007**, *450*, 566–569. [CrossRef] [PubMed]

162. Niedbala, W.; Wei, X.q.; Cai, B.; Hueber, A.J.; Leung, B.P.; McInnes, I.B.; Liew, F.Y. Il-35 is a novel cytokine with therapeutic effects against collagen-induced arthritis through the expansion of regulatory t cells and suppression of th17 cells. *Eur. J. Immunol.* **2007**, *37*, 3021–3029. [CrossRef] [PubMed]

163. Wirtz, S.; Billmeier, U.; Mchedlidze, T.; Blumberg, R.S.; Neurath, M.F. Interleukin-35 mediates mucosal immune responses that protect against t-cell–dependent colitis. *Gastroenterology* **2011**, *141*, 1875–1886. [CrossRef] [PubMed]

164. Liu, J.-Q.; Liu, Z.; Zhang, X.; Shi, Y.; Talebian, F.; Carl, J.W.; Yu, C.; Shi, F.-D.; Whitacre, C.C.; Trgovcich, J. Increased th17 and regulatory T cell responses in ebv-induced gene 3-deficient mice lead to marginally enhanced development of autoimmune encephalomyelitis. *J. Immunol.* **2012**, *188*, 3099–3106. [CrossRef] [PubMed]

165. Mirlekar, B.; Michaud, D.; Searcy, R.; Greene, K.; Pylayeva-Gupta, Y. Il35 hinders endogenous antitumor t-cell immunity and responsiveness to immunotherapy in pancreatic cancer. *Cancer Immunol. Res.* **2018**, *6*, 1014–1024. [CrossRef] [PubMed]

166. Turnis, M.E.; Sawant, D.V.; Szymczak-Workman, A.L.; Andrews, L.P.; Delgoffe, G.M.; Yano, H.; Beres, A.J.; Vogel, P.; Workman, C.J.; Vignali, D.A. Interleukin-35 limits anti-tumor immunity. *Immunity* **2016**, *44*, 316–329. [CrossRef] [PubMed]

167. Jiang, H.; Zhang, T.; Yan, M.-X.; Wu, W. Il-35 inhibits cd8 (+) T cells activity by suppressing expression of costimulatory molecule cd28 and th1 cytokine production. *Transl. Cancer Res.* **2019**, *8*, 1319–1325. [CrossRef]

168. Yang, L.; Shao, X.; Jia, S.; Zhang, Q.; Jin, Z. Interleukin-35 dampens cd8+ T cells activity in patients with non-viral hepatitis-related hepatocellular carcinoma. *Front. Immunol.* **2019**, *10*, 1032. [CrossRef]

169. Mirlekar, B.; Michaud, D.; Lee, S.J.; Kren, N.P.; Harris, C.; Greene, K.; Goldman, E.C.; Gupta, G.P.; Fields, R.C.; Hawkins, W.G. B cell–derived il35 drives stat3-dependent cd8+ T-cell exclusion in pancreatic cancer. *Cancer Immunol. Res.* **2020**, *8*, 292–308. [CrossRef]

170. Wang, K.; Liu, J.; Li, J. Il-35-producing b cells in gastric cancer patients. *Medicine* **2018**, *97*, e0710. [CrossRef]

171. Collison, L.W.; Delgoffe, G.M.; Guy, C.S.; Vignali, K.M.; Chaturvedi, V.; Fairweather, D.; Satoskar, A.R.; Garcia, K.C.; Hunter, C.A.; Drake, C.G. The composition and signaling of the il-35 receptor are unconventional. *Nat. Immunol.* **2012**, *13*, 290–299. [CrossRef] [PubMed]

172. Collison, L.W.; Chaturvedi, V.; Henderson, A.L.; Giacomin, P.R.; Guy, C.; Bankoti, J.; Finkelstein, D.; Forbes, K.; Workman, C.J.; Brown, S.A. Il-35-mediated induction of a potent regulatory t cell population. *Nat. Immunol.* **2010**, *11*, 1093–1101. [CrossRef] [PubMed]

173. Dambuza, I.M.; He, C.; Choi, J.K.; Yu, C.-R.; Wang, R.; Mattapallil, M.J.; Wingfield, P.T.; Caspi, R.R.; Egwuagu, C.E. Il-12p35 induces expansion of il-10 and il-35-expressing regulatory B cells and ameliorates autoimmune disease. *Nat. Commun.* **2017**, *8*, 1–12.

174. Wang, R.-X.; Yu, C.-R.; Dambuza, I.M.; Mahdi, R.M.; Dolinska, M.B.; Sergeev, Y.V.; Wingfield, P.T.; Kim, S.-H.; Egwuagu, C.E. Interleukin-35 induces regulatory B cells that suppress autoimmune disease. *Nat. Med.* **2014**, *20*, 633–641. [CrossRef] [PubMed]

175. Tao, Q.; Pan, Y.; Wang, Y.; Wang, H.; Xiong, S.; Li, Q.; Wang, J.; Tao, L.; Wang, Z.; Wu, F. Regulatory T cells-derived il-35 promotes the growth of adult acute myeloid leukemia blasts. *Int. J. Cancer* **2015**, *137*, 2384–2393. [CrossRef]

176. Wang, H.-M.; Zhang, X.-H.; Feng, M.-M.; Qiao, Y.-J.; Ye, L.-Q.; Chen, J.; Fan, F.-F.; Guo, L.-L. Interleukin-35 suppresses the antitumor activity of T cells in patients with non-small cell lung cancer. *Cell. Physiol. Biochem.* **2018**, *47*, 2407–2419. [CrossRef]

177. Zou, J.-M.; Qin, J.; Li, Y.-C.; Wang, Y.; Li, D.; Shu, Y.; Luo, C.; Wang, S.-S.; Chi, G.; Guo, F. Il-35 induces n2 phenotype of neutrophils to promote tumor growth. *Oncotarget* **2017**, *8*, 33501–33514. [CrossRef]
178. Zhang, J.; Lin, Y.; Li, C.; Zhang, X.; Cheng, L.; Dai, L.; Wang, Y.; Wang, F.; Shi, G.; Li, Y. Il-35 decelerates the inflammatory process by regulating inflammatory cytokine secretion and m1/m2 macrophage ratio in psoriasis. *J. Immunol.* **2016**, *197*, 2131–2144. [CrossRef]
179. Ye, J.; Huang, Y.; Que, B.; Chang, C.; Liu, W.; Hu, H.; Liu, L.; Shi, Y.; Wang, Y.; Wang, M. Interleukin-12p35 knock out aggravates doxorubicin-induced cardiac injury and dysfunction by aggravating the inflammatory response, oxidative stress, apoptosis and autophagy in mice. *EBioMedicine* **2018**, *35*, 29–39. [CrossRef]
180. Haller, S.; Duval, A.; Migliorini, R.; Stevanin, M.; Mack, V.; Acha-Orbea, H. Interleukin-35-producing cd8α+ dendritic cells acquire a tolerogenic state and regulate t cell function. *Front. Immunol.* **2017**, *8*, 98. [CrossRef]
181. Dixon, K.O.; van der Kooij, S.W.; Vignali, D.A.; van Kooten, C. Human tolerogenic dendritic cells produce il-35 in the absence of other il-12 family members. *Eur. J. Immunol.* **2015**, *45*, 1736–1747. [CrossRef] [PubMed]
182. Liu, X.; Sun, Y.; Zheng, Y.; Zhang, M.; Jin, X.; Kang, K.; Wang, Y.; Li, S.; Zhang, H.; Zhao, Q. Administration of interleukin-35-conditioned autologous tolerogenic dendritic cells prolong allograft survival after heart transplantation. *Cell. Physiol. Biochem.* **2018**, *49*, 1221–1237. [CrossRef] [PubMed]
183. Xue, W.; Yan, D.; Kan, Q. Interleukin-35 as an emerging player in tumor microenvironment. *J. Cancer* **2019**, *10*, 2074–2082. [CrossRef]
184. Zhu, J.; Yang, X.; Wang, Y.; Zhang, H.; Guo, Z. Interleukin-35 is associated with the tumorigenesis and progression of prostate cancer. *Oncol. Lett.* **2019**, *17*, 5094–5102. [CrossRef] [PubMed]
185. Heim, L.; Kachler, K.; Siegmund, R.; Trufa, D.I.; Mittler, S.; Geppert, C.-I.; Friedrich, J.; Rieker, R.J.; Sirbu, H.; Finotto, S. Increased expression of the immunosuppressive interleukin-35 in patients with non-small cell lung cancer. *Br. J. Cancer* **2019**, *120*, 903–912. [CrossRef]
186. Ma, Y.; Chen, L.; Xie, G.; Zhou, Y.; Yue, C.; Yuan, X.; Zheng, Y.; Wang, W.; Deng, L.; Shen, L. Elevated level of interleukin-35 in colorectal cancer induces conversion of t cells into itr35 by activating stat1/stat3. *Oncotarget* **2016**, *7*, 73003–73015. [CrossRef]
187. Zhang, J.; Mao, T.; Wang, S.; Wang, D.; Niu, Z.; Sun, Z.; Zhang, J. Interleukin-35 expression is associated with colon cancer progression. *Oncotarget* **2017**, *8*, 71563–71573. [CrossRef]
188. Sun, M.; Zheng, X.; Meng, Q.; Dong, Y.; Zhang, G.; Rao, D.; An, X.; Yang, Z.; Pan, L.; Zhang, S. Interleukin-35 expression in non-small cell lung cancer is associated with tumor progression. *Cell. Physiol. Biochem.* **2018**, *51*, 1839–1851. [CrossRef]
189. Jiang, Q.; Ma, L.; Li, R.; Sun, J. Colon cancer-induced interleukin-35 inhibits beta-catenin-mediated pro-oncogenic activity. *Oncotarget* **2018**, *9*, 11989–11998. [CrossRef]
190. Long, J.; Guo, H.; Cui, S.; Zhang, H.; Liu, X.; Li, D.; Han, Z.; Xi, L.; Kou, W.; Xu, J. Il-35 expression in hepatocellular carcinoma cells is associated with tumor progression. *Oncotarget* **2016**, *7*, 45678–45686. [CrossRef]
191. Chatrabnous, N.; Ghaderi, A.; Ariafar, A.; Razeghinia, M.S.; Nemati, M.; Jafarzadeh, A. Serum concentration of interleukin-35 and its association with tumor stages and foxp3 gene polymorphism in patients with prostate cancer. *Cytokine* **2019**, *113*, 221–227. [CrossRef]
192. Chen, G.; Liang, Y.; Guan, X.; Chen, H.; Liu, Q.; Lin, B.; Chen, C.; Huang, M.; Chen, J.; Wu, W. Circulating low il-23: Il-35 cytokine ratio promotes progression associated with poor prognosisin breast cancer. *Am. J. Transl. Res.* **2016**, *8*, 2255–2264.
193. Larousserie, F.; Kebe, D.; Huynh, T.; Audebourg, A.; Tamburini, J.; Terris, B.; Devergne, O. Evidence for il-35 expression in diffuse large b-cell lymphoma and impact on the patient's prognosis. *Front. Oncol.* **2019**, *9*, 563. [CrossRef]
194. Wang, J.; Tao, Q.; Wang, H.; Wang, Z.; Wu, F.; Pan, Y.; Tao, L.; Xiong, S.; Wang, Y.; Zhai, Z. Elevated il-35 in bone marrow of the patients with acute myeloid leukemia. *Hum. Immunol.* **2015**, *76*, 681–686. [CrossRef]
195. Huang, C.; Li, N.; Li, Z.; Chang, A.; Chen, Y.; Zhao, T.; Li, Y.; Wang, X.; Zhang, W.; Wang, Z. Tumour-derived interleukin 35 promotes pancreatic ductal adenocarcinoma cell extravasation and metastasis by inducing icam1 expression. *Nat. Commun.* **2017**, *8*, 1–15.
196. Nicholl, M.B.; Ledgewood, C.L.; Chen, X.; Bai, Q.; Qin, C.; Cook, K.M.; Herrick, E.J.; Diaz-Arias, A.; Moore, B.J.; Fang, Y. Il-35 promotes pancreas cancer growth through enhancement of proliferation and inhibition of apoptosis: Evidence for a role as an autocrine growth factor. *Cytokine* **2014**, *70*, 126–133. [CrossRef]
197. Jin, P.; Ren, H.; Sun, W.; Xin, W.; Zhang, H.; Hao, J. Circulating il-35 in pancreatic ductal adenocarcinoma patients. *Hum. Immunol.* **2014**, *75*, 29–33. [CrossRef]
198. Wang, X.; Wei, Y.; Xiao, H.; Liu, X.; Zhang, Y.; Han, G.; Chen, G.; Hou, C.; Ma, N.; Shen, B. A novel il-23p19/ebi3 (il-39) cytokine mediates inflammation in lupus-like mice. *Eur. J. Immunol.* **2016**, *46*, 1343–1350. [CrossRef]
199. Wang, X.; Liu, X.; Zhang, Y.; Wang, Z.; Zhu, G.; Han, G.; Chen, G.; Hou, C.; Wang, T.; Ma, N. Interleukin (il)-39 [il-23p19/epstein–barr virus-induced 3 (ebi3)] induces differentiation/expansion of neutrophils in lupus-prone mice. *Clin. Exp. Immunol.* **2016**, *186*, 144–156. [CrossRef] [PubMed]
200. Manning, A.A.; Zhao, L.; Zhu, Z.; Xiao, H.; Redington, C.G.; Ding, V.A.; Stewart-Hester, T.; Bai, Q.; Dunlap, J.; Wakefield, M.R. Il-39 acts as a friend to pancreatic cancer. *Med. Oncol.* **2019**, *36*, 22. [CrossRef]
201. Hawkes, J.E.; Yan, B.Y.; Chan, T.C.; Krueger, J.G. Discovery of the il-23/il-17 signaling pathway and the treatment of psoriasis. *J. Immunol.* **2018**, *201*, 1605–1613. [CrossRef]

202. Hasegawa, H.; Mizoguchi, I.; Chiba, Y.; Ohashi, M.; Xu, M.; Yoshimoto, T. Expanding diversity in molecular structures and functions of the il-6/il-12 heterodimeric cytokine family. *Front. Immunol.* **2016**, *7*, 479. [CrossRef]
203. Floss, D.; Schönberg, M.; Franke, M.; Horstmeier, F.; Engelowski, E.; Schneider, A.; Rosenfeldt, E.; Scheller, J. Il-6/il-12 cytokine receptor shuffling of extra-and intracellular domains reveals canonical stat activation via synthetic il-35 and il-39 signaling. *Sci. Rep.* **2017**, *7*, 1–13.
204. Hu, J.; Sun, C.; Bernatchez, C.; Xia, X.; Hwu, P.; Dotti, G.; Li, S. T-cell homing therapy for reducing regulatory T cells and preserving effector t-cell function in large solid tumors. *Clin. Cancer Res.* **2018**, *24*, 2920–2934. [CrossRef]
205. Berraondo, P.; Etxeberria, I.; Ponz-Sarvise, M.; Melero, I. Revisiting interleukin-12 as a cancer immunotherapy agent. *Clin. Cancer Res.* **2018**, *24*, 2716–2718. [CrossRef]

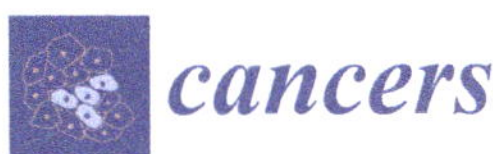

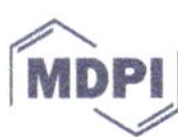

Review

Immunocyte Membrane-Coated Nanoparticles for Cancer Immunotherapy

Ping Gong [1,2,*], Yifan Wang [2], Pengfei Zhang [1], Zhaogang Yang [2], Weiye Deng [2], Zhihong Sun [1,3], Mingming Yang [2], Xuefeng Li [2], Gongcheng Ma [1], Guanjun Deng [1], Shiyan Dong [2], Lintao Cai [1] and Wen Jiang [2,*]

[1] Guangdong Key Laboratory of Nanomedicine, Shenzhen Engineering Laboratory of Nanomedicine and Nanoformulations, CAS-HK Joint Lab for Biomaterials, CAS Key Laboratory of Health Informatics, Institute of Biomedicine and Biotechnology, Shenzhen Institute of Advanced Technology, Chinese Academy of Sciences, Shenzhen 518055, China; pf.zhang@siat.ac.cn (P.Z.); zh.sun@siat.ac.cn (Z.S.); gc.ma@siat.ac.cn (G.M.); gj.deng@siat.ac.cn (G.D.); lt.cai@siat.ac.cn (L.C.)

[2] Department of Radiation Oncology, University of Texas Southwestern Medical Center, 2280 Inwood Road, Dallas, TX 75235, USA; yifan.wang@utsouthwestern.edu (Y.W.); zhaogang.yang@utsouthwestern.edu (Z.Y.); weiye.deng@utsouthwestern.edu (W.D.); mingming.yang@utsouthwestern.edu (M.Y.); xuefeng.li@utsouthwestern.edu (X.L.); shiyan.dong@utsouthwestern.edu (S.D.)

[3] Yantai Yuhuangding Hospital, Yantai 264000, China

[*] Correspondence: ping.gong@siat.ac.cn (P.G.); wen.jiang@utsouthwestern.edu (W.J.); Tel.: +86-755-8639-2223 (P.G.); +1-214-648-8893 (W.J.); Fax: +86-755-8658-5222 (P.G.); +1-214-645-7622 (W.J.)

Simple Summary: Cancer immunotherapy is a breakthrough in cancer treatment. Unfortunately, despite the encouraging results in clinical treatment, cancer immunotherapy such as CAR-T, PD-1 still faces lots of challenges. Therefore, it is necessary to develop new methods to improve the effectiveness and safety of tumor immunotherapy. In recent years, cell membrane-coated nanomaterial is one of the most promising drug delivery systems and is receiving a great deal of attention due to its naturally biocompatible characteristics. This review summarizes the latest research progress, the advantages, the disadvantages, and the application of immunocyte membrane-coated nanoparticles in cancer immunotherapy.

Abstract: Despite the advances in surface bioconjugation of synthetic nanoparticles for targeted drug delivery, simple biological functionalization is still insufficient to replicate complex intercellular interactions naturally. Therefore, these foreign nanoparticles are inevitably exposed to the immune system, which results in phagocytosis by the reticuloendothelial system and thus, loss of their biological significance. Immunocyte membranes play a key role in intercellular interactions, and can protect foreign nanomaterials as a natural barrier. Therefore, biomimetic nanotechnology based on cell membranes has developed rapidly in recent years. This paper summarizes the development of immunocyte membrane-coated nanoparticles in the immunotherapy of tumors. We will introduce several immunocyte membrane-coated nanocarriers and review the challenges to their large-scale preparation and application.

Keywords: immunocyte membrane-coated nanoparticles; biomimicry; cancer immunotherapy; macrophage; T-cell; natural killer; dendritic cell

Citation: Gong, P.; Wang, Y.; Zhang, P.; Yang, Z.; Deng, W.; Sun, Z.; Yang, M.; Li, X.; Ma, G.; Deng, G.; Dong, S.; et al. Immunocyte Membrane-Coated Nanoparticles for Cancer Immunotherapy. *Cancers* **2021**, *13*, 77. https://doi.org/10.3390/cancers13010077

Received: 17 November 2020
Accepted: 17 December 2020
Published: 30 December 2020

Publisher's Note: MDPI stays neutral with regard to jurisdictional claims in published maps and institutional affiliations.

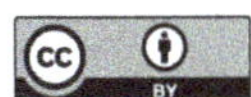

1. Introduction

Cancer immunotherapy (immuno-oncology) is a kind of treatment that aims to restore the capacity of the immune system to identify and reject cancer. Immunotherapy is considered to be a promising new generation of therapy, since immunotherapy can eliminate cancer cells by activating adaptive immunity and innate immunity of patients, with higher specificity and less toxicity, Compared with traditional therapies, such as chemotherapy and radiotherapy [1,2]. Presently, cancer immunotherapy mainly includes cellular immunotherapy (Provenge, CAR-T), antibody therapy (Alemtuzumab, Durvalumab), cytokine therapy (interferon, interleukin) and oncolytic viruses. However, despite the encouraging results in tumor treatment, cancer immunotherapy still faces lots of challenges, which may be mainly attributed to tumor heterogeneity, immune cell dysfunction, tumor microenvironment, acquired resistance to immunotherapy, and immunotoxicity [3]. Therefore, it is necessary to improve the effectiveness and safety of tumor immunotherapy. Recent trends in cancer immunotherapy have focused on developing immunocyte membrane-based nanomaterials.

Cell membranes are composed primarily of lipids, proteins and carbohydrates, and they give cells their structure, protect intracellular components from the extracellular environment, and regulate the materials that enter and leave the cell [4–7]. The cell membrane also plays an important role in cell-cell contact, surface recognition, and cell signaling and communication [8,9]. The protein content of cell membrane is very high, usually about 50% of membrane volume [10]. These membrane proteins are crucial to the cellular survival and function because they are responsible for many vital biological events, such as energy storage, cytoskeleton contact, signaling, enzymatic activity, substance transport, and information transduction [11,12]. Moreover, the membrane proteins can differ substantially across different cell types, and even the same type of cells from different individuals can have completely different glycosylation modifications [10,13]. Hence, as membrane markers, membrane proteins and their glycosylation, which allow cells to recognize each another, are of great importance for cell-to-cell communication. On the one hand, cell-cell recognition is critical for cellular signaling processes that can affect formation and development of tissues and organs in early stage of ontogeny. On the other hand, cell-to-cell communication based on membrane proteins plays a very key role in the distinction between "self" and "non-self" in subsequent immune responses [14].

As a lipid bilayer mixed with proteins, the cell membrane is actually a perfect two-dimensional nanomaterial with various functions, since the thickness of cell membrane is only about 10 nm [15]. Moreover, owing to the lipid bilayer's spontaneously "self-sealing" behavior, broken cell membranes can also naturally form nearly spherical nanovesicles with an internal, aqueous lumen [10]. It is feasible and would be significant to use cell membranes to coat nanomaterials for more effective drug delivery. Numerous nanomaterials coated with cell membrane have been fabricated from many different types of cells, such as red blood cells [16–20], cancer cells, immunocytes, stem cells, platelets [21], and bacteria. These cell membrane-based biomimetic nanomaterials not only retain the complex biological functions of natural cell membranes, but they also maintain the highly adjustable physicochemical properties of the synthesized nanomaterials [22–24].

Natural cell membranes that camouflage the nanoparticles' antigenic diversity from the source cells can have a variety of source cell-relevant functions, such as "self" markers, biological targeting, communication and negotiation with the immune system, and homing to specific regions [25–27]. Cell membrane-coated nanoparticles' unique abilities to biomimic and biointerface with cell membranes not only give them certain physiochemical properties, such as high cargo loading and great stability under high shear-stress conditions [24,28,29], but also make them tunable to have certain biological functions, such as long circulation, targeted recognition, enhanced accumulation in disease sites, and deep tumor penetration [30–32].

In addition, bare nanoparticles usually adsorb biomolecules in plasma and/or intracellular fluid in vivo and form a biological coating on their surface, namely protein corona owing to high surface free energy of nanomaterials [33]. The composition of protein corona varies depending on the composition, size, and surface modification of the nanomaterial, as well as the environment surrounding the nanomaterial. This protein corona may shield the specific surface structure and cover the targeting ligand, thus hindering the specific reaction between the nanoparticle and its target, which greatly affects the nanoparticles' fate and may results in removal of nanoparticles from the bloodstream [34–36]. Therefore, it is crucial to avoid the formation of protein corona in the development of nanomaterials for biological or biomedical application. However, having a cell membrane coating around the nanoparticles can successfully prevent nanomaterials from forming a protein corona. As the interface between the cell and the outside world, the cell membrane is perfectly compatible with biofluids, effectively blocking the interactions between the nanomaterials and biological system. This strategy allows nanoparticles to navigate more effectively within the body, thereby limiting off-target side effects, significantly regulating immune responses and, ultimately, enhancing treatment efficacy and expanding the application range of nanomaterials [37,38].

Herein, we summarize the recent progress in research on biomimetic immunocyte membrane-coated nanoparticles for cancer immunotherapy. This article will introduce macrophage membrane, T-cell membrane, Natural killer membrane and dendritic cell membrane-based nanoparticles (neutrophil membrane and platelet membrane-based nano-materials have been introduced in a recent review, so this article will not discuss these in detail). We will highlight their novelty, analyze their potential prospects in the biomedical field, and finally discuss the challenges in their large-scale preparation and application.

2. Immunocyte Membrane Molecules Contributing to Nanomaterials' Anti-Tumor Immune Effects

Immune response depends on the communication and mutual recognition between immunocytes, and between immunocytes and other cells. Immunocyte recognition is based on immunocyte membrane molecules, usually known as cell surface markers. There is a wide variety of immunocyte surface markers related to tumor immunity, including receptors, antigens, adhesion molecules, and other molecules on the cell surface. Table 1 summarizes some of the major cell membrane surface markers that may contribute to nanomaterials' anti-tumor immune effects. Because of these specific surface markers, immunocyte membranes have unique functions and can play a special role in assisting drug delivery, especially in tumor cell recognition and anti-tumor immunity.

Because nanoparticles are foreign substances, one of the fundamental problems and technical barriers to using them is uptake by the reticuloendothelial system (RES) or the mononuclear phagocytic system (MPS), which is part of the immune system and consists of phagocytic cells such as monocytes, macrophages in lymph nodes and spleen, and Kupffer cells in liver [39–41]. When nanoparticles enter the body, they are first "opsonized" and coated by non-specific proteins that make them more recognizable to phagocytic cells such as macrophages, monocytes, and dendritic cells. Once opsonization, phagocytosis will occur, by which the nanoparticles are engulfed and eventually destroyed or removed from the bloodstream [42]. The most common strategy to reduce RES uptake is to shield nanoparticles with polyethylene glycols (PEGs) or other polymers. This is effective, but it cannot avoid uptake completely [43]. However, when nanoparticles are covered with immunocyte membranes, especially macrophage membranes, the RES system can be completely avoided, because the immune system recognizes nanoparticles camouflaged with macrophage membranes as "self" rather than "foreign."

In addition, some specific receptors and adhesion molecules on macrophage membranes, such as C-C chemokine receptor 2 (CCR2), vascular cell adhesion molecule-1 (VCAM-1, CD106), and intercellular adhesion molecule-1 (ICAM-1; CD54), can guide nanoparticles coated with membranes to inflammatory and tumor sites. Notably, the binding of ICAM-1with macrophage adhesion ligand-1 (Mac-1; ITGAM), leukocyte function-associated antigen-1 (LFA-1), and fibrinogen can facilitate the transmigration of leukocytes across vascular endothelia [44,45]. ICAM-1 and soluble ICAM-1 also have antagonistic effects on the tight junctions and thus promote nanoparticles coated with membranes to cross the blood–brain barrier (BBB) [46,47].

The second valuable cell membrane is natural killer (NK) cell membranes. NK cells are unique lymphocytes that can recognize and kill aberrant cells without antibodies or major histocompatibility complex (MHC) [48]. Therefore, NK cells are key for tumor cell surveillance, because tumor cells that are missing MHC I markers cannot be detected and destroyed by other immune cells, such as T-cells [49]. Although NK cells lack antigen-specific cell surface receptors, they have many alternative receptors that can recognize tumor cells, including NKG2D, NKp44, NKp46, NKp30, and DNAM [50,51]. NKG2D, for example, is a disulfide-linked homodimer that recognizes several ligands, including

UL16-binding protein (ULBP) and MHC class I chain-related gene A (MICA), which are typically expressed on tumor cells [52].

T-cell membranes are helpful for recognizing and targeting tumor cells because of the T-cell receptor (TCR) on the cell surface. As a protein complex, TCR recognizes fragments of antigens as peptides bound to MHC molecules, thus allowing T-cells to target both surface and intracellular tumor neoantigens [53,54]. Neoantigens are mutated antigens specifically expressed by tumor tissue, but not expressed on the surface of normal cells, so they are highly specific for individuals [55]. Since TCRs can recognize neoantigens and then target tumor cells or tumor tissue, nanoparticles coated with T-cell membranes could target tumor cells or tumor tissue with highly specificity for individuals.

Furthermore, PD-1, CTLA4, and other specific checkpoint inhibitory receptors on T-cells are harmful to tumor immunotherapy, but these checkpoint inhibitory receptors can also identify the corresponding ligands, such as PDL-1, on tumor cells [56,57]. Hence, TCRs are beneficial to the delivery of nanodrugs, because they can target tumor cells.

The greatest advantage of mature dendritic cell (DC) membranes is that they possess the antigen presentation function of whole DCs and can specifically activate T-cells, because they have a broad spectrum of peptide/MHC complexes on their surface [58,59]. DCs can also express co-stimulatory molecules and adhesion molecules, such as ICAM-3/CD50, CD40, CD44, and integrin family members [60,61]. These markers can reduce the negative charge on the cell surface and mediate cell adhesion, thus promoting the interaction between DCs and T-cells [62].

Table 1. Immunocyte Membrane Surface Markers That May Contribute to Nanomaterials' Anti-Tumor Immune Effects.

Cell Type	Marker	Ligand	Function
Macrophage	CCR2	CCL2	Induces a strong chemotactic response, guides immune cells to inflammatory and tumor sites
	VCAM-1	4VLA-4) or integrin $\alpha 4\beta 1$	Cell adhesion, cell signal transduction
	ICAM-1	LFA-1, Mac-1	Facilitates transmigration of leukocytes across vascular endothelia, intercellular adhesion
T-cell	TCR	peptide/MHC complex	Antigen recognition and presentation
	CD28	CD80, CD86	Brings T-cell and antigen-presenting cell membranes into close proximity
	CTLA-4	CD80, CD86	Immune checkpoint and down-regulates immune responses
	PD-1	PD-l, B7	Immune checkpoint and down-regulates immune responses
	LFA-1	ICAM	Cell adhesion and co-stimulator
	LFA-2	LFA-3, CD48	Cell adhesion and co-stimulator
NK cell	NK p46	CD247, FCER1G.	Activates NK cells, mediates tumor cell lysis
	NKp44	NKp44L, 21spe-MLL5, PCNA, HSPGs	Activates NK cells, mediates tumor cell lysis. Transmembrane Signaling Receptor Activity
	NCAM1	rabies virus glycoprotein	MAPK cascade, cell adhesion, host-virus interaction
	FCGR3	immunoglobulin gamma Fc region	Binds to the Fc portion of igg antibodies and activates antibody-dependent cell mediated cytotoxicity (ADCC)
	DNAM-1	PVR, NECTIN2	Signal transducing adhesion involved in the adhesion of certain tumor cells to CTL and NK cells, mediates their cytotoxicity
DC	peptide/MHC complex	TCR	Antigen recognition and presentation
	INAM	IRF3	Stimulates NK cell activation
	ICAM	LFA-1	Cell adhesion and co-stimulator

3. Macrophage Membranes

Macrophages express a wide variety of surface membrane receptors that recognize a wide range of endogenous and exogenous ligands [63]. It is through the mediation of these membrane receptors that macrophages can interact not only with natural and varied self-components of the host, but also with foreign components, such as microbes, and then induce appropriate responses [64,65]. Hence, nanoparticles coated with macrophage membranes is really useful for innate and acquired immunity.

3.1. Immune Evasion and Tumor Targeting

Su et al. [66] have developed Saikosaponin D loaded macrophage membrane-biomimetic nanoparticles (SCMNPs) for breast cancer therapy. This nano-drug system consists of a poly (latic-co-glycolic acid) nanoparticles and macrophage membrane hybridized with T7 peptide. The presence of receptors and ligands on macrophage membranes endowed SCMNPs with the ability to macrophage-homing, while the presence of T7 peptide enabled the nanoparticles to recognize tumor cells overexpressing transferrin receptors. SCM-NPs thus could escape phagocytosis by the RES system and selectively accumulate into tumor tissues. The drug Saikosaponin D encapsulated in SCMNP could inhibit tumor neovascularization by regulating angiogenic pathway related factors such as vascular endothelial growth factor (VEGF), Phosphatidylinositol 3-kinase (PI3K)/protein kinase B (AKT), and extracellular-regulated kinase (ERK), thus effectively inhibiting tumor growth and metastasis of breast cancer. This biomimetic strategy based on macrophage membranes provided a target anti-angiogenic therapeutic model for the precise and effective treatment of breast cancer.

In addition, Yan et al. [67] developed macrophage membrane-cloaked luminescence nanoparticle@MOF-derived mesoporous carbon nano-drug delivery system to escape the RES system. This multiple drug co-loaded nano-drug delivery system exhibited potential for autofluorescence-free, long-lasting persistent fluorescence imaging-guided drug targeted delivery and cancer therapy. Li et al. [68] subsequently reported that liposomes coated with isolated macrophage membranes could enhance delivery to metastatic sites via α4 integrin−VCAM-1 interactions and then target lung metastasis of breast cancer. Jiang et al. [69] collected macrophage membranes to encapsulate cskc-PPiP/PTX@Ma nanoparticles and found that this delivery system exhibited a favorable tumor-homing ability in systemic circulation and high biocompatibility because of its membrane coating.

Recently, Liu et al. [70] used macrophage membrane-coated iron oxide nanoparticles (Fe_3O_4@MM) to enhance photothermal tumor therapy. Because they were derived from an Fe_3O_4 core and had a macrophage membrane shell, the Fe_3O_4@MM NPs exhibited good biocompatibility, immune evasion, cancer targeting, and light-to-heat conversion capabilities. Quercetin-loaded hollow bismuth selenide nanoparticles are another example of nanoparticles coated with macrophage membranes. Compared with bare nanoparticles, macrophage membrane-camouflaged nanoparticles prolonged circulation life and accelerated and enhanced tumor tropic accumulation, thus showing promise in suppressing breast cancer lung metastasis in vivo [71]. Recently, Deng et al. [72] constructed a multifunctional biomimetic superparticle, termed as DOX-QDs-Lip@M nanoparticle for enhanced cancer imaging and anti-metastasis treatment. Due to the presence of α4 integrins in macrophage membrane, the nanocarrier had the ability to bind VCAM-1 on cancer cell and escape the immune system's response. Furthermore, the bionic membranes could stabilize the synthetic liposome structure and thus avoid the leakage of the loaded content such as DOX and ZAISe/ZnS QDs in the liposome.

Mesoporous silica nanocapsules camouflaged by macrophage cell membranes actively targeted tumors because of the guidance of the surface proteins on the macrophage cell membranes [73]. Because coating with macrophage cell membranes is a simple and effective surface engineering method that can activate tumor targeting, these membranes have also been used to disguise conversion nanoparticles (UCNPs) [74]. Xia et al. [75] developed albumin nanoparticles coated with macrophage plasma membranes loaded with paclitaxel to prolong blood circulation and achieve targeted therapy against malignant melanoma.

3.2. Penetrating the Blood–Brain Barrier (BBB) and Targeting Glioblastoma

BBB is a crucial selective semi-permeable border, which composed of endothelial cells adjoined continuously by the tight junctions and can restricts the passage of solutes. However, BBB also limits beneficial drug delivery to the central nervous system. Thus, overcoming the obstacle of BBB is the primary challenge in the treatment for central nervous system disorders. We developed IR-792 nanoparticles (MDINPs) decorated with macrophage plasma membranes for NIR-Ib fluorescence imaging-guided photothermal therapy (PTT) on orthotopic glioblastoma [76]. The macrophage membrane proteins (Integrin α4 and Mac-1) in the outer layer of MDINPs bind to the corresponding receptors, such as VCAM-1 and ICAM-1, on brain vascular endothelial cells, which activate the signaling pathway, reduce the expression of tight junction-related proteins (zonula occludens 1), and finally break down the tight junction, so that MDINPs can easily pass through the BBB. MDINPs also selectively accumulated at the tumor site because of the tumor targeting effect of the macrophage membranes. In animal experiments, MDINPs-mediated NIR-Ib fluorescence imaging-guided PTT prolonged the survival of mice. These results show a new strategy for integrating diagnosis and therapeutics in glioblastoma.

3.3. Anti-Proliferation

As a precursor of the soluble form of TNFα, transmembrane TNFα is expressed on the membrane of some cells such as lymphocytes and activated macrophages [77]. Since the 1980s, studies have shown that transmembrane TNFα expressed on human macrophages and lymphocytes induces strong and long-term tumor regression [78–81]. A good example is that tumor cells could be lysed by incubating them with transmembrane TNFα on paraformaldehyde-fixed activated macrophages [80]. Based on macrophages' ability to easily produce TNFα by the induction with lipopolysaccharide or other agents, a unique therapeutic nano-drug delivery system had been prepared by cloaking a degradable, biosafety, chitosan nanocarrier with bioengineered TNFα-binding macrophage membrane [82]. In this paper, THP-1 cells (a human monocytic cell line derived from an acute monocytic leukemia patient) differentiated with phorbol 12-myristate 13-acetate (PMA) were induced by bacterial lipopolysaccharide to produce macrophage membrane-tethered TNFα first. Then, the TNFα-binding macrophage membrane were decorated onto the surface of polymeric nanoparticles. In vitro experiments have shown that the membrane-cloaked nanocarriers have high stability and biocompatibility, and have the potential to significantly prevent the proliferation of tumor cells.

3.4. Macrophage Hybrid Membrane

Although macrophage-based tumor immunotherapy approaches have many advantages, they also face some challenges. First, tumor cells in general express CD47 molecule, an inhibitory receptor, which interacts with the signal-regulated protein alpha (SIRPα) on macrophages to prevent phagocytosis of tumor cells by macrophages. Second, an immunosuppressive microenvironment in tumors polarize macrophages from the anti-tumor M1 phenotype to the tumorigenic M2 phenotype. M2 macrophages can promote tumorigenesis, vascular regeneration, and metastasis. However, a hybrid cellular membrane nanovesicle (hNVs) reported by Chen et al. could overcome these drawbacks of macrophage-based immunotherapy and amplify macrophage immune responses against tumor recurrence and metastasis (Figure 1) [83]. hNVs, originated from three types of membranes, macrophage, platelet, and cancer cell, could interact with circulating tumor cells, accumulate in surgical sites, and then repolarize tumor-associated macrophages towards M1 phenotype. At the same time, hNVs also could bind to macrophages via CD47 and block CD47–SIRPα interaction between tumor cells and macrophages. As a result, hNVs could promote macrophages phagocytosis of tumor cells and significantly enhance the efficiency of cancer immunotherapy.

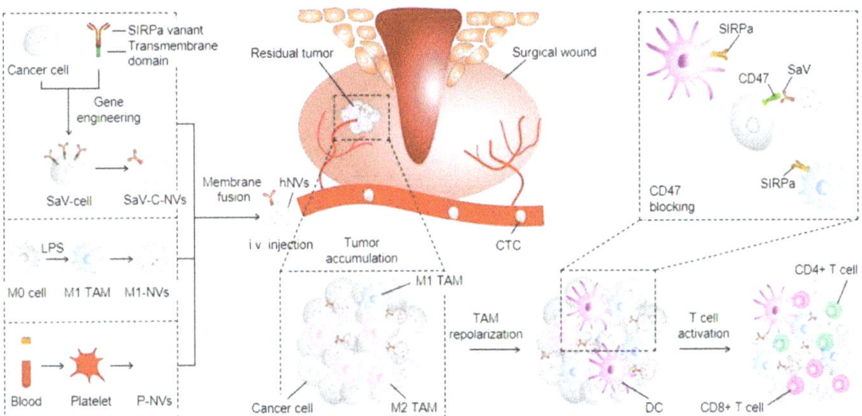

Figure 1. Schematic showing the formation of hNVs and the mechanism by which hNVs amplify macrophage immune responses against cancer recurrence and metastasis [83].

Yuan et al. [84] also explored macrophage-cancer hybrid membrane-coated nanoparticles for targeted treatment of lung metastases from breast cancer. Owing to the presence of macrophage and cancer cell membranes, these nanodrugs had a multi-targeting capability, and consequently they could accumulate to sites of inflammation, as well as target homogenous metastatic tumor. The doxorubicin-loaded nanodrugs were highly effective in the treatment of cancer, with nearly 88.9% cure rate in breast cancer-derived lung metastasis model.

4. T-Cell Membranes

T lymphocytes play a central role in the immune response. T-cells can attack and destroy tumor cells by their highly specific TCR, which bind to antigens present on the surface of other cells [85–89]. Each T-cell recognizes only a single antigen, but collectively, T-cells have a wide array of receptors targeting millions of antigens [90]. Many immunotherapy approaches have been developed to get rid of cancer cells by activating TCR-peptide-MHC interactions. Adoptive T-cell therapies such as chimeric antigen receptor (CAR) T-cell therapy have been a huge clinical success in hematological cancer treatment. However, such methods are generally not clinically effective in solid tumor treatment because of the lack of tumor-specific biomarkers on the surface of solid tumor cells [91].

4.1. Targeting Tumors through TCRs

Recently, Nguyen et al. [92] explored a new approach: coating Trametinib-loaded PLGA nanoparticles with melanoma-specific T-cell membranes (T-MNPs) to improve the therapeutic efficiency of chemo-drugs and overcome the non-specific targeting of anti-cancer drugs. The T-cell membranes on the surface of T-MNPs were derived from the T-cell hybridoma, which could express gp100 antigen-MHC molecule, could specifically bind melanoma cells expressing gp100 peptide, and enhance the uptake of T-MNPs. The T-cell membrane also gave the nanoparticles high stability and hemo-compatibility and cyto-compatibility. Membrane-coated NPs were taken up by a melanoma cell line in vitro three times as much as bare nanoparticles. Moreover, in vivo biodistribution studies displayed the theragnostic capabilities of these NPs, the tumor retention of which was more than twice as high as the uncoated and non-specific membrane-coated groups. Hepatocellular carcinoma (HCC)—specific CAR-T cell membrane-coated nanoparticles have been developed by Yuan et al. [93] for the treatment of HCC. The nanosystem packed with CAR-T cell membranes showed a superior ability to target HCC cells and improved therapeutic effect compared to naked nanosystem, because the CAR-T cell membranes specifically recognize GPC3+ HCC cells.

4.2. The Dual-Targeting Strategy

Since T-cell membranes have a variety of specific recognition receptors, these membranes are ideally suited for biomimetic nano-drug systems to tumors. This single-targeted therapy strategy is not so effective because of tumors' inter- and intra-heterogeneity. Hence, dual or multi-targeting is a promising approach to tackle either target antigen loss or down-regulation [94]. Cai et al. [95] employed a dual-targeting strategy based on azide (N_3)-labeled T-cell membrane-coated nanoparticles to enhance PTT for tumor. In this work, the bicyclononyne (BCN) group as artificial receptors were introduced into the tumor via natural glycometabolic labeling by pretreating the tumor with Ac_4ManN-BCN group first. Then, T-cell membranes were modified with N_3. Therefore, the nanoparticles coated with N_3-labeled T-cell membranes (N_3-TINPs) could dual-target tumor cells via both N_3-BCN bio-orthogonal click reaction and TCR-peptide/MHC recognition. The fluorescence intensity of the mouse tumors treated with N_3-TINPs was 1.5-fold that of unlabeled nanoparticles. The accumulation of N_3-TINPs in the tumor obviously increased the photothermal curative efficacy, yet virtually no side effects. Thus, dual-targeting N_3-TINPs-based click chemistry approach could offer an alternative dual-targeting strategy for advancing cancer treatment.

5. NK Cell Membranes

NK cells can lead to immune surveillance against cancer and eliminate small tumors early. Because they can engage tumor targets without needing specific antigens, NK cells' therapeutic potential has been broadly explored to control the metastatic dissemination of malignancies [96]. NK cells lack genetically rearranged antigen receptors [97], but they can still recognize and directly lyse abnormal cells without prior sensitization [98,99]. This occurs through a well-established and unique set of receptors expressed on NK cells' surface, which trigger cell lysis activity by interacting with ligands on infected and transformed cells [100]. The receptors on NK membranes, especially activated receptors such as NKp30, NKp44 NKp46, DNAM-1 (CD226), and NKG2D, are closely associated with tumor recognition and tumor killing [101]. NKp30 recognizes B7-H6 tumor antigens, while NKp44 binds proliferating cell nuclear antigen (PCNA) and other tumor-associated ligands [100,102]. NKp46 inhibits metastatic growth in mice [103]. DNAM-1 is an adhesion and co-stimulatory molecule that promotes NK cell cytotoxic activity upon binding to its ligands, CD112 and CD155 [104]. The NKG2D form transduces activating signals to initiate cytotoxic activity upon binding to specific stress-induced ligands, MICA and MHC class I polypeptide-related sequence B (MICB), which are selectively expressed on tumor cells [105–107].

5.1. Targeting Tumors

Aryal Murali et al. developed an NK cell membrane-cloaked fusogenic liposomal delivery system (NKsome) for targeted cancer therapy [108]. The engineered NKsomes have a variety of receptor proteins on their surface, thus they exhibited not only high binding ability to tumor cells in vitro, but also powerful tumor-homing efficiency in vivo. They also have outstanding biocompatibility and long blood circulation time (18 h). Further in vivo experiments showed that NKsome had promising therapeutic effects on MCF-7 tumor xenograft models. This study demonstrated that biomimetic nanocarriers based on NK cell membrane can partly communicate like immune cells and thus have therapeutic advantages through enhancing tumor drug delivery.

5.2. M1 Polarization and Induction of Immunogenic Cell Death (ICD)

Our group reported on NK cell membrane-cloaked photosensitizer TCPP-loaded nanoparticles (NK-NPs) that could eliminate primary tumors and inhibit distant tumors [109]. NK cell membranes on the surface of NPs enabled the NK-NPs to target 4T1 tumors via NK cell membrane receptors, such as NKG2D and DNAM-1 (Figure 2). Furthermore, NK cell membrane proteins such as RAB-10, IRGM1, RANKL Galectin-12, and CB1, can interact with macrophage surface receptors such as tumor necrosis factor or receptor toll-like receptor 4, to prompt or increase pro-inflammatory M1 macrophage polarization, which would kill tumor cells directly by secreting reactive oxygen species (ROS) and nitrogen radicals [110–112].

At the same time, the photosensitizer TCPP inside the NPs, after being irradiated with light, can destroy the cancer cells and induces immunogenic cell death (ICD). These dying cancer cells secrete damage-associated molecular patterns (DAMPs), promote activation of DCs and initiate an adaptive immune response. Results from animal experiments confirmed that NK-NPs selectively accumulate in 4T1 tumors and could eliminate primary tumor growth and produce an abscopal effect (a distant anti-tumor activity induced by local treatments), and then inhibit distant tumors. Thus, this NK cell membrane-based method offers a promising strategy for tumor immunotherapy.

5.3. Penetrating the BBB

Treating brain tumors with drugs is extremely difficult because the BBB hinders the delivery of systemic therapies into the tumor. Many strategies have been proposed for improving drug delivery across the BBB [113,114]. Since immunocytes, such as macrophages, neutrophils, T-cells, and NK cells, use specialized mechanisms to penetrate the BBB without compromising their structural integrity [115,116], using these immune cells as vehicles to deliver drugs through the BBB has recently become a research hotspot in this field.

Our group developed aggregation-induced emission (AIE) characteristic nanodots decorated with NK membranes (NK@AIEdots) for near-infrared-II fluorescence-guided glioma theranostics [117]. The binding of NK@AIEdots with cell adhesion molecules (CAMs) on brain microvascular endothelial cells by LFA-1 (lymphocyte function-associated antigen 1) and VLA-4 (very late antigen-4) on NK cell membranes could trigger an intracellular signaling cascade, which would disrupt tight junctions and reorganize actin cytoskeletons to form intercellular gaps at the BBB. Then, NK@AIEdots could cross the BBB through the paracellular pathway. Furthermore, NK@AIEdots could target malignant glioma cells (U-87 MG) through the receptors (DNAM-1 and NKG2D) on the NK membrane. The sufficient accumulation and high quantum yield of NK@AIEdots, on the one hand, allow them to perform high contrast and through-skull tumor NIR-II fluorescent imaging, and on the other hand, create NK@AIEdots-induced localized hyperthermia effects with laser irradiation, which could effectively inhibit glioma growth.

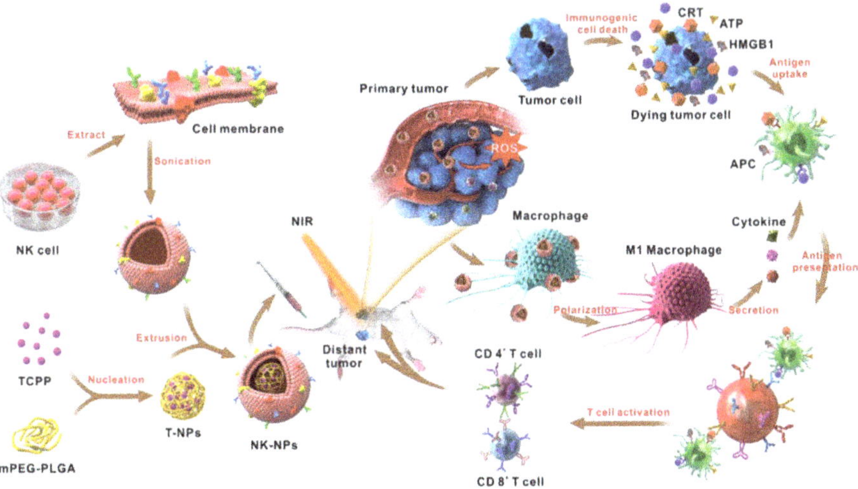

Figure 2. Schematic illustration of NK cell membrane-cloaked nanoparticles for PDT-enhanced cell membrane immunotherapy [109].

6. Dendritic Cell Membrane

As the most potent of all professional antigen-presenting cells (APCs), dendritic cells (DCs) can activate not only resting helper T-cells, but also memory and naive T-cells [60,61,118–120]. DCs act as immune sentinels that survey the body and collect information for responding to challenges, and they play a central role in initiating and regulating adaptive immune responses [121]. The generation of tolerogenic DCs induces anergy and contributes to tumor cells escaping immune surveillance, so it would be significant to artificially manipulate DCs to promote T-cells [122]. There are several approaches used in clinical trials to generate DCs, for example, in vivo expansion of circulating DCs, differentiation from CD34$^+$ hematopoietic precursors or monocyte precursors, and more recently, isolation and enrichment of circulating blood DC subpopulations. However, the clinical efficacy of most of these methods remains unsubstantiated. There is great potential for the development of a new DC-based cancer immunotherapy. At present, a DC membrane-based therapeutic method has been developed.

6.1. Activation and Maintenance of Antigen-Specific T-cells

Moon et al. [123] developed nanosized dendritic cell membrane vesicles (DC-MVs) capable of activating APCs and delivering peptide antigens. DC-MVs successfully led to maturation of dendritic cells and promoted T-cell survival and proliferation in vitro. These effects were also observed in vivo, where antigen-specific T-cells adoptively transferred into mice exhibited greater proliferation after vaccination with DC-MVs and peptide antigen than after peptide antigen alone. Additionally, vaccination with DC-MVs enhanced levels of endogenous T-cell responses against model antigen ovalbumin in an OVA-expressing tumor model. These results suggest that DC-MVs are a potentially attractive platform for further development as a peptide-based vaccine for cancer immunotherapy.

Zhang et al. [124] reported on DC-cancer fused membrane-based nanoparticles (NP@FMs) for targeted tumor therapy. The fused membranes (FMs) not only endowed NP@FMs with targeting capability to homologous tumors (breast cancer cell line 4T1), but also provided them with the capability to locate the lymph node and induce immune response. NP@FMs could trigger innate immunity and initiate adaptive immunity, they also could induce death of cancer cells by photodynamic therapy (PDT). Owing to the combination of PDT and immunotherapy, NP@FMs displayed powerful ability to inhibit the proliferation of distant tumors without radiation exposure. Furthermore, the primary and distant tumors were almost completely eliminated.

6.2. Intelligent Nano-DCs

Our group developed intelligent nano-DCs (iDCs), which consist of nanoparticles loaded with photothermal agents (IR-797) and coated with a mature DC membrane. The DC membrane on the iDCs maintains the antigen presentation and T-cell priming capabilities of native DCs (Figure 3). The iDCs can enter the lymph node and stimulate T-cells, which migrate to the tumor site. The activated T-cells reduce the expression of heat shock proteins (HSPs) in tumor cells, thereby rendering them more sensitive to heat stress. Adding mild PTT (42–45 °C) can enhance the tumoricidal effect. Consequently, dying tumor cells and surviving immune cells can induce ICD, reinitiate the self-sustaining cycle of cancer immunity, and contribute to a synergistic anti-tumor effect. Furthermore, unlike the adoptive transfer of activated DCs, iDCs as a refined and precise system in combination with DC-based immunotherapy and thermal therapy can be stored long-term and at a large scale, so they can be applied in different patients [125].

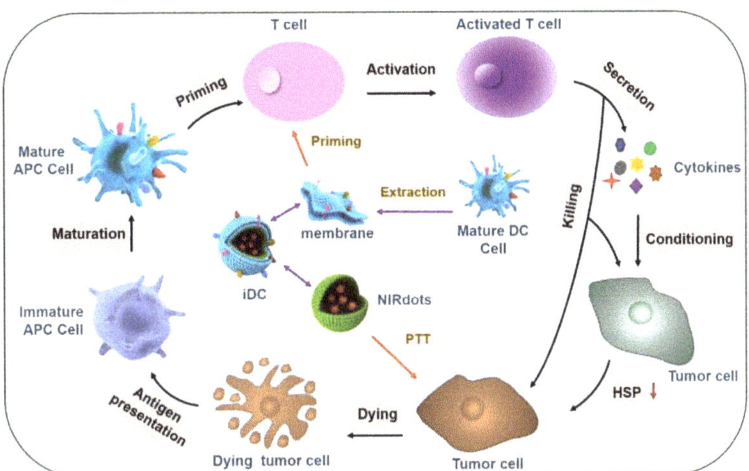

Figure 3. Schematic illustration of the preparation of intelligent dendritic cells (iDCs) and the mechanism of synergy between iDCs and mild photothermal-immunotherapy.

7. Conclusions

We have summarized the current research on immunocyte membrane-coated nanoparticles (Table 2). As a new biomimetic drug delivery platform, the immunocyte membrane covering approach is a feasible way to overcome the limitations of introducing foreign materials into the immune system by providing a unique biological interface, and would thus have a wide range of advantages for activating the innate and adaptive immune responses. The cell membranes discussed herein include those originating from macrophages, NK cells, T-cells, and dendritic cells. Macrophages are the main component cell of the RES, so macrophage membranes can help nanoparticles escape the phagocytosis of RES perfectly. In addition, some specific receptors and adhesion molecules can guide nanoparticles camouflaged with macrophage membranes to inflammatory and tumor sites. NK membranes can guide particles to target tumor sites and cross the BBB by a well-established and unique set of receptors expressed on the surface of NK cells. T-cell membranes display some distinctive properties, including binding to neoantigens and displaying specific receptors, which endow biomimetic nanoparticles with immune escape and good targeting abilities. Modified DC membranes enable the membrane-based nanocarriers to present antigens and then activate T-cells. Moreover, by combining with other therapeutic agents such as chemotherapeutic drugs or photosensitizers to treat tumors, cell membrane-coating approaches could enhance cancer therapy.

However, there are some critical issues that must be addressed for the further development and translation of immunocyte membrane-based nanocarriers. First, there is an urgent need for a standard protocol to guide the preparation of immunocyte membrane-based carriers, owing to the difficulty of controlling the parameters of natural materials. Since the functional proteins on cell membranes are susceptible to inactivation, the extraction of cell membranes needs to be done carefully. The whole membrane extraction mainly includes cell lysis, removal of intracellular contents, purification of membranes, and coating cell membrane onto nanoparticle core. The detailed preparation parameters vary according to the cell type. To generate cell membranes-derived nanoparticles with reproducibility and scalability, a more standard protocol needs to be proposed to guide the synthesis of biomimetic nanomaterials.

Table 2. The functions, advantages and disadvantages of different immunocyte membrane-coated nanoparticles.

Source of Cell Membranes	Functions	Advantages	Disadvantages	References
Macrophage	Prolonged circulation time; penetrating the blood–brain barrier (BBB); anti-proliferation; tumor targeting; inflammation targeting	Immune evasion; targeting glioblastoma; enhanced intratumoral penetration	Only targeting to limited types of tumor	[66–82]
T-cell	Prolonged circulation time; targeting to specific tumors through TCRs;	Dual-targeting; improved tumoritropic accumulation of drug	MHC Restriction; only targeting to limited types of tumor	[92,95]
NK cell	Prolonged circulation time; tumor targeting; penetrating the blood–brain barrier (BBB); M1 polarization and induction of immunogenic cell death (ICD)	targeting glioblastoma; broad spectrum tumor targeting	Limited multiplication of primary NK cells	[108,109,117]
DC	Antigen-presenting; tumor vaccine; promote T-cells; lymph node targeting	Activation and maintenance of antigen-specific T-cells; providing immunological co-stimulatory molecules	MHC restriction;	[123–125]

Second, more researchers should study the integrity of membranes on artificial particles in vivo. The incomplete membrane may lead to the exposure of naked nanomaterials, which in turn may affect the biological effectiveness of cell membranes-derived nanoparticles. There are no relevant research data concerning the extent to which the non-integrity of cell membrane actually affects the function of cell membranes-derived nanomaterials. Therefore, more research should be done in the integrity of membranes on nanoparticles.

Third, measures should be taken to further transform and functionalize immunocyte membranes to broaden the application of membrane-derived nanoparticles. These methods, such as membrane hybridization, lipid insertion, metabolic engineering, and genetic modification, would contribute diverse functions in a nondisruptive fashion while preserving the natural function of the cell membranes. In addition, Immunocyte-derived exosomes also are considered to be very promising system for drug delivery and are receiving a great deal of attention due to their naturally biocompatible characteristics [126]. The exosomes based on monocytes and macrophages could prolong blood circulation time and avoid immune phagocytosis [127]. DC-derived exosomes show attractive application prospects in vaccine delivery, and they have been proven safe in multiple phase I trials in different types of cancers [128]. Nevertheless, the difficulty in purifying exosomes maybe restrict their large-scale application.

Finally, the biological safety of immunocyte membranes in nanoparticles in vivo should be investigated carefully. First, the accumulation of nanomaterials with a large proportion in normal tissues can be harmful. Second, mismatch of allogeneic MHC between donor and recipient of immunocyte membranes may lead to serious safety problems. Thirdly, modified membranes may also raise health risks, such as TNF α-binding macrophage membranes, which maybe induce hyperinflammation.

Funding: This work was supported by the National Natural Science Foundation of China (81671758 and 32000982), a Guangdong Basic and Applied Basic Research Fund Project (2019A1515110222), the China Postdoctoral Science Foundation (2019M660219), a Special Research Assistant Project of the Chinese Academy of Sciences (Y959101001), the Chinese Academy of Sciences (Y959101001), the Guangdong Natural Science Foundation of Research Team (2016A030312006).

Acknowledgments: The authors thank Jonathan Feinberg from the Department of Radiation Oncology, UT Southwestern Medical Center for professional editorial assistance.

Conflicts of Interest: The authors declare no conflict of interest. The funders had no role in the design of the study; in the collection, analyses, or interpretation of data; in the writing of the manuscript, or in the decision to publish the results.

References

1. Sharma, P.; Wagner, K.; Wolchok, J.D.; Allison, J.P. Novel cancer immunotherapy agents with survival benefit: Recent successes and next steps. *Nat. Rev. Cancer* **2011**, *11*, 805–812. [CrossRef] [PubMed]
2. Finck, A.; Gill, S.I.; June, C.H. Cancer immunotherapy comes of age and looks for maturity. *Nat. Commun.* **2020**, *11*, 1–4. [CrossRef] [PubMed]
3. Mellman, I.; Coukos, G.; Dranoff, G. Cancer immunotherapy comes of age. *Nature* **2011**, *480*, 480–489. [CrossRef] [PubMed]
4. Policard, A. Cell Membranes and Their Role in the Cell Function. *Pathol. Biol.* **1968**, *16*, 973–977. [PubMed]
5. Bentrup, F.W. Function of Cell Membranes in Cytomorphogenesis. *Ber. Deut. Bot. Ges.* **1968**, *81*, 311–314.
6. Obrien, J.S. Cell Membranes—Composition—Structure—Function. *J. Theor. Biol.* **1967**, *15*, 307–324. [CrossRef]
7. Murti, C.R.K. Biochemical Function of Cell Membranes. *J. Sci. Ind. Res. India* **1963**, *22*, 123–128.
8. Zingaretti, G.; Nunez, C.; Rubiano, F.; Heymsfield, S.B. Cell membrane function modeled using bioimpedance analysis. *Faseb. J.* **2000**, *14*, A486.
9. Whittaker, V.P. Structure and Function of Animal-Cell Membranes. *Br. Med. Bull.* **1968**, *24*, 101–106. [CrossRef]
10. Alberts, B.; Johnson, A.; Lewis, J.; Raff, M.; Roberts, K.; Walter, P. *Molecular Biology of the Cell*; Garland Science: New York, NY, USA, 2002.
11. Sackmann, E. Thermo-elasticity and adhesion as regulators of cell membrane architecture and function. *J. Phys. Condens. Matter* **2006**, *18*, R785–R825. [CrossRef]
12. Takakuwa, Y. Regulation of red cell membrane protein interactions: Implications for red cell function. *Curr. Opin. Hematol.* **2001**, *8*, 80–84. [CrossRef] [PubMed]
13. Brandley, B.K.; Schnaar, R.L. Cell-surface carbohydrates in cell recognition and response. *J. Leukoc. Biol.* **1986**, *40*, 97–111. [CrossRef] [PubMed]
14. Coers, J. Self and Non-self Discrimination of Intracellular Membranes by the Innate Immune System. *PLoS Pathog.* **2013**, *9*, e1003538. [CrossRef] [PubMed]
15. Heyden, S.; Ortiz, M. Investigation of the influence of viscoelasticity on oncotripsy. *Comput. Method Appl. Mech. Eng.* **2017**, *314*, 314–322. [CrossRef]
16. Biagiotti, S.; Paoletti, M.F.; Fraternale, A.; Rossi, L.; Magnani, M. Drug delivery by red blood cells. *IUBMB Life* **2011**, *63*, 621–631. [CrossRef]
17. Kim, J.S.; Kang, M.; Bagyinszky, E.; Thanavel, R.; An, S.A. Mimicking red blood cells for drug delivery. *Nanomedicine* **2011**, *6*, 420.
18. Piergiovanni, M.; Casagrande, G.; Taverna, F.; Corridori, I.; Frigerio, M.; Bianchi, E.; Arienti, F.; Mazzocchi, A.; Dubini, G.; Costantino, M.L. Shear-Induced Encapsulation into Red Blood Cells: A New Microfluidic Approach to Drug Delivery. *Ann. Biomed. Eng.* **2020**, *48*, 236–246. [CrossRef]
19. Glassman, P.M.; Villa, C.H.; Ukidve, A.; Zhao, Z.; Smith, P.; Mitragotri, S.; Russell, A.J.; Brenner, J.S.; Muzykantov, V.R. Vascular Drug Delivery Using Carrier Red Blood Cells: Focus on RBC Surface Loading and Pharmacokinetics. *Pharmaceutics* **2020**, *12*, 440. [CrossRef]
20. Kolesnikova, T.A.; Skirtach, A.G.; Mohwald, H. Red blood cells and polyelectrolyte multilayer capsules: Natural carriers versus polymer-based drug delivery vehicles. *Expert Opin. Drug Deliv.* **2013**, *10*, 47–58. [CrossRef]
21. Hu, C.M.J.; Fang, R.H.; Wang, K.C.; Luk, B.T.; Thamphiwatana, S.; Dehaini, D.; Nguyen, P.; Angsantikul, P.; Wen, C.H.; Kroll, A.V.; et al. Nanoparticle biointerfacing by platelet membrane cloaking. *Nature* **2015**, *526*, 118–121. [CrossRef]
22. Zhen, X.; Cheng, P.; Pu, K. Recent Advances in Cell Membrane-Camouflaged Nanoparticles for Cancer Phototherapy. *Small* **2019**, *15*, e1804105. [CrossRef] [PubMed]
23. Fang, R.H.; Kroll, A.V.; Zhang, L. Nanoparticle-Based Manipulation of Antigen-Presenting Cells for Cancer Immunotherapy. *Small* **2015**, *11*, 5483–5496. [CrossRef] [PubMed]
24. He, Z.; Zhang, Y.; Feng, N. Cell membrane-coated nanosized active targeted drug delivery systems homing to tumor cells: A review. *Mater. Sci. Eng. C Mater. Biol. Appl.* **2020**, *106*, 110298. [CrossRef] [PubMed]
25. Zou, S.; Wang, B.; Wang, C.; Wang, Q.; Zhang, L. Cell membrane-coated nanoparticles: Research advances. *Nanomedicine* **2020**, *15*, 625–641. [CrossRef]
26. Muzykantov, V.R. Drug delivery by red blood cells: Vascular carriers designed by mother nature. *Expert Opin. Drug Deliv.* **2010**, *7*, 403–427. [CrossRef]
27. Magnani, M.; Rossi, L.; Casabianca, A.; Fraternale, A.; Schiavano, G.; Brandi, G.; Mannello, F.; Piedimonte, G. Red blood cells as advanced drug delivery systems for antiviral nucleoside analogues. *Adv. Exp. Med. Biol.* **1992**, *326*, 239–245. [CrossRef]
28. Wang, S.; Gao, J.; Wang, Z. Outer membrane vesicles for vaccination and targeted drug delivery. *Wiley Interdiscip. Rev. Nanomed. Nanobiotechnol.* **2019**, *11*, e1523. [CrossRef]
29. Ai, X.; Wang, S.; Duan, Y.; Zhang, Q.; Chen, M.S.; Gao, W.; Zhang, L. Emerging Approaches to Functionalizing Cell Membrane-Coated Nanoparticles. *Biochemistry* **2020**. [CrossRef]
30. Xuan, M.J.; Shao, J.X.; Li, J.B. Cell membrane-covered nanoparticles as biomaterials. *Natl. Sci. Rev.* **2019**, *6*, 551–561. [CrossRef]

31. Li, R.X.; He, Y.W.; Zhang, S.Y.; Qin, J.; Wang, J.X. Cell membrane-based nanoparticles: A new biomimetic platform for tumor diagnosis and treatment. *Acta Pharm. Sin. B* **2018**, *8*, 14–22. [CrossRef]

32. Bose, R.J.C.; Paulmurugan, R.; Moon, J.; Lee, S.H.; Park, H. Cell membrane-coated nanocarriers: The emerging targeted delivery system for cancer theranostics. *Drug Discov. Today* **2018**, *23*, 891–899. [CrossRef] [PubMed]

33. Oh, J.Y.; Kim, H.S.; Palanikumar, L.; Go, E.M.; Jana, B.; Park, S.A.; Kim, H.Y.; Kim, K.; Seo, J.K.; Kwak, S.K.; et al. Cloaking nanoparticles with protein corona shield for targeted drug delivery. *Nat. Commun.* **2018**, *9*, 4548. [CrossRef] [PubMed]

34. Tekie, F.S.M.; Hajiramezanali, M.; Geramifar, P.; Raoufi, M.; Dinarvand, R.; Soleimani, M.; Atyabi, F. Controlling evolution of protein corona: A prosperous approach to improve chitosan-based nanoparticle biodistribution and half-life. *Sci. Rep.* **2020**, *10*, 9664. [CrossRef] [PubMed]

35. Ritz, S.; Schottler, S.; Kotman, N.; Baier, G.; Musyanovych, A.; Kuharev, J.; Landfester, K.; Schild, H.; Jahn, O.; Tenzer, S.; et al. Protein corona of nanoparticles: Distinct proteins regulate the cellular uptake. *Biomacromolecules* **2015**, *16*, 1311–1321. [CrossRef]

36. Kroll, A.V.; Fang, R.H.; Zhang, L.F. Biointerfacing and Applications of Cell Membrane-Coated Nanoparticles. *Bioconjugate Chem.* **2017**, *28*, 23–32. [CrossRef]

37. Chai, Z.L.; Hu, X.F.; Lu, W.Y. Cell membrane-coated nanoparticles for tumor-targeted drug delivery. *Sci. China Mater.* **2017**, *60*, 504–510. [CrossRef]

38. Wang, H.J.; Liu, Y.; He, R.Q.; Xu, D.L.; Zang, J.; Weeranoppanant, N.; Dong, H.Q.; Li, Y.Y. Cell membrane biomimetic nanoparticles for inflammation and cancer targeting in drug delivery. *Biomater. Sci.* **2020**, *8*, 552–568. [CrossRef]

39. Chow, A.; Brown, B.D.; Merad, M. Studying the mononuclear phagocyte system in the molecular age. *Nat. Rev. Immunol.* **2011**, *11*, 788–798. [CrossRef]

40. Hume, D.A. The mononuclear phagocyte system. *Curr. Opin. Immunol.* **2006**, *18*, 49–53. [CrossRef]

41. Nezelof, C. Cells of the Mononuclear Phagocyte System—Origin, Lifetime, Function. *Arch. Pediatrie* **1995**, *2*, S28–S31. [CrossRef]

42. Nie, S.M. Understanding and overcoming major barriers in cancer nanomedicine. *Nanomedicine-UK* **2010**, *5*, 523–528. [CrossRef] [PubMed]

43. Sathyamoorthy, N.; Dhanaraju, M.D. Shielding Therapeutic Drug Carriers from the Mononuclear Phagocyte System: A Review. *Crit. Rev. Ther. Drug* **2016**, *33*, 489–567. [CrossRef] [PubMed]

44. Rothlein, R.; Dustin, M.L.; Marlin, S.D.; Springer, T.A. A human intercellular adhesion molecule (ICAM-1) distinct from LFA-1. *J. Immunol.* **1986**, *137*, 1270–1274. [PubMed]

45. Barreiro, O.; Yanez-Mo, M.; Serrador, J.M.; Montoya, M.C.; Vicente-Manzanares, M.; Tejedor, R.; Furthmayr, H.; Sanchez-Madrid, F. Dynamic interaction of VCAM-1 and ICAM-1 with moesin and ezrin in a novel endothelial docking structure for adherent leukocytes. *J. Cell. Biol.* **2002**, *157*, 1233–1245. [CrossRef] [PubMed]

46. Polin, R.S.; Bavbek, M.; Shaffrey, M.E.; Billups, K.; Bogaev, C.A.; Kassell, N.F.; Lee, K.S. Detection of soluble E-selectin, ICAM-1, VCAM-1, and L-selectin in the cerebrospinal fluid of patients after subarachnoid hemorrhage. *J. Neurosurg.* **1998**, *89*, 559–567. [CrossRef] [PubMed]

47. Nordal, R.A.; Wong, C.S. Intercellular adhesion molecule-1 and blood-spinal cord barrier disruption in central nervous system radiation injury. *J. Neuropathol. Exp. Neurol.* **2004**, *63*, 474–483. [CrossRef]

48. Vivier, E.; Raulet, D.H.; Moretta, A.; Caligiuri, M.A.; Zitvogel, L.; Lanier, L.L.; Yokoyama, W.M.; Ugolini, S. Innate or adaptive immunity? The example of natural killer cells. *Science* **2011**, *331*, 44–49. [CrossRef]

49. Pfefferle, A.; Jacobs, B.; Haroun-Izquierdo, A.; Kveberg, L.; Sohlberg, E.; Malmberg, K.J. Deciphering Natural Killer Cell Homeostasis. *Front. Immunol.* **2020**, *11*, 812. [CrossRef]

50. Parodi, M.; Favoreel, H.; Candiano, G.; Gaggero, S.; Sivori, S.; Mingari, M.C.; Moretta, L.; Vitale, M.; Cantoni, C. NKp44-NKp44 Ligand Interactions in the Regulation of Natural Killer Cells and Other Innate Lymphoid Cells in Humans. *Front. Immunol.* **2019**, *10*, 719. [CrossRef]

51. Smyth, M.J.; Hayakawa, Y.; Takeda, K.; Yagita, H. New aspects of natural-killer-cell surveillance and therapy of cancer. *Nat. Rev. Cancer* **2002**, *2*, 850–861. [CrossRef]

52. Terunuma, H.; Deng, X.W.; Dewan, Z.; Fujimoto, S.; Yamamoto, N. Potential role of NK cells in the induction of immune responses: Implications for NK cell-based immunotherapy for cancers and viral infections. *Int. Rev. Immunol.* **2008**, *27*, 93–110. [CrossRef] [PubMed]

53. Katz, S.G.; Rabinovich, P.M. T Cell Reprogramming Against Cancer. *Methods Mol. Biol.* **2020**, *2097*, 3–44. [CrossRef] [PubMed]

54. Raskov, H.; Orhan, A.; Christensen, J.P.; Gogenur, I. Cytotoxic CD8(+) T cells in cancer and cancer immunotherapy. *Br. J. Cancer* **2020**, 1–9. [CrossRef] [PubMed]

55. Jiang, T.; Shi, T.; Zhang, H.; Hu, J.; Song, Y.; Wei, J.; Ren, S.; Zhou, C. Tumor neoantigens: From basic research to clinical applications. *J. Hematol. Oncol.* **2019**, *12*, 93. [CrossRef]

56. Brunet, J.F.; Denizot, F.; Luciani, M.F.; Roux-Dosseto, M.; Suzan, M.; Mattei, M.G.; Golstein, P. A new member of the immunoglobulin superfamily—CTLA-4. *Nature* **1987**, *328*, 267–270. [CrossRef]

57. Lorusso, D.; Ceni, V.; Muratore, M.; Salutari, V.; Nero, C.; Pietragalla, A.; Ciccarone, F.; Carbone, V.; Daniele, G.; Scambia, G. Emerging role of immune checkpoint inhibitors in the treatment of ovarian cancer. *Expert Opin. Emerg. Drugs* **2020**, *10*, 1–9. [CrossRef]

58. Wang, Y.; Xiang, Y.; Xin, V.W.; Wang, X.W.; Peng, X.C.; Liu, X.Q.; Wang, D.; Li, N.; Cheng, J.T.; Lyv, Y.N.; et al. Dendritic cell biology and its role in tumor immunotherapy. *J. Hematol. Oncol.* **2020**, *13*, 107. [CrossRef]

59. Apostolopoulos, V.; Thalhammer, T.; Tzakos, A.G.; Stojanovska, L. Targeting antigens to dendritic cell receptors for vaccine development. *J. Drug. Deliv.* **2013**, *2013*, 869718. [CrossRef]
60. Steinman, R.M. Dendritic cells and the control of immunity: Enhancing the efficiency of antigen presentation. *Mt. Sinai. J. Med.* **2001**, *68*, 160–166.
61. Banchereau, J.; Steinman, R.M. Dendritic cells and the control of immunity. *Nature* **1998**, *392*, 245–252. [CrossRef]
62. Rhee, I.; Zhong, M.C.; Reizis, B.; Cheong, C.; Veillette, A. Control of dendritic cell migration, T cell-dependent immunity, and autoimmunity by protein tyrosine phosphatase PTPN12 expressed in dendritic cells. *Mol. Cell. Biol.* **2014**, *34*, 888–899. [CrossRef] [PubMed]
63. Gordon, S. Pattern recognition receptors: Doubling up for the innate immune response. *Cell* **2002**, *111*, 927–930. [CrossRef]
64. Liu, H.; Mi, Z.; Wang, Z.; Zhang, F. Revealing of Pattern recognition receptors mediated macrophage immune response network induced by Mycobacterium leprae. *J. Invest. Dermatol.* **2020**, *140*, S42. [CrossRef]
65. Taylor, P.R.; Martinez-Pomares, L.; Stacey, M.; Lin, H.H.; Brown, G.D.; Gordon, S. Macrophage receptors and immune recognition. *Annu. Rev. Immunol.* **2005**, *23*, 901–944. [CrossRef] [PubMed]
66. Sun, K.J.; Yu, W.J.; Ji, B.; Chen, C.B.; Yang, H.M.; Du, Y.Y.; Song, M.Y.; Cai, H.Q.; Yan, F.; Su, R. Saikosaponin D loaded macrophage membrane-biomimetic nanoparticles target angiogenic signaling for breast cancer therapy. *Appl. Mater. Today* **2020**, *18*, 100505. [CrossRef]
67. Chen, L.J.; Zhao, X.; Liu, Y.Y.; Yan, X.P. Macrophage membrane coated persistent luminescence nanoparticle@MOF-derived mesoporous carbon core-shell nanocomposites for autofluorescence-free imaging-guided chemotherapy. *J. Mater. Chem. B* **2020**, *8*, 8071–8083. [CrossRef]
68. Cao, H.; Dan, Z.; He, X.; Zhang, Z.; Yu, H.; Yin, Q.; Li, Y. Liposomes Coated with Isolated Macrophage Membrane Can Target Lung Metastasis of Breast Cancer. *ACS Nano* **2016**, *10*, 7738–7748. [CrossRef]
69. Zhang, Y.; Cai, K.; Li, C.; Guo, Q.; Chen, Q.; He, X.; Liu, L.; Zhang, Y.; Lu, Y.; Chen, X.; et al. Macrophage-Membrane-Coated Nanoparticles for Tumor-Targeted Chemotherapy. *Nano Lett.* **2018**, *18*, 1908–1915. [CrossRef]
70. Meng, Q.F.; Rao, L.; Zan, M.; Chen, M.; Yu, G.T.; Wei, X.; Wu, Z.; Sun, Y.; Guo, S.S.; Zhao, X.Z.; et al. Macrophage membrane-coated iron oxide nanoparticles for enhanced photothermal tumor therapy. *Nanotechnology* **2018**, *29*, 134004. [CrossRef]
71. Zhao, H.; Li, L.; Zhang, J.; Zheng, C.; Ding, K.; Xiao, H.; Wang, L.; Zhang, Z. C-C Chemokine Ligand 2 (CCL2) Recruits Macrophage-Membrane-Camouflaged Hollow Bismuth Selenide Nanoparticles To Facilitate Photothermal Sensitivity and Inhibit Lung Metastasis of Breast Cancer. *ACS Appl. Mater. Interfaces* **2018**, *10*, 31124–31135. [CrossRef]
72. Liang, B.; Deng, T.; Li, J.; Ouyang, X.; Na, W.; Deng, D. Biomimetic theranostic strategy for anti-metastasis therapy of breast cancer via the macrophage membrane camouflaged superparticles. *Mater. Sci. Eng. C Mater. Biol. Appl.* **2020**, *115*, 111097. [CrossRef] [PubMed]
73. Xuan, M.; Shao, J.; Dai, L.; He, Q.; Li, J. Macrophage Cell Membrane Camouflaged Mesoporous Silica Nanocapsules for In Vivo Cancer Therapy. *Adv. Healthc. Mater.* **2015**, *4*, 1645–1652. [CrossRef] [PubMed]
74. Rao, L.; He, Z.; Meng, Q.F.; Zhou, Z.; Bu, L.L.; Guo, S.S.; Liu, W.; Zhao, X.Z. Effective cancer targeting and imaging using macrophage membrane-camouflaged upconversion nanoparticles. *J. Biomed. Mater. Res. A* **2017**, *105*, 521–530. [CrossRef] [PubMed]
75. Cao, X.; Tan, T.; Zhu, D.; Yu, H.; Liu, Y.; Zhou, H.; Jin, Y.; Xia, Q. Paclitaxel-Loaded Macrophage Membrane Camouflaged Albumin Nanoparticles for Targeted Cancer Therapy. *Int. J. Nanomed.* **2020**, *15*, 1915–1928. [CrossRef] [PubMed]
76. Lai, J.; Deng, G.; Sun, Z.; Peng, X.; Li, J.; Gong, P.; Zhang, P.; Cai, L. Scaffolds biomimicking macrophages for a glioblastoma NIR-Ib imaging guided photothermal therapeutic strategy by crossing Blood-Brain Barrier. *Biomaterials* **2019**, *211*, 48–56. [CrossRef] [PubMed]
77. Horiuchi, T.; Mitoma, H.; Harashima, S.; Tsukamoto, H.; Shimoda, T. Transmembrane TNF-alpha: Structure, function and interaction with anti-TNF agents. *Rheumatology* **2010**, *49*, 1215–1228. [CrossRef]
78. Decker, T.; Lohmannmatthes, M.L.; Gifford, G.E. Cell-Associated Tumor-Necrosis-Factor (Tnf) as a Killing Mechanism of Activated Cytotoxic Macrophages. *J. Immunol.* **1987**, *138*, 957–962.
79. Peck, R.; Brockhaus, M.; Frey, J.R. Cell-Surface Tumor Necrosis Factor (Tnf) Accounts for Monocyte-Mediated and Lymphocyte-Mediated Killing of Tnf-Resistant Target-Cells. *Cell. Immunol.* **1989**, *122*, 1–10. [CrossRef]
80. Fishman, M. Cytolytic Activities of Activated Macrophages Versus Paraformaldehyde-Fixed Macrophages—Soluble Versus Membrane-Associated Tnf. *Cell. Immunol.* **1991**, *137*, 164–174. [CrossRef]
81. Caron, G.; Delneste, Y.; Aubry, J.P.; Magistrellli, G.; Herbault, N.; Blaecke, A.; Meager, A.; Bonnefoy, J.Y.; Jeannin, P. Human NK cells constitutively express membrane TNF-alpha (mTNF alpha) and present mTNF alpha-dependent cytotoxic activity. *Eur. J. Immunol.* **1999**, *29*, 3588–3595. [CrossRef]
82. Bhattacharyya, S.; Ghosh, S.S. Transmembrane TNFalpha-Expressed Macrophage Membrane-Coated Chitosan Nanoparticles as Cancer Therapeutics. *ACS Omega* **2020**, *5*, 1572–1580. [CrossRef] [PubMed]
83. Rao, L.; Wu, L.; Liu, Z.; Tian, R.; Yu, G.; Zhou, Z.; Yang, K.; Xiong, H.G.; Zhang, A.; Yu, G.T.; et al. Hybrid cellular membrane nanovesicles amplify macrophage immune responses against cancer recurrence and metastasis. *Nat. Commun.* **2020**, *11*, 4909. [CrossRef] [PubMed]
84. Gong, C.; Yu, X.; You, B.; Wu, Y.; Wang, R.; Han, L.; Wang, Y.; Gao, S.; Yuan, Y. Macrophage-cancer hybrid membrane-coated nanoparticles for targeting lung metastasis in breast cancer therapy. *J. Nanobiotechnol.* **2020**, *18*, 92. [CrossRef] [PubMed]

85. Wang, R.F.; Rosenberg, S.A. Human tumor antigens recognized by T lymphocytes: Implications for cancer therapy. *J. Leukoc. Biol.* **1996**, *60*, 296–309. [CrossRef]
86. Boon, T.; van der Bruggen, P. Human tumor antigens recognized by T lymphocytes. *J. Exp. Med.* **1996**, *183*, 725–729. [CrossRef]
87. Boon, T.; Cerottini, J.C.; Van den Eynde, B.; van der Bruggen, P.; Van Pel, A. Tumor antigens recognized by T lymphocytes. *Annu. Rev. Immunol.* **1994**, *12*, 337–365. [CrossRef]
88. Van der Bruggen, P.; Van den Eynde, B. Molecular definition of tumor antigens recognized by T lymphocytes. *Curr. Opin. Immunol.* **1992**, *4*, 608–612. [CrossRef]
89. Plata, F.; Langlade-Demoyen, P.; Abastado, J.P.; Berbar, T.; Kourilsky, P. Retrovirus antigens recognized by cytolytic T lymphocytes activate tumor rejection in vivo. *Cell* **1987**, *48*, 231–240. [CrossRef]
90. Reinherz, E.L. alphabeta TCR-mediated recognition: Relevance to tumor-antigen discovery and cancer immunotherapy. *Cancer Immunol. Res.* **2015**, *3*, 305–312. [CrossRef]
91. He, Q.H.; Jiang, X.H.; Zhou, X.K.; Weng, J.S. Targeting cancers through TCR-peptide/MHC interactions. *J. Hematol. Oncol.* **2019**, *12*, 1–17. [CrossRef]
92. Yaman, S.; Ramachandramoorthy, H.; Oter, G.; Zhukova, D.; Nguyen, T.; Sabnani, M.K.; Weidanz, J.A.; Nguyen, K.T. Melanoma Peptide MHC Specific TCR Expressing T-Cell Membrane Camouflaged PLGA Nanoparticles for Treatment of Melanoma Skin Cancer. *Front Bioeng. Biotech.* **2020**, *8*, 943. [CrossRef] [PubMed]
93. Ma, W.J.; Zhu, D.M.; Li, J.H.; Chen, X.; Xie, W.; Jiang, X.; Wu, L.; Wang, G.G.; Xiao, Y.S.; Liu, Z.S.; et al. Coating biomimetic nanoparticles with chimeric antigen receptor T cell-membrane provides high specificity for hepatocellular carcinoma photothermal therapy treatment. *Theranostics* **2020**, *10*, 1281–1295. [CrossRef] [PubMed]
94. Van der Schans, J.J.; van de Donk, N.W.C.J.; Mutis, T. Dual Targeting to Overcome Current Challenges in Multiple Myeloma CAR T-Cell Treatment. *Front. Oncol.* **2020**, *10*, 1362. [CrossRef] [PubMed]
95. Han, Y.T.; Pan, H.; Li, W.J.; Chen, Z.; Ma, A.Q.; Yin, T.; Liang, R.J.; Chen, F.M.; Ma, N.; Jin, Y.; et al. T Cell Membrane Mimicking Nanoparticles with Bioorthogonal Targeting and Immune Recognition for Enhanced Photothermal Therapy. *Adv. Sci.* **2019**, *6*, 1362. [CrossRef] [PubMed]
96. Choucair, K.; Duff, J.R.; Cassidy, C.S.; Albrethsen, M.T.; Kelso, J.D.; Lenhard, A.; Staats, H.; Patel, R.; Brunicardi, F.C.; Dworkin, L.; et al. Natural killer cells: A review of biology, therapeutic potential and challenges in treatment of solid tumors. *Future Oncol.* **2019**, *15*, 3053–3069. [CrossRef] [PubMed]
97. Chiossone, L.; Dumas, P.Y.; Vienne, M.; Vivier, E. Natural killer cells and other innate lymphoid cells in cancer. *Nat. Rev. Immunol.* **2018**, *18*, 671–688. [CrossRef]
98. Kiessling, R.; Klein, E.; Wigzell, H. "Natural" killer cells in the mouse. I. Cytotoxic cells with specificity for mouse Moloney leukemia cells. Specificity and distribution according to genotype. *Eur. J. Immunol.* **1975**, *5*, 112–117. [CrossRef]
99. Herberman, R.B.; Nunn, M.E.; Lavrin, D.H. Natural cytotoxic reactivity of mouse lymphoid cells against syngeneic acid allogeneic tumors. I. Distribution of reactivity and specificity. *Int. J. Cancer* **1975**, *16*, 216–229. [CrossRef]
100. Koch, J.; Steinle, A.; Watzl, C.; Mandelboim, O. Activating natural cytotoxicity receptors of natural killer cells in cancer and infection. *Trends Immunol.* **2013**, *34*, 182–191. [CrossRef]
101. Moretta, A.; Bottino, C.; Vitale, M.; Pende, D.; Cantoni, C.; Mingari, M.C.; Biassoni, R.; Moretta, L. Activating receptors and coreceptors involved in human natural killer cell-mediated cytolysis. *Annu. Rev. Immunol.* **2001**, *19*, 197–223. [CrossRef]
102. Schlecker, E.; Fiegler, N.; Arnold, A.; Altevogt, P.; Rose-John, S.; Moldenhauer, G.; Sucker, A.; Paschen, A.; von Strandmann, E.P.; Textor, S.; et al. Metalloprotease-mediated tumor cell shedding of B7-H6, the ligand of the natural killer cell-activating receptor NKp30. *Cancer Res.* **2014**, *74*, 3429–3440. [CrossRef] [PubMed]
103. Pessino, A.; Sivori, S.; Bottino, C.; Malaspina, A.; Morelli, L.; Moretta, L.; Biassoni, R.; Moretta, A. Molecular cloning of NKp46: A novel member of the immunoglobulin superfamily involved in triggering of natural cytotoxicity. *J. Exp. Med.* **1998**, *188*, 953–960. [CrossRef] [PubMed]
104. Stannard, K.A.; Lemoine, S.; Waterhouse, N.J.; Vari, F.; Chatenoud, L.; Gandhi, M.K.; Martinet, L.; Smyth, M.J.; Guillerey, C. Human peripheral blood DNAM-1(neg) NK cells are a terminally differentiated subset with limited effector functions. *Blood Adv.* **2019**, *3*, 1681–1694. [CrossRef] [PubMed]
105. Fionda, C.; Soriani, A.; Zingoni, A.; Santoni, A.; Cippitelli, M. NKG2D and DNAM-1 Ligands: Molecular Targets for NK Cell-Mediated Immunotherapeutic Intervention in Multiple Myeloma. *BioMed Res. Int.* **2015**, *2015*, 178698. [CrossRef] [PubMed]
106. Soriani, A.; Fionda, C.; Ricci, B.; Iannitto, M.L.; Cippitelli, M.; Santoni, A. Chemotherapy-elicited upregulation of NKG2D and DNAM-1 ligands as a therapeutic target in multiple myeloma. *Oncoimmunology* **2013**, *2*, e26663. [CrossRef] [PubMed]
107. Zingoni, A.; Ardolino, M.; Santoni, A.; Cerboni, C. NKG2D and DNAM-1 activating receptors and their ligands in NK-T cell interactions: Role in the NK cell-mediated negative regulation of T cell responses. *Front. Immunol.* **2012**, *3*, 408. [CrossRef] [PubMed]
108. Pitchaimani, A.; Nguyen, T.D.T.; Aryal, S. Natural killer cell membrane infused biomimetic liposomes for targeted tumor therapy. *Biomaterials* **2018**, *160*, 124–137. [CrossRef]
109. Deng, G.; Sun, Z.; Li, S.; Peng, X.; Li, W.; Zhou, L.; Ma, Y.; Gong, P.; Cai, L. Cell-Membrane Immunotherapy Based on Natural Killer Cell Membrane Coated Nanoparticles for the Effective Inhibition of Primary and Abscopal Tumor Growth. *ACS Nano* **2018**, *12*, 12096–12108. [CrossRef]

110. Huang, R.; Wang, X.; Zhou, Y.; Xiao, Y. RANKL-induced M1 macrophages are involved in bone formation. *Bone Res.* **2017**, *5*, 17019. [CrossRef]
111. Wan, L.; Lin, H.J.; Huang, C.C.; Chen, Y.C.; Hsu, Y.A.; Lin, C.H.; Lin, H.C.; Chang, C.Y.; Huang, S.H.; Lin, J.M.; et al. Galectin-12 enhances inflammation by promoting M1 polarization of macrophages and reduces insulin sensitivity in adipocytes. *Glycobiology* **2016**, *26*, 732–744. [CrossRef]
112. Wang, D.; Lou, J.; Ouyang, C.; Chen, W.; Liu, Y.; Liu, X.; Cao, X.; Wang, J.; Lu, L. Ras-related protein Rab10 facilitates TLR4 signaling by promoting replenishment of TLR4 onto the plasma membrane. *Proc. Natl. Acad. Sci. USA* **2010**, *107*, 13806–13811. [CrossRef] [PubMed]
113. Arvanitis, C.D.; Ferraro, G.B.; Jain, R.K. The blood-brain barrier and blood-tumour barrier in brain tumours and metastases. *Nat. Rev. Cancer* **2020**, *20*, 26–41. [CrossRef] [PubMed]
114. Bhowmik, A.; Khan, R.; Ghosh, M.K. Blood brain barrier: A challenge for effectual therapy of brain tumors. *Biomed Res. Int.* **2015**, *2015*, 320941. [CrossRef] [PubMed]
115. Takeshita, Y.; Ransohoff, R.M. Inflammatory cell trafficking across the blood-brain barrier: Chemokine regulation and in vitro models. *Immunol. Rev.* **2012**, *248*, 228–239. [CrossRef] [PubMed]
116. Von Wedel-Parlow, M.; Schrot, S.; Lemmen, J.; Treeratanapiboon, L.; Wegener, J.; Galla, H.J. Neutrophils cross the BBB primarily on transcellular pathways: An in vitro study. *Brain Res.* **2011**, *1367*, 62–76. [CrossRef] [PubMed]
117. Deng, G.; Peng, X.; Sun, Z.; Zheng, W.; Yu, J.; Du, L.; Chen, H.; Gong, P.; Zhang, P.; Cai, L.; et al. Natural-Killer-Cell-Inspired Nanorobots with Aggregation-Induced Emission Characteristics for Near-Infrared-II Fluorescence-Guided Glioma Theranostics. *ACS Nano* **2020**, *14*, 11452–11462. [CrossRef]
118. Lee, H.K.; Iwasaki, A. Innate control of adaptive immunity: Dendritic cells and beyond. *Semin. Immunol.* **2007**, *19*, 48–55. [CrossRef]
119. Schroder, J.M.; Reich, K.; Kabashima, K.; Liu, F.T.; Romani, N.; Metz, M.; Kerstan, A.; Lee, P.H.; Loser, K.; Schon, M.P.; et al. Who is really in control of skin immunity under physiological circumstances—Lymphocytes, dendritic cells or keratinocytes? *Exp. Dermatol.* **2006**, *15*, 913–929. [CrossRef]
120. Zitvogel, L. Dendritic and natural killer cells cooperate in the control/switch of innate immunity. *J. Exp. Med.* **2002**, *195*, F9–F14. [CrossRef]
121. Wculek, S.K.; Cueto, F.J.; Mujal, A.M.; Melero, I.; Krummel, M.F.; Sancho, D. Dendritic cells in cancer immunology and immunotherapy. *Nat. Rev. Immunol.* **2020**, *20*, 7–24. [CrossRef]
122. Fucikova, J.; Palova-Jelinkova, L.; Bartunkova, J.; Spisek, R. Induction of Tolerance and Immunity by Dendritic Cells: Mechanisms and Clinical Applications. *Front. Immunol.* **2019**, *10*, 2393. [CrossRef] [PubMed]
123. Ochyl, L.J.; Moon, J.J. Dendritic Cell Membrane Vesicles for Activation and Maintenance of Antigen-Specific T Cells. *Adv. Healthc Mater.* **2019**, *8*, e1801091. [CrossRef] [PubMed]
124. Liu, W.L.; Zou, M.Z.; Liu, T.; Zeng, J.Y.; Li, X.; Yu, W.Y.; Li, C.X.; Ye, J.J.; Song, W.; Feng, J.; et al. Expandable Immunotherapeutic Nanoplatforms Engineered from Cytomembranes of Hybrid Cells Derived from Cancer and Dendritic Cells. *Adv. Mater.* **2019**, *31*, e1900499. [CrossRef] [PubMed]
125. Sun, Z.; Deng, G.; Peng, X.; Xu, X.; Liu, L.; Xu, Z.; Peng, J.; Ma, Y.; Zhang, P.; Wang, Y.; et al. Intelligent Photothermal Dendritic Cells Restart the Cancer Immunity Cycle. *Cell Rep.* **2020**, under review. [CrossRef]
126. Luan, X.; Sansanaphongpricha, K.; Myers, I.; Chen, H.W.; Yuan, H.B.; Sun, D.X. Engineering exosomes as refined biological nanoplatforms for drug delivery. *Acta Pharmacol. Sin.* **2017**, *38*, 754–763. [CrossRef]
127. Shenoda, B.B.; Ajit, S.K. Modulation of Immune Responses by Exosomes Derived from Antigen-Presenting Cells. *Clin. Med. Insights Pathol.* **2016**, *9*, 1–8. [CrossRef]
128. Escudier, B.; Dorval, T.; Chaput, N.; Andre, F.; Caby, M.P.; Novault, S.; Flament, C.; Leboulaire, C.; Borg, C.; Amigorena, S.; et al. Vaccination of metastatic melanoma patients with autologous dendritic cell (DC) derived-exosomes: Results of thefirst phase I clinical trial. *J. Transl. Med.* **2005**, *3*, 10. [CrossRef]

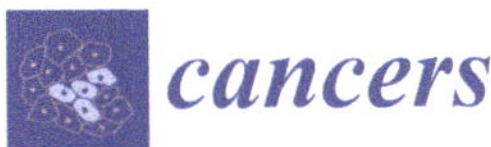

Review

Randomized Controlled Immunotherapy Clinical Trials for GBM Challenged

Stefaan W. Van Gool [1,*], Jennifer Makalowski [1], Simon Fiore [1], Tobias Sprenger [1], Lothar Prix [2], Volker Schirrmacher [1] and Wilfried Stuecker [1]

[1] Immun-Onkologisches Zentrum Köln, Hohenstaufenring 30-32, 50674 Koln, Germany; makalowski@iozk.de (J.M.); fiore@iozk.de (S.F.); tobias@sprenger-praxis.de (T.S.); v.schirrmacher@web.de (V.S.); stuecker@iozk.de (W.S.)

[2] Biofocus, Berghäuser Strasse 295, 45659 Recklinghausen, Germany; l.prix@ladr.de

[*] Correspondence: vangool@iozk.de; Tel.: +49-221-420-39925

Simple Summary: Although multiple meta-analyses on active specific immunotherapy treatment for glioblastoma multiforme (GBM) have demonstrated a significant prolongation of overall survival, no single research group has succeeded in demonstrating the efficacy of this type of treatment in a prospective, double-blind, placebo-controlled, randomized clinical trial. In this paper, we explain how the complexity of the tumor biology and tumor–host interactions make proper stratification of a control group impossible. The individualized characteristics of advanced therapy medicinal products for immunotherapy contribute to heterogeneity within an experimental group. The dynamics of each tumor and in each patient aggravate comparative stable patient groups. Finally, combinations of immunotherapy strategies should be integrated with first-line treatment. We illustrate the complexity of a combined first-line treatment with individualized multimodal immunotherapy in a group of 70 adults with GBM and demonstrate that the integration of immunogenic cell death treatment within maintenance chemotherapy followed by dendritic cell vaccines and maintenance immunotherapy might provide a step towards improving the overall survival rate of GBM patients.

Citation: Van Gool, S.W.; Makalowski, J.; Fiore, S.; Sprenger, T.; Prix, L.; Schirrmacher, V.; Stuecker, W. Randomized Controlled Immunotherapy Clinical Trials for GBM Challenged. *Cancers* **2021**, *13*, 32. https://dx.doi.org/10.3390/cancers13010032

Received: 28 October 2020
Accepted: 21 December 2020
Published: 24 December 2020

Publisher's Note: MDPI stays neutral with regard to jurisdictional claims in published maps and institutional affiliations.

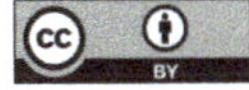

Abstract: Immunotherapies represent a promising strategy for glioblastoma multiforme (GBM) treatment. Different immunotherapies include the use of checkpoint inhibitors, adoptive cell therapies such as chimeric antigen receptor (CAR) T cells, and vaccines such as dendritic cell vaccines. Antibodies have also been used as toxin or radioactive particle delivery vehicles to eliminate target cells in the treatment of GBM. Oncolytic viral therapy and other immunogenic cell death-inducing treatments bridge the antitumor strategy with immunization and installation of immune control over the disease. These strategies should be included in the standard treatment protocol for GBM. Some immunotherapies are individualized in terms of the medicinal product, the immune target, and the immune tumor–host contact. Current individualized immunotherapy strategies focus on combinations of approaches. Standardization appears to be impossible in the face of complex controlled trial designs. To define appropriate control groups, stratification according to the Recursive Partitioning Analysis classification, MGMT promotor methylation, epigenetic GBM sub-typing, tumor microenvironment, systemic immune functioning before and after radiochemotherapy, and the need for/type of symptom-relieving drugs is required. Moreover, maintenance of a fixed treatment protocol for a dynamic, deadly cancer disease in a permanently changing tumor–host immune context might be inappropriate. This complexity is illustrated using our own data on individualized multimodal immunotherapies for GBM. Individualized medicines, including multimodal immunotherapies, are a rational and optimal yet also flexible approach to induce long-term tumor control. However, innovative methods are needed to assess the efficacy of complex individualized treatments and implement them more quickly into the general health system.

Keywords: GBM; newcastle disease virus; modulated electrohyperthermia; dendritic cell vaccination; clinical trial; individualized multimodal immunotherapy

1. Introduction

Cancer is the second leading cause of death, accounting for about 1 in 6 human deaths. Worldwide, in 2018, about 9.6 million deaths were due to cancer [1]. Between 2013 and 2017, the cancer death rate (mortality rate) in the US was 158/100,000 individuals per year. The rate of new cases (incidence) in a similar period was 442/100,000 individuals per year [2]. Intensive preclinical and clinical research is being performed to find solutions. In some domains, like pediatric hemato-oncology, major progress has been realized towards a cure through systematic randomized controlled clinical trials (RCTs). In each trial, a new experimental arm is assessed versus the best current treatment as the control arm [3,4], in combination with careful monitoring of (long-term) side effects [5].

Despite being an orphan disease, brain tumors are the leading cause of cancer death in males aged 20 to 39 years and the fourth most common cause of cancer death in females in the same age range [6]. Glioblastoma Multiforme (GBM) is the most frequently diagnosed malignant brain cancer in adults and has the worst prognosis [7,8]. The cause of GBM formation is not known. Ageing that progressively suppresses normal immune surveillance has been mentioned to contribute to GBM cell initiation and/or outgrowth [9]. Irradiation is certainly a cause for GBM formation, and the prognosis of a second malignant GBM is extremely poor [10]. Long-term exposure to higher doses of non-ionising irradiation has been associated with the formation of GBM [11]. Finally, viral infections like CMV (variants) have been mentioned as being potential triggers for GBM formation [12]. The classic pillars of treatment for GBM nowadays are neurosurgery, radiochemotherapy, and maintenance chemotherapy [13,14]. In recent years, the standard of care has not changed. Intensive research in different domains has been performed to improve the prognosis of GBM patients, including research in tumor-treating fields, anti-angiogenic treatments, targeted therapies, oncolytic virus therapy, and immunotherapies. The latter term covers different approaches, like restorative immunotherapy, modulating immunotherapy, passive immunotherapy, adoptive immunotherapy, and active-specific immunotherapy with vaccines [15]. For the development and production of mostly personalized cell-based therapies, Good Manufacturing Practice (GMP) facilities are required.

On the occasion of a regulatory audit in July 2019, in connection with the installation of a new GMP facility at the Immune Oncologic Centre in Köln (IOZK, www.iozk.de) and the running GMP-compatible production of IO-Vac® Dendritic cell (DC) vaccines, a discussion was raised with respect to RCTs within the spectrum of delivered individualized multimodal immunotherapy (IMI) activities. The background of this question is a subject of current global debate regarding the future use of controlled RCTs to obtain evidence of the efficacy of immunotherapies. This was exemplified by the symposium organized in Brussels on 22 April 2020, entitled "are randomized trials obsolete?" [16]. On 27 May 2015, the IOZK received a certificate of GMP manufacturing compliance (DE_NW_04_GMP_2015_0030) and approval to produce specific autologous anti-tumor DC vaccines for intradermal injection (DE_NW_04_MIA_2015_0033). Since then, multimodal immunotherapy has been implemented in several domains of cancer. Both certificates were renewed on 20 May 2020 (i.e., DE-NW-04-GMP-2020-0054 and DE-NW-04-MIA-2020-0017).

The IOZK is a translational immune-oncology center specializing in the fast translation of emerging novel insights derived from multiple domains of immunotherapy into clinical applications for use on a compassionate basis ("Individueller Heilversuch") for patients with cancer. The key medicinal product is IO-Vac®, which is an approved Advanced Therapy Medicinal Product (ATMP). The IO-Vac® vaccine consists of autologous mature DCs loaded with autologous tumor antigens and matured with danger signals including the Newcastle Disease Virus (NDV). Over the years, the IOZK has established its value for the treatment of cancer patients. Several case reports and retrospective analyses of patient groups have been published [17–20]. For the current retrospective analysis, the database was fixed at 28 June 2020, including all records registered from 1 June 2015 to 31 May 2020. Over this 5-year time period, 1456 medical records were initiated at the IOZK. The patients came from 69 countries (with 46% from Germany). From this group of patients, 1098 patients agreed to go through an immune-oncologic evaluation and immunodiagnostic blood sampling in order to study the cell numbers and functioning of their immune compartment, the tumor–host immune interactions, their general health status, and their infection status. Ultimately, 651 were able to, and individually consented to, starting multimodal immunotherapy, after being extensively informed about all aspects of the treatment. These patients belonged to all categories of cancer disease. The three most frequent cancer disease categories were neuro-oncology (42%), digestive oncology (18%), and breast cancer (11%). The domain of neuro-oncology represents almost half of all patients effectively treated at the IOZK. This group of patients is still a very heterogeneous group, including multiple types of brain cancer disease, and including patients at different stages of disease. From the 276 patients, 171 patients (62%) were recorded as having GBM.

Based on this large number of patients and the presence of extensive preclinical, translational, and clinical expertise in immunotherapy for GBM, the discussion about the challenges in setting up RCTs for immunotherapy herein will be focused on IMI for GBM, in particular to demonstrate why RCTs to prove the efficacy of this type of treatment are lacking, despite several meta-analyses pointing to a significant shift in overall survival (OS) rates due to the use of active specific immunotherapy with DC vaccines [21–25]. We aim to discuss this complex problem by reviewing the literature (Sections 2–7). Afterwards, we illustrate elements from this narrative review with our own data obtained by a retrospective analysis of our patient records (Sections 8–10).

2. Current Anti-Cancer Treatment Strategies for GBM

GBM is one of the leading causes of death due to cancer in humans and is a major burden for the community [26,27]. Earlier, in the period of poor imaging possibilities, neurosurgery was the only treatment for GBM, and this was mostly performed to make pathological diagnoses and to temporarily relieve symptoms. Only during the last century other treatment modalities became available, of which radiotherapy was the first approach. Radiotherapy became part of the standard care for GBM in the 1940s. The authors could not find any RCTs from that period. Evidence of the efficacy of radiotherapy was certainly created by the demonstration of a dose–response relationship [28]. An RCT, including radiotherapy, chemotherapy, or best available care for anaplastic astrocytoma, was realized around the same period, clearly demonstrating the effect of radiotherapy on OS [29]. Radiotherapy was shown to improve the median OS of GBM patients by some months, and 60 Gy appeared to be the most efficacious and safe dose [30]. More recently, chemotherapeutic agents and combination treatments have been implemented. The addition of temozolomide (TMZ) during radiotherapy, followed by TMZ maintenance chemotherapy (TMZm), further improved the median OS (again, by some months). Proof of evidence was generated through a prospective RCT. In this trial, patients were stratified by World Health Organization (WHO) performance status, type of surgery, and institution [13]. Later on, the data were presented according to an adapted Recursive Partitioning Analysis (RPA) classification, which included age, WHO performance status, extent of surgery, and mental status as variables, resulting in Class III, Class IV, and Class V patients [14].

The MGMT promotor methylation status of the tumor was rapidly recognized as a key factor in the efficacy of TMZ [31]. Retrospective analyses of available MGMT promotor methylation data in relation to the survival data in the RCT have shed new light on such data [14]. The progression-free survival (PFS) benefit attained through the addition of TMZ to surgery and radiotherapy lost its significance in MGMT promotor unmethylated patients, and the gain in median OS was only 0.8 months (i.e., 24 to 25 days), albeit still being significant. Although the results of the original prospective RCT were published 15 years ago, this so-called Stupp regimen is still the standard of care world-wide for both MGMT promotor-methylated and unmethylated patients. Due to its major effect, even in multivariate analyses, the MGMT promotor methylation status has become part of the in/exclusion criteria for RCTs or is used in the stratification of the randomization. Step by step, more insight into the transcriptomic and genomic dimensions were found, and

GBM molecular stratification appeared, pointing to EGFR, NF1, and PDGFRA/IDH1 as playing roles in triggering intracellular pathways but also in influencing the response to anti-GBM treatments, formation of the tumor microenvironment, and tumor spread [32]. A further molecular biological analysis including epigenetic profiling unraveled at least six sub-types of GBM, all having different disease characteristics and prognoses [33].

Radiotherapy and chemotherapy treatment modalities are directed against the cancer itself, but cause acute and long-term side effects to the body. These treatments might, however, also have important effects on the immune system. It is already well-known that neurosurgical removal of the tumor transiently "relieves" the systemic immune system from tumor-induced immunosuppression [34], which returns upon disease progression [35]. Both radiotherapy and TMZ have effects on inflammation and the systemic immune compartment but may also influence the tumor microenvironment [36–40].

The improvement in therapeutic approaches has been paralleled by improvements in imaging technologies. Furthermore, knowledge of the molecular biology domain has increased rapidly, thereby introducing new approaches to the development of targeted treatments with less toxicity. A whole series of targeted therapies have been investigated for GBM, as single drugs in relapsed patients or as add-ons to the Stupp regimen [41–46]. Fast molecular biological diagnostic procedures and initiation of adapted drug combinations have opened the door to so-called personalized medicine. For the first time, a particular tumor entity is no longer treated according to pre-designed treatments or study protocols but may become adapted to the individual tumor biology profile of each individual patient. Along the same line, targeted therapies can be implemented to treat any type of cancer, regardless of where in the body it started or the type of tissue from which it developed, pointing to the term "tumor-agnostic treatment" [47].

3. Challenges for RCTs

RCTs, originally conceived as a study concept by Sir Austin Bradford Hill (who also developed the criteria for determining a causal association) and applied for the first time in 1948 [48], aim to control for selection bias and allocation bias by balancing patient groups based on known and unknown prognostic factors. Blinding further reduces experimenter and subject biases. The study methodology allows the efficacy of an intervention under investigation to be demonstrated with the greatest amount of evidence in a defined patient population compared to a control population without this particular intervention. RCTs are the gold standard for proving the efficacy of an intervention. Nevertheless, over the years, research has neglected the additional value of observational studies, demonstrating the effectiveness of interventions [49–54].

Evolution towards the personalization of medicine is challenging for classic RCTs, especially when related to GBM [55]. Stratification is a requirement to avoid differences between patients treated in an experimental arm versus patients treated in a control arm. The need for larger patient groups has resulted in longer recruitment periods and more expensive clinical trials. The rapid introduction of new drugs has forced clinical researchers to form innovative statistical designs for clinical trials, such as Continual Reassessment Method designs, Sequential Multiple Assignment Randomized Trial designs, and Multi-Arm Multi-Stage clinical designs [56].

At present, most (if not all) single-drug-targeted therapy trials for GBM have failed [57], and a new challenge has emerged. Indeed, GBM is a mixture of different tumor cell clones, including glioma cancer stem cells, and there are dynamic changes in emerging and disappearing clones during the course of the disease and in relation to the treatment(s) given [58,59]. Keeping a patient under a fixed treatment protocol over time, eventually in clinical trials, to treat a dynamically and rapidly changing deadly tumor might no longer be considered appropriate in light of advances in modern medicine. Much more effort should be put into studies on liquid biopsies in patients with GBM [60]. These tests should be performed repeatedly during treatment in order to monitor changes in tumor biology during treatment, as has been shown for other cancer diseases [61].

Inflammatory reactions occurring in the context of immunotherapy might necessitate medical intervention, such as the use of steroids or Bevacizumab, for a short period of time. Due to the deadly nature of the disease, changes over time should be taken into account when treating the patient using a study protocol. Such changes during the protocol might induce drop-out of the trial, which is—from a medical perspective—an emotional burden for the patient. Otherwise, changes in treatment have to be taken as data within the protocol, which creates statistical conflicts with the control group of patients, who must then be treated differently.

One of the particular statistical challenges in demonstrating the efficacy of an active specific immunotherapy is the need to assess the increase of percentage long-term OS, rather than the shift of PFS [62], the latter being the usual primary read-out for testing new drugs in late stage phase II RCTs. A phenomenon of GBM pseudo-progression due to immunotherapy makes the read-out of PFS virtually impossible. Similar to the change in using the MacDonald's criteria [63] to the RANO criteria [64] to define progression at a time when TMZ was implemented in routine clinical treatment, iRANO criteria have been developed to assess the progression of GBM disease in the context of immunotherapy [65,66]. The increase in the percentage of long-term OS due to DC vaccines as a primary read-out necessitates the use of a much higher number of patients in a RCT, as compared with examining a shift in the median PFS, to yield results showing a significant difference with high enough power. Still, long-term OS is the only relevant read-out from immunotherapy trials.

4. Immunotherapy for GBM

Immunotherapy was called a "break-through for cancer" by Science in 2013. In 2011 and 2018, Nobel Prizes for Medicine were devoted to researchers who discovered important insights into the use of immunotherapy for cancer. At present, immunotherapy is definitively an important pillar in anticancer treatment in general, including GBM. Immunotherapy is a very broad term, comprising several technologies. Immunomodulation with checkpoint inhibitors is considered to belong to the domain of tumor-agnostic treatments [47]. Immunotherapies generally do not point to the molecular biological characteristics inside tumor cells, but, rather, to the surface of tumor cells, including a heterogeneous number of known and unknown tumor antigens [67] and immune costimulatory and inhibitory molecules on the surface [68–70], as well as the production of cytokines and chemokines that influence the immune system and the inflammatory response [71]. Terms like "cold" versus "hot" tumors, describing differences in lymphocyte infiltration in the tumor microenvironment, have become highly relevant [72]. The tumor mutational burden might be related to the presence of more or less tumor antigens on the surface [73,74]. Some genetic abnormalities, such as the p53 mutation, affect the extent of the expression of MHC molecules on the tumor cell surface [75]. An immunogram is created using the tumor foreignness, general immune status, immune cell infiltration, absence/presence of checkpoints, absence/presence of soluble inhibitors, absence/presence of inhibitory tumor metabolism, and sensitivity of the tumor to immune effectors [76]. The recognition that almost half of GBM tumors consist of cells belonging to the myeloid compartment (e.g., M1/M2 macrophages, tumor-associated macrophages, myeloid-derived suppressor cells, microglia) makes the understanding of the response to treatment and the ultimate outcome of patients more difficult [77,78]. Overall, the tumor microenvironment can be categorized into three functional sub-types that play significant roles in the outcomes of patients [79]. Interestingly, Hallaert et al. [80] also observed that the connection of GBM to the sub-ventricular zone appears to be a novel, independent risk factor leading to a worse prognosis. An association between sub-ventricular zone contact and markers related to the epithelial–mesenchymal transition was discovered [81]. Moreover, there is a definite influence of the tumor and the response to treatment on the systemic immune and inflammatory compartments [34]. Finally, steroids, radiotherapy, and chemotherapy all influence antitumor immune responses [39]; this, again, differs from patient to patient. A strong correlation was found between OS and the systemic immune profile after neurosurgical resection and after radiochemotherapy when the extent of resection and timing of immunotherapy were taken into account [40].

5. Risk Factors and Levels of Personalized Medicine

All in all, in addition to the clinical risk profile, the intracellular molecular biology, and the epigenetic profiling of tumor cells, the anatomic location of the tumor, tumor–host interactions in the tumor microenvironment, the systemic immune system, the combination treatment design and the reaction of the body, and dynamic changes in the tumor should be taken into account and used as mandatory stratification tools in the design of RCTs with experimental versus control groups (Table 1). Some of these have been included in novel molecular RPA classification (GBM-molRPA) systems [82].

Table 1. Risk factors for stratification in randomization or for in/exclusion criteria.

1. Recursive Partitioning Analysis (RPA) clinical classification
- Grading
- Extent of resection
- Age
- Karnofsky performance index
- Mental status
- Dose of radiotherapy

2. Molecular biology of tumor
- Tumor mutational burden
- Epigenetic sub-typing
- Molecular machinery of tumor cell clones
- Metabolic features of tumor

3. Load of glioma cancer stem cells in connection to periventricular zones of the brain
4. Tumor–host immune reaction
- Tumor antigen expression
- Check point expression
- Inflammatory response, M1/M2 balance, Tumor-associated macrophages, myeloid-derived suppressor cells, microglia reactivity
- T-cell infiltration
- Vascularization and oxidative stress

5. Systemic immune compartment
- Cell numbers under standard of care treatment
- Th1/Th2 balance
- Presence of Treg
- Presence of MDSC
- Level of natural killer cell reactivity

6. Systemic treatments outside standard of care
- Steroids
- Anti-angiogenic drugs
- Complementary medicines

Immunotherapy covers many treatment modalities. Some of these treatment modalities, such as cytokines, are not personalized to each patient. Other drugs, like antibodies, are themselves not personalized, but are directed against personalized targets on the tumor cell surface. For adoptive cell therapies with chimeric antigen receptor (CAR) T-cells or T cell receptor-transduced T-cells, both the ATMP itself and the target are personalized [83–85]. In the domain of active specific immunotherapy with vaccines, the vaccine itself can be an individual product at the level of the antigen carrier (like autologous DCs) and/or at the level of the antigen, such as tumor-derived antigens and, especially, highly individualized tumor-specific epitopes [86–88]. Extensive individualization of the treatment drug and target makes the design of a homogeneous experimental arm versus control arm very challenging. By introducing immunotherapy into a first-line treatment combination, new dimensions of personalization for the treatment of GBM have become clear (Table 2).

Table 2. Levels of personalized medicine for Glioblastoma Multiforme (GBM).

1. Molecular biology of tumor

- Tumor mutational burden
- Epigenetic sub-typing
- Molecular machinery of tumor cell clones
- Metabolic features of the tumor

2. Tumor–host immune reaction

- Tumor antigen expression
- Check point expression
- Inflammatory response, M1/M2 balance, TAM, MDSC, microglia reactivity
- T-cell infiltration
- Vascularization and oxidative stress
- Load of glioma cancer stem cells in connection to periventricular zones of the brain

3. Immune reactivity against the tumor

- Th1/Th2 balance
- Presence of Treg
- Presence of MDSC
- Level of NK cell reactivity

4. Reaction of the immune system upon other treatments

- Sensitivity to radiotherapy
- Sensitivity to chemotherapy
- Use of steroids
- Use of anti-angiogenic drugs

5. Response to treatment
6. Immunotherapy components

- Tumor antigens
- Patient-derived cell products

Overwhelming evidence of the efficacy of DC vaccination for GBM has been presented in preclinical models [89–101], as well as in phase I and early phase II non-controlled clinical trials [88,102–164]. The observation of long-term OS in patients after DC vaccination, noting that the intervention abruptly changes the 100% lethality of disease, has generated strong evidence of its efficacy. Several meta-analyses have demonstrated a significant improvement in long-term OS when GBM patients were treated with DC vaccines as compared with patients given a control treatment [21–25]. Of note, the latter meta-analysis also demonstrated a lack of additional toxicity due to immunotherapy in comparison with the standard of care. This means that the set-up of new phase I or phase IIa clinical trials is no longer innovative.

As has already been pointed out for the changes in molecular sub-clones over time during treatment, evidence that tumor–host immune interactions can also change over time has been obtained. Examples are the downregulation of specific target antigens [165] or the upregulation of PDL1 on tumor cells, allowing them to escape from immune attack during immunotherapy [19]. Dynamic changes in the expression of tumor-associated antigens and immunosuppressive factors in the tumor microenvironment during treatment have also been described [164].

6. Current Landscape

On 12 October 2020, we performed a search of Clinicaltrials.gov using the terms "dendritic cell", "interventional studies" "glioblastoma", and "interventional phase 2 phase 3 phase 4". Twenty-nine studies were available, with 12 of them reporting to be recruiting (Table 3). Seven of these studies were RCTs, with six having OS in the read-out analysis. Only one study (NCT04277221) was a phase 3 study. NCT03395587, NCT04115761, and NCT01567202 integrated DC vaccination into the primary standard of care for IDH1wt GBM. Similarly, NCT03548571 integrated DC vaccination into the primary standard of care, but only for MGMT promotor non-methylated patients. The RCTs NCT02465268 and NCT03688178 integrated DC vaccination into the standard of care, but did not mention the requirement of IDH1 wild-type status.

Hence, at the moment of writing, seven RCTs are recruiting and studying DC vaccination for patients with initial diagnosis of GBM. None of these studies mentioned further stratification. The median number of patients used for randomization was 106, ranging from 24 to 136. Nevertheless, based on the analysis above, stratification at multiple levels (as summarized in Table 1) should be used in order to design a proper control group. Such stratification affects the number of patients recruited, and this number seems, in all running trials, to be too small to yield a significant difference with sufficient power in the efficacy of DC vaccination to increase the percentage of patients with long-term OS versus an appropriate control group.

Table 3. ClinicalTrials.gov Search Results on 12/10/2020 for "dendritic cell", "interventional studies" "glioblastoma", and "interventional phase 2 phase 3 phase 4".

Label	Phase	Number of Patients	Randomized	Status	Primary Outcome	Estimated Study Completion
NCT00576537	2	50	No	Completed	Safety/Toxicity	10/2011
NCT02649582	1 + 2	20	No	Recruiting	OS, Safety/Toxicity Feasibility	12/2020
NCT00846456	1 + 2	20	No	Completed	Toxicity, Immune response	02/2013
NCT00323115	2	11	No	Completed	Immune response, Toxicity, PFS	07/2013
NCT02366728	2	100	RCT	Active, not recruiting	OS, DC migration	08/2020
NCT01204684	2	60	RCT	Active, not recruiting	PFS, OS	01/2021
NCT03927222	2	48	No	Recruiting	OS, DC migration	12/2023
NCT01006044	2	26	No	Completed	PFS, Toxicity	08/2014
NCT03395587	2	136	RCT	Recruiting	OS, PFS	06/2023
NCT04523688	2	28	No	Not recruiting	PFS	12/2025
NCT03548571	2 + 3	60	RCT	Recruiting	PFS, OS	05/2023
NCT04115761	2	24	RCT	Recruiting	PSF	06/2022
NCT03014804	2	0	RCT	Withdrawn		
NCT03879512	1 + 2	25	No	Recruiting	OS, PFS	01/2022
NCT02772094	2	50	No	Unknown	OS, Toxicity	12/2016
NCT01567202	2	100	RCT	Recruiting	Response, PFS, OS	02/2020
NCT01213407	2	87	RCT	Completed	PFS, OS	11/2015
NCT01291420	1 + 2	10	No	Unknown	Immune response	Unknown
NCT02465268	2	120	RCT	Recruiting	OS, Immune response, PFS	06/2024
NCT04277221	3	118	RCT	Recruiting	OS, PFS	12/2022
NCT00323115	2	11	No	Completed	T-cell response	07/2013
NCT03400917	2	55	No	Completed	OS	02/2023
NCT02546102	3	414	RCT	Suspended	OS	12/2021
NCT01280552	2	124	RCT	Completed	OS	12/2015
NCT00045968	3	348	RCT	Unknown	PFS	11/2016
NCT03688178	2	112	RCT	Recruiting	OS, Varlimumab safety, Treg level	03/2025
NCT01759810	2 + 3	60	No	Enrolling by invitation	OS	12/2020
NCT02754362	2	10	No	Withdrawn	Immune response	06/2019
NCT04388033	1 + 2	10	No	Recruiting	Safety, PFS	12/2023

DC: dendritic cell; OS: overall survival; PFS: progression free survival; RCT: randomized controlled trial.

7. Non-Scientific Challenges

In the design of larger RCTs with a control arm, clinical researchers have run into new problems. GBM is a deadly disease. The first interest of the patient is the prolongation of a good-quality life. As DC vaccination has already been shown to significantly prolong long-term OS with a good quality of life, it eventually became unethical to prevent patients in the control arm from being given this innovative fourth anti-GBM immunotherapy modality. Therefore, some RCTs published with PFS as the primary endpoint used a cross-over protocol from the control group to the DC vaccination group, either structurally within the trial design (EudraCT 2009-018228-14) [151] or after reaching the primary end-point (NCT00045968) [160]. By doing so, the OS assessment was, in fact, no longer controlled. In the former study, stratification of RPA classification was used. In the latter study, stratification for MGMT methylation was used.

It is notable that the three largest RCTs initiated to date have faced huge logistic/financial problems, as follows: (1) The EudraCT 2009-018228-14 trial aimed to include 146 study objects but was abruptly closed by the sponsor after the inclusion of 135 patients. The reasons for this were kept confidential. Nevertheless, the scientific data were made available, were extremely well-documented, and were partially transferred onto the platform of the EU Project Computational Horizons in Cancer (www.chic-vph.eu). Data on 132 patients were finally brought into a new study, named the Glioma Translat Study, and published [166,167]; (2) NCT00045968 was designed to include 348 study objects with PFS as the primary read-out and OS as the secondary read-out. Eighty sites in four countries were used for recruitment. The study screened 1268 patients and ended up with 331 randomizations into the main study [160]. Patient recruitment was initiated in 2007 but was paused from 2009 to 2011 for economic reasons. The final patient was enrolled in November 2015. This resulted in a recruitment period of nine years, an effective inclusion period of six years, and a mean of four patients per recruiting site at an effective rate of less than one patient per year per site. Five years later, at the time of writing, the final results regarding the randomized data collected on these patients and the answer to the primary question (PFS) have not yet been published; (3) NCT02546102 suspended further patient randomization due to financial reasons [168]. It is not clear how many patients had already been recruited into the trial.

Finally, patients have started searching on blogs and in social media communities for solutions to surviving GBM. An impressive list of complementary medicines and diets is available and freely accessible to patients. Some of these complementary medicines surely influence the course of the disease or the reactivity of the host [169–173]. It seems impossible to control for this when setting up and running RCTs at present.

8. Individualized Multimodal Immunotherapy for GBM

Two conclusions have become clear: (1) Individualized treatment at multiple levels, with strategies that follow the dynamic changes in both the tumor and host (e.g., immunity, inflammation) during treatment, is needed for the treatment of GBM; and (2) IMI is becoming part of the first-line treatment for GBM, integrated into the standard of care. The potential inherent immunization component of standard anti-GBM strategies (e.g., neurosurgery, radiotherapy, and chemotherapy) and the proven induction of immunogenic cell death (ICD) through the use of innovative anti-cancer treatments (e.g., modulated electrohyperthermia, oncolytic virus therapy) [174,175] should be exploited and strengthened with active immunization strategies and further optimized with immunomodulatory strategies in the context of optimized complementary medicine. Only broad and long-term immune control over GBM is able to induce long-term OS. The rationale of such a strategy has been published [176]. In Sections 8–10, we aim to illustrate several elements discussed in the former narrative review with observational data obtained by a retrospective analysis of our own patient records. Over the years, we have developed a multistep treatment approach, in which ICD is induced by the combination of bolus injections with NDV and modulated electrohyperthermia (mEHT) integrated as an add-in treatment during the alkylating mode of tumor cell killing induced by TMZm chemotherapy, followed by IO-Vac® DC vaccination, in order to actively induce an antitumor immune response in combination with individually adapted immunomodulatory strategies. Finally, ICD treatment is maintained with immunomodulation [19].

Of the 171 recorded patients with GBM in the IOZK database, 90 patients (53%) received IMI in combination with first-line treatment for compassionate use ("individueller Heilversuch"). For the current retrospective analysis, we excluded all patients below 18 and above 75 years of age, patients with a proven pre-history of low-grade glioma and/or proven IDH1 mutation, patients with proven histone mutations, and patients with radiotherapy-induced GBM as a second malignancy, leaving 70 patients for analysis.

The final patient group consisted of 70 patients (33 females, 37 males). The median age of the patients was 50 years (range 18–69 years). The median Karnofsky performance index score was 90 (range 50–100). Clinical patient characteristics are shown in Figure 1. The patients presented for immune diagnostic blood sampling at IOZK at a median of three months after operation (range 0.5–23 months); hence, most sampling was done after radiochemotherapy. General blood counts and immune cell counts and functioning, as analyzed in the routine clinical laboratory, are shown in Figure 2A. A large proportion of patients were lymphopenic at that time—caused by the radiochemotherapy—a finding compatible with published data [39].

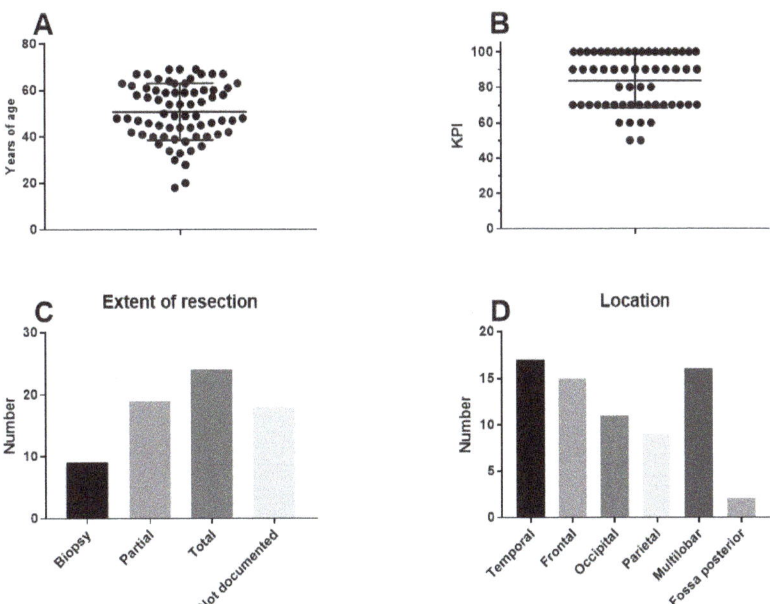

Figure 1. Clinical characteristics of the patients. Seventy adults with primary GBM receiving first-line standard of care in combination with individualized multimodal immunotherapy were included in this retrospective analysis: (**A**) age distribution; (**B**) distribution of Karnofsky performance index scores; (**C**) reported resection (number of patients); and (**D**) reported location (number of patients).

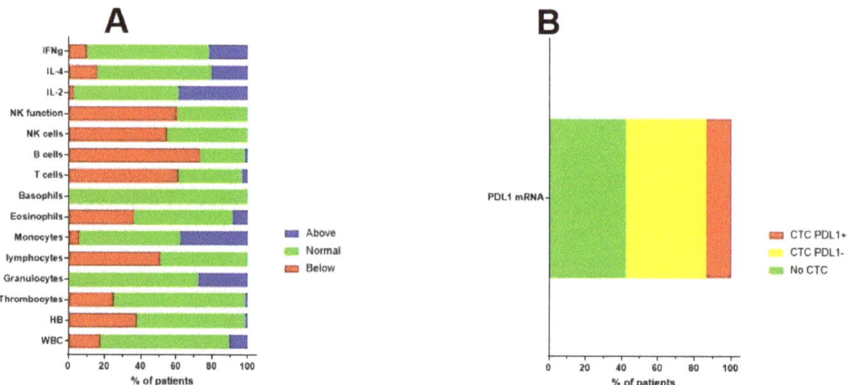

Figure 2. Immune variables before the start of immunotherapy. (**A**) Before the start of individualized multimodal immunotherapy, blood was drawn and sent to the routine clinical lab for analysis. Different immune variables are shown. The percentages of patients with values above (blue), within (normal, green), or below (red) the normal range are shown. (**B**) Blood was also sent to Biofocus in order to detect circulating tumor cells based on mRNA expression of GBM-related oncogenes. When cells were detected, the RNA expression for PDL1 was subsequently analyzed and cells were defined as negative (yellow) or positive (red) for the expression of mRNA for PDL1.

The MGMT promotor methylation status of the resected tumor was documented in 52 cases, from which 32 patients were categorized as unmethylated. In 67 patients, the presence of circulating tumor cells (CTCs) was investigated at the time of immune diagnostic blood sampling. Blood samples were sent to Biofocus (https://www.biofocus.de/) for analysis. In 28 patients, no CTCs were detected. CTCs were detected in 39 patients, based on the presence of large cells with mRNA expression for specific oncogenes (EGFR, ERBB2, C-kit, and Telomerase) above a cut-off in comparison with house-keeping mRNA expression. In nine patients, mRNA expression for PDL1 was above the cut-off value of 2 (Figure 2B). In 11 patients, increased mRNA expression for MGMT was observed, of which seven patients were histologically classified as being MGMT promotor unmethylated, while three patients were classified as being methylated (one patient had an unknown histology result). For 16 patients who had CTC without increased mRNA for MGMT, six samples matched with a histologic classification as MGMT promotor methylated, while nine samples mismatched with the histologic classification and were classified as MGMT promotor unmethylated. It should be noted that the categories for both histology-based MGMT promotor methylation and the mRNA expression of MGMT in CTCs were derived from continuous variables linked with methylated versus unmethylated status. Moreover, GBM might depict heterogeneity for MGMT promotor methylation, such that histology sampling errors cannot be excluded. Finally, the presence of CTCs was investigated at a median of three months after operation, thereby potentially illustrating clonal evolution during the first period of radiochemotherapy.

To further illustrate the biological evolutions that occurred during treatment, we looked at the evolution of mRNA expressions in CTCs for the oncogenes EGFR, ERBB2, C-kit, and Telomerase, as well as the mRNA for MGMT and PDL1 over time. For this, available data on mRNA expression in CTCs were sampled and put on a time line for each patient starting from neurosurgery. As mentioned earlier, the patients started immunotherapy at different time points and were treated individually. This is reflected by the use of an individual monitoring schedule for each patient. Figure 3A shows the evolution of the EGFR mRNA expression over time for individual patients. Changes in mRNA expression were only observed in three patients. On the contrary, as shown in Figure 3B, mRNA expression for ERBB2, C-kit, Telomerase, MGMT, and PDL1, in comparison to mRNA expression for the house-keeping gene NADPH, clearly changed over time and was often visible around the appearance of relapse. As an example, the mRNA expression for PDL1 in the CTCs of patients 22,731 and 23,346 was low at the start of immunotherapy treatment. These values, however, increased during treatment and were ultimately accompanied by relapse. Patient 23,346 was treated with pembrolizumab. Patient 24,005 also had a very high level of mRNA expression for PDL1 when the CTCs became positive for the first time. This patient also received four doses of pembrolizumab, after which the CTCs became negative for the PDL1 marker. These descriptive data indirectly demonstrate the possible relative changes in sub-clones during the disease process, which might contribute to the occurrence of relapse and which might be monitored for timely intervention. GBM is thus a dynamic tumoral process. The descriptive analysis illustrates the heterogeneity within these 70 patients at the levels of clinical risk factors, immune variables in the peripheral blood, and molecular tumor biology data, as well as the dynamic processes occurring in the molecular biology of the tumor.

The patients received IMI within the first-line treatment. Table 4 shows the details of the IMI treatment. A median of two (range 0–5) IO-Vac® DC vaccines, 25 (range 0–77) NDV administrations, and 30 (range 0–77) sessions of modulated electrohyperthermia were given to each patient. One IO-Vac® DC vaccine consisted of a median of 12.2×10^6 autologous mature IO-Vac® DCs loaded with autologous tumor proteins derived from tumor lysate (when available and appropriate to the GMP requirements) or obtained as ICD-therapy-induced, serum-derived, antigenic, extracellular microvesicles, and apoptotic bodies.

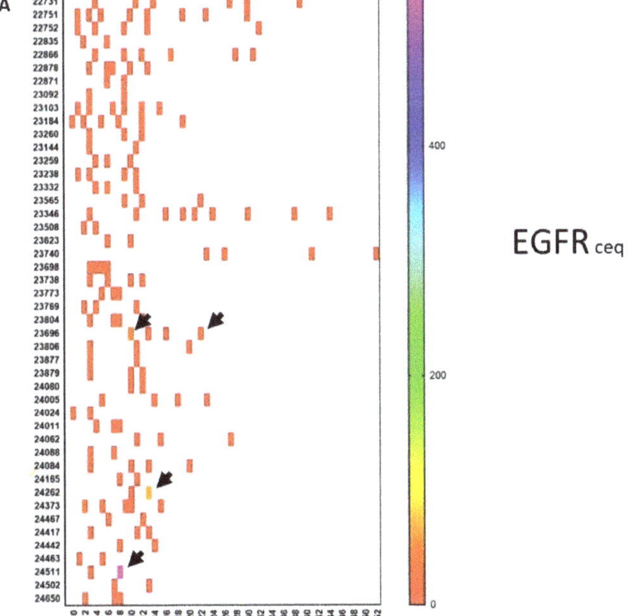

Figure 3. *Cont.*

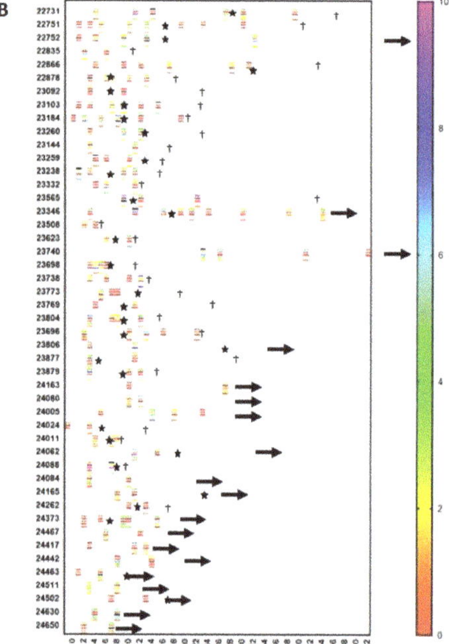

Figure 3. Evolution of oncogene expression in circulating tumor cells. Circulating tumor cells were measured repetitively in 46 patients. Each patient is referenced with a number on the *y*-axis. Time in months is indicated on the *x*-axis. The scale of the color of each test is shown on the right-hand side. (**A**) The level of mRNA expression for EGFR is expressed as the ceq (cell equivalent). Most of the values are negative (red). However, as indicated by the arrows, some patients showed an upregulation of EGFR during the disease course. (**B**) This shows a similar data set-up as in panel A. For each patient, data on mRNA expression are relative to the house-keeping gene GADPH and are shown in a particular color, for which the scale is shown on the right-hand side. For each patient, up to five lines are shown at different moments during the disease course. From top to bottom, values for ERBB2, c-Kit, telomerase, MGMT, and PDL1 are shown for each patient. Stars indicate new events. A † indicates when the patient died. An arrow to the right indicates the time at which the patient was censored in the analysis.

Table 4. Treatment details.

	Vaccine	**Local Hyperthermia**	**NDV**	**DC Total**	**DC/Vaccine**
N	69	70	69	70	112
Minimum	0	0	0	0	2,400,000
25%P	1	13	17	6,950,000	8,075,000
Median	2	25	30	20,115,000	12,200,000
75%	2	42	42	34,200,000	19,145,000

NDV: Newcastle Disease Virus.

9. A Case of Complete Remission and Specific T-Cell Response

In our retrospective analysis of these 70 patients, one particular innovative finding emerged. As the tumor-specific antigens were not known when using tumor lysate or serum-derived, extracellular vesicles and apoptotic bodies, the immune monitoring in our clinical setting was not a major focus. Nevertheless, proof of principle of ICD therapy in combination with TMZ maintenance chemotherapy followed by vaccination with IO-Vac® DC vaccines loaded with ICD therapy-induced, serum-derived, antigenic, extracellular microvesicles, and apoptotic bodies [19] for the induction of a tumor-neo-epitope-specific immune response was demonstrated in one patient. This 18-year-old patient had an incomplete resection of a left frontal lobe IDH1 wild-type and MGMT unmethylated GBM. The tumor mutational burden was low (0.5 variants/megabase), and there was no evidence for microsatellite instability or germline variants. She was treated with radiochemotherapy and, subsequently, five cycles of TMZm chemotherapy (Figure 4). At presentation, her Karnofsky performance index was 90. She was lymphopenic with 279/uL CD3+ T-cells, 78/uL CD19+ B-cells, and 56/uL CD16+CD56+ NK cells. Her NK cell functioning was below the reference value. She had Th2/Th17 skewing. Her CTCs showed upregulated expression (3.44) of mRNA for MGMT, which was compatible with the known unmethylated MGMT promotor status. The expression of mRNA for PDL1 was 1.13 (cut-off for positivity = 2). She continued treatment for another seven TMZm chemotherapy cycles combined with 5-day ICD treatments, which were given during each TMZm cycle at days 8 to 12. Afterwards, she received two IO-Vac® DC vaccinations loaded with ICD treatment-induced, serum-derived, antigenic, extracellular microvesicles, and apoptotic bodies. Later on, she received two IO-Vac® DC vaccines loaded with tumor-specific peptides based on the individualized tumor-specific neo-antigen detection tests performed at CeGaT (www.CeGaT.de). At the time of writing, she receives monthly maintenance ICD treatments and is still in complete remission. Interestingly, we were able to monitor the tumor antigen-specific T-cell responses as, in this case, the neo-antigens were known. A first sample was available after the fifth TMZm cycle, prior to the addition of multimodal immunotherapy. A second sample was available at the time of blood sampling to prepare the second IO-Vac® DC vaccine (Figure 4). From the data, it is clear that surgery, radiochemotherapy, and five cycles of TMZm did not induce a tumor-specific T-cell response. However, the addition of seven ICD treatments to the last seven TMZm treatments and the first IO-Vac® DC vaccine loaded with ICD-treatment-induced, serum-derived, antigenic, extracellular microvesicles, and apoptotic bodies generated a clear tumor antigen-specific CD4+ and CD8+ T-cell response. The impact of this observation might be meaningful. First, it is not mandatory to have fresh frozen tumor material to prepare a tumor lysate as an antigenic source. This avoids the critical challenges of yielding, freezing, transporting, analyzing, and preparing tumor material within a GMP context. Secondly, and even more importantly, if molecular subclones can change over time, their antigenic profiles can change as well. ICD treatment allows the yield of tumor antigens that are expressed within the body at the time of treatment and makes it possible for the vaccine to immunize against the antigens that are actually present, instead of tumor antigens identified at the time of tumor resection prior to radiotherapy and chemotherapy and hence prior to eventual treatment-induced tumor clone changes.

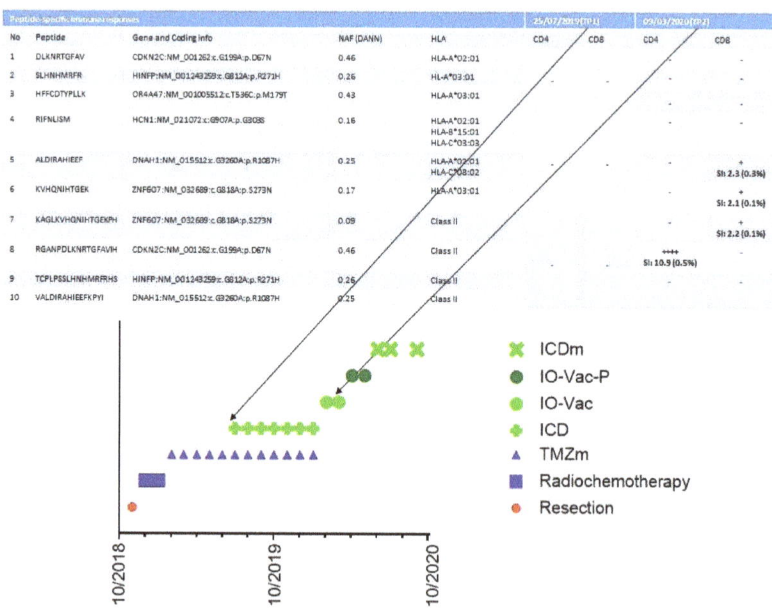

Figure 4. Detection of tumor-specific T-cell clones. The treatment timeline for patient 24442 and its multiple components are shown in the bottom part of the figure. TMZm indicates five days of temozolomide maintenance treatment in cycles (every 28 days). ICD indicates immunogenic cell death (ICD) treatment consisting of the combination of five injections with Newcastle Disease Virus and five sessions of modulated electrohyperthermia. IO-Vac indicates a vaccination cycle including six ICD treatments and an injection of IO-Vac® DC vaccine, consisting of autologous mature dendritic cells loaded with ICD-treatment-induced, serum-derived, antigenic, extracellular microvesicles and apoptotic bodies. IO-Vac-P vaccination cycles are equal to IO-Vac vaccination cycles, but the DCs are loaded with tumor-specific neo-peptides. The upper part of the curve shows the specific peptide sequences, the respective gene and coding information, the Novel Allele Frequency (NAF), and the HLA phenotype. TP1 and TP2 indicate the two respective time points at which T-cells were frozen for immune monitoring purposes. SI is the stimulation index, the ratio of polyfunctional activated CD4+ or CD8+ T-cells (positive for at least two activation markers from CD154, IFN-g, TNF, and/or IL-2) in the peptide-stimulated sample, compared with the unstimulated control. Additionally, the percentage of activated CD4+ or CD8+ T-cells (positive for at least one activation marker of CD154, IFN-g, TNF, and/or IL2) above the background and after in vitro amplification is given. This percentage does not directly reflect the frequencies in vivo. SI ≥ 2: weak response (+); SI ≥ 3: positive response (++); SI > 5: strong response (+++); SI > 10: very strong response (++++). Peptides 1–3, 4–6, and 7–10 were pooled for the analysis of TP1. Peptides 9 and 10 were pooled for the analysis of TP2.

10. Results in Term of OS

As we did not have reference radiology for the independent assessment of new events, given the need to follow the iRANO criteria [65,66] and as OS is certainly the most important outcome in the context of immunotherapy, we focused on the OS of the patients. As described earlier in Section 8, the retrospectively analyzed group of 70 patients was a heterogeneous group of patients. They best reflected adapted RPA class 4 patients, as published by Stupp et al. [14]. This reference was used as a historical control. Data were analyzed using GraphPad Prism version 7.00 for Windows (GraphPad Software, La Jolla, CA, USA, www.graphpad.com). One patient was lost during follow up. The median OS was 20.03 months (Figure 5A) with a 2-year OS of 38.83% (CI95%: +13.04, −13.25) and a 3-year OS of 31.41% (CI95%: +13.35, −12.55). Patients younger than 50 years (21 MGMT promoter unmethylated, 7 methylated, and 7 unknown) had a median OS of 22.07 months, which was not statistically different from the median OS of 18.07 months observed for patients older than 50 years (11 unmethylated, 13 methylated, and 11 unknown). We found MGMT promotor methylation status to be a significant factor (Figure 5B, log-rank test: p = 0.0004): patients (n = 20) with patients with MGMT promotor methylation having a median OS of 42.85 months versus 11.77 months for patients with unmethylated MGMT promotor status (n = 32).

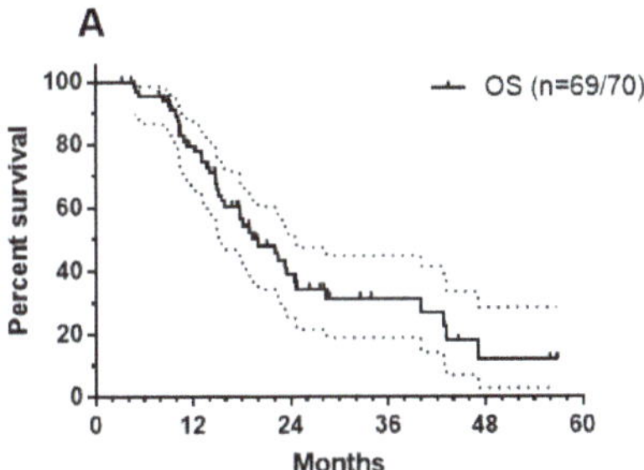

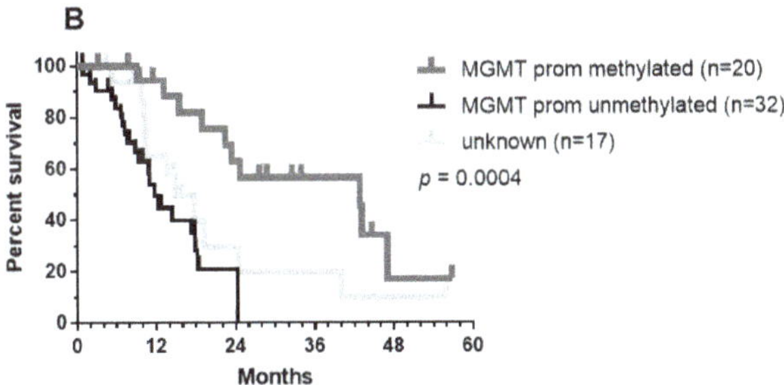

Figure 5. OS data: (**A**) OS data of the total patient group (CI95% values are shown). One patient out of 70 was lost during the follow up period and (**B**) the patient group was divided according to MGMT promotor methylation status—methylated (grey), unmethylated (black), data not registered (light grey). The p-values show significance using the Log-rank (Mantel–Cox) test.

For 16 patients, local therapy (neurosurgery, radiochemotherapy) was followed by IMI (Group 1). ICD therapy (the combination of IV bolus injections of NDV together with mEHT [19]) integrated into the TMZm chemotherapy cycles followed by IO-Vac® DC vaccines and maintenance ICD therapy was given to 46 patients (Group 2). Eight patients started with IMI after the last TMZ maintenance chemotherapy cycle (Group 3). The OS data were significantly different for the three treatment groups: 13.08 months for group 1, 22.46 months for group 2, and undefined for group 3 (median follow-up of surviving patients: 28.59 months, range 26.3–55.9 months; Figure 6A). The latter likely points to favorable selection of a small group of patients who experienced no events until after the end of the maintenance chemotherapy and profited from subsequent IMI treatment. The median OS of the patients with unmethylated MGMT promotor status was 11.25 months for group 1 (n = 7) and 18.07 months for group 2 (n = 21), with a 2-year OS of 0% in group 1 versus 17.18% (CI95% +31.65, −15.86) in group 2 (Figure 6B, log-rank test: p = 0.0273). The median OS of the patients with methylated MGMT promotor status was 42.85 months for group 2 (n = 15) with a 2-year OS of 66.66% (CI95%: +19.3, −32.96). There were only three patients in group 1 who had a tumor with MGMT promotor methylation status. Within treatment group 2, the differences in the OS curve due to MGMT promotor methylation status were significant (Figure 6C, Log-rank test: p = 0.0036).

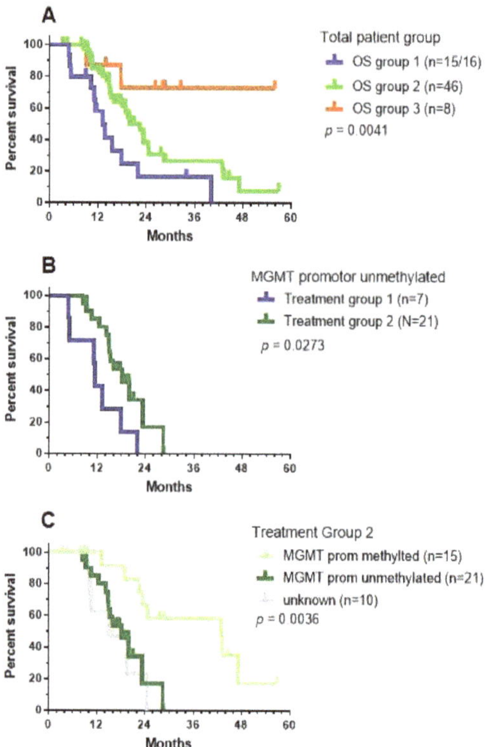

Figure 6. OS data for the treatment groups. As explained in the text, patients were categorized into three different treatment groups: (**A**) OS data for the three different patient groups; (**B**) OS data for the patients without MGMT promotor methylation belonging to treatment groups 1 (blue) and 2 (green); and (**C**) OS data of patients from treatment group 2, divided according to MGMT promotor methylation status. The *p*-values show the significance calculated using the Log-rank (Mantel–Cox) test.

Considering these data and the data published by Stupp et al. [14], patients with MGMT promotor unmethylated status have no relevant benefit from the addition of TMZ [14] or from treatment with IMI alone. However, the data from treatment group 2 suggest the potential benefit of the integration of ICD treatment within TMZm chemotherapy followed by IO-Vac® DC vaccinations, which was found to increase the median OS by about six months. On the other hand, treatment with IMI after local therapy for patients with MGMT promotor methylated GBM yielded similar median OS data as treatment with TMZm chemotherapy, while the integration of ICD treatment with TMZm chemotherapy followed by IO-Vac® DC vaccinations increased the median OS further—by about 18 months. These data are worth validating in prospective clinical research.

11. Conclusions

In this paper, we reviewed the multiple challenges related to the use of immunotherapy RCTs for GBM (Sections 2–7) and illustrated these challenges in a retrospective analysis of GBM patients treated at IOZK (Sections 8–10). GBM treatment is affected by the complexity of the tumor, the complexity of the immune and inflammatory micro-environment, the complexity of combined treatment approaches, and the complexity of dynamic changes occurring within the tumor, the tumor microenvironment, and the immune system. The set-up of immunotherapy RCTs for GBM is affected by the need for multiple stratifications to create an appropriate control group. Both stratification and the read-out of OS necessitate the use of a large number of study participants. The costs to run such RCTs are related not only to the Good Clinical Practice (GCP) documentation but also to the production of the ATMP in a GMP environment. As already mentioned, there has been an abundance of smaller phase I and phase II single-arm clinical trials, and several meta-analyses have shown the efficacy and safety of DC vaccination for GBM treatment. The high cost of non-innovative small RCTs with predicted negative outcomes due to a lack of appropriate stratification makes them not appropriate at this time due to limited resources. Models for OS and immunotherapy responses in patients with GBM based on DNA-methylation-driven, gene-based, molecular classifications and multi-omic analyses may be better tools for predicting the efficacy individually for each patient [177]. However, patients suffering today from GBM need better treatments, including the use of first-line immunotherapy to fight their cancers.

The multimodality of immunotherapy, besides the standard of care, presents a further challenge to the classic step-wise research methodology used in clinical research. IOZK aims to contribute to the general knowledge and communicate their gained experiences to the wider scientific community. The ATMP IO-Vac® DC vaccine has been used as part of IMI treatment in the framework of "Individueller Heilversuch". Each patient is treated at all personalized levels necessary. For each individual patient, the best possible solution for their medical needs is worked out. Prospective medical research questions on groups of patients are not generated. Nevertheless, the IOZK aims to repetitively freeze the database at certain time points and sample patient data to carry out scientifically correct retrospective analyses. The current analysis suggests that the addition of ICD treatment with NDV and mEHT during the application of TMZ maintenance chemotherapy, followed by IO-Vac® DC vaccinations and maintenance ICD treatment, may be beneficial for both MGMT promotor unmethylated and methylated GBM patients.

A final challenge in the broad implementation of innovative therapies like IMI, given that its effectiveness has been accepted without the use of RCTs, is the expected cost versus the length of additional survival. The production of personalized ATMPs under GMP conditions is expensive. The control over the ATMP quality, and hence over the costs, belongs to the authorities, who are also responsible for health policies in general. This topic points to the need for a cost-effectiveness analysis to compare the costs and outcomes of treatment options. The aim is to ensure the greatest possible health benefits are attained with a given budget. For macroeconomic considerations, cost-effectiveness thresholds (CETs) are usually related to the gross domestic product (GDP) per capita [178]. To the best of our knowledge, no representative data related to the integration of IMI into standard of care treatment of GBM are available. Single studies have appraised the additional cost of targeted therapies per year of survival if combined with chemotherapy. In non-small-cell lung cancer, for example, the additional cost for using atezolizumab in combination with carboplatin/nab-paclitaxel amounts to 333,199 USD per quality-adjusted life year [179]. Understandably, the respective costs are difficult to calculate and depend heavily on the type of cancer, the treatment in question, and the parameters used in the cost-effectiveness study. Accordingly, different methods have been described [180]. What we can say is that overall spending on cancer drugs has been increasing. For example, spending on cancer drugs rose from €7.6 billion in 2005 to €19.1 billion in 2014 in the EU [181]. For some types of cancer, calculations are available. Between 2007 and 2012, the mean amounts of money spent in the first year after diagnosis was $35,849, $26,295, $55,597, and $63,063 for breast, prostate, lung, and colorectal cancers, respectively [182]. In view of the overall increase in costs, even higher expenditure must be expected today. A more recent study on breast cancer reported the average cost per patient in the year after diagnosis as being between $60,637 and $134,682, depending on the cancer stage [183]. Newly approved pharmaceuticals easily cost more than $100,000 US per year. Costs are driven by various factors that are not proportional to their often modest additional benefits [184,185], exceeding the cost-effectiveness thresholds. In comparison, the addition of modulated electrohyperthermia to dose-dense temozolomide for the treatment of recurrent GBM has proven to be cost-effective [186]. Taken together, it is methodically difficult to compare the cost–benefit ratio of the integration of IMI into standard of care treatment. Considering the far higher overall costs of targeted therapies, one may expect that the ratio would not be unfavorable.

Author Contributions: Ideation, S.W.V.G., T.S., V.S. and W.S.; literature search, S.W.V.G., J.M. and T.S.; data analysis, S.W.V.G., S.F. and L.P.; Writing—original draft preparation, S.W.V.G.; Writing—review & editing, J.M., S.F., T.S., L.P., V.S. and W.S. All authors have read and agreed to the published version of the manuscript.

Funding: This research received no external funding.

Informed Consent Statement: All patients gave written informed consent for individualized multimodal immunotherapy as compassionate use treatment ("individueller Heilversuch").

Data Availability Statement: The data presented in Sections 8–10 are available on request from the corresponding author. The data are not publicly available due to privacy reasons.

Acknowledgments: The authors thank the clinical team, the team from the immune-diagnostic laboratory, and the team from the GMP laboratory at the IOZK for their excellent work in making this complex treatment possible for patients with GBM.

Conflicts of Interest: The authors declare no conflict of interest.

References

1. Available online: https://www.who.int/news-room/fact-sheets/detail/cancer (accessed on 18 December 2020).
2. Available online: https://www.cancer.gov (accessed on 18 December 2020).
3. Creutzig, U.; Zimmermann, M.; Dworzak, M.N.; Ritter, J.; Schellong, G.; Reinhardt, D. Development of a curative treatment within the AML-BFM studies. *Klin. Padiatr.* **2013**, *225* (Suppl. 1), S79–S86. [CrossRef]
4. Schrappe, M.; Reiter, A.; Ludwig, W.D.; Harbott, J.; Zimmermann, M.; Hiddemann, W.; Niemeyer, C.; Henze, G.; Feldges, A.; Zintl, F.; et al. Improved outcome in childhood acute lymphoblastic leukemia despite reduced use of anthracyclines and cranial radiotherapy: Results of trial ALL-BFM 90. German-Austrian-Swiss ALL-BFM Study Group. *Blood* **2000**, *95*, 3310–3322.
5. Loning, L.; Zimmermann, M.; Reiter, A.; Kaatsch, P.; Henze, G.; Riehm, H.; Schrappe, M. Secondary neoplasms subsequent to Berlin-Frankfurt-Munster therapy of acute lymphoblastic leukemia in childhood: Significantly lower risk without cranial radiotherapy. *Blood* **2000**, *95*, 2770–2775. [CrossRef]
6. Siegel, R.L.; Miller, K.D.; Jemal, A. Cancer Statistics, 2020. *Ca Cancer J. Clin.* **2020**, *70*, 7–30. [CrossRef]
7. Thakkar, J.P.; Dolecek, T.A.; Horbinski, C.; Ostrom, Q.T.; Lightner, D.D.; Barnholtz-Sloan, J.S.; Villano, J.L. Epidemiologic and molecular prognostic review of glioblastoma. *Cancer Epidemiol. Biomark. Prev.* **2014**, *23*, 1985–1996. [CrossRef] [PubMed]
8. Louis, D.N.; Perry, A.; Reifenberger, G.; von Deimling, A.; Figarella-Branger, D.; Cavenee, W.K.; Ohgaki, H.; Wiestler, O.D.; Kleihues, P.; Ellison, D.W. The 2016 World Health Organization Classification of Tumors of the Central Nervous System: A summary. *Acta Neuropathol.* **2016**, *131*, 803–820. [CrossRef]
9. Ladomersky, E.; Scholtens, D.M.; Kocherginsky, M.; Hibler, E.A.; Bartom, E.T.; Otto-Meyer, S.; Zhai, L.; Lauing, K.L.; Choi, J.; Sosman, J.A.; et al. The Coincidence between Increasing Age, Immunosuppression, and the Incidence of Patients with Glioblastoma. *Front. Pharm.* **2019**, *10*, 200. [CrossRef] [PubMed]
10. Izycka-Swieszewska, E.; Bien, E.; Stefanowicz, J.; Szurowska, E.; Szutowicz-Zielinska, E.; Koczkowska, M.; Sigorski, D.; Kloc, W.; Rogowski, W.; Adamkiewicz-Drozynska, E. Malignant Gliomas as Second Neoplasms in Pediatric Cancer Survivors: Neuropathological Study. *Biomed. Res. Int.* **2018**, *2018*, 4596812. [CrossRef] [PubMed]
11. Hardell, L.; Carlberg, M.; Hansson Mild, K. Use of mobile phones and cordless phones is associated with increased risk for glioma and acoustic neuroma. *Pathophysiology* **2013**, *20*, 85–110. [CrossRef] [PubMed]
12. Soderberg-Naucler, C.; Johnsen, J.I. Cytomegalovirus infection in brain tumors: A potential new target for therapy? *Oncoimmunology* **2012**, *1*, 739–740. [CrossRef]
13. Stupp, R.; Mason, W.P.; van den Bent, M.J.; Weller, M.; Fisher, B.; Taphoom, M.J.; Belanger, K.; Brandes, A.A.; Marosi, C.; Bogdahn, U.; et al. Radiotherapy plus concomitant and adjuvant temozolomide for glioblastoma. *New Eng. J. Med.* **2005**, *352*, 987–996. [CrossRef] [PubMed]
14. Stupp, R.; Hegi, M.E.; Mason, W.P.; van den Bent, M.J.; Taphoorn, M.J.; Janzer, R.C.; Ludwin, S.K.; Allgeier, A.; Fisher, B.; Belanger, K.; et al. Effects of radiotherapy with concomitant and adjuvant temozolomide versus radiotherapy alone on survival in glioblastoma in a randomised phase III study: 5-year analysis of the Eortc-Ncic trial. *Lancet Oncol.* **2009**, *10*, 459–466. [CrossRef]
15. De Vleeschouwer, S.; Van Gool, S.W.; Van Calenbergh, F. Immunotherapy for malignant gliomas: Emphasis on strategies of active specific immunotherapy using autologous dendritic cells. *Childs Nerv. Syst.* **2005**, *21*, 7–18. [CrossRef] [PubMed]
16. Available online: https://www.iddi.com/news/news-events/symposium-are-randomized-trials-still-needed-in-2020/ (accessed on 18 December 2020).

17. Schirrmacher, V.; Bihari, A.S.; Stucker, W.; Sprenger, T. Long-term remission of prostate cancer with extensive bone metastases upon immuno- and virotherapy: A case report. *Oncol. Lett.* **2014**, *8*, 2403–2406. [CrossRef] [PubMed]

18. Schirrmacher, V.; Stucker, W.; Lulei, M.; Bihari, A.S.; Sprenger, T. Long-term survival of a breast cancer patient with extensive liver metastases upon immune and virotherapy: A case report. *Immunotherapy* **2015**, *7*, 855–860. [CrossRef]

19. Van Gool, S.W.; Makalowski, J.; Feyen, O.; Prix, L.; Schirrmacher, V.; Stuecker, W. The induction of immunogenic cell death (ICD) during maintenance chemotherapy and subsequent multimodal immunotherapy for glioblastoma (GBM). *Austin Oncol. Case Rep.* **2018**, *3*, 1010.

20. Van Gool, S.W.; Makalowski, J.; Bonner, E.R.; Feyen, O.; Domogalla, M.P.; Prix, L.; Schirrmacher, V.; Nazarian, J.; Stuecker, W. Addition of Multimodal Immunotherapy to Combination Treatment Strategies for Children with DIPG: A Single Institution Experience. *Medicines* **2020**, *7*, 29. [CrossRef]

21. Cao, J.X.; Zhang, X.Y.; Liu, J.L.; Li, D.; Li, J.L.; Liu, Y.S.; Wang, M.; Xu, B.L.; Wang, H.B.; Wang, Z.X. Clinical efficacy of tumor antigen-pulsed DC treatment for high-grade glioma patients: Evidence from a meta-analysis. *PLoS ONE* **2014**, *9*, e107173. [CrossRef]

22. Wang, X.; Zhao, H.Y.; Zhang, F.C.; Sun, Y.; Xiong, Z.Y.; Jiang, X.B. Dendritic cell-based vaccine for the treatment of malignant glioma: A systematic review. *Cancer Investig.* **2014**, *32*, 451–457. [CrossRef]

23. Eagles, M.E.; Nassiri, F.; Badhiwala, J.H.; Suppiah, S.; Almenawer, S.A.; Zadeh, G.; Aldape, K.D. Dendritic cell vaccines for high-grade gliomas. *Clin. Risk Manag.* **2018**, *14*, 1299–1313. [CrossRef]

24. Vatu, B.I.; Artene, S.A.; Staicu, A.G.; Turcu-Stiolica, A.; Folcuti, C.; Dragoi, A.; Cioc, C.; Baloi, S.C.; Tataranu, L.G.; Silosi, C.; et al. Assessment of efficacy of dendritic cell therapy and viral therapy in high grade glioma clinical trials. A meta-analytic review. *J. Immunoass. Immunochem.* **2019**, *40*, 70–80. [CrossRef] [PubMed]

25. Lv, L.; Huang, J.; Xi, H.; Zhou, X. Efficacy and safety of dendritic cell vaccines for patients with glioblastoma: A meta-analysis of randomized controlled trials. *Int. Immunopharmacol.* **2020**, *83*, 106336. [CrossRef] [PubMed]

26. Burnet, N.G.; Jefferies, S.J.; Benson, R.J.; Hunt, D.P.; Treasure, F.P. Years of life lost (YLL) from cancer is an important measure of population burden–and should be considered when allocating research funds. *Br. J. Cancer* **2005**, *92*, 241–245. [CrossRef] [PubMed]

27. Rouse, C.; Gittleman, H.; Ostrom, Q.T.; Kruchko, C.; Barnholtz-Sloan, J.S. Years of potential life lost for brain and CNS tumors relative to other cancers in adults in the United States, 2010. *Neuro Oncol.* **2016**, *18*, 70–77. [CrossRef]

28. Walker, M.D.; Strike, T.A.; Sheline, G.E. An analysis of dose-effect relationship in the radiotherapy of malignant gliomas. *Int. J. Radiat. Oncol. Biol. Phys.* **1979**, *5*, 1725–1731. [CrossRef]

29. Walker, M.D.; Alexander, E., Jr.; Hunt, W.E.; MacCarty, C.S.; Mahaley, M.S., Jr.; Mealey, J., Jr.; Norrell, H.A.; Owens, G.; Ransohoff, J.; Wilson, C.B.; et al. Evaluation of BCNU and/or radiotherapy in the treatment of anaplastic gliomas. A cooperative clinical trial. *J. Neurosurg.* **1978**, *49*, 333–343. [CrossRef]

30. Gzell, C.; Back, M.; Wheeler, H.; Bailey, D.; Foote, M. Radiotherapy in Glioblastoma: The Past, the Present and the Future. *Clin. Oncol. R Coll. Radiol.* **2017**, *29*, 15–25. [CrossRef]

31. Hegi, M.E.; Diserens, A.C.; Gorlia, T.; Hamou, M.F.; de Tribolet, N.; Weller, M.; Kros, J.M.; Hainfellner, J.A.; Mason, W.; Mariani, L.; et al. MGMT gene silencing and benefit from temozolomide in glioblastoma. *New Engl. J. Med.* **2005**, *352*, 997–1003. [CrossRef]

32. Verhaak, R.G.; Hoadley, K.A.; Purdom, E.; Wang, V.; Qi, Y.; Wilkerson, M.D.; Miller, C.R.; Ding, L.; Golub, T.; Mesirov, J.P.; et al. Integrated genomic analysis identifies clinically relevant subtypes of glioblastoma characterized by abnormalities in PDGFRA, IDH1, EGFR, and NF1. *Cancer Cell.* **2010**, *17*, 98–110. [CrossRef]

33. Sturm, D.; Witt, H.; Hovestadt, V.; Khuong-Quang, D.A.; Jones, D.T.; Konermann, C.; Pfaff, E.; Tonjes, M.; Sill, M.; Bender, S.; et al. Hotspot mutations in H3F3A and IDH1 define distinct epigenetic and biological subgroups of glioblastoma. *Cancer Cell.* **2012**, *22*, 425–437. [CrossRef]

34. Dix, A.R.; Brooks, W.H.; Roszman, T.L.; Morford, L.A. Immune defects observed in patients with primary malignant brain tumors. *J. Neuroimmunol.* **1999**, *100*, 216–232. [CrossRef]

35. Grabowski, M.M.; Sankey, E.W.; Ryan, K.J.; Chongsathidkiet, P.; Lorrey, S.J.; Wilkinson, D.S.; Fecci, P.E. Immune suppression in gliomas. *J. Neurooncol.* **2020**. [CrossRef]

36. North, R.J. Gamma-irradiation facilitates the expression of adoptive immunity against established tumors by eliminating suppressor T cells. *Cancer Immunol. Immunother.* **1984**, *16*, 175–181. [CrossRef] [PubMed]

37. Jordan, J.T.; Sun, W.; Hussain, S.F.; DeAngulo, G.; Prabhu, S.S.; Heimberger, A.B. Preferential migration of regulatory T cells mediated by glioma-secreted chemokines can be blocked with chemotherapy. *Cancer Immunol. Immunother.* **2008**, *57*, 123–131. [CrossRef] [PubMed]

38. Fadul, C.E.; Fisher, J.L.; Gui, J.; Hampton, T.H.; Cote, A.L.; Ernstoff, M.S. Immune modulation effects of concomitant temozolomide and radiation therapy on peripheral blood mononuclear cells in patients with glioblastoma multiforme. *Neuro Oncol.* **2011**, *13*, 393–400. [CrossRef]

39. Dutoit, V.; Philippin, G.; Widmer, V.; Marinari, E.; Vuilleumier, A.; Migliorini, D.; Schaller, K.; Dietrich, P.Y. Impact of Radiochemotherapy on Immune Cell Subtypes in High-Grade Glioma Patients. *Front. Oncol.* **2020**, *10*, 89. [CrossRef]

40. Antonopoulos, M.; Van Gool, S.W.; Dionysiou, D.; Graf, N.; Stamatakos, G. Immune phenotype correlates with survival in patients with GBM treated with standard temozolomide-based therapy and immunotherapy. *Anticancer Res.* **2019**, *39*, 2043–2051. [CrossRef]

41. Sathornsumetee, S.; Rich, J.N. Designer therapies for glioblastoma multiforme. *Ann. N. Y. Acad. Sci.* **2008**, *1142*, 108–132. [CrossRef]

42. Chen, R.; Cohen, A.L.; Colman, H. Targeted Therapeutics in Patients with High-Grade Gliomas: Past, Present, and Future. *Curr. Treat. Options Oncol.* **2016**, *17*, 42. [CrossRef]

43. Dos Santos, M.A.; Pignon, J.P.; Blanchard, P.; Lefeuvre, D.; Levy, A.; Touat, M.; Louvel, G.; Dhermain, F.; Soria, J.C.; Deutsch, E.; et al. Systematic review and meta-analysis of phase I/II targeted therapy combined with radiotherapy in patients with glioblastoma multiforme: Quality of report, toxicity, and survival. *J. Neurooncol.* **2015**, *123*, 307–314. [CrossRef]

44. Su, J.; Cai, M.; Li, W.; Hou, B.; He, H.; Ling, C.; Huang, T.; Liu, H.; Guo, Y. Molecularly Targeted Drugs Plus Radiotherapy and Temozolomide Treatment for Newly Diagnosed Glioblastoma: A Meta-Analysis and Systematic Review. *Oncol. Res.* **2016**, *24*, 117–128. [CrossRef] [PubMed]

45. Cihoric, N.; Tsikkinis, A.; Minniti, G.; Lagerwaard, F.J.; Herrlinger, U.; Mathier, E.; Soldatovic, I.; Jeremic, B.; Ghadjar, P.; Elicin, O.; et al. Current status and perspectives of interventional clinical trials for glioblastoma-analysis of ClinicalTrials.gov. *Radiat. Oncol.* **2017**, *12*, 63. [CrossRef]

46. Sim, H.W.; Morgan, E.R.; Mason, W.P. Contemporary management of high-grade gliomas. *Cns Oncol.* **2018**, *7*, 51–65. [CrossRef] [PubMed]

47. Lavacchi, D.; Roviello, G.; D'Angelo, A. Tumor-Agnostic Treatment for Cancer: When How is Better than Where. *Clin. Drug Investig.* **2020**, *40*, 519–527. [CrossRef] [PubMed]

48. Medical Research Council Streptomycin in Tuberculosis Trials Committee. Streptomycin treatment of pulmonary tuberculosis. *Br. Med. J.* **1948**, *2*, 769–782. [CrossRef]

49. Sorensen, H.T.; Lash, T.L.; Rothman, K.J. Beyond randomized controlled trials: A critical comparison of trials with nonrandomized studies. *Hepatology* **2006**, *44*, 1075–1082. [CrossRef]

50. Shikata, S.; Nakayama, T.; Noguchi, Y.; Taji, Y.; Yamagishi, H. Comparison of effects in randomized controlled trials with observational studies in digestive surgery. *Ann. Surg.* **2006**, *244*, 668–676. [CrossRef]

51. Vincent, J.L. We should abandon randomized controlled trials in the intensive care unit. *Crit. Care Med.* **2010**, *38*, S534–S538. [CrossRef]

52. Jones, D.S.; Podolsky, S.H. The history and fate of the gold standard. *Lancet* **2015**, *385*, 1502–1503. [CrossRef]

53. Trentino, K.; Farmer, S.; Gross, I.; Shander, A.; Isbister, J. Observational studies-should we simply ignore them in assessing transfusion outcomes? *BMC Anesth.* **2016**, *16*, 96. [CrossRef]

54. Sharma, M.; Nazareth, I.; Petersen, I. Observational studies of treatment effectiveness: Worthwhile or worthless? *Clin. Epidemiol.* **2019**, *11*, 35–42. [CrossRef] [PubMed]

55. Aldape, K.; Brindle, K.M.; Chesler, L.; Chopra, R.; Gajjar, A.; Gilbert, M.R.; Gottardo, N.; Gutmann, D.H.; Hargrave, D.; Holland, E.C.; et al. Challenges to curing primary brain tumours. *Nat. Rev. Clin. Oncol.* **2019**. [CrossRef] [PubMed]

56. Halabi, S.; Michiels, S. (Eds.) *Textbook of Clinical trials in Oncology. A Statistical Perspective*; CRC Press: Boca Raton, FL, USA, 2019.

57. Stepanenko, A.A.; Chekhonin, V.P. Recent Advances in Oncolytic Virotherapy and Immunotherapy for Glioblastoma: A Glimmer of Hope in the Search for an Effective Therapy? *Cancers* **2018**, *10*, 492. [CrossRef] [PubMed]

58. Jain, K.K. A Critical Overview of Targeted Therapies for Glioblastoma. *Front. Oncol.* **2018**, *8*, 419. [CrossRef] [PubMed]

59. Suter, R.; Rodriguez-Blanco, J.; Ayad, N.G. Epigenetic pathways and plasticity in brain tumors. *Neurobiol. Dis.* **2020**, 105060. [CrossRef] [PubMed]

60. Muller Bark, J.; Kulasinghe, A.; Chua, B.; Day, B.W.; Punyadeera, C. Circulating biomarkers in patients with glioblastoma. *Br. J. Cancer* **2020**, *122*, 295–305. [CrossRef]

61. Fiegl, H.; Millinger, S.; Mueller-Holzner, E.; Marth, C.; Ensinger, C.; Berger, A.; Klocker, H.; Goebel, G.; Widschwendter, M. Circulating tumor-specific DNA: A marker for monitoring efficacy of adjuvant therapy in cancer patients. *Cancer Res.* **2005**, *65*, 1141–1145. [CrossRef]

62. Sharma, P.; Allison, J.P. Immune checkpoint targeting in cancer therapy: Toward combination strategies with curative potential. *Cell* **2015**, *161*, 205–214. [CrossRef]

63. Macdonald, D.R.; Cascino, T.L.; Schold, S.C., Jr.; Cairncross, J.G. Response criteria for phase II studies of supratentorial malignant glioma. *J. Clin. Oncol.* **1990**, *8*, 1277–1280. [CrossRef]

64. Jaspan, T.; Morgan, P.S.; Warmuth-Metz, M.; Sanchez Aliaga, E.; Warren, D.; Calmon, R.; Grill, J.; Hargrave, D.; Garcia, J.; Zahlmann, G. Response Assessment in Pediatric Neuro-Oncology: Implementation and Expansion of the RANO Criteria in a Randomized Phase II Trial of Pediatric Patients with Newly Diagnosed High-Grade Gliomas. *Am. J. Neuroradiol.* **2016**, *37*, 1581–1587. [CrossRef]

65. Okada, H.; Weller, M.; Huang, R.; Finocchiaro, G.; Gilbert, M.R.; Wick, W.; Ellingson, B.M.; Hashimoto, N.; Pollack, I.F.; Brandes, A.A.; et al. Immunotherapy response assessment in neuro-oncology: A report of the RANO working group. *Lancet Oncol.* **2015**, *16*, e534–e542. [CrossRef]

66. Aquino, D.; Gioppo, A.; Finocchiaro, G.; Bruzzone, M.G.; Cuccarini, V. MRI in Glioma Immunotherapy: Evidence, Pitfalls, and Perspectives. *J. Immunol. Res.* **2017**, *2017*, 5813951. [CrossRef]

67. Sharma, P.; Debinski, W. Receptor-Targeted Glial Brain Tumor Therapies. *Int. J. Mol. Sci.* **2018**, *19*, 3326. [CrossRef]

68. Huang, J.; Liu, F.; Liu, Z.; Tang, H.; Wu, H.; Gong, Q.; Chen, J. Immune Checkpoint in Glioblastoma: Promising and Challenging. *Front. Pharm.* **2017**, *8*, 242. [CrossRef]

69. Wang, X.; Guo, G.; Guan, H.; Yu, Y.; Lu, J.; Yu, J. Challenges and potential of PD-1/PD-L1 checkpoint blockade immunotherapy for glioblastoma. *J. Exp. Clin. Cancer Res.* **2019**, *38*, 87. [CrossRef]
70. Ameratunga, M.; Coleman, N.; Welsh, L.; Saran, F.; Lopez, J. CNS cancer immunity cycle and strategies to target this for glioblastoma. *Oncotarget* **2018**, *9*, 22802–22816. [CrossRef]
71. Zhu, C.; Zou, C.; Guan, G.; Guo, Q.; Yan, Z.; Liu, T.; Shen, S.; Xu, X.; Chen, C.; Lin, Z.; et al. Development and validation of an interferon signature predicting prognosis and treatment response for glioblastoma. *Oncoimmunology* **2019**, *8*, e1621677. [CrossRef]
72. Kmiecik, J.; Poli, A.; Brons, N.H.; Waha, A.; Eide, G.E.; Enger, P.O.; Zimmer, J.; Chekenya, M. Elevated CD3+ and CD8+ tumor-infiltrating immune cells correlate with prolonged survival in glioblastoma patients despite integrated immunosuppressive mechanisms in the tumor microenvironment and at the systemic level. *J. Neuroimmunol.* **2013**, *264*, 71–83. [CrossRef]
73. Bouffet, E.; Larouche, V.; Campbell, B.B.; Merico, D.; de Borja, R.; Aronson, M.; Durno, C.; Krueger, J.; Cabric, V.; Ramaswamy, V.; et al. Immune Checkpoint Inhibition for Hypermutant Glioblastoma Multiforme Resulting from Germline Biallelic Mismatch Repair Deficiency. *J. Clin. Oncol.* **2016**, *34*, 2206–2211. [CrossRef]
74. Adhikaree, J.; Moreno-Vicente, J.; Kaur, A.P.; Jackson, A.M.; Patel, P.M. Resistance Mechanisms and Barriers to Successful Immunotherapy for Treating Glioblastoma. *Cells* **2020**, *9*, 263. [CrossRef]
75. Wang, B.; Niu, D.; Lai, L.; Ren, E.C. p53 increases MHC class I expression by upregulating the endoplasmic reticulum aminopeptidase ERAP1. *Nat. Commun.* **2013**, *4*, 2359. [CrossRef]
76. Blank, C.U.; Haanen, J.B.; Ribas, A.; Schumacher, T.N. Cancer Immunology. The cancer immunogram. *Science* **2016**, *352*, 658–660. [CrossRef] [PubMed]
77. Tomaszewski, W.; Sanchez-Perez, L.; Gajewski, T.F.; Sampson, J.H. Brain Tumor Micro-environment and Host State-Implications for Immunotherapy. *Clin. Cancer Res.* **2019**. [CrossRef] [PubMed]
78. Pires-Afonso, Y.; Niclou, S.P.; Michelucci, A. Revealing and Harnessing Tumour-Associated Microglia/Macrophage Heterogeneity in Glioblastoma. *Int. J. Mol. Sci.* **2020**, *21*, 689. [CrossRef] [PubMed]
79. Zhang, B.; Shen, R.; Cheng, S.; Feng, L. Immune microenvironments differ in immune characteristics and outcome of glioblastoma multiforme. *Cancer Med.* **2019**, *8*, 2897–2907. [CrossRef] [PubMed]
80. Hallaert, G.; Pinson, H.; Van den Broecke, C.; Vanhauwaert, D.; Van Roost, D.; Boterberg, T.; Kalala, J.P. Subventricular zone contacting glioblastoma: Tumor size, molecular biological factors and patient survival. *Acta Oncol.* **2020**. [CrossRef]
81. Berendsen, S.; van Bodegraven, E.; Seute, T.; Spliet, W.G.M.; Geurts, M.; Hendrikse, J.; Schoysman, L.; Huiszoon, W.B.; Varkila, M.; Rouss, S.; et al. Adverse prognosis of glioblastoma contacting the subventricular zone: Biological correlates. *PLoS ONE* **2019**, *14*, e0222717. [CrossRef]
82. Wee, C.W.; Kim, I.H.; Park, C.K.; Kim, J.W.; Dho, Y.S.; Ohka, F.; Aoki, K.; Motomura, K.; Natsume, A.; Kim, N.; et al. Validation of a novel molecular RPA classification in glioblastoma (GBM-molRPA) treated with chemoradiation: A multi-institutional collaborative study. *Radiother. Oncol.* **2018**, *129*, 347–351. [CrossRef]
83. Brown, C.E.; Badie, B.; Barish, M.E.; Weng, L.; Ostberg, J.R.; Chang, W.C.; Naranjo, A.; Starr, R.; Wagner, J.; Wright, C.; et al. Bioactivity and Safety of IL13Ralpha2-Redirected Chimeric Antigen Receptor CD8+ T Cells in Patients with Recurrent Glioblastoma. *Clin. Cancer Res.* **2015**, *21*, 4062–4072. [CrossRef]
84. O'Rourke, D.M.; Nasrallah, M.P.; Desai, A.; Melenhorst, J.J.; Mansfield, K.; Morrissette, J.J.D.; Martinez-Lage, M.; Brem, S.; Maloney, E.; Shen, A.; et al. A single dose of peripherally infused EGFRvIII-directed CAR T cells mediates antigen loss and induces adaptive resistance in patients with recurrent glioblastoma. *Sci. Transl. Med.* **2017**, *9*. [CrossRef]
85. Golinelli, G.; Grisendi, G.; Prapa, M.; Bestagno, M.; Spano, C.; Rossignoli, F.; Bambi, F.; Sardi, I.; Cellini, M.; Horwitz, E.M.; et al. Targeting GD2-positive glioblastoma by chimeric antigen receptor empowered mesenchymal progenitors. *Cancer Gene.* **2018**. [CrossRef] [PubMed]
86. Rammensee, H.G.; Singh-Jasuja, H. HLA ligandome tumor antigen discovery for personalized vaccine approach. *Expert Rev. Vaccines* **2013**, *12*, 1211–1217. [CrossRef] [PubMed]
87. Sahin, U.; Derhovanessian, E.; Miller, M.; Kloke, B.P.; Simon, P.; Lower, M.; Bukur, V.; Tadmor, A.D.; Luxemburger, U.; Schrors, B.; et al. Personalized RNA mutanome vaccines mobilize poly-specific therapeutic immunity against cancer. *Nature* **2017**. [CrossRef] [PubMed]
88. Johanns, T.M.; Miller, C.A.; Liu, C.J.; Perrin, R.J.; Bender, D.; Kobayashi, D.K.; Campian, J.L.; Chicoine, M.R.; Dacey, R.G.; Huang, J.; et al. Detection of neoantigen-specific T cells following a personalized vaccine in a patient with glioblastoma. *Oncoimmunology* **2019**, *8*, e1561106. [CrossRef] [PubMed]
89. De Vleeschouwer, S.; Arredouani, M.; Ade, M.; Cadot, P.; Vermassen, E.; Ceuppens, J.L.; Van Gool, S.W. Uptake and presentation of malignant glioma tumor cell lysates by monocyte-derived dendritic cells. *Cancer Immunol. Immunother.* **2005**, *54*, 372–382. [CrossRef] [PubMed]
90. De Vleeschouwer, S.; Spencer, L.I.; Ceuppens, J.L.; Van Gool, S.W. Persistent IL-10 production is required for glioma growth suppressive activity by Th1-directed effector cells after stimulation with tumor lysate-loaded dendritic cells. *J. Neurooncol.* **2007**, *84*, 131–140. [CrossRef]
91. Maes, W.; Deroose, C.; Reumers, V.; Krylyshkina, O.; Gijsbers, R.; Ceuppens, J.; Baekelandt, V.; Debyser, Z.; Van Gool, S. In vivo bioluminescence imaging in an experimental mouse model for dendritic cell based immunotherapy against malignant glioma. *J. Neuro Oncol.* **2009**, *91*, 127–139. [CrossRef]

92. Maes, W.; Galicia Rosas, G.; Verbinnen, B.; Boon, L.; De Vleeschouwer, S.; Ceuppens, J.L.; Van Gool, S.W. DC vaccination with anti-CD25 treatment leads to long-term immunity against experimental glioma. *Neuro Oncol.* **2009**, *11*, 529–542. [CrossRef]

93. Ardon, H.; Verbinnen, B.; Maes, W.; Beez, T.; Van Gool, S.; De Vleeschouwer, S. Technical advancement in regulatory T cell isolation and characterization using CD127 expression in patients with malignant glioma treated with autologous dendritic cell vaccination. *J. Immunol. Methods* **2010**, *352*, 169–173. [CrossRef]

94. Maes, W.; Van Gool, S.W. Experimental immunotherapy for malignant glioma: Lessons from two decades of research in the GL261 model. *Cancer Immunol. Immunother.* **2011**, *60*, 153–160. [CrossRef]

95. Vandenberk, L.; Van Gool, S.W. Treg infiltration in glioma: A hurdle for antiglioma immunotherapy. *Immunotherapy* **2012**, *4*, 675–678. [CrossRef] [PubMed]

96. Koks, C.A.E.; Garg, A.D.; Ehrhardt, M.; Riva, M.; De Vleeschouwer, S.; Agostinis, P.; Graf, N.; Van Gool, S.W. Newcastle disease virotherapy induces long-term survival and tumor-specific immune memory in orthotopic glioma through the induction of immunogenic cell death. *Int. J. Cancer* **2014**, *136*, e313–e325. [CrossRef]

97. Koks, C.A.; De Vleeschouwer, S.; Graf, N.; Van Gool, S.W. Immune Suppression during Oncolytic Virotherapy for High-Grade Glioma; Yes or No? *J. Cancer* **2015**, *6*, 203–217. [CrossRef]

98. Vandenberk, L.; Belmans, J.; Van Woensel, M.; Riva, M.; Van Gool, S.W. Exploiting the Immunogenic Potential of Cancer Cells for Improved Dendritic Cell Vaccines. *Front. Immunol.* **2015**, *6*, 663. [CrossRef]

99. Garg, A.D.; Vandenberk, L.; Koks, C.; Verschuere, T.; Boon, L.; Van Gool, S.W.; Agostinis, P. Dendritic cell vaccines based on immunogenic cell death elicit danger signals and T cell-driven rejection of high-grade glioma. *Sci. Transl. Med.* **2016**, *8*, 328ra327. [CrossRef] [PubMed]

100. Vandenberk, L.; Garg, A.D.; Verschuere, T.; Koks, C.; Belmans, J.; Beullens, M.; Agostinis, P.; De Vleeschouwer, S.; Van Gool, S.W. Irradiation of necrotic cancer cells, employed for pulsing dendritic cells (DCs), potentiates DC vaccine-induced antitumor immunity against high-grade glioma. *Oncoimmunology* **2016**, *5*, e1083669. [CrossRef] [PubMed]

101. Belmans, J.; Van Woensel, M.; Creyns, B.; Dejaegher, J.; Bullens, D.M.; Van Gool, S.W. Immunotherapy with subcutaneous immunogenic autologous tumor lysate increases murine glioblastoma survival. *Sci. Rep.* **2017**, *7*, 13902. [CrossRef]

102. Liau, L.M.; Black, K.L.; Martin, N.A.; Sykes, S.N.; Bronstein, J.M.; Jouben-Steele, L.; Mischel, P.S.; Belldegrun, A.; Cloughesy, T.F. Treatment of a patient by vaccination with autologous dendritic cells pulsed with allogeneic major histocompatibility complex class I-matched tumor peptides. Case Report. *Neurosurg. Focus* **2000**, *9*, e8. [CrossRef]

103. Yu, J.S.; Wheeler, C.J.; Zeltzer, P.M.; Ying, H.; Finger, D.N.; Lee, P.K.; Yong, W.H.; Incardona, F.; Thompson, R.C.; Riedinger, M.S.; et al. Vaccination of malignant glioma patients with peptide-pulsed dendritic cells elicits systemic cytotoxicity and intracranial T-cell infiltration. *Cancer Res.* **2001**, *61*, 842–847.

104. Kikuchi, T.; Akasaki, Y.; Irie, M.; Homma, S.; Abe, T.; Ohno, T. Results of a phase I clinical trial of vaccination of glioma patients with fusions of dendritic and glioma cells. *Cancer Immunol. Immunother.* **2001**, *50*, 337–344. [CrossRef]

105. Wheeler, C.J.; Black, K.L.; Liu, G.; Ying, H.; Yu, J.S.; Zhang, W.; Lee, P.K. Thymic CD8(+) T cell production strongly influences tumor antigen recognition and age-dependent glioma mortality. *J. Immunol.* **2003**, *171*, 4927–4933. [CrossRef] [PubMed]

106. Yamanaka, R.; Abe, T.; Yajima, N.; Tsuchiya, N.; Homma, J.; Kobayashi, T.; Narita, M.; Takahashi, M.; Tanaka, R. Vaccination of recurrent glioma patients with tumour lysate-pulsed dendritic cells elicits immune responses: Results of a clinical phase I/II trial. *Br. J. Cancer* **2003**, *89*, 1172–1179. [CrossRef] [PubMed]

107. Caruso, D.A.; Orme, L.M.; Neale, A.M.; Radcliff, F.J.; Amor, G.M.; Maixner, W.; Downie, P.; Hassall, T.E.; Tang, M.L.; Ashley, D.M. Results of a phase 1 study utilizing monocyte-derived dendritic cells pulsed with tumor RNA in children and young adults with brain cancer. *Neuro. Oncol.* **2004**, *6*, 236–246. [CrossRef] [PubMed]

108. De Vleeschouwer, S.; Van Calenbergh, F.; Demaerel, P.; Flamen, P.; Rutkowski, S.; Kaempgen, E.; Wolff, J.E.A.; Plets, C.; Sciot, R.; Van Gool, S.W. Transient local response and persistent tumor control of recurrent malignant glioma treated with combination therapy including dendritic cell therapy. *J. Neurosurg.* **2004**, *100*, 492–497. [PubMed]

109. Kikuchi, T.; Akasaki, Y.; Abe, T.; Fukuda, T.; Saotome, H.; Ryan, J.L.; Kufe, D.W.; Ohno, T. Vaccination of glioma patients with fusions of dendritic and glioma cells and recombinant human interleukin 12. *J. Immunother.* **2004**, *27*, 452–459. [CrossRef]

110. Rutkowski, S.; De Vleeschouwer, S.; Kaempgen, E.; Wolff, J.E.A.; Kuhl, J.; Demaerel, P.; Warmuth-Metz, M.; Flamen, P.; Van Calenbergh, F.; Plets, C.; et al. Surgery and adjuvant dendritic cell-based tumour vaccination for patients with relapsed malignant glioma, a feasibility study. *Br. J. Cancer* **2004**, *91*, 1656–1662. [CrossRef]

111. Wheeler, C.J.; Das, A.; Liu, G.; Yu, J.S.; Black, K.L. Clinical responsiveness of glioblastoma multiforme to chemotherapy after vaccination. *Clin. Cancer Res.* **2004**, *10*, 5316–5326. [CrossRef]

112. Yu, J.S.; Liu, G.; Ying, H.; Yong, W.H.; Black, K.L.; Wheeler, C.J. Vaccination with tumor lysate-pulsed dendritic cells elicits antigen-specific, cytotoxic T-cells in patients with malignant glioma. *Cancer Res.* **2004**, *64*, 4973–4979. [CrossRef]

113. Liau, L.M.; Prins, R.M.; Kiertscher, S.M.; Odesa, S.K.; Kremen, T.J.; Giovannone, A.J.; Lin, J.W.; Chute, D.J.; Mischel, P.S.; Cloughesy, T.F.; et al. Dendritic cell vaccination in glioblastoma patients induces systemic and intracranial T-cell responses modulated by the local central nervous system tumor microenvironment. *Clin. Cancer Res.* **2005**, *11*, 5515–5525. [CrossRef]

114. Yamanaka, R.; Honma, J.; Tsuchiya, N.; Yajima, N.; Kobayashi, T.; Tanaka, R. Tumor lysate and IL-18 loaded dendritic cells elicits Th1 response, tumor-specific CD8+ cytotoxic T cells in patients with malignant glioma. *J. Neurooncol.* **2005**, *72*, 107–113. [CrossRef] [PubMed]

115. Yamanaka, R.; Homma, J.; Yajima, N.; Tsuchiya, N.; Sano, M.; Kobayashi, T.; Yoshida, S.; Abe, T.; Narita, M.; Takahashi, M.; et al. Clinical evaluation of dendritic cell vaccination for patients with recurrent glioma: Results of a clinical phase I/II trial. *Clin. Cancer Res.* **2005**, *11*, 4160–4167. [CrossRef]

116. Khan, J.A.; Yaqin, S. Dendritic cell therapy with improved outcome in glioma multiforme—A case report. *J. Zhejiang Univ. Sci. B* **2006**, *7*, 114–117. [CrossRef]

117. Okada, H.; Lieberman, F.S.; Walter, K.A.; Lunsford, L.D.; Kondziolka, D.S.; Bejjani, G.K.; Hamilton, R.L.; Torres-Trejo, A.; Kalinski, P.; Cai, Q.; et al. Autologous glioma cell vaccine admixed with interleukin-4 gene transfected fibroblasts in the treatment of patients with malignant gliomas. *J. Transl. Med.* **2007**, *5*, 67. [CrossRef]

118. De Vleeschouwer, S.; Fieuws, S.; Rutkowski, S.; Van Calenbergh, F.; Van Loon, J.; Goffin, J.; Sciot, R.; Wilms, G.; Demaerel, P.; Warmuth-Metz, M.; et al. Postoperative adjuvant dendritic cell-based immunotherapy in patients with relapsed glioblastoma multiforme. *Clin. Cancer Res.* **2008**, *14*, 3098–3104. [CrossRef]

119. Prins, R.M.; Cloughesy, T.F.; Liau, L.M. Cytomegalovirus immunity after vaccination with autologous glioblastoma lysate. *New Engl. J. Med.* **2008**, *359*, 539–541. [CrossRef]

120. Walker, D.G.; Laherty, R.; Tomlinson, F.H.; Chuah, T.; Schmidt, C. Results of a phase I dendritic cell vaccine trial for malignant astrocytoma: Potential interaction with adjuvant chemotherapy. *J. Clin. Neurosci.* **2008**, *15*, 114–121. [CrossRef]

121. Wheeler, C.J.; Black, K.L.; Liu, G.; Mazer, M.; Zhang, X.X.; Pepkowitz, S.; Goldfinger, D.; Ng, H.; Irvin, D.; Yu, J.S. Vaccination elicits correlated immune and clinical responses in glioblastoma multiforme patients. *Cancer Res.* **2008**, *68*, 5955–5964. [CrossRef]

122. Sampson, J.H.; Archer, G.E.; Mitchell, D.A.; Heimberger, A.B.; Herndon, J.E.; Lally-Goss, D.; McGehee-Norman, S.; Paolino, A.; Reardon, D.A.; Friedman, A.H.; et al. An epidermal growth factor receptor variant III-targeted vaccine is safe and immunogenic in patients with glioblastoma multiforme. *Mol. Cancer* **2009**, *8*, 2773–2779. [CrossRef]

123. Ardon, H.; Van Gool, S.; Lopes, I.S.; Maes, W.; Sciot, R.; Wilms, G.; Demaerel, P.; Bijttebier, P.; Claes, L.; Goffin, J.; et al. Integration of autologous dendritic cell-based immunotherapy in the primary treatment for patients with newly diagnosed glioblastoma multiforme: A pilot study. *J. Neurooncol.* **2010**, *99*, 261–272. [CrossRef]

124. Ardon, H.; De Vleeschouwer, S.; Van Calenbergh, F.; Claes, L.; Kramm, C.M.; Rutkowski, S.; Wolff, J.E.; Van Gool, S.W. Adjuvant dendritic cell-based tumour vaccination for children with malignant brain tumours. *Pediatr. Blood Cancer* **2010**, *54*, 519–525. [CrossRef]

125. Chang, C.N.; Huang, Y.C.; Yang, D.M.; Kikuta, K.; Wei, K.J.; Kubota, T.; Yang, W.K. A phase I/II clinical trial investigating the adverse and therapeutic effects of a postoperative autologous dendritic cell tumor vaccine in patients with malignant glioma. *J. Clin. Neurosci.* **2011**, *18*, 1048–1054. [CrossRef]

126. Fadul, C.E.; Fisher, J.L.; Hampton, T.H.; Lallana, E.C.; Li, Z.; Gui, J.; Szczepiorkowski, Z.M.; Tosteson, T.D.; Rhodes, C.H.; Wishart, H.A.; et al. Immune response in patients with newly diagnosed glioblastoma multiforme treated with intranodal autologous tumor lysate-dendritic cell vaccination after radiation chemotherapy. *J. Immunother.* **2011**, *34*, 382–389. [CrossRef]

127. Okada, H.; Kalinski, P.; Ueda, R.; Hoji, A.; Kohanbash, G.; Donegan, T.E.; Mintz, A.H.; Engh, J.A.; Bartlett, D.L.; Brown, C.K.; et al. Induction of CD8+ T-cell responses against novel glioma-associated antigen peptides and clinical activity by vaccinations with {alpha}-type 1 polarized dendritic cells and polyinosinic-polycytidylic acid stabilized by lysine and carboxymethylcellulose in patients with recurrent malignant glioma. *J. Clin. Oncol.* **2011**, *29*, 330–336. [CrossRef] [PubMed]

128. Prins, R.M.; Soto, H.; Konkankit, V.; Odesa, S.K.; Eskin, A.; Yong, W.H.; Nelson, S.F.; Liau, L.M. Gene expression profile correlates with T-cell infiltration and relative survival in glioblastoma patients vaccinated with dendritic cell immunotherapy. *Clin. Cancer Res.* **2011**, *17*, 1603–1615. [CrossRef]

129. Akiyama, Y.; Oshita, C.; Kume, A.; Iizuka, A.; Miyata, H.; Komiyama, M.; Ashizawa, T.; Yagoto, M.; Abe, Y.; Mitsuya, K.; et al. alpha-type-1 polarized dendritic cell-based vaccination in recurrent high-grade glioma: A phase I clinical trial. *BMC Cancer* **2012**, *12*, 623. [CrossRef]

130. Ardon, H.; Van Gool, S.W.; Verschuere, T.; Maes, W.; Fieuws, S.; Sciot, R.; Wilms, G.; Demaerel, P.; Goffin, J.; Van Calenbergh, F.; et al. Integration of autologous dendritic cell-based immunotherapy in the standard of care treatment for patients with newly diagnosed glioblastoma: Results of the HGG-2006 phase I/II trial. *Cancer Immunol. Immunother.* **2012**, *61*, 2033–2044. [CrossRef] [PubMed]

131. Cho, D.Y.; Yang, W.K.; Lee, H.C.; Hsu, D.M.; Lin, H.L.; Lin, S.Z.; Chen, C.C.; Harn, H.J.; Liu, C.L.; Lee, W.Y.; et al. Adjuvant immunotherapy with whole-cell lysate dendritic cells vaccine for glioblastoma multiforme: A phase II clinical trial. *World Neurosurg.* **2012**, *77*, 736–744. [CrossRef] [PubMed]

132. De Vleeschouwer, S.; Ardon, H.; van Calenbergh, F.; Sciot, R.; Wilms, G.; van Loon, J.; Goffin, J.; van Gool, S. Stratification according to Hgg-Immuno Rpa model predicts outcome in a large group of patients with relapsed malignant glioma treated by adjuvant postoperative dendritic cell vaccination. *Cancer Immunol. Immunother.* **2012**, *61*, 2105–2112. [CrossRef]

133. Elens, I.; De Vleeschouwer, S.; Pauwels, F.; Van Gool, S.W. Resection and immunotherapy for recurrent grade III glioma. *Isrn Immunol.* **2012**, *2012*, 530179. [CrossRef]

134. Fong, B.; Jin, R.; Wang, X.; Safaee, M.; Lisiero, D.N.; Yang, I.; Li, G.; Liau, L.M.; Prins, R.M. Monitoring of regulatory T cell frequencies and expression of CTLA-4 on T cells, before and after DC vaccination, can predict survival in GBM patients. *PLoS ONE* **2012**, *7*, e32614. [CrossRef]

135. Iwami, K.; Shimato, S.; Ohno, M.; Okada, H.; Nakahara, N.; Sato, Y.; Yoshida, J.; Suzuki, S.; Nishikawa, H.; Shiku, H.; et al. Peptide-pulsed dendritic cell vaccination targeting interleukin-13 receptor alpha2 chain in recurrent malignant glioma patients with HLA-A*24/A*02 allele. *Cytotherapy* **2012**. [CrossRef]
136. Jie, X.; Hua, L.; Jiang, W.; Feng, F.; Feng, G.; Hua, Z. Clinical application of a dendritic cell vaccine raised against heat-shocked glioblastoma. *Cell Biochem. Biophys.* **2012**, *62*, 91–99. [CrossRef]
137. Qin, K.; Tian, G.; Li, P.; Chen, Q.; Zhang, R.; Ke, Y.Q.; Xiao, Z.C.; Jiang, X.D. Anti-glioma response of autologous T cells stimulated by autologous dendritic cells electrofused with CD133(+) or CD133(-) glioma cells. *J. Neuroimmunol.* **2012**, *242*, 9–15. [CrossRef]
138. Sampson, J.H.; Schmittling, R.J.; Archer, G.E.; Congdon, K.L.; Nair, S.K.; Reap, E.A.; Desjardins, A.; Friedman, A.H.; Friedman, H.S.; Herndon, J.E.; et al. A Pilot Study of IL-2Ralpha Blockade during Lymphopenia Depletes Regulatory T-cells and Correlates with Enhanced Immunity in Patients with Glioblastoma. *PLoS ONE* **2012**, *7*, e31046. [CrossRef]
139. Valle, R.D.; de Cerio, A.L.; Inoges, S.; Tejada, S.; Pastor, F.; Villanueva, H.; Gallego, J.; Espinos, J.; Aristu, J.; Idoate, M.A.; et al. Dendritic cell vaccination in glioblastoma after fluorescence-guided resection. *World J. Clin. Oncol.* **2012**, *3*, 142–149. [CrossRef]
140. Lasky, J.L., III; Panosyan, E.H.; Plant, A.; Davidson, T.; Yong, W.H.; Prins, R.M.; Liau, L.M.; Moore, T.B. Autologous Tumor Lysate-pulsed Dendritic Cell Immunotherapy for Pediatric Patients with Newly Diagnosed or Recurrent High-grade Gliomas. *Anticancer Res.* **2013**, *33*, 2047–2056.
141. Pellegatta, S.; Eoli, M.; Frigerio, S.; Antozzi, C.; Bruzzone, M.G.; Cantini, G.; Nava, S.; Anghileri, E.; Cuppini, L.; Cuccarini, V.; et al. The natural killer cell response and tumor debulking are associated with prolonged survival in recurrent glioblastoma patients receiving dendritic cells loaded with autologous tumor lysates. *Oncoimmunology* **2013**, *2*, e23401. [CrossRef] [PubMed]
142. Phuphanich, S.; Wheeler, C.J.; Rudnick, J.D.; Mazer, M.; Wang, H.; Nuno, M.A.; Richardson, J.E.; Fan, X.; Ji, J.; Chu, R.M.; et al. Phase I trial of a multi-epitope-pulsed dendritic cell vaccine for patients with newly diagnosed glioblastoma. *Cancer Immunol. Immunother.* **2013**, *62*, 125–135. [CrossRef]
143. Prins, R.M.; Wang, X.; Soto, H.; Young, E.; Lisiero, D.N.; Fong, B.; Everson, R.; Yong, W.H.; Lai, A.; Li, G.; et al. Comparison of glioma-associated antigen peptide-loaded versus autologous tumor lysate-loaded dendritic cell vaccination in malignant glioma patients. *J. Immunother.* **2013**, *36*, 152–157. [CrossRef]
144. Vik-Mo, E.O.; Nyakas, M.; Mikkelsen, B.V.; Moe, M.C.; Due-Tonnesen, P.; Suso, E.M.; Saeboe-Larssen, S.; Sandberg, C.; Brinchmann, J.E.; Helseth, E.; et al. Therapeutic vaccination against autologous cancer stem cells with mRNA-transfected dendritic cells in patients with glioblastoma. *Cancer Immunol. Immunother.* **2013**. [CrossRef]
145. Eyrich, M.; Schreiber, S.C.; Rachor, J.; Krauss, J.; Pauwels, F.; Hain, J.; Wolfl, M.; Lutz, M.B.; De, V.S.; Schlegel, P.G.; et al. Development and validation of a fully GMP-compliant production process of autologous, tumor-lysate-pulsed dendritic cells. *Cytotherapy* **2014**, *16*, 946–964. [CrossRef]
146. Ishikawa, E.; Muragaki, Y.; Yamamoto, T.; Maruyama, T.; Tsuboi, K.; Ikuta, S.; Hashimoto, K.; Uemae, Y.; Ishihara, T.; Matsuda, M.; et al. Phase I/IIa trial of fractionated radiotherapy, temozolomide, and autologous formalin-fixed tumor vaccine for newly diagnosed glioblastoma. *J. Neurosurg.* **2014**, *121*, 543–553. [CrossRef]
147. Hunn, M.K.; Bauer, E.; Wood, C.E.; Gasser, O.; Dzhelali, M.; Ancelet, L.R.; Mester, B.; Sharples, K.J.; Findlay, M.P.; Hamilton, D.A.; et al. Dendritic cell vaccination combined with temozolomide retreatment: Results of a phase I trial in patients with recurrent glioblastoma multiforme. *J. Neurooncol.* **2015**, *121*, 319–329. [CrossRef]
148. Mitchell, D.A.; Batich, K.A.; Gunn, M.D.; Huang, M.N.; Sanchez-Perez, L.; Nair, S.K.; Congdon, K.L.; Reap, E.A.; Archer, G.E.; Desjardins, A.; et al. Tetanus toxoid and CCL3 improve dendritic cell vaccines in mice and glioblastoma patients. *Nature* **2015**, *519*, 366–369. [CrossRef]
149. Muller, K.; Henke, G.; Pietschmann, S.; van Gool, S.; De Vleeschouwer, S.; von Bueren, A.O.; Compter, I.; Friedrich, C.; Matuschek, C.; Klautke, G.; et al. Re-irradiation or re-operation followed by dendritic cell vaccination? Comparison of two different salvage strategies for relapsed high-grade gliomas by means of a new prognostic model. *J. Neurooncol.* **2015**, *124*, 325–332. [CrossRef]
150. Sakai, K.; Shimodaira, S.; Maejima, S.; Udagawa, N.; Sano, K.; Higuchi, Y.; Koya, T.; Ochiai, T.; Koide, M.; Uehara, S.; et al. Dendritic cell-based immunotherapy targeting Wilms' tumor 1 in patients with recurrent malignant glioma. *J. Neurosurg.* **2015**, *123*, 989–997. [CrossRef]
151. Van Gool, S.W. Brain tumor immunotherapy: What have we learned so far? *Front. Oncol.* **2015**, *5*, 98. [CrossRef]
152. Akasaki, Y.; Kikuchi, T.; Homma, S.; Koido, S.; Ohkusa, T.; Tasaki, T.; Hayashi, K.; Komita, H.; Watanabe, N.; Suzuki, Y.; et al. Phase I/II trial of combination of temozolomide chemotherapy and immunotherapy with fusions of dendritic and glioma cells in patients with glioblastoma. *Cancer Immunol. Immunother.* **2016**, *65*, 1499–1509. [CrossRef]
153. Pollack, I.F.; Jakacki, R.I.; Butterfield, L.H.; Hamilton, R.L.; Panigrahy, A.; Normolle, D.P.; Connelly, A.K.; Dibridge, S.; Mason, G.; Whiteside, T.L.; et al. Antigen-specific immunoreactivity and clinical outcome following vaccination with glioma-associated antigen peptides in children with recurrent high-grade gliomas: Results of a pilot study. *J. Neurooncol.* **2016**, *130*, 517–527. [CrossRef]
154. Inoges, S.; Tejada, S.; de Cerio, A.L.; Gallego Perez-Larraya, J.; Espinos, J.; Idoate, M.A.; Dominguez, P.D.; de Eulate, R.G.; Aristu, J.; Bendandi, M.; et al. A phase II trial of autologous dendritic cell vaccination and radiochemotherapy following fluorescence-guided surgery in newly diagnosed glioblastoma patients. *J. Transl. Med.* **2017**, *15*, 104. [CrossRef]
155. Sakai, K.; Shimodaira, S.; Maejima, S.; Sano, K.; Higuchi, Y.; Koya, T.; Sugiyama, H.; Hongo, K. Clinical effect and immunological response in patients with advanced malignant glioma treated with WT1-pulsed dendritic cell-based immunotherapy: A report of two cases. *Interdiscip. Neurosurg. Adv. Tech. Case Manag.* **2017**, *9*, 24–29. [CrossRef]

156. Benitez-Ribas, D.; Cabezon, R.; Florez-Grau, G.; Molero, M.C.; Puerta, P.; Guillen, A.; Paco, S.; Carcaboso, A.M.; Santa-Maria Lopez, V.; Cruz, O.; et al. Immune Response Generated with the Administration of Autologous Dendritic Cells Pulsed with an Allogenic Tumoral Cell-Lines Lysate in Patients with Newly Diagnosed Diffuse Intrinsic Pontine Glioma. *Front. Oncol.* **2018**, *8*, 127. [CrossRef] [PubMed]

157. Buchroithner, J.; Erhart, F.; Pichler, J.; Widhalm, G.; Preusser, M.; Stockhammer, G.; Nowosielski, M.; Iglseder, S.; Freyschlag, C.F.; Oberndorfer, S.; et al. Audencel Immunotherapy Based on Dendritic Cells Has No Effect on Overall and Progression-Free Survival in Newly Diagnosed Glioblastoma: A Phase II Randomized Trial. *Cancers* **2018**, *10*, 372. [CrossRef] [PubMed]

158. Jan, C.I.; Tsai, W.C.; Harn, H.J.; Shyu, W.C.; Liu, M.C.; Lu, H.M.; Chiu, S.C.; Cho, D.Y. Predictors of Response to Autologous Dendritic Cell Therapy in Glioblastoma Multiforme. *Front. Immunol.* **2018**, *9*, 727. [CrossRef] [PubMed]

159. Erhart, F.; Buchroithner, J.; Reitermaier, R.; Fischhuber, K.; Klingenbrunner, S.; Sloma, I.; Hibsh, D.; Kozol, R.; Efroni, S.; Ricken, G.; et al. Immunological analysis of phase II glioblastoma dendritic cell vaccine (Audencel) trial: Immune system characteristics influence outcome and Audencel up-regulates Th1-related immunovariables. *Acta Neuropathol. Commun.* **2018**, *6*, 135. [CrossRef] [PubMed]

160. Liau, L.M.; Ashkan, K.; Tran, D.D.; Campian, J.L.; Trusheim, J.E.; Cobbs, C.S.; Heth, J.A.; Salacz, M.; Taylor, S.; D'Andre, S.D.; et al. First results on survival from a large Phase 3 clinical trial of an autologous dendritic cell vaccine in newly diagnosed glioblastoma. *J. Transl. Med.* **2018**, *16*, 142. [CrossRef]

161. Pellegatta, S.; Eoli, M.; Cuccarini, V.; Anghileri, E.; Pollo, B.; Pessina, S.; Frigerio, S.; Servida, M.; Cuppini, L.; Antozzi, C.; et al. Survival gain in glioblastoma patients treated with dendritic cell immunotherapy is associated with increased NK but not CD8(+) T cell activation in the presence of adjuvant temozolomide. *Oncoimmunology* **2018**, *7*, e1412901. [CrossRef]

162. Yao, Y.; Luo, F.; Tang, C.; Chen, D.; Qin, Z.; Hua, W.; Xu, M.; Zhong, P.; Yu, S.; Chen, D.; et al. Molecular subgroups and B7-H4 expression levels predict responses to dendritic cell vaccines in glioblastoma: An exploratory randomized phase II clinical trial. *Cancer Immunol. Immunother.* **2018**. [CrossRef]

163. Rudnick, J.D.; Sarmiento, J.M.; Uy, B.; Nuno, M.; Wheeler, C.J.; Mazer, M.J.; Wang, H.; Hu, J.L.; Chu, R.M.; Phuphanich, S.; et al. A phase I trial of surgical resection with Gliadel Wafer placement followed by vaccination with dendritic cells pulsed with tumor lysate for patients with malignant glioma. *J. Clin. Neurosci.* **2020**, *74*, 187–193. [CrossRef]

164. Wang, Q.T.; Nie, Y.; Sun, S.N.; Lin, T.; Han, R.J.; Jiang, J.; Li, Z.; Li, J.Q.; Xiao, Y.P.; Fan, Y.Y.; et al. Tumor-associated antigen-based personalized dendritic cell vaccine in solid tumor patients. *Cancer Immunol. Immunother.* **2020**, *69*, 1375–1387. [CrossRef]

165. Sampson, J.H.; Heimberger, A.B.; Archer, G.E.; Aldape, K.D.; Friedman, A.H.; Friedman, H.S.; Gilbert, M.R.; Herndon, J.E.; McLendon, R.E.; Mitchell, D.A.; et al. Immunologic escape after prolonged progression-free survival with epidermal growth factor receptor variant III peptide vaccination in patients with newly diagnosed glioblastoma. *J. Clin. Oncol.* **2010**, *28*, 4722–4729. [CrossRef] [PubMed]

166. Dejaegher, J.; Solie, L.; Hunin, Z.; Sciot, R.; Capper, D.; Siewert, C.; Van Cauter, S.; Wilms, G.; van Loon, J.; Ectors, N.; et al. Methylation based glioblastoma subclassification is related to tumoral T cell infiltration and survival. *Neuro Oncol.* **2020**. [CrossRef] [PubMed]

167. Dejaegher, J. *Local and Systemic Immune Interactions in Malignant Gliomas*; KU Leuven: Leuven, Belgium, 2017.

168. Available online: https://immuno-oncologynews.com/2017/06/26/glioblastoma-potential-therapy-ict-107-trial-suspended-cash-strapped-immunocellular/ (accessed on 18 December 2020).

169. Kast, R.E.; Karpel-Massler, G.; Halatsch, M.E. CUSP9* treatment protocol for recurrent glioblastoma: Aprepitant, artesunate, auranofin, captopril, celecoxib, disulfiram, itraconazole, ritonavir, sertraline augmenting continuous low dose temozolomide. *Oncotarget* **2014**, *5*, 8052–8082. [CrossRef] [PubMed]

170. Lissoni, P.; Messina, G.; Lissoni, A.; Franco, R. The psychoneuroendocrine-immunotherapy of cancer: Historical evolution and clinical results. *J. Res. Med. Sci.* **2017**, *22*, 45. [CrossRef] [PubMed]

171. Santos, J.G.; Da Cruz, W.M.S.; Schonthal, A.H.; Salazar, M.D.; Fontes, C.A.P.; Quirico-Santos, T.; Da Fonseca, C.O. Efficacy of a ketogenic diet with concomitant intranasal perillyl alcohol as a novel strategy for the therapy of recurrent glioblastoma. *Oncol. Lett.* **2018**, *15*, 1263–1270. [CrossRef]

172. Lopez-Valero, I.; Torres, S.; Salazar-Roa, M.; Garcia-Taboada, E.; Hernandez-Tiedra, S.; Guzman, M.; Sepulveda, J.M.; Velasco, G.; Lorente, M. Optimization of a preclinical therapy of cannabinoids in combination with temozolomide against glioma. *Biochem. Pharm.* **2018**, *157*, 275–284. [CrossRef]

173. Friesen, C.; Hormann, I.; Roscher, M.; Fichtner, I.; Alt, A.; Hilger, R.; Debatin, K.M.; Miltner, E. Opioid receptor activation triggering downregulation of cAMP improves effectiveness of anti-cancer drugs in treatment of glioblastoma. *Cell Cycle* **2014**, *13*, 1560–1570. [CrossRef]

174. Galluzzi, L.; Vitale, I.; Aaronson, S.A.; Abrams, J.M.; Adam, D.; Agostinis, P.; Alnemri, E.S.; Altucci, L.; Amelio, I.; Andrews, D.W.; et al. Molecular mechanisms of cell death: Recommendations of the Nomenclature Committee on Cell Death 2018. *Cell Death Differ.* **2018**. [CrossRef]

175. Galluzzi, L.; Vitale, I.; Warren, S.; Adjemian, S.; Agostinis, P.; Martinez, A.B.; Chan, T.A.; Coukos, G.; Demaria, S.; Deutsch, E.; et al. Consensus guidelines for the definition, detection and interpretation of immunogenic cell death. *J. Immunother. Cancer* **2020**, *8*. [CrossRef]

176. Van Gool, S.W.; Makalowski, J.; Domogalla, M.P.; Marko, M.; Feyen, O.; Sprenger, K.; Schirrmacher, V.; Stuecker, W. Personalised medicine in glioblastoma multiforme. In *Challenges and Solutions of Oncological Hyperthermia*; Szasz, A., Ed.; Cambridge Scholars Publishing: Newcastle upon Tyne, UK, 2020; pp. 126–158.
177. Wang, Z.; Gao, L.; Guo, X.; Lian, W.; Deng, K.; Xing, B. Development and Validation of a Novel DNA Methylation-Driven Gene Based Molecular Classification and Predictive Model for Overall Survival and Immunotherapy Response in Patients with Glioblastoma: A Multiomic Analysis. *Front. Cell Dev. Biol.* **2020**, *8*, 576996. [CrossRef]
178. Bertram, M.Y.; Lauer, J.A.; De Joncheere, K.; Edejer, T.; Hutubessy, R.; Kieny, M.P.; Hill, S.R. Cost-effectiveness thresholds: Pros and cons. *Bull. World Health Organ.* **2016**, *94*, 925–930. [CrossRef] [PubMed]
179. Lin, S.; Luo, S.; Zhong, L.; Lai, S.; Zeng, D.; Rao, X.; Huang, P.; Weng, X. Cost-effectiveness of atezolizumab plus chemotherapy for advanced non-small-cell lung cancer. *Int. J. Clin. Pharm.* **2020**, *42*, 1175–1183. [CrossRef] [PubMed]
180. Aguiar, P.; Barreto, C.M.N.; Bychkovsky, B.L.; de Lima Lopes, G. Cost-effectiveness studies in oncology. In *Mehods and Biostatistics in Oncology*; Araujo, R., Riechelmann, R., Eds.; Springer: Berlin/Heidelberg, Germany, 2018. [CrossRef]
181. Jonsson, B.; Hofmarcher, T.; Lindgren, P.; Wilking, N. The cost and burden of cancer in the European Union 1995-2014. *Eur. J. Cancer* **2016**, *66*, 162–170. [CrossRef] [PubMed]
182. Chen, C.T.; Li, L.; Brooks, G.; Hassett, M.; Schrag, D. Medicare Spending for Breast, Prostate, Lung, and Colorectal Cancer Patients in the Year of Diagnosis and Year of Death. *Health Serv. Res.* **2018**, *53*, 2118–2132. [CrossRef] [PubMed]
183. Blumen, H.; Fitch, K.; Polkus, V. Comparison of Treatment Costs for Breast Cancer, by Tumor Stage and Type of Service. *Am. Health Drug Benefits* **2016**, *9*, 23–32. [PubMed]
184. Vivot, A.; Jacot, J.; Zeitoun, J.D.; Ravaud, P.; Crequit, P.; Porcher, R. Clinical benefit, price and approval characteristics of FDA-approved new drugs for treating advanced solid cancer, 2000–2015. *Ann. Oncol.* **2017**, *28*, 1111–1116. [CrossRef] [PubMed]
185. Prasad, V.; De Jesus, K.; Mailankody, S. The high price of anticancer drugs: Origins, implications, barriers, solutions. *Nat. Rev. Clin. Oncol.* **2017**, *14*, 381–390. [CrossRef]
186. Roussakow, S.V. Clinical and economic evaluation of modulated electrohyperthermia concurrent to dose-dense temozolomide 21/28 days regimen in the treatment of recurrent glioblastoma: A retrospective analysis of a two-centre German cohort trial with systematic comparison and effect-to-treatment analysis. *BMJ Open* **2017**, *7*, e017387. [CrossRef]

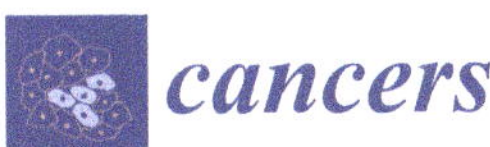

Review

Immunocompetent Mouse Models in the Search for Effective Immunotherapy in Glioblastoma

Roxanne Wouters [1,2,†], Sien Bevers [1,3,†], Matteo Riva [1,4], Frederik De Smet [3] and An Coosemans [1,*]

[1] Laboratory of Tumor Immunology and Immunotherapy, Department of Oncology, Leuven Cancer Institute, KU Leuven, 3000 Leuven, Belgium; roxanne.wouters@kuleuven.be (R.W.); sien.bevers@kuleuven.be (S.B.); matteo.riva@kuleuven.be (M.R.)

[2] Oncoinvent, A.S., 0484 Oslo, Norway

[3] The Laboratory for Precision Cancer Medicine, Translational Cell and Tissue Research Unit, Department of Imaging and Pathology, KU Leuven, 3000 Leuven, Belgium; frederik.desmet@kuleuven.be

[4] Department of Neurosurgery, Mont-Godinne Hospital, UCL Namur, 5530 Yvoir, Belgium

[*] Correspondence: an.coosemans@kuleuven.be

[†] These authors contributed equally to this paper.

Simple Summary: Glioblastoma (GBM) remains the most aggressive brain tumor. Treatment typically includes surgery and radio/chemotherapy, but in spite of intensive treatment, virtually all tumors recur within the time-frame of months with insufficient and unsuccessful second line options. This clinical reality is in contrast to preclinical animal experiments, which often show successful outcomes of novel immunotherapeutic approaches. This discrepancy is largely explained by the small number of animal models and their limited capacity to mimic the complexity of the human disease. Moreover, new treatment options are typically administered as single treatments in animal models, whereas patients receive them in combination with standard-of-care. In this review, we provide an overview of the existing mouse models for GBM research and how each of them mimic (parts of) the human disease spectrum. As such we provide an overview of the advantages and limitations of the currently available options for in vivo drug testing for GBM.

Citation: Wouters, R.; Bevers, S.; Riva, M.; De Smet, F.; Coosemans, A. Immunocompetent Mouse Models in the Search for Effective Immunotherapy in Glioblastoma. *Cancers* **2021**, *13*, 19. https://dx.doi.org/10.3390/cancers13010019

Received: 30 November 2020
Accepted: 20 December 2020
Published: 23 December 2020

Publisher's Note: MDPI stays neutral with regard to jurisdictional claims in published maps and institutional affiliations.

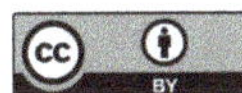

Abstract: Glioblastoma (GBM) is the most aggressive intrinsic brain tumor in adults. Despite maximal therapy consisting of surgery and radio/chemotherapy, GBM remains largely incurable with a median survival of less than 15 months. GBM has a strong immunosuppressive nature with a multitude of tumor and microenvironment (TME) derived factors that prohibit an effective immune response. To date, all clinical trials failed to provide lasting clinical efficacy, despite the relatively high success rates of preclinical studies to show effectivity of immunotherapy. Various factors may explain this discrepancy, including the inability of a single mouse model to fully recapitulate the complexity and heterogeneity of GBM. It is therefore critical to understand the features and limitations of each model, which should probably be combined to grab the full spectrum of the disease. In this review, we summarize the available knowledge concerning immune composition, stem cell characteristics and response to standard-of-care and immunotherapeutics for the most commonly available immunocompetent mouse models of GBM.

Keywords: glioblastoma; immunotherapy; model; animal model; preclinical; murine; immune response

1. Introduction

Glioblastoma (GBM), is the most lethal brain tumor in adults, despite all therapeutic efforts [1,2]. After standard-of-care treatment, consisting of maximal surgical resection followed by radiotherapy (RT) and adjuvant temozolomide (TMZ), the median overall survival generally does not exceed 15 months [3–5]. This underscores the unmet medical need for the development of more efficient treatments. Several immunotherapeutic strategies, such as immune checkpoint inhibitors, cellular therapies and oncolytic viral therapies, have been explored in GBM [6,7]. However, to date all randomized clinical trials failed to provide lasting clinical efficacy [8–12], despite the many successes of pre-clinical studies [13–15]. We are therefore facing an important translational gap.

We believe that the discrepancy between preclinical and clinical results for immunotherapy in GBM can be explained by several factors, two of which play a pivotal role. First, current experimental models probably insufficiently mimic the complex situation in the human brain and are therefore unable to adequately predict the clinical scenario. In particular, the immune suppressive tumor microenvironment and its impact on immunotherapy has been mostly ignored or insufficiently characterized in previous preclinical studies [16,17]. Second, preclinical studies have rarely implemented the standard-of-care treatment (surgery, RT and TMZ) when testing the effect of immune modulators. This issue is particularly relevant for immunotherapy, since conventional treatments can modify the immune biology of GBM thereby altering the response to additional immunotherapy [8,18–21].

We believe that addressing these two problems would strongly boost the translational impact of GBM preclinical studies. However, integrating the full standard-of-care in preclinical research is challenging and require specific neurosurgical skills and equipment, which are not always available. Conversely, preclinical testing with multiple immunocompetent mouse models in order to better recapitulate multiple aspects of GBM biology and inter-patient heterogeneity is relatively straightforward. Nevertheless, to this end it is essential to know all relevant features of the available tumor models [22–29], in order to make an appropriate evaluation of which are the most adequate for each specific research question.

In this review, we will summarize the main features of the most relevant immunocompetent GBM mouse models (Tables 1 and 2). For each model, we collected the available information on tumor immunity, cancer stemness, response to standard-of-care treatment and the effect of immunotherapeutics. The final goal will be to provide a useful tool for model selection and combination for the preclinical testing of new immunotherapeutic approaches against GBM.

2. Oldest Available Immunocompetent Mouse Models for GBM

The development and characterization of these oldest models has already been reviewed in detail in a previous publication by Oh et al. in 2014 [30]. Therefore, for these older models we will mainly focus on their most recent developments. An overview of these mouse models and relevant information can be found in Figure 1 and Table 1.

Table 1. Overview of the different characteristics of the GL26, GL261, ML/CT-2A, SMA-560 and 4C8 mouse models.

Model	Host	Induction	Histology	Immune Composition	Stem Cells	Effect of Standard-of-Care Therapy	Response to Immunotherapy	Reference
GL261	C57BL/6	Chemical induction with methylcholanthrene	GBM, ependymoblastoma	Immunogenic profile with high of frequency activated microglia and CD3$^+$ T cells, low frequency of Tregs, presence of TAMs, low frequency of APCs	Stem cell like phenotype with Nestin and CD133 expression	RT: +/− TMZ: +	Survival benefit with several immunotherapeutic strategies in single and combination treatment (ICB, vaccination, virotherapy, …)	Ausman 1970 [15,21,31–115]
GL26	C57BL/6	Chemical induction with carcinogen implantation	GBM, ependymoblastoma	CD8$^+$ T cell and myeloid cell infiltration with high expression of PD-1 and TIGIT immune checkpoints	Gene expression profile of glioma stem cells	TMZ: +	Generally positive	Sugiura 1969 [116–130]
ML/CT-2A	C57BL/6	Chemical induction with methylcholanthrene	Anaplastic astrocytoma	Overall immune suppressive microenvironment with low numbers of microglia, high numbers of resident macrophages and exhausted CD8$^+$ T cells with TIM-3 and LAG-3 expression	Positive for CD133, Nestin and Oct4 stem cell markers	RT: -	Generally positive	Seyfried 1992 [26,33,77,131–147]
SMA-560	VM/Dk	Spontaneous	Anaplastic astrocytoma	Upregulation immunoregulatory pathways, TGF-β signaling	CD44 and Nestin expression when cultured in spheres	RT: - TMZ: -	Generally positive	Fraser 1971 [134,148–160]
4C8	B6D2F1	Clonal cell lines of a glial tumor from a transgenic mouse	Oligodendroglioma, astrocytoma	Large number of macrophages at the tumor periphery instead of in the tumor core	Not assessed	Not assessed	Generally positive (limited amount of data available)	Weiner 1999 [161–165]

GBM: glioblastoma, Treg: regulatory T cell, DC: dendritic cell, MHC-I/II: major histocompatibility complex I or II, TAM: tumor associated macrophage, APC: antigen presenting cell, PD-1: programmed cell death protein 1, TIGIT: T cell immunoglobulin and ITIM domain, TGF-β: transforming growth factor β, TIM-3: T cell immunoglobulin and mucin-domain containing 3, LAG-3: lymphocyte activation gene 3, RT: radiotherapy, TMZ: Temozolomide, ICB: immune checkpoint blockade. Bold: highlight.

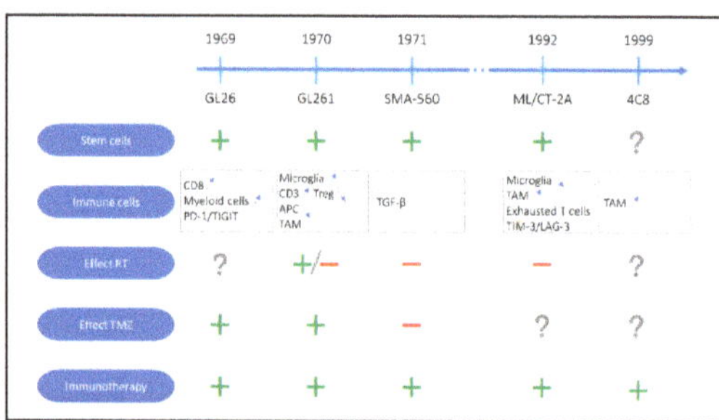

Figure 1. Schematic and chronological presentation of the old preclinical immunocompetent mouse models for glioblastoma with information about stemness, immune cell composition, the effects of standard of care and the efficiency of immunotherapy. RT: radiotherapy, TMZ: Temozolomide, PD-1: programmed cell death protein 1, TIGIT: T cell immunoglobulin and ITIM domain, Treg: regulatory T cell, TAM: tumor associated macrophage, TGF-β: transforming growth factor β, TIM-3: T cell immunoglobulin and mucin-domain containing 3, LAG-3: lymphocyte activation gene 3, (+) presence of stem cell populations and/or positive effect of treatment administration, (-) no effect of treatment administration and (?) data not available in literature.

2.1. GL261

2.1.1. Origins and Tumor Characteristics

This chemically induced model was first developed in 1970 by Ausman et al. [116]. and has by far been the most widely used in glioblastoma research. In vivo, GL261 cells have been shown to express different general stem cell markers such as CD133 and nestin [31] while exhibiting infiltrative capacity of brain-tumor derived mesenchymal stem cells positive for Sox2, nestin, Sca-1, CD9, CD44 and CD166 [32]. Khalsa et al. performed a bulk RNA sequencing analysis on GL261 tumors which showed a strong enrichment of differentially expressed genes related to several immune pathways compared to naïve control mice, especially related to genes relevant for T cells, macrophages and eosinophils [33]. The same study also indicated a higher frequency of activated microglia, more total T cells, a lower frequency of regulatory T cells and antigen presenting cells compared to the ML/CT-2A tumor model [33]. All findings point towards the fact that the GL261 tumor model is more immunogenic than other models, such as the ML/CT-2A tumor model.

2.1.2. Effect of Standard-of-Care

Both whole brain and focal beam irradiation strategies have been evaluated in the GL261 model. While whole brian irradiation was able to prolong survival and deliver long-term surviving mice, focal beam irradiation didn't show the same potential [34–37]. Administration of TMZ was able to provide similar survival benefits in the GL261 model as is seen in GBM patients [38–40].

2.1.3. Immunotherapeutic Approaches

Many different immunotherapies have been tested in the GL261 model. These include studies investigating programmed cell death protein 1 (PD-1) checkpoint blockade or other immune checkpoint inhibitors, oncolytic virotherapy, chimeric antigen receptor (CAR) T cell therapy, dendritic cell vaccination and many others [15,35,41–84]. In addition, the efficacy of many other less common immunotherapeutic approaches have been investigated in the GL261 models [85–109]. The vast majority of these therapies showed promising results, with a stronger anti-tumor response and improved survival rates. These immunotherapeutic strategies have been investigated as single treatments, in combination with other types of immunotherapies or in combination with the standard-of-care treatment. However, only part of the standard-of-care (usually TMZ, less commonly RT or RT-TMZ) was taken into consideration [39,40,78,79,110–114]. Interestingly, the efficacy of checkpoint inhibition directed against PD-1 or its ligand (PD-L1) in combination with TMZ, RT, or both was tested in six, two or one preclinical studies, respectively. Out of these eight combinatorial studies, seven were conducted with the GL261 tumor model [21].

The effects of steroids, largely used in the clinic to reduce brain oedema in GBM patients, were analyzed in one study using the GL261 tumor model. This study demonstrates that steroids have an inhibitory effect on anti-tumor immunity and that blocking cytotoxic T-lymphocyte-associated protein 4 (CTLA-4), but not PD-1, could partially prevent such negative modulation [115].

2.2. GL26

2.2.1. Origins and Tumor Characteristics

The GL26 model is the oldest immunocompetent preclinical model for GBM and has been developed in 1969 by chemical induction [116]. It has been less extensively used than the (similar) GL261 model. Although both models show a great histological resemblance, the main difference is that GL26 tumors show a large extent of necrosis and vascularity and therefore tend to be more hemorrhagic [116]. Crommentuijn et al. [117] described the presence of a tumor antigen-specific CD8$^+$ T cell population which displays a tolerogenic phenotype with a high expression of several immune checkpoints such as PD-1 and T cell immunoglobulin and ITIM domain (TIGIT). The infiltration of myeloid cells expressing these immune checkpoint ligands was also observed [117]. Furthermore, the importance of galactokinase (Gal1) in the immune suppression of the GL26 model was described, since it masks tumor cells from immune recognition [118,119]. The importance of glial toll-like receptor 2 (TLR2) as a bridge between the innate and the adaptive immune response was also reported, which is crucial in providing an effective immune response against the tumor [120]. Genetic analysis of GL26 tumors also revealed a specific acquisition of several stem cell markers that were correlated to anti-tumor T cell activity [121].

2.2.2. Effect of Standard-of-Care

Radiotherapy (also if as whole body irradiation) and TMZ as a monotherapies have both been proven to be effective in prolonging survival in the GL26 mouse model [122–126]. Furthermore, TMZ treatment was able to increase cross-priming of tumor antigen-specific CD4$^+$ T cells and CD8$^+$ T cells and suppressed the frequency of regulatory T cells (Tregs) [125].

2.2.3. Immunotherapeutic Approaches

GBM is strongly invasive and tumor cells can be found embedded in the normal parenchyma at great distance from the main tumor. This makes a complete resection not feasible [117]. Yadav et al. analyzed this problem with the GL26 model, and they found that down regulation of C-X-C chemokine receptor type 4 (CXCR4) led to less perivascular invasion and increased survival. Furthermore, CXCR4 knockdown sensitizes the tumors to irradiation, making this molecule an interesting therapeutic target [127]. Another novel therapeutic strategy targets the proton/H$^+$ eflux mechanism important for the maintance of the intracellular pH. The inhibition of the H+ eflux mechanism (NHE1) reduced tumor volume, invasion and prolonged overall survival in GL26 (and SB28) glioma models. This type of treatment resulted in an accumulation of CD8$^+$ T cells and sensitized animals to anti-PD-1 therapy [128]. Also the mTOR pathway is a frequent target of anti-glioma therapy. Targeting this pathway with rapamycin in combination with immunotherapy had a synergistic effect and a long term survival advantage. Rapamycin administration also resulted in a long lasting central memory CD8$^+$ T cell response and a stronger anti-tumor response after a second tumor challenge [129]. The combination of TMZ with interferon (IFN)-β was also tested in the GL26 model and showed enhanced anti-tumor effects compared to TMZ alone [130].

2.3. ML/CT-2A

2.3.1. Origins and Tumor Characteristics

The CT-2A model was first described by Seyfried et al. in 1992 [131] and accurately represents numerous GBM characteristics, including the intra-tumoral cellular heterogeneity and the proliferative and metabolic profiles [132]. CT-2A cells cultured as monolayer cells (ML/CT-2A) in vitro express different stem cell markers such as CD133, nestin and Oct4 [26]. Also in vivo the expression of CD133 and Nestin is observed in ML/CT-2A tumors [133], indicating that the cells keep their stemness during tumor growth in mice. Khalsa et al. performed RNA sequencing to identify the ML/CT-2A immune profile in vitro [33]. In contrast to the highly immunogenic GL261 model, ML/CT-2A cells showed no enrichment of any immune response-related pathway. In vivo, ML/CT-2A tumors had lower numbers of $CD45^{low}CD11b^{low}CX3CR1^+$ microglial cells (considered activated or resting based on MHCII positive or negative staining, respectively), but higher numbers of $CD11b^+F4/80^+CD64^+Ly6C^-$ resident macrophages and $CD39^+Tim3^+Lag3^+CD8^+$ exhausted cytotoxic T cells compared to other glioblastoma tumor models. Furthermore, 70–80% of T cells in the tumor microenvironment of ML/CT-2A tumors exhibit prolonged expression of T cell immunoglobulin and mucin domain-containing protein 3 (TIM-3) and lymphocyte-activation gene 3 (LAG-3), both markers for dysfunctional T cells [33]. Overall, the ML/CT-2A model is characterized by an immune suppressive tumor microenvironment and exhausted effector T cell function, making it a very suitable tumor model for GBM research in the field of immunotherapy since a similar immune phenotype is observed in GBM patients [134].

2.3.2. Effect of Standard-of-Care

The ML/CT-2A model has not been widely used in preclinical studies assessing the effects of the standard-of-care treatment. Only one study described the effects of RT in the model [135], where whole brain irradiation was ineffective in prolonging survival in mice. As already mentioned, the surgical removal has an influence on the immune composition of the remaining/recurrent tumor, with obvious implications for immunotherapies. Nevertheless, this treatment has only occasionally been assessed in preclinical studies. Khalsa et al. performed an immunophenotyping of the ML/CT-2A mouse model before and after surgical resection of the tumor [33]. After tumor resection, an increase of $CD4^+$ and $CD8^+$ T cells and activated microglia was observed with a decrease of resting macrophages and resident microglia. Furthermore, PD-1 expression decreased and CD25 expression increased on $CD4^+$ T cells post-tumor resection [33]. These data suggest that tumor resection in the ML/CT-2A model partially removes the immune suppressive microenvironment and promotes immune activation, possibly creating a favorable momentum for administration of immunotherapies.

2.3.3. Immunotherapeutic Approaches

Given the disappointing results of checkpoint blockade in GBM patients, the current focus of preclinical research in this field is on combining checkpoint blockade with newly identified targets such as interleukin 6 (IL-6), IL-7, IL-12 or phagocytosis pathways, in order to overcome T cell exhaustion [136–138]. In the ML/CT-2A tumor model, the combination of PD-1 checkpoint inhibition with anti-CD137 decreased TIL exhaustion, improved TIL functionality and resulted in 50% long term survivors [139]. Another novel combination treatment recently tested was the combination of anti-PD-L1 with gene-mediated cytotoxic immunotherapy which resulted in more long term survivors as compared to the monotherapies [140]. One last focus of interest has been to improve the delivery of checkpoint inhibitors via lipid nanoparticles. In combination with RT, this strategy led to a depletion of tumor-associated myeloid cells and a significantly improved survival in ML/CT-2A and GL261 models [135].

Oncolytic virus (OV) therapy has great potential for success, however the best balance between maximal anti-tumor activity and acceptable toxicity is difficult to find, especially following direct intracranial infusion. Certain OVs based on herpes simplex virus (HSV) are safe but have only little anti-tumor response. To overcome this limitation Passaro et al. engineered an HSV to express an antibody against PD-1 and injected it intratumorally. This resulted in an increased median survival and immune memory against the both ML/CT-2A and GL261 tumors [141]. The combination of OV therapy with PD-1/PD-L1 immunotherapy provided a synergistic effect leading to an improved overall survival and an activation of the immune response capable to reverse the tumor-induced immune suppression [142,143]. On the other hand, OVs based on vesicular stomatitis virus (VSV) have a very robust anti-tumor effect but are extremely neurotoxic when injected in the brain. Therefore, Balathasan et al. [144] used an intravenous pretreatment of VSVΔ51 as a way to induce peripheral immunization before intracranial injection of an otherwise lethal dose of VSVΔ51. This resulted in complete tumor regression in 20% of ML/CT-2A tumor bearing mice. Also OVs based on Semliki Forest Virus (SFV) have been developed [145,146]. When injected intravenously, they resulted in a prolonged survival with 27% of the mice bearing ML/CT-2A tumors cured, whereas there was no significant effect in the GL261 model [146].

In an interesting study, Ladomersky et al. used the ML/CT-2A model to demonstrate increased immune suppression, decreased immunotherapeutic efficacy and decreased survival in old age animals (75 week old mice, corresponding to 58–59 year old humans) [77]. The impact of age on GBM development and treatment has been ignored most of times: in the majority of studies, animals of young age (6–12 weeks, corresponding to early adulthood in humans) are used for preclinical GBM research [147]. Given that the median age at diagnosis for GBM is 65 years, the age difference between tumor models and patients is extremely relevant.

2.4. SMA-560

2.4.1. Origins and Tumor Characteristics

The SMA-560 model is one of the few models that spontaneously arose in VM/Dk mice as initially described by Fraser et al. in 1971 [148]. It was established as a cell line in 1980 by Serano and colleagues [149]. The fact that the model developed spontaneously in immunocompetent mice, makes it a very interesting model to study. A genetic characterization of the model revealed an upregulation of genes involved in antigen presentation, interferon-related protein expression and a general increase in genes related to immunoregulatory pathways indicating the presence of an ineffective immune response in the tumor microenvironment of the SMA-560 model [150]. Furthermore, the immune suppressive protein transforming growth factor beta (TGF-β) has been shown to play an important role in SMA-560 tumor development [151]. The expression of PD-1, TIM-3 and LAG-3 on tumor infiltrating lymphocytes is also increased in SMA-560 tumors [134]. In terms of stemness characteristics, it has been described that in vitro SMA-560 cells express only a limited amount of CD44 and nestin stem cell markers. However, when cultured in sphere cultures the cells seem to increase their CD44 and Nestin expression, which was correlated with a more aggressive tumor behaviour in vivo [152]. Schneider and colleagues described the difference in tumorigeneic potential in young and old VM/Dk mice. Interestingly at baseline, older SMA-560 mice had a significantly worse survival as compared to younger mice, in contrast to the GL261 model where this difference was not observed [153].

2.4.2. Effect of Standard-of-Care

In vitro, SMA-560 cells were highly resistant to TMZ treatment and only responded to high doses of irradiation [152]. However, only a few studies assessed these effects in vivo [154]. Whole brain irradiation as a single treatment or combined with TMZ was either ineffective or provided only a limited and non-significant improvement in survival compared to control mice [154,155]. This indicates that the standard-of-care used in GBM patients is ineffective in prolonging survival of the SMA-560 mouse model. Therefore, the translational potential of the model should be considered carefully when translating results to the whole GBM patient population. However, a tumor model that does not respond to RT or TMZ can be relevant in studying treatment options for patients who respond poorly to this standard-of-care treatment regimen or for the recurrent situation where resistance appeared.

2.4.3. Immunotherapeutic Approaches

An important immunological therapeutic target studied in the SMA-560 model is excessive TGF-β signaling [156,157]. As such, the administration of phosphorothioate-locked nucleic acid (LNA)-modified antisense oligonucleotide gapmers targetting TGF-β resulted in prolonged survival and increased CD3$^+$ and CD8$^+$ cytotoxic T cell infiltration [158]. Another emerging treatment strategy that has been tested in this model is CAR T cell therapy, which was shown to generate a pro-inflammatory tumor microenvironment and to significantly extend survival in the SMA-560 model [159]. Furthermore, anti-angiogenic treatment has a positive effect on survival in the SMA-560 model [155]. One of the problems in GBM treatment is the delivery of the compound trough the blood brain barrier. In this regard, microbubbles have been tested to increase the local concentration of certain types of treatments. This strategy was succesfully tested for doxorubicin in the SMA-560 model [160].

2.5. C8

2.5.1. Origins and Tumor Characteristics

The 4C8 model was established in 1999 from clonal cell lines of a glial tumor (MOCH-1) in B6D2F1 mice [161]. Gazdzinski et al. [162] compared the characteristics of this model with the GL261 model. The 4C8 model is less aggressive, the tumor has higher cell density, less necrosis and invasiveness with a more normal vasculature and less mitotic cells as compared to the GL261 model. Both models have a large number of infiltrating macrophages; however, these cells are located at the tumor periphery in the 4C8 model [162]. All these features, consistently pointing towards a lower aggressiveness in comparison to the GL261 model, have strongly limited the used of the 4C8 tumor model.

2.5.2. Immunotherapeutic Approaches

This model has been used very limitedly in immunotherapeutic or anti-angiogenic research [163,164]. The combination of an anti-angiogenic receptor tyrosine kinase inhibitor with a proteasome inhibitor resulted in a significantly improved survival and an induction of anti-angiogenic effects which leads to vascular normalization [164]. The effects of oncolytic virotherapy were assessed in the model as well. In vitro, 4C8 cells showed the same sensitivity as human glioma cells to a series of type HSV-1 [165]. In vivo studies showed a prolongation of survival with an intracranial injection of an IL-12-expressing HSV [165].

3. Recently Developed Immunocompetent Mouse Models for GBM

Various new GBM models have been developed in the last years. In most cases, this has been done by means of viral vectors which were either used to manipulate isolated mouse cells (mGB2, NSCL61 and bTiTs-G3) or injected directly into the animals' brain (SB28, 005 GSC and NFpp10 models). Additionally, tumor models have been generated from spontaneously developed tumors in genetically altered mice (KR158B and Mut3) or by culturing older cell lines in a different way (CT-2A). In all cases, stable cells lines amenable of standard intracranial injection have been obtained [22–25,27,28,166]. An overview of these mouse models and relevant information can be found in Figure 2 and Table 2.

Table 2. Overview of the different characteristics of the KR158B, Mut3, 005 GSCs, NSCL61, bRiTs-G3, NFpp10-GBM, NS/CT-2A, SB28 and mGB2 mouse models.

Model	Host	Induction	Histology	Immune Composition	Stem Cells	Effect of Standard-of-Care Therapy	Response to Immunotherapy	Reference
KR158B	C57BL/6	Spontaneous tumor development in Nf1 and p53 mutant mice	Secondary GBM	Not assessed	Not assessed	RT/TMZ: +	Resistance to ICB	Reilly 2000 [12,29,65,166–168]
Mut3	C57BL/6	Spontaneous tumor development in Nf1, p53 and Pten mutant mice	GBM, high-grade astrocytoma	High levels of classical and exhausted CD8$^+$ T cells, CD4$^+$ T cells, Tregs and resting microglia and low levels of DC infiltration	Increased GFAP and Nestin expression	Not assessed	Not assessed	Kwon 2008 [33,169,170]
005 GSCs	C57BL/6	Transduction in hippocampus of adult mice with vectors with activated HRas en AKT	GBM, heterogeneous	Relatively non-immunogenic, absence of MHC-I and down regulation of co-stimulatory molecules, limited T cell activation, strong correlation with human tumor immune microenvironment	Glioma stem cell tumor model	Not assessed	Resistance to ICB	Marumoto 2008 [24,33,168,171–175]
NSCL61	BALB/c	HrasL61 overexpression in p53 deficient neural stem cells	GBM, heterogeneous	Not assessed	Tumor model is derived from neural stem cells	Not assessed	Generally positive (limited amount of data available)	Hide 2009 [27,68,72]
bRiTs-G3	C57BL/6	Overexpression of HRasV12 in neural stem cells from mice with homozygous deletion of the Ink4a/Arf locus	GBM, mesenchymal	Not assessed	Tumor model is derived from neural stem cells	RT: + RT resistance develops after repeated exposure	Generally positive (limited amount of data available)	Sampetrean 2011 [28,68,176]
NFpp10-GBM	C57BL/6	Embryonic stem cells infected with shp53-shNf1 and shPten lentiviral vector	GBM	Lack of T cell infiltration	Tumor model is derived from neural stem cells	Not assessed	Resistance to ICB	Allen 2017 [13,24,25,177]

Table 2. *Cont.*

Model	Host	Induction	Histology	Immune Composition	Stem Cells	Effect of Standard-of-Care Therapy	Response to Immunotherapy	Reference
NS/CT-2A	C57BL/6	Culturing of CT-2A cells in serum-free stem cell culture medium	Astrocytoma	Decrease in number of Tregs and increased CD8+ T cells compared to ML/CT-2A	Increased expression of Nestin and CD133 expression compared to ML/CT-2A	RT: + TMZ: + RT/TMZ: +	Resistance to ICB	Binello 2012 [21,26,30,133,178]
SB28	C57BL/6	Intraventricular transfection of Nras, PDGF and shp53 in neonates	GBM, proneural	Weakly immunogenic: few infiltrating T cells, abundant macrophage and microglial infiltration, absence of MHC-I and MHC-II expression	Not assessed	Not assessed	Resistance to ICB	Kosaka 2014 [9,12,23,58]
mGB2	C57BL/6	p53 and Pten deficient neural stem cells in adult mice	GBM, mesenchymal	Strong presence of myeloid cells and only few lymphocytes	Tumor model is derived from neural stem cells	Not assessed	Not assessed	Costa 2019 [22,179]

GBM: glioblastoma, Treg: regulatory T cell, DC: dendritic cell, MHC-I/II: major histocompatibility complex I or II, RT: radiotherapy, TMZ: Temozolomide, ICB: immune checkpoint blockade, GFAP: glial fibrillary acidic protein, PDGF: platelet-derived growth factor, Pten: phosphatase and tensin homolog, Nf1: neurofibromin 1, Nras: neuroblastoma reticular activating system, Hras: Harvey rat sarcoma viral oncogene homolog. Bold: highlight.

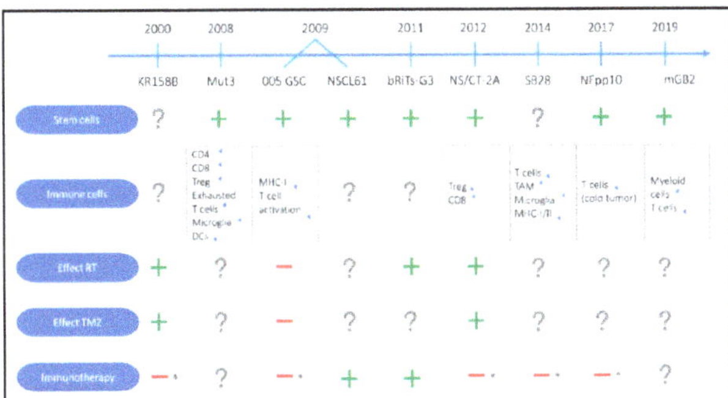

Figure 2. Schematic and chronological presentation of the more recent preclinical immunocompetent mouse models for glioblastoma with information about stemness, immune cell composition, the effects of standard of care and the efficiency of immunotherapy. RT: radiotherapy, TMZ: Temozolomide, Treg: regulatory T cell, DC: dendritic cell, MHC-I/II: major histocompatibility complex I or II, TAM: tumor associated macrophage, (+) presence of stem cell populations and/or positive effect of treatment administration, (−) no effect of treatment administration, (?) data not available in literature and (*) resistance to immune checkpoint blockade.

3.1. KR158B

3.1.1. Origins and Tumor Characteristics

This mouse model was developed in 2000 by Reilly et al. and it is the first astrocytoma mouse model that was generated by knocking-down neurofibromin 1 (Nf1) and tumor protein p53 in mice which then spontaneously developed brain tumors with variable histology from low grade astrocytoma to GBM [29]. KR158B is the cell line derived from the most aggressive variants, which recapitulate the main features of human GBM [166]. To date, information on the immune and stemness characterization of this model is not available yet.

3.1.2. Effect of Standard-of-Care

The administration of whole brain irradiation and TMZ as single treatments wasn't able to positively affect survival in the KR158B model, and the combination of both resulted in a small median survival benefit of only five days, in line with results in the most aggressive human GBMs and making this a promising model for future preclinical research [166].

3.1.3. Immunotherapeutic Approaches

In the KR158B model, the combination of myeloablative conditioning, dendritic cell (DC) vaccination and adoptive cellular therapy resulted in a doubeling of the median survival and 30% of cured mice [166]. This model has also been used to test alternative TMZ treatment schedules in combination with immunotherapy [65,167,168]. The combination of TMZ and anti-PD-1 treatment has been shown to decrease the expression of T cell exhaustion markers. However, this had no effect on survival indicating that the model can develop resistance mechanisms to both these treatments [65]. However, the combined inhibition of PD-1 and C-C chemokine receptor type 2 (CCR2) lead to a synergistic effect and improved mouse survival, overvcoming the resistance to anti-PD-1 monotherapy [168]. The recent failure of clinical trials involving anti-PD-1 treatment [12] has demonstrated that human GBM are able to promote strong resistance mechanisms hampering the efficacy of checkpoint inhibitors. Therefore, performing preclinical research in models showing the same type of resistance, such as the KR158B, is of the utmost importance for an appropriate design of future clinical trials.

3.2. Mut3

The Mut3 tumor model was developed by Kwon et al. [169] in 2008 by generating *Nf1*, *p53* and *Pten* deficient mice which subsequently developed spontaneous high-grade astrocytomas. Neural stem cells (NSCs) from presymptomatic mice already showed aberrant stem cell features including higher proliferation levels, increased glial fibrillary acidic protein (GFAP) and increased Nestin expression [170]. The Mut3 cell line was generated by isolating the spontaneously developed tumors and bringing them in culture where they are maintained in neurosphere conditions [169]. Mut3 tumors are immunologically characterized by high levels of both classical and exhausted infiltrating CD8+ T cells, CD4+ T cells, Tregs, and resting microglia, and by low levels of DC infiltration [33]. At this moment, no data is available on effects of standard-of-care or immunotherapeutics in the model.

3.3. 005 GSCs

3.3.1. Origins and Tumor Characteristics

Marumoto et al. [24] developed this mouse model by injecting Cre-*loxP*–controlled lentiviral vectors expressing activated oncogenes AKT and Harvey-Ras in the hippocampus of GFAP-Cre Tp53+/− mice. Subsequently, the obtained tumor cells were cultured as neurospheres and the 005 GSCs cell line was established [24,171]. Next, Saha et al. developed an immunocompetent model by reinjecting the 005 GSC cells in C57BL/6 mice [172,173]. 005 GSC-derived tumors show the same features as the primary tumor. Furthermore, 005 GSC cells express several stem cell markers such as Nestin, CD133 and Sox2 and proangiogenic vascular endothelial growth factor (VEGF) both in vitro and in vivo [173]. Even though RNA seq analysis performed by Khalsa et al. [33] showed that 005 GSC tumors exhibit a more immunologically active profile, Cheema et al. [173] described the tumors as non-immunogenic with the absence of major histocompatibility complex (MHC)-I expression and down regulation of co-stimulatory molecules. Nonetheless, Khalsa et al. showed that 005 GSC tumors had large amounts of activated and resting microglia and CD4+ Tregs, but low numbers of classical and exhausted CD8+ T cells [33]. This immunological phenotype strongly correlates with the immune microenvironment of GBM tumors in patients, making it a highly translational mouse model to be used for preclinical studies involving immunotherapeutic GBM research [33].

3.3.2. Effect of Standard-of-Care

Saha et al. [174] demonstrated that both low and high doses of TMZ treatment were ineffective in providing a survival benefit in the 005 GSC tumor model. In combination with OV, TMZ even counteracted the OVs positive effect on survival, indicating the chemoresistant nature of the 005 GSC tumor model and the importance of implementing standard-of-care treatment in preclinical research. The effects of RT on 005 GSC tumors have not yet been described.

3.3.3. Immunotherapeutic Approaches

005 GSC model has experienced occasional use in immunotherapy research to evaluate the effect of combination treatments with OV, VEGF receptor (VEGFR) tyrosine kinase inhibitors (TKI) and immune checkpoint blockade [172,173,175]. Cheema et al. [173] showed the effect of a genetically engineered oncolytic HSV armed with IL-12 (G47Δ-mIL12). Median survival was prolonged after intratumoral injection of G47Δ-mIL12. Treatment with G47Δ-mIL12 doesn't only target GSCs but also increases IFN-γ release, inhibits angiogenesis, and reduces the number of Tregs in the tumor [173]. The combination of G47Δ-mIL12 with the VEGFR TKI axitinib, anti-CTLA-4, anti-PD-1 or anti-PD-L1 further enhanced the positive effects on survival [172,175] while monotherapy of checkpoint inhibition with anti-CTLA-4, anti-PD-1 or anti-PD-L1 only showed positive but modest effects [172]. Interestingly, a triple combination of G47Δ-mIL12 with anti-CTLA-4 and anti-PD-1 showed a synergistic curative effect that was accompanied with M1 macrophage

polarization and an increased CD8$^+$ T cell / Treg ratio [172]. Additionally, targeting myeloid-derived suppressor cells (MDSCs) by using a CCR2 antagonist was able to sensitize 005 GSC tumors to anti-PD-1 therapy [168].

3.4. NSCL61

3.4.1. Origins and Tumor Characteristics

The NSCL61 model was originally developed by Hide et al. [27] in 2009 by the overexpression of oncogenic Harvey rat sarcoma viral oncogene homolog (HRas)^{L61} in p53 deficient NSCs that subsequently formed tumors in nude mice after stereotactic injection. These tumors were grown in culture as the NSCL61 cells and consist of an heterogenous population of both glioma initiating and non-tumorigenic cells [27]. An immunocompetent tumor model can be established by injecting NSCL61 cells stereotactically in C57BL/6 mice [68]. An immunological evaluation of NSCL61 tumors has not yet been performed.

3.4.2. Immunotherapeutic Approaches

The NSCL61 has only been sparsly used in preclinical GBM research [68,72]. Tumor cell lysate-based vaccination therapy in combination with immunotherapy targeting CD40 resulted in the induction of IFN-γ secretion from CD4$^+$ T cells and prolonged survival [72]. The local delivery of anti-CD40 monoclonal antibodies resulted in an increased apoptosis, T cell infiltration and significantly prolonged survival in the NSCL61 and bRiTs-G3 model, but not in the GL261 model due to a lower CD40 expression [68].

3.5. bRiTs-G3

3.5.1. Origins and Tumor Characteristics

Sampetrean et al. [28] developed the bRiTs-G3 model in 2011 by retroviral transduction of constitutively active HRas^{V12} in normal neural stem/progenitor cells isolated from the subventricular zone of adult mice with a homozygous deletion of the *Ink4a/Arf* locus. Brain tumor-initiating cells were subsequently cultured as neurospheres. Molecular characterization of bRiTs-G3 tumors showed expression of mesenchymal and stem cell markers indicating a mesenchymal GBM subtype [28].

3.5.2. Effect of Standard-of-Care

The bRiTs-G3 tumor model was used to study resistance to RT by exposing the cells in vitro to repeated cycles of irradiation. After stereotactic injection of the pretreated cells, bRiTs-G3 tumors were resistant to subsequent treatment with RT, indicating the bRiTs-G3 cells acquire a radio-resistant phenotype after repeated exposure to irradiation [176].

3.5.3. Immunotherapeutic Approaches

When the bRiTs-G3 cells acquire their radioresistant phenotype, this also results in upregulation of insulin-like growth factor 1 receptor (IGF1R). Therefore, IGF1R blockade has been proposed as treatment option to prevent RT resistance and recurrence after RT [176]. Additionally, the bRiTs-G3 models has been used in immunotherapy research with anti-CD40 treatment where it significantly prolonged survival compared to control mice [68].

3.6. NFpp10-GBM

3.6.1. Origins and Tumor Characteristics

NFpp10-GBM cells were created in 2017 by infecting embryonic C57Bl/6 NSCs with lentiviral vectors containing shP53-shNF1 and shPten [13,24,25]. To date, this model has not yet been fully characterized and has only experienced very limited use in preclinical GBM research.

3.6.2. Immunotherapeutic Approaches

The NFpp10-GBM model is mainly used to study tumor vasculature and angiogenesis [13,177]. The combination treatment of VEGF inhibition and anti-PD-L1 had no significant effect on survival. The ineffectiveness of the combination treatment was not due to the lack of PD-L1 expression of the cells, but rather the lack of T cell infiltration into the tumor [13]. To increase treatment efficacy a vascular targeting peptide (VTP) was developed containing the tumor necrosis factor (TNF) superfamily cytokine LIGHT which stimulates T cells, promotes vascular inflammation and is involved in lymph node neogenesis. Triple treatment with LIGHT-VTP, anti-VEGF and anti-PD-L1 resulted in a significantly reduced tumor burden as compared to untreated controls. Additionally, this combination treatment amplified high endothelial venules' frequency and T cell accumulation [177].

3.7. NS/CT-2A

3.7.1. Origins and Tumor Characteristics

As highlighted in the already mentioned review by Oh et al. [30], culturing CT-2A cells in neurospheres (NS/CT-2A) results in an increase of their stemness features. However, the difference in immunogenicity between CT-2A cells cultured in ML and NS was not described yet [26]. In a study performed by our group in 2019, NS/CT-2A tumors have been shown to induce a shorter survival and a higher expression of stemness and vascular markers compared with their ML counterpart. Furthermore, NS/CT-2A tumors showed an increase in CD8$^+$ T cells and a decrease in the number of Tregs compared to ML/CT-2A tumors [133]. These features of the NS/CT-2A tumor model make it suitable for preclinical research aimed at developing therapeutic strategies against tumor stem cells and immune suppression.

3.7.2. Effect of Standard-of-Care

In the NS/CT-2A model, TMZ and stereotactic RT were able to prolong survival when administered as monotherapies or in combination. As monotherapy, stereotactic RT positively modulated both the adaptive and the innate immune system (increased CD8$^+$ T cells and decreased M2 macrophages and monocytic MDSCs (mMDSCs)) while TMZ only improved innate immunity (reduced mMDSCs) and to a lower extent than stereotactic RT [21]. Interestingly, the combination of these two treatments, despite prolonging survival, was immunologically detrimental compared to RT alone. This model was also used to assess the effects of stereotactic RT dose-escalation and dose-fractionation. RT dose-escalation was associated with prolonged survival, improved anti-tumor immunity and reduced expression of stem cell markers. Conversely, RT dose-fractionation drastically reduced this positive effect [178]. Given the fact that GBM patients are currently treated with a fractionated RT schedule, these results highlight the need for studies aimed at identifying new RT schedules capable to induce a better immune modulation and a more efficient combination with immunotherapeutics.

3.7.3. Immunotherapeutic Approaches

As already mentioned, the combination of stereotactic RT and TMZ in the NS/CT-2A model induced a less favorable immune microenvironment compared to RT alone. The model also appeared quite resistant to anti-PD-1 since this treatment could only induce minor modifications of survival and tumor immunity when administered alone or following RT-TMZ [21].

3.8. SB28

3.8.1. Origins and Tumor Characteristics

The SB28 cell line was developed by Kosaka et al. [23] via intraventricular injection of the oncogenes neuroblastoma reticular activating system (NRas), platelet-derived growth factor (PDGF) and short hairpin p53 in neonate C56BL/6 mice. Seven weeks following glioma induction, brain tissue was harvested, minced and seeded. The clone with the highest luciferase activity was selected and the SB28 cell-line was established [23]. There was an inverse correlation between the number of injected SB28 cells and the median survival [58]. The tumors can be classified as proneural, as indicated by the presence of PDGF alterations, and they are weakly immunogenic, as is the case for human GBMs [23, 58]. High cellularity of the tumor area, invasion of the normal brain parenchyma and areas of hypervascularization are also common characteristics of SB28 tumors and human GBM. Very few infiltrating T cells can be found, in contrast to abundant macrophage and microglial infiltration. Due to the absence of constitutive MHC-I and MHC-II expression, SB28 tumors are less susceptible of T cell immunosurveillance compared to GL261 tumors. SB28 tumors exhibit a very low mutational load (50-fold less than GL261 tumors), resulting in only a few neoepitopes and explaining the weak immunogenicity. The mutated genes were equally distributed across several pathways, but 10% of all mutations were found in the PDGF signaling pathway, confirming the proneural classification [58].

3.8.2. Immunotherapeutic Approaches

The use of combined anti-PD-1 and anti-CTLA-4 was curative in over 50% of GL261 bearing mice, whereas it was ineffective in SB28 tumors [58]. This indicates that the SB28 model is more representative to human disease where immune checkpoint blockade provided unsatisfactory results so far [9,12]. Another study investigated the modulation of CD40 signaling and cyclooxygenase (COX)-2 blockade in the SB28 and GL261 models. The combination strategy promoted M1 cells, enhanced T cell effectors and prolonged survival [23].

3.9. mGB2

The mGB2 tumor model was generated by Costa et al. [22] in 2019 by means of a double knockout (DKO) of *Pten* and *p53* specifically in NSCs. Histopathological analysis of the developed tumors showed microvascular proliferation, necrotic areas and positivity for markers such as GFAP, oligodendrocyte transcription factor (OLIG2) and Ki67, all characteristics of human high-grade gliomas [22]. Subsequently, NSCs were isolated from the DKO mice and grown in culture. Reinjection of the cells in adult C57Bl/6 mice resulted in tumor induction 6–8 months later with a median survival of 170 days and with similar characteristics as the original tumor [22]. In order to try to reduce the survival time, tumor cells from a fully established invasive high-grade glioma (murine glioblastoma 0; mGB0) were isolated. Cells were serially implanted for two in vivo passages (mGB1 and mGB2) resulting in tumor development in all mice and a progressive shortening of the median survival. Based on genomic and transcriptomic data, mGB0 can be classified as the classical subtype, mGB1 as the proneural subtype and mGB2 as the mesenchymal subtype. mGB2 was selected as the most representative cell line compared to human disease with the worst prognosis and many histopathological features of high-grade gliomas. Also similar to what is observed in human GBMs, abundant myeloid cells and only few lymphocytes were found [179]. No therapies have been tested so far.

4. Conclusions

Immunocompetent mouse models are essential in preclinical GBM research, especially in the search for new immunotherapeutic strategies. When we compare all relevant mouse models based on their stemness, immune characteristics and response to standard-of-care treatment, it is clear that there is not one mouse model that perfectly recapitulates the heterogeneity of a human GBM tumor. However, the overview we present here can help in deciding which model is best suited for which type of research. For instance, the translational impact of research involving immune checkpoint blockade might not be recommended for a mouse model such as GL261 that is very sensitive to this type of immunotherapy (which is not compatible with the clinical situation). A better choice would be to use mouse models that show a certain degree of resistance to immune checkpoint blockade such as KR158B, 005 GSC, Nfpp10-GBM or SB28. In addition, if we want to take into account any type of model-intrinsic response to certain treatments, it would be even better to evaluate new treatment modalities in multiple models. Furthermore, different tumor models might correlate to different patient populations of GBM. Therefore, the heterogeneity of GBM would be better addressed in preclinical research if a heterogeneous composition of tumor models is used. Interestingly, a recent study highlighted a variable response to immune checkpoint inhibitors in syngeneic mice inoculated with the same type of cells (GL261) [180]. If individual factors are relevant in a standardize situation such as a syngeneic model, it is reasonable to expect that they play a dramatic role in actual patients. For all these reasons, we believe that understanding and modelling patients' heterogeneity in preclinical research will be one of the most relevant challenges in future preclinical research for GBM.

Another outstanding question relates to how the genomic aberrations of each tumor model correlate to aberrations in its microenvironment, and, even more importantly, how this compares to the human situation. Indeed, ongoing trials for targeted therapies are mainly based on genomic matching; however, the identification of those patient populations with similar immunologic features as observed in the mouse models is still lacking, but could be key in targeting the right approaches to the right patients.

Lastly, it is striking that only very few preclinical studies have incorporated the standard-of-care regimen when testing new treatments. Moreover, in the limited cases where standard-of-care is taken into account, this usually only consisted of RT and/or TMZ and rarely included a surgical resection of the tumor, nevertheless the corner stone of the clinical treatment. It is well known that GBMs at first diagnosis and at recurrence (therefore, after the whole standard of care treatment) harbor important differences in term of molecular features and druggable targets [181]. In this view, it is of paramount importance to integrate in the pipeline of preclinical studies surgery, focal radiotherapy and TMZ-based chemotherapy in order to model such longitudinal neoplastic evolution. A paradigm shift is necessary: preclinical research should not only be aimed at discovering new treatments, but also at identifying the most appropriate momentum for their administration in order to maximize their effect in synergy with standard therapies.

Author Contributions: Conceptualization, M.R. and A.C.; methodology, S.B.; investigation, S.B., R.W. and F.D.S.; writing—original draft preparation, S.B. and R.W.; writing—review and editing, M.R., A.C. and F.D.S.; visualization, M.R. and R.W.; supervision, A.C.; project administration, A.C.; funding acquisition, A.C. All authors have read and agreed to the published version of the manuscript.

Funding: This research received no external funding.

Conflicts of Interest: The authors declare no conflict of interest.

References

1. Cloughesy, T.F.; Mochizuki, A.Y.; Orpilla, J.R.; Hugo, W.; Lee, A.H.; Davidson, T.B.; Wang, A.C.; Ellingson, B.M.; Rytlewski, J.A.; Sanders, C.M.; et al. Neoadjuvant anti-PD-1 immunotherapy promotes a survival benefit with intratumoral and systemic immune responses in recurrent glioblastoma. *Nat. Med.* **2019**, *25*, 477–486. [CrossRef] [PubMed]
2. Bianco, J.; Bastiancich, C.; Jankovski, A.; Rieux, A.D.; Préat, V.; Danhier, F. On glioblastoma and the search for a cure: Where do we stand? *Cell. Mol. Life Sci.* **2017**, *74*, 2451–2466. [CrossRef] [PubMed]
3. Prados, M.D.; Byron, S.A.; Tran, N.L.; Phillips, J.J.; Molinaro, A.M.; Ligon, K.L.; Wen, P.Y.; Kuhn, J.G.; Mellinghoff, I.K.; de Groot, J.F.; et al. Toward precision medicine in glioblastoma: The promise and the challenges. *Neuro. Oncol.* **2015**, *17*, 1051–1063. [CrossRef]
4. Jackson, C.M.; Choi, J.; Lim, M. Mechanisms of immunotherapy resistance: Lessons from glioblastoma. *Nat. Immunol.* **2019**, *20*, 1100–1109. [CrossRef] [PubMed]
5. Ostrom, Q.T.; Bauchet, L.; Davis, F.G.; Deltour, I.; Fisher, J.L.; Langer, C.E.; Pekmezci, M.; Schwartzbaum, J.A.; Turner, M.C.; Walsh, K.M.; et al. The epidemiology of glioma in adults: A state of the science review. *Neuro-Oncol.* **2014**, *16*, 896–913. [CrossRef]
6. Bagley, S.J.; Desai, A.S.; Linette, G.P.; June, C.H.; O'Rourke, D.M. CAR T-cell therapy for glioblastoma: Recent clinical advances and future challenges. *Neuro. Oncol.* **2018**, *20*, 1429–1438. [CrossRef]
7. Wang, J.; Shen, F.; Yao, Y.; Wang, L.L.; Zhu, Y.; Hu, J. Adoptive Cell Therapy: A Novel and Potential Immunotherapy for Glioblastoma. *Front. Oncol.* **2020**, *10*, 59. [CrossRef]

8. Lim, M.; Xia, Y.; Bettegowda, C.; Weller, M. Current state of immunotherapy for glioblastoma. *Nat. Rev. Clin. Oncol.* **2018**, *15*, 422–442. [CrossRef]

9. Liau, L.M.; Ashkan, K.; Tran, D.D.; Campian, J.L.; Trusheim, J.E.; Cobbs, C.S.; Heth, J.A.; Salacz, M.; Taylor, S.; D'Andre, S.D.; et al. First results on survival from a large Phase 3 clinical trial of an autologous dendritic cell vaccine in newly diagnosed glioblastoma. *J. Transl. Med.* **2018**, *16*, 142. [CrossRef]

10. Wen, P.Y.; Reardon, D.A.; Armstrong, T.S.; Phuphanich, S.; Aiken, R.D.; Landolfi, J.C.; Curry, W.T.; Zhu, J.J.; Glantz, M.; Peereboom, D.M.; et al. A randomized double-blind placebo-controlled phase II trial of dendritic cell vaccine ICT-107 in newly diagnosed patients with glioblastoma. *Clin. Cancer Res.* **2019**, *25*, 5799–5807. [CrossRef]

11. Sprooten, J.; Ceusters, J.; Coosemans, A.; Agostinis, P.; De Vleeschouwer, S.; Zitvogel, L.; Kroemer, G.; Galluzzi, L.; Garg, A.D. Trial watch: Dendritic cell vaccination for cancer immunotherapy. *Oncoimmunology* **2019**, *8*, 1638212. [CrossRef]

12. Reardon, D.A.; Brandes, A.A.; Omuro, A.; Mulholland, P.; Lim, M.; Wick, A.; Baehring, J.; Ahluwalia, M.S.; Roth, P.; Bähr, O.; et al. Effect of Nivolumab vs Bevacizumab in Patients with Recurrent Glioblastoma: The CheckMate 143 Phase 3 Randomized Clinical Trial. *JAMA Oncol.* **2020**, *6*, 1003–1010. [CrossRef] [PubMed]

13. Allen, E.; Jabouille, A.; Rivera, L.B.; Lodewijckx, I.; Missiaen, R.; Steri, V.; Feyen, K.; Tawney, J.; Hanahan, D.; Michael, I.P.; et al. Combined antiangiogenic and anti-PD-L1 therapy stimulates tumor immunity through HEV formation. *Sci. Transl. Med.* **2017**, *9*, eaak9679. [CrossRef]

14. Verreault, M.; Schmitt, C.; Goldwirt, L.; Pelton, K.; Haidar, S.; Levasseur, C.; Guehennec, J.; Knoff, D.; Labussière, M.; Marie, Y.; et al. Preclinical efficacy of the MDM2 inhibitor RG7112 in MDM2-amplified and TP53 wild-type glioblastomas. *Clin. Cancer Res.* **2016**, *22*, 1185–1196. [CrossRef] [PubMed]

15. Wu, A.; Maxwell, R.; Xia, Y.; Cardarelli, P.; Oyasu, M.; Belcaid, Z.; Kim, E.; Hung, A.; Luksik, A.S.; Garzon-Muvdi, T.; et al. Combination anti-CXCR4 and anti-PD-1 immunotherapy provides survival benefit in glioblastoma through immune cell modulation of tumor microenvironment. *J. Neurooncol.* **2019**, *143*, 241–249. [CrossRef]

16. Gupta, S.K.; Kizilbash, S.H.; Carlson, B.L.; Mladek, A.C.; Boakye-Agyeman, F.; Bakken, K.K.; Pokorny, J.L.; Schroeder, M.A.; Decker, P.A.; Cen, L.; et al. Delineation of MGMT Hypermethylation as a Biomarker for Veliparib-Mediated Temozolomide-Sensitizing Therapy of Glioblastoma. *J. Natl. Cancer Inst.* **2016**, *108*, 1–10. [CrossRef]

17. Zahonero, C.; Aguilera, P.; Ramírez-Castillejo, C.; Pajares, M.; Bolós, M.V.; Cantero, D.; Perez-Nuñez, A.; Hernández-Laín, A.; Sánchez-Gómez, P.; Sepúlveda, J.M. Preclinical test of dacomitinib, an irreversible EGFR inhibitor, confirms its effectiveness for glioblastoma. *Mol. Cancer Ther.* **2015**, *14*, 1548–1558. [CrossRef]

18. Guishard, A.F.; Yakisich, J.S.; Azad, N.; Iyer, A.K.V. Translational gap in ongoing clinical trials for glioma. *J. Clin. Neurosci.* **2018**, *47*, 28–42. [CrossRef]

19. Coosemans, A.; Vankerckhoven, A.; Baert, T.; Boon, L.; Ruts, H.; Riva, M.; Blagden, S.; Delforge, M.; Concin, N.; Mirza, M.R.; et al. Combining conventional therapy with immunotherapy: A risky business? *Eur. J. Cancer* **2019**, *113*, 41–44. [CrossRef]

20. Kumar-Sinha, C.; Chinnaiyan, A.M. Precision oncology in the age of integrative genomics. *Nat. Biotechnol.* **2018**, *36*, 46–60. [CrossRef]

21. Riva, M.; Wouters, R.; Sterpin, E.; Giovannoni, R.; Boon, L.; Himmelreich, U.; Gsell, W.; Van Ranst, M.; Coosemans, A. Radiotherapy, Temozolomide and anti-programmed cell death protein 1 treatments modulate the immune microenvironment in experimental high-grade glioma. *Neurosurgery* **2020**. [CrossRef] [PubMed]

22. Costa, B.; Eisemann, T.; Strelau, J.; Spaan, I.; Korshunov, A.; Liu, H.K.; Bugert, P.; Angel, P.; Peterziel, H. Intratumoral platelet aggregate formation in a murine preclinical glioma model depends on podoplanin expression on tumor cells. *Blood Adv.* **2019**, *3*, 1092–1102. [CrossRef] [PubMed]

23. Kosaka, A.; Ohkuri, T.; Okada, H. Combination of an agonistic anti-CD40 monoclonal antibody and the COX-2 inhibitor celecoxib induces anti-glioma effects by promotion of type-1 immunity in myeloid cells and T-cells. *Cancer Immunol. Immunother.* **2014**, *63*, 847–857. [CrossRef] [PubMed]

24. Marumoto, T.; Tashiro, A.; Friedmann-morvinski, D.; Soda, Y.; Gage, F.H.; Verma, I.M. Development of a novel mouse glioma model using lentiviral vectors. *Nat. Med.* **2009**, *15*, 110–116. [CrossRef]

25. Friedmann-Morvinski, D.; Bushong, E.A.; Ke, E.; Soda, Y.; Marumoto, T.; Singer, O.; Ellisman, M.H.; Verma, I.M. Dedifferentiation of Neurons and Astrocytes by Oncogenes Can Induce Gliomas in Mice. *Science* **2012**, *338*, 1080–1084. [CrossRef]

26. Binello, E.; Qadeer, Z.A.; Kothari, H.P.; Emdad, L.; Germano, I.M. Stemness of the CT-2A immunocompetent mouse brain tumor model: Characterization in vitro. *J. Cancer* **2012**, *3*, 166–174. [CrossRef]

27. Hide, T.; Takezaki, T.; Nakatani, Y.; Nakamura, H.; Kuratsu, J.I.; Kondo, T. Sox11 prevents tumorigenesis of glioma-initiating cells by inducing neuronal differentiation. *Cancer Res.* **2009**, *69*, 7953–7959. [CrossRef]

28. Sampetrean, O.; Saga, I.; Nakanishi, M.; Sugihara, E.; Fukaya, R.; Onishi, N.; Osuka, S.; Akahata, M.; Kai, K.; Sugimoto, H.; et al. Invasion precedes tumor mass formation in a malignant brain tumor model of genetically modified neural stem cells. *Neoplasia* **2011**, *13*, 784–791. [CrossRef]

29. Reilly, K.M.; Loisel, D.A.; Bronson, R.T.; McLaughlin, M.E.; Jacks, T. Nf1;Trp53 mutant mice develop glioblastoma with evidence of strain-specific effects. *Nat. Genet.* **2000**, *26*, 109–113. [CrossRef]

30. Oh, T.; Fakurnejad, S.; Sayegh, E.T.; Clark, A.J.; Ivan, M.E.; Sun, M.Z.; Safaee, M.; Bloch, O.; James, C.D.; Parsa, A.T. Immunocompetent murine models for the study of glioblastoma immunotherapy. *J. Transl. Med.* **2014**, *12*, 107. [CrossRef]

31. Wu, A.; Oh, S.; Wiesner, S.M.; Ericson, K.; Chen, L.; Hall, W.A.; Champoux, P.E.; Low, W.C.; Ohlfest, J.R. Persistence of CD133+ cells in human and mouse glioma cell lines: Detailed characterization of GL261 glioma cells with cancer stem cell-like properties. *Stem Cells Dev.* **2008**, *17*, 173–184. [CrossRef] [PubMed]

32. Behnan, J.; Isakson, P.; Joel, M.; Cilio, C.; Langmoen, I.A.; Vik-Mo, E.O.; Badn, W. Recruited brain tumor-derived mesenchymal stem cells contribute to brain tumor progression. *Stem Cells* **2014**, *32*, 1110–1123. [CrossRef] [PubMed]

33. Khalsa, J.K.; Cheng, N.; Keegan, J.; Chaudry, A.; Driver, J.; Bi, W.L.; Lederer, J.; Shah, K. Immune phenotyping of diverse syngeneic murine brain tumors identifies immunologically distinct types. *Nat. Commun.* **2020**, *11*, 3912. [CrossRef] [PubMed]

34. Miller, I.S.; Didier, S.; Murray, D.W.; Turner, T.H.; Issaivanan, M.; Ruggieri, R.; Al-Abed, Y.; Symons, M. Semapimod sensitizes glioblastoma tumors to ionizing radiation by targeting microglia. *PLoS ONE* **2014**, *9*, e95885. [CrossRef] [PubMed]

35. Tran, T.A.T.; Kim, Y.H.; Duong, T.H.; Jung, S.; Kim, I.Y.; Moon, K.S.; Jang, W.Y.; Lee, H.J.; Lee, J.J.; Jung, T.Y. Peptide Vaccine Combined Adjuvants Modulate Anti-tumor Effects of Radiation in Glioblastoma Mouse Model. *Front. Immunol.* **2020**, *11*, 1165. [CrossRef]

36. Durant, S.T.; Zheng, L.; Wang, Y.; Chen, K.; Zhang, L.; Zhang, T.; Yang, Z.; Riches, L.; Trinidad, A.G.; Fok, J.H.L.; et al. The brain-penetrant clinical ATM inhibitor AZD1390 radiosensitizes and improves survival of preclinical brain tumor models. *Sci. Adv.* **2018**, *4*, eaat1719. [CrossRef]

37. Zeng, J.; See, A.P.; Phallen, J.; Jackson, C.M.; Belcaid, Z.; Ruzevick, J.; Durham, N.; Meyer, C.; Harris, T.J.; Albesiano, E.; et al. Anti-PD-1 blockade and stereotactic radiation produce long-term survival in mice with intracranial gliomas. *Int. J. Radiat. Oncol. Biol. Phys.* **2013**, *86*, 343–349. [CrossRef]

38. Dai, B.; Qi, N.; Li, J.; Zhang, G. Temozolomide combined with PD-1 Antibody therapy for mouse orthotopic glioma model. *Biochem. Biophys. Res. Commun.* **2018**, *501*, 871–876. [CrossRef]

39. Ferrer-Font, L.; Arias-Ramos, N.; Lope-Piedrafita, S.; Julià-Sapé, M.; Pumarola, M.; Arús, C.; Candiota, A.P. Metronomic treatment in immunocompetent preclinical GL261 glioblastoma: Effects of cyclophosphamide and temozolomide. *NMR Biomed.* **2017**, *30*, e3748. [CrossRef]

40. Hanihara, M.; Kawataki, T.; Oh-Oka, K.; Mitsuka, K.; Nakao, A.; Kinouchi, H. Synergistic antitumor effect with indoleamine 2,3-dioxygenase inhibition and temozolomide in a murine glioma model. *J. Neurosurg.* **2016**, *124*, 1594–1601. [CrossRef]

41. Malo, C.S.; Renner, D.N.; Huseby Kelcher, A.M.; Jin, F.; Hansen, M.J.; Pavelko, K.D.; Johnson, A.J. The effect of vector silencing during picornavirus vaccination against experimental melanoma and glioma. *PLoS ONE* **2016**, *11*, e0162064. [CrossRef] [PubMed]

42. Bu, N.; Wu, H.; Zhang, G.; Zhan, S.; Zhang, R.; Sun, H.; Du, Y.; Yao, L.; Wang, H. Exosomes from Dendritic Cells Loaded with Chaperone-Rich Cell Lysates Elicit a Potent T Cell Immune Response Against Intracranial Glioma in Mice. *J. Mol. Neurosci.* **2015**, *56*, 631–643. [CrossRef]

43. Yan, Y.; Fang, M.; Xuan, W.; Wu, X.; Meng, X.; Wang, L.; Yu, Y. The therapeutic potency of HSP65-GTL in GL261 Glioma-bearing Mice. *J. Immunother.* **2015**, *38*, 341–349. [CrossRef] [PubMed]

44. Durant, S.T.; Zheng, L.; Wang, Y.; Chen, K.; Zhang, L.; Zhang, T.; Yang, Z.; Riches, L.; Trinidad, A.G.; Fok, J.H.; et al. Survivin Monoclonal Antibodies Detect Survivin Cell Surface Expression and Inhibit Tumor Growth in vivo. *Clin. Cancer Res.* **2018**, *176*, 139–148.

45. Chen, M.; Sun, R.; Shi, B.; Wang, Y.; Di, S.; Luo, H.; Sun, Y.; Li, Z.; Zhou, M.; Jiang, H. Antitumor efficacy of chimeric antigen receptor T cells against EGFRvIII-expressing glioblastoma in C57BL/6 mice. *Biomed. Pharmacother.* **2019**, *113*, 108734. [CrossRef]

46. Cockle, J.V.; Rajani, K.; Zaidi, S.; Kottke, T.; Thompson, J.; Diaz, R.M.; Shim, K.; Peterson, T.; Parney, I.F.; Short, S.; et al. Combination viroimmunotherapy with checkpoint inhibition to treat glioma, based on location-specific tumor profiling. *Neuro. Oncol.* **2016**, *18*, 518–527. [CrossRef]

47. Jiang, H.; Clise-Dwyer, K.; Ruisaard, K.E.; Fan, X.; Tian, W.; Gumin, J.; Lamfers, M.L.; Kleijn, A.; Lang, F.F.; Yung, W.K.; et al. Delta-24-RGD oncolytic adenovirus elicits anti-glioma immunity in an immunocompetent mouse model. *PLoS ONE* **2014**, *9*, e97407. [CrossRef]

48. Tang, B.; Guo, Z.S.; Bartlett, D.L.; Yan, D.Z.; Schane, C.P.; Thomas, D.L.; Liu, J.; McFadden, G.; Shisler, J.L.; Roy, E.J. Synergistic Combination of Oncolytic Virotherapy and Immunotherapy for Glioma. *Clin. Cancer Res.* **2020**, *26*, 2216–2230. [CrossRef]

49. Koks, C.A.; Garg, A.D.; Ehrhardt, M.; Riva, M.; Vandenberk, L.; Boon, L.; De Vleeschouwer, S.; Agostinis, P.; Graf, N.; Van Gool, S.W. Newcastle disease virotherapy induces long-term survival and tumor-specific immune memory in orthotopic glioma through the induction of immunogenic cell death. *Int. J. Cancer* **2015**, *136*, E313–E325. [CrossRef]

50. Kleijn, A.; van den Bossche, W.; Haefner, E.S.; Belcaid, Z.; Burghoorn-Maas, C.; Kloezeman, J.J.; Pas, S.D.; Leenstra, S.; Debets, R.; de Vrij, J.; et al. The Sequence of Delta24-RGD and TMZ Administration in Malignant Glioma Affects the Role of CD8+T Cell Anti-tumor Activity. *Mol. Ther. Oncolytics* **2017**, *5*, 11–19. [CrossRef]

51. Zhu, S.; Lv, X.; Zhang, X.; Li, T.; Zang, G.; Yang, N.; Wang, X.; Wu, J.; Chen, W.; Liu, Y.J.; et al. An effective dendritic cell-based vaccine containing glioma stem-like cell lysate and CpG adjuvant for an orthotopic mouse model of glioma. *Int. J. Cancer* **2019**, *144*, 2867–2879. [CrossRef] [PubMed]

52. Hardcastle, J.; Mills, L.; Malo, C.S.; Jin, F.; Kurokawa, C.; Geekiyanage, H.; Schroeder, M.; Sarkaria, J.; Johnson, A.J.; Galanis, E. Immunovirotherapy with measles virus strains in combination with anti-PD-1 antibody blockade enhances antitumor activity in glioblastoma treatment. *Neuro. Oncol.* **2017**, *19*, 493–502. [CrossRef] [PubMed]

53. Jahan, N.; Talat, H.; Alonso, A.; Saha, D.; Curry, W.T. Triple combination immunotherapy with GVAX, anti-PD-1 monoclonal antibody, and agonist anti-OX40 monoclonal antibody is highly effective against murine intracranial glioma. *Oncoimmunology* **2019**, *8*, e1577108. [CrossRef] [PubMed]
54. Patel, M.A.; Kim, J.E.; Theodros, D.; Tam, A.; Velarde, E.; Kochel, C.M.; Francica, B.; Nirschl, T.R.; Ghasemzadeh, A.; Mathios, D.; et al. Agonist anti-GITR monoclonal antibody and stereotactic radiation induce immune-mediated survival advantage in murine intracranial glioma. *J. Immunother. Cancer* **2016**, *4*, 28. [CrossRef] [PubMed]
55. Belcaid, Z.; Phallen, J.A.; Zeng, J.; See, A.P.; Mathios, D.; Gottschalk, C.; Nicholas, S.; Kellett, M.; Ruzevick, J.; Jackson, C.; et al. Focal radiation therapy combined with 4-1BB activation and CTLA-4 blockade yields long-term survival and a protective antigen-specific memory response in a murine glioma model. *PLoS ONE* **2014**, *9*, e101764. [CrossRef] [PubMed]
56. Hung, A.L.; Maxwell, R.; Theodros, D.; Belcaid, Z.; Mathios, D.; Luksik, A.S.; Kim, E.; Wu, A.; Xia, Y.; Garzon-Muvdi, T.; et al. TIGIT and PD-1 dual checkpoint blockade enhances antitumor immunity and survival in GBM. *Oncoimmunology* **2018**, *7*, e1466769. [CrossRef]
57. Kim, J.E.; Patel, M.A.; Mangraviti, A.; Kim, E.S.; Theodros, D.; Velarde, E.; Liu, A.; Sankey, E.W.; Tam, A.; Xu, H.; et al. Combination Therapy with Anti-PD-1, Anti-TIM-3, and Focal Radiation Results in Regression of Murine Gliomas. *Clin. Cancer Res.* **2017**, *23*, 124–136. [CrossRef]
58. Genoud, V.; Marinari, E.; Nikolaev, S.I.; Castle, J.C.; Bukur, V.; Dietrich, P.Y.; Okada, H.; Walker, P.R. Responsiveness to anti-PD-1 and anti-CTLA-4 immune checkpoint blockade in SB28 and GL261 mouse glioma models. *Oncoimmunology* **2018**, *7*, e1501137. [CrossRef]
59. Qian, J.; Wang, C.; Wang, B.; Yang, J.; Wang, Y.; Luo, F.; Xu, J.; Zhao, C.; Liu, R.; Chu, Y. The IFN-γ/PD-L1 axis between T cells and tumor microenvironment: Hints for glioma anti-PD-1/PD-L1 therapy. *J. Neuroinflamm.* **2018**, *15*, 290. [CrossRef]
60. Garg, A.D.; Vandenberk, L.; Van Woensel, M.; Belmans, J.; Schaaf, M.; Boon, L.; De Vleeschouwer, S.; Agostinis, P. Preclinical efficacy of immune-checkpoint monotherapy does not recapitulate corresponding biomarkers-based clinical predictions in glioblastoma. *Oncoimmunology* **2017**, *6*, e1295903. [CrossRef]
61. Shevtsov, M.; Pitkin, E.; Ischenko, A.; Stangl, S.; Khachatryan, W.; Galibin, O.; Edmond, S.; Lobinger, D.; Multhoff, G. Ex vivo Hsp70-activated NK cells in combination with PD-1 inhibition significantly increase overall survival in preclinical models of glioblastoma and lung cancer. *Front. Immunol.* **2019**, *10*, 454. [CrossRef] [PubMed]
62. Kim, J.W.; Kane, J.R.; Panek, W.K.; Young, J.S.; Rashidi, A.; Yu, D.; Kanojia, D.; Hasan, T.; Miska, J.; Gómez-Lim, M.A.; et al. A Dendritic Cell-Targeted Adenoviral Vector Facilitates Adaptive Immune Response Against Human Glioma Antigen (CMV-IE) and Prolongs Survival in a Human Glioma Tumor Model. *Neurotherapeutics* **2018**, *15*, 1127–1138. [CrossRef] [PubMed]
63. Maggio, D.; Ho, W.S.; Breese, R.; Walbridge, S.; Wang, H.; Cui, J.; Heiss, J.D.; Gilbert, M.R.; Kovach, J.S.; Lu, R.O.; et al. Inhibition of protein phosphatase-2A with LB-100 enhances antitumor immunity against glioblastoma. *J. Neurooncol.* **2020**, *148*, 231–244. [CrossRef] [PubMed]
64. Mathios, D.; Park, C.K.; Marcus, W.D.; Alter, S.; Rhode, P.R.; Jeng, E.K.; Wong, H.C.; Pardoll, D.M.; Lim, M. Therapeutic administration of IL-15 superagonist complex ALT-803 leads to long-term survival and durable antitumor immune response in a murine glioblastoma model. *Int. J. Cancer* **2016**, *138*, 187–194. [CrossRef] [PubMed]
65. Karachi, A.; Yang, C.; Dastmalchi, F.; Sayour, E.J.; Huang, J.; Azari, H.; Long, Y.; Flores, C.; Mitchell, D.A.; Rahman, M. Modulation of temozolomide dose differentially affects T-cell response to immune checkpoint inhibition. *Neuro. Oncol.* **2019**, *21*, 730–741. [CrossRef] [PubMed]
66. Li, J.; Liu, X.; Duan, Y.; Liu, Y.; Wang, H.; Lian, S.; Zhuang, G.; Fan, Y. Combined blockade of Ts cell immunoglobulin and mucin domain 3 and carcinoembryonic antigen-related cell adhesion molecule 1 results in durable therapeutic efficacy in mice with intracranial gliomas. *Med. Sci. Monit.* **2017**, *23*, 3593–3602. [CrossRef]
67. Jahan, N.; Talat, H.; Curry, W.T. Agonist OX40 immunotherapy improves survival in glioma-bearing mice and is complementary with vaccination with irradiated GM-CSF-expressing tumor cells. *Neuro. Oncol.* **2018**, *20*, 44–54. [CrossRef] [PubMed]
68. Shoji, T.; Saito, R.; Chonan, M.; Shibahara, I.; Sato, A.; Kanamori, M.; Sonoda, Y.; Kondo, T.; Ishii, N.; Tominaga, T. Local convection-enhanced delivery of an anti-CD40 agonistic monoclonal antibody induces antitumor effects in mouse glioma models. *Neuro. Oncol.* **2016**, *18*, 1120–1128. [CrossRef]
69. Eberstå, S.; Sandén, E.; Fritzell, S.; Darabi, A.; Visse, E.; Siesjö, P. Intratumoral COX-2 inhibition enhances GM-CSF immunotherapy against established mouse GL261 brain tumors. *Int. J. Cancer* **2014**, *134*, 2748–2753. [CrossRef]
70. Miska, J.; Rashidi, A.; Chang, A.L.; Muroski, M.E.; Han, Y.; Zhang, L.; Lesniak, M.S. Anti-GITR therapy promotes immunity against malignant glioma in a murine model. *Cancer Immunol. Immunother.* **2016**, *65*, 1555–1567. [CrossRef]
71. Zheng, H.; Yang, B.; Xu, D.; Wang, W.; Tan, J.; Sun, L.; Li, Q.; Sun, L.; Xia, X. Induction of specific T helper-9 cells to inhibit glioma cell growth. *Oncotarget* **2017**, *8*, 4864–4874. [CrossRef] [PubMed]
72. Chonan, M.; Saito, R.; Shoji, T.; Shibahara, I.; Kanamori, M.; Sonoda, Y.; Watanabe, M.; Kikuchi, T.; Ishii, N.; Tominaga, T. CD40/CD40L expression correlates with the survival of patients with glioblastomas and an augmentation in CD40 signaling enhances the efficacy of vaccinations against glioma models. *Neuro. Oncol.* **2015**, *17*, 1453–1462. [CrossRef] [PubMed]
73. Vandenberk, L.; Garg, A.D.; Verschuere, T.; Koks, C.; Belmans, J.; Beullens, M.; Agostinis, P.; De Vleeschouwer, S.; Van Gool, S.W. Irradiation of necrotic cancer cells, employed for pulsing dendritic cells (DCs), potentiates DC vaccine-induced antitumor immunity against high-grade glioma. *Oncoimmunology* **2016**, *5*, e1083669. [CrossRef] [PubMed]

74. Moertel, C.L.; Xia, J.; LaRue, R.; Waldron, N.N.; Andersen, B.M.; Prins, R.M.; Okada, H.; Donson, A.M.; Foreman, N.K.; Hunt, M.A.; et al. CD200 in CNS tumor-induced immunosuppression: The role for CD200 pathway blockade in targeted immunotherapy. *J. Immunother. Cancer* **2014**, *2*, 46. [CrossRef] [PubMed]

75. Jordan, M.; Waxman, D.J. CpG-1826 immunotherapy potentiates chemotherapeutic and anti-tumor immune responses to metronomic cyclophosphamide in a preclinical glioma model. *Physiol. Behav.* **2018**, *176*, 139–148. [CrossRef] [PubMed]

76. Zhang, Y.; Luo, F.; Li, A.; Qian, J.; Yao, Z.; Feng, X.; Chu, Y. Systemic injection of TLR1/2 agonist improves adoptive antigen-specific T cell therapy in glioma-bearing mice. *Clin. Immunol.* **2014**, *154*, 26–36. [CrossRef]

77. Ladomersky, E.; Zhai, L.; Lauing, K.L.; Bell, A.; Xu, J.; Kocherginsky, M.; Zhang, B.; Wu, J.D.; Podojil, J.R.; Platanias, L.C.; et al. Advanced Age Increases Immunosuppression in the Brain and Decreases Immunotherapeutic Efficacy in Subjects with Glioblastoma. *Clin. Cancer Res.* **2020**, *26*, 5232–5245. [CrossRef]

78. Azambuja, J.H.; da Silveira, E.F.; de Carvalho, T.R.; Oliveira, P.S.; Pacheco, S.; do Couto, C.T.; Beira, F.T.; Stefanello, F.M.; Spanevello, R.M.; Braganhol, E. Glioma sensitive or chemoresistant to temozolomide differentially modulate macrophage protumor activities. *Biochim. Biophys. Acta Gen. Subj.* **2017**, *1861*, 2652–2662. [CrossRef]

79. Wu, S.; Calero-Pérez, P.; Villamañan, L.; Arias-Ramos, N.; Pumarola, M.; Ortega-Martorell, S.; Julià-Sapé, M.; Arús, C.; Candiota, A.P. Anti-tumour immune response in GL261 glioblastoma generated by Temozolomide Immune-Enhancing Metronomic Schedule monitored with MRSI-based nosological images. *NMR Biomed.* **2020**, *33*, e4229. [CrossRef]

80. Dey, M.; Chang, A.L.; Miska, J.; Wainwright, D.A.; Ahmed, A.U.; Balyasnikova, I.V.; Pytel, P.; Han, Y.; Tobias, A.; Zhang, L.; et al. Dendritic Cell-Based Vaccines that Utilize Myeloid Rather than Plasmacytoid Cells Offer a Superior Survival Advantage in Malignant Glioma. *Physiol. Behav.* **2017**, *176*, 139–148. [CrossRef]

81. Kindy, M.S.; Yu, J.; Zhu, H.; Smith, M.T.; Gattoni-Celli, S. A therapeutic cancer vaccine against GL261 murine glioma. *J. Transl. Med.* **2016**, *14*, 1–9. [CrossRef] [PubMed]

82. Dong, B.; Wang, L.; Nie, S.; Li, X.; Xiao, Y.; Yang, L.; Meng, X.; Zhao, P.; Cui, C.; Tu, L.; et al. Anti-glioma effect of intracranial vaccination with tumor cell lysate plus flagellin in mice. *Vaccine* **2018**, *36*, 8148–8157. [CrossRef]

83. Renner, D.N.; Jin, F.; Litterman, A.J.; Balgeman, A.J.; Hanson, L.M.; Gamez, J.D.; Chae, M.; Carlson, B.L.; Sarkaria, J.N.; Parney, I.F.; et al. Effective treatment of established GL261 murine gliomas through picornavirus vaccination-enhanced tumor antigen-specific CD8+ T cell responses. *PLoS ONE* **2015**, *10*, e0125565. [CrossRef] [PubMed]

84. Gattoni-Celli, S.; Young, M.R.I. Restoration of immune responsiveness to glioma by vaccination of mice with established brain gliomas with a semi-allogeneic vaccine. *Int. J. Mol. Sci.* **2016**, *17*, 1465. [CrossRef] [PubMed]

85. Barrett, J.A.; Cai, H.; Miao, J.; Khare, P.D.; Gonzalez, P.; Dalsing-Hernandez, J.; Sharma, G.; Chan, T.; Cooper, L.J.N.; Lebel, F. Regulated intratumoral expression of IL-12 using a RheoSwitch Therapeutic System® (RTS®) gene switch as gene therapy for the treatment of glioma. *Cancer Gene Ther.* **2018**, *25*, 106–116. [CrossRef] [PubMed]

86. Riccadonna, C.; Yacoub Maroun, C.; Vuillefroy de Silly, R.; Boehler, M.; Calvo Tardón, M.; Jueliger, S.; Taverna, P.; Barba, L.; Marinari, E.; Pellegatta, S.; et al. Decitabine treatment of glioma-initiating cells enhances immune recognition and killing. *PLoS ONE* **2016**, *11*, e0162105. [CrossRef]

87. Hsu, S.P.C.; Chen, Y.C.; Chiang, H.C.; Huang, Y.C.; Huang, C.C.; Wang, H.E.; Wang, Y.S.; Chi, K.H. Rapamycin and hydroxychloroquine combination alters macrophage polarization and sensitizes glioblastoma to immune checkpoint inhibitors. *J. Neurooncol.* **2020**, *146*, 417–426. [CrossRef]

88. Ciesielski, M.J.; Bu, Y.; Munich, S.A.; Teegarden, P.; Smolinski, M.P.; Clements, J.L.; Lau, J.Y.N.; Hangauer, D.G.; Fenstermaker, R.A. KX2-361: A novel orally bioavailable small molecule dual Src/tubulin inhibitor that provides long term survival in a murine model of glioblastoma. *J. Neurooncol.* **2018**, *140*, 519–527. [CrossRef]

89. Su, Y.-T.; Butler, M.; Zhang, M.; Zhang, W.; Song, H.; Hwang, L.; Tran, A.D.; Bash, R.E.; Schorzman, A.N.; Pang, Y.; et al. MerTK inhibition decreases immune suppressive glioblastoma-associated macrophages and neoangiogenesis in glioblastoma microenvironment. *Neuro-Oncol. Adv.* **2020**, *2*, 1–13. [CrossRef]

90. McFarland, B.C.; Marks, M.P.; Rowse, A.L.; Fehling, S.C.; Gerigk, M.; Qin, H.; Benveniste, E.N. Loss of SOCS3 in myeloid cells prolongs survival in a syngeneic model of glioma. *Oncotarget* **2016**, *7*, 20621–20635. [CrossRef]

91. Leten, C.; Trekker, J.; Struys, T.; Dresselaers, T.; Gijsbers, R.; Vande Velde, G.; Lambrichts, I.; Van Der Linden, A.; Verfaillie, C.M.; Himmelreich, U. Assessment of bystander killing-mediated therapy of malignant brain tumors using a multimodal imaging approach. *Stem Cell Res. Ther.* **2015**, *6*, 163. [CrossRef] [PubMed]

92. Tong, L.; Li, J.; Li, Q.; Wang, X.; Medikonda, R.; Zhao, T.; Li, T.; Ma, H.; Yi, L.; Liu, P.; et al. ACT001 reduces the expression of PD-L1 by inhibiting the phosphorylation of STAT3 in glioblastoma. *Theranostics* **2020**, *10*, 5943–5956. [CrossRef] [PubMed]

93. Wu, J.; Waxman, D.J. Metronomic cyclophosphamide eradicates large implanted GL261 gliomas by activating antitumor Cd8+ T-cell responses and immune memory. *Oncoimmunology* **2015**, *4*, e1005521. [CrossRef]

94. Wu, J.; Jordan, M.; Waxman, D.J. Metronomic cyclophosphamide activation of anti-tumor immunity: Tumor model, mouse host, and drug schedule dependence of gene responses and their upstream regulators. *BMC Cancer* **2016**, *16*, 623. [CrossRef]

95. Wu, J.; Waxman, D.J. Metronomic cyclophosphamide schedule-dependence of innate immune cell recruitment and tumor regression in an implanted glioma model. *Cancer Lett.* **2014**, *353*, 272–280. [CrossRef]

96. Pérez, J.E.; Fritzell, S.; Kopecky, J.; Visse, E.; Darabi, A.; Siesjö, P. The effect of locally delivered cisplatin is dependent on an intact immune function in an experimental glioma model. *Sci. Rep.* **2019**, *9*, 5632. [CrossRef]

97. Wei, J.; Nduom, E.K.; Kong, L.Y.; Hashimoto, Y.; Xu, S.; Gabrusiewicz, K.; Ling, X.; Huang, N.; Qiao, W.; Zhou, S.; et al. MiR-138 exerts anti-glioma efficacy by targeting immune checkpoints. *Neuro. Oncol.* **2016**, *18*, 639–648. [CrossRef]

98. Strong, A.D.; Indart, M.C.; Hill, N.R.; Daniels, R.L. GL261 glioma tumor cells respond to ATP with an intracellular calcium rise and glutamate release. *Physiol. Behav.* **2017**, *176*, 139–148. [CrossRef] [PubMed]

99. Han, C.J.; Zheng, J.Y.; Sun, L.; Yang, H.C.; Cao, Z.Q.; Zhang, X.H.; Zheng, L.T.; Zhen, X.C. The oncometabolite 2-hydroxyglutarate inhibits microglial activation via the AMPK/mTOR/NF-κB pathway. *Acta Pharmacol. Sin.* **2019**, *40*, 1292–1302. [CrossRef] [PubMed]

100. Panek, W.K.; Pituch, K.C.; Miska, J.; Kim, J.W.; Rashidi, A.; Kanojia, D.; Lopez-Rosas, A.; Han, Y.; Yu, D.; Chang, C.L.; et al. Local Application of Autologous Platelet Rich Fibrin Patch (PRF- P) Suppresses Regulatory T cell Recruitment in a Murine Glioma Model. *Mol. Neurobiol.* **2019**, *176*, 139–148. [CrossRef] [PubMed]

101. Bongiorno, E.K.; Garcia, S.A.; Sauma, S.; Hooper, D.C. Type 1 immune mechanisms driven by the response to infection with attenuated rabies virus result in changes in the immune bias of the tumor microenvironment and necrosis of mouse GL261 brain tumors. *J. Immunol.* **2017**, *176*, 139–148. [CrossRef]

102. Roberts, N.B.; Alqazzaz, A.; Hwang, J.R.; Qi, X.; Keegan, A.D.; Kim, A.J.; Winkles, J.A.; Woodworth, G.F. Oxaliplatin disrupts pathological features of glioma cells and associated macrophages independent of apoptosis induction. *J. Neurooncol.* **2018**, *140*, 497–507. [CrossRef] [PubMed]

103. Xu, S.; Wei, J.; Wang, F.; Kong, L.Y.; Ling, X.Y.; Nduom, E.; Gabrusiewicz, K.; Doucette, T.; Yang, Y.; Yaghi, N.K.; et al. Effect of miR-142-3p on the M2 macrophage and therapeutic efficacy against murine glioblastoma. *J. Natl. Cancer Inst.* **2014**, *106*, 1–11. [CrossRef] [PubMed]

104. Yang, J.; Liu, R.; Deng, Y.; Qian, J.; Lu, Z.; Wang, Y.; Zhang, D.; Luo, F.; Chu, Y. MiR-15a/16 deficiency enhances anti-tumor immunity of glioma-infiltrating CD8+ T cells through targeting mTOR. *Int. J. Cancer* **2017**, *141*, 2082–2092. [CrossRef] [PubMed]

105. Mukherjee, S.; Baidoo, J.N.E.; Sampat, S.; Mancuso, A.; David, L.; Cohen, L.S.; Zhou, S.; Banerjee, P. Liposomal tricurin, a synergistic combination of curcumin, epicatechin gallate and resveratrol, repolarizes tumor-associated microglia/macrophages, and eliminates glioblastoma (GBM) and GBM Stem Cells. *Molecules* **2018**, *23*, 201. [CrossRef] [PubMed]

106. Mukherjee, S.; Fried, A.; Hussaini, R.; White, R.; Baidoo, J.; Yalamanchi, S.; Banerjee, P. Phytosomal curcumin causes natural killer cell-dependent repolarization of glioblastoma (GBM) tumor-associated microglia/macrophages and elimination of GBM and GBM stem cells. *J. Exp. Clin. Cancer Res.* **2018**, *37*, 168. [CrossRef] [PubMed]

107. Lepore, F.; D'Alessandro, G.; Antonangeli, F.; Santoro, A.; Esposito, V.; Limatola, C.; Trettel, F. CXCL16/CXCR6 axis drives microglia/macrophages phenotype in physiological conditions and plays a crucial role in glioma. *Front. Immunol.* **2018**, *9*, 2750. [CrossRef]

108. Yan, J.; Kong, L.Y.; Hu, J.; Gabrusiewicz, K.; Dibra, D.; Xia, X.; Heimberger, A.B.; Li, S. FGL2 as a Multimodality Regulator of Tumor-Mediated Immune Suppression and Therapeutic Target in Gliomas. *J. Natl. Cancer Inst.* **2015**, *107*, djv137. [CrossRef]

109. Turubanova, V.D.; Balalaeva, I.V.; Mishchenko, T.A.; Catanzaro, E.; Alzeibak, R.; Peskova, N.N.; Efimova, I.; Bachert, C.; Mitroshina, E.V.; Krysko, O.; et al. Immunogenic cell death induced by a new photodynamic therapy based on photosens and photodithazine. *J. Immunother. Cancer* **2019**, *7*, 350. [CrossRef]

110. Sun, S.; Du, G.; Xue, J.; Ma, J.; Ge, M.; Wang, H.; Tian, J. PCC0208009 enhances the anti-tumor effects of temozolomide through direct inhibition and transcriptional regulation of indoleamine 2,3-dioxygenase in glioma models. *Int. J. Immunopathol. Pharmacol.* **2018**, *32*, 2058738418787991. [CrossRef]

111. Ferrer-Font, L.; Villamañan, L.; Arias-Ramos, N.; Vilardell, J.; Plana, M.; Ruzzene, M.; Pinna, L.A.; Itarte, E.; Arús, C.; Candiota, A.P. Targeting protein kinase CK2: Evaluating CX-4945 potential for GL261 glioblastoma therapy in immunocompetent mice. *Pharmaceuticals* **2017**, *10*, 24. [CrossRef] [PubMed]

112. Proske, J.; Walter, L.; Bumes, E.; Hutterer, M.; Vollmann-Zwerenz, A.; Eyüpoglu, I.Y.; Savaskan, N.E.; Seliger, C.; Hau, P.; Uhl, M. Adaptive immune response to and survival effect of temozolomide-and valproic acid-induced autophagy in glioblastoma. *Anticancer Res.* **2016**, *36*, 899–906. [PubMed]

113. Ott, M.; Kassab, C.; Marisetty, A.; Hashimoto, Y.; Wei, J.; Zamler, D.; Leu, J.S.; Tomaszowski, K.H.; Sabbagh, A.; Fang, D.; et al. Radiation with STAT3 blockade triggers dendritic cell-T cell interactions in the glioma microenvironment and therapeutic efficacy. *Clin. Cancer Res.* **2020**, *26*, 4983–4994. [CrossRef] [PubMed]

114. Li, M.; Bolduc, A.R.; Hoda, M.N.; Gamble, D.N.; Dolisca, S.B.; Bolduc, A.K.; Hoang, K.; Ashley, C.; McCall, D.; Rojiani, A.M.; et al. The indoleamine 2,3-dioxygenase pathway controls complement-dependent enhancement of chemo-radiation therapy against murine glioblastoma. *J. Immunother. Cancer* **2014**, *2*, 21. [CrossRef] [PubMed]

115. Giles, A.J.; Hutchinson, M.N.D.; Sonnemann, H.M.; Jung, J.; Fecci, P.E.; Ratnam, N.M.; Zhang, W.; Song, H.; Bailey, R.; Davis, D.; et al. Dexamethasone-induced immunosuppression: Mechanisms and implications for immunotherapy. *J. Immunother. Cancer* **2018**, *6*, 51. [CrossRef] [PubMed]

116. Ausman, J.I.; Shapiro, W.R.; Rall, D.P. Studies on the Chemotherapy of Experimental Brain Tumors: Development of an Experimental Model. *Cancer Res.* **1970**, *30*, 2394–2400. [PubMed]

117. Crommentuijn, M.H.W.; Schetters, S.T.T.; Dusoswa, S.A.; Kruijssen, L.J.W.; Garcia-Vallejo, J.J.; van Kooyk, Y. Immune involvement of the contralateral hemisphere in a glioblastoma mouse model. *J. Immunother. Cancer* **2020**, *8*, e000323. [CrossRef]

118. Baker, G.J.; Castro, M.G.; Lowenstein, P.R. Isolation and flow cytometric analysis of glioma-infiltrating peripheral blood mononuclear cells. *J. Vis. Exp.* **2015**, *2015*, e53676. [CrossRef]

119. Baker, G.J.; Chockley, P.; Zamler, D.; Castro, M.G.; Lowenstein, P.R. Natural killer cells require monocytic Gr-1+/CD11b+ myeloid cells to eradicate orthotopically engrafted glioma cells. *Oncoimmunology* **2016**, *5*, e1163461. [CrossRef]

120. Chang, C.Y.; Jeon, S.B.; Yoon, H.J.; Choi, B.K.; Kim, S.S.; Oshima, M.; Park, E.J. Glial TLR2-driven innate immune responses and CD8 + T cell activation against brain tumor. *Glia* **2019**, *67*, 1179–1195. [CrossRef]

121. Irvin, D.K.; Jouanneau, E.; Duvall, G.; Zhang, X.X.; Zhai, Y.; Sarayba, D.; Seksenyan, A.; Panwar, A.; Black, K.L.; Wheeler, C.J. T cells enhance stem-like properties and conditional malignancy in gliomas. *PLoS ONE* **2010**, *5*, e10974. [CrossRef] [PubMed]

122. Candolfi, M.; Yagiz, K.; Wibowo, M.; Ahlzadeh, G.E.; Puntel, M.; Ghiasi, H.; Kamran, N.; Paran, C.; Lowenstein, P.R.; Castro, M.G. Temozolomide does not impair gene therapy-mediated antitumor immunity in syngeneic brain tumor models. *Clin. Cancer Res.* **2014**, *20*, 1555–1565. [CrossRef] [PubMed]

123. Luo, L.; Guan, X.; Begum, G.; Ding, D.; Gayden, J.; Hasan, M.N.; Fiesler, V.M.; Dodelson, J.; Kohanbash, G.; Hu, B.; et al. Blockade of Cell Volume Regulatory Protein NKCC1 Increases TMZ-Induced Glioma Apoptosis and Reduces Astrogliosis. *Mol. Cancer Ther.* **2020**, *19*, 1550–1561. [CrossRef] [PubMed]

124. Safdie, F.; Brandhorst, S.; Wei, M.; Wang, W.; Lee, C.; Hwang, S.; Conti, P.S.; Chen, T.C.; Longo, V.D. Fasting Enhances the Response of Glioma to Chemo- and Radiotherapy. *PLoS ONE* **2012**, *7*, e44603. [CrossRef] [PubMed]

125. Kim, T.G.; Kim, C.H.; Park, J.S.; Park, S.D.; Kim, C.K.; Chung, D.S.; Hong, Y.K. Immunological factors relating to the antitumor effect of temozolomide chemoimmunotherapy in a murine glioma model. *Clin. Vaccine Immunol.* **2010**, *17*, 143–153. [CrossRef]

126. Guan, X.; Hasan, M.N.; Begum, G.; Kohanbash, G.; Carney, K.E.; Pigott, V.M.; Persson, A.I.; Castro, M.G.; Jia, W.; Sun, D. Blockade of Na/H exchanger stimulates glioma tumor immunogenicity and enhances combinatorial TMZ and anti-PD-1 therapy. *Cell Death Dis.* **2018**, *9*, 1010. [CrossRef]

127. Yadav, V.N.; Zamler, D.; Baker, G.J.; Kadiyala, P.; Erdreich-Epstein, A.; DeCarvalho, A.C.; Mikkelsen, T.; Castro, M.G.; Lowenstein, P.R. CXCR4 increases in-vivo glioma perivascular invasion, and reduces radiation induced apoptosis: A genetic knockdown study. *Oncotarget* **2016**, *7*, 83701–83719. [CrossRef]

128. Guan, X.; Luo, L.; Begum, G.; Kohanbash, G.; Song, Q.; Rao, A.; Amankulor, N.; Sun, B.; Sun, D.; Jia, W. Elevated Na/H exchanger 1 (SLC9A1) emerges as a marker for tumorigenesis and prognosis in gliomas. *J. Exp. Clin. Cancer Res.* **2018**, *37*, 255. [CrossRef]

129. Mineharu, Y.; Kamran, N.; Lowenstein, P.R.; Castro, M.G. Blockade of mTOR Signaling via Rapamycin Combined with Immunotherapy Augments Anti-glioma Cytotoxic and Memory T cells' Functions. *Mol. Cancer Ther.* **2014**, *13*, 3024–3036. [CrossRef]

130. Park, J.H.; Ryu, C.H.; Kim, M.J.; Jeun, S.S. Combination therapy for gliomas using temozolomide and interferon-beta secreting human bone marrow derived mesenchymal stem cells. *J. Korean Neurosurg. Soc.* **2015**, *57*, 323–328. [CrossRef]

131. Seyfried, T.N.; El-Abbadi, M.; Roy, M.L. Ganglioside distribution in murine neural tumors. *Mol. Chem. Neuropathol.* **1992**, *17*, 147–167. [CrossRef]

132. Martínez-Murillo, R.; Martínez, A. Standardization of an orthotopic mouse brain tumor model following transplantation of CT-2A astrocytoma cells. *Histol. Histopathol.* **2007**, *22*, 1309–1326. [PubMed]

133. Riva, M.; Wouters, R.; Weerasekera, A.; Belderbos, S.; Nittner, D.; Thal, D.R.; Baert, T.; Giovannoni, R.; Gsell, W.; Himmelreich, U.; et al. CT-2A neurospheres-derived high-grade glioma in mice: A new model to address tumor stem cells and immunosuppression. *Biol. Open* **2019**, *8*, bio044552. [CrossRef] [PubMed]

134. Woroniecka, K.; Chongsathidkiet, P.; Rhodin, K.; Kemeny, H.; Dechant, C.; Farber, S.H.; Elsamadicy, A.A.; Cui, X.; Koyama, S.; Jackson, C.; et al. T-cell exhaustion signatures vary with tumor type and are severe in glioblastoma. *Clin. Cancer Res.* **2018**, *24*, 4175–4186. [CrossRef] [PubMed]

135. Zhang, P.; Miska, J.; Lee-Chang, C.; Rashidi, A.; Panek, W.K.; An, S.; Zannikou, M.; Lopez-Rosas, A.; Han, Y.; Xiao, T.; et al. Therapeutic targeting of tumor-associated myeloid cells synergizes with radiation therapy for glioblastoma. *Proc. Natl. Acad. Sci. USA* **2019**, *116*, 23714–23723. [CrossRef] [PubMed]

136. Mohme, M.; Maire, C.L.; Geumann, U.; Schliffke, S.; Dührsen, L.; Fita, K.; Akyüz, N.; Binder, M.; Westphal, M.; Guenther, C.; et al. Local Intracerebral Immunomodulation Using Interleukin-Expressing Mesenchymal Stem Cells in Glioblastoma. *Clin. Cancer Res.* **2020**, *26*, 2626–2639. [CrossRef]

137. von Roemeling, C.A.; Wang, Y.; Qie, Y.; Yuan, H.; Zhao, H.; Liu, X.; Yang, Z.; Yang, M.; Deng, W.; Bruno, K.A.; et al. Therapeutic modulation of phagocytosis in glioblastoma can activate both innate and adaptive antitumour immunity. *Nat. Commun.* **2020**, *11*, 1508. [CrossRef]

138. Lamano, J.B.; Lamano, J.B.; Li, Y.D.; DiDomenico, J.D.; Choy, W.; Veliceasa, D.; Oyon, D.E.; Fakurnejad, S.; Ampie, L.; Kesavabhotla, K.; et al. Glioblastoma-derived IL6 induces immunosuppressive peripheral myeloid cell PD-L1 and promotes tumor growth. *Clin. Cancer Res.* **2019**, *25*, 3643–3657. [CrossRef]

139. Woroniecka, K.I.; Rhodin, K.E.; Dechant, C.; Cui, X.; Chongsathidkiet, P.; Wilkinson, D.; Waibl-Polania, J.; Sanchez-Perez, L.; Fecci, P.E. 4-1BB agonism averts Til exhaustion and licenses PD-1 blockade in glioblastoma and other intracranial cancers. *Clin. Cancer Res.* **2020**, *26*, 1349–1358. [CrossRef]

140. Speranza, M.C.; Passaro, C.; Ricklefs, F.; Kasai, K.; Klein, S.R.; Nakashima, H.; Kaufmann, J.K.; Ahmed, A.K.; Nowicki, M.O.; Obi, P.; et al. Preclinical investigation of combined gene-mediated cytotoxic immunotherapy and immune checkpoint blockade in glioblastoma. *Neuro. Oncol.* **2018**, *20*, 225–235. [CrossRef]

141. Passaro, C.; Alayo, Q.; DeLaura, I.; McNulty, J.; Grauwet, K.; Ito, H.; Bhaskaran, V.; Mineo, M.; Lawler, S.E.; Shah, K.; et al. Erratum: Arming an oncolytic herpes simplex virus type 1 with a single-chain fragment variable antibody against PD-1 for experimental glioblastoma therapy. *Clin. Cancer Res.* **2020**, *26*, 758. [CrossRef] [PubMed]

142. Belcaid, Z.; Berrevoets, C.; Choi, J.; van Beelen, E.; Stavrakaki, E.; Pierson, T.; Kloezeman, J.; Routkevitch, D.; van der Kaaij, M.; van der Ploeg, A.; et al. Low-dose oncolytic adenovirus therapy overcomes tumor-induced immune suppression and sensitizes intracranial gliomas to anti-PD-1 therapy. *Neuro-Oncology Adv.* **2020**, *2*, vdaa011. [CrossRef] [PubMed]

143. Liu, C.J.; Schaettler, M.; Blaha, D.T.; Bowman-Kirigin, J.A.; Kobayashi, D.K.; Livingstone, A.J.; Bender, D.; Miller, C.A.; Kranz, D.M.; Johanns, T.M.; et al. Treatment of an aggressive orthotopic murine glioblastoma model with combination checkpoint blockade and a multivalent neoantigen vaccine. *Neuro. Oncol.* **2020**, *22*, 1276–1288. [CrossRef] [PubMed]

144. Balathasan, L.; Tang, V.A.; Yadollahi, B.; Brun, J.; Labelle, M.; Lefebvre, C.; Swift, S.L.; Stojdl, D.F. Activating Peripheral Innate Immunity Enables Safe and Effective Oncolytic Virotherapy in the Brain. *Mol. Ther. Oncolytics* **2017**, *7*, 45–56. [CrossRef]

145. Sarén, T.; Ramachandran, M.; Martikainen, M.; Yu, D. Insertion of the Type-I IFN Decoy Receptor B18R in a miRNA-Tagged Semliki Forest Virus Improves Oncolytic Capacity but Results in Neurotoxicity. *Mol. Ther. Oncolytics* **2017**, *7*, 67–75. [CrossRef]

146. Ramachandran, M.; Yu, D.; Dyczynski, M.; Baskaran, S.; Zhang, L.; Lulla, A.; Lulla, V.; Saul, S.; Nelander, S.; Dimberg, A.; et al. Safe and effective treatment of experimental neuroblastoma and glioblastoma using systemically delivered triple microrna-detargeted oncolytic semliki forest virus. *Clin. Cancer Res.* **2017**, *23*, 1519–1530. [CrossRef]

147. Dutta, S.; Sengupta, P. Men and mice: Relating their ages. *Life Sci.* **2016**, *152*, 244–248. [CrossRef]

148. Fraser, H. Astrocytomas in an inbred mouse strain. *J. Pathol.* **1971**, *103*, 266–270. [CrossRef]

149. Serano, R.D.; Pegram, C.N.; Bigner, D.D. Tumorigenic cell culture lines from a spontaneous VM/Dk murine astrocytoma (SMA). *Acta Neuropathol.* **1980**, *51*, 53–64. [CrossRef]

150. Learn, C.A.; Grossi, P.M.; Schmittling, R.J.; Xie, W.; Mitchell, D.A.; Karikari, I.; Wei, Z.; Dressman, H.; Sampson, J.H. Genetic analysis of intracranial tumors in a murine model of glioma demonstrate a shift in gene expression in response to host immunity. *J. Neuroimmunol.* **2007**, *182*, 63–72. [CrossRef]

151. Tran, T.T.; Uhl, M.; Ma, J.Y.; Janssen, L.; Sriram, V.; Aulwurm, S.; Kerr, I.; Lam, A.; Webb, H.K.; Kapoun, A.M.; et al. Inhibiting TGF-β signaling restores immune surveillance in the SMA-560 glioma model. *Neuro. Oncol.* **2007**, *9*, 259–270. [CrossRef] [PubMed]

152. Ahmad, M.; Frei, K.; Willscher, E.; Stefanski, A.; Kaulich, K.; Roth, P.; Stühler, K.; Reifenberger, G.; Binder, H.; Weller, M. How stemlike are sphere cultures from long-term cancer cell lines? Lessons from mouse glioma models. *J. Neuropathol. Exp. Neurol.* **2014**, *73*, 1062–1077. [CrossRef] [PubMed]

153. Schneider, H.; Lohmann, B.; Wirsching, H.G.; Hasenbach, K.; Rushing, E.J.; Frei, K.; Pruschy, M.; Tabatabai, G.; Weller, M. Age-associated and therapy-induced alterations in the cellular microenvironment of experimental gliomas. *Oncotarget* **2017**, *8*, 87124–87135. [CrossRef] [PubMed]

154. Schötterl, S.; Huber, S.M.; Lentzen, H.; Mittelbronn, M.; Naumann, U. Adjuvant Therapy Using Mistletoe Containing Drugs Boosts the T-Cell-Mediated Killing of Glioma Cells and Prolongs the Survival of Glioma Bearing Mice. *Evidence-Based Complement. Altern. Med.* **2018**, *2018*, 3928572. [CrossRef] [PubMed]

155. Schneider, H.; Szabo, E.; Machado, R.A.; Broggini-Tenzer, A.; Walter, A.; Lobell, M.; Heldmann, D.; Süssmeier, F.; Grünewald, S.; Weller, M. Novel TIE-2 inhibitor BAY-826 displays in vivo efficacy in experimental syngeneic murine glioma models. *J. Neurochem.* **2017**, *140*, 170–182. [CrossRef]

156. Seystahl, K.; Papachristodoulou, A.; Burghardt, I.; Schneider, H.; Hasenbach, K.; Janicot, M.; Roth, P.; Weller, M. Biological role and therapeutic targeting of TGF-β$_3$ in glioblastoma. *Mol. Cancer Ther.* **2017**, *16*, 1177–1186. [CrossRef]

157. Silginer, M.; Weller, M.; Ziegler, U.; Roth, P. Integrin inhibition promotes atypical anoikis in glioma cells. *Cell Death Dis.* **2014**, *5*, e1012–e1013. [CrossRef]

158. Papachristodoulou, A.; Silginer, M.; Weller, M.; Schneider, H.; Hasenbach, K.; Janicot, M.; Roth, P. Therapeutic targeting of TGFb ligands in glioblastoma using novel antisense oligonucleotides reduces the growth of experimental gliomas. *Clin. Cancer Res.* **2019**, *25*, 7189–7201. [CrossRef]

159. Pituch, K.C.; Miska, J.; Krenciute, G.; Panek, W.K.; Li, G.; Rodriguez-Cruz, T.; Wu, M.; Han, Y.; Lesniak, M.S.; Gottschalk, S.; et al. Adoptive Transfer of IL13Rα2-Specific Chimeric Antigen Receptor T Cells Creates a Pro-inflammatory Environment in Glioblastoma. *Mol. Ther.* **2018**, *26*, 986–995. [CrossRef]

160. Kovacs, Z.; Werner, B.; Rassi, A.; Sass, J.O.; Martin-Fiori, E.; Bernasconi, M. Prolonged survival upon ultrasound-enhanced doxorubicin delivery in two syngenic glioblastoma mouse models. *J. Control. Release* **2014**, *187*, 74–82. [CrossRef]

161. Weiner, N.; Pyles, R.B.; Chalk, C.L.; Balko, M.G.; Miller, M.A.; Dyer, C.A.; Warnick, R.E.; Parysek, L.M. A syngeneic mouse glioma model for study of glioblastoma therapy. *J. Neuropathol. Exp. Neurol.* **1999**, *58*, 54–60. [CrossRef] [PubMed]

162. Gazdzinski, L.M.; Nieman, B.J. Cellularimaging and texture analysis distinguish differences in cellular dynamics in mouse brain tumors. *Magn. Reson. Med.* **2014**, *71*, 1531–1541. [CrossRef] [PubMed]

163. Lobo, M.R.; Wang, X.; Gillespie, G.Y.; Woltjer, R.L.; Pike, M.M. Combined efficacy of cediranib and quinacrine in glioma is enhanced by hypoxia and causally linked to autophagic vacuole accumulation. *PLoS ONE* **2014**, *9*, e114110. [CrossRef] [PubMed]

164. Lobo, M.R.; Kukino, A.; Tran, H.; Schabel, M.C.; Springer, C.S., Jr.; Gillespie, G.Y.; Grafe, M.R.; Woltjer, R.L.; Pike, M.M. Synergistic antivascular and antitumor efficacy with combined cediranib and SC6889 in intracranial mouse glioma. *PLoS ONE* **2015**, *10*, e0144488. [CrossRef]

165. Hellums, E.K.; Markert, J.M.; Parker, J.N.; He, B.; Perbal, B.; Roizman, B.; Whitley, R.J.; Langford, C.P.; Bharara, S.; Gillespie, G.Y. Increased efficacy of an interleukin-12-secreting herpes simplex virus in a syngeneic intracranial murine glioma model. *Neuro. Oncol.* **2005**, *7*, 213–224. [CrossRef]

166. Flores, C.; Pham, C.; Snyder, D.; Yang, S.; Sanchez-Perez, L.; Sayour, E.; Cui, X.; Kemeny, H.; Friedman, H.; Bigner, D.D.; et al. Novel role of hematopoietic stem cells in immunologic rejection of malignant gliomas. *Oncoimmunology* **2015**, *4*, e994374. [CrossRef] [PubMed]

167. Pérez, J.E.; Kopecky, J.; Visse, E.; Darabi, A.; Siesjö, P. Convection-enhanced delivery of temozolomide and whole cell tumor immunizations in GL261 and KR158 experimental mouse gliomas. *BMC Cancer* **2020**, *20*, 7.

168. Flores-Toro, J.A.; Luo, D.; Gopinath, A.; Sarkisian, M.R.; Campbell, J.J.; Charo, I.F.; Singh, R.; Schall, T.J.; Datta, M.; Jain, R.K.; et al. CCR2 inhibition reduces tumor myeloid cells and unmasks a checkpoint inhibitor effect to slow progression of resistant murine gliomas. *Proc. Natl. Acad. Sci. USA* **2020**, *117*, 1129–1138. [CrossRef]

169. Kwon, C.H.; Zhao, D.; Chen, J.; Alcantara, S.; Li, Y.; Burns, D.K.; Mason, R.P.; Lee, E.Y.; Wu, H.; Parada, L.F. Pten haploinsufficiency accelerates formation of high-grade astrocytomas. *Cancer Res.* **2008**, *68*, 3286–3294. [CrossRef]

170. Llaguno, S.A.; Chen, J.; Kwon, C.H.; Jackson, E.L.; Li, Y.; Burns, D.K.; Alvarez-Buylla, A.; Parada, L.F. Malignant Astrocytomas Originate from Neural Stem/Progenitor Cells in a Somatic Tumor Suppressor Mouse Model. *Cancer Cell* **2009**, *15*, 45–56. [CrossRef]

171. Soda, Y.; Marumoto, T.; Friedmann-Morvinski, D.; Soda, M.; Liu, F.; Michiue, H.; Pastorino, S.; Yang, M.; Hoffman, R.M.; Kesari, S.; et al. Transdifferentiation of glioblastoma cells into vascular endothelial cells. *Proc. Natl. Acad. Sci. USA* **2011**, *108*, 4274–4280. [CrossRef] [PubMed]

172. Saha, D.; Martuza, R.L.; Rabkin, S.D. Macrophage Polarization Contributes to Glioblastoma Eradication by Combination Immunovirotherapy and Immune Checkpoint Blockade. *Cancer Cell* **2017**, *32*, 253–267. [CrossRef] [PubMed]

173. Cheema, T.A.; Wakimoto, H.; Fecci, P.E.; Ning, J.; Kuroda, T.; Jeyaretna, D.S.; Martuza, R.L.; Rabkin, S.D. Multifaceted oncolytic virus therapy for glioblastoma in an immunocompetent cancer stem cell model. *Proc. Natl. Acad. Sci. USA* **2013**, *110*, 12006–12011. [CrossRef] [PubMed]

174. Saha, D.; Rabkin, S.D.; Martuza, R.L. Temozolomide antagonizes oncolytic immunovirotherapy in glioblastoma. *J. Immunother. Cancer* **2020**, *8*, 345. [CrossRef]

175. Saha, D.; Wakimoto, H.; Peters, C.W.; Antoszczyk, S.J.; Rabkin, S.D.; Martuza, R.L. Combinatorial effects of vegfr kinase inhibitor axitinib and oncolytic virotherapy in mouse and human glioblastoma stem-like cell models. *Clin. Cancer Res.* **2018**, *24*, 3409–3422. [CrossRef]

176. Osuka, S.; Sampetrean, O.; Shimizu, T.; Saga, I.; Onishi, N.; Sugihara, E.; Okubo, J.; Fujita, S.; Takano, S.; Matsumura, A.; et al. IGF1 receptor signaling regulates adaptive radioprotection in glioma stem cells. *Stem Cells* **2013**, *31*, 627–640. [CrossRef]

177. He, B.; Jabouille, A.; Steri, V.; Johansson-Percival, A.; Michael, I.P.; Kotamraju, V.R.; Junckerstorff, R.; Nowak, A.K.; Hamzah, J.; Lee, G.; et al. Vascular targeting of LIGHT normalizes blood vessels in primary brain cancer and induces intratumoural high endothelial venules. *J. Pathol.* **2018**, *245*, 209–221. [CrossRef]

178. Riva, M.; Wouters, R.; Nittner, D.; Ceuster, J.; Sterpin, E.; Giovannoni, R.; Himmelreich, U.; Gsell, W.; Van Ranst, M.; Coosemans, A. Radiation dose-escalation and dose-fractionation modulate the immune microenvironment, cancer stem cells and vasculature in experimental high-grade gliomas. *J. Neurosurg. Sci.* **2020**. [CrossRef]

179. Costa, B.; Fletcher, M.; Boskovic, P.; Ivanova, E.L.; Eisemann, T.; Lohr, S.; Bunse, L.; Löwer, M.; Burchard, S.; Korshunov, A.; et al. A novel neural stem cell-derived immunocompetent mouse model of glioblastoma for preclinical studies. *bioRxiv* **2020**. [CrossRef]

180. Aslan, K.; Turco, V.; Blobner, J.; Sonner, J.K.; Liuzzi, A.R.; Núñez, N.G.; De Feo, D.; Kickingereder, P.; Fischer, M.; Green, E.; et al. Heterogeneity of response to immune checkpoint blockade in hypermutated experimental gliomas. *Nature Comm* **2020**, *11*, 931. [CrossRef]

181. Schafer, N.; Gielen, G.H.; Rauschenbach, L.; Kebir, S.; Till, A.; Reinartz, R.; Simon, M.; Niehusmann, P.; Kleinschnitz, C.; Herrlinger, U.; et al. Longitudinal heterogeneity in glioblastoma: Moving targets in recurrent versus primary tumors. *J. Transl. Med.* **2019**, *17*, 96. [CrossRef] [PubMed]

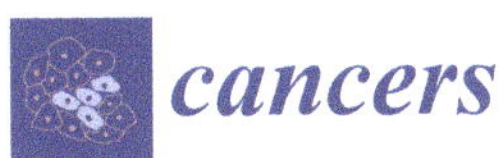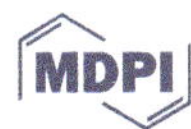

Review

Convergent Evolution by Cancer and Viruses in Evading the NKG2D Immune Response

Richard Baugh, Hena Khalique and Leonard W. Seymour *

Anticancer Viruses and Cancer Vaccines Research Group, Department of Oncology, University of Oxford, Oxford OX3 7DQ, UK; richard.baugh@oncology.ox.ac.uk (R.B.); hena.khalique@oncology.ox.ac.uk (H.K.)
* Correspondence: len.seymour@oncology.ox.ac.uk; Tel.: +44-01865-617331

Received: 13 November 2020; Accepted: 16 December 2020; Published: 18 December 2020

Simple Summary: Cells undergoing stress, viral infection, and malignant transformation express natural killer group 2 member D (NKG2D) ligands on their surface, rendering them susceptible to immunosurveillance. Given this selective pressure exerted on viruses and cancer cells, many viruses and several cancers have evolved means of evading NKG2D recognition. This review highlights the various ways in which stresses, viruses and cancers induce the expression of NKG2D ligands, before comparing the similarities and differences between viral and cancer mechanisms to subsequently prevent recognition by the NKG2D system.

Abstract: The natural killer group 2 member D (NKG2D) receptor and its family of NKG2D ligands (NKG2DLs) are key components in the innate immune system, triggering NK, $\gamma\delta$ and CD8$^+$ T cell-mediated immune responses. While surface NKG2DL are rarely found on healthy cells, expression is significantly increased in response to various types of cellular stress, viral infection, and tumour cell transformation. In order to evade immune-mediated cytotoxicity, both pathogenic viruses and cancer cells have evolved various mechanisms of subverting immune defences and preventing NKG2DL expression. Comparisons of the mechanisms employed following virus infection or malignant transformation reveal a pattern of converging evolution at many of the key regulatory steps involved in NKG2DL expression and subsequent immune responses. Exploring ways to target these shared steps in virus- and cancer-mediated immune evasion may provide new mechanistic insights and therapeutic opportunities, for example, using oncolytic virotherapy to re-engage the innate immune system towards cancer cells.

Keywords: NKG2D ligands; NKG2D receptor; NK cells; immune evasion; convergent evolution; cancer; viruses; immunotherapy

---

1. Introduction

Cancer cells have long been defined with a set of characteristics, known as the 'hallmarks of cancer', with immune evasion rapidly emerging as a key player in cancer progression [1]. Viruses share several of these hallmarks with cancer cells to achieve a successful infection, as immune evasion is also critically important for viruses.

1.1. NKG2D Receptor and NK Cell Activation

Natural killer (NK) cells play a critical role in the innate immunosurveillance of both virally infected cells and tumours. They possess an extensive repertoire of both activatory and inhibitory receptors that recognise a range of ligands on target cells [2]. In contrast to T cell activation by clonotypic T cell receptor (TCR) interacting with specific peptides presented in the context of major histocompatibility complex (MHC), NK cells are inhibited by MHC molecules, and are instead activated by the lack of MHC, referred to as 'missing-self' [3]. NK cells also interpret other positive and negative signals from their environment and the target cell. Some of the activatory receptors responsible for processing positive signals include NKp46, NKp44 and NKp30 [2]. One of the most well-documented activatory receptors is the natural killer group 2 member D (NKG2D) receptor. NKG2D receptor and its ligands (NKG2DLs) are part of the early warning signals for the innate immune system; flagging up cells that may represent danger to the host organism. NKG2D receptor is an activatory receptor expressed on the surface of NK cells, CD8[+] T cells, natural killer T (NKT) cells, γδ T cells and some CD4[+] T cell subsets [4–6]. NKG2D is an invariant homodimeric receptor, with each monomer consisting of a type-II transmembrane domain and a C-type lectin-like extracellular domain, and is associated with DNAX activating protein 10 (DAP10) or DAP12 in mice, and DAP10 only in humans [4] (Figure 1a).

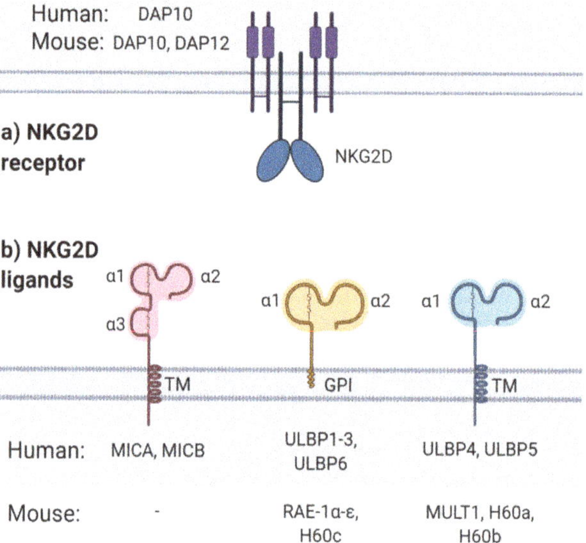

Figure 1. NKG2D receptor and ligands. (**a**) The natural killer group 2 member D (NKG2D) receptor is expressed by natural killer (NK) cells, γδ T cells, CD8[+] T cells, and some CD4[+] T cells. The NKG2D receptor is associated with DNAX activating protein (DAP) 10 in humans, but DAP10 and DAP12 in mice. (**b**) NKG2D ligands (NKG2DLs) include MHC-class-I-polypeptide-related sequence (MIC) A and MICB, and UL16 binding protein (ULBP) 1-6 in humans, and retinoic acid early inducible (RAE-1) α-ε, H60a-c, and murine UL16 binding protein-like transcript (MULT) 1 in mice. All NKG2DLs feature MHC-class-I-like α1 and α2 domains, whilst MICA and MICB also have an α3-like domain but do not bind to β2-microglobulin. Some NKG2DLs are transmembrane proteins (TM), while others are linked to the membrane via glycophosphatidylinositol (GPI) anchors. Diagram created with BioRender.com.

NKG2D binding to NKG2DLs can directly activate NK cells that have already been stimulated with interleukin (IL) -2 or IL-15 [7,8], whereas additional costimulatory signals are required to activate T cells and freshly isolated NK cells [9,10]. Binding of NKG2D to its ligands recruits phosphatidylinositol 3-kinase (PI3K) and growth factor receptor-bound protein 2 (GRB2), triggering a subsequent phosphorylation cascade. If the balance of the overall signalling favours NK cell activation, it can stimulate effector functions including cytokine release and perforin/granzyme-mediated cytotoxicity [11].

1.2. NKG2D Ligands

Although the NKG2D receptor is germline-encoded, it can recognise a diverse range of MHC-class-I-related ligands. In humans, these NKG2DLs include MHC-class-I-polypeptide-related sequence A (MIC) A and MICB, and UL16 binding protein (ULBP) 1-6, also known as retinoic acid early inducible transcript 1 (RAET1) proteins [6,12–17]. In contrast, murine NKG2DLs include retinoic acid early inducible (RAE-1) α-ε, H60a-c, and murine UL16 binding protein-like transcript (MULT) 1 [18,19]. All NKG2DLs share homology with MHC class I molecules, featuring α1 and α2 domains, while MICA and MICB also have an α3 domain. However, unlike MHC class I molecules, they cannot bind and present antigenic peptides and are not associated with β_2-microglobulin. Despite their overall similarities, NKG2DLs vary from each other in sequence; binding affinity to NKG2D; and membrane anchorage, either transmembrane proteins or glycophosphatidylinositol (GPI)-linked [20] (Figure 1b). NKG2DLs also display a high degree of polymorphism in humans, with 104 and 37 distinct alleles currently assigned for MICA and MICB genes, respectively [21]. These polymorphisms can vary certain properties of the NKG2DLs, such as binding affinity to NKG2D receptor [22,23] or protein length [24,25].

The expression of NKG2DLs on normal, healthy cells is low or absent. However, expression dramatically increases during events of cellular stress, virus infection or malignant transformation. This expression pattern in stressed, virus-infected or cancer cells is often referred to as 'induced self'; whereby germline-encoded NKG2DLs are upregulated, enabling NK or T cell recognition, and often occurs in parallel with viral- or cancer-mediated downregulation of MHC class I expression (i.e., 'missing-self') [26]. Upregulation of NKG2DLs allows for rapid NK or T cell-mediated immunosurveillance and elimination of cells that may pose as a threat to the organism: cells that have undergone DNA damage after heat or oxidative shock, and may therefore have acquired oncogenic mutations; cells that have been infected by a viral pathogen, and may lead to a larger-scale infection if left unchecked; or rapidly proliferating cells that may progress to become cancer.

1.3. Evading Detection by NKG2D

In the constant battle between the host immune system and cancer or viruses, a plethora of mechanisms are employed by both cancer cells and virus-infected cells to counteract the NKG2D-mediated immune response. A detailed insight into regulatory mechanisms for NKG2DL expression is reviewed by Raulet et al. [20]. This review covers in detail the various mechanisms in which stresses, viruses and cancers can induce the expression of NKG2DLs, before discussing the strategies employed by viruses and cancers to subsequently evade the NKG2D response. Finally, this review highlights the converging evolution displayed by both viruses and cancers to target the critical stages in its regulation.

2. NKG2DL Expression in Healthy Cells and Autoimmunity

NKG2DL expression can lead to NK and T cell-mediated cytotoxicity and inflammation. Therefore, surface expression of these ligands is minimal in healthy quiescent cells to prevent autoimmunity. For example, although MICA is expressed at a low level by healthy intestinal epithelial cells (IECs), patients with Crohn's Disease demonstrate increased MICA expression on these IECs compared to healthy controls, leading to activation and autoimmunity from a subset of CD4+NKG2D+ T cells [5]. Interestingly, Schrambach and colleagues revealed MICA and MICB mRNA transcripts in healthy organ tissue as well as various tumours [27], suggesting regulation of surface NKG2DL expression is not solely controlled at a transcriptional level.

2.1. Cell Stress Induces NKG2DL mRNA and Protein Expression

NKG2DL expression in normal cells is increased following a variety of cellular insults. Human IECs exposed to heat shock demonstrated increased MICA and MICB mRNAs and surface protein expression, along with an increase in heat shock protein (hsp) 70 mRNA [28]. The heat shock-induced upregulation of MICA and MICB also sensitised the target cells to lysis by γδ T cells [28]. A study using human colorectal carcinoma cell lines demonstrated that MICA and MICB mRNA and surface protein expression were low when cells were at high confluency and quiescent. However, the expression of both mRNAs and surface protein was greatly increased in response to oxidative or heat stress, or when cells were proliferating [29]. This stress response is thought to be mediated, at least initially, at the level of transcription, since the promoter regions for MICA and MICB contained conserved heat shock elements (HSE), which are capable of binding heat shock factor 1 (HSF1) in response to heat shock and oxidative stress in a manner similar to regulation of hsp70 expression [12,29]. In a similar study performed on the human colorectal carcinoma cell line CaCo-2, oxidative stress induced by H_2O_2 also increased MICA and MICB mRNA expression, although surface protein levels were not measured [30].

Other forms of cell stress have also been reported to induce NKG2DL expression. Endoplasmic reticulum (ER) stress, induced with an inhibitor of the ER Ca^{2+} pump, increased ULBP1, 2, 5, and 6 mRNAs and surface protein in a range of human intestinal epithelial cell lines, as well as MULT1 in murine cells in vivo [31].

DNA damage is another form of cellular stress capable of upregulating surface NKG2DL expression. Gasser et al. demonstrated that activation of the DNA damage response (DDR) by chemotherapeutic agents, ionising radiation or stalling of DNA replication cycles increased NKG2DL expression. This increased NKG2DL expression was found to occur in an ataxia telangiectasia, mutated- (ATM), ATM- and Rad3-related- (ATR) and checkpoint kinase (Chk) 1-dependent manner, sensitising cells to lysis by NK cells [32]. Further evidence towards the link between reactive oxygen species, DNA damage and NKG2DL upregulation was demonstrated by using sublethal doses of chemotherapeutic agents which cause oxidative stress, such as doxorubicin and melphalan, which triggered MICA upregulation in multiple myeloma cells. This transcriptional increase in MICA was attributed to DDR-dependent activity of the transcription factor E2F1 [33]. Additionally, the *ULBP1* and *ULBP2* genes have a response element for the tumour suppressor protein p53, which is stabilised during the DDR. Hence p53 stabilisation during the DDR directly causes an increase in ULBP1 and ULBP2 transcription [34,35].

2.2. Post-Transcriptional Regulation of NKG2DL Expression During Cell Stress

Protein expression is not only controlled at the level of transcription; mRNA stability, protein stability and intracellular localisation also play a significant role in regulating functional protein expression. As mentioned earlier, Schrambach et al. observed that MICA and MICB mRNA transcripts were expressed in various healthy human tissues [27], which appears in contrast to the concept that NKG2DL proteins are not expressed by healthy cells, indicating that other regulatory mechanisms are involved beyond gene transcription.

Interestingly, Vantourout et al. describe a mechanism in which ultraviolet B (UVB) radiation upregulated MICA, MICB and ULBP2 in human epithelial cells via stress-induced epidermal growth factor receptor (EGFR) signalling, rather than due to the DDR [36]. They found that under normal conditions, AU-rich element/poly(U)-binding/degradation factor 1 (AUF1) protein targets AU-rich elements (AREs) in the 3′ untranslated region (UTR) of human NKG2DL mRNAs. AUF1 binding to NKG2DL transcripts causes mRNA destabilisation and degradation. However, stress-induced EGFR signalling prevents AUF1 binding and NKG2DL mRNA destabilisation, thus, allowing translation and NKG2DL protein expression.

MicroRNAs (miRNAs) have also been implicated in the regulation of many genes, including MICA and MICB. A particular set of miRNAs found to be expressed in normal human cells can bind to the 3′ UTR of MICA and MICB mRNA transcripts, resulting in their destabilisation and degradation, hence preventing protein translation [37]. It has been hypothesised that these miRNAs play a critical part in the regulation of MICA and MICB protein expression and preventing unwanted autoimmunity. During normal conditions, these miRNAs are expressed, establishing a threshold for MICA and MICB mRNA to reach for protein expression and NKG2D recognition and subsequent cell lysis. During transient cell stress, such as heat shock, the MICA and MICB mRNA levels dramatically increase, while the miRNA expression remains relatively unchanged, enabling a saturation of the miRNAs and for some MICA/B mRNA transcripts to escape miRNA-mediated degradation, and thus, allow protein translation. It has been speculated that this system endows several advantages, such as rapid increases in protein expression, while preventing NKG2D recognition of otherwise healthy cells, due to small fluctuations in MICA or MICB expression [37].

In contrast to the findings regarding p53-mediated increase in *ULBP1* and *ULBP2* transcription mentioned earlier [34,35], p53 also induces expression of miR-34a and miR-34c, which target ULBP2 mRNA for destabilisation [38]. These observations suggest two possibly contrasting roles for p53 in NKG2DL expression and requires more investigation into how the regulation is fine-tuned.

Additionally, healthy primary human bronchial epithelial cells constitutively expressed NKG2DL mRNA transcripts but lacked surface protein expression. However, increased surface NKG2DL expression was detected upon exposure to oxidative stress in the form of H_2O_2, although the mRNA and total protein levels remained consistent, indicating a stress-mediated activation of protein translocation to the surface [39]. This rapid method of protein translocation and increased surface expression may allow quicker responses and immunological detection of oxidatively-stressed cells within the well-oxygenated pulmonary environment.

Protein stability has also been reported to play a role in regulating murine NKG2DL expression [40]. Nice et al. report that during normal conditions, MULT1 is targeted by membrane-associated RING-CH (MARCH) 4 and MARCH9 E3 ubiquitin ligases and is subsequently degraded. Upon heat shock treatment, however, this degradation was inhibited, and surface MULT1 increased [40].

3. NKG2DL Expression Is Induced in Virally Infected Cells

Viral infection of a cell and the subsequent virus-mediated change of the cellular phenotype to enable viral genome replication, immune evasion and proliferation leads to a highly stressful environment for the host cell. Viral genomic replication [41–43], production of viral proteins [42,44], altering cellular metabolism [45], and manipulating signalling pathways to support the infection [46–48] are all common traits shared by many viruses during infection, all of which can induce some degree of stress to the host cell. Therefore, the process of viral infection is likely to trigger many of the cellular stresses mentioned in the previous section, such as DDR activation [41], oxidative stress [49,50], and heat shock [51], which would induce the expression of NKG2DLs. However, as described below, viruses also employ a variety of mechanisms to subsequently downregulate these ligands.

As mentioned earlier, the DDR is one of the major regulators of NKG2DL expression in stressed cells, but it is also heavily involved in upregulation of NKG2DL expression in virus-infected cells. Many viruses, especially double-stranded DNA (dsDNA) viruses, have been demonstrated to trigger the DDR during early stages of infection. Some examples include herpes simplex virus (HSV) [52], Epstein-Barr virus (EBV) [43], adenovirus [53], and human immunodeficiency virus (HIV) [42]. Given that DDR activation induces NKG2DL expression [32], viruses that do trigger the DDR during early stages of virus infection subsequently induce NKG2DL expression [54]. Furthermore, if left unrestrained, the DDR would likely concatemerise the nascent virus DNA genomes together. Accordingly, most viruses have also evolved means to inhibit the prolonged activation of the DDR during infection by inhibiting various proteins involved in the response [55].

Other viruses, or viral gene products have also been implicated in directly increasing NKG2DL expression, including: adenovirus serotype 5 (Ad5) E1A oncogene, which binds to a transcriptional co-adaptor protein p300, resulting in increased NKG2DL expression in mice and human tumour cells [44]; the HIV-1 viral gene product Vpr specifically increases expression ULBP1 and ULBP2 on $CD4^+$ T cells by activating ATR [42]; influenza virus increases surface expression of ULBP1, 2 and 3 on infected dendritic cells [56]; and ectromelia virus (ECTV) induces MULT1 expression in murine embryonic fibroblasts [57].

Viruses modulate cell signalling pathways upon infection to enable productive replication and biosynthesis, while preventing the host cell from undergoing apoptosis. One important pathway which is commonly hijacked by many viruses is the PI3K-Akt-mammalian target of rapamycin (mTOR) pathway, whereby, activation promotes cell survival, pro-viral metabolism and biosynthesis [46,58]. Several viruses have been shown to activate PI3K, including adenovirus [48],

HSV-1 [59], human cytomegalovirus (HCMV) [47] and murine cytomegalovirus (MCMV) [60]. MCMV-induced PI3K activation has been demonstrated to increase expression of RAE-1 ligands in mouse cells [60]. However, PI3K activation alone was not sufficient to induce expression without viral infection, suggesting other additional signals and virus-induced stresses were also required for NKG2DL expression [60].

4. Virus Immune Evasion

Much of our understanding of how cell biology and immunology works has been gained from studying how viruses exploit, inhibit, or subvert these mechanisms for their own gain. Investigations into the viral attempts to inhibit the NKG2D system to achieve immune evasion have revealed the importance of the NKG2D response and helped to uncover various mechanistic details. Comparing the evolution of viruses from a range of distinct viral families reveals that many have independently converged on interfering with the NKG2D immune response [61].

Some viruses result in persistent infections, such as those from the *Herpesviridae* family including HCMV and HSV. Herpesviruses are enveloped dsDNA viruses with large genomes. The HCMV genome contains over 150 open reading frames (ORFs), enabling the virus to encode a wide array of proteins, each with distinct and specific functions. This large genome size endows herpesviruses with the potential to modulate the infected host cell, enabling immune evasion and persistent infections via a host of different viral proteins. In light of this, herpesviruses represent a significant proportion of the examples mentioned below in their strategies to interfere with the NKG2D immune response by using a variety of viral gene products [62].

4.1. Viral Proteins Use a Range of Strategies to Downregulate NKG2DL Expression

Much of the early work investigating the effects of viral modulation of NKG2DLs was conducted using cytomegaloviruses, MCMV and HCMV. MCMV has been shown to downregulate surface expression of each of the murine NKG2DLs through a variety of means: (1) MCMV glycoprotein gp40, encoded by the gene *m152*, resulted in the specific downregulation of surface expression of RAE-1α, β, δ, ε and γ [63]; (2) a protein encoded by MCMV gene *m155* was found to target H60 for lysosomal degradation, thus reducing surface expression [64]; (3) an MCMV glycoprotein encoded by gene *m145* downregulates MULT1 [65]; (4) fcr-1 protein, encoded by the gene *m138,* rapidly decreased surface expression of both MULT1 and H60 [66].

Early studies investigating the immune evasion mechanisms of HCMV demonstrated that HCMV membrane glycoprotein UL16 is capable of binding to MICB, ULBP1 and ULBP2, and that exogenous addition of soluble UL16 was able to block the binding of these ligands to the NKG2D receptor on NK cells [13]. Further investigations demonstrated enhanced NK cell-mediated killing of fibroblasts infected with UL16-deleted HCMV compared to the wild type virus, and was attributed to the downregulation of surface MICB, ULBP1 and ULBP2 [67]. Two studies by Welte et al. and Dunn et al. later demonstrated the mechanism of HCMV UL16-mediated downregulation of MICB, ULBP1 and ULBP2. They showed that UL16 is retained in the ER and cis-Golgi apparatus membranes, whilst simultaneously sequestering the NKG2DLs intracellularly by binding via the UL16 ectodomain [68,69]. Wu et al. were able to demonstrate that the intracellular retention of MICB was due to a tyrosine-based motif in the cytoplasmic domain of UL16, and deletion of this motif restored MICB trafficking to the cell surface [70].

Beyond UL16, HCMV also has other mechanisms to downregulate NKG2DLs. HCMV protein UL142 blocks surface expression of full-length MICA protein, again by retaining it in the cis-Golgi apparatus [71]. Interestingly however, not all alleles of MICA were affected equally. The MICA*008 allele has a truncated transmembrane region and has no cytoplasmic tail, masking it from UL142 binding and enabling surface expression in HCMV-infected cells [25,72]. This suggests a possible evolutionary pressure for this mutant allele to be selected for human resistance to HCMV infection, as MICA*008 is the most prevalent allele in several populations, including North American Caucasians [24]. However, recently evidence has emerged to suggest HCMV has since co-evolved alongside the

MICA*008 allele, as the US9 protein has been found to specifically target MICA*008 for proteasomal degradation [73].

After performing a genome-wide screen for other HCMV proteins that may interact with NKG2DLs, Fielding et al. further identified a number of proteins in the US12 family [74,75]. They revealed that US18 and US20 were capable of targeting MICA for lysosomal degradation, and functioned either independently or together in concert [74]. They also reported that US12, US13 and US20 were involved in downregulating MICB and ULBP2 [75].

Other herpesviruses, such as HSV-1 and varicella-zoster virus (VZV), also downregulate NKG2DLs, although precise mechanistic details remain uncertain. For example, VZV upregulates MICA, but downregulates ULBP2 and ULBP3 surface expression, whereas HSV-1 decreases total MICA, ULPB2 and ULBP3 protein, and downregulates surface ULBP1 surface expression only [76]. However, Schepis et al. reported a downregulation in surface expression of MICA and ULBP2 only, with total protein remaining unchanged, and attributed this to a late viral gene product retaining the proteins intracellularly [77]. The discrepancies observed here may be due to the different cell lines tested, as Campbell et al. noted similar decreases in ARPE-19 epithelial cells, human foreskin fibroblasts and 293T human embryonic kidney cells, whereas Schepis et al. used tumour cell lines including U373 astroglioma cell line and HeLa epithelial tumour cell line.

Human herpesvirus (HHV)-7 U21 gene product has been demonstrated to bind and direct ULBP1 for lysosomal degradation, and downregulate surface MICA and MICB expression via an unknown mechanism [78]. Similarly, an unknown early viral gene product of HHV-6 downregulates surface MICB, ULBP1 and ULBP3 by targeting them for degradation [79]. Meanwhile, Kaposi's sarcoma-associated herpesvirus (KSHV) expresses the protein K5 which has E3 ubiquitin ligase activity, resulting in ubiquitinylation of MICA (and other immunoreceptors including MHC class I) and the redistribution of MICA away from the cell surface and into intracellular compartments [80].

Other viruses have also evolved proteins to downregulate NKG2DL expression. Hepatitis C virus (HCV) non-structural protease NS3/4A has been implicated in reduced MICA and MICB expression, although the mechanism remains unclear [81].

Adenovirus also uses proteins to enable immune evasion. Although the Ad5 early gene E1A alone is capable of inducing expression of NKG2DLs when expressed by human cancer cells [44], Ad5 also has evolved other mechanisms to negate this effect and avoid NK cell killing. The Ad5 E3/19K gene not only downregulates HLA-1 during infection, but has also been demonstrated to directly cause retention of MICA and MICB in the ER, thus countering the immunogenic effects of the E1A gene and enabling immune evasion [82].

Hepatitis B virus (HBV) uses viral proteins to downregulate NKG2DLs via yet another mechanism. The HBV protein HBx promotes increased expression of the transcription factors GATA-2 and GATA-3 and forms a trimeric protein complex with HBx and GATA-2/3. This protein complex then binds to the promoter region for MICA and MICB and represses transcription [83]. Additionally, the HBV protein HBc also binds to CpG islands in the MICA/B promoters to further repress MICA/B transcription [83].

While the HIV-1 Vpr protein increases ULBP1 and ULBP2 expression in infected CD4$^+$ T cells via induction of DNA damage sensors [42], HIV-1 also expresses a protein called Nef which subsequently downregulates MICA, ULBP1 and especially ULBP2 [84]. The Nef protein has already been implicated in its role in directing various immune receptors away from the cell surface such as CD4, CD28 and MHC class I molecules [85], however the precise mechanism for how Nef downregulates surface NKG2DLs appears to differ compared to other surface receptors [84].

Vesicular stomatitis virus (VSV) has been shown to dramatically increase MICA mRNA expression upon infection of Jurkat T cells; however, surface MICA protein expression is decreased on infected Jurkat T cells and melanoma cell lines [86]. Investigation into the possible mechanism of this MICA protein downregulation revealed that it was not dependent on: the matrix (M) protein, which is responsible for VSV immune evasion of type I interferon (IFN); or VSV-mediated global inhibition of host translation; or intracellular retention of MICA, as seen in HCMV-infected cells [86]. Although the exact mechanism and protein responsible could not be elucidated, the authors concluded the downregulation likely occurs at an early post-transcriptional level [86].

The sheer number and variety of examples outlined above of different viral proteins capable of limiting NKG2DL expression highlights the importance of evading the NKG2D immune response for viruses. Herpesviruses, in particular, represent a large proportion of these examples, with multiple distinct viral proteins responsible for limiting NKG2DL protein stability or surface localisation. The diversity of examples suggests that intracellular retention or degradation of NKG2DLs is a highly effective immune evasion strategy.

4.2. Viral Strategies to Evade Pattern Recognition Receptors

Double-stranded RNA (dsRNA) or dsDNA viral genomes present in the cytoplasm are sensed by the pattern recognition receptors (PRRs) such as retinoic acid-inducible gene (RIG)-1, melanoma differentiation-associated protein (MDA)-5 and cyclic-GMP-AMP synthase (cGAS). These PRRs can trigger increases in NKG2DL expression upon infection with cytoplasmic DNA viruses, such as vaccinia virus (VV). To counter this, the VV gene *EL3* encodes a dsRNA binding protein, which shields dsRNA produced during infection from recognition by PRRs. Avoiding detection by PRRs is a surprisingly effective mechanism, as infection of fibroblasts with *EL3*-deleted VVs shows increased surface NKG2DL expression and sensitises them to NK cell lysis [87].

HIV-1 also has an indirect method of avoiding detection by the host cell and thus preventing the expression of NKG2DLs. Apolipoprotein B-editing complex 3G (APOBEC3G or A3G) is an antiviral factor which forms part of the innate immune defence system against viruses, by deaminating cytidine residues in viral genomes and causing viral hypermutation and inactivation. The activity of A3G induces the DDR in infected cells, thus triggering NKG2DL expression and sensitivity to NK cell lysis [88]. To counteract this however, the HIV-1 viral infectivity factor (Vif) targets A3G for proteasomal degradation and thus prevents DDR-induced NKG2DL expression [88].

4.3. Viruses Can Use miRNAs to Regulate NKG2DL Expression at a Post-Transcriptional Level

The 3' UTRs of MICA and MICB mRNAs have conserved sites that are targeted by cellular miRNAs that destabilise the transcripts and trigger mRNA degradation. miRNA destabilisation is believed to be part of the normal regulation of MICA/B expression in healthy cells [37]. Interestingly, HCMV also exploits this system of regulation. HCMV miRNA-UL112 targets the same 3' UTR of MICA and MICB mRNA transcripts as the cellular miRNAs, resulting in destabilisation and degradation of MICA and MICB mRNAs and preventing protein translation [37,89]. Other herpesviruses like KSHV and EBV also express miRNAs, miR-K12-7 and miR-BART2-5p respectively, that target the 3' UTR of MICB transcripts similarly to HCMV [90]. These miRNAs share no sequence homology between HCMV, KSHV and EBV however, and bind to different sites within the 3' UTR, suggesting a degree of convergent evolution between different herpesviruses to target MICB [90].

Self-defence using miRNAs targeting NKG2DLs is also observed in other families of virus. For example, human polyomaviruses (PyVs) JCV and BK strains both express an identical miRNA, miR-J1-3p, which reduces surface ULBP3 expression [91]. However, the authors reported that the ULBP3 mRNA transcripts were not degraded, suggesting an alternative post-transcriptional means of repression, such as translation inhibition.

HSV-1 has developed an alternative, indirect method of using miRNAs to downregulate NKG2DLs at a post-transcriptional level. HSV-1 miR-H8 does not bind to NKG2DL mRNA transcripts directly; instead, it targets mRNA transcripts for one of the key proteins involved in covalently attaching proteins to GPI anchors at the cell surface [92]. Therefore, by preventing translation of part of the GPI-anchoring machinery, it reduces surface expression of some of the GPI-anchored NKG2DLs such as ULBP2 and ULBP3 [92].

4.4. Virus-Mediated Shedding of NKG2DL

HCMV miRNAs have been further implicated in downregulation of surface NKG2DL, albeit via a different and indirect mechanism. HCMV miRNA-US25-2-3p binds to the 3′ UTR of mRNA transcripts encoding for tissue inhibitor of metalloproteinases-3 (TIMP-3) and leads to degradation of the mRNA. TIMP-3 is an inhibitor of metalloproteinases on the surface of cells such as a disintegrin and metalloprotease (ADAM) 17 and matrix metalloprotease (MMP) 14. The subsequent reduction in TIMP-3 protein results in enhanced activity of such metalloproteases, leading to an increased cleavage and shedding of MICA and MICB from the surface of HCMV infected cells [93].

Patients with chronic HIV-1 infections have been reported to have increased levels of soluble NKG2DLs in their sera, and HIV-1 infection of CD4$^+$ T cells in vitro lead to increased MICA, MICB and ULBP2 surface expression but also increased protein shedding, [94]. Furthermore, the shedding of NKG2DLs in HIV-1 infected lymphocytes could be prevented with the addition of MMP inhibitors, implying possible a link between viral upregulation of cellular MMPs [94].

4.5. Virus-Mediated Immune Subversion

While many viruses have evolved mechanisms to downregulate the NKG2DLs on the infected host cells to achieve immune evasion, some viruses instead use other mechanisms to avoid destruction. For example, zoonotic orthopoxviruses (ZPXVs), such as cowpox and monkeypox have evolved an entirely alternative strategy to evade NKG2D mediated detection. These ZPXVs express a highly conserved orthopox MHC class I-like protein (OMCP), which is secreted from infected cells and antagonises NKG2D receptors themselves with high affinity [95]. Alternatively, HCV non-structural protein NS5A stimulates monocytes to shift their cytokine profile via binding to Toll-like receptor (TLR4), increasing IL-10 whilst decreasing IL-12 secretion levels. The increased IL-10 secretion leads to a concomitant increase in transforming growth factor (TGF) β, which downregulates NKG2D receptor expression on circulating NK cells [96].

Other cytokines produced in response to viral infection have also been identified. Muntasell et al. revealed that peripheral blood mononuclear cells (PBMCs) infected with HCMV in vitro caused a selective decrease in NKG2D receptor on NK cells [97]. However, this downregulation was found to be transient, with normal expression returning 7 days after infection. Interestingly, this effect could be abrogated by antagonising type I IFN, IL-12 or IFN-γ, indicating that these proinflammatory cytokines were responsible. The authors suggested that this cytokine-mediated downregulation of NKG2D receptor may be part of a physiological negative feedback system to limit NK cell responses against healthy cells expressing NKG2DLs during inflammatory responses [97].

As mentioned above, elevated levels of soluble NKG2DLs in patient sera have been observed in HIV$^+$ patients, attributed to shedding of ligands from HIV-1 infected lymphocytes [94]. Furthermore, in vitro experiments using plasma from HIV-1-infected patients caused a significant downregulation of NKG2D receptor on NK cells and CD8$^+$ T cells obtained from healthy donors [94]. Compared to patients receiving highly active antiretroviral therapy (HAART) with lower soluble NKG2DL levels, naïve HIV$^+$ patients with elevated soluble NKG2DL levels displayed reduced NKG2D receptor expression on circulating NK cells and CD8$^+$ T cells [94]. These findings suggest that soluble NKG2DLs not only decrease target ligands on the infected cell surface, but also affect the capacity for an NKG2D-mediated immune response on a systemic level by downregulating NKG2D receptor. Following these findings, it not unlikely that shedding of MICA and MICB due to HCMV miRNA-US25-2-3p mentioned above [93] may also cause a systemic decrease in NKG2D receptor levels on immune cells, although this has not yet been investigated. The mechanism of soluble NKG2DL-mediated downregulation of NKG2D receptor expression will be discussed later in Section 6.2.

4.6. Evolution of Viral Immune Evasion Has Converged on Disrupting the NKG2D System

The NKG2D system appears to be a critical component in immune control of viral infection, given the examples of multiple viruses from entirely distinct families deploying various strategies to prevent NKG2D signalling (Table 1). While some viruses directly reduce the expression of NKG2DLs of the infected host cell, others achieve the same results via different means instead, by targeting the NKG2D receptor itself either directly or subverting the immune response indirectly. These examples of convergent evolution by multiple related and unrelated viruses demonstrate the importance of the NKG2D system in controlling viral infection.

Table 1. Summary of viral mechanisms of NKG2D immune evasion.

Virus	Immunoevasin	Mechanism	Reference
MCMV	gp40	Downregulation of surface RAE-1α-γ expression	[63]
	m155	Targets H60 for degradation	[64]
	m145	Downregulation of MULT1 surface expression	[65]
	Fcr-1	Downregulation of MULT1 and H60 surface expression	[66]
HCMV	UL16	Retention of MICB, ULBP2 and ULBP3 in ER and cis-Golgi apparatus	[13,67–70]
	UL142	Retention of MICA in cis-Golgi apparatus	[25,71,72]
	US9	Targets MICA *008 for degradation	[73]
	US12, US13, US18, US20	Target MICA, MICB and ULBP2 for degradation	[74,75]
	miR-UL112	Targets 3′ UTR of MICA and MICB transcripts, causing mRNA destabilisation	[37,89]
	miR-US25-2-3p	Downregulation of TIMP3, causing increasing shedding by ADAM17 and MMP14 Shedding	[93]
VZV	Unknown	Downregulation of ULBP2 and ULBP3 by unknown mechanism	[76]
HSV-1	Late viral gene product(s)	Downregulation of MICA, ULBP1, ULBP2 and ULBP3 (cell-dependent) at a post-translational stage	[76,77]
	miR-H8	Disrupts expression of GPI-anchoring machinery, reducing ULBP2 and ULBP3 surface expression	[92]
HHV-7	U21	Targets ULBP1 for degradation and downregulates MICA and MICB by unknown mechanism	[78]
HHV-6	Early viral gene product(s)	Targets MICB, ULBP1 and ULBP3 for degradation	[79]

Table 1. *Cont.*

Virus	Immunoevasin	Mechanism	Reference
KSHV	K5	Ubiquitinylates MICA, causing redistribution from surface	[80]
	miR-K12-7	Targets 3′ UTR of MICB transcripts, causing mRNA destabilisation	[90]
EBV	miR-BART2-5p	Targets 3′ UTR of MICB transcripts, causing mRNA destabilisation	[90]
HBV	HBx	Forms complex with GATA-2/3 to repress MICA and MICB transcription	[83]
	HBc	Binds to CpG islands in MICA/B promoters to repress transcription	[83]
HCV	NS3/4a	Decreases MICA and MICB by unknown mechanism	[81]
	NS5a	Stimulates immunosuppressive cytokine production and NKG2D receptor downregulation	[96]
Ad5	E3/19K	Retention of MICA and MICB in ER	[82]
HIV-1	Nef	Downregulation of MICA, ULBP1 and ULBP2	[84]
	Vif	Degradation of A3G, preventing DDR-mediated NKG2DL expression	[88]
	Unknown	Shedding of MICA, MICB and ULBP2 by host MMP shedding	[94]
VSV	Unknown	Unknown (post-transcriptional)	[86]
VV	EL3	Prevents detection of dsRNA viral genome from PRRs	[87]
PyVs (JCV and BK)	miR-J1-3p	Targets 3′ UTR of ULBP3 mRNA and prevents translation	[91]
ZPXV	OMCP	Antagonism of NKG2D receptor	[95]

Murine cytomegalovirus (MCMV), human cytomegalovirus (HCMV), varicella-zoster virus (VZV), herpes simplex virus-1 (HSV-1), human herpesvirus (HHV), Kaposi's sarcoma-associated herpesvirus (KSHV), Epstein-Barr virus (EBV), hepatitis B virus (HBV), hepatitis C virus (HCV), adenovirus serotype 5 (Ad5), human immunodeficiency virus-1 (HIV-1), vesicular stomatitis virus (VSV), vaccinia virus (VV), polyomavirus (PyV), zoonotic orthopoxvirus (ZPXV).

5. NKG2DL Expression in Transformed Cells

Early observations that tumour cell lines were killed by NK cells and T cells lead to the discovery of the NKG2D receptor and its ligands [6]. Various studies revealed tumour cells induced to express RAE-1 and H60 proteins resulted in tumour rejection in mice in an NK cell-dependent manner [18,98–100]. The importance of NKG2D immune surveillance has been made clear in NKG2D-deficient mouse models, which spontaneously developed cancer much more than wild type mice [101].

5.1. Tumours Upregulate NKG2DLs via Chronic DDR

Increased NKG2DL expression has been reported in many human cancers including leukaemia [102], colorectal carcinoma [103], hepatocellular carcinoma [104], melanoma [105], pancreatic carcinoma [106], breast carcinoma [107] and glioma [108].

Active DNA damage responses have been identified in cells undergoing the early stages of tumourigenesis in precursor lesions, including phosphorylated histone H2AX, p53 and kinases ATM and Chk2 [109,110]. These activated proteins are part of the DNA damage checkpoint, which can trigger cell cycle arrest or apoptosis of these cells undergoing the first stages of transformation to prevent tumourigenesis. Gasser et al. provided a mechanistic link between this DNA damage response and immune surveillance of premalignant lesions by the upregulation of NKG2DLs. By using various genotoxic stressors on both mouse and human non-tumour cell lines to induce an ATM/ATR-mediated DNA damage checkpoint, they demonstrated increased NKG2DL expression. This upregulation could be abrogated by specific inhibition of this DNA damage checkpoint. Furthermore, they suggest that established tumour cells sustain their increased NKG2DL expression due to chronic activation of the DNA damage checkpoint [32].

A further link between DNA damage in cancer cells and NKG2DL expression was later made with the observation that doxycyclin-inducible wild type (but not a DNA-binding mutant variant) p53 mediated ULBP1 and ULBP2 surface upregulation via increased levels of mRNA transcription in p53-null human non-small cell lung cancer cells [35].

Detection of cytosolic dsDNA by PRRs is critical in triggering the innate immune response towards cytosolic DNA, either of viral origin, or because of DNA damage associated with cancer cells. Cytosolic dsDNA is detected and bound to by the enzyme cGAS, which synthesises the soluble secondary messenger cyclic-GMP-AMP (cGAMP). cGAMP molecules then potently activate stimulator of interferon genes protein (STING), leading to phosphorylation of IFN regulatory factor (IRF) 3. Activated pIRF3 then causes transcriptional upregulation of type I IFN genes and triggers innate immune responses [111]. A study using mouse lymphoma cell lines demonstrated that the DDR in cancer cells resulted in cytosolic dsDNA, which activated the cGAS-STING pathway, triggering an IRF3-dependent induction of RAE-1 ligands [112].

5.2. NKG2DLs Are Upregulated in Tumours through Deregulation of the Cell Cycle and Activated Cell Signalling

Excessive and dysregulated cell cycle entry is a feature of cancer cells. E2F transcription factors play a crucial role in regulating the transition from G1 phase to S phase and entering the cell cycle. Studies using proliferating mouse cancer cells, as well as normal primary murine fibroblasts induced to proliferate, and other highly proliferative tissues demonstrated that the proliferative signals in these cells induced increased transcription of *Raet1e* [113]. This increased transcription was dependent on E2F transcription factors, which have binding sites in the *Raet1e* promoter [113].

The PI3K pathway is a key regulator of cell survival and proliferation, and is commonly activated in the early stages of tumourigenesis [114]. PI3K activation is involved in maintaining sustained expression of RAE-1 and MULT1 in transformed mouse cell lines [60]. However, the activation of the PI3K pathway alone was not sufficient to induce expression in cells, suggesting other factors also influenced expression [60]. In line with this evidence, c-Myc activity (downstream of PI3K pathway) is involved in NKG2DL expression during early stages of tumourigenesis in a spontaneously developing murine lymphoma model [115].

As mentioned earlier, UVB stress-induced EGFR signalling can cause MICA, MICB and ULBP2 upregulation in human epithelial cells [36]. Given the EGFR signalling pathway is commonly hyperactivated in human cancers, and the positive correlation between EGFR and NKG2DL expression in human carcinomas [36]. This may highlight another mechanism in which cancer cell phenotypes induce NKG2DL expression.

6. Cancer Strategies to Evade NKG2D

As observed with a variety of different viruses, there is also a significant selective pressure for immune evasion in to cells undergoing malignant transformation, and effective immune evasion is now recognised as one of the hallmarks of cancer [1].

Given this selective pressure applied to cancer cells, it is unsurprising that, similarly to several viral infections, many cancers also acquire mechanisms to promote immune escape by modulating the NKG2D response. For example, experimentally induced tumour cells were positive for RAE-1 protein expression in perforin-deficient mice, whereas expression was low or absent in WT mice [116], indicating a selection pressure exerted by the immune system for cancer cells to reduce or lose expression of NKG2DLs.

6.1. Loss of NKG2DLs May Be Involved in Metastatic Progression

Cancer stage progression has also been linked to NKG2DL expression in uveal melanoma patients. In a study by Vetter et al., half of the primary tumours sampled were positive for MICA/B, yet all metastatic lesions were absent for MICA/B, suggesting an involvement of the loss of MIC expression in tumour progression and metastasis [117].

6.2. Downregulation of NKG2Ds on Immune Cells by Cell-Bound and Soluble NKG2DLs

Groh and colleagues made an early observation in patients with a range of human epithelial tumours, including breast, lung, ovarian, colon and melanoma, that NKG2D receptor expression was significantly decreased on $CD8^+$ tumour-infiltrating lymphocytes (TILs), NK cells and $\gamma\delta$ T cells in patients with tumours positive for MIC [118]. By coculturing PBMCs with B cells transfected with MICA or MICB, they noted that surface NKG2D expression was significantly decreased on $CD8^+$ T cells compared to PBMCs cocultured with un-transfected controls after 48 h. Additionally, they noted that total NKG2D receptor expression was decreased in these PBMCs, suggesting protein recycling from the cell surface and degradation. Subsequent treatments with bafilomycin A1 or chloroquine (inhibitors of lysosomal acidification and protein degradation) prevented the decrease in total protein. They concluded that surface NKG2D protein was recycled and degraded upon interaction with MICA or MICB positive cells, in a process of ligand-induced recycling in a manner similar to CD28 and TCR-CD3 complexes, following antigenic stimulation [119,120].

However, Groh and colleagues observed a similar decrease in surface and total NKG2D receptor expression in circulating PBMCs, not just those in the tumour, in patients with MIC-positive tumours. This observation ruled out the possibility that this downregulation was solely due to interactions with NKG2DL-expressing cancer cells. They subsequently discovered that the patients with MIC-positive tumours and low NKG2D receptor expression on TILs and PBMCs had soluble MIC (sMIC) A and sMICB in their blood sera, but patients with MIC-negative tumours did not. Treatment of $CD8^+$ T cells with recombinant sMICA recreated the NKG2D receptor decrease [118]. This observation of epithelial tumours shedding NKG2DLs was one of the first immune evasion mechanisms of the NKG2D system to be discovered.

Shed NKG2DLs in the form of sMICA and sMICB have not only been observed in epithelial cancer patients, but also haematopoietic malignancies such as leukaemia [102]. Strikingly, in a comprehensive analysis of 205 leukaemia patients, all patient sera contained soluble NKG2DLs [121].

6.3. Mechanisms of NKG2DL Shedding by Tumour Cells

Investigations into the mechanisms of NKG2DL shedding have revealed this process is mediated by metalloproteases on the surface of the cancer cells, and that shedding can be inhibited with the addition of metalloprotease inhibitors [122]. Various metalloproteases have been implicated in NKG2DL shedding, particularly enzymes from the ADAM family, specifically ADAM10 and ADAM17 being responsible for MICA [123] and MICB cleavage [124]. Additional evidence suggests the thioreductase activity of ER protein 5 (ERp5) is also required for MICA shedding [125]. Furthermore, MICA and MICB shedding from a range of tumour cell lines was attributed to either or both ADAM10 and ADAM17, but the regulation of this process was different depending on the cancer cell lines tested [126]. Additionally, genotoxic stressors such as doxorubicin and melphalan have been demonstrated to upregulate ADAM10 activity on multiple myeloma cells, resulting in increased MIC shedding [127].

In contrast to the reported ADAM10 and ADAM17 activity for MICA/B shedding, MMP14 has been demonstrated to cause MICA shedding in prostate and breast cancer cell lines, independent of ADAM activity [128]. Additionally, studies on malignant glioma cells revealed that only ULBP2 was shed via ADAM10 and ADAM17 activity [129]. Similar observations have also been seen with glioma stem-like cells, with ADAM10- and ADAM17-dependent shedding of ULBP2 [130].

These discrepancies observed in the precise mechanisms and enzymes involved in NKG2DL shedding are likely to be due to the heterogeneities between the various cancer cells and cell lines used in the experimental models, as well as the allelic heterogeneity within the population. However, it does reveal a degree of complexity in the regulation of NKG2DL shedding.

Interestingly, the most common allele for MICA, MICA*008, which features a different transmembrane region and a truncated cytoplasmic tail compared to other alleles, is shed in a protease-independent manner. Instead of being shed by proteolytic cleavage at the cell surface, MICA*008 is released from cancer cells within the membranes of exosomes. These MICA*008-containing exosomes are still able to downregulate the NKG2D receptor on NK cells [131]. The selection of an allele for MICA in the population, which is resistant both to viral MICA-binding proteins as well as proteolytic cleavage by host cell metalloproteases upregulated in cancers, may highlight another example of human evolution to bypass cancer and virus-mediated immune evasion. However, cancer shedding of MICA*008 via exosome secretion appears to be one way in which cancers have adapted to circumvent this.

6.4. Soluble NKG2DLs Affect Other Immune Cell Types

While sMIC has been shown to decrease surface expression of NKG2D receptors on CD8$^+$ T cells and NK cells, Xiao et al. demonstrated that mouse bone marrow cells differentiated into myeloid-derived suppressor cells (MSDCs) when treated with sMIC, while macrophages differentiated into 'alternatively' activated immunosuppressive macrophages [132]. This suggests tumour shedding of MIC not only directly enables immune evasion on a systemic level by global downregulation of NKG2D receptors on PBMCs and TILs, but also helps to establish an immunosuppressive tumour microenvironment through the repolarisation of myeloid cells.

Interestingly, Deng et al. provided evidence in contrast to the concept that soluble NKG2DLs exclusively suppress NK cell activity by downregulating NKG2D receptor [133]. These new findings led to the proposal that soluble MULT1 (sMULT1) actually enhanced NK cell-mediated tumour rejection. This was attributed to high affinity sMULT1 being able to bind to NKG2D receptors on NK cells, out-competing the binding of lower affinity NKG2DLs expressed by tumour-associated myeloid cells which would trigger NKG2D receptor downregulation, similarly to sNKG2DLs [133].

6.5. Tumours Use miRNAs to Downregulate NKG2DL Expression at the Post-Transcriptional Level

The use of miRNAs to regulate the stability of MICA/B mRNA transcripts has already been mentioned in the context of healthy and stressed cells, and that HCMV miRNA-UL112 exploits this system to enable immune evasion. This strategy has also been implicated in cancer immune evasion. Cellular miRNAs such as miR-20a, miR-93 and miR-106b which bind to the 3′ UTRs of MICA/B transcripts are upregulated in many human cancers, and are responsible for the downregulation in MICA and MICB protein [37]. Interestingly, some of these same cellular miRNAs had already been identified as cancer-associated miRNAs, with involvement in other pro-tumour processes in cancers, including breast cancer [134] and leukaemia [135]. Various other examples include: miR-10b, a metastasis-associated miRNA, which targets MICB transcripts in breast cancer cell lines [136]; miR-20a targets MICA and MICB transcripts, and also inhibits the MAPK/ERK pathway to downregulate ULBP2 in breast cancer [137]; miR-34a and miR-34c downregulate ULBP2 [38]; miR-93, miR-20a and miR-106b reduced expression of MICA, MICB, ULBP2 and ULBP3 in glioma cells [138]; and miR-889 which targets MICB transcripts in hepatocellular carcinoma cells [139]. Interestingly, both miR-20a [137] and miR-889 [139] expression decreased upon treatment with histone deacetylase (HDAC) inhibitors, resulting in an increase in NKG2DLs. These findings may provide some mechanistic insight as to why HDAC inhibitors increase cancer cell susceptibility to NK cell lysis [140].

6.6. Other Strategies Used by Tumours Subvert the NKG2D Immune Response

Other mechanisms to downregulate NKG2DL expression by cancer cells have also been observed. Isocitrate dehydrogenase (IDH) is mutated in many glioma patients and results in the production of the oncometabolite 2-hydroxyglutarate (2-HG). 2-HG inhibits histone demethylases and can cause epigenetic hypermethylation [141]. In primary human glioma stem-like cell lines, IDH mutated cells led to NKG2DLs becoming transcriptionally silenced as a result of 2-HG accumulation [142].

While some tumours intervene in NKG2DL expression before the protein translation stage, examples from melanoma cell lines and patient-derived metastases revealed a strategy more similar to that observed by viruses: intracellular retention of NKG2DL proteins [143]. These cells lacked surface MICA expression but still expressed intracellular protein, which was accumulated in the ER before being transported back to the cytoplasm for proteasomal degradation [143].

Cytokines in the tumour microenvironment can also influence immune evasion via the NKG2D system. TGF-β expressed by glioma cells enables immune evasion from the NKG2D system in several ways: (1) downregulation of NKG2DLs on the surface of glioma cells by inhibiting MICA, ULBP2 and ULBP4 transcription [144,145], (2) increased expression of inhibitory receptor CD94/NKG2A to prevent NK cell activation [144], and (3) downregulation of NKG2D receptors on CD8$^+$ T cells and NK cells [146]. These findings suggest that TGF-β produced by glioma cells acts in both an autocrine and paracrine modality to mediate immune evasion from NK cells and CD8$^+$ T cells. Additionally, Eisele et al. demonstrated by immunohistochemistry of gliomas that MICA and ULBP2 expression is inversely correlated with WHO grade of malignancy, although tumour expression was significantly higher than normal brain [145]. Furthermore, although TGF-β signalling increases metalloproteinase expression on glioma cells [147], the increased shedding of MICA and ULBP2 by glioma cells was not due to TGF-β-dependent metalloproteinases [145].

Further examples of cancer cells subverting the anti-cancer immune response by secretion of soluble factors have been observed in glioblastoma patients. Glioblastoma cells were found to express lactate dehydrogenase (LDH) isoform 5, which induced the expression of NKG2DLs on autologous tumour infiltrating myeloid cells and circulating monocytes in patients, as well as on monocytes isolated from healthy individuals [148]. These myeloid cells expressing NKG2DLs behaved similarly to soluble ligands upon interaction with NK cells and resulted in NKG2D receptor downregulation [148].

Surprisingly, pro-inflammatory IFNs appear to play a role in NKG2DL expression. Bui et al. reported that either IFN-γ or IFN-α reduced H60 expression on 3′methylchloanthrene sarcomas in mice [149]. Additionally, Zhang et al. reported IFN-α increased MICA expression, meanwhile IFN-γ decreased MICA expression in various human cancer cell lines, including cervical cancer and erythroleukemia, by promoting MMP-mediated shedding of MICA [150]. Furthermore, IFN-γ decreased transcription of MICA, ULBP1 and ULBP2 in patient-derived melanoma and glioma cell lines in a dose- and time-dependent fashion [151]. Investigations into the mechanism of this IFN-γ-mediated downregulation revealed that IFN-γ induced the expression of miR-520b, a miRNA that targets the 3′ UTR of MICA mRNA transcripts in a range of cancer cell lines including melanoma, HeLa, breast and colorectal [152]. It has been speculated that the downregulation of NKG2DLs in response to IFN-γ may be a regulatory mechanism that allows switching from innate immune surveillance via NKG2DLs to adaptive immune responses via MHC and T cells [149].

7. Viral and Cancer Immune Evasion Strategies Converge on the NKG2D Response

The focus of this review is to bring attention to the similarities between virus and cancer immune evasion via the NKG2D system. Several viruses from a wide range of viral families use strategies to interfere with the key stages in the pathway, ranging from avoiding initial detection by PRRs, to transcriptional repression, mRNA stabilisation, NKG2DL protein stability and cellular localisation, shedding from the protein surface and subversion of the subsequent immune response. Several different cancers also interfere with many of these critical stages, sharing a striking similarity with viral immune evasion (Figure 2).

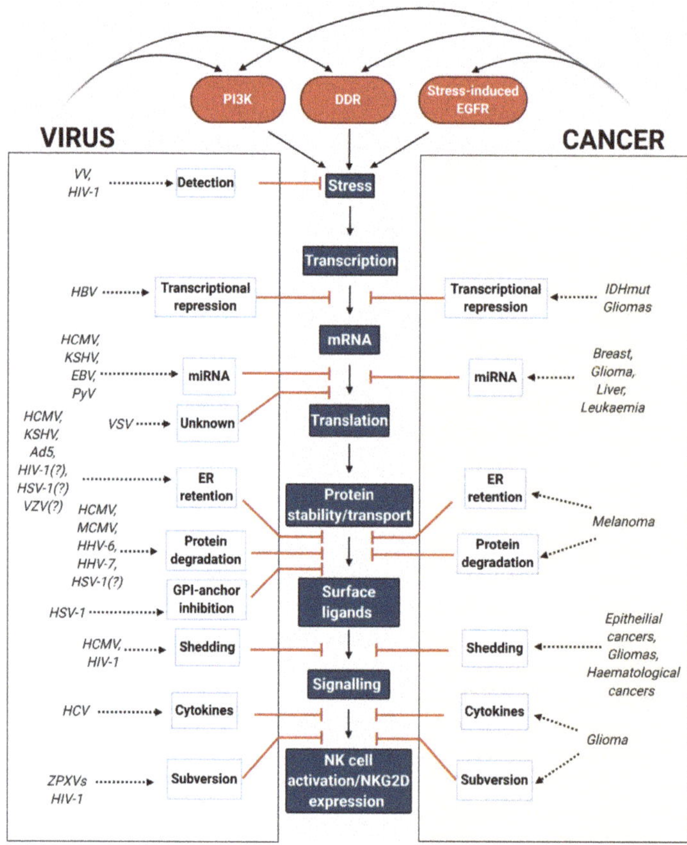

Figure 2. Converging evolution of viruses and cancers to interfere with the NKG2D immune response. Viruses and cancers induce various signalling pathways that induce natural killer group 2 member D ligand (NKG2DL) expression, including the phosphatidylinositol 3-kinase (PI3K) pathway, DNA damage response (DDR) and stress-induced epidermal growth factor receptor (EGFR) signalling. Various viruses and cancers interfere with the key stages in NKG2DL expression, including detection of stress, transcription, mRNA stability, translation, protein stability and transport, surface protein levels, NKG2D signalling and immune cell subversion. Vaccinia virus (VV), human immunodeficiency virus-1 (HIV-1), hepatitis B virus (HBV), human cytomegalovirus (HCMV), murine cytomegalovirus (MCMV), Kaposi's sarcoma-associated herpesvirus (KSHV), Epstein-Barr virus (EBV), polyomavirus (PyV), vesicular stomatitis virus (VSV), adenovirus serotype 5 (Ad5), herpes simplex virus-1 (HSV-1), varicella-zoster virus (VZV), human herpesvirus (HHV), hepatitis C virus (HCV), zoonotic orthopoxvirus (ZPXV). Diagram created with BioRender.com.

Viruses can use an expansive toolkit to achieve immune evasion, using wholly new proteins or miRNAs acquired through countless generations of evolution that are well-suited to carry out their specific task. However, cancers must make use of a relatively limited toolkit in comparison to achieve the same goal, as they are constrained by a shorter evolutionary timeframe, and must rely on proteins or miRNAs already encoded in their genomes, or slight variations thereof. Therefore, cancers must find ways to manipulate their toolkit, turning tools which normally serve the cell, tissue, and organism, into tools which enable cancer survival. This observation is highlighted by the abundance and variety of viral proteins that are unique to those viruses, which directly bind to, interfere with, or degrade NKG2DLs. Meanwhile, cancers appear to have a reliance on the tools already available to them, albeit by dysregulating them, such as upregulating cellular miRNAs to destabilise mRNA transcripts, or by activating surface proteases to increase NKG2DL shedding. Given the differences in the tools available at their disposal, is perhaps surprising to see such a high degree of functional convergence between the immune evasion strategies of both viruses and cancers.

8. Strategies Employed by the Immune System to Counter Viral and Tumour Immune Evasion

In parallel to the selection pressures exerted on viral and tumour evolution, they impart their own selection pressure on the immune system, driven by the necessity to constantly adapt and counter immune evasion tactics employed by pathogens and cancers. While viruses and cancer cells develop ways to downregulate or subvert the NKG2D response, the immune system has developed various means to counteract.

For example, using a family of multiple different ligands that are all capable of binding to the NKG2D receptor endows certain advantages to the organism. It enables a degree of functional redundancy, in which various signals and pathways induce the expression of different ligands, all of which converge on binding to NKG2D and bringing about a similar immune response [153]. However, evidence is emerging to suggest that NKG2DLs are non-redundant, and that induced expression of certain ligands reflects a specific danger signal and threat [154]. For example, ULBP1 expression positively correlates with leukaemia sensitivity to NKG2D-mediated lysis by $\gamma\delta$ T cells, and loss of ULBP1 conferred resistance to lysis, whereas MICA downregulation did not [155]. Although specific pathways may induce the expression of certain ligands, the pathways themselves tend to be shared by a general cellular phenotype that reflects danger: either stress, infection, or neoplastic transformation. Furthermore, ligand diversity makes total immune evasion as a result of viral gene products or a mutation during malignant transformation far more unlikely [153,154].

In addition to the range of different NKG2DLs, they are also some of the most polymorphic genes in humans. Different ligands, and even different alleles can change the extent of NKG2D receptor signalling. For example, the MICA-129Met variant has a far greater binding affinity to NKG2D compared to the MICA 129Val isoform, and results in stronger signalling and faster activation kinetics [22]. Conversely however, the ULBP0602 isoform has a greater binding affinity compared to other isoforms, but resulted in reduced NKG2D-mediated activation [23]. These findings suggest different polymorphisms of NKG2DLs in the population that differ in binding affinities may influence the intensity of the immune response towards the target cell.

Further evidence for the evolution of the NKG2D system being driven by viruses is the MICA*008 allele, which lacks the cytoplasmic tail and thus cannot be bound and downregulated by HCMV UL142 protein [25,72]. The prevalence of this allele in the human population may highlight the selective advantage of this allele in conferring resistance to HCMV infection.

9. Conclusions and Outlook

Cancer immunotherapy is a rapidly advancing field, with vast potential for using the patient's own immune system, or genetically engineered immune cells to eradicate the tumours at multiple sites throughout the body. Given NKG2DLs are expressed by many different cancer cells, they appear as an attractive 'pan-cancer' antigen to target using immunotherapies, and could circumvent issues with other immunotherapies associated with tumour heterogeneity and loss of MHC class I expression in tumours. This strategy has already been pursued, such as by the use of NKG2D chimeric antigen receptor (CAR) T cells, with evidence of efficacy even in heterogeneous tumours in vivo [156]. Furthermore, NKG2D-targeted immunotherapies may combine advantageously with conventional therapies which further induce NKG2DL expression. For example, Weiss and colleagues demonstrated synergy between radiotherapy and NKG2D CAR T cells in murine glioblastoma models [157]. However, more understanding of NKG2DL expression in non-tumour cells is needed, given some on-target, off-tumour toxicities have been observed using NKG2D-CAR T cells [158].

Asides from using engineered immune cells, other strategies have been investigated to enhance natural innate immune responses towards tumour cells expressing NKG2DLs. Techniques to inhibit proteolytic shedding of NKG2DLs, using chemical inhibitors [159,160] or antibodies which block the proteolytic cleavage site [161], have been explored. Additionally, antibodies to neutralise sMIC, preventing NKG2D receptor downregulation have also been investigated [162]. These are particularly attractive strategies and may work together in concert with NKG2D CAR T cells or other NKG2D-targeting cell therapies.

Oncolytic virotherapy (OVT) is a rapidly developing area for cancer immunotherapy. OVT uses modified viruses that selectively infect and replicate within cancer cells, causing lytic cancer cell death [163]. Many different viruses are being investigated for use as OVT, including adenovirus [164], HSV-1 [165] and VSV [86]. A notable example being an oncolytic HSV-1, Talimogene laherparevec (T-VEC), which gained FDA approval in 2015 [166]. As well as their ability for direct tumour lysis [167], oncolytic viruses can also be used as gene therapy vectors, delivering therapeutic agents in situ in the tumour. OVT for the treatment of cancer represents a cross-over between viruses and cancers. Targeting shared strategies of viral and cancer immune evasion of the NKG2D immune response could therefore provide significant, or even synergistic efficacy. One specific example could be to use the oncolytic virus as a gene therapy vector to deliver small interfering RNA (siRNA) within the cancer cell, knocking down ADAM10 and ADAM17 expression, and thus prevent NKG2DL shedding. The cumulative effects of heightened NKG2DL expression normally associated with cancer cells, alongside virus-induced NKG2DL expression, with further siRNA-mediated inhibition of NKG2DL shedding could drastically increase the likelihood of immune detection and cancer cell lysis.

As the field of immunology ever advances and we understand more about the similarities between viral and cancer immune evasion, we may gain further insight into new potential strategies to exploit the NKG2D system for anti-cancer therapy. Furthermore, NKG2DL-targeting therapies used for cancer treatment may even have a possible benefit for antiviral therapy.

Author Contributions: Conceptualization, R.B.; writing—original draft preparation, R.B.; writing—review and editing, R.B., H.K. and L.W.S.; supervision, L.W.S. All authors have read and agreed to the published version of the manuscript.

Funding: This research was funded by Brain Research UK, grant number STU1617-02 (doctoral studentship to R.B) and Cancer Research UK, grant number C552/A29106 (to H.K.).

Acknowledgments: The author is grateful to past and present members of the Seymour lab for their helpful discussion, feedback, and advice during the writing of this review.

Conflicts of Interest: The authors declare no conflict of interest.

References

1. Hanahan, D.; Weinberg, R.A. Hallmarks of Cancer: The Next Generation. *Cell* **2011**, *144*, 646–674. [CrossRef]
2. Barrow, A.D.; Martin, C.J.; Colonna, M. The natural cytotoxicity receptors in health and disease. *Front. Immunol.* **2019**, *10*, 1–20. [CrossRef] [PubMed]
3. Kärre, K.; Ljunggren, H.G.; Piontek, G.; Kiessling, R. Selective rejection of H–2-deficient lymphoma variants suggests alternative immune defence strategy. *Nature* **1986**, *319*, 675–678. [CrossRef] [PubMed]
4. Raulet, D.H. Roles of the NKG2D immunoreceptor and its ligands. *Nat. Rev. Immunol.* **2003**, *3*, 781–790. [CrossRef] [PubMed]

5. Allez, M.; Tieng, V.; Nakazawa, A.; Treton, X.; Pacault, V.; Dulphy, N.; Caillat–Zucman, S.; Paul, P.; Gornet, J.; Douay, C.; et al. CD4+NKG2D+ T Cells in Crohn's Disease Mediate Inflammatory and Cytotoxic Responses Through MICA Interactions. *Gastroenterology* **2007**, *132*, 2346–2358. [CrossRef]

6. Bauer, S. Activation of NK Cells and T Cells by NKG2D, a Receptor for Stress-Inducible MICA. *Science* **1999**, *285*, 727–729. [CrossRef] [PubMed]

7. Mukherjee, S.; Jensen, H.; Stewart, W.; Stewart, D.; Ray, W.C.; Chen, S.-Y.; Nolan, G.P.; Lanier, L.L.; Das, J. In silico modeling identifies CD45 as a regulator of IL-2 synergy in the NKG2D-mediated activation of immature human NK cells. *Sci. Signal.* **2017**, *10*, eaai9062. [CrossRef]

8. Horng, T.; Bezbradica, J.S.; Medzhitov, R. NKG2D signaling is coupled to the interleukin 15 receptor signaling pathway. *Nat. Immunol.* **2007**, *8*, 1345–1352. [CrossRef]

9. Groh, V.; Rhinehart, R.; Randolph-Habecker, J.; Topp, M.S.; Riddell, S.R.; Spies, T. Costimulation of CD8αβ T cells by NKG2D via engagement by MIC induced on virus-infected cells. *Nat. Immunol.* **2001**, *2*, 255–260. [CrossRef]

10. Bryceson, Y.T.; Ljunggren, H.-G.; Long, E.O. Minimal requirement for induction of natural cytotoxicity and intersection of activation signals by inhibitory receptors. *Blood* **2009**, *114*, 2657–2666. [CrossRef]

11. Lanier, L.L. NK CELL RECOGNITION. *Annu. Rev. Immunol.* **2005**, *23*, 225–274. [CrossRef] [PubMed]

12. Groh, V.; Bahram, S.; Bauer, S.; Herman, A.; Beauchamp, M.; Spies, T. Cell stress-regulated human major histocompatibility complex class I gene expressed in gastrointestinal epithelium. *Proc. Natl. Acad. Sci. USA* **1996**, *93*, 12445–12450. [CrossRef] [PubMed]

13. Cosman, D.; Müllberg, J.; Sutherland, C.L.; Chin, W.; Armitage, R.; Fanslow, W.; Kubin, M.; Chalupny, N.J. ULBPs, Novel MHC Class I–Related Molecules, Bind to CMV Glycoprotein UL16 and Stimulate NK Cytotoxicity through the NKG2D Receptor. *Immunity* **2001**, *14*, 123–133. [CrossRef]

14. Jan Chalupny, N.; Sutherland, C.L.; Lawrence, W.A.; Rein-Weston, A.; Cosman, D. ULBP4 is a novel ligand for human NKG2D. *Biochem. Biophys. Res. Commun.* **2003**, *305*, 129–135. [CrossRef]

15. Cao, W.; Xi, X.; Wang, Z.; Dong, L.; Hao, Z.; Cui, L.; Ma, C.; He, W. Four novel ULBP splice variants are ligands for human NKG2D. *Int. Immunol.* **2008**, *20*, 981–991. [CrossRef] [PubMed]

16. Bacon, L.; Eagle, R.A.; Meyer, M.; Easom, N.; Young, N.T.; Trowsdale, J. Two Human ULBP/RAET1 Molecules with Transmembrane Regions Are Ligands for NKG2D. *J. Immunol.* **2004**, *173*, 1078–1084. [CrossRef]

17. Eagle, R.A.; Traherne, J.A.; Hair, J.R.; Jafferji, I.; Trowsdale, J. ULBP6/RAET1L is an additional human NKG2D ligand. *Eur. J. Immunol.* **2009**, *39*, 3207–3216. [CrossRef]

18. Cerwenka, A.; Bakker, A.B.; McClanahan, T.; Wagner, J.; Wu, J.; Phillips, J.H.; Lanier, L.L. Retinoic Acid Early Inducible Genes Define a Ligand Family for the Activating NKG2D Receptor in Mice. *Immunity* **2000**, *12*, 721–727. [CrossRef]

19. Carayannopoulos, L.N.; Naidenko, O.V.; Fremont, D.H.; Yokoyama, W.M. Cutting Edge: Murine UL16-Binding Protein-Like Transcript 1: A Newly Described Transcript Encoding a High-Affinity Ligand for Murine NKG2D. *J. Immunol.* **2002**, *169*, 4079–4083. [CrossRef]

20. Raulet, D.H.; Gasser, S.; Gowen, B.G.; Deng, W.; Jung, H. Regulation of Ligands for the NKG2D Activating Receptor. *Annu. Rev. Immunol.* **2013**, *31*, 413–441. [CrossRef]

21. HLA Nomenclature @ hla.alleles.org. Available online: http://hla.alleles.org/proteins/classo.html (accessed on 10 November 2020).

22. Isernhagen, A.; Malzahn, D.; Bickeböller, H.; Dressel, R. Impact of the MICA-129Met/val dimorphism on NKG2D-mediated biological functions and disease risks. *Front. Immunol.* **2016**, *7*, 1–9. [CrossRef] [PubMed]

23. Zuo, J.; Willcox, C.R.; Mohammed, F.; Davey, M.; Hunter, S.; Khan, K.; Antoun, A.; Katakia, P.; Croudace, J.; Inman, C.; et al. A disease-linked ULBP6 polymorphism inhibits NKG2D-mediated target cell killing by enhancing the stability of NKG2D ligand binding. *Sci. Signal.* **2017**, *10*, eaai8904. [CrossRef] [PubMed]

24. Zhang, Y.; Lazaro, A.M.; Lavingia, B.; Stastny, P. Typing for all known MICA alleles by group-specific PCR and SSOP. *Hum. Immunol.* **2001**, *62*, 620–631. [CrossRef]

25. Chalupny, N.J.; Rein-Weston, A.; Dosch, S.; Cosman, D. Down-regulation of the NKG2D ligand MICA by the human cytomegalovirus glycoprotein UL142. *Biochem. Biophys. Res. Commun.* **2006**, *346*, 175–181. [CrossRef]

26. Lodoen, M.B.; Lanier, L.L. Viral modulation of NK cell immunity. *Nat. Rev. Microbiol.* **2005**, *3*, 59–69. [CrossRef]

27. Schrambach, S.; Ardizzone, M.; Leymarie, V.; Sibilia, J.; Bahram, S. In Vivo Expression Pattern of MICA and MICB and Its Relevance to Auto-Immunity and Cancer. *PLoS ONE* **2007**, *2*, e518. [CrossRef]

28. Groh, V. Recognition of Stress-Induced MHC Molecules by Intestinal Epithelial T Cells. *Science* **1998**, *279*, 1737–1740. [CrossRef]

29. Venkataraman, G.M.; Suciu, D.; Groh, V.; Boss, J.M.; Spies, T. Promoter Region Architecture and Transcriptional Regulation of the Genes for the MHC Class I-Related Chain A and B Ligands of NKG2D. *J. Immunol.* **2007**, *178*, 961–969. [CrossRef]

30. Yamamoto, K. Oxidative stress increases MICA and MICB gene expression in the human colon carcinoma cell line (CaCo-2). *Biochim. Biophys. Acta—Gen. Subj.* **2001**, *1526*, 10–12. [CrossRef]

31. Hosomi, S.; Grootjans, J.; Tschurtschenthaler, M.; Krupka, N.; Matute, J.D.; Flak, M.B.; Martinez-Naves, E.; del Moral, M.G.; Glickman, J.N.; Ohira, M.; et al. Intestinal epithelial cell endoplasmic reticulum stress promotes MULT1 up-regulation and NKG2D-mediated inflammation. *J. Exp. Med.* **2017**, *214*, 2985–2997. [CrossRef]

32. Gasser, S.; Orsulic, S.; Brown, E.J.; Raulet, D.H. The DNA damage pathway regulates innate immune system ligands of the NKG2D receptor. *Nature* **2005**, *436*, 1186–1190. [CrossRef] [PubMed]

33. Soriani, A.; Iannitto, M.L.; Ricci, B.; Fionda, C.; Malgarini, G.; Morrone, S.; Peruzzi, G.; Ricciardi, M.R.; Petrucci, M.T.; Cippitelli, M.; et al. Reactive Oxygen Species– and DNA Damage Response–Dependent NK Cell Activating Ligand Upregulation Occurs at Transcriptional Levels and Requires the Transcriptional Factor E2F1. *J. Immunol.* **2014**, *193*, 950–960. [CrossRef] [PubMed]

34. Li, H.; Lakshmikanth, T.; Garofalo, C.; Enge, M.; Spinnler, C.; Anichini, A.; Szekely, L.; Kärre, K.; Carbone, E.; Selivanova, G. Pharmacological activation of p53 triggers anticancer innate immune response through induction of ULBP2. *Cell Cycle* **2011**, *10*, 3346–3358. [CrossRef] [PubMed]

35. Textor, S.; Fiegler, N.; Arnold, A.; Porgador, A.; Hofmann, T.G.; Cerwenka, A. Human NK Cells Are Alerted to Induction of p53 in Cancer Cells by Upregulation of the NKG2D Ligands ULBP1 and ULBP2. *Cancer Res.* **2011**, *71*, 5998–6009. [CrossRef]

36. Vantourout, P.; Willcox, C.; Turner, A.; Swanson, C.M.; Haque, Y.; Sobolev, O.; Grigoriadis, A.; Tutt, A.; Hayday, A. Immunological Visibility: Posttranscriptional Regulation of Human NKG2D Ligands by the EGF Receptor Pathway. *Sci. Transl. Med.* **2014**, *6*, 231ra49. [CrossRef]

37. Stern-Ginossar, N.; Gur, C.; Biton, M.; Horwitz, E.; Elboim, M.; Stanietsky, N.; Mandelboim, M.; Mandelboim, O. Human microRNAs regulate stress-induced immune responses mediated by the receptor NKG2D. *Nat. Immunol.* **2008**, *9*, 1065–1073. [CrossRef]

38. Heinemann, A.; Zhao, F.; Pechlivanis, S.; Eberle, J.; Steinle, A.; Diederichs, S.; Schadendorf, D.; Paschen, A. Tumor suppressive microRNAs miR-34a/c control cancer cell expression of ULBP2, a stress-induced ligand of the natural killer cell receptor NKG2D. *Cancer Res.* **2012**, *72*, 460–471. [CrossRef]

39. Borchers, M.T.; Harris, N.L.; Wesselkamper, S.C.; Vitucci, M.; Cosman, D. NKG2D ligands are expressed on stressed human airway epithelial cells. *Am. J. Physiol. Cell. Mol. Physiol.* **2006**, *291*, L222–L231. [CrossRef]

40. Nice, T.J.; Deng, W.; Coscoy, L.; Raulet, D.H. Stress-Regulated Targeting of the NKG2D Ligand Mult1 by a Membrane-Associated RING-CH Family E3 Ligase. *J. Immunol.* **2010**, *185*, 5369–5376. [CrossRef]

41. Sinclair, A.; Yarranton, S.; Schelcher, C. DNA-damage response pathways triggered by viral replication. *Expert Rev. Mol. Med.* **2006**, *8*, 1–11. [CrossRef]

42. Ward, J.; Davis, Z.; DeHart, J.; Zimmerman, E.; Bosque, A.; Brunetta, E.; Mavilio, D.; Planelles, V.; Barker, E. HIV-1 Vpr Triggers Natural Killer Cell–Mediated Lysis of Infected Cells through Activation of the ATR-Mediated DNA Damage Response. *PLoS Pathog.* **2009**, *5*, e1000613. [CrossRef] [PubMed]

43. Kudoh, A.; Fujita, M.; Zhang, L.; Shirata, N.; Daikoku, T.; Sugaya, Y.; Isomura, H.; Nishiyama, Y.; Tsurumi, T. Epstein-Barr Virus Lytic Replication Elicits ATM Checkpoint Signal Transduction While Providing an S-phase-like Cellular Environment. *J. Biol. Chem.* **2005**, *280*, 8156–8163. [CrossRef] [PubMed]

44. Routes, J.M.; Ryan, S.; Morris, K.; Takaki, R.; Cerwenka, A.; Lanier, L.L. Adenovirus serotype 5 E1A sensitizes tumor cells to NKG2D-dependent NK cell lysis and tumor rejection. *J. Exp. Med.* **2005**, *202*, 1477–1482. [CrossRef] [PubMed]

45. Thai, M.; Graham, N.A.; Braas, D.; Nehil, M.; Komisopoulou, E.; Kurdistani, S.K.; McCormick, F.; Graeber, T.G.; Christofk, H.R. Adenovirus E4ORF1-Induced MYC Activation Promotes Host Cell Anabolic Glucose Metabolism and Virus Replication. *Cell Metab.* **2014**, *19*, 694–701. [CrossRef]

46. Cooray, S. The pivotal role of phosphatidylinositol 3-kinase-Akt signal transduction in virus survival. *J. Gen. Virol.* **2004**, *85*, 1065–1076. [CrossRef]

47. Johnson, R.A.; Wang, X.; Ma, X.-L.; Huong, S.-M.; Huang, E.-S. Human Cytomegalovirus Up-Regulates the Phosphatidylinositol 3-Kinase (PI3-K) Pathway: Inhibition of PI3-K Activity Inhibits Viral Replication and Virus-Induced Signaling. *J. Virol.* **2001**, *75*, 6022–6032. [CrossRef]

48. Kong, K.; Kumar, M.; Taruishi, M.; Javier, R.T. The Human Adenovirus E4-ORF1 Protein Subverts Discs Large 1 to Mediate Membrane Recruitment and Dysregulation of Phosphatidylinositol 3-Kinase. *PLoS Pathog.* **2014**, *10*, e1004102. [CrossRef]

49. Ren, J.H.; Chen, X.; Zhou, L.; Tao, N.N.; Zhou, H.Z.; Liu, B.; Li, W.Y.; Huang, A.L.; Chen, J. Protective role of Sirtuin3 (SIRT3) in oxidative stress mediated by hepatitis B virus X protein expression. *PLoS ONE* **2016**, *11*, 1–15. [CrossRef]

50. Camini, F.C.; da Silva Caetano, C.C.; Almeida, L.T.; de Brito Magalhães, C.L. Implications of oxidative stress on viral pathogenesis. *Arch. Virol.* **2017**, *162*, 907–917. [CrossRef]

51. Filone, C.M.; Caballero, I.S.; Dower, K.; Mendillo, M.L.; Cowley, G.S.; Santagata, S.; Rozelle, D.K.; Yen, J.; Rubins, K.H.; Hacohen, N.; et al. The Master Regulator of the Cellular Stress Response (HSF1) Is Critical for Orthopoxvirus Infection. *PLoS Pathog.* **2014**, *10*. [CrossRef]

52. Shirata, N.; Kudoh, A.; Daikoku, T.; Tatsumi, Y.; Fujita, M.; Kiyono, T.; Sugaya, Y.; Isomura, H.; Ishizaki, K.; Tsurumi, T. Activation of Ataxia Telangiectasia-mutated DNA Damage Checkpoint Signal Transduction Elicited by Herpes Simplex Virus Infection. *J. Biol. Chem.* **2005**, *280*, 30336–30341. [CrossRef] [PubMed]

53. Carson, C.T. The Mre11 complex is required for ATM activation and the G2/M checkpoint. *EMBO J.* **2003**, *22*, 6610–6620. [CrossRef] [PubMed]

54. Cerboni, C.; Fionda, C.; Soriani, A.; Zingoni, A.; Doria, M.; Cippitelli, M.; Santoni, A. The DNA Damage Response: A Common Pathway in the Regulation of NKG2D and DNAM-1 Ligand Expression in Normal, Infected, and Cancer Cells. *Front. Immunol.* **2014**, *4*, 1–7. [CrossRef] [PubMed]

55. Turnell, A.S.; Grand, R.J. DNA viruses and the cellular DNA-damage response. *J. Gen. Virol.* **2012**, *93*, 2076–2097. [CrossRef]

56. Draghi, M.; Pashine, A.; Sanjanwala, B.; Gendzekhadze, K.; Cantoni, C.; Cosman, D.; Moretta, A.; Valiante, N.M.; Parham, P. NKp46 and NKG2D Recognition of Infected Dendritic Cells Is Necessary for NK Cell Activation in the Human Response to Influenza Infection. *J. Immunol.* **2007**, *178*, 2688–2698. [CrossRef]

57. Fang, M.; Lanier, L.L.; Sigal, L.J. A Role for NKG2D in NK Cell–Mediated Resistance to Poxvirus Disease. *PLoS Pathog.* **2008**, *4*, e30. [CrossRef]

58. Buchkovich, N.J.; Yu, Y.; Zampieri, C.A.; Alwine, J.C. The TORrid affairs of viruses: Effects of mammalian DNA viruses on the PI3K–Akt–mTOR signalling pathway. *Nat. Rev. Microbiol.* **2008**, *6*, 266–275. [CrossRef]

59. Hsu, M.J.; Wu, C.Y.; Chiang, H.H.; Lai, Y.L.; Hung, S.L. PI3K/Akt signaling mediated apoptosis blockage and viral gene expression in oral epithelial cells during herpes simplex virus infection. *Virus Res.* **2010**, *153*, 36–43. [CrossRef]

60. Tokuyama, M.; Lorin, C.; Delebecque, F.; Jung, H.; Raulet, D.H.; Coscoy, L. Expression of the RAE-1 Family of Stimulatory NK-Cell Ligands Requires Activation of the PI3K Pathway during Viral Infection and Transformation. *PLoS Pathog.* **2011**, *7*, e1002265. [CrossRef]

61. Lanier, L.L. Evolutionary struggles between NK cells and viruses. *Nat. Rev. Immunol.* **2008**, *8*, 259–268. [CrossRef]

62. De Pelsmaeker, S.; Romero, N.; Vitale, M.; Favoreel, H.W. Herpesvirus Evasion of Natural Killer Cells. *J. Virol.* **2018**, *92*, 1–19. [CrossRef] [PubMed]

63. Lodoen, M.; Ogasawara, K.; Hamerman, J.A.; Arase, H.; Houchins, J.P.; Mocarski, E.S.; Lanier, L.L. NKG2D-mediated Natural Killer Cell Protection Against Cytomegalovirus Is Impaired by Viral gp40 Modulation of Retinoic Acid Early Inducible 1 Gene Molecules. *J. Exp. Med.* **2003**, *197*, 1245–1253. [CrossRef] [PubMed]

64. Lodoen, M.B.; Abenes, G.; Umamoto, S.; Houchins, J.P.; Liu, F.; Lanier, L.L. The Cytomegalovirus m155 Gene Product Subverts Natural Killer Cell Antiviral Protection by Disruption of H60–NKG2D Interactions. *J. Exp. Med.* **2004**, *200*, 1075–1081. [CrossRef] [PubMed]

65. Krmpotic, A.; Hasan, M.; Loewendorf, A.; Saulig, T.; Halenius, A.; Lenac, T.; Polic, B.; Bubic, I.; Kriegeskorte, A.; Pernjak-Pugel, E.; et al. NK cell activation through the NKG2D ligand MULT-1 is selectively prevented by the glycoprotein encoded by mouse cytomegalovirus gene m145. *J. Exp. Med.* **2005**, *201*, 211–220. [CrossRef] [PubMed]

66. Lenac, T.; Budt, M.; Arapovic, J.; Hasan, M.; Zimmermann, A.; Simic, H.; Krmpotic, A.; Messerle, M.; Ruzsics, Z.; Koszinowski, U.H.; et al. The herpesviral Fc receptor fcr-1 down-regulates the NKG2D ligands MULT-1 and H60. *J. Exp. Med.* **2006**, *203*, 1843–1850. [CrossRef]

67. Valés-Gómez, M.; Browne, H.; Reyburn, H.T. Expression of the UL16 glycoprotein of Human Cytomegalovirus protects the virus-infected cell from attack by natural killer cells. *BMC Immunol.* **2003**, *4*, 4. [CrossRef]

68. Welte, S.A.; Sinzger, C.; Lutz, S.Z.; Singh-Jasuja, H.; Sampaio, K.L.; Eknigk, U.; Rammensee, H.-G.; Steinle, A. Selective intracellular retention of virally induced NKG2D ligands by the human cytomegalovirus UL16 glycoprotein. *Eur. J. Immunol.* **2003**, *33*, 194–203. [CrossRef]

69. Dunn, C.; Chalupny, N.J.; Sutherland, C.L.; Dosch, S.; Sivakumar, P.V.; Johnson, D.C.; Cosman, D. Human Cytomegalovirus Glycoprotein UL16 Causes Intracellular Sequestration of NKG2D Ligands, Protecting Against Natural Killer Cell Cytotoxicity. *J. Exp. Med.* **2003**, *197*, 1427–1439. [CrossRef]

70. Wu, J.; Chalupny, N.J.; Manley, T.J.; Riddell, S.R.; Cosman, D.; Spies, T. Intracellular Retention of the MHC Class I-Related Chain B Ligand of NKG2D by the Human Cytomegalovirus UL16 Glycoprotein. *J. Immunol.* **2003**, *170*, 4196–4200. [CrossRef]

71. Ashiru, O.; Bennett, N.J.; Boyle, L.H.; Thomas, M.; Trowsdale, J.; Wills, M.R. NKG2D Ligand MICA Is Retained in the cis-Golgi Apparatus by Human Cytomegalovirus Protein UL142. *J. Virol.* **2009**, *83*, 12345–12354. [CrossRef]

72. Zou, Y.; Bresnahan, W.; Taylor, R.T.; Stastny, P. Effect of Human Cytomegalovirus on Expression of MHC Class I-Related Chains A. *J. Immunol.* **2005**, *174*, 3098–3104. [CrossRef] [PubMed]

73. Seidel, E.; Le, V.T.K.; Bar-On, Y.; Tsukerman, P.; Enk, J.; Yamin, R.; Stein, N.; Schmiedel, D.; OiknineDjian, E.; Weisblum, Y.; et al. Dynamic Co-evolution of Host and Pathogen: HCMV Downregulates the Prevalent Allele MICA*008 to Escape Elimination by NK Cells. *Cell Rep.* **2015**, *10*, 968–982. [CrossRef] [PubMed]

74. Fielding, C.A.; Aicheler, R.; Stanton, R.J.; Wang, E.C.Y.; Han, S.; Seirafian, S.; Davies, J.; McSharry, B.P.; Weekes, M.P.; Antrobus, P.R.; et al. Two Novel Human Cytomegalovirus NK Cell Evasion Functions Target MICA for Lysosomal Degradation. *PLoS Pathog.* **2014**, *10*, e1004058. [CrossRef]

75. Fielding, C.A.; Weekes, M.P.; Nobre, L.V.; Ruckova, E.; Wilkie, G.S.; Paulo, J.A.; Chang, C.; Suárez, N.M.; Davies, J.A.; Antrobus, R.; et al. Control of immune ligands by members of a cytomegalovirus gene expansion suppresses natural killer cell activation. *Elife* **2017**, *6*, 1–27. [CrossRef]

76. Campbell, T.M.; McSharry, B.P.; Steain, M.; Slobedman, B.; Abendroth, A. Varicella-Zoster Virus and Herpes Simplex Virus 1 Differentially Modulate NKG2D Ligand Expression during Productive Infection. *J. Virol.* **2015**, *89*, 7932–7943. [CrossRef]

77. Schepis, D.; D'Amato, M.; Studahl, M.; Bergström, T.; Kärre, K.; Berg, L. Herpes simplex virus infection downmodulates NKG2D ligand expression. *Scand. J. Immunol.* **2009**, *69*, 429–436. [CrossRef] [PubMed]

78. Schneider, C.L.; Hudson, A.W. The human herpesvirus-7 (HHV-7) U21 immunoevasin subverts NK-mediated cytoxicity through modulation of MICA and MICB. *PLoS Pathog.* **2011**, *7*. [CrossRef]

79. Schmiedel, D.; Tai, J.; Levi-Schaffer, F.; Dovrat, S.; Mandelboim, O. Human Herpesvirus 6B Downregulates Expression of Activating Ligands during Lytic Infection To Escape Elimination by Natural Killer Cells. *J. Virol.* **2016**, *90*, 9608–9617. [CrossRef]

80. Thomas, M.; Boname, J.M.; Field, S.; Nejentsev, S.; Salio, M.; Cerundolo, V.; Wills, M.; Lehner, P.J. Down-regulation of NKG2D and NKp80 ligands by Kaposi's sarcoma-associated herpesvirus K5 protects against NK cell cytotoxicity. *Proc. Natl. Acad. Sci. USA* **2008**, *105*, 1656–1661. [CrossRef]

81. Wen, C.; He, X.; Ma, H.; Hou, N.; Wei, C.; Song, T.; Zhang, Y.; Sun, L.; Ma, Q.; Zhong, H. Hepatitis C Virus Infection Downregulates the Ligands of the Activating Receptor NKG2D. *Cell. Mol. Immunol.* **2008**, *5*, 475–478. [CrossRef]

82. McSharry, B.P.; Burgert, H.-G.; Owen, D.P.; Stanton, R.J.; Prod'homme, V.; Sester, M.; Koebernick, K.; Groh, V.; Spies, T.; Cox, S.; et al. Adenovirus E3/19K Promotes Evasion of NK Cell Recognition by Intracellular Sequestration of the NKG2D Ligands Major Histocompatibility Complex Class I Chain-Related Proteins A and B. *J. Virol.* **2008**, *82*, 4585–4594. [CrossRef] [PubMed]

83. Guan, Y.; Li, W.; Hou, Z.; Han, Q.; Lan, P.; Zhang, J.; Tian, Z.; Zhang, C. HBV suppresses expression of MICA/B on hepatoma cells through up-regulation of transcription factors GATA2 and GATA3 to escape from NK cell surveillance. *Oncotarget* **2016**, *7*, 56107–56119. [CrossRef] [PubMed]

84. Cerboni, C.; Neri, F.; Casartelli, N.; Zingoni, A.; Cosman, D.; Rossi, P.; Santoni, A.; Doria, M. Human immunodeficiency virus 1 Nef protein downmodulates the ligands of the activating receptor NKG2D and inhibits natural killer cell-mediated cytotoxicity. *J. Gen. Virol.* **2007**, *88*, 242–250. [CrossRef] [PubMed]

85. Roeth, J.F.; Collins, K.L. Human Immunodeficiency Virus Type 1 Nef: Adapting to Intracellular Trafficking Pathways. *Microbiol. Mol. Biol. Rev.* **2006**, *70*, 548–563. [CrossRef]

86. Jensen, H.; Andresen, L.; Nielsen, J.; Christensen, J.P.; Skov, S. Vesicular stomatitis virus infection promotes immune evasion by preventing NKG2D-ligand surface expression. *PLoS ONE* **2011**, *6*, 1–8. [CrossRef]

87. Esteso, G.; Guerra, S.; Valés-Gómez, M.; Reyburn, H.T. Innate immune recognition of double-stranded RNA triggers increased expression of NKG2D ligands after virus infection. *J. Biol. Chem.* **2017**, *292*, 20472–20480. [CrossRef]

88. Norman, J.M.; Mashiba, M.; McNamara, L.A.; Onafuwa-Nuga, A.; Chiari-Fort, E.; Shen, W.; Collins, K.L. The antiviral factor APOBEC3G enhances the recognition of HIV-infected primary T cells by natural killer cells. *Nat. Immunol.* **2011**, *12*, 975–983. [CrossRef]

89. Stern-Ginossar, N.; Elefant, N.; Zimmermann, A.; Wolf, D.G.; Saleh, N.; Biton, M.; Horwitz, E.; Prokocimer, Z.; Prichard, M.; Hahn, G.; et al. Host Immune System Gene Targeting by a Viral miRNA. *Science* **2007**, *317*, 376–381. [CrossRef]

90. Nachmani, D.; Stern-Ginossar, N.; Sarid, R.; Mandelboim, O. Diverse Herpesvirus MicroRNAs Target the Stress-Induced Immune Ligand MICB to Escape Recognition by Natural Killer Cells. *Cell Host Microbe* **2009**, *5*, 376–385. [CrossRef]

91. Bauman, Y.; Nachmani, D.; Vitenshtein, A.; Tsukerman, P.; Drayman, N.; Stern-Ginossar, N.; Lankry, D.; Gruda, R.; Mandelboim, O. An Identical miRNA of the Human JC and BK Polyoma Viruses Targets the Stress-Induced Ligand ULBP3 to Escape Immune Elimination. *Cell Host Microbe* **2011**, *9*, 93–102. [CrossRef]

92. Enk, J.; Levi, A.; Weisblum, Y.; Yamin, R.; Charpak-Amikam, Y.; Wolf, D.G.; Mandelboim, O. HSV1 MicroRNA Modulation of GPI Anchoring and Downstream Immune Evasion. *Cell Rep.* **2016**, *17*, 949–956. [CrossRef] [PubMed]

93. Esteso, G.; Luzón, E.; Sarmiento, E.; Gómez-Caro, R.; Steinle, A.; Murphy, G.; Carbone, J.; Valés-Gómez, M.; Reyburn, H.T. Altered MicroRNA Expression after Infection with Human Cytomegalovirus Leads to TIMP3 Downregulation and Increased Shedding of Metalloprotease Substrates, Including MICA. *J. Immunol.* **2014**, *193*, 1344–1352. [CrossRef] [PubMed]

94. Matusali, G.; Tchidjou, H.K.; Pontrelli, G.; Bernardi, S.; D'Ettorre, G.; Vullo, V.; Buonomini, A.R.; Andreoni, M.; Santoni, A.; Cerboni, C.; et al. Soluble ligands for the NKG2D receptor are released during HIV-1 infection and impair NKG2D expression and cytotoxicity of NK cells. *FASEB J.* **2013**, *27*, 2440–2450. [CrossRef] [PubMed]

95. Campbell, J.A.; Trossman, D.S.; Yokoyama, W.M.; Carayannopoulos, L.N. Zoonotic orthopoxviruses encode a high-affinity antagonist of NKG2D. *J. Exp. Med.* **2007**, *204*, 1311–1317. [CrossRef]

96. Sène, D.; Levasseur, F.; Abel, M.; Lambert, M.; Camous, X.; Hernandez, C.; Pène, V.; Rosenberg, A.R.; Jouvin-Marche, E.; Marche, P.N.; et al. Hepatitis C Virus (HCV) Evades NKG2D-Dependent NK Cell Responses through NS5A-Mediated Imbalance of Inflammatory Cytokines. *PLoS Pathog.* **2010**, *6*, e1001184. [CrossRef]

97. Muntasell, A.; Magri, G.; Pende, D.; Angulo, A.; López-Botet, M. Inhibition of NKG2D expression in NK cells by cytokines secreted in response to human cytomegalovirus infection. *Blood* **2010**, *115*, 5170–5179. [CrossRef]

98. Diefenbach, A.; Jamieson, A.M.; Liu, S.D.; Shastri, N.; Raulet, D.H. Ligands for the murine NKG2D receptor: Expression by tumor cells and activation of NK cells and macrophages. *Nat. Immunol.* **2000**, *1*, 119–126. [CrossRef]

99. Diefenbach, A.; Jensen, E.R.; Jamieson, A.M.; Raulet, D.H. Rae1 and H60 ligands of the NKG2D receptor stimulate tumour immunity. *Nature* **2001**, *413*, 165–171. [CrossRef]

100. Cerwenka, A.; Baron, J.L.; Lanier, L.L. Ectopic expression of retinoic acid early inducible-1 gene (RAE-1) permits natural killer cell-mediated rejection of a MHC class I-bearing tumor in vivo. *Proc. Natl. Acad. Sci. USA* **2001**, *98*, 11521–11526. [CrossRef]

101. Guerra, N.; Tan, Y.X.; Joncker, N.T.; Choy, A.; Gallardo, F.; Xiong, N.; Knoblaugh, S.; Cado, D.; Greenberg, N.R.; Raulet, D.H. NKG2D-Deficient Mice Are Defective in Tumor Surveillance in Models of Spontaneous Malignancy. *Immunity* **2008**, *28*, 571–580. [CrossRef]

102. Salih, H.R.; Antropius, H.; Gieseke, F.; Lutz, S.Z.; Kanz, L.; Rammensee, H.-G.; Steinle, A. Functional expression and release of ligands for the activating immunoreceptor NKG2D in leukemia. *Blood* **2003**, *102*, 1389–1396. [CrossRef] [PubMed]

103. Watson, N.F.S.; Spendlove, I.; Madjd, Z.; McGilvray, R.; Green, A.R.; Ellis, I.O.; Scholefield, J.H.; Durrant, L.G. Expression of the stress-related MHC class I chain-related protein MICA is an indicator of good prognosis in colorectal cancer patients. *Int. J. Cancer* **2006**, *118*, 1445–1452. [CrossRef] [PubMed]

104. Jinushi, M.; Takehara, T.; Tatsumi, T.; Kanto, T.; Groh, V.; Spies, T.; Kimura, R.; Miyagi, T.; Mochizuki, K.; Sasaki, Y.; et al. Expression and role of MICA and MICB in human hepatocellular carcinomas and their regulation by retinoic acid. *Int. J. Cancer* **2003**, *104*, 354–361. [CrossRef] [PubMed]

105. Vetter, C.S.; Groh, V.; thor Straten, P.; Spies, T.; Bröcker, E.-B.; Becker, J.C. Expression of Stress-induced MHC Class I Related Chain Molecules on Human Melanoma. *J. Investig. Dermatol.* **2002**, *118*, 600–605. [CrossRef] [PubMed]

106. Duan, X.; Deng, L.; Chen, X.; Lu, Y.; Zhang, Q.; Zhang, K.; Hu, Y.; Zeng, J.; Sun, W. Clinical significance of the immunostimulatory MHC class I chain-related molecule A and NKG2D receptor on NK cells in pancreatic cancer. *Med. Oncol.* **2011**, *28*, 466–474. [CrossRef]

107. de Kruijf, E.M.; Sajet, A.; van Nes, J.G.H.; Putter, H.; Smit, V.T.H.B.M.; Eagle, R.A.; Jafferji, I.; Trowsdale, J.; Liefers, G.J.; van de Velde, C.J.H.; et al. NKG2D ligand tumor expression and association with clinical outcome in early breast cancer patients: An observational study. *BMC Cancer* **2012**, *12*, 24. [CrossRef]

108. Friese, M.A.; Platten, M.; Lutz, S.Z.; Naumann, U.; Aulwurm, S.; Bischof, F.; Bühring, H.-J.; Dichgans, J.; Rammensee, H.-G.; Steinle, A.; et al. MICA/NKG2D-mediated immunogene therapy of experimental gliomas. *Cancer Res.* **2003**, *63*, 8996–9006.

109. Bartkova, J.; Hořejší, Z.; Koed, K.; Krämer, A.; Tort, F.; Zieger, K.; Guldberg, P.; Sehested, M.; Nesland, J.M.; Lukas, C.; et al. DNA damage response as a candidate anti-cancer barrier in early human tumorigenesis. *Nature* **2005**, *434*, 864–870. [CrossRef]

110. Gorgoulis, V.G.; Vassiliou, L.-V.F.; Karakaidos, P.; Zacharatos, P.; Kotsinas, A.; Liloglou, T.; Venere, M.; DiTullio, R.A.; Kastrinakis, N.G.; Levy, B.; et al. Activation of the DNA damage checkpoint and genomic instability in human precancerous lesions. *Nature* **2005**, *434*, 907–913. [CrossRef]

111. Corrales, L.; McWhirter, S.M.; Dubensky, T.W.; Gajewski, T.F. The host STING pathway at the interface of cancer and immunity. *J. Clin. Investig.* **2016**, *126*, 2404–2411. [CrossRef]

112. Lam, A.R.; Le Bert, N.; Ho, S.S.W.; Shen, Y.J.; Tang, M.L.F.; Xiong, G.M.; Croxford, J.L.; Koo, C.X.; Ishii, K.J.; Akira, S.; et al. RAE1 Ligands for the NKG2D Receptor Are Regulated by STING-Dependent DNA Sensor Pathways in Lymphoma. *Cancer Res.* **2014**, *74*, 2193–2203. [CrossRef] [PubMed]

113. Jung, H.; Hsiung, B.; Pestal, K.; Procyk, E.; Raulet, D.H. RAE-1 ligands for the NKG2D receptor are regulated by E2F transcription factors, which control cell cycle entry. *J. Exp. Med.* **2012**, *209*, 2409–2422. [CrossRef] [PubMed]

114. Cully, M.; You, H.; Levine, A.J.; Mak, T.W. Beyond PTEN mutations: The PI3K pathway as an integrator of multiple inputs during tumorigenesis. *Nat. Rev. Cancer* **2006**, *6*, 184–192. [CrossRef]

115. Unni, A.M.; Bondar, T.; Medzhitov, R. Intrinsic sensor of oncogenic transformation induces a signal for innate immunosurveillance. *Proc. Natl. Acad. Sci. USA* **2008**, *105*, 1686–1691. [CrossRef]

116. Smyth, M.J.; Swann, J.; Cretney, E.; Zerafa, N.; Yokoyama, W.M.; Hayakawa, Y. NKG2D function protects the host from tumor initiation. *J. Exp. Med.* **2005**, *202*, 583–588. [CrossRef] [PubMed]

117. Vetter, C.S.; Lieb, W.; Bröcker, E.-B.; Becker, J.C. Loss of nonclassical MHC molecules MIC-A/B expression during progression of uveal melanoma. *Br. J. Cancer* **2004**, *91*, 1495–1499. [CrossRef]

118. Groh, V.; Wu, J.; Yee, C.; Spies, T. Tumour-derived soluble MIC ligands impair expression of NKG2D and T-cell activation. *Nature* **2002**, *419*, 734–738. [CrossRef]

119. Linsley, P.S.; Bradshaw, J.; Urnes, M.; Grosmaire, L.; Ledbetter, J.A. CD28 engagement by B7/BB-1 induces transient down-regulation of CD28 synthesis and prolonged unresponsiveness to CD28 signaling. *J. Immunol.* **1993**, *150*, 3161–3169.

120. Valitutti, S.; Müller, S.; Salio, M.; Lanzavecchia, A. Degradation of T Cell Receptor (TCR)–CD3-ζ Complexes after Antigenic Stimulation. *J. Exp. Med.* **1997**, *185*, 1859–1864. [CrossRef]

121. Hilpert, J.; Grosse-Hovest, L.; Grünebach, F.; Buechele, C.; Nuebling, T.; Raum, T.; Steinle, A.; Salih, H.R. Comprehensive Analysis of NKG2D Ligand Expression and Release in Leukemia: Implications for NKG2D-Mediated NK Cell Responses. *J. Immunol.* **2012**, *189*, 1360–1371. [CrossRef]

122. Salih, H.R.; Rammensee, H.-G.; Steinle, A. Cutting Edge: Down-Regulation of MICA on Human Tumors by Proteolytic Shedding. *J. Immunol.* **2002**, *169*, 4098–4102. [CrossRef] [PubMed]

123. Waldhauer, I.; Goehlsdorf, D.; Gieseke, F.; Weinschenk, T.; Wittenbrink, M.; Ludwig, A.; Stevanovic, S.; Rammensee, H.G.; Steinle, A. Tumor-associated MICA is shed by ADAM proteases. *Cancer Res.* **2008**, *68*, 6368–6376. [CrossRef] [PubMed]

124. Boutet, P.; Agüera-González, S.; Atkinson, S.; Pennington, C.J.; Edwards, D.R.; Murphy, G.; Reyburn, H.T.; Valés-Gómez, M. Cutting Edge: The Metalloproteinase ADAM17/TNF-α-Converting Enzyme Regulates Proteolytic Shedding of the MHC Class I-Related Chain B Protein. *J. Immunol.* **2009**, *182*, 49–53. [CrossRef] [PubMed]

125. Kaiser, B.K.; Yim, D.; Chow, I.-T.; Gonzalez, S.; Dai, Z.; Mann, H.H.; Strong, R.K.; Groh, V.; Spies, T. Disulphide-isomerase-enabled shedding of tumour-associated NKG2D ligands. *Nature* **2007**, *447*, 482–486. [CrossRef]

126. Chitadze, G.; Lettau, M.; Bhat, J.; Wesch, D.; Steinle, A.; Fürst, D.; Mytilineos, J.; Kalthoff, H.; Janssen, O.; Oberg, H.-H.; et al. Shedding of endogenous MHC class I-related chain molecules A and B from different human tumor entities: Heterogeneous involvement of the "a disintegrin and metalloproteases" 10 and 17. *Int. J. Cancer* **2013**, *133*, 1557–1566. [CrossRef]

127. Zingoni, A.; Cecere, F.; Vulpis, E.; Fionda, C.; Molfetta, R.; Soriani, A.; Petrucci, M.T.; Ricciardi, M.R.; Fuerst, D.; Amendola, M.G.; et al. Genotoxic Stress Induces Senescence-Associated ADAM10-Dependent Release of NKG2D MIC Ligands in Multiple Myeloma Cells. *J. Immunol.* **2015**, *195*, 736–748. [CrossRef]

128. Liu, G.; Atteridge, C.L.; Wang, X.; Lundgren, A.D.; Wu, J.D. Cutting Edge: The Membrane Type Matrix Metalloproteinase MMP14 Mediates Constitutive Shedding of MHC Class I Chain-Related Molecule A Independent of A Disintegrin and Metalloproteinases. *J. Immunol.* **2010**, *184*, 3346–3350. [CrossRef]

129. Chitadze, G.; Lettau, M.; Luecke, S.; Wang, T.; Janssen, O.; Fürst, D.; Mytilineos, J.; Wesch, D.; Oberg, H.-H.; Held-Feindt, J.; et al. NKG2D- and T-cell receptor-dependent lysis of malignant glioma cell lines by human γδ T cells: Modulation by temozolomide and A disintegrin and metalloproteases 10 and 17 inhibitors. *Oncoimmunology* **2016**, *5*, e1093276. [CrossRef]

130. Wolpert, F.; Tritschler, I.; Steinle, A.; Weller, M.; Eisele, G. A disintegrin and metalloproteinases 10 and 17 modulate the immunogenicity of glioblastoma-initiating cells. *Neuro Oncol.* **2014**, *16*, 382–391. [CrossRef]

131. Ashiru, O.; Boutet, P.; Fernandez-Messina, L.; Aguera-Gonzalez, S.; Skepper, J.N.; Vales-Gomez, M.; Reyburn, H.T. Natural Killer Cell Cytotoxicity Is Suppressed by Exposure to the Human NKG2D Ligand MICA*008 That Is Shed by Tumor Cells in Exosomes. *Cancer Res.* **2010**, *70*, 481–489. [CrossRef]

132. Xiao, G.; Wang, X.; Sheng, J.; Lu, S.; Yu, X.; Wu, J.D. Soluble NKG2D ligand promotes MDSC expansion and skews macrophage to the alternatively activated phenotype. *J. Hematol. Oncol.* **2015**, *8*, 13. [CrossRef] [PubMed]

133. Deng, W.; Gowen, B.G.; Zhang, L.; Wang, L.; Lau, S.; Iannello, A.; Xu, J.; Rovis, T.L.; Xiong, N.; Raulet, D.H. A shed NKG2D ligand that promotes natural killer cell activation and tumor rejection. *Science* **2015**, *348*, 136–139. [CrossRef] [PubMed]

134. Huang, Q.; Gumireddy, K.; Schrier, M.; le Sage, C.; Nagel, R.; Nair, S.; Egan, D.A.; Li, A.; Huang, G.; Klein-Szanto, A.J.; et al. The microRNAs miR-373 and miR-520c promote tumour invasion and metastasis. *Nat. Cell Biol.* **2008**, *10*, 202–210. [CrossRef] [PubMed]

135. Landais, S.; Landry, S.; Legault, P.; Rassart, E. Oncogenic Potential of the miR-106-363 Cluster and Its Implication in Human T-Cell Leukemia. *Cancer Res.* **2007**, *67*, 5699–5707. [CrossRef] [PubMed]

136. Tsukerman, P.; Stern-Ginossar, N.; Gur, C.; Glasner, A.; Nachmani, D.; Bauman, Y.; Yamin, R.; Vitenshtein, A.; Stanietsky, N.; Bar-Mag, T.; et al. MiR-10b Downregulates the Stress-Induced Cell Surface Molecule MICB, a Critical Ligand for Cancer Cell Recognition by Natural Killer Cells. *Cancer Res.* **2012**, *72*, 5463–5472. [CrossRef] [PubMed]

137. Shen, J.; Pan, J.; Du, C.; Si, W.; Yao, M.; Xu, L.; Zheng, H.; Xu, M.; Chen, D.; Wang, S.; et al. Silencing NKG2D ligand-targeting miRNAs enhances natural killer cell-mediated cytotoxicity in breast cancer. *Cell Death Dis.* **2017**, *8*, e2740. [CrossRef] [PubMed]

138. Codo, P.; Weller, M.; Meister, G.; Szabo, E.; Steinle, A.; Wolter, M.; Reifenberger, G.; Roth, P. MicroRNA-mediated down-regulation of NKG2D ligands contributes to glioma immune escape. *Oncotarget* **2014**, *5*, 7651–7662. [CrossRef]

139. Xie, H.; Zhang, Q.; Zhou, H.; Zhou, J.; Zhang, J.; Jiang, Y.; Wang, J.; Meng, X.; Zeng, L.; Jiang, X. microRNA-889 is downregulated by histone deacetylase inhibitors and confers resistance to natural killer cytotoxicity in hepatocellular carcinoma cells. *Cytotechnology* **2018**, *70*, 513–521. [CrossRef]

140. Armeanu, S.; Bitzer, M.; Lauer, U.M.; Venturelli, S.; Pathil, A.; Krusch, M.; Kaiser, S.; Jobst, J.; Smirnow, I.; Wagner, A.; et al. Natural Killer Cell–Mediated Lysis of Hepatoma Cells via Specific Induction of NKG2D Ligands by the Histone Deacetylase Inhibitor Sodium Valproate. *Cancer Res.* **2005**, *65*, 6321–6329. [CrossRef]

141. Lu, C.; Ward, P.S.; Kapoor, G.S.; Rohle, D.; Turcan, S.; Abdel-Wahab, O.; Edwards, C.R.; Khanin, R.; Figueroa, M.E.; Melnick, A.; et al. IDH mutation impairs histone demethylation and results in a block to cell differentiation. *Nature* **2012**, *483*, 474–478. [CrossRef]

142. Zhang, X.; Rao, A.; Sette, P.; Deibert, C.; Pomerantz, A.; Kim, W.J.; Kohanbash, G.; Chang, Y.; Park, Y.; Engh, J.; et al. IDH mutant gliomas escape natural killer cell immune surveillance by downregulation of NKG2D ligand expression. *Neuro Oncol.* **2016**, *18*, 1402–1412. [CrossRef] [PubMed]

143. Fuertes, M.B.; Girart, M.V.; Molinero, L.L.; Domaica, C.I.; Rossi, L.E.; Barrio, M.M.; Mordoh, J.; Rabinovich, G.A.; Zwirner, N.W. Intracellular Retention of the NKG2D Ligand MHC Class I Chain-Related Gene A in Human Melanomas Confers Immune Privilege and Prevents NK Cell-Mediated Cytotoxicity. *J. Immunol.* **2008**, *180*, 4606–4614. [CrossRef] [PubMed]

144. Friese, M.A.; Wischhusen, J.; Wick, W.; Weiler, M.; Eisele, G.; Steinle, A.; Weller, M. RNA Interference Targeting Transforming Growth Factor-β Enhances NKG2D-Mediated Antiglioma Immune Response, Inhibits Glioma Cell Migration and Invasiveness, and Abrogates Tumorigenicity In vivo. *Cancer Res.* **2004**, *64*, 7596–7603. [CrossRef] [PubMed]

145. Eisele, G. TGF- and metalloproteinases differentially suppress NKG2D ligand surface expression on malignant glioma cells. *Brain* **2006**, *129*, 2416–2425. [CrossRef] [PubMed]

146. Crane, C.A.; Han, S.J.; Barry, J.J.; Ahn, B.J.; Lanier, L.L.; Parsa, A.T. TGF- downregulates the activating receptor NKG2D on NK cells and CD8$^+$ T cells in glioma patients. *Neuro-Oncology* **2010**, *12*, 7–13. [CrossRef]

147. Wick, W.; Platten, M.; Weller, M. Glioma cell invasion: Regulation of metalloproteinase activity by TGF-beta. *J. Neurooncol.* **2001**, *53*, 177–185. [CrossRef]

148. Crane, C.A.; Austgen, K.; Haberthur, K.; Hofmann, C.; Moyes, K.W.; Avanesyan, L.; Fong, L.; Campbell, M.J.; Cooper, S.; Oakes, S.A.; et al. Immune evasion mediated by tumor-derived lactate dehydrogenase induction of NKG2D ligands on myeloid cells in glioblastoma patients. *Proc. Natl. Acad. Sci. USA* **2014**, *111*, 12823–12828. [CrossRef]

149. Bui, J.D.; Carayannopoulos, L.N.; Lanier, L.L.; Yokoyama, W.M.; Schreiber, R.D. IFN-Dependent Down-Regulation of the NKG2D Ligand H60 on Tumors. *J. Immunol.* **2006**, *176*, 905–913. [CrossRef]

150. Zhang, C.; Niu, J.; Zhang, J.; Wang, Y.; Zhou, Z.; Zhang, J.; Tian, Z. Opposing effects of interferon-α and interferon-γ on the expression of major histocompatibility complex class I chain-related A in tumors. *Cancer Sci.* **2008**, *99*, 1279–1286. [CrossRef]

151. Schwinn, N.; Vokhminova, D.; Sucker, A.; Textor, S.; Striegel, S.; Moll, I.; Nausch, N.; Tuettenberg, J.; Steinle, A.; Cerwenka, A.; et al. Interferon-γ down-regulates NKG2D ligand expression and impairs the NKG2D-mediated cytolysis of MHC class I-deficient melanoma by natural killer cells. *Int. J. Cancer* **2009**, *124*, 1594–1604. [CrossRef]

152. Yadav, D.; Ngolab, J.; Lim, R.S.; Krishnamurthy, S.; Bui, J.D. Cutting Edge: Down-Regulation of MHC Class I-Related Chain A on Tumor Cells by IFN-γ-Induced MicroRNA. *J. Immunol.* **2009**, *182*, 39–43. [CrossRef] [PubMed]

153. Eagle, R.A.; Trowsdale, J. Promiscuity and the single receptor: NKG2D. *Nat. Rev. Immunol.* **2007**, *7*, 737–744. [CrossRef] [PubMed]

154. Zingoni, A.; Molfetta, R.; Fionda, C.; Soriani, A.; Paolini, R.; Cippitelli, M.; Cerboni, C.; Santoni, A. NKG2D and Its Ligands: "One for All, All for One". *Front. Immunol.* **2018**, *9*. [CrossRef] [PubMed]

155. Lança, T.; Correia, D.V.; Moita, C.F.; Raquel, H.; Neves-Costa, A.; Ferreira, C.; Ramalho, J.S.; Barata, J.T.; Moita, L.F.; Gomes, A.Q.; et al. The MHC class Ib protein ULBP1 is a nonredundant determinant of leukemia/lymphoma susceptibility to γδ T-cell cytotoxicity. *Blood* **2010**, *115*, 2407–2411. [CrossRef] [PubMed]

156. Spear, P.; Barber, A.; Rynda-Apple, A.; Sentman, C.L. NKG2D CAR T-cell therapy inhibits the growth of NKG2D ligand heterogeneous tumors. *Immunol. Cell Biol.* **2013**, *91*, 435–440. [CrossRef] [PubMed]

157. Weiss, T.; Weller, M.; Guckenberger, M.; Sentman, C.L.; Roth, P. NKG2D-based CAR T cells and radiotherapy exert synergistic efficacy in glioblastoma. *Cancer Res.* **2018**, *78*, 1031–1043. [CrossRef]

158. Sentman, M.-L.; Murad, J.M.; Cook, W.J.; Wu, M.-R.; Reder, J.; Baumeister, S.H.; Dranoff, G.; Fanger, M.W.; Sentman, C.L. Mechanisms of Acute Toxicity in NKG2D Chimeric Antigen Receptor T Cell–Treated Mice. *J. Immunol.* **2016**, *197*, 4674–4685. [CrossRef]

159. Arai, J.; Goto, K.; Tanoue, Y.; Ito, S.; Muroyama, R.; Matsubara, Y.; Nakagawa, R.; Kaise, Y.; Lim, L.A.; Yoshida, H.; et al. Enzymatic inhibition of MICA sheddase ADAM17 by lomofungin in hepatocellular carcinoma cells. *Int. J. Cancer* **2018**, *143*, 2575–2583. [CrossRef]

160. Shiraishi, K.; Mimura, K.; Kua, L.-F.; Koh, V.; Siang, L.K.; Nakajima, S.; Fujii, H.; Shabbir, A.; Yong, W.-P.; So, J.; et al. Inhibition of MMP activity can restore NKG2D ligand expression in gastric cancer, leading to improved NK cell susceptibility. *J. Gastroenterol.* **2016**, *51*, 1101–1111. [CrossRef]

161. Ferrari de Andrade, L.; Tay, R.E.; Pan, D.; Luoma, A.M.; Ito, Y.; Badrinath, S.; Tsoucas, D.; Franz, B.; May, K.F.; Harvey, C.J.; et al. Antibody-mediated inhibition of MICA and MICB shedding promotes NK cell–driven tumor immunity. *Science* **2018**, *359*, 1537–1542. [CrossRef]

162. Lu, S.; Zhang, J.; Liu, D.; Li, G.; Staveley-O'Carroll, K.F.; Li, Z.; Wu, J.D. Nonblocking Monoclonal Antibody Targeting Soluble MIC Revamps Endogenous Innate and Adaptive Antitumor Responses and Eliminates Primary and Metastatic Tumors. *Clin. Cancer Res.* **2015**, *21*, 4819–4830. [CrossRef] [PubMed]

163. Seymour, L.W.; Fisher, K.D. Oncolytic viruses: Finally delivering. *Br. J. Cancer* **2016**, *114*, 357–361. [CrossRef] [PubMed]

164. Kuhn, I.; Harden, P.; Bauzon, M.; Chartier, C.; Nye, J.; Thorne, S.; Reid, T.; Ni, S.; Lieber, A.; Fisher, K.; et al. Directed evolution generates a novel oncolytic virus for the treatment of colon cancer. *PLoS ONE* **2008**, *3*, 1–11. [CrossRef] [PubMed]

165. Mineta, T.; Rabkin, S.D.; Yazaki, T.; Hunter, W.D.; Martuza, R.L. Attenuated multi-mutated herpes simplex virus-1 for the treatment of malignant gliomas. *Nat. Med.* **1995**, *1*, 938–943. [CrossRef] [PubMed]

166. Conry, R.M.; Westbrook, B.; McKee, S.; Norwood, T.G. Talimogene laherparepvec: First in class oncolytic virotherapy. *Hum. Vaccines Immunother.* **2018**, *14*, 839–846. [CrossRef] [PubMed]

167. Dyer, A.; Di, Y.; Calderon, H.; Illingworth, S.; Kueberuwa, G.; Tedcastle, A.; Jakeman, P.; Chia, S.L.; Brown, A.; Silva, M.A.; et al. Oncolytic Group B Adenovirus Enadenotucirev Mediates Non-apoptotic Cell Death with Membrane Disruption and Release of Inflammatory Mediators. *Mol. Ther. Oncolytics* **2017**, *4*, 18–30. [CrossRef]

Publisher's Note: MDPI stays neutral with regard to jurisdictional claims in published maps and institutional affiliations.

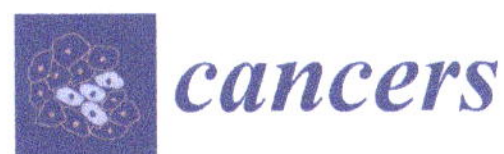 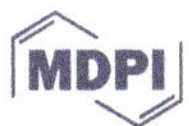

Review

Modulating the Tumour Microenvironment by Intratumoural Injection of Pattern Recognition Receptor Agonists

Olivia K. Burn [1,2]**, Kef K. Prasit** [1,2] **and Ian F. Hermans** [1,2,*]

[1] Malaghan Institute of Medical Research, P.O. Box 7060, Wellington 6042, New Zealand;
   oburn@malaghan.org.nz (O.K.B.); kprasit@malaghan.org.nz (K.K.P.)
[2] Maurice Wilkins Centre, Private Bag 92019, Auckland 1042, New Zealand
*   Correspondence: ihermans@malaghan.org.nz; Tel.: +64-44-996-914

Received: 30 November 2020; Accepted: 16 December 2020; Published: 18 December 2020

Simple Summary: The immune system is capable of eliminating solid cancers through the action of immune cells that recognise antigens that are unique to tumour tissue. However, the activity of tumour-specific immune cells is often blunted by the immunosuppressive environment within the tumour core. One strategy to overcome this limitation is to inject immune modulators directly into the tumour bed to stimulate the local network of immune cells. Not only does this promote local antitumour activity, but also facilitates the infiltration of immune cells with antitumour activity at distant tumour sites. A major class of compounds used for this purpose are recognised by pattern recognition receptors (PRR), providing molecular cues typically associated with infection or tissue damage to inflate the response. In this review, we summarise research into the use of such compounds in preclinical studies, including promising studies conducted in combination with conventional cancer therapies and other immunotherapies.

Abstract: Signalling through pattern recognition receptors (PRRs) leads to strong proinflammatory responses, enhancing the activity of antigen presenting cells and shaping adaptive immune responses against tumour associated antigens. Unfortunately, toxicities associated with systemic administration of these agonists have limited their clinical use to date. Direct injection of PRR agonists into the tumour can enhance immune responses by directly modulating the cells present in the tumour microenvironment. This can improve local antitumour activity, but importantly, also facilitates systemic responses that limit tumour growth at distant sites. As such, this form of therapy could be used clinically where metastatic tumour lesions are accessible, or as neoadjuvant therapy. In this review, we summarise current preclinical data on intratumoural administration of PRR agonists, including new strategies to optimise delivery and impact, and combination studies with current and promising new cancer therapies.

Keywords: pattern-recognition receptors; toll-like receptors; intratumoural; tumour microenvironment

---

1. Introduction

There have been significant advances in the development and use of immunomodulatory compounds to reverse immune tolerance and exhaustion in order to facilitate anti-tumour immune responses. While the most clinically relevant advance has been the development of immune checkpoint inhibitors to block negative signalling in anti-tumour T cells, other approaches have focused on delivering stimulatory signals, either to T cells directly, or to the antigen-presenting cells (APCs) that ultimately orchestrate adaptive immunity. One broad class of such immunostimulatory compounds are agonists for patter recognition receptors (PRRs), a series of innate receptors that screen the environment for molecular cues associated with infection or tissue distress [1]. Integration of signals facilitated by these innate immune-sensing pathways plays a significant role in regulating immediate host innate immunity, and also shaping the quality of induced adaptive responses featuring T cells and B cells [2].

It is now recognised that a critical barrier to effective immunity against solid tumours is the local tumour microenvironment (TME), with its unique local milieu of immunosuppressive cells and hypoxia-induced factors that ultimately serve to limit the activity of infiltrating immune effector cells [3–5]. By administering PRR agonists to the host, it is possible to deliver positive signals that can overcome some of these immunosuppressive networks [6–8]. Furthermore, the administration of PRR agonists into an environment where APCs have captured tumour antigens can create an immunopermissive environment where antigen-specific adaptive responses can be initiated, or existing ones given an effective boost [9]. To maximise the likelihood of stimulating appropriate antigen-loaded APCs, it may be necessary to introduce the PRR agonists directly into the TME. This can be achieved in some clinical situations by intratumoural administration, the focus of this review.

Many PRRs have been described, with the main families explored in the context of intratumoural administration being the Toll-like receptors (TLR), retinoic acid-inducible gene I (RIG-I)-like receptors (RLRs), and DNA sensors such as stimulator of interferon genes (STING). All of these receptors transmit signals when they encounter agonists in the form of pathogen-associated molecular patterns (PAMPs) or damage-associated molecular patterns (DAMPs) [10,11]. PAMPs are structures typically observed in pathogenic prokaryotes, such as lipopolysaccharide (LPS), peptidoglycans, and lipoproteins derived from bacterial cell walls, bacterial structural proteins such as flagellin, nucleic structures such the unmethylated deoxyribonucleic acid (DNA) associated with bacteria and some fungi and parasites, or double stranded ribonucleic acid (dsRNA) typically seen in viral species [12]. DAMPs result from cellular stress, apoptosis, and necrosis, such as chromatin-associated protein high-mobility group box 1 (HMGB1) [13], heat shock proteins (HSPs) [14], extracellular adenosine triphosphate (ATP) [15], and proteolytically digested fragments of the extracellular matrix, such as biglycan and fibrinogen [16,17]. Although their intracellular signalling pathways are often distinct, they ultimately lead (alone or in combination) to increased transcription of genes involved in inflammatory responses. These include proinflammatory cytokines such as IL-1, IL-6, IL-12, and tumour necrosis factor (TNF), type-I interferons (IFNs) that promote APC maturation and the cytotoxic activity of macrophages and natural killer (NK) cells [18–22], and chemokines that recruit lymphocytes and neutrophils [23,24]. Combined, these factors contribute to the mobilisation of adaptive immune responses. While PRR agonists have been investigated as systemic therapies, advancement to the clinic has been hampered by systemic toxicities [25–27]. However, studies suggest that an intratumoural route of administration can lead to high local concentrations of PRR agonists in the TME while limiting systemic exposure that can potentially lead to toxicity [6,28], even when used in a repetitive dosing regimen [29–31].

While PRRs are highly expressed by APC lineages that are known to infiltrate the TME, including conventional myeloid dendritic cells (cDC), plasmacytoid dendritic cells (pDC), and tumour associated macrophages (TAMs), they can also be expressed on CD8$^+$ and CD4$^+$ T cells, regulatory T cells (Treg), and B cells [32]. The impact of PRR agonism on the adaptive immune response can therefore be indirect, through the activation of APCs, or direct, through direct stimulation of adaptive effectors cells. Importantly, although the immediate response to intratumoural delivery of an agonist is to alter the function of cells in the local TME, numerous studies have shown that it is possible to create an environment that supports a systemic immune response that can initiate tumour regression in non-injected distal tumour sites, referred to as an abscopal effect. Here we discuss the recent advances in our understanding of how the TME can be shaped by intratumoural PRR agonists (Figure 1). In much of this preclinical work, PRR agonists have been studied in combination with other immunomodulatory strategies, such as with checkpoint inhibitors, or with conventional therapies such as radiation and chemotherapy, in order to promote long-term tumour eradication (summarised in Table 1).

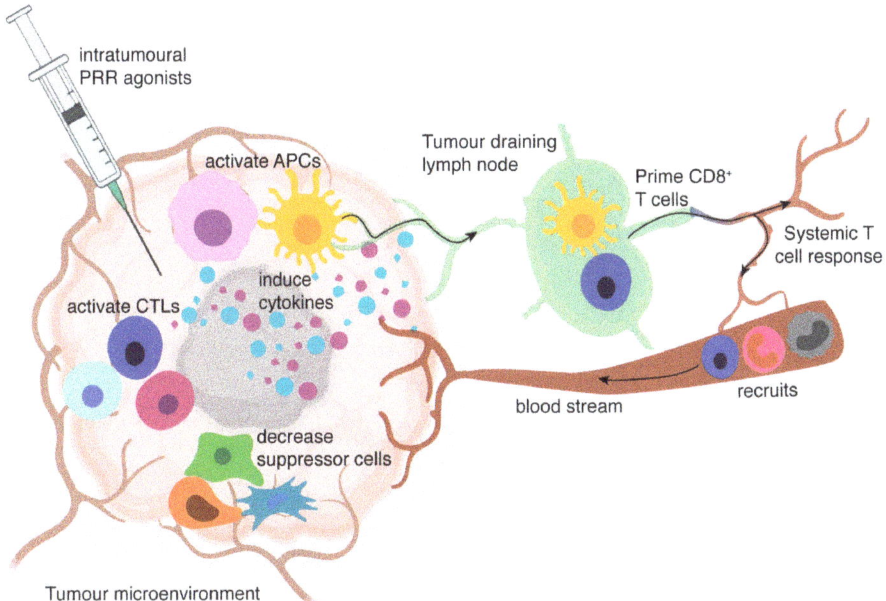

Figure 1. Intratumoural pattern recognition receptors (PRR) agonists induce a proinflammatory tumour microenvironment. PRR engagement on antigen-presenting cells (APCs) results in the activation of APCs including conventional myeloid dendritic cells (cDCs), plasmacytoid dendritic cells (pDCs) and macrophages. These activated APCs produce cytokine profiles mostly dominated by type I interferons (IFN) as well as proinflammatory cytokines, such as IL-12p70, IL-6, IL-1 and tumour necrosis factor (TNF). This creates an environment that favours the activation or restimulation of T cells, decreases the activity of myeloid-derived suppressor cells (MDSCs) and regulatory T cells (Tregs), and polarises macrophages to an anti-tumoural M1-type phenotype. Activated APCs also appear in tumour-draining lymph nodes, where they can contribute to presentation of tumour-associated antigens to T cells. Chemokines released in the tumour help recruit circulating T cells, natural killer (NK) cells, monocytes, and neutrophils. Ultimately, a systemic immune response is generated that can be capable of inducing regression at distant tumours.

Table 1. Intratumoural PRR agonists and effective treatment combinations in a preclinical setting.

Intratumoural Agonist	Analogues	PRR Receptors	Notable Cytokines	Effects on APCs	Critical Effector Cells	Beneficial Combinations
Pam$_3$CSK$_4$		TLR1 TLR2	IFN-γ	Limited effects alone	Limited effects alone	Anti-CTLA-4 [33]
acGM-1.8		TLR2	TNF, IL-12p70 and IFN-γ	Increased M1/M2 macrophage ratio	Increased Teff/Treg ratio	
Poly I:C	BO-112	TLR3 RIG-I	Type I IFN	Dependent on cDC1	Increased Teff/Treg ratio	Flt3 ligand with anti-PD-L1 mAb and BRAF inhibition [34]; CpG-ODN [35]
Poly A:U		TLR3	Type I IFN	Activate cDCs	Increased Teff/Treg ratio and granzyme B-producing CD8$^+$ T cells	
LPS	MPL G100	TLR4	Type I IFN	Activate cDC1s Increased M1/M2 macrophage ratio	Increased Teff Increased NK cells	Anti-CD40 mAb [36]; anti-PD1 or anti-PD-L1 [37]
Resiquimod (R848)		TLR7 TLR8	Type I IFN	Activate pDCs Activation of cDCs Increased M1/M2 macrophage ratio	Increased Teff	

Table 1. *Cont.*

Intratumoural Agonist	Analogues	PRR Receptors	Notable Cytokines	Effects on APCs	Critical Effector Cells	Beneficial Combinations
Telratolimod		TLR7 TLR8	Type I IFN	Activate pDCs Activation of cDCs Increased M1/M2 macrophage ratio	Increased Teff	Anti-PD-L1 mAb [29]; anti-PD-1 mAb [38]; anti-CTLA-4 and anti-PD-L1 mAb [39]; anti-OX40 mAb [29]
CpG ODN	SD-101 CMP-001 IMO-2125	TLR9	Type I IFN	Macrophages responsible for early rejection phase Activate pDCs Accumulation and activation of cDCs Reduced MDSC function	Increased infiltration of antigen-specific T cells Increased NK cells	Anti-CD40 antibody [40]; anti-CTLA4 [41]; anti-OX40 mAb alone [42] or in combination with anti-CTLA-4 [43]; anti-PD-1 mAb alone [44] or in combination with local radiotherapy [45]; metronomic cyclophosphamide [31], doxorubicin [46]; ibrutinib [47]; poly I:C [35]; 3M-052 [48]
MK461		RIG-I	Type I IFN		Dependent on T and NK cells	
SLR14		RIG-I	Type I IFN	Phagocytosed by CD11b$^+$ myeloid cells	Increased Teff/Treg ratio	Anti-PD-1 [49]
Murine CDNs	DMXAA CDG	STING	Type I IFN	Dependent on cDC1	Dependent on T cells	Anti-CTLA-4, anti-PD-1 and agonistic anti-CD137 [50]; carboplatin and anti-PD1 [51]
Synthetic human CDNs	ADU-S100 cGAMP GSK532	STING	Type I IFN	Activate cDCs	Dependent on CD8$^+$ T cells	VEGFR2 blockade and anti-CTLA-4 or anti-PD1 mAb [52]; anti-PD-1 with anti-CTLA4 [53]

2. Intratumoural PRR Ligands and the TME

2.1. TLR Agonists

Downstream TLR signalling involves the recruitment of adapter proteins, with myeloid differentiation factor 88 (MyD88) utilised by all TLRs excluding TLR3, and TIR domain-containing adapter inducing interferon β (TRIF) used by both TLR3 and TLR4. Engagement of these adapters ultimately transmits signals through nuclear factor-κB (NF-κB), mitogen-activated protein (MAP) kinases, and interferon-regulatory factors (IRFs) to influence the expression of genes relevant to inflammation (reviewed extensively elsewhere; [54]). When considering APCs such as DCs, signalling through TLRs expressed on the cell surface (TLR1, 2, 4, 5, 6) generally induces a cytokine profile featuring IL-1, IL-12, and TNF, while TLRs within the endosomal compartment (TLR3, 7, 8, 9) promote significant type I IFN release [55–57]. Through direct signalling, or via the cytokines induced, TLRs can regulate essential processes for initiating T cell immunity, including altering rates of antigen uptake, processing and presentation of antigen by APCs, as well as inducing enhanced expression of molecules required for T cell activation, including the critical co-stimulatory molecules of the B7 family (e.g., CD80 and CD86) and TNFR family (e.g., CD40, OX40L) [58–62]. Below, we review the effect of agonists for the different TLRs in the context of intratumoural cancer treatment. Although TLR signalling occurs in cells that are not regarded as APCs, much of the data indicates a critical role for enhancing APC function in the efficacy of these treatments.

2.1.1. TLR9

Perhaps the most clinically advanced of the PRR agonists evaluated target TLR9 (reviewed in [63,64]). In general, monotherapy with intratumoural administration has shown to be safe, but with limited clinical efficacy observed to date, although more promising results have been observed when injected in combination with other cancer therapies. Further preclinical studies, like those described below, are needed to optimise this therapy for the clinic.

Primarily expressed on B cells and pDCs, TLR9 is located in intracellular vesicles, where it detects the presence of unmethylated cytidine phosphate guanosine (CpG) dinucleotides associated with the genomes of most bacteria and DNA viruses, inducing signalling via the MyD88 pathway [65]. Synthetic TLR9 agonists have been developed based on CpG-oligodinucleotides (ODN) containing hexamer CpG motifs that are not common in vertebrate DNA. Early studies with intratumoural CpG-ODNs in Lewis rats implanted with syngeneic glioma cells showed increased tumour infiltration with macrophage/microglial cells, $CD8^+$ T cells, and NK cells, and protection against a second tumour challenge. In follow-up studies in mice, the effect was lost in nude mice, suggesting that CpG-ODN was not directly cytotoxic and required immunostimulation for the antitumour effect [66]. Specific cell depletion studies showed that macrophages played a critical role in the early phase of tumour rejection, capable of controlling growth temporarily in nude mice, but full rejection required a later phase only seen in T cell-replete animals [67]. Several studies in different tumour models in mice confirmed a critical role for $CD8^+$ T cells, and establishment of a memory response [68], with transfer of activated T cells sufficient to mount fully protective responses in RAG-1 knockout mice (which are otherwise deficient in adaptive immune cells) [69]. Initial priming was shown to involve modulation of DC function in a CT26 colon carcinoma model, with CpG-ODN treatment shown to induce the expression of CCL20 in the tumour, attracting large numbers of circulating DCs into the tumour mass. Whereas the TME typically caused inhibition of DC activation in this model, CPG-ODN treatment enabled tumoural DCs to effectively cross-present tumour antigens to activate $CD8^+$ T cells. This local effect on tumoural DC number and function was critical, as systemic delivery of the DC growth factor, Flt3 ligand could increase circulating DCs, but had no effect on the number of tumoural DCs or impact on tumour growth [70]. More mechanistic insight came from studies comparing intratumoural CpG-ODN to intravenous treatment, where intratumoural treatment was shown to lead to more extensive infiltration of antigen-specific T cells, which was attributed to significantly higher levels of inflammatory chemokines (RANTES, IP-10, MCP-1, MCP5, MIP1α, and MIP1β) in the TME. In vivo, depletion of pDCs, which are known to express TLR9 [71,72], greatly reduced the levels of chemokines induced, and impaired T cell accumulation and the antitumour effect [73]. Given the known capacity for pDCs to produce type I IFNs, this cytokine response was likely key to the improved T cell activity, through its effects on APC function, including improved cross-priming [74–76], and also its direct effect on T cell memory formation [77,78]. Indeed, a type I IFN response is now a feature used in developing this intratumoural therapy. For example, in a recent study, twenty novel CpG-C ODNs were screened for their ability to induce secretion of IFN-α (along with IL-6 and TNF) in human peripheral blood mononuclear cells (PBMCs) to select new efficacious agonists for further evaluation [79]. Interestingly, one study did not show a role for pDC in response to CpG-ODN in a mouse model of T cell lymphoma; instead, CpG-B ODN stimulation recruited neutrophils into the milieu, resulting in the activation of cDCs, with subsequent increased antitumour T cell priming in draining lymph nodes [80]. Another important facet of the intratumoural effect of CpG-ODN is the impact on myeloid-derived suppressor cells (MDSC), which represents an important constituent of the immunosuppressive TME. Delivery of CpG-ODN directly into the tumour has been shown to reduce the immunosuppressive activity of monocytic MDSC (which express TLR9) and cause their differentiation into macrophages with direct tumouricidal capability [81].

Intratumoural CpG-ODN treatment has been evaluated in combination with evolving new therapies based on antibody-mediated modulation of T cells. Intravenously administered monoclonal antibodies against OX40, which enhance T cell activation, or against CTLA4 to block a cell-intrinsic negative regulatory immune checkpoint in T cells, combined effectively with the intratumoural CpG-ODN treatment in a mouse model of B cell lymphoma [40]. In fact, B cell lymphoma may represent an unusual case, as it was unexpectedly found that tumour rejection did not require host expression of TLR9, and was associated with increased expression of the co-stimulatory molecules CD80 and CD86 on the lymphoma cells; the lymphoma cells themselves may therefore be acting as APCs [82]. In some studies, CpG-ODN induced the upregulation of PD-1 expression on immune cells [83], making this an obvious, clinically relevant combination to explore. Durable rejection of injected tumours, and activity against un-injected distant tumours, was observed when CpG-ODN was combined with anti-PD-1 in models of CT26 colon carcinoma, TSA mammary adenocarcinoma, and MCA38 colon carcinoma—all models that showed little response to PD-1 blockade alone [44]. The effect of PD-1 blockade was to alter CpG-ODN-mediated differentiation of tumour-specific CD8$^+$ T cells into short-lived effector cells, and preferentially expand long-lived memory precursors, which likely accounted for the increased durability of the combination [44]. Studies of CpG-ODN treatment with anti-CTLA-4 in B16 melanoma were also encouraging, although when evaluated further, only the more immunogenic model, B16.OVA, resulted in full synergy with abscopal effect, whereas in the less immunogenic B16.F10 melanoma model, only the locally injected site responded to the combination [41]. Combining with a CTLA-4 antibody of increased potency improved the distant response. Interestingly, in some studies, CpG-ODN administration was found to increase OX40 co-stimulatory receptor expression on CD4$^+$ T cells, and combining intratumoural treatment with intravenous agonistic anti-OX40 antibody was found to be particularly effective [42]. Successful combination therapy with anti-OX40 and anti-CTLA-4 could be achieved by administering the antibodies intratumourally, which helped deplete immunosuppressive Tregs in the TME [43]. The upregulation of OX40 has been investigated as an early predictor of response to CpG-ODN, with increased uptake of a near-infrared (NIR) fluorescence probe affixed to an antibody for OX40 seen with CpG-ODN treatment in a model of hepatocellular carcinoma [84]. In the clinic, checkpoint blockade is currently being evaluated in combination with other conventional therapies, such as radiation treatment [85]. However, promising preclinical studies indicate that intratumoural CpG-ODN treatment could be added to the mix. For example, local radiotherapy, intratumoural CpG-ODN, and systemic PD-1 blockade were shown to be particularly effective in lung cancer models, associated with increased DC activation and infiltration of cytokine-producing CD8$^+$ T cells [45].

Low-dose metronomic cyclophosphamide complements the actions of an intratumoural CpG-ODN to potentiate innate immunity and drive anti-tumour responses [31]. In this setting, the chemotherapy shaped the immune response, with a reduction in Tregs, and an increase in M1-type macrophages, a phenotype typically associated with antitumour effects through direct tumouricidal activity and release of factors such as IL-12, CXCL9, and CXCL10 that enhance T cell and NK cell function and migration to the tumour. A corresponding decrease in M2-type macrophages was observed. These pro-tumourigenic cells produce the immunosuppressive cytokine IL-10, are able to recruit Tregs, and express PD-L1, which triggers negative signalling via PD-1 in T cells; they also promote angiogenesis and tumour progression through the production of VEGF and the release of chemokines such as CCL18 and CCL22, and enzymes like matrix metalloproteinase [86–88]. Another way to exploit chemotherapeutic agents in combination therapy is to use agents such as doxorubicin and oxaliplatin that induce immunogenic cell death (ICD) to release antigens and broaden the immune response. A recent study used intratumoural injection of an ICD inducer in combination with a cell-labelling version of CpG-ODN that is retained at the injection site to generate an in situ apoptotic cell-adjuvant complex to drive antitumour responses [46]. Ibrutinib, an irreversible inhibitor of Bruton's tyrosine kinase, that is an effective treatment against many types of B cell lymphomas, also causes ICD and was shown to combine effectively with intratumoural CpG-ODN in a mouse model of lymphoma [47].

Many recent preclinical studies have focused on improving the delivery of CpG-ODN to the TME and have often been conducted in combination with other therapies. Potent anti-tumour responses were observed in mice by incorporating CpG-ODN and anti-CD40 agonist antibody into liposomal carriers, with elimination of systemic toxic side effects achieved by focused sequestration in the TME [89]. As the phosphodiester-backbones of CpG-ODN can be susceptible to nuclease activity, encapsulation into liposomes has been used to improve stability in vivo [90]. This was also achieved using a poly(L-glutamic acid)-modified CpG-ODN [91], or modified with polyethyleneimine [92]. Conjugating CpG-ODN to carbon nanotubes proved to be effective in intracranial treatment, abrogating tumour growth not only in the brain, but also subcutaneous tumours [93]. In a recent study, the challenge of delivering a payload into the compressed TME was overcome by loading CpG onto apoptotic bodies, which were phagocytosed by inflammatory monocytes that actively infiltrate the tumour centre [94]. Others have utilised delivery on synthetic high density lipoproteins (together with a chemotherapeutic agent) [95] or used the specific targeting of some peptide moieties for the TME to direct uptake into the tumour [96]. An albumin-binding analogue of CpG-ODN was shown to accumulate in tumours after the local tumour area was subjected to radiation therapy [97]. In some studies, the delivery vehicles were functionalised to provide additional antitumour activity. For example, CpG-ODN and tumour antigens were integrated with gold nanorods capable of photo-heat conversion, so that illumination of the tumour area with NIR light resulted in a local rise in temperature that caused additional tumour destruction [98]. CpG-ODN has also been incorporated into carbon nanotubes, which have a photohyperthermic effect induced by NIR irradiation [99], and a similar concept has been used with a hydrogel containing gold nanoparticles exposed to laser irradiation at 780 nm to cause the local temperature rise [100]. Tumour elimination with a low radioactivity dose was achieved by intratumoural injection of a sodium alginate formulation containing CpG-ODN and a catalase labelled with the therapeutic ^{131}I radioisotope [101].

The CpG-ODNs evaluated preclinically fall into three general classes. Class-A CpG ODNs stimulate pDC to produce high quantities of IFN-α, induce maturation of APC, and activate NK cells indirectly via the IFN-α produced. Class-B CpG-ODNs activate B cells and NK cells, but are associated with lower levels of DC activation and IFN-α induction, while Class-C CpG-ODNs combine the properties of class-A and Class-B. Toxicities associated with repeated administration (with systemic access) can cause splenomegaly, lymphoid follicle destruction, and hepatotoxicity in mice [102–104]. Some hematologic adverse events and influenza-like symptoms have been observed in human cancer clinical trials [105,106], and some adverse events, such as platelet activation, complement activation, and clotting time prolongation are caused by the unnatural phosphorothioate backbone used in Class-B CpG-ODNs [107–109]. In contrast, Class-A CpG-ODNs are composed of mostly natural phosphodiester backbones, but as such are susceptible to degradation [110]. To address this, in a recent study Class-A CpG-ODN was encapsulated into lipid nanoparticles, which showed potential as a safe and effective alternative formulation for cancer immunotherapy [111]. Another downside of Class-B CpG-ODNs is that they can limit their immune stimulatory activity through activation of the signal transducer and activator of transcription 3 (STAT3), which is responsible for orchestrating immunosuppressive networks in the TME. A recent study showed in vitro that while Class-B CpG-ODN alone can induce activation of DCs, combined inhibition of the JAK2/STAT3 pathway resulted in superior DC activity [112].

Another strategy to improve intratumoural responses to intratumoural administration involves combining TLR signalling via both the TRIF and MyD88 pathways to activate separate kinetics. It has been shown that combining CpG-ODN with the TLR3 agonist poly I:C can synergistically upregulate the expression of IL-12p40 in murine peritoneal macrophages, and potentially lead to enhanced antigen cross-presentation [113]. Intratumoural administration of both poly I:C and CpG-ODN, combined with systemic transfer of melanoma-specific T cells, led to the eradication of established tumours [35], which was attributed to improved activity of host DCs. The improved T cell activity was lost in Tap-deficient mice, suggesting an enhanced capacity for cross-presentation was essential to the response. In another study involving co-delivery of agonists, concurrent targeting of TLRs 7, 8, and 9 by intratumoural injection increased the number and tumouricidal activity of tumour infiltrating CD8^{+} T cells and NK cells, and reduced the frequency of immunosuppressive MDSCs [48].

2.1.2. TLR2

TLR2 recognises bacterial-derived lipopeptides and signals as a heterodimer with either TLR1 or TLR6. The activity of Bacillus Calmette-Guerin (BCG), a clinically approved intratumoural therapy for bladder cancer, has been attributed to a number of PAMPs, including the activation of TLR1/TLR2 signalling via recognition of lipopeptides within the cell wall [114]. Pam$_3$CysSerLys$_4$ (Pam$_3$CSK$_4$) is a triacylated lipopeptide that mimics the acylated amino terminus of bacterial lipoproteins and is commonly used as a synthetic TLR1/TLR2 agonist [115]. Intratumoural administration of Pam_3CSK_4 alone has been attempted, but had no significant effect on tumour growth in a B16.F10 melanoma model [33]. A recently described TLR2-specific agonist based on a glucomannan polysaccharide modified with acetyl groups (acGM-1.8) displayed a much higher safety profile than Pam_3CSK_4, with some antitumour activity as a single agent [116]. Following intratumoural administration of acGM-1.8 into mice with established sarcoma lesions on both flanks, strong anti-tumour responses were observed against both the treated and untreated bilateral tumours. The local response was abrogated by intratumoural clodronate liposome injection, highlighting a role for macrophage activity. In support of this, large changes in the phenotype of TAMs were observed, with an increase in M1-type macrophages and decrease in M2-type macrophages. In fact, intratumoural acGM-1.8 changed the overall cytokine profile within the tumour, with an increase in levels of TNF, IL-12p70, and IFN-γ, and an increased ratio of effector T cells (Teff) to Tregs. Furthermore, the antitumour response was not induced in $Rag^{-/-}$ mice, suggesting induction of a crucial adaptive immune response [116].

Studies in mice conducted with intratumoural Pam_3CSK_4 combined with systemic administration of anti-CTLA-4 showed enhanced efficacy in a B16.F10 melanoma model [33]. Interestingly, in this combination setting, there was an increase in Fcγ receptor IV expression on macrophages, resulting in greater antibody-dependent macrophage-mediated depletion of CTLA-4-positive Tregs in the tumour [33,117]. Thus, intratumoural delivery of PRR agonists can play unexpected supporting roles in established treatments, and carefully selected combinations can result in synergistic effects.

2.1.3. TLR3

TLR3 recognises exogenous and endogenous dsRNA in endosomes, stimulating a signalling pathway via TRIF that culminates with the secretion of inflammatory cytokines and type I IFN. Poly I:C is an analogue of viral dsRNA that acts as an agonist of endosomal TLR3 [118]. In mice, intratumoural administration of poly I:C delayed B16.OVA melanoma and E0771 breast cancer outgrowth [83]. Moreover, intratumoural administration of a nanoparticle form of poly I:C, BO-112, induced strong anti-tumour activity in multiple mouse tumour models where subcutaneous administration failed [119]. The antitumour effects were associated with enhanced infiltration of antigen-specific T cells into the tumour and tumour-draining lymph nodes, with an increased Teff/Treg ratio. The protection provided by either intratumoural BO-112 or poly I:C was lost in $Batf3^{-/-}$ mice, which lack conventional DC-1 cells (cDC1), a population with a heightened propensity for cross-priming $CD8^+$ T cells, that was shown to be the major TLR3-positive DC population in the tumour tissue in wild-type animals [34,119,120]. The anti-tumour effects of the TLR3 agonists were also abolished in IFNAR1 knockout mice [34,119,120], highlighting a key role for type I IFN signalling.

Intratumoural administration of poly A:U, a double-stranded polyribonucleotide that is less toxic (but also less potent) than poly I:C, could also delay the growth of B16 melanomas, which was again associated with an increased Teff/Treg ratio, and also a greater number of $CD8^+$ T cells expressing the effector molecule granzyme B [120–122]. There was also increased expression of PD-1 on $CD8^+$ T cells and PD-L1 on myeloid cell populations including M2-type macrophages, suggesting combinations of poly A:U with inhibitors to neutralise this immune checkpoint may enhance the response [120]. Combining intratumoural poly I:C with systemic administration of Flt3 ligand resulted in enhanced cDC1 accumulation in the tumour and was associated with an increased tumour antigen-specific $CD8^+$ T cell response. Taking this a step further, responses were improved again when Flt3 and poly I:C were used in conjunction with PD-L1 blockade and B-Raf proto-oncogene (BRAF) blockade [34], two commonly used treatments in the clinic. Overall, given that combination treatments have been more effective in preclinical studies, intratumoural TLR3 agonists like BO-112 are currently being investigated in patients with solid tumours in combination with systemic anti-PD-1 (NCT02828098; NCT04508140; NCT02423863) [123].

2.1.4. TLR4

Agonists for TLR4 are already clinically approved for use as immune adjuvants in vaccine therapy, as exemplified by the use of monophosphoryl lipid A (MPL), a detoxified version of the well-known TLR4 agonist LPS, in the human papillomavirus (HPV) vaccine, Cervarix[TM] [124,125]. Preclinical studies in mice have shown that intratumoural administration of LPS can result in antitumour effects, with more consistent tumour control observed compared to subcutaneous administration at a contralateral site or intraperitoneal administration [36,126,127]. Assessment of tumours after intratumoural treatment with LPS, or with a synthetic lipid A derivative (formulated glucopyranosyl lipid A; G100), revealed an inflamed tumour milieu, with an influx of effector T cells and NK cells and increased expression of activation markers on tumour-resident cDC1s [30,128]. Interestingly, as seen with CpG-ODN, in a model of B cell lymphoma, G100 induced a protective CD8[+] T cell response that was dependent on tumour cell expression of TLR4 [129].

It is widely known that exposure to LPS can polarise macrophages to an M1 phenotype [130–132]. Others have shown that TLR4 signalling in the TME can promote the recruitment of macrophages from the systemic circulation into the tumour environment [133–135]. However, these effects have not been consistently seen with intratumoural treatment. A minor increase in macrophage infiltrate within the TME was observed following G100 administration, but not with LPS [30,128]. Interestingly, low dose LPS resulted in increased infiltration of M1-type macrophages and elevated type I IFN, but failed to control tumour growth in a model of 4T1 breast cancer [136]. Instead, this treatment enhanced tumour growth, resulting in larger primary tumour volume and greater metastasis to the lungs. As intratumourally LPS treated mice displayed elevated systemic inflammatory cytokines, including IL-1α, IL-1β, and TNF, it was suggested that systemic inflammation hindered the antitumour response. Indeed, in a separate study, intratumoural LPS was found to enhance the antitumour response of an oncolytic virus targeting OVA in a model of B16.OVA melanoma, but this combination actually resulted in rapid morbidity and mortality in the majority of mice [137]. Together these findings suggest that strategies to improve sequestration in the tumour with limited leakage are needed, or perhaps the evaluation of TLR4 agonists with less potent activity.

Combination treatments may be required to extract benefit from intratumoural treatment with TLR4 agonists. The combination of intratumoural MPL and agonistic anti-CD40, which is known to activate macrophages, enhanced macrophage-induced killing of tumour cells, resulting in a significant increase in anti-tumour activity in mice compared to either treatment alone [36]. The alarmin, HMGN1, has been identified as a TLR4 ligand, and when injected intratumourally with cyclophosphamide and the TLR7/8 ligand, resiquimod (R848), caused the elimination of established CT26 colon carcinomas [138]. This response correlated with an increase in tumour infiltrating T cells and increased activation and homing of tumour DCs to the draining lymph node. Systemic administration of G100 has been reported to enhance the antitumour response when combined with either anti-PD1 or anti-PDL1 in a model of B16.F10 melanoma [37]. However, the impact of intratumoural delivery has not to our knowledge been reported. Despite this, numerous clinical trials are currently investigating the intratumoural effects of G100 as a monotherapy or in combination with checkpoint inhibitors, radiotherapy, and antigen (NCT02035657, NCT02180698, NCT02320305, NCT02501473).

2.1.5. TLR7/8

The intracellular TLR7/TLR8 receptors recognise single-stranded RNA and RNA viruses, and induce signalling via the MyD88 pathway. The activation of TLR7/8 on cDCs leads to their maturation and improves antigen cross-presentation via increased formation of MHC-peptide complexes, up-regulation of costimulatory molecules (CD80/86, CD40), and release of IL-12, while ligation by TLR7/8 agonists on pDCs induces the production of type I IFNs, further amplifying antigen cross-presentation [139].

The two dual TLR7/8 agonists, resiquimod and telratolimod (also known as MEDI9197 and 3M-052), have been observed to delay tumour growth when administered intratumourally in models of squamous cell carcinoma [140], melanoma [39], colon adenocarcinoma [29], breast cancer [38], and glioma [141]. Both promote polarisation of the TME towards a Th1 phenotype, with increases in effector T cells and M1-type macrophages and the production of IFN-α by pDCs alongside DC maturation. Intratumoural PD-1/PD-L1 expression was increased following telratolimod administration and consequently, the combination of telratolimod and systemic anti-PD-L1 led to increases in median survival in a B16.OVA model and induced tumour regression [29]. Furthermore, combination with anti-PD1 increased survival and prevented metastases in the triple negative 4T1 breast cancer model [38]. Combining telratolimod with both anti-CTLA-4 and anti-PD-L1 resulted in superior activity against treated and untreated tumours than single agents in B16.F10 melanomas, with both tumours displaying an increase in antigen-specific CD8$^+$ T cells [39]. Significant tumour growth inhibition was achieved when combining intratumoural telratolimod with systemic agonistic anti-OX40 compared to either agent given alone, which may be due to observed increases in OX40 receptor expression in treated tumours as a result of TLR7/8 agonism [29]. As observed with TLR9 agonists, attempts to improve the retention of TLR7/8 agonists in the tumour by formulating resiquimod into thermosensitive liposomes have been investigated [142].

Telratolimod has been evaluated in a phase I trial in patients with advanced solid tumours either as a monotherapy or in combination with anti-PD-L1 therapy and/or palliative radiation therapy. However, no patient responses were observed, despite both systemic and intratumoural immune activation, suggesting further investigation into the patient populations or combinations that best work with TLR7/8 agonists is needed [143].

2.2. STING, RIG-I, or NLR Agonists

2.2.1. RIG-I

RIG-I is a cytosolic PRR that plays a prominent role in antiviral defence by detecting viral and endogenous RNA and triggering binding to the mitochondrial antiviral signalling protein MAVS [144]. Its activation induces apoptosis preferentially in tumour cells and simultaneously activates the innate immune system via type I IFN signalling [145,146]. Intratumoural administration of the RIG-I agonist, MK461, resulted in a rapid antitumour response dependent on NK cells followed by long-term tumour control, most likely mediated by T cells [74,147]. In support, the RIG-I agonist stem loop RNA 14 (SLR14) was found to induce a strong anti-tumour response at both treated and untreated tumour sites, with residual antitumour activity observed in RAG$^{-/-}$ mice [49]. Therefore, both T cells and non-T cells appear to be involved in the response triggered by intratumoural RIG-I signalling. Interestingly, fluorescence-labelled SLR14 is mainly taken up by CD11b$^+$ myeloid cells in the TME, however, further investigation into what subtype of myeloid cells and how this enhanced the inflammatory profile in the tumour is required.

An identified advantage of therapy utilising RLR signalling is that tumour cells are highly sensitive to RLR-induced apoptosis, whereas non-malignant cells are protected by endogenous B-cell lymphoma-extra large (Bcl-xL) expression [145,148]. Therefore, RIG-I agonists have been combined with checkpoint inhibitors, with the addition of the agonist overcoming tumour resistance to anti-PD-1 and anti-CTLA4 by enhancing tumour cell death and cross-priming by cDC1s to potentiate systemic cytotoxic T lymphocyte (CTL) antitumour responses [49,149].

2.2.2. STING

STING is a transmembrane receptor that responds to cyclic dinucleotide (CDN) binding, resulting in downstream signalling involving TBK1 activation, IRF-3 phosphorylation, and the production primarily of IFN-β, as well as IFN-α, TNF, and IL-1β [150–153]. Intratumoural administration of a mouse-selective STING agonist, 5,6-dimethylxanthenone-4acetic acid (DMXAA), was shown to generate potent T cell responses in multiple tumour models, including B16.SIY and methylcholanthrene (MCA)-induced sarcomas, resulting in tumour rejection in the majority of mice [154,155]. A significant portion of the anti-tumour response induced by DMXAA was lost in IFNAR-deficient mice and Batf3$^{-/-}$ mice, supporting the role of cDC1s and type I IFN signalling in STING agonist activity [155]. The response was abrogated in Rag$^{-/-}$ mice, indicating a crucial antitumour T cell response [52].

STING activation increases expression of OX40 and CD27 in the TME, while also upregulating inhibitory immune checkpoints such as the PD-1/PD-L1 axis and CTLA-4 [52], suggesting STING agonists should be used in combination with immune checkpoint inhibitors. Indeed, one study found that the agonist, cyclic di-GMP (CDG), potentiated the effects of a triple combination including anti-CTLA-4, anti-PD-1, and agonistic anti-CD137, in a model of prostate cancer [50]. Effective therapy was correlated with increased Teff/Treg ratio and increased M1-type macrophages. A separate study found that STING agonism in a combination with chemotherapeutic carboplatin and anti-PD1 significantly increased survival in an ovarian carcinoma model relative to the carboplatin and anti-PD-1 double combination [51].

The synthetic CDNs, 2'3'-c-di-AM(PS)2 (ADU-S100, also called MIW815 or RR-CDA) and 3'3'-cGAMP (cGAMP) and GSK532, and CDN-unrelated STING agonists, TTI-10001 and CRD5500 (also called LB-061), activate human STING alleles and have exhibited antitumour efficacy when administered intratumourally in several mouse tumour models including CT26 colon [53,156,157], MC-38 colon [158], Lewis lung carcinoma [52], and 4T1 breast carcinomas [159]. Similar to studies with murine agonists, induction of a strong type I IFN signal within the TME was central to the response alongside an increase in the Teff/Treg ratio. The dosing regimen was found to important in one study, with repetitive low doses of ADU-S100 shown to be more effective than a high dose regimen at inducing a tumour-specific CD8$^+$ T cell response and durable anti-tumour immunity [53]. When used in combination therapy, STING agonists were found to help remodel the tumour vasculature, with the triple combination of ADU-S100 with vascular endothelial growth factor receptor 2 (VEGFR2) blockade and either anti-PD1 or anti-CTLA4 resulting in improved antitumour activity and overall survival [52]. These strong antitumour effects have provided the rationale for clinical assessment of intratumoural STING agonists alone (NCT03937141; NCT04220866; NCT03843359) or in combination with anti-PD1 and anti-CTLA4 (NCT03172936; NCT02675439; NCT03010176).

2.3. Available Local Antigen Dose—The Missing Ingredient?

The key threshold in determining the efficacy of intratumoural treatment with PRR agonists is the initial priming (or boosting) of sufficient numbers of T cells to elicit an effective response. Efficacy may, therefore, be down to the antigen dose released within the immunostimulatory environment that is created by treatment. As already noted, antigen dose can be enhanced with the use of agents that induce ICD, and this is likely to be the reason intratumoural PRR agonists often work in synergy with conventional treatments, such as chemotherapy or radiation therapy. This also likely explains the success in preclinical models in combining intratumoural PRR agonists with antibodies that cause antibody-dependent cellular cytotoxicity, such as anti-CD20 and anti-Mucin-1 [160–162]. In exploring the concept of raising local antigen dose, an early study showed enhanced antitumour activity with intratumoural CpG-ODN in combination with tumour lysate-pulsed DCs [163]. In another study, CpG-ODNs were combined with a recombinant adenovirus encoding tumour necrosis factor-related apoptosis-inducing ligand (TRAIL) to induce tumour cell apoptosis and thereby release antigens [164]. Absorption of LPS onto a GM-CSF-secreting whole tumour cell vaccine (GVAX) enhanced the therapeutic efficacy when injected intratumourally compared to GVAX alone in a CT26 colon carcinoma model [165]. Where tumour antigens are known, it may be possible to inject specific tumour antigens to increase the local dose. A recombinant adenovirus encoding a tumour-associated antigen was used successfully with CpG-ODN to increase survival times [166], and CpG-ODN also supported induction of antigen-specific responses following injection of a fusion protein containing a viral oncoprotein antigen [167]. Studies incorporating CpG-ODN and antigen into an injectable hydrogel were recently followed up with the additional incorporation of immune cells, which enhanced the antitumour effect [168]. In another study of note, tumours were injected with CpG-ODN and antigen that was not even expressed in the tumour [169]. In this case, the choice of a particularly immunodominant epitope may have generated memory CD8$^+$ T cells that performed immunologic helper functions. The authors speculated that other irrelevant antigens may be used similarly, and had previously shown that injecting the pan MHC class II-binding peptide (pan HLA-DR reactive epitope; PADRE) helped control tumours through the generation of CD4$^+$ T helper cells [170]. As there have been significant advances in using bioinformatics to quickly develop personalised vaccines against patient-specific neoantigens [171], it is possible that in the future these vaccines could be repurposed for intratumoural delivery with PRR agonists.

With adoptive T cell therapies finding clinical application, current protocols may also be increased by timely intratumoural administration of PRR agonists. In mouse models, the efficacy of transfer of melanoma-specific CTL therapy was increased in this manner, with the PRR agonists activating host cells to enhance the IFN-γ production and killing by adoptively transferred T cells [35]. Intratumoural injection may also be used to help increase tumour-specific T cell numbers in vivo for subsequent ex vivo expansion and transfer [172].

We note that anti-tumour responses to PRR agonists alone have tended to be observed in tumour models known to respond to checkpoint inhibitors, such as CT26, MC38, and 4T1 [29,147,173], suggesting that some level of pre-existing immunity is advantageous. However, as noted earlier, combining checkpoint blockade with PRR agonists can often result in more animals responding, suggesting that the PRR agonists can to some extent turn a "cold" tumour, with limited immune infiltration, into a "hot" one with increased infiltration. While this is could be a major benefit of the combined approach, a potential side effect could be increased toxicity, which is not insignificant with checkpoint blockade alone. However, increased toxicity has not been noted in the clinical application of intratumoural CpG-ODN and anti-PD1 [174], suggesting that the localised effect of intratumoural administration may limit deleterious effects. Nonetheless, the dose of PRR agonists used in the clinic should be considered carefully, especially where repeated dosing in the context of combined treatment could potentially amplify risks.

3. Concluding Statement

Preclinical studies have highlighted the unique added benefit of delivering PRR agonists directly into the tumour bed. However, full regression is rarely seen with this treatment alone, which has also been seen in clinical studies. The future of this form of treatment is therefore likely to be in combination with other cancer therapies, whether this is chemotherapy, radiation therapy, or recently developed immunotherapies based on T cell modulation. The major advantage of such "in situ vaccination" with PRR agonists is that the tumour antigens targeted do not have to be defined. Nonetheless, it may be possible to incorporate this untargeted element of the treatment with targeted therapies, be they antigen-specific or personalised vaccines, or adoptive T cell therapies.

Author Contributions: Conceptualisation, writing, and editing: O.K.B., K.K.P., and I.F.H. All authors have read and agreed to the published version of the manuscript.

Funding: O.K.B., K.K.P., and I.F.H. were financially supported by the Malaghan Institute of Medical Research and Maurice Wilkins Centre.

Acknowledgments: The authors were supported by an Independent Research Organisation grant from the Health Research Council of New Zealand to the Malaghan Institute (grant number HRC14/1003), and the New Zealand Ministry of Business Innovation and Employment (RTVU1603). Figure created with BioRender.com.

Conflicts of Interest: I.F.H. is CSO of biotech start-up Avalia Immunotherapies Limited. The other authors declare no conflict of interest.

References

1. Janeway, C. Approaching the asymptote? Evolution and revolution in immunology. *Cold Spring Harb. Symp. Quant. Biol.* **1989**, *54*, 1–13. [CrossRef] [PubMed]
2. Iwasaki, A.; Medzhitov, R. Control of adaptive immunity by the innate immune system. *Nat. Immunol.* **2015**, *16*, 343–353. [CrossRef] [PubMed]
3. Kerkar, S.P.; Restifo, N.P. Cellular constituents of immune escape within the tumor microenvironment. *Cancer Res.* **2012**, *72*, 3125–3130. [CrossRef]
4. Junttila, M.R.; de Sauvage, F.J. Influence of tumour micro-environment heterogeneity on therapeutic response. *Nature* **2013**, *501*, 346–354. [CrossRef] [PubMed]
5. Vaupel, P.; Thews, O.; Hoeckel, M. Treatment resistance of solid tumors. *Med. Oncol.* **2001**, *18*, 243–260. [CrossRef]
6. Bourquin, C.; Pommier, A.; Hotz, C. Harnessing the immune system to fight cancer with Toll-like receptor and RIG-I-like receptor agonists. *Pharmacol. Res.* **2020**, *154*, 104192. [CrossRef] [PubMed]
7. Peng, G. Toll-like receptor 8-mediated reversal of CD4+ regulatory T cell function. *Science* **2005**, *309*, 1380–1384. [CrossRef]
8. Li, S.; Sun, R.; Chen, Y.; Wei, H.; Tian, Z. TLR2 limits development of hepatocellular carcinoma by reducing IL18-mediated immunosuppression. *Cancer Res.* **2015**, *75*, 986–995. [CrossRef]
9. Van Mierlo, G.J.D.; Boonman, Z.F.H.M.; Dumortier, H.M.H.; den Boer, A.T.; Fransen, M.F.; Nouta, J.; van der Voort, E.I.H.; Offringa, R.; Toes, R.E.M.; Melief, C.J.M. Activation of dendritic cells that cross-present tumor-derived antigen licenses CD8+ CTL to cause tumor eradication. *J. Immunol.* **2004**, *173*, 6753–6759. [CrossRef]
10. Janeway, C.A., Jr.; Medzhitov, R. Innate immune recognition. *Annu. Rev. Immunol.* **2002**, *20*, 197–216. [CrossRef]
11. Matzinger, P. Tolerance, danger, and the extended family. *Annu. Rev. Immunol.* **1994**, *12*, 991–1045. [CrossRef] [PubMed]
12. Takeuchi, O.; Akira, S. Pattern recognition receptors and inflammation. *Cell* **2010**, *140*, 805–820. [CrossRef] [PubMed]
13. Scaffidi, P.; Misteli, T.; Bianchi, M.E. Release of chromatin protein HMGB1 by necrotic cells triggers inflammation. *Nature* **2002**, *418*, 191–195. [CrossRef] [PubMed]
14. Pockley, A.G.; Shepherd, J.; Corton, J.M. Detection of heat shock protein 70 (HSP70) and anti-HSP70 antibodies in the serum of normal individuals. *Immunol. Investig.* **1998**, *27*, 367–377. [CrossRef]
15. Khakh, B.S.; Burnstock, G. The double life of ATP. *Sci. Am.* **2009**, *301*, 84–92. [CrossRef]
16. Schaefer, L.; Babelova, A.; Kiss, E.; Hausser, H.-J.; Baliova, M.; Krzyzankova, M.; Marsche, G.; Young, M.F.; Mihalik, D.; Götte, M.; et al. The matrix component biglycan is proinflammatory and signals through Toll-like receptors 4 and 2 in macrophages. *J. Clin. Investig.* **2005**, *115*, 2223–2233. [CrossRef]
17. Smiley, S.T.; King, J.A.; Hancock, W.W. Fibrinogen stimulates macrophage chemokine secretion through Toll-like receptor. *J. Immunol.* **2001**, *167*, 2887–2894. [CrossRef]
18. Bekeredjian-Ding, I.; Roth, S.I.; Gilles, S.; Giese, T.; Ablasser, A.; Hornung, V.; Endres, S.; Hartmann, G. T cell-independent, TLR-induced IL-12p70 production in primary human monocytes. *J. Immunol.* **2006**, *176*, 7438–7446. [CrossRef]
19. Hayashi, F.; Smith, K.D.; Ozinsky, A.; Hawn, T.R.; Yi, E.C.; Goodlett, D.R.; Eng, J.K.; Akira, S.; Underhill, D.M.; Aderem, A. The innate immune response to bacterial flagellin is mediated by Toll-like receptor. *Nature* **2001**, *410*, 1099–1103. [CrossRef]
20. Le Bon, A.; Etchart, N.; Rossmann, C.; Ashton, M.; Hou, S.; Gewert, D.; Borrow, P.; Tough, D.F. Cross-priming of CD8+ T cells stimulated by virus-induced type I interferon. *Nat. Immunol.* **2003**, *4*, 1009–1015. [CrossRef]
21. Stetson, D.B.; Medzhitov, R. Type I Interferons in host defense. *Immunity* **2006**, *25*, 373–381. [CrossRef] [PubMed]
22. Lebon, A.; Tough, D.F. Type I interferon as a stimulus for cross-priming. *Cytokine Growth Factor Rev.* **2008**, *19*, 33–40. [CrossRef] [PubMed]
23. De Filippo, K.; Dudeck, A.; Hasenberg, M.; Nye, E.; van Rooijen, N.; Hartmann, K.; Gunzer, M.; Roers, A.; Hogg, N. Mast cell and macrophage chemokines CXCL1/CXCL2 control the early stage of neutrophil recruitment during tissue inflammation. *Blood* **2013**, *121*, 4930–4937. [CrossRef] [PubMed]

24. Sokol, C.L.; Luster, A.D. The chemokine system in innate immunity. *Cold Spring Harb. Perspect. Biol.* **2015**, *7*, a016303. [CrossRef] [PubMed]

25. Kaczanowska, S.; Joseph, A.M.; Davila, E. TLR agonists: Our best frenemy in cancer immunotherapy. *J. Leukoc. Biol.* **2013**, *93*, 847–863. [CrossRef] [PubMed]

26. Garay, R.P.; Viens, P.; Bauer, J.; Normier, G.; Bardou, M.; Jeannin, J.-F.; Chiavaroli, C. Cancer relapse under chemotherapy: Why TLR2/4 receptor agonists can help. *Eur. J. Pharmacol.* **2007**, *563*, 1–17. [CrossRef]

27. Vacchelli, E.; Galluzzi, L.; Eggermont, A.; Fridman, W.H.; Galon, J.; Sautès-Fridman, C.; Tartour, E.; Zitvogel, L.; Kroemer, G. Trial watch: FDA-approved Toll-like receptor agonists for cancer therapy. *OncoImmunology* **2012**, *1*, 894–907. [CrossRef]

28. Engel, A.L.; Holt, G.; Lu, H. The pharmacokinetics of Toll-like receptor agonists and the impact on the immune system. *Expert Rev. Clin. Pharmacol.* **2011**, *4*, 275–289. [CrossRef]

29. Mullins, S.R.; Vasilakos, J.P.; Deschler, K.; Grigsby, I.; Gillis, P.; John, J.; Elder, M.J.; Swales, J.; Timosenko, E.; Cooper, Z.; et al. Intratumoral immunotherapy with TLR7/8 agonist MEDI9197 modulates the tumor microenvironment leading to enhanced activity when combined with other immunotherapies. *J. Immunother. Cancer* **2019**, *7*, 244. [CrossRef]

30. Albershardt, T.C.; LeLeux, J.; Parsons, A.J.; Krull, J.E.; Berglund, P.; Ter Meulen, J. Intratumoral immune activation with TLR4 agonist synergizes with effector T cells to eradicate established murine tumors. *NPJ Vaccines* **2020**, *5*, 50. [CrossRef]

31. Leong, W.I.; Ames, R.Y.; Haverkamp, J.M.; Torres, L.; Kline, J.; Bans, A.; Rocha, L.; Gallotta, M.; Guiducci, C.; Coffman, R.L.; et al. Low-dose metronomic cyclophosphamide complements the actions of an intratumoral C-class CpG TLR9 agonist to potentiate innate immunity and drive potent T cell-mediated anti-tumor responses. *Oncotarget* **2019**, *10*, 7220–7237. [CrossRef] [PubMed]

32. Iwasaki, A.; Medzhitov, R. Toll-like receptor control of the adaptive immune responses. *Nat. Immunol.* **2004**, *5*, 987–995. [CrossRef] [PubMed]

33. Sharma, N.; Vacher, J.; Allison, J.P. TLR1/2 ligand enhances antitumor efficacy of CTLA-4 blockade by increasing intratumoral Treg depletion. *Proc. Natl. Acad. Sci. USA* **2019**, *116*, 10453–10462. [CrossRef] [PubMed]

34. Salmon, H.; Idoyaga, J.; Rahman, A.; Leboeuf, M.; Remark, R.; Jordan, S.; Casanova-Acebes, M.; Khudoynazarova, M.; Agudo, J.; Tung, N.; et al. Expansion and activation of CD103+ dendritic cell progenitors at the tumor site enhances tumor responses to therapeutic PD-L1 and BRAF inhibition. *Immunity* **2016**, *44*, 924–938. [CrossRef]

35. Amos, S.M.; Pegram, H.J.; Westwood, J.A.; John, L.B.; Devaud, C.; Clarke, C.J.; Restifo, N.P.; Smyth, M.J.; Darcy, P.K.; Kershaw, M.H. Adoptive immunotherapy combined with intratumoral TLR agonist delivery eradicates established melanoma in mice. *Cancer Immunol. Immunother.* **2011**, *60*, 671–683. [CrossRef]

36. Van De Voort, T.J.; Felder, M.A.R.; Yang, R.K.; Sondel, P.M.; Rakhmilevich, A.L. Intratumoral delivery of low doses of anti-CD40 mAb combined with monophosphoryl lipid A induces local and systemic antitumor effects in immunocompetent and T cell-deficient mice. *J. Immunother.* **2013**, *36*, 29–40. [CrossRef]

37. Albershardt, T.C.; Parsons, A.J.; ter Meulen, J.; Berglund, P. Checkpoint inhibitors synergize with therapeutic platforms, ZVex™ and GLAAS™ by enhancing lentiviral vector-induced tumor-specific immunity and adjuvant-mediated anti-tumor efficacy. *J. Immunother. Cancer* **2015**, *3*, P346. [CrossRef]

38. Zanker, D.J.; Spurling, A.J.; Brockwell, N.K.; Owen, K.L.; Zakhour, J.M.; Robinson, T.; Duivenvoorden, H.M.; Hertzog, P.J.; Mullins, S.R.; Wilkinson, R.W.; et al. Intratumoral administration of the Toll-like receptor 7/8 agonist 3M-052 enhances interferon-driven tumor immunogenicity and suppresses metastatic spread in preclinical triple-negative breast cancer. *Clin. Transl. Immunol.* **2020**, *9*, e1177. [CrossRef]

39. Singh, M.; Khong, H.; Dai, Z.; Huang, X.-F.; Wargo, J.A.; Cooper, Z.; Vasilakos, J.P.; Hwu, P.; Overwijk, W.W. Effective innate and adaptive antimelanoma immunity through localized TLR7/8 activation. *J. Immunol.* **2014**, *193*, 4722–4731. [CrossRef]

40. Houot, R.; Levy, R. T-cell modulation combined with intratumoral CpG cures lymphoma in a mouse model without the need for chemotherapy. *Blood* **2009**, *113*, 3546–3552. [CrossRef]

41. Reilley, M.J.; Morrow, B.; Ager, C.R.; Liu, A.; Hong, D.S.; Curran, M.A. TLR9 activation cooperates with T cell checkpoint blockade to regress poorly immunogenic melanoma. *J. Immunother. Cancer* **2019**, *7*, 1–9. [CrossRef] [PubMed]

42. Sagiv-Barfi, I.; Czerwinski, D.K.; Levy, S.; Alam, I.S.; Mayer, A.T.; Gambhir, S.S.; Levy, R. Eradication of spontaneous malignancy by local immunotherapy. *Sci. Transl. Med.* **2018**, *10*, eaan4488. [CrossRef] [PubMed]

43. Marabelle, A.; Kohrt, H.; Sagiv-Barfi, I.; Ajami, B.; Axtell, R.C.; Zhou, G.; Rajapaksa, R.; Green, M.R.; Torchia, J.; Brody, J.; et al. Depleting tumor-specific Tregs at a single site eradicates disseminated tumors. *J. Clin. Investig.* **2013**, *123*, 2447–2463. [CrossRef] [PubMed]

44. Wang, S.; Campos, J.; Gallotta, M.; Gong, M.; Crain, C.; Naik, E.; Coffman, R.L.; Guiducci, C. Intratumoral injection of a CpG oligonucleotide reverts resistance to PD-1 blockade by expanding multifunctional CD8+ T cells. *Proc. Natl. Acad. Sci. USA* **2016**, *113*, E7240–E7249. [CrossRef] [PubMed]

45. Zhuang, Y.; Li, S.; Wang, H.; Pi, J.; Xing, Y.; Li, G. PD-1 blockade enhances radio-immunotherapy efficacy in murine tumor models. *J. Cancer Res. Clin. Oncol.* **2018**, *144*, 1909–1920. [CrossRef]

46. Walters, A.A.; Wang, J.T.-W.; Al-Jamal, K.T. Evaluation of cell surface reactive immuno-adjuvant in combination with immunogenic cell death inducing drug for in situ chemo-immunotherapy. *J. Control. Release* **2020**, *322*, 519–529. [CrossRef]

47. Sagiv-Barfi, I.; Kohrt, H.E.; Burckhardt, L.; Czerwinski, D.K.; Levy, R. Ibrutinib enhances the antitumor immune response induced by intratumoral injection of a TLR9 ligand in mouse lymphoma. *Blood* **2015**, *125*, 2079–2086. [CrossRef]

48. Zhao, B.G.; Vasilakos, J.P.; Tross, D.; Smirnov, D.; Klinman, D.M. Combination therapy targeting toll like receptors 7, 8 and 9 eliminates large established tumors. *J. Immunother. Cancer* **2014**, *2*, 12. [CrossRef]

49. Jiang, X.; Muthusamy, V.; Fedorova, O.; Kong, Y.; Kim, D.J.; Bosenberg, M.; Pyle, A.M.; Iwasaki, A. Intratumoral delivery of RIG-I agonist SLR14 induces robust antitumor responses. *J. Exp. Med.* **2019**, *216*, 2854–2868. [CrossRef]

50. Ager, C.R.; Reilley, M.J.; Nicholas, C.; Bartkowiak, T.; Jaiswal, A.R.; Curran, M.A. Intratumoral STING activation with T-cell checkpoint modulation generates systemic antitumor immunity. *Cancer Immunol. Res.* **2017**, *5*, 676–684. [CrossRef] [PubMed]

51. Ghaffari, A.; Peterson, N.; Khalaj, K.; Vitkin, N.; Robinson, A.; Francis, J.-A.; Koti, M. STING agonist therapy in combination with PD-1 immune checkpoint blockade enhances response to carboplatin chemotherapy in high-grade serous ovarian cancer. *Br. J. Cancer* **2018**, *119*, 440–449. [CrossRef] [PubMed]

52. Yang, H.; Lee, W.S.; Kong, S.J.; Kim, C.G.; Kim, J.H.; Chang, S.K.; Kim, S.; Kim, G.; Chon, H.J.; Kim, C. STING activation reprograms tumor vasculatures and synergizes with VEGFR2 blockade. *J. Clin. Investig.* **2019**, *129*, 4350–4364. [CrossRef] [PubMed]

53. Sivick, K.E.; Desbien, A.L.; Glickman, L.H.; Reiner, G.L.; Corrales, L.; Surh, N.H.; Hudson, T.E.; Vu, U.T.; Francica, B.J.; Banda, T.; et al. Magnitude of therapeutic STING activation determines CD8+ T cell-mediated anti-tumor immunity. *Cell Rep.* **2018**, *25*, 3074–3085.e5. [CrossRef]

54. O'Neill, L.A.; Golenbock, D.T.; Bowie, A.G. The history of Toll-like receptors—Redefining innate immunity. *Nat. Rev. Immunol.* **2013**, *13*, 453–460. [CrossRef]

55. Osmond, T.L.; Farrand, K.J.; Painter, G.F.; Ruedl, C.; Petersen, T.R.; Hermans, I.F. Activated NKT cells can condition different splenic dendritic cell subsets to respond more effectively to TLR engagement and enhance cross-priming. *J. Immunol.* **2015**, *195*, 821–831. [CrossRef]

56. Blasius, A.L.; Beutler, B.A. Intracellular toll-like receptors. *Immunity* **2010**, *32*, 305–315. [CrossRef]

57. Mukherjee, S.; Karmakar, S.; Babu, S.P.S. TLR2 and TLR4 mediated host immune responses in major infectious diseases: A review. *Braz. J. Infect. Dis.* **2016**, *20*, 193–204. [CrossRef]

58. Horrevorts, S.K.; Duinkerken, S.; Bloem, K.; Secades, P.; Kalay, H.; Musters, R.J.; van Vliet, S.J.; Garcia-Vallejo, J.J.; van Kooyk, Y. Toll-like receptor 4 triggering promotes cytosolic routing of DC-SIGN-targeted antigens for presentation on MHC class I. *Front. Immunol.* **2018**, *9*, 1231. [CrossRef]

59. Mazzoni, A.; Segal, D.M. Controlling the Toll road to dendritic cell polarization. *J. Leukoc. Biol.* **2004**, *75*, 721–730. [CrossRef]

60. E Sousa, C.R. Toll-like receptors and dendritic cells: For whom the bug tolls. *Semin. Immunol.* **2004**, *16*, 27–34. [CrossRef]

61. Jacquemin, C.; Schmitt, N.; Contin-Bordes, C.; Liu, Y.; Narayanan, P.; Seneschal, J.; Maurouard, T.; Dougall, D.; Davizon, E.S.; Dumortier, H.; et al. OX40 ligand contributes to human lupus pathogenesis by promoting T follicular helper response. *Immunity* **2015**, *42*, 1159–1170. [CrossRef] [PubMed]

62. Cheever, M.A. Twelve immunotherapy drugs that could cure cancers. *Immunol. Rev.* **2008**, *222*, 357–368. [CrossRef] [PubMed]

63. Adamus, T.; Kortylewski, M. The revival of CpG oligonucleotide-based cancer immunotherapies. *Współczesna Onkol.* **2018**, *2018*, 56–60. [CrossRef]

64. Karapetyan, L.; Luke, J.J.; Davar, D. Toll-like receptor 9 agonists in cancer. *Onco Targets Ther.* **2020**, *13*, 10039–10061. [CrossRef] [PubMed]

65. Kaisho, T.; Akira, S. Regulation of dendritic cell function through Toll-like receptors. *Curr. Mol. Med.* **2003**, *3*, 373–385. [CrossRef]

66. Carpentier, A.F.; Xie, J.; Mokhtari, K.; Delattre, J.-Y. Successful treatment of intracranial gliomas in rat by oligodeoxynucleotides containing CpG motifs. *Clin. Cancer Res.* **2000**, *6*, 2469–2473. [PubMed]

67. Auf, G.; Carpentier, A.F.; Chen, L.; Le Clanche, C.; Delattre, J.Y. Implication of macrophages in tumor rejection induced by CpG-oligodeoxynucleotides without antigen. *Clin. Cancer Res.* **2001**, *7*, 3540–3543. [PubMed]

68. Sharma, S.; Karakousis, C.P.; Takita, H.; Shin, K.; Brooks, S.P. Intra-tumoral injection of CpG results in the inhibition of tumor growth in murine Colon-26 and B-16 tumors. *Biotechnol. Lett.* **2003**, *25*, 149–153. [CrossRef]

69. Lonsdorf, A.S.; Kuekrek, H.; Stern, B.V.; Boehm, B.O.; Lehmann, P.V.; Tary-Lehmann, M. Intratumor CpG-oligodeoxynucleotide injection induces protective antitumor T cell immunity. *J. Immunol.* **2003**, *171*, 3941–3946. [CrossRef]

70. Furumoto, K.; Soares, L.; Engleman, E.G.; Merad, M. Induction of potent antitumor immunity by in situ targeting of intratumoral DCs. *J. Clin. Investig.* **2004**, *113*, 774–783. [CrossRef]

71. Bao, M.; Liu, Y.-J. Regulation of TLR7/9 signaling in plasmacytoid dendritic cells. *Protein Cell* **2012**, *4*, 40–52. [CrossRef] [PubMed]

72. Rothenfusser, S.; Tuma, E.; Endres, S.; Hartmann, G. Plasmacytoid dendritic cells: The key to CpG. *Hum. Immunol.* **2002**, *63*, 1111–1119. [CrossRef]

73. Lou, Y.; Liu, C.; Lizée, G.; Peng, W.; Xu, C.; Ye, Y.; Rabinovich, B.A.; Hailemichael, Y.; Gelbard, A.; Zhou, D.; et al. Antitumor activity mediated by CpG. *J. Immunother.* **2011**, *34*, 279–288. [CrossRef]

74. Lorenzi, S.; Mattei, F.; Sistigu, A.; Bracci, L.; Spadaro, F.; Sanchez, M.; Spada, M.; Belardelli, F.; Gabriele, L.; Schiavoni, G. Type I IFNs control antigen retention and survival of CD8α+ dendritic cells after uptake of tumor apoptotic cells leading to cross-priming. *J. Immunol.* **2011**, *186*, 5142–5150. [CrossRef]

75. Diamond, M.S.; Kinder, M.; Matsushita, H.; Mashayekhi, M.; Dunn, G.P.; Archambault, J.M.; Lee, H.; Arthur, C.D.; White, J.M.; Kalinke, U.; et al. Type I interferon is selectively required by dendritic cells for immune rejection of tumors. *J. Exp. Med.* **2011**, *208*, 1989–2003. [CrossRef]

76. Fuertes, M.B.; Kacha, A.K.; Kline, J.; Woo, S.-R.; Kranz, D.M.; Murphy, K.M.; Gajewski, T.F. Host type I IFN signals are required for antitumor CD8+ T cell responses through CD8α+ dendritic cells. *J. Exp. Med.* **2011**, *208*, 2005–2016. [CrossRef]

77. Huber, J.P.; Farrar, J.D. Regulation of effector and memory T-cell functions by type I interferon. *Immunology* **2011**, *132*, 466–474. [CrossRef]

78. Xiao, Z.; Casey, K.A.; Jameson, S.C.; Curtsinger, J.M.; Mescher, M.F. Programming for CD8 T cell memory development requires IL-12 or type I IFN. *J. Immunol.* **2009**, *182*, 2786–2794. [CrossRef]

79. Li, T.; Wu, J.; Zhu, S.; Zang, G.; Li, S.; Lv, X.; Yue, W.; Qiao, Y.; Cui, J.; Shao, Y.; et al. A novel C type CpG oligodeoxynucleotide exhibits immunostimulatory activity in vitro and enhances antitumor effect in vivo. *Front. Pharmacol.* **2020**, *11*, 8. [CrossRef]

80. Humbert, M.; Guery, L.; Brighouse, D.; Lemeille, S.; Hugues, S. Intratumoral CpG-B promotes anti-tumoral neutrophil, cDC, and T cell cooperation without reprograming tolerogenic pDC. *Cancer Res.* **2018**, *78*, 3280–3292. [CrossRef]

81. Shirota, Y.; Shirota, H.; Klinman, D.M. Intratumoral injection of CpG oligonucleotides induces the differentiation and reduces the immunosuppressive activity of myeloid-derived suppressor cells. *J. Immunol.* **2012**, *188*, 1592–1599. [CrossRef] [PubMed]

82. Li, J.; Song, W.; Czerwinski, D.K.; Varghese, B.; Uematsu, S.; Akira, S.; Krieg, A.M.; Levy, R. Lymphoma immunotherapy with CpG oligodeoxynucleotides requires TLR9 either in the host or in the tumor itself. *J. Immunol.* **2007**, *179*, 2493–2500. [CrossRef]

83. Yin, P.; Liu, X.; Mansfield, A.S.; Harrington, S.M.; Li, Y.; Yan, Y.; Dong, H. CpG-induced antitumor immunity requires IL-12 in expansion of effector cells and down-regulation of PD-1. *Oncotarget* **2016**, *7*, 70223–70231. [CrossRef] [PubMed]

84. Chen, X.; Li, D.; Cao, Y.; Gao, J.; Jin, H.-J.; Shan, H. Early therapeutic vaccination prediction of hepatocellular carcinoma via imaging OX40-mediated tumor infiltrating lymphocytes. *Mol. Pharm.* **2019**, *16*, 4252–4259. [CrossRef] [PubMed]

85. Yan, Y.; Kumar, A.B.; Finnes, H.; Markovic, S.N.; Park, S.; Dronca, R.S.; Dong, H. Combining immune checkpoint inhibitors with conventional cancer therapy. *Front. Immunol.* **2018**, *9*, 1739. [CrossRef] [PubMed]

86. Mantovani, A.; Sica, A.; Sozzani, S.; Allavena, P.; Vecchi, A.; Locati, M. The chemokine system in diverse forms of macrophage activation and polarization. *Trends Immunol.* **2004**, *25*, 677–686. [CrossRef] [PubMed]

87. Mantovani, A.; Sozzani, S.; Locati, M.; Allavena, P.; Sica, A. Macrophage polarization: Tumor-associated macrophages as a paradigm for polarized M2 mononuclear phagocytes. *Trends Immunol.* **2002**, *23*, 549–555. [CrossRef]

88. Ostrand-Rosenberg, S.; Sinha, P. Macrophages and tumor development. In *Tumor Induced Immune Suppression: Mechanisms and Therapeutic Reversal*; Gavrilovich, D.I., Hurwitz, A.A., Eds.; Springer: New York, NY, USA, 2008; pp. 131–155. ISBN 9780387691183.

89. Kwong, B.; Liu, H.; Irvine, D.J. Induction of potent anti-tumor responses while eliminating systemic side effects via liposome-anchored combinatorial immunotherapy. *Biomaterials* **2011**, *32*, 5134–5147. [CrossRef]

90. Kim, D.H.; Moon, C.; Oh, S.-S.; Park, S.; Jeong, J.-W.; Kim, S.; Lee, H.G.; Kwon, H.-J.; Kim, K.D. Liposome-encapsulated CpG enhances antitumor activity accompanying the changing of lymphocyte populations in tumor via intratumoral administration. *Nucleic Acid Ther.* **2015**, *25*, 95–102. [CrossRef]

91. Ma, Q.; Zhou, D.; DeLyria, E.S.; Wen, X.; Lu, W.; Thapa, P.; Liu, C.; Li, D.; Bassett, R.L.; Overwijk, W.W.; et al. Synthetic poly(L-glutamic acid)-conjugated CpG exhibits antitumor efficacy with increased retention in tumor and draining lymph nodes after intratumoral injection in a mouse model of melanoma. *J. Immunother.* **2017**, *40*, 11–20. [CrossRef]

92. Xu, Y.; Ma, S.; Si, X.; Zhao, J.; Yu, H.; Ma, L.; Song, W.; Tang, Z. Polyethyleneimine-CpG nanocomplex as an in situ vaccine for boosting anticancer immunity in melanoma. *Macromol. Biosci.* **2020**, e2000207. [CrossRef] [PubMed]

93. Fan, H.; Zhang, I.; Chen, X.; Zhang, L.; Wang, H.; da Fonseca, A.C.C.; Manuel, E.R.; Diamond, D.J.; Raubitschek, A.; Badie, B. Intracerebral CpG immunotherapy with carbon nanotubes abrogates growth of subcutaneous melanomas in mice. *Clin. Cancer Res.* **2012**, *18*, 5628–5638. [CrossRef] [PubMed]

94. Zheng, L.; Hu, X.; Wu, H.; Mo, L.; Xie, S.; Li, J.; Peng, C.; Xu, S.; Qiu, L.; Tan, W. In vivo monocyte/macrophage-hitchhiked intratumoral accumulation of nanomedicines for enhanced tumor therapy. *J. Am. Chem. Soc.* **2019**, *142*, 382–391. [CrossRef] [PubMed]

95. Scheetz, L.; Yu, M.; Li, D.; Castro, M.G.; Moon, J.J.; Schwendeman, A.S. Synthetic HDL nanoparticles delivering docetaxel and CpG for chemoimmunotherapy of colon adenocarcinoma. *Int. J. Mol. Sci.* **2020**, *21*, 1777. [CrossRef]

96. Buss, C.G.; Bhatia, S.N. Nanoparticle delivery of immunostimulatory oligonucleotides enhances response to checkpoint inhibitor therapeutics. *Proc. Natl. Acad. Sci. USA* **2020**, *117*, 13428–13436. [CrossRef]

97. Appelbe, O.K.; Moynihan, K.D.; Flor, A.; Rymut, N.; Irvine, D.J.; Kron, S.J. Radiation-enhanced delivery of systemically administered amphiphilic-CpG oligodeoxynucleotide. *J. Control. Release* **2017**, *266*, 248–255. [CrossRef]

98. Li, Y.; He, L.; Dong, H.; Liu, Y.; Wang, K.; Li, A.; Ren, T.; Shi, D.; Li, Y. Fever-inspired immunotherapy based on photothermal CpG nanotherapeutics: The critical role of mild heat in regulating tumor microenvironment. *Adv. Sci.* **2018**, *5*, 1700805. [CrossRef]

99. Zhou, S.; Hashida, Y.; Kawakami, S.; Mihara, J.; Umeyama, T.; Imahori, H.; Murakami, T.; Yamashita, F.; Hashida, M. Preparation of immunostimulatory single-walled carbon nanotube/CpG DNA complexes and evaluation of their potential in cancer immunotherapy. *Int. J. Pharm.* **2014**, *471*, 214–223. [CrossRef]

100. Yata, T.; Takahashi, Y.; Tan, M.; Nakatsuji, H.; Ohtsuki, S.; Murakami, T.; Imahori, H.; Umeki, Y.; Shiomi, T.; Takakura, Y.; et al. DNA nanotechnology-based composite-type gold nanoparticle-immunostimulatory DNA hydrogel for tumor photothermal immunotherapy. *Biomaterials* **2017**, *146*, 136–145. [CrossRef]

101. Chao, Y.; Xu, L.; Liang, C.; Feng, L.; Xu, J.; Dong, Z.; Tian, L.; Yi, X.; Yang, K.; Liu, Z. Combined local immunostimulatory radioisotope therapy and systemic immune checkpoint blockade imparts potent antitumour responses. *Nat. Biomed. Eng.* **2018**, *2*, 611–621. [CrossRef]

102. Heikenwalder, M.; Polymenidou, M.; Junt, T.; Sigurdson, C.; Wagner, H.; Akira, S.; Zinkernagel, R.; Aguzzi, A. Lymphoid follicle destruction and immunosuppression after repeated CpG oligodeoxynucleotide administration. *Nat. Med.* **2004**, *10*, 187–192. [CrossRef] [PubMed]

103. Behrens, E.M.; Canna, S.W.; Slade, K.; Rao, S.; Kreiger, P.A.; Paessler, M.; Kambayashi, T.; Koretzky, G.A. Repeated TLR9 stimulation results in macrophage activation syndrome–like disease in mice. *J. Clin. Investig.* **2011**, *121*, 2264–2277. [CrossRef]

104. Sparwasser, T.; Hültner, L.; Koch, E.S.; Luz, A.; Lipford, G.B.; Wagner, H. Immunostimulatory CpG-oligodeoxynucleotides cause extramedullary murine hemopoiesis. *J. Immunol.* **1999**, *162*, 2368–2374. [PubMed]

105. Manegold, C.; van Zandwijk, N.; Szczesna, A.; Zatloukal, P.; Au, J.S.K.; Blasinska-Morawiec, M.; Serwatowski, P.; Krzakowski, M.; Jassem, J.; Tan, E.H.; et al. A phase III randomized study of gemcitabine and cisplatin with or without PF-3512676 (TLR9 agonist) as first-line treatment of advanced non-small-cell lung cancer. *Ann. Oncol.* **2012**, *23*, 72–77. [CrossRef] [PubMed]

106. Hirsh, V.; Paz-Ares, L.; Boyer, M.; Rosell, R.; Middleton, G.; Eberhardt, W.E.; Szczesna, A.; Reiterer, P.; Saleh, M.; Arrieta, O.; et al. Randomized phase III trial of paclitaxel/carboplatin with or without PF-3512676 (Toll-like receptor 9 agonist) as first-line treatment for advanced non–small-cell lung cancer. *J. Clin. Oncol.* **2011**, *29*, 2667–2674. [CrossRef] [PubMed]

107. Flierl, U.; Nero, T.L.; Lim, B.; Arthur, J.F.; Yao, Y.; Jung, S.M.; Gitz, E.; Pollitt, A.Y.; Zaldivia, M.T.; Jandrot-Perrus, M.; et al. Phosphorothioate backbone modifications of nucleotide-based drugs are potent platelet activators. *J. Exp. Med.* **2015**, *212*, 129–137. [CrossRef]

108. Henry, S.P.; Beattie, G.; Yeh, G.; Chappel, A.; Giclas, P.; Mortari, A.; Jagels, M.A.; Kornbrust, U.J.; Levin, A.A. Complement activation is responsible for acute toxicities in rhesus monkeys treated with a phosphorothioate oligodeoxynucleotide. *Int. Immunopharmacol.* **2002**, *2*, 1657–1666. [CrossRef]

109. Shaw, D.R.; Rustagi, P.K.; Kandimalla, E.R.; Manning, A.N.; Jiang, Z.; Agrawal, S. Effects of synthetic oligonucleotides on human complement and coagulation. *Biochem. Pharmacol.* **1997**, *53*, 1123–1132. [CrossRef]

110. Hanagata, N. Structure-dependent immunostimulatory effect of CpG oligodeoxynucleotides and their delivery system. *Int. J. Nanomed.* **2012**, *7*, 2181–2195. [CrossRef]

111. Munakata, L.; Tanimoto, Y.; Osa, A.; Meng, J.; Haseda, Y.; Naito, Y.; Machiyama, H.; Kumanogoh, A.; Omata, D.; Maruyama, K.; et al. Lipid nanoparticles of Type-A CpG D35 suppress tumor growth by changing tumor immune-microenvironment and activate CD8 T cells in mice. *J. Control. Release* **2019**, *313*, 106–119. [CrossRef]

112. Van Pul, K.M.; Vuylsteke, R.J.C.L.M.; de Beijer, M.T.A.; van de Ven, R.; van den Tol, M.P.; Stockmann, H.B.A.C.; de Gruijl, T.D. Breast cancer-induced immune suppression in the sentinel lymph node is effectively countered by CpG-B in conjunction with inhibition of the JAK2/STAT3 pathway. *J. Immunother. Cancer* **2020**, *8*, e000761. [CrossRef] [PubMed]

113. Ouyang, X.; Negishi, H.; Takeda, R.; Fujita, Y.; Taniguchi, T.; Honda, K. Cooperation between MyD88 and TRIF pathways in TLR synergy via IRF5 activation. *Biochem. Biophys. Res. Commun.* **2007**, *354*, 1045–1051. [CrossRef] [PubMed]

114. Simons, M.P.; O'Donnell, M.A.; Griffith, T.S. Role of neutrophils in BCG immunotherapy for bladder cancer. *Urol. Oncol. Semin. Orig. Investig.* **2008**, *26*, 341–345. [CrossRef] [PubMed]

115. Jin, M.S.; Kim, S.E.; Heo, J.Y.; Lee, M.E.; Kim, H.M.; Paik, S.-G.; Lee, H.; Lee, J.-O. Crystal structure of the TLR1-TLR2 heterodimer induced by binding of a tri-acylated lipopeptide. *Cell* **2007**, *130*, 1071–1082. [CrossRef] [PubMed]

116. Feng, Y.; Mu, R.; Wang, Z.; Xing, P.; Zhang, J.; Dong, L.; Wang, C. A toll-like receptor agonist mimicking microbial signal to generate tumor-suppressive macrophages. *Nat. Commun.* **2019**, *10*, 1–14. [CrossRef] [PubMed]

117. Simpson, T.R.; Li, F.; Montalvo-Ortiz, W.; Sepulveda, M.A.; Bergerhoff, K.; Arce, F.; Roddie, C.; Henry, J.Y.; Yagita, H.; Wolchok, J.D.; et al. Fc-dependent depletion of tumor-infiltrating regulatory T cells co-defines the efficacy of anti-CTLA-4 therapy against melanoma. *J. Exp. Med.* **2013**, *210*, 1695–1710. [CrossRef] [PubMed]

118. Kawai, T.; Akira, S. The role of pattern-recognition receptors in innate immunity: Update on Toll-like receptors. *Nat. Immunol.* **2010**, *11*, 373–384. [CrossRef]

119. Aznar, M.A.; Planelles, L.; Perez-Olivares, M.; Molina, C.; Garasa, S.; Etxeberria, I.; Perez, G.; Rodriguez, I.; Bolaños, E.; Lopez-Casas, P.; et al. Immunotherapeutic effects of intratumoral nanoplexed poly I:C. *J. Immunother. Cancer* **2019**, *7*, 116. [CrossRef]

120. Roselli, E.; Araya, P.; Núñez, N.G.; Gatti, G.; Graziano, F.; Sedlik, C.; Benaroch, P.; Piaggio, E.; Maccioni, M. TLR3 activation of intratumoral CD103+ dendritic cells modifies the tumor infiltrate conferring anti-tumor immunity. *Front. Immunol.* **2019**, *10*, 503. [CrossRef]

121. Nocera, D.A.; Roselli, E.; Araya, P.; Nuñez, N.G.; Lienenklaus, S.; Jablonska, J.; Lienenklaus, S.; Gatti, G.; Brinkmann, M.M.; Kröger, A.; et al. In vivo visualizing the IFN-β response required for tumor growth control in a therapeutic model of polyadenylic-polyuridylic acid administration. *J. Immunol.* **2016**, *196*, 2860–2869. [CrossRef]

122. Nowacki, T.M.; Kuerten, S.; Zhang, W.; Shive, C.L.; Kreher, C.R.; Boehm, B.O.; Lehmann, P.V.; Tary-Lehmann, M. Granzyme B production distinguishes recently activated CD8+ memory cells from resting memory cells. *Cell. Immunol.* **2007**, *247*, 36–48. [CrossRef]

123. Marquez-Rodas, I.; Longo, F.; Aix, S.P.; Jove, M.; Rubio, B.; Blanco, A.C.; Rodriguez-Ruiz, M.; Ponz-Sarvise, M.; Castañon, E.; Gajate, P.; et al. Combination of intratumoural double-stranded RNA (dsRNA) BO-112 with systemic anti-PD-1 in patients with anti-PD-1 refractory cancer. *Ann. Oncol.* **2019**, *30*, xi37–xi38. [CrossRef]

124. World Health Organization. Human papillomavirus vaccines: WHO position paper, May 2017—Recommendations. *Vaccine* **2017**, *35*, 5753–5755. [CrossRef]

125. Cheng, L.; Wang, Y.; Du, J. Human papillomavirus vaccines: An updated review. *Vaccines* **2020**, *8*, 391. [CrossRef]

126. Chicoine, M.R.; Won, E.K.; Zahner, M.C. Intratumoral injection of lipopolysaccharide causes regression of subcutaneously implanted mouse glioblastoma multiforme. *Neurosurgery* **2001**, *48*, 607–615. [CrossRef]

127. Chicoine, M.R.; Zahner, M.; Won, E.K.; Kalra, R.R.; Kitamura, T.; Perry, A.; Higashikubo, R. The in vivo antitumoral effects of lipopolysaccharide against glioblastoma multiforme are mediated in part by Toll-like receptor 4. *Neurosurgery* **2007**, *60*, 372–381. [CrossRef]

128. Maito, F.L.D.M.; De Souza, A.P.D.; Pereira, L.; Smithey, M.; Hinrichs, D.J.; Bouwer, A.; Bonorino, C. Intratumoral TLR-4 agonist injection is critical for modulation of tumor microenvironment and tumor rejection. *ISRN Immunol.* **2012**, *2012*, 1–11. [CrossRef]

129. Lu, H.; Betancur, A.; Chen, M.; ter Meulen, J.H. Toll-like receptor 4 expression on lymphoma cells is critical for therapeutic activity of intratumoral therapy with synthetic TLR4 agonist glucopyranosyl lipid A. *Front. Oncol.* **2020**, *10*, 1438. [CrossRef]

130. Grassin-Delyle, S.; Abrial, C.; Salvator, H.; Brollo, M.; Naline, E.; DeVillier, P. The role of Toll-like receptors in the production of cytokines by human lung macrophages. *J. Innate Immun.* **2020**, *12*, 63–73. [CrossRef]

131. Genin, M.; Clement, F.; Fattaccioli, A.; Raes, M.; Michiels, C. M1 and M2 macrophages derived from THP-1 cells differentially modulate the response of cancer cells to etoposide. *BMC Cancer* **2015**, *15*, 1–14. [CrossRef]

132. Zheng, X.-F.; Hong, Y.-X.; Feng, G.-J.; Zhang, G.-F.; Rogers, H.; Lewis, M.A.O.; Williams, D.W.; Xia, Z.-F.; Song, B.; Wei, X. Lipopolysaccharide-induced M2 to M1 macrophage transformation for IL-12p70 production is blocked by *Candida albicans* mediated up-regulation of EBI3 expression. *PLoS ONE* **2013**, *8*, e63967. [CrossRef]

133. Wang, X.; Li, X.; Zhang, X.; Zang, L.; Yang, H.; Zhao, W.; Zhao, H.; Li, Q.; Xia, B.; Yu, Y.; et al. Toll-like receptor 4–induced inflammatory responses contribute to the tumor-associated macrophages formation and infiltration in patients with diffuse large B-cell lymphoma. *Ann. Diagn. Pathol.* **2015**, *19*, 232–238. [CrossRef]

134. Hakim, F.; Wang, Y.; Zhang, S.X.; Zheng, J.; Yolcu, E.S.; Carreras, A.; Khalyfa, A.; Shirwan, H.; Almendros, I.; Gozal, D. Fragmented sleep accelerates tumor growth and progression through recruitment of tumor-associated macrophages and TLR4 signaling. *Cancer Res.* **2014**, *74*, 1329–1337. [CrossRef]

135. Kelly, M.G.; Alvero, A.B.; Chen, R.; Silasi, D.-A.; Abrahams, V.M.; Chan, S.; Visintin, I.; Rutherford, T.; Mor, G. TLR-4 signaling promotes tumor growth and paclitaxel chemoresistance in ovarian cancer. *Cancer Res.* **2006**, *66*, 3859–3868. [CrossRef]

136. Shen, H.; Sun, C.C.; Kang, L.; Tan, X.; Shi, P.; Wang, L.; Liu, E.; Gong, J. Low-dose salinomycin inhibits breast cancer metastasis by repolarizing tumor hijacked macrophages toward the M1 phenotype. *Eur. J. Pharm. Sci.* **2020**, 105629. [CrossRef]

137. Rommelfanger, D.M.; Grau, M.C.; Diaz, R.M.; Ilett, E.; Alvarez-Vallina, L.; Thompson, J.M.; Kottke, T.J.; Melcher, A.; Vile, R. The efficacy versus toxicity profile of combination virotherapy and TLR immunotherapy highlights the danger of administering TLR agonists to oncolytic virus-treated mice. *Mol. Ther.* **2013**, *21*, 348–357. [CrossRef]

138. Nie, Y.; Yang, D.; Trivett, A.; Han, Z.; Xin, H.; Chen, X.; Oppenheim, J.J. Development of a curative therapeutic vaccine (TheraVac) for the treatment of large established tumors. *Sci. Rep.* **2017**, *7*, 14186. [CrossRef]

139. Larangé, A.; Antonios, D.; Pallardy, M.; Kerdine-Römer, S. TLR7 and TLR8 agonists trigger different signaling pathways for human dendritic cell maturation. *J. Leukoc. Biol.* **2009**, *85*, 673–683. [CrossRef]

140. Gadkaree, S.K.; Fu, J.; Sen, R.; Korrer, M.J.; Allen, C.; Kim, Y.J. Induction of tumor regression by intratumoral STING agonists combined with anti-programmed death-L1 blocking antibody in a preclinical squamous cell carcinoma model. *Head Neck* **2017**, *39*, 1086–1094. [CrossRef]

141. Grauer, O.M.; Molling, J.W.; Bennink, E.; Toonen, L.W.J.; Sutmuller, R.P.M.; Nierkens, S.; Adema, G.J. TLR ligands in the local treatment of established intracerebral murine gliomas. *J. Immunol.* **2008**, *181*, 6720–6729. [CrossRef]

142. Zhang, H.; Tang, W.-L.; Kheirolomoom, A.; Fite, B.Z.; Wu, B.; Lau, K.; Baikoghli, M.; Raie, M.N.; Tumbale, S.K.; Foiret, J.; et al. Development of thermosensitive resiquimod-loaded liposomes for enhanced cancer immunotherapy. *J. Control. Release* **2020**. [CrossRef]

143. Siu, L.L.; Brody, J.; Gupta, S.; Marabelle, A.; Jimeno, A.; Munster, P.; Grilley-Olson, J.; Rook, A.H.; Hollebecque, A.; Wong, R.K.S.; et al. Safety and clinical activity of intratumoral MEDI9197 alone and in combination with durvalumab and/or palliative radiation therapy in patients with advanced solid tumors. *J. Immunother. Cancer* **2020**, *8*, e001095. [CrossRef]

144. Yoneyama, M.; Onomoto, K.; Fujita, T. Cytoplasmic recognition of RNA. *Adv. Drug Deliv. Rev.* **2008**, *60*, 841–846. [CrossRef]

145. Besch, R.; Poeck, H.; Hohenauer, T.; Senft, D.; Häcker, G.; Berking, C.; Hornung, V.; Endres, S.; Ruzicka, T.; Rothenfusser, S.; et al. Proapoptotic signaling induced by RIG-I and MDA-5 results in type I interferon–independent apoptosis in human melanoma cells. *J. Clin. Investig.* **2009**, *119*, 2399–2411. [CrossRef]

146. Takeuchi, O.; Akira, S. Innate immunity to virus infection. *Immunol. Rev.* **2009**, *227*, 75–86. [CrossRef]

147. Barsoum, J.; Renn, M.; Schuberth, C.; Jakobs, C.; Schwickart, A.; Schlee, M.; Boorn, J.V.D.; Hartmann, G. Abstract B44: Selective stimulation of RIG-I with a novel synthetic RNA induces strong anti-tumor immunity in mouse tumor models. *Cancer Immunol Res* **2017**, *5*, B44. [CrossRef]

148. Bhoopathi, P.; Quinn, B.A.; Gui, Q.; Shen, X.-N.; Grossman, S.R.; Das, S.K.; Sarkar, D.; Fisher, P.B.; Emdad, L. Pancreatic cancer-specific cell death induced in vivo by cytoplasmic-delivered polyinosine-polycytidylic Acid. *Cancer Res.* **2014**, *74*, 6224–6235. [CrossRef]

149. Heidegger, S.; Wintges, A.; Stritzke, F.; Bek, S.; Steiger, K.; Koenig, P.-A.; Göttert, S.; Engleitner, T.; Öllinger, R.; Nedelko, T.; et al. RIG-I activation is critical for responsiveness to checkpoint blockade. *Sci. Immunol.* **2019**, *4*, eaau8943. [CrossRef]

150. Burdette, D.L.; Monroe, K.M.; Sotelo-Troha, K.; Iwig, J.S.; Eckert, B.; Hyodo, M.; Hayakawa, Y.; Vance, R.E. STING is a direct innate immune sensor of cyclic di-GMP. *Nature* **2011**, *478*, 515–518. [CrossRef]

151. Burdette, D.L.; Vance, R.E. STING and the innate immune response to nucleic acids in the cytosol. *Nat. Immunol.* **2012**, *14*, 19–26. [CrossRef]

152. Ishikawa, H.; Barber, G.N. STING is an endoplasmic reticulum adaptor that facilitates innate immune signalling. *Nature.* **2008**, *455*, 674–678. [CrossRef]

153. Diner, E.J.; Burdette, D.L.; Wilson, S.C.; Monroe, K.M.; Kellenberger, C.A.; Hyodo, M.; Hayakawa, Y.; Hammond, M.C.; Vance, R.E. The innate immune DNA sensor cGAS produces a noncanonical cyclic dinucleotide that activates human STING. *Cell Rep.* **2013**, *3*, 1355–1361. [CrossRef]

154. Woo, S.-R.; Fuertes, M.B.; Corrales, L.; Spranger, S.; Furdyna, M.J.; Leung, M.Y.; Duggan, R.; Wang, Y.; Barber, G.N.; Fitzgerald, K.A.; et al. STING-dependent cytosolic DNA sensing mediates innate immune recognition of immunogenic tumors. *Immunity* **2014**, *41*, 830–842. [CrossRef] [PubMed]

155. Corrales, L.; Glickman, L.H.; McWhirter, S.M.; Kanne, D.B.; Sivick, K.E.; Katibah, G.E.; Woo, S.-R.; Lemmens, E.; Banda, T.; Leong, J.J.; et al. Direct activation of STING in the tumor microenvironment leads to potent and systemic tumor regression and immunity. *Cell Rep.* **2015**, *11*, 1018–1030. [CrossRef]

156. Yang, J.; Adam, M.; Clemens, J.; Creech, K.; Schneck, J.; Pasikanti, K.; Tran, J.-L.; Joglekar, D.; Hopson, C.; Pesiridis, S.; et al. Abstract 5554: Preclinical characterization of GSK532, a novel STING agonist with potent anti-tumor activity. *Cancer Res* **2018**, *78*, 13. [CrossRef]

157. Banerjee, M.; Basu, S.; Middya, S.; Shrivastava, R.; Ghosh, R.; Pryde, D.C.; Yadav, D.; Bhattacharya, G.; Soram, T.; Puniya, K.; et al. CRD5500: A versatile small molecule STING agonist amenable to bioconjugation as an ADC. In Proceedings of the AACR Annual Meeting 2019, Atlanta, GA, USA, 23 March–3 April 2019. *Cancer Res.* **2019**, *79*. [CrossRef]

158. Viller, N.N.; Dove, P.; Rosa, D.; Bossen, B.; Truong, T.; Mutukura, T.; Jin, D.; Charbonneau, M.; Brinen, L.; Dodge, K.; et al. Poster 668: TTI-10001, a next generation small molecule STING agonist, demonstrates potent anti-tumor activity in mice following oral or intravenous administration. In 34th Annual Meeting & Pre-Conference Programs of the Society for Immunotherapy of Cancer (SITC 2019): Part 2. *J. Immunother. Cancer* **2019**, *7*, 283. [CrossRef]

159. Wang, F.; Su, H.; Xu, D.; Dai, W.; Zhang, W.; Wang, Z.; Anderson, C.F.; Zheng, M.; Oh, R.; Wan, F.; et al. Tumour sensitization via the extended intratumoural release of a STING agonist and camptothecin from a self-assembled hydrogel. *Nat. Biomed. Eng.* **2020**, *4*, 1090–1101. [CrossRef] [PubMed]

160. Betting, D.J.; Yamada, R.E.; Kafi, K.; Said, J.; van Rooijen, N.; Timmerman, J.M. Intratumoral but not systemic delivery of CpG oligodeoxynucleotide augments the efficacy of anti-CD20 monoclonal antibody therapy against B cell lymphoma. *J. Immunother.* **2009**, *32*, 622–631. [CrossRef]

161. Betting, D.J.; Hurvitz, S.A.; Steward, K.K.; Yamada, R.E.; Kafi, K.; van Rooijen, N.; Timmerman, J.M. Combination of cyclophosphamide, rituximab, and intratumoral CpG oligodeoxynucleotide successfully eradicates established B cell lymphoma. *J. Immunother.* **2012**, *35*, 534–543. [CrossRef]

162. Schettini, J.; Kidiyoor, A.; Besmer, D.M.; Tinder, T.L.; Das Roy, L.; Lustgarten, J.; Gendler, S.J.; Mukherjee, P. Intratumoral delivery of CpG-conjugated anti-MUC1 antibody enhances NK cell anti-tumor activity. *Cancer Immunol. Immunother.* **2012**, *61*, 2055–2065. [CrossRef] [PubMed]

163. Pilon-Thomas, S.A.; Li, W.; Briggs, J.J.; Djeu, J.; Mulé, J.J.; Riker, A.I. Immunostimulatory effects of CpG-ODN upon dendritic cell-based immunotherapy in a murine melanoma model. *J. Immunother.* **2006**, *29*, 381–387. [CrossRef] [PubMed]

164. VanOosten, R.L.; Griffith, T.S. Activation of tumor-specific CD8+ T cells after intratumoral Ad5-TRAIL/CpG oligodeoxynucleotide combination therapy. *Cancer Res.* **2007**, *67*, 11980–11990. [CrossRef] [PubMed]

165. Davis, M.B.; Vasquez-Dunddel, D.; Fu, J.; Albesiano, E.; Pardoll, E.; Kim, Y. Intratumoral administration of TLR4 agonist absorbed into a cellular vector improves antitumor responses. *Clin. Cancer Res.* **2011**, *17*, 3984–3992. [CrossRef]

166. Geary, S.M.; Lemke, C.D.; Lubaroff, D.M.; Salem, A.K. Tumor immunotherapy using adenovirus vaccines in combination with intratumoral doses of CpG ODN. *Cancer Immunol. Immunother.* **2011**, *60*, 1309–1317. [CrossRef]

167. Mansilla, C.; Berraondo, P.; Durantez, M.; Martínez, M.; Casares, N.; Arribillaga, L.; Rudilla, F.; Fioravanti, J.; Lozano, T.; Villanueva, L.; et al. Eradication of large tumors expressing human papillomavirus E7 protein by therapeutic vaccination with E7 fused to the extra domain a from fibronectin. *Int. J. Cancer* **2011**, *131*, 641–651. [CrossRef]

168. Umeki, Y.; Saito, M.; Kusamori, K.; Tsujimura, M.; Nishimura, M.; Takahashi, Y.; Takakura, Y.; Nishikawa, M. Combined encapsulation of a tumor antigen and immune cells using a self-assembling immunostimulatory DNA hydrogel to enhance antigen-specific tumor immunity. *J. Control. Release* **2018**, *288*, 189–198. [CrossRef]

169. Song, L.; Yang, M.-C.; Knoff, J.; Sun, Z.-Y.; Wu, T.-C.; Hung, C.-F. Cancer immunotherapy using a potent immunodominant CTL epitope. *Vaccine* **2014**, *32*, 6039–6048. [CrossRef]

170. Song, L.; Yang, M.-C.; Knoff, J.; Wu, T.-C.; Hung, C.-F. Cancer immunotherapy employing an innovative strategy to enhance CD4+ T cell help in the tumor microenvironment. *PLoS ONE* **2014**, *9*, e115711. [CrossRef]

171. Hu, Z.; Ott, P.A.; Wu, C.J. Towards personalized, tumour-specific, therapeutic vaccines for cancer. *Nat. Rev. Immunol.* **2018**, *18*, 168–182. [CrossRef]

172. Brody, J.D.; Goldstein, M.J.; Czerwinski, D.K.; Levy, R. Immunotransplantation preferentially expands T-effector cells over T-regulatory cells and cures large lymphoma tumors. *Blood* **2009**, *113*, 85–94. [CrossRef] [PubMed]

173. Kim, K.; Skora, A.D.; Li, Z.; Liu, Q.; Tam, A.J.; Blosser, R.L.; Diaz, L.A.; Papadopoulos, N.; Kinzler, K.W.; Vogelstein, B.; et al. Eradication of metastatic mouse cancers resistant to immune checkpoint blockade by suppression of myeloid-derived cells. *Proc. Natl. Acad. Sci. USA* **2014**, *111*, 11774–11779. [CrossRef] [PubMed]

174. Ribas, A.; Medina, T.; Kummar, S.; Amin, A.; Kalbasi, A.; Drabick, J.J.; Barve, M.; Daniels, G.A.; Wong, D.J.; Schmidt, E.V.; et al. SD-101 in combination with pembrolizumab in advanced melanoma: Results of a phase Ib, multicenter study. *Cancer Discov.* **2018**, *8*, 1250–1257. [CrossRef] [PubMed]

Publisher's Note: MDPI stays neutral with regard to jurisdictional claims in published maps and institutional affiliations.

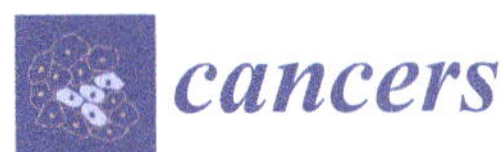 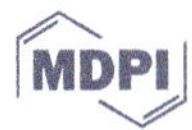

Review

The Origin and Immune Recognition of Tumor-Specific Antigens

Anca Apavaloaei, Marie-Pierre Hardy, Pierre Thibault * and Claude Perreault *

Institute for Research in Immunology and Cancer, Université de Montréal, Montréal, QC H3T 1J4, Canada; anca.apavaloaei@umontreal.ca (A.A.); marie-pierre.hardy@umontreal.ca (M.-P.H.)

* Correspondence: pierre.thibault@umontreal.ca (P.T.); claude.perreault@umontreal.ca (C.P.); Tel.: +1-514-343-6910 (P.T.); +1-514-343-6126 (C.P.)

Received: 27 August 2020; Accepted: 11 September 2020; Published: 12 September 2020

Simple Summary: Cancer immunology is a rapidly evolving field. In this context, this review article has three objectives. First, to explain the genomic origin of tumor antigens and to emphasize that many of them are encoded by unconventional RNAs. Second, to discuss the inherent limitations of all strategies aimed at discovering tumor antigens, and to highlight the importance of using mass spectrometry validation for each antigen considered for clinical trials. Third, to explain that many tumor antigens are not spontaneously detected by the immune system, because they are not presented adequately by dendritic cells. Concepts presented in this article must be taken into account in the design of cancer immunotherapies and of cancer vaccines in particular.

Abstract: The dominant paradigm holds that spontaneous and therapeutically induced anti-tumor responses are mediated mainly by CD8 T cells and directed against tumor-specific antigens (TSAs). The presence of specific TSAs on cancer cells can only be proven by mass spectrometry analyses. Bioinformatic predictions and reverse immunology studies cannot provide this type of conclusive evidence. Most TSAs are coded by unmutated non-canonical transcripts that arise from cancer-specific epigenetic and splicing aberrations. When searching for TSAs, it is therefore important to perform mass spectrometry analyses that interrogate not only the canonical reading frame of annotated exome but all reading frames of the entire translatome. The majority of aberrantly expressed TSAs (aeTSAs) derive from unstable short-lived proteins that are good substrates for direct major histocompatibility complex (MHC) I presentation but poor substrates for cross-presentation. This is an important caveat, because cancer cells are poor antigen-presenting cells, and the immune system, therefore, depends on cross-presentation by dendritic cells (DCs) to detect the presence of TSAs. We, therefore, postulate that, in the untreated host, most aeTSAs are undetected by the immune system. We present evidence suggesting that vaccines inducing direct aeTSA presentation by DCs may represent an attractive strategy for cancer treatment.

Keywords: antigen processing and presentation; cancer immunotherapy; cross-priming; immunogenicity; major histocompatibility complex; T lymphocyte; tumor-infiltrating lymphocytes; tumor microenvironment; tumor-specific antigen

---

1. Introduction

The introduction of immune checkpoint therapy in the treatment of several cancer types has dramatically changed the landscape of oncology [1,2]. The success of this approach is based on the paradigm that T lymphocytes, and in particular the CD8 subset [3], recognize tumor antigens that can elicit vigorous immune responses and tumor rejection [4]. Attention has focused on major histocompatibility complex (MHC)-associated peptides (MAPs), which are the ligands recognized by classic T cells. However, the precise nature of the MAPs capable of causing tumor rejection remains unclear. Seen as promising for decades, tumor-associated antigens (TAAs) have recently fallen into disfavor. TAAs are MAPs that are not cancer-specific but are overexpressed in cancer cells (Table 1). Since they are part of the normal immune self, TAAs are not highly immunogenic and TAA vaccines have yielded disappointing results [5,6]. Strong evidence suggests that anti-tumor immune responses potentiated by immune checkpoint therapy are directed against tumor-specific antigens (TSAs); that is, MAPs found only on cancer cells [4,7,8]. Nonetheless the molecular landscape of actionable TSAs remains largely elusive.

Table 1. Features of tumor antigens.

Feature	TAAs	mTSAs	aeTSAs
Cancer-specific	No	Yes	Yes
Mutation	No	Yes	No
Shared among tumors	Yes	No	Yes
Number per tumor	Medium-High	Very low	Medium-High
Selected studies containing MS analyses	[9–12]	[13–17]	[18,19]

aeTSA, aberrantly expressed tumor-specific antigen; MS, mass spectrometry; mTSA, mutated tumor-specific antigen; TAA, tumor-associated antigen.

2. Misconceptions about TSAs

2.1. Neoantigens and the Fallacy of the Converse

Efforts seeking to discover TSAs initially focused on MAPs coded by mutated exons. This makes sense, because the cancer specificity of mutated MAPs is unquestionable, and exons have long been considered the sole protein-coding genomic sequences. These efforts led to the discovery of mutated TSAs (mTSAs), only a few of which were validated by mass spectrometry [4,20]. Furthermore, in several cases, tumor-infiltrating lymphocytes specific for mTSAs were shown to have the ability to mediate tumor regression [21,22]. Unfortunately, excitement over the discovery of exonic mTSAs led to a misconception with major implications. As exonic mTSAs were, in selected cases, sufficient to elicit anti-tumor responses, it was assumed that they were necessary to elicit anti-tumor responses (fallacy of the converse). In other words, it was postulated that exonic mTSAs were the sole actionable TSAs. This reasoning was incorrect, because the term TSA should designate any cancer-specific MAP, whatever its genomic origin (exonic or not) and irrespective of its mutational status (i.e., mutated or not). This concept has important implications. First, annotated exons represent only 2% of the genome and many allegedly non-protein coding (non exonic) sequences are coding for proteins and do generate MAPs [23–26]. Second, epigenetic and splicing aberrations as well as frameshift translation in cancer cells lead to the appearance of numerous proteins and MAPs that are not found in normal cells. Cancer-specific MAPs resulting from translation of any open reading frames not expressed in normal adult cells are referred to as aberrantly expressed TSAs (aeTSAs) (Table 1). aeTSAs can derive from i) canonical (annotated) onco-fetal genes that are normally repressed in the adult organism (e.g., MAGEA3) or ii) from non-canonical transcripts that arise from cancer-specific epigenetic changes, frameshift translation, or splicing aberrations. Notably, translation of a whole cancer-specific transcript can yield more numerous TSAs than a single base pair substitution [27]. When compared to mTSAs, aeTSAs display two advantageous features. First, they are more numerous [18]. Indeed, in a recent study of 23 ovarian cancers, 103 TSAs were identified of which only three were exonic mTSAs [19]. Second, whereas mTSAs are generally unique to individual patients, aeTSAs are shared by many tumors. In ovarian cancer, 78% of transcripts coding for individual aeTSAs were found in at least 10% of tumors and 18% in at least 80% of tumors [19].

When exonic mTSAs were discovered, they were frequently labeled as neoantigens. In fact, the terms TSA and neoantigens should be synonymous. Accordingly, we would have no objection to talk of neoantigens and to classify them into mutated and aberrantly expressed neoantigens. However, many scientists still believe that neoantigens means exonic mTSAs. Therefore, as recommended by Haen et al. [5], we will refrain from using the term neoantigen in order to avoid any ambiguity.

2.2. Can mTSAs Be Identified without Mass Spectrometry Analyses?

Mass spectrometry remains the only method that allows direct and definitive identification of the amino acid sequence of MAPs and TSAs [5,28–30]. However, mass spectrometry analyses require (i) large tumor samples and (ii) specialized equipment and expertise, which are not widely available. Hence, research teams have tried to identify TSAs using genomic data (exome and/or transcriptome sequencing) and algorithms to predict MHC-binding affinity. Unfortunately, two types of evidence suggest that most "predicted TSAs" are false discoveries: one type is based on mass spectrometry validation of predicted TSAs, the second on in-depth genomic analyses. Almost all studies have focused exclusively on exonic mTSAs.

2.2.1. Mass Spectrometry Validation of Predicted mTSAs

In 16 primary human hepatocellular carcinomas, Löffler et al. predicted the occurrence of 1888 exonic mTSAs (a mean of 118 per tumor), none of which was validated by mass spectrometry [13]. In colorectal carcinomas, Newey et al. predicted the occurrence of 304 mTSAs, of which only three were validated by mass spectrometry. In smaller scale studies, not a single mTSA was validated by mass spectrometry analyses of four acute lymphoblastic leukemias [18] and three pancreatic adenocarcinomas [16].

2.2.2. In-Depth Genomic Analyses

According to the tenets of immunoediting [31], exonic mTSAs should be under negative selection pressure (enforced by TSA-responsive T cells). This negative selection should decrease the ratio of non-synonymous over synonymous mutations in mTSA-coding sequences. However, no such decrease was found in analyses of genomic data from 8,683 tumor samples [32]. Likewise, comprehensive analyses of over 1,000 melanoma exomes revealed no evidence of HLA-restricted negative selection against exonic mutations [33]. Furthermore, response to immune checkpoint therapy in patients with lung cancer did not correlate more with predicted mTSAs than with the global mutation load [34]. These data mean that the number of exonic mTSAs has been grossly overestimated in many studies and that the mTSA repertoire of a tumor cannot be predicted with current algorithms. The reason for this is that while these algorithms can accurately predict with reasonable accuracy the MHC-binding affinity of a peptide, they fail to take into account the numerous translational and post-translational events that regulate MAP biogenesis and presentation [35–37].

2.2.3. Can Reverse Immunology Eliminate False Positive TSA Predictions?

Testing the immunogenicity of validated TSAs using various in vitro methods (MHC-MAP multimers binding, cytokine production, etc.) provides useful information. It shows which TSAs are more likely to stimulate anti-tumor responses in vivo. However, it is commonly assumed that if a predicted mTSA (not validated by mass spectrometry) can elicit T-cell responses from peripheral blood mononuclear cells, it is more likely to be a genuine TSA. We disagree with this assumption. The fact that a predicted TSA is immunogenic simply means that it can be recognized by some T cells; this does not increase the likelihood that this predicted TSA is a genuine TSA (present on cancer cells). Two "peptide stories" illustrate this point: those of *ELAGIGILTV* and *RIAECILGM*. The *ELAGIGILTV* peptide is an in vitro modified version of the wild-type *EAAGIGILTV* MART-1/Melan-A26-35 decamer. Hence, for the immune system, *ELAGIGILTV* is akin to an mTSA. While this peptide is not found on cancer cells, it is so immunogenic that it is commonly used as a positive control in ex vivo immunogenicity assays [38,39]. The TEL-AML1 fusion protein results from a 12:21 chromosomal translocation and is frequently found in B-cell precursor acute lymphoblastic leukemia. A peptide resulting from this fusion protein, *RIAECILGM*, was predicted to be presented by HLA-A*02:01, and priming of T cells against this peptide generated cytotoxic T cells that killed autologous leukemic cells [40]. Further in-depth studies showed that this epitope is not presented by leukemic cells; it is not endogenously processed, because it is cleaved by proteasomes [41]. Killing of leukemic cells by T cells primed against RIAECILGM was most likely due to the inherent cross-reactivity of T cells, which is further amplified in T-cell lines [42]. Indeed, positive selection in the thymus preferentially rescues cross-reactive T cells [43], and a single T-cell receptor may recognize more than a million different MAPs [44].

3. Strategies for Mass Spectrometry-Based Identification of aeTSAs

aeTSAs present several attractive features. They are more common than mTSAs, and they are shared by many tumors of a given type (Table 1). Furthermore, in pre-clinical models, they were shown to elicit curative anti-tumor responses [18,45]. Since aeTSAs can be coded by any reading frame of the entire genome, their search space is greater than that of mTSAs [8,46,47]. Therefore, it is currently impossible to rely on available bioinformatic tools to predict the aeTSA landscape of a tumor, and mass spectrometry analyses are mandatory for aeTSA identification. The key question here is: once a putative aeTSA is identified, how do we demonstrate its cancer-specificity? In other words, how can we prove that an unmutated MAP is not expressed by any normal cell type? Three approaches have been developed, each with pros and cons.

The first approach postulates that a MAP is a TSA if it is found in cancer cells but not in an atlas of MAPs identified in normal tissue extracts [9,10]. The problem here is that this atlas does not contain the MAP repertoire of all cell types. Thus, since most epithelial cells express lower levels of MHC molecules than hematopoietic cells [48,49], whole tissue extracts are enriched in hematopoietic relative to epithelial MAPs. Furthermore, several cell types in the organism are not present in numbers sufficient for mass spectrometry analyses. Hence, some TSAs identified with this approach may be false positives.

In the second approach, normal adjacent tissue (not tumor-infiltrated) is used as a negative control [50]. Once again, the absence of a MAP in the normal adjacent tissue does not guarantee that it is not present in other cell types in the organism. We speculate that this approach can also lead to dismissal of genuine TSAs. Our assumption is based on the notion that normal tumor-adjacent tissue may in fact not be normal but rather pre-neoplastic and, therefore, share TSAs with the tumor [51]. Indeed, as we age, physiologically healthy tissues such as skin [52,53], colon [54,55], esophagus [56,57], and blood [58–65] acquire mutations in cancer-associated genes. Timing analyses suggest that driver mutations often precede diagnosis by many years, if not decades. A notable example is ovarian adenocarcinoma, which appears to have a median latency of more than 10 years [66].

The third approach is based on the assumption that a TSA cannot be present in cells that do not express TSA-coding transcripts. In contrast to mass spectrometry analyses, transcriptomic analyses have been performed in many subjects on practically all cell types. Hence, when we identify aeTSA candidates, we evaluate whether its coding transcript is found in normal tissues from the GTEx database (https://gtexportal.org/home/) or in our datasets of medullary thymic epithelial cells [26]. We believe that inclusion of medullary thymic epithelial cells in the "negative controls" is important for three reasons: (i) they orchestrate central immune tolerance [67], (ii) they express much higher levels of MHC I molecules than other epithelial cell types [49], and (iii) they promiscuously express more genes than other types of somatic cells [68,69]. Promiscuous gene expression in medullary thymic epithelial cells involves not only classic genes, but also other genomic regions such as endogenous retroelements [26]. The downside of this approach is that it can lead to the dismissal of genuine aeTSAs. Indeed, expression of a transcript in some normal cell does not necessarily lead to expression processing and presentation of the corresponding TSA.

It must nonetheless be acknowledged that mass spectrometry studies come with intrinsic challenges and limitations [5]. First and foremost, in discovery mode, "shotgun mass spectrometry" has limited sensitivity and, therefore, requires large amounts of starting material for in-depth coverage of the immunopeptidome (e.g., 1 g of tumor tissue). Second, relative to transcriptome sequencing, mass spectrometry has a relatively low throughput and is not quantitative. Finally, mass spectrometry fails to differentiate between isobaric amino acids (Leucine vs. Isoleucine) and is relatively costly in terms of reagents and resources. Several technical innovations are being developed in order to overcome these limitations [30,70].

4. Immune Recognition of TSAs

4.1. Cancer Cells Are Poor T-Cell Activators

The general rules of T-cell priming also apply to cancer cells. Indeed, T-cell recognition of tumors requires both signal 1 (TCR ligands such as TSAs) and signal 2 (co-stimulation) [71]. The most critical positive co-stimulatory signal is provided by CD28 upon interaction with its ligands of the B7 family (CD80/86) on antigen-presenting cells (APCs) [72]. Tumor cells are poor APCs: they express no/low levels of CD28 ligands, and carcinomas (90% of cancers) derive from epithelial cells expressing 10 to 100-fold less MHC I molecules than DCs [49]. As a result, tumor cells are inefficient at directly priming naïve CD8 T cells, and activation of T cells against tumor antigens depends on cross-presentation by professional APCs [73]. Accordingly, anti-tumor responses, either spontaneous or induced with immune checkpoint therapy, correlate with intratumoral infiltration and maturation of cross-presenting $CD8\alpha^+CD103^+$ dendritic cells (DCs) [20,74,75]. These specialized DCs internalize and cross-present tumor antigens to T cells and induce a CD28-dependent proliferation of tumor-specific T cells, which regulates the strength of the immune response [76–79].

4.2. Cross-Presentation Yields a Biased Representation of the TSA Repertoire

The rules governing direct presentation and cross-presentation are different. Direct presentation favors short-lived and rapidly degraded proteins, many of which represent unstable defective ribosomal products that may derive from specialized ribosomes (immunoribosomes) [80–82]. In contrast, cross-presentation of exogenous antigens preferentially samples long-lived, stable proteins [83,84]. Thus, direct presentation correlates with the rate of protein translation and proteasomal degradation, whereas cross-presentation correlates with steady-state protein amounts [85]. APCs acquire proteins from donor cells (e.g., cancer cells) through endocytic mechanisms of which the most efficient is phagocytosis [86]. Internalized proteins can then be degraded by proteasomes, either in endocytic organelles or in the cytosol [86,87]. A key implication is that cross-presentation can only display a fraction of TSAs; that is, TSAs derived from highly abundant and stable proteins. Hence, the immune system remains ignorant of TSAs found in unstable and rapidly degraded proteins.

4.3. The Strength of Effector T-Cell Responses

The amplitude of anti-tumor T-cell responses depends on two factors: (i) epitope density on APCs and cancer cells, and (ii) the frequency of antigen-responsive T cells in the pre-immune repertoire. Epitope density (number of MAPs per cell) on APCs during initial priming regulates not only the magnitude but also the avidity and functionality of the effector T-cell population [88,89]. For most—though not all—antigens, cross-presentation yields a lower epitope density than direct presentation [90]. In addition, epitope density on tumor cells dictates their susceptibility to CD8 T-cell cytotoxicity. At this point, intratumoral heterogeneity has to be taken into consideration, because it is a hallmark of all cancers. For immuno-oncologists, this means that individual tumor cells may display different levels of TSA expression. Both in mice and humans, the proportion of TSA-positive tumor cells positively regulates the outcome of interactions between CD8 T cells and the tumor [91–93]. The presence of some TSA-negative tumor cells does not necessarily lead to immunotherapy failure. Indeed, TSA-negative tumor cells can be eradicated by T-cell targeting of the tumor stroma and, in particular, endothelial cells [94]. Intratumoral T cells can damage the tumor vasculature via two mechanisms: (i) killing of endothelial cells that cross-present TSAs and (ii) via the potent angiostatic effect of IFN-γ and TNF-α [89,95,96]. Nonetheless, these data suggest that chances of success of immunotherapy should be improved by selecting clonal TSAs (present on most/all cancer cells) and targeting multiple TSAs.

4.4. Vaccination-Induced T-Cell Priming

DC-based vaccines can elicit strong anti-tumor responses against TSAs that are ignored when presented solely by cancer cells (Figure 1). This is illustrated well by the aeTSA VNYLHRNV. While this peptide is expressed at high levels on EL4 cells (908 copies per cell), immunization with irradiated EL4 cells does not prolong the survival of mice upon subsequent injection of unirradiated EL4 cells. However, 100% of mice immunized with DCs coated with VNYLHRNV survive when injected with EL4 cells [18]. Moreover, immunization generates TSA-responsive memory CD8 T cells, since mice survive a novel injection of EL4 cells 100 days later. Hence, VNYLHRNV is highly immunogenic when presented by DCs, but in the absence of therapeutic vaccination, this EL4 TSA is not cross-presented by DCs in vivo.

Properly designed nanoparticulate liposomal RNA vaccines are efficiently taken up by DCs in secondary lymphoid organs in vivo [97]. In these conditions, since the DC-targeted RNAs drive synthesis of antigenic peptides inside DCs, their processing follows the rule of direct presentation as opposed to cross-presentation. A phase I trial evaluating a nanoparticulate liposomal RNA vaccine in immune checkpoint therapy-experienced melanoma patients (stage III B, C and stage IV) recently provided suggestive evidence that, when presented by DCs, aeTSAs can elicit anti-tumor responses [98]. This vaccine contained four antigens that were originally labeled as TAAs. However, while one of these antigens is clearly a TAA (*TYR*), the other three are probably aeTSAs coded by conventional annotated genes: *MAGEA3, CTAG1B (NY-ESO-1)*, and *TPTE*. Indeed, while *TYR* is expressed in the normal skin, the three putative aeTSAs are not expressed in normal extra-thymic tissues (except for the testis). However, *MAGEA3, CTAG1B*, and *TPTE* RNAs are expressed at very low levels in medullary thymic epithelial cells (<0.5 transcripts per kilobase million [26]). The probability that transcripts expressed at such levels might generate MAPs is very low [35,99] but cannot be formally excluded in the absence of immunopeptidomic studies on medullary thymic epithelial cells. We, therefore, consider that these three antigens are probably, but not certainly, aeTSAs. Notably, objective anti-tumor response correlated more closely with the expansion of T cells recognizing MAGEA3 and CTAG1B [98]. This study, therefore, (i) supports the immunogenicity of aeTSAs in humans and (ii) suggests that direct aeTSA presentation by DCs activates and expands a pool of complementary aeTSA-specific T cells that were insensitive to immune checkpoint therapy and likely tumor-naïve.

4.5. Combining Vaccines and Immune Checkpoint Therapy

In general, a high density of tumor-infiltrating lymphocytes positively correlates response to immune checkpoint therapy [100]. This suggests that immune checkpoint therapy works at least in part by invigorating T cells responding to cross-presented TSAs. Likewise, preliminary evidence suggests that immune checkpoint therapy may potentiate T-cell response to aeTSAs directly presented by DCs [98]. The idea of combining vaccines and immune checkpoint therapy, therefore, appears very attractive.

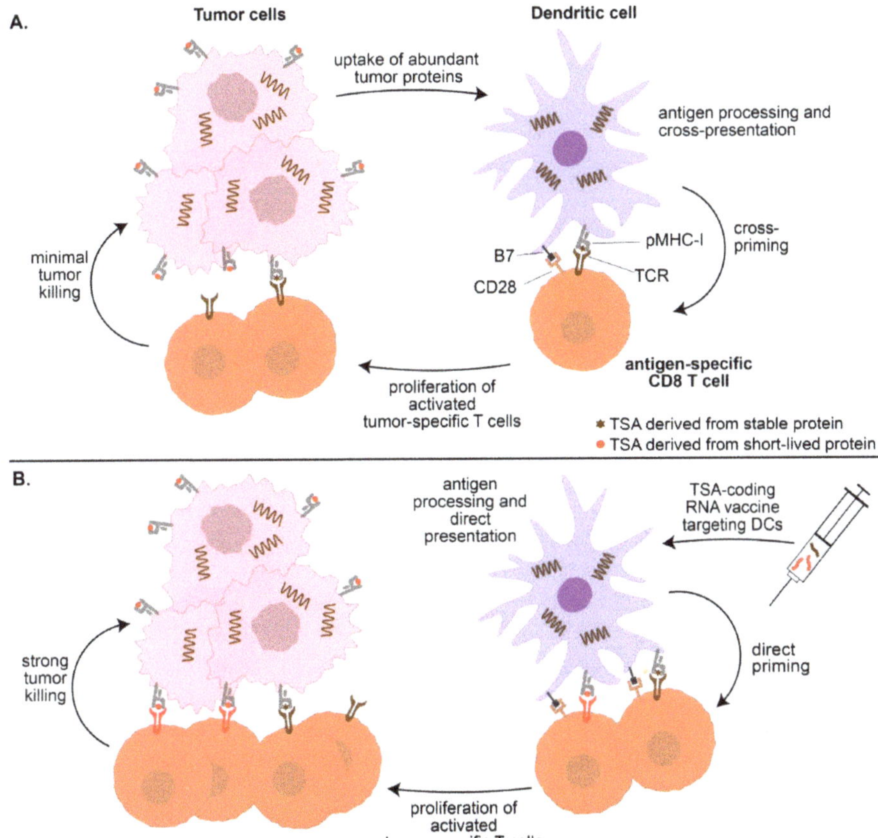

Figure 1. Priming of anti-tumor CD8$^+$ T cells by dendritic cells (DCs). (**A**) Most cancer cells are poor antigen-presenting cells (APCs) that are not efficient at direct antigen presentation. DCs are potent APCs, but under basal conditions, they can cross-present only a fraction of the tumor-specific antigens (TSA) repertoire generated by cancer cells. TSAs derived from unstable rapidly degraded proteins (the most common of TSAs) are not cross-presented by DCs and are, therefore, ignored by the immune system. (**B**) Therapeutic mRNA vaccines can deliver any TSA-coding transcripts to DCs for direct presentation to CD8 T cells. In this way, TSAs derived from both short-lived proteins and stable proteins can be detected by CD8 T cells.

5. Conclusions

Therapeutic vaccines can induce durable regressions of premalignant oncogenic human papilloma virus type 16-induced anogenital lesions [101]. To the best of our knowledge, this vaccine containing viral peptides remains the sole therapeutic TSA-based vaccine that has shown reliable efficacy. The first non-viral TSA vaccines tested in clinical trials were based on predicted mTSAs not validated by mass spectrometry [102–105]. Evidence that most predicted mTSAs not validated by mass spectrometry may be false discoveries does not bode well for the success of these studies. aeTSAs present attractive features and give encouraging results in pre-clinical models. However, evidence supporting their value or superiority over TAAs in humans remains anecdotal and has yet to be formally assessed. For cancer immunologists wishing to develop therapeutic vaccines, the time is not for celebrations but rather to develop innovative research strategies in a climate tinged with both optimism and critical thinking. We also propose that TSAs should be validated by mass spectrometry analyses of primary human tumors before they are tested in clinical trials. Finally, we strongly encourage the sharing of mass spectrometry datasets via the SysteMHC Atlas whose primary objective is to provide a systems-level definition of MAP and TSA repertoires presented by normal and neoplastic cells [30,106].

Author Contributions: Conceptualization, writing, and editing: A.A., M.-P.H., P.T., C.P. All authors have read and agreed to the published version of the manuscript.

Funding: This research was funded by The Canadian Cancer Society, grant numbers 705604 and 705714, and The Oncopole (EMC^2 grant).

Acknowledgments: The authors also thank the staff of the following core facilities at the Institute for Research in Immunology and Cancer: Proteomics, Genomics and Bioinformatics.

Conflicts of Interest: M.P.H., P.T. and C.P. are named inventors on patents related to tumor-specific antigens filed by Université de Montréal. The funders had no role in the design of the study; in the collection, analyses, or interpretation of data; in the writing of the manuscript, or in the decision to publish the results.

References

1. Sharma, P.; Allison, J.P. The future of immune checkpoint therapy. *Science* **2015**, *348*, 56–61. [CrossRef]
2. Chowdhury, P.S.; Chamoto, K.; Honjo, T. Combination therapy strategies for improving PD-1 blockade efficacy: A new era in cancer immunotherapy. *J. Intern. Med.* **2018**, *283*, 110–120. [CrossRef]
3. Galon, J.; Bruni, D. Tumor Immunology and Tumor Evolution: Intertwined Histories. *Immunity* **2020**, *52*, 55–81. [CrossRef]
4. Schumacher, T.N.; Scheper, W.; Kvistborg, P. Cancer Neoantigens. *Annu. Rev. Immunol.* **2019**, *37*, 173–200. [CrossRef]
5. Haen, S.P.; Loffler, M.W.; Rammensee, H.G.; Brossart, P. Towards new horizons: Characterization, classification and implications of the tumour antigenic repertoire. *Nat. Rev. Clin. Oncol.* **2020**. [CrossRef]
6. Bezu, L.; Kepp, O.; Cerrato, G.; Pol, J.; Fucikova, J.; Spisek, R.; Zitvogel, L.; Kroemer, G.; Galluzzi, L. Trial watch: Peptide-based vaccines in anticancer therapy. *Oncoimmunology* **2018**, *7*, e1511506. [CrossRef]
7. Tran, E.; Robbins, P.F.; Rosenberg, S.A. 'Final common pathway' of human cancer immunotherapy: Targeting random somatic mutations. *Nat. Immunol.* **2017**, *18*, 255–262. [CrossRef]
8. Smith, C.C.; Selitsky, S.R.; Chai, S.; Armistead, P.M.; Vincent, B.G.; Serody, J.S. Alternative tumour-specific antigens. *Nat. Rev. Cancer* **2019**, *19*, 465–478. [CrossRef]
9. Reustle, A.; Di Marco, M.; Meyerhoff, C.; Nelde, A.; Walz, J.S.; Winter, S.; Kandabarau, S.; Buttner, F.; Haag, M.; Backert, L.; et al. Integrative -omics and HLA-ligandomics analysis to identify novel drug targets for ccRCC immunotherapy. *Genome Med.* **2020**, *12*, 32. [CrossRef]
10. Schuster, H.; Peper, J.K.; Bosmuller, H.C.; Rohle, K.; Backert, L.; Bilich, T.; Ney, B.; Loffler, M.W.; Kowalewski, D.J.; Trautwein, N.; et al. The immunopeptidomic landscape of ovarian carcinomas. *Proc. Natl. Acad. Sci. USA* **2017**, *114*, E9942–E9951. [CrossRef]
11. Shraibman, B.; Barnea, E.; Kadosh, D.M.; Haimovich, Y.; Slobodin, G.; Rosner, I.; Lopez-Larrea, C.; Hilf, N.; Kuttruff, S.; Song, C.; et al. Identification of Tumor Antigens Among the HLA Peptidomes of Glioblastoma Tumors and Plasma. *Mol. Cell. Proteom.* **2019**, *18*, 1255–1268. [CrossRef]
12. Loffler, M.W.; Kowalewski, D.J.; Backert, L.; Bernhardt, J.; Adam, P.; Schuster, H.; Dengler, F.; Backes, D.; Kopp, H.G.; Beckert, S.; et al. Mapping the HLA Ligandome of Colorectal Cancer Reveals an Imprint of Malignant Cell Transformation. *Cancer Res.* **2018**, *78*, 4627–4641. [CrossRef]
13. Löffler, M.W.; Mohr, C.; Bichmann, L.; Freudenmann, L.K.; Walzer, M.; Schroeder, C.M.; Trautwein, N.; Hilke, F.J.; Zinser, R.S.; Mühlenbruch, L.; et al. Multi-omics discovery of exome-derived neoantigens in hepatocellular carcinoma. *Genome Med.* **2019**, *11*, 1–16. [CrossRef]
14. Newey, A.; Griffiths, B.; Michaux, J.; Pak, H.S.; Stevenson, B.J.; Woolston, A.; Semiannikova, M.; Spain, G.; Barber, L.J.; Matthews, N.; et al. Immunopeptidomics of colorectal cancer organoids reveals a sparse HLA class I neoantigen landscape and no increase in neoantigens with interferon or MEK-inhibitor treatment. *J. Immunother. Cancer* **2019**, *7*, 309. [CrossRef]
15. Bassani-Sternberg, M.; Braunlein, E.; Klar, R.; Engleitner, T.; Sinitcyn, P.; Audehm, S.; Straub, M.; Weber, J.; Slotta-Huspenina, J.; Specht, K.; et al. Direct identification of clinically relevant neoepitopes presented on native human melanoma tissue by mass spectrometry. *Nat. Commun.* **2016**, *7*, 13404. [CrossRef]

16. Bassani-Sternberg, M.; Digklia, A.; Huber, F.; Wagner, D.; Sempoux, C.; Stevenson, B.J.; Thierry, A.C.; Michaux, J.; Pak, H.; Racle, J.; et al. A Phase Ib Study of the Combination of Personalized Autologous Dendritic Cell Vaccine, Aspirin, and Standard of Care Adjuvant Chemotherapy Followed by Nivolumab for Resected Pancreatic Adenocarcinoma—A Proof of Antigen Discovery Feasibility in Three Patients. *Front. Immunol* **2019**, *10*. [CrossRef]

17. Khodadoust, M.S.; Olsson, N.; Wagar, L.E.; Haabeth, O.A.; Chen, B.; Swaminathan, K.; Rawson, K.; Liu, C.L.; Steiner, D.; Lund, P.; et al. Antigen presentation profiling reveals recognition of lymphoma immunoglobulin neoantigens. *Nature* **2017**, *543*, 723–727. [CrossRef]

18. Laumont, C.M.; Vincent, K.; Hesnard, L.; Audemard, E.; Bonneil, E.; Laverdure, J.P.; Gendron, P.; Courcelles, M.; Hardy, M.P.; Côté, C.; et al. Non-coding regions are the main source of targetable tumor-specific antigens. *Sci. Transl. Med.* **2018**, *10*, eaau5516. [CrossRef]

19. Zhao, Q.; Laverdure, J.P.; Lanoix, J.; Durette, C.; Coté, C.; Bonneil, E.; Laumont, C.M.; Gendron, P.; Vincent, K.; Courcelles, M.; et al. Proteogenomics uncovers a vast repertoire of shared tumor-specific antigens in ovarian cancer. *Cancer Immunol. Res.* **2020**, *8*, 544–555. [CrossRef]

20. Gubin, M.M.; Zhang, X.; Schuster, H.; Caron, E.; Ward, J.P.; Noguchi, T.; Ivanova, Y.; Hundal, J.; Arthur, C.D.; Krebber, W.J.; et al. Checkpoint blockade cancer immunotherapy targets tumour-specific mutant antigens. *Nature* **2014**, *515*, 577–581. [CrossRef]

21. Tran, E.; Robbins, P.F.; Lu, Y.C.; Prickett, T.D.; Gartner, J.J.; Jia, L.; Pasetto, A.; Zheng, Z.; Ray, S.; Groh, E.M.; et al. T-Cell Transfer Therapy Targeting Mutant KRAS in Cancer. *N. Engl. J. Med.* **2016**, *375*, 2255–2262. [CrossRef]

22. Yamamoto, T.N.; Kishton, R.J.; Restifo, N.P. Developing neoantigen-targeted T cell-based treatments for solid tumors. *Nat. Med.* **2019**, *25*, 1488–1499. [CrossRef]

23. Wei, L.H.; Guo, J.U. Coding functions of "noncoding" RNAs. *Science* **2020**, *367*, 1074–1075. [CrossRef]

24. Chen, J.; Brunner, A.D.; Cogan, J.Z.; Nunez, J.K.; Fields, A.P.; Adamson, B.; Itzhak, D.N.; Li, J.Y.; Mann, M.; Leonetti, M.D.; et al. Pervasive functional translation of noncanonical human open reading frames. *Science* **2020**, *367*, 1140–1146. [CrossRef]

25. Laumont, C.M.; Daouda, T.; Laverdure, J.P.; Bonneil, E.; Caron-Lizotte, O.; Hardy, M.P.; Granados, D.P.; Durette, C.; Lemieux, S.; Thibault, P.; et al. Global proteogenomic analysis of human MHC class I-associated peptides derived from non-canonical reading frames. *Nat. Commun.* **2016**, *7*, 10238. [CrossRef]

26. Larouche, J.D.; Trofimov, A.; Hesnard, L.; Ehx, G.; Zhao, Q.; Vincent, K.; Durette, C.; Gendron, P.; Laverdure, J.P.; Bonneil, E.; et al. Widespread and tissue-specific expression of endogenous retroelements in human somatic tissues. *Genome Med.* **2020**, *12*, 40. [CrossRef]

27. Koster, J.; Plasterk, R.H.A. A library of Neo Open Reading Frame peptides (NOPs) as a sustainable resource of common neoantigens in up to 50% of cancer patients. *Sci. Rep.* **2019**, *9*, 6577. [CrossRef]

28. Schmidt, M.; Lill, J.R. MHC class I presented antigens from malignancies: A perspective on analytical characterization & immunogenicity. *J. Proteom.* **2018**. [CrossRef]

29. Hardy, M.P.; Vincent, K.; Perreault, C. The Genomic Landscape of Antigenic Targets for T Cell-Based Leukemia Immunotherapy. *Front. Immunol.* **2019**, *10*, 2934. [CrossRef]

30. Vizcaino, J.A.; Kubiniok, P.; Kovalchik, K.; Ma, Q.; Duquette, J.D.; Mongrain, I.; Deutsch, E.W.; Peters, B.; Sette, A.; Sirois, I.; et al. The Human Immunopeptidome Project: A roadmap to predict and treat immune diseases. *Mol. Cell. Proteom.* **2020**, *19*, 31–49. [CrossRef]

31. Schreiber, R.D.; Old, L.J.; Smyth, M.J. Cancer immunoediting: Integrating immunity's roles in cancer suppression and promotion. *Science* **2011**, *331*, 1565–1570. [CrossRef]

32. Van den Eynden, J.; Jimenez-Sanchez, A.; Miller, M.L.; Larsson, E. Lack of detectable neoantigen depletion signals in the untreated cancer genome. *Nat. Genet.* **2019**, *51*, 1741–1748. [CrossRef]

33. Alkallas, R.; Lajoie, M.; Hoang, K.V.; Lefrancois, P.; Lingrand, M.; Ahanfeshar-Adams, M.; Watters, K.; Spatz, A.; Zippin, J.H.; Najafabadi, H.S.; et al. Multi-omic analysis reveals significantly mutated genes and DDX3X as a sex-specific tumor suppressor in cutaneous melanoma. *Nat. Cancer* **2020**, *1*, 635–652. [CrossRef]

34. Hellmann, M.D.; Nathanson, T.; Rizvi, H.; Creelan, B.C.; Sanchez-Vega, F.; Ahuja, A.; Ni, A.; Novik, J.B.; Mangarin, L.M.B.; Abu-Akeel, M.; et al. Genomic Features of Response to Combination Immunotherapy in Patients with Advanced Non-Small-Cell Lung Cancer. *Cancer Cell* **2018**, *33*, 843–852. [CrossRef]

35. Pearson, H.; Daouda, T.; Granados, D.P.; Durette, C.; Bonneil, E.; Courcelles, M.; Rodenbrock, A.; Laverdure, J.P.; Cote, C.; Mader, S.; et al. MHC class I-associated peptides derive from selective regions of the human genome. *J. Clin. Investig.* **2016**, *126*, 4690–4701. [CrossRef]

36. Editorial, N.B. The problem with neoantigen prediction. *Nat. Biotechnol.* **2017**, *35*, 97. [CrossRef]

37. Granados, D.P.; Sriranganadane, D.; Daouda, T.; Zieger, A.; Laumont, C.M.; Caron-Lizotte, O.; Boucher, G.; Hardy, M.P.; Gendron, P.; Cote, C.; et al. Impact of genomic polymorphisms on the repertoire of human MHC class I-associated peptides. *Nat. Commun.* **2014**, *5*, 3600. [CrossRef]

38. Dutoit, V.; Rubio-Godoy, V.; Pittet, M.J.; Zippelius, A.; Dietrich, P.Y.; Legal, F.A.; Guillaume, P.; Romero, P.; Cerottini, J.C.; Houghten, R.A.; et al. Degeneracy of antigen recognition as the molecular basis for the high frequency of naive A2/Melan-a peptide multimer(+) CD8(+) T cells in humans. *J. Exp. Med.* **2002**, *196*, 207–216. [CrossRef]

39. Hesnard, L.; Legoux, F.; Gautreau, L.; Moyon, M.; Baron, O.; Devilder, M.C.; Bonneville, M.; Saulquin, X. Role of the MHC restriction during maturation of antigen-specific human T cells in the thymus. *Eur. J. Immunol.* **2016**, *46*, 560–569. [CrossRef]

40. Yotnda, P.; Garcia, F.; Peuchmaur, M.; Grandchamp, B.; Duval, M.; Lemonnier, F.; Vilmer, E.; Langlade-Demoyen, P. Cytotoxic T cell response against the chimeric ETV6-AML1 protein in childhood acute lymphoblastic leukemia. *J. Clin. Investig.* **1998**, *102*, 455–462. [CrossRef]

41. Popovic, J.; Li, L.P.; Kloetzel, P.M.; Leisegang, M.; Uckert, W.; Blankenstein, T. The only proposed T-cell epitope derived from the TEL-AML1 translocation is not naturally processed. *Blood* **2011**, *118*, 946–954. [CrossRef]

42. Sewell, A.K. Why must T cells be cross-reactive? *Nat. Rev. Immunol* **2012**, *12*, 669–677. [CrossRef]

43. Khosravi-Maharlooei, M.; Obradovic, A.; Misra, A.; Motwani, K.; Holzl, M.; Seay, H.R.; DeWolf, S.; Nauman, G.; Danzl, N.; Li, H.; et al. Crossreactive public TCR sequences undergo positive selection in the human thymic repertoire. *J. Clin. Investig.* **2019**, *129*, 2446–2462. [CrossRef]

44. Wooldridge, L.; Ekeruche-Makinde, J.; van den Berg, H.A.; Skowera, A.; Miles, J.J.; Tan, M.P.; Dolton, G.; Clement, M.; Llewellyn-Lacey, S.; Price, D.A.; et al. A single autoimmune T cell receptor recognizes more than a million different peptides. *J. Biol. Chem.* **2012**, *287*, 1168–1177. [CrossRef]

45. Probst, P.; Kopp, J.; Oxenius, A.; Colombo, M.P.; Ritz, D.; Fugmann, T.; Neri, D. Sarcoma Eradication by Doxorubicin and Targeted TNF Relies upon CD8+ T-cell Recognition of a Retroviral Antigen. *Cancer Res.* **2017**, *77*, 3644–3654. [CrossRef]

46. Laumont, C.M.; Perreault, C. Exploiting non-canonical translation to identify new targets for T-cell based cancer immunotherapy. *Cell. Mol Life Sci.* **2017**, *75*, 607–621. [CrossRef]

47. Frankiw, L.; Baltimore, D.; Li, G. Alternative mRNA splicing in cancer immunotherapy. *Nat. Rev. Immunol.* **2019**, *19*, 675–687. [CrossRef]

48. Boegel, S.; Lower, M.; Bukur, T.; Sorn, P.; Castle, J.C.; Sahin, U. HLA and proteasome expression body map. *BMC Med. Genom.* **2018**, *11*, 36. [CrossRef]

49. Benhammadi, M.; Mathé, J.; Dumont-Lagace, M.; Kobayashi, K.S.; Gaboury, L.; Brochu, S.; Perreault, C. IFN lambda enhances constitutive expression of MHC class I molecules on thymic epithelial cells. *J. Immunol.* **2020**, *205*, 1268–1280. [CrossRef]

50. Chong, C.; Muller, M.; Pak, H.; Harnett, D.; Huber, F.; Grun, D.; Leleu, M.; Auger, A.; Arnaud, M.; Stevenson, B.J.; et al. Integrated proteogenomic deep sequencing and analytics accurately identify non-canonical peptides in tumor immunopeptidomes. *Nat. Commun.* **2020**, *11*, 1293. [CrossRef]

51. Reuben, A.; Zhang, J.; Chiou, S.H.; Gittelman, R.M.; Li, J.; Lee, W.C.; Fujimoto, J.; Behrens, C.; Liu, X.; Wang, F.; et al. Comprehensive T cell repertoire characterization of non-small cell lung cancer. *Nat. Commun.* **2020**, *11*, 603. [CrossRef]

52. Martincorena, I.; Roshan, A.; Gerstung, M.; Ellis, P.; Van Loo, P.; McLaren, S.; Wedge, D.C.; Fullam, A.; Alexandrov, L.B.; Tubio, J.M.; et al. High burden and pervasive positive selection of somatic mutations in normal human skin. *Science* **2015**, *348*, 880–886. [CrossRef]

53. Jonason, A.S.; Kunala, S.; Price, G.J.; Restifo, R.J.; Spinelli, H.M.; Persing, J.A.; Leffell, D.J.; Tarone, R.E.; Brash, D.E. Frequent clones of p53-mutated keratinocytes in normal human skin. *Proc. Natl. Acad. Sci. USA* **1996**, *93*, 14025–14029. [CrossRef]

54. Blokzijl, F.; de Ligt, J.; Jager, M.; Sasselli, V.; Roerink, S.; Sasaki, N.; Huch, M.; Boymans, S.; Kuijk, E.; Prins, P.; et al. Tissue-specific mutation accumulation in human adult stem cells during life. *Nature* **2016**, *538*, 260–264. [CrossRef]

55. Lee-Six, H.; Olafsson, S.; Ellis, P.; Osborne, R.J.; Sanders, M.A.; Moore, L.; Georgakopoulos, N.; Torrente, F.; Noorani, A.; Goddard, M.; et al. The landscape of somatic mutation in normal colorectal epithelial cells. *Nature* **2019**, *574*, 532–537. [CrossRef]

56. Martincorena, I.; Fowler, J.C.; Wabik, A.; Lawson, A.R.J.; Abascal, F.; Hall, M.W.J.; Cagan, A.; Murai, K.; Mahbubani, K.; Stratton, M.R.; et al. Somatic mutant clones colonize the human esophagus with age. *Science* **2018**, *362*, 911–917. [CrossRef]

57. Yokoyama, A.; Kakiuchi, N.; Yoshizato, T.; Nannya, Y.; Suzuki, H.; Takeuchi, Y.; Shiozawa, Y.; Sato, Y.; Aoki, K.; Kim, S.K.; et al. Age-related remodelling of oesophageal epithelia by mutated cancer drivers. *Nature* **2019**, *565*, 312–317. [CrossRef]

58. Acuna-Hidalgo, R.; Sengul, H.; Steehouwer, M.; van de Vorst, M.; Vermeulen, S.H.; Kiemeney, L.; Veltman, J.A.; Gilissen, C.; Hoischen, A. Ultra-sensitive Sequencing Identifies High Prevalence of Clonal Hematopoiesis-Associated Mutations throughout Adult Life. *Am. J. Hum. Genet.* **2017**, *101*, 50–64. [CrossRef]

59. Zink, F.; Stacey, S.N.; Norddahl, G.L.; Frigge, M.L.; Magnusson, O.T.; Jonsdottir, I.; Thorgeirsson, T.E.; Sigurdsson, A.; Gudjonsson, S.A.; Gudmundsson, J.; et al. Clonal hematopoiesis, with and without candidate driver mutations, is common in the elderly. *Blood* **2017**, *130*, 742–752. [CrossRef]

60. Desai, P.; Mencia-Trinchant, N.; Savenkov, O.; Simon, M.S.; Cheang, G.; Lee, S.; Samuel, M.; Ritchie, E.K.; Guzman, M.L.; Ballman, K.V.; et al. Somatic mutations precede acute myeloid leukemia years before diagnosis. *Nat. Med.* **2018**, *24*, 1015–1023. [CrossRef]

61. Xie, M.; Lu, C.; Wang, J.; McLellan, M.D.; Johnson, K.J.; Wendl, M.C.; McMichael, J.F.; Schmidt, H.K.; Yellapantula, V.; Miller, C.A.; et al. Age-related mutations associated with clonal hematopoietic expansion and malignancies. *Nat. Med.* **2014**, *20*, 1472–1478. [CrossRef]

62. Loh, P.R.; Genovese, G.; Handsaker, R.E.; Finucane, H.K.; Reshef, Y.A.; Palamara, P.F.; Birmann, B.M.; Talkowski, M.E.; Bakhoum, S.F.; McCarroll, S.A.; et al. Insights into clonal haematopoiesis from 8342 mosaic chromosomal alterations. *Nature* **2018**, *559*, 350–355. [CrossRef]

63. Bowman, R.L.; Busque, L.; Levine, R.L. Clonal Hematopoiesis and Evolution to Hematopoietic Malignancies. *Cell Stem Cell* **2018**, *22*, 157–170. [CrossRef] [PubMed]

64. Abelson, S.; Collord, G.; Ng, S.W.K.; Weissbrod, O.; Mendelson Cohen, N.; Niemeyer, E.; Barda, N.; Zuzarte, P.C.; Heisler, L.; Sundaravadanam, Y.; et al. Prediction of acute myeloid leukaemia risk in healthy individuals. *Nature* **2018**, *559*, 400–404. [CrossRef] [PubMed]

65. Watson, C.J.; Papula, A.L.; Poon, G.Y.P.; Wong, W.H.; Young, A.L.; Druley, T.E.; Fisher, D.S.; Blundell, J.R. The evolutionary dynamics and fitness landscape of clonal hematopoiesis. *Science* **2020**, *367*, 1449–1454. [CrossRef] [PubMed]

66. Gerstung, M.; Jolly, C.; Leshchiner, I.; Dentro, S.C.; Gonzalez, S.; Rosebrock, D.; Mitchell, T.J.; Rubanova, Y.; Anur, P.; Yu, K.; et al. The evolutionary history of 2,658 cancers. *Nature* **2020**, *578*, 122–128. [CrossRef]

67. Kadouri, N.; Nevo, S.; Goldfarb, Y.; Abramson, J. Thymic epithelial cell heterogeneity: TEC by TEC. *Nat. Rev. Immunol.* **2019**. [CrossRef]

68. Sansom, S.N.; Shikama-Dorn, N.; Zhanybekova, S.; Nusspaumer, G.; Macaulay, I.C.; Deadman, M.E.; Heger, A.; Ponting, C.P.; Hollander, G.A. Population and single-cell genomics reveal the Aire dependency, relief from Polycomb silencing, and distribution of self-antigen expression in thymic epithelia. *Genome Res.* **2014**, *24*, 1918–1931. [CrossRef]

69. St-Pierre, C.; Brochu, S.; Vanegas, J.R.; Dumont-Lagace, M.; Lemieux, S.; Perreault, C. Transcriptome sequencing of neonatal thymic epithelial cells. *Sci. Rep.* **2013**, *3*, 1860. [CrossRef]

70. Pfammatter, S.; Bonneil, E.; Lanoix, J.; Vincent, K.; Hardy, M.P.; Courcelles, M.; Perreault, C.; Thibault, P. Extending the Comprehensiveness of Immunopeptidome Analyses Using Isobaric Peptide Labeling. *Anal. Chem.* **2020**, *92*, 9194–9204. [CrossRef]

71. Chen, L.; McGowan, P.; Ashe, S.; Johnston, J.; Li, Y.; Hellstrom, I.; Hellstrom, K.E. Tumor immunogenicity determines the effect of B7 costimulation on T cell-mediated tumor immunity. *J. Exp. Med.* **1994**, *179*, 523–532. [CrossRef] [PubMed]

72. Esensten, J.H.; Helou, Y.A.; Chopra, G.; Weiss, A.; Bluestone, J.A. CD28 Costimulation: From Mechanism to Therapy. *Immunity* **2016**, *44*, 973–988. [CrossRef] [PubMed]

73. Ochsenbein, A.F. Immunological ignorance of solid tumors. *Springer Semin. Immunopathol.* **2005**, *27*, 19–35. [CrossRef] [PubMed]

74. Salmon, H.; Idoyaga, J.; Rahman, A.; Leboeuf, M.; Remark, R.; Jordan, S.; Casanova-Acebes, M.; Khudoynazarova, M.; Agudo, J.; Tung, N.; et al. Expansion and Activation of CD103(+) Dendritic Cell Progenitors at the Tumor Site Enhances Tumor Responses to Therapeutic PD-L1 and BRAF Inhibition. *Immunity* **2016**, *44*, 924–938. [CrossRef]

75. Spranger, S.; Bao, R.; Gajewski, T.F. Melanoma-intrinsic beta-catenin signalling prevents anti-tumour immunity. *Nature* **2015**, *523*, 231–235. [CrossRef]

76. Kamphorst, A.O.; Pillai, R.N.; Yang, S.; Nasti, T.H.; Akondy, R.S.; Wieland, A.; Sica, G.L.; Yu, K.; Koenig, L.; Patel, N.T.; et al. Proliferation of PD-1+ CD8 T cells in peripheral blood after PD-1-targeted therapy in lung cancer patients. *Proc. Natl. Acad. Sci. USA* **2017**, *114*, 4993–4998. [CrossRef]

77. Topalian, S.L.; Taube, J.M.; Pardoll, D.M. Neoadjuvant checkpoint blockade for cancer immunotherapy. *Science* **2020**, *367*. [CrossRef]

78. Tumeh, P.C.; Harview, C.L.; Yearley, J.H.; Shintaku, I.P.; Taylor, E.J.; Robert, L.; Chmielowski, B.; Spasic, M.; Henry, G.; Ciobanu, V.; et al. PD-1 blockade induces responses by inhibiting adaptive immune resistance. *Nature* **2014**, *515*, 568–571. [CrossRef]

79. Rizvi, N.A.; Hellmann, M.D.; Snyder, A.; Kvistborg, P.; Makarov, V.; Havel, J.J.; Lee, W.; Yuan, J.; Wong, P.; Ho, T.S.; et al. Cancer immunology. Mutational landscape determines sensitivity to PD-1 blockade in non-small cell lung cancer. *Science* **2015**, *348*, 124–128. [CrossRef]

80. Yewdell, J.W.; Holly, J. DRiPs get molecular. *Curr. Opin. Immunol.* **2020**, *64*, 130–136. [CrossRef]

81. Cosma, G.L.; Lobby, J.L.; Fay, E.J.; Siciliano, N.A.; Langlois, R.A.; Eisenlohr, L.C. Kinetically distinct processing pathways diversify the CD8(+) T cell response to a single viral epitope. *Proc. Natl. Acad. Sci. USA* **2020**, *117*, 19399–19407. [CrossRef] [PubMed]

82. Wei, J.; Kishton, R.J.; Angel, M.; Conn, C.S.; Dalla-Venezia, N.; Marcel, V.; Vincent, A.; Catez, F.; Ferre, S.; Ayadi, L.; et al. Ribosomal Proteins Regulate MHC Class I Peptide Generation for Immunosurveillance. *Mol. Cell* **2019**, *73*, 1162–1173.e5. [CrossRef] [PubMed]

83. Shen, L.; Rock, K.L. Cellular protein is the source of cross-priming antigen in vivo. *Proc. Natl. Acad. Sci. USA* **2004**, *101*, 3035–3040. [CrossRef]

84. Norbury, C.C.; Basta, S.; Donohue, K.B.; Tscharke, D.C.; Princiotta, M.F.; Berglund, P.; Gibbs, J.; Bennink, J.R.; Yewdell, J.W. CD8+ T cell cross-priming via transfer of proteasome substrates. *Science* **2004**, *304*, 1318–1321. [CrossRef] [PubMed]

85. Yewdell, J.W. Designing CD8+ T cell vaccines: It's not rocket science (yet). *Curr. Opin. Immunol.* **2010**, *22*, 402–410. [CrossRef]

86. Colbert, J.D.; Cruz, F.M.; Rock, K.L. Cross-presentation of exogenous antigens on MHC I molecules. *Curr. Opin. Immunol.* **2020**, *64*, 1–8. [CrossRef]

87. Sengupta, D.; Graham, M.; Liu, X.; Cresswell, P. Proteasomal degradation within endocytic organelles mediates antigen cross-presentation. *EMBO J.* **2019**, *38*, e99266. [CrossRef]

88. Cosma, G.L.; Eisenlohr, L.C. Impact of epitope density on CD8(+) T cell development and function. *Mol. Immunol.* **2019**, *113*, 120–125. [CrossRef]

89. Meunier, M.C.; Delisle, J.S.; Bergeron, J.; Rineau, V.; Baron, C.; Perreault, C. T cells targeted against a single minor histocompatibility antigen can cure solid tumors. *Nat. Med.* **2005**, *11*, 1222–1229. [CrossRef]

90. Wu, T.; Guan, J.; Handel, A.; Tscharke, D.C.; Sidney, J.; Sette, A.; Wakim, L.M.; Sng, X.Y.X.; Thomas, P.G.; Croft, N.P.; et al. Quantification of epitope abundance reveals the effect of direct and cross-presentation on influenza CTL responses. *Nat. Commun.* **2019**, *10*, 2846. [CrossRef]

91. Gejman, R.S.; Chang, A.Y.; Jones, H.F.; DiKun, K.; Hakimi, A.A.; Schietinger, A.; Scheinberg, D.A. Rejection of immunogenic tumor clones is limited by clonal fraction. *eLife* **2018**, *7*. [CrossRef] [PubMed]

92. Leisegang, M.; Engels, B.; Schreiber, K.; Yew, P.Y.; Kiyotani, K.; Idel, C.; Arina, A.; Duraiswamy, J.; Weichselbaum, R.R.; Uckert, W.; et al. Eradication of Large Solid Tumors by Gene Therapy with a T-Cell Receptor Targeting a Single Cancer-Specific Point Mutation. *Clin. Cancer Res.* **2016**, *22*, 2734–2743. [CrossRef] [PubMed]

93. McGranahan, N.; Swanton, C. Neoantigen quality, not quantity. *Sci. Transl. Med.* **2019**, *11*. [CrossRef] [PubMed]

94. Schietinger, A.; Philip, M.; Liu, R.B.; Schreiber, K.; Schreiber, H. Bystander killing of cancer requires the cooperation of CD4(+) and CD8(+) T cells during the effector phase. *J. Exp. Med.* **2010**, *207*, 2469–2477. [CrossRef]

95. Spiotto, M.T.; Rowley, D.A.; Schreiber, H. Bystander elimination of antigen loss variants in established tumors. *Nat. Med.* **2004**, *10*, 294–298. [CrossRef]

96. Blankenstein, T. The role of tumor stroma in the interaction between tumor and immune system. *Curr. Opin. Immunol.* **2005**, *17*, 180–186. [CrossRef]

97. Kranz, L.M.; Diken, M.; Haas, H.; Kreiter, S.; Loquai, C.; Reuter, K.C.; Meng, M.; Fritz, D.; Vascotto, F.; Hefesha, H.; et al. Systemic RNA delivery to dendritic cells exploits antiviral defence for cancer immunotherapy. *Nature* **2016**, *534*, 396–401. [CrossRef]

98. Sahin, U.; Oehm, P.; Derhovanessian, E.; Jabulowsky, R.A.; Vormehr, M.; Gold, M.; Maurus, D.; Schwarck-Kokarakis, D.; Kuhn, A.N.; Omokoko, T.; et al. An RNA vaccine drives immunity in checkpoint-inhibitor-treated melanoma. *Nature* **2020**, *585*, 107–112. [CrossRef]

99. Bassani-Sternberg, M.; Pletscher-Frankild, S.; Jensen, L.J.; Mann, M. Mass spectrometry of human leukocyte antigen class I peptidomes reveals strong effects of protein abundance and turnover on antigen presentation. *Mol. Cell. Proteom.* **2015**, *14*, 658–673. [CrossRef]

100. Havel, J.J.; Chowell, D.; Chan, T.A. The evolving landscape of biomarkers for checkpoint inhibitor immunotherapy. *Nat. Rev. Cancer* **2019**, *19*, 133–150. [CrossRef]

101. Melief, C.J.M.; Welters, M.J.P.; Vergote, I.; Kroep, J.R.; Kenter, G.G.; Ottevanger, P.B.; Tjalma, W.A.A.; Denys, H.; van Poelgeest, M.I.E.; Nijman, H.W.; et al. Strong vaccine responses during chemotherapy are associated with prolonged cancer survival. *Sci. Transl. Med.* **2020**, *12*. [CrossRef] [PubMed]

102. Hilf, N.; Kuttruff-Coqui, S.; Frenzel, K.; Bukur, V.; Stevanovic, S.; Gouttefangeas, C.; Platten, M.; Tabatabai, G.; Dutoit, V.; van der Burg, S.H.; et al. Actively personalized vaccination trial for newly diagnosed glioblastoma. *Nature* **2019**, *565*, 240–245. [CrossRef] [PubMed]

103. Keskin, D.B.; Anandappa, A.J.; Sun, J.; Tirosh, I.; Mathewson, N.D.; Li, S.; Oliveira, G.; Giobbie-Hurder, A.; Felt, K.; Gjini, E.; et al. Neoantigen vaccine generates intratumoral T cell responses in phase Ib glioblastoma trial. *Nature* **2019**, *565*, 234–239. [CrossRef] [PubMed]

104. Sahin, U.; Derhovanessian, E.; Miller, M.; Kloke, B.P.; Simon, P.; Lower, M.; Bukur, V.; Tadmor, A.D.; Luxemburger, U.; Schrors, B.; et al. Personalized RNA mutanome vaccines mobilize poly-specific therapeutic immunity against cancer. *Nature* **2017**, *547*, 222–226. [CrossRef] [PubMed]

105. Ott, P.A.; Hu, Z.; Keskin, D.B.; Shukla, S.A.; Sun, J.; Bozym, D.J.; Zhang, W.; Luoma, A.; Giobbie-Hurder, A.; Peter, L.; et al. An immunogenic personal neoantigen vaccine for patients with melanoma. *Nature* **2017**, *547*, 217–221. [CrossRef]

106. Shao, W.; Pedrioli, P.G.A.; Wolski, W.; Scurtescu, C.; Schmid, E.; Vizcaino, J.A.; Courcelles, M.; Schuster, H.; Kowalewski, D.; Marino, F.; et al. The SysteMHC Atlas project. *Nucleic Acids Res.* **2018**, *46*, D1237–D1247. [CrossRef]

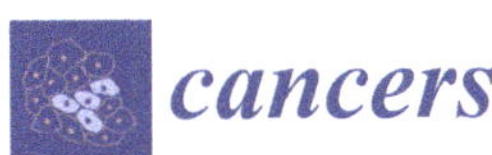

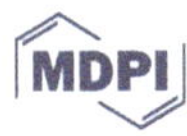

Commentary

Immune Checkpoint Blockade in HER2-Positive Breast Cancer: What Role in Early Disease Setting?

Cinzia Solinas [1,*], Debora Fumagalli [2] and Maria Vittoria Dieci [3]

[1]   Medical Oncology, Azienda Tutela della Salute Sardegna, San Francesco Hospital, 08100 Nuoro, Italy
[2]   Breast International Group, 1000 Brussels, Belgium; debora.fumagalli@gmail.com
[3]   Medical Oncology 2, Veneto Institute of Oncology IOV-IRCCS, 35128 Padova, Italy;
      mariavittoriadieci@gmail.com
*   Correspondence: czsolinas@gmail.com or ci.solinas@atssardegna.it

Simple Summary: This work aims to discuss how an anti- or pro-tumor immune response could be manipulated through immune checkpoint blockade in patients with early stage HER2-positive breast cancer. By summarizing previously published evidence in the field, authors present their personal view on how immune checkpoint blockade could be implemented in the neoadjuvant setting in this patient population. The hypothesis being presented is that an appropriate and effective administration of immune checkpoint blockade could assure a lasting control of the disease, by preventing relapses. One of the research priorities should be the identification of the patients who could benefit more by this strategy.

Abstract: The present commentary synthesizes the current evidence on the role of the immune response in HER2-positive breast cancer. It points out the strengths and weaknesses of the findings observed so far, particularly in the early setting, including the clinical significance of scoring tumor-infiltrating lymphocytes. A figure proposing research hypotheses for the implementation of immune checkpoint blockade use for patient candidates to neoadjuvant treatment is presented.

Keywords: HER2-positive; breast cancer; immune checkpoint blockade; immune checkpoint molecules; PD-1/PD-L1; immunotherapy

Citation: Solinas, C.; Fumagalli, D.; Dieci, M.V. Immune Checkpoint Blockade in HER2-Positive Breast Cancer: What Role in Early Disease Setting? *Cancers* **2021**, *13*, 1655. https://doi.org/10.3390/cancers13071655

Academic Editors: Michael Kershaw and Clare Slaney

Received: 8 March 2021
Accepted: 22 March 2021
Published: 1 April 2021

Publisher's Note: MDPI stays neutral with regard to jurisdictional claims in published maps and institutional affiliations.

1. Introduction

Immune checkpoint blockade represents a successful immunotherapy strategy aimed at boosting a pre-existing adaptive anti-tumor immune response with a potential lasting control of the disease [1]. The latter could be achieved because adaptive immunity is characterized by memory and by the possibility to simultaneously target the tumor-associated antigens that can be generated as cancer develops. This innovative treatment approach is revolutionary for the durable responses it can induce. Further, stimulating the immune system could potentially target multiple neo-antigens over time. All these peculiar aspects have generated a great interest in identifying the patient subsets that benefit more from immune checkpoint blockade, particularly in early settings, where the chances of cure are higher for cancer patients.

After the introduction of effective anti-human epidermal growth factor receptor-2 (HER2) agents, early-stage HER2-positive breast cancer patients have experienced improved survival [2]. Some of these patients achieve excellent outcomes and are ideal candidates for de-escalation treatment strategies aimed at sparing toxicities from chemotherapy, as explored in studies like CompassHER2-pCR (NCT04266249) and Decrescendo (NCT04675827) [3]. However, up to 20% of early stage HER2-positive breast cancer patients still relapse and develop an advanced disease [2]. For these patients, innovative add-on strategies should be developed. Upfront use of immune checkpoint blockade could be useful in this context, but it is not known which patients could benefit more from this approach.

The aim of this commentary is to briefly summarize evidence on the relationship between a spontaneous immune response (i.e., the one present in inflamed tumors that are characterized by a detectable immune infiltration) and outcome and/or responses to standard treatments in HER2-positive breast cancer. In addition, some research hypotheses for the experimental use of immune checkpoint blockade in the neoadjuvant setting are proposed, which take into account the implementation of immune-related biomarkers and add-on or de-escalation treatment strategies. Further, research priorities are identified.

2. HER2-Positive Breast Cancer Patients and Tumor-Infiltrating Lymphocytes: Clinical Significance

The HER2-positive subtype represents up to 20% of breast cancer diagnoses [4]. Its main oncogenic driver is represented by the amplification and over expression of HER2, whose activity is inhibited by a variety of anti-HER2 agents that are nowadays being used in the clinic, with relevant clinical benefit in all the settings of the disease [2]. This subtype is characterized by heterogeneity, mostly driven by the presence or absence of the hormone receptors' expression, which identifies distinct subgroups with different prognoses and responses to treatments [5].

Gene-expression data reveal that up to 50–60% of HER2-positive breast cancers have a HER2-enriched PAM50 molecular profile, particularly hormone receptor-negative (75%) compared to hormone receptor-positive (30%) cancers [6–9]. This molecular subtype is characterized by high activity in HER2 signaling, rendering these tumors HER2 hypersensitive, thus particularly responsive to anti-HER2 targeted agents [10]. Other predictors of benefit from these drugs are: high expression of the *ERBB2* gene [10] and of immune gene signatures [11], the latter being able to predict a higher likelihood of pathological complete response after neoadjuvant treatments (an intermediate endpoint for survival [12]), and a longer event-free survival [13]. In addition, a high extent of tumor-infiltrating lymphocytes (TIL) evaluated on hematoxylin and eosin (HE)-stained slides has been associated with better outcomes (pathological complete response, event-free survival and disease-free survival) in several trials, confirming the relevant role played by the host immunity during the course of this disease [14,15].

TIL represent a well recognized biomarker in the cancer field, particularly in this new era of cancer immunotherapy. TIL are easily, reproducibly and cheaply scored by pathologists on HE slides used in clinical routine [16]. In the HER2-positive breast cancer subtype, higher TIL levels were observed in the hormone receptor-negative with respect to the hormone receptor-positive subgroup [17,18].

Immunohistochemical (IHC) analysis allows to identify the various immune cell subsets that are globally scored as TIL on HE slides (based on morphological features). These include: Helper T cells (Th, CD4$^+$), cytotoxic T cells (CTL, CD8$^+$), B cells (CD20$^+$) from the adaptive immunity; macrophages, neutrophils, myeloid derived suppressor cells, natural killer (NK) from the innate immunity [19]. Among the cells of the adaptive immunity (characterized by immunological memory), Th lymphocytes contribute to the development of a response by activating tumor antigen-specific effector lymphocytes (CTL) and through the recruitment of various cells of the innate immunity. There are several subpopulations of Th, such as the anti-tumor Th1 (able to kill tumor cells by releasing cytokines that activate death receptors on target cells, and to produce cytokines that activate CTL), and the Th2 that promote a pro-tumor microenvironment. CTL kill tumor cells, and B cells are able to secrete antibodies and cytokines, assuring an effective anti-tumor immune response in breast cancer [20].

Of interest, the prognostic relevance of TIL scored on HE slides in neoadjuvant and adjuvant trials of HER2-positive breast cancer has been shown to be independent both of other clinicopathological characteristics [21,22] and of the administered treatment [15]. The various anti-HER2 compounds exert in fact different immune effects [5] through complex interactions between the various cells of the tumor microenvironment (particularly those from innate immunity) and the treatments (including chemotherapy) co-administered. Specifically, (1) the anti-HER2 monoclonal antibody trastuzumab increases the antibody-dependent cell-mediated cytotoxicity (ADCC) since its Fc portion (the tail region of an antibody that does not recognize the antigen) interacts with the Fcγ receptors expressed on the effector cells of the innate immunity (NK cells, neutrophils and γδT-cells) and with some proteins of the complement system [5]. Similar effects are seen with (2) the anti-HER2 monoclonal antibody pertuzumab that induces ADCC and augments the density of Fcγ receptor binding sites on HER2-positive cells, potentiating NK cell activity [5], and with (3) the antibody drug conjugate trastuzumab emtasine (T-DM1), which increases ADCC [5]. The (4) tyrosine kinase inhibitor lapatinib raises the density of HER2 receptors on the surface of tumor cells, potentiating the ADCC associated with trastuzumab [5]. Anthracyclines, taxanes, cyclophosphamide and other cytotoxic agents employed in breast cancer can also mediate immune effects [23].

Thus, it is expected that stratification of patients on the basis of the level of immune infiltration of their tumors (reflected by the extent of baseline TIL on HE slides) should allow to identify patients that are more likely to benefit from standard treatments and/or experience better outcomes. Further, it could be helpful in identifying those patients at higher risk of relapse (those having lower TIL) who might have the opportunity to be treated with immune checkpoint blockade as an add-on strategy.

3. Potential Role of Immune Checkpoint Blockade in HER2-Positive Breast Cancer

A growing interest in manipulating the patient's own immune response against cancer has followed the introduction of immune checkpoint blockade strategies. One of the crucial steps for further exploration of this treatment strategy is represented by the identification of the target patient population.

Evidence from studies in triple negative breast cancer, the breast cancer subtype showing the highest levels of TIL infiltration, reveals that programmed cell death-1 or its ligand (PD-(L)1) immune checkpoint blockade is more active in early settings, independent of PD-L1 expression on tumor cells, lymphocytes and macrophages [24]. In contrast, in the advanced disease the presence of PD-L1 expression by immune cells identifies the subgroup that benefits more from the association of an anti-PD-L1 plus chemotherapy [25].

In HER2-positive breast cancer limited efficacy of immune checkpoint blockade combined with T-DM1 or trastuzumab has been observed in the advanced setting in patients previously treated with trastuzumab and expressing PD-L1 on immune cells and/or having higher levels of TIL [26,27]. However, these results derive from hypothesis-generating trials and deserve further confirmation, also considering that early and late diseases appear to have a different biological profile. For example, the levels of TIL on metastatic HER2-positive samples may be lower than matched primary tumors [28] and the infiltration by CTL may be lower in metastatic samples from patients pre-treated with chemotherapy and anti-HER2 therapy [29].

So far, not much is known about the role of immune checkpoint blockade in early settings in this subtype, also considering the variety and efficacy of the anti-HER2 drugs now available (i.e., trastuzumab +/− pertuzumab as part of the (neo)adjuvant treatment and T-DM1 as part of the post surgical treatment in patients with a residual disease after neoadjuvant treatment).

Biologically, a mouse model revealed that the efficacy of immune checkpoint blockade in early settings was higher in the presence of tumor antigens (i.e., as in the case of a neoadjuvant approach), rather than in their absence [30]. Ideally, administration of immune checkpoint blockade would be more efficacious as part of the upfront neoadjuvant treatment space, which in HER2-positive breast cancer currently looks crowded with several treatment strategies being explored [31].

However, some studies have shown that tumors with high TIL (the most infiltrated that traditionally benefit most from immune checkpoint blockade) are also characterized by excellent responses to neoadjuvant treatments with anti-HER2 agents plus taxane

+/− anthracycline-based chemotherapy regimens and by excellent prognosis (event-free survival) [15,17].

Whether patients with highly infiltrated tumors really need a boost to their immunity with immune checkpoint blockade, considering that standard treatments are very efficacious, is still a crucial point that needs to be addressed.

4. Potential Use of Immune Checkpoint Blockade in the Neoadjuvant Setting for HER2-Positive Breast Cancer Patients

The neoadjuvant setting represents an ideal scenario to test drug sensitivity, characterize the biology of the disease, identify reliable predictive biomarkers and to guide treatment decisions based on the presence of a residual disease [32]. Current guidelines suggest that neoadjuvant treatment in HER2-positive breast cancer patients should be administered for clinical ≥ T2 or ≥N1 (Figure 1) [33]. Figure 1 summarizes various research hypotheses that could be tested upfront (panel A) or in the presence of a residual disease after neoadjuvant therapy (panel B) in HER2-positive breast cancer patients stratified based on the extent of baseline TIL assessed on HE slides from pre-treatment biopsies. Of note, frequencies of pathological complete response achievement based on baseline TIL levels refer to HER2-positive breast cancer patients treated with trastuzumab plus anthracyclines and taxanes in the pre-pertuzumab era [15].

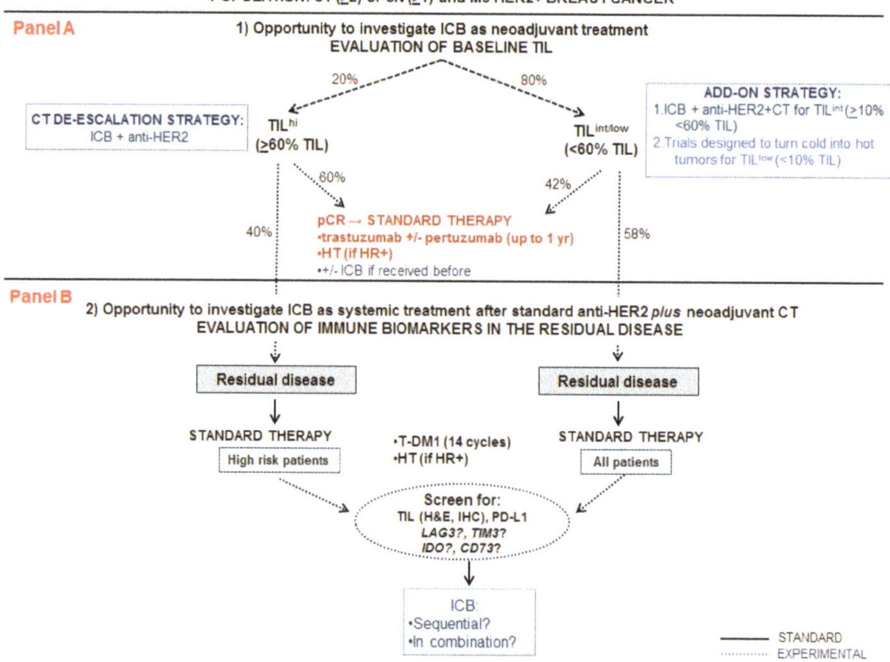

Figure 1. Figure 1 represents proposed research hypotheses for the use of immune checkpoint blockade (ICB) in early-stage HER2-positive breast cancer patients who are candidates for neoadjuvant therapy (≥cT2 or ≥cN1 and M0) with the employment of tumor-infiltrating lymphocytes (TIL) assessed on diagnostic biopsies as an additional biomarker to guide treatment decisions. Panel (**A**) shows upfront treatment strategies whereas panel (**B**) proposes the treatment strategies to be administered in the presence of a residual disease after neoadjuvant therapy (panel (**B**)). References: [15,34]. Legend: CT, chemotherapy; HE, hematoxylin and eosin; HR, hormone receptor; HT, hormone therapy; ICB, immune checkpoint blockade; IHC, immunohistochemistry; M, metastasis; N, nodal status; pCR, pathologic complete response; T, tumor size; T-DM1, trastuzumab emtansine; TIL, tumor-infiltrating lymphocytes; TIL^{hi}, ≥60% tumor-infiltrating lymphocytes; TIL^{int}, ≥10% <60% tumor-infiltrating lymphocytes; TIL^{lo}, <10% tumor-infiltrating lymphocytes.

Baseline high TIL infiltration (with a TIL cut-off of $\geq$60% from previously published randomized controlled trials [15]) is found in around 20% of patients with early stage HER2-positive breast cancers and has been associated with a higher likelihood of pathological complete response (Figure 1, left side). Previous studies showed in fact that up to 60% of these patients achieve a pathological complete response (Figure 1) [15]. The remaining 40% present a residual disease, and become candidates to receive standard T-DM1 [25] +/− hormone therapy (according to the baseline hormone receptors status). In this patient population, upfront anti-PD-(L)1-based immune checkpoint blockade could be administered in association with dual anti-HER2 blockade (trastuzumab plus pertuzumab) as a chemotherapy de-escalation strategy (Figure 1, panel A, left side).

The remaining 80% of HER2-positive breast cancer patients treated in the neoadjuvant setting (Figure 1, right side) represent a highly heterogeneous group including tumors with either a very low (TIL^{lo} usually below 10%) or with an intermediate TIL (TIL^{int} ranging from 10% up to 60%) infiltration. Around half of these patients achieve a pathological complete response after standard anti-HER2 therapy, whereas the other half have a residual disease [15] and will be candidates for T-DM1 +/− hormonotherapy. Upfront anti-PD-(L)1-based immune checkpoint blockade could be associated with chemotherapy and standard anti-HER2 treatments (pertuzumab plus trastuzumab), particularly in the group of patients with baseline intermediate TIL, as an add-on strategy (Figure 1, panel A, right side). The group of patients with low TIL should theoretically be ideal candidates for strategies aimed at increasing immune infiltration, such as vaccines [35] or adoptive T cell transfer [36] though these treatments need further investigations in breast cancer.

Patients from both groups (Figure 1, panel A, left and right side) who have achieved a pathological complete response could be candidates to receive immune checkpoint blockade plus standard anti-HER2 treatment if immunotherapy was previously administered (Figure 1, panel A).

5. Potential Use of Immune Checkpoint Blockade in the Presence of a Residual Disease after Neoadjuvant Therapy

Even though HER2-positive breast cancer patients with baseline high TIL achieve a better event-free survival [17], it is not clear whether this also applies to patients who have a residual disease after neoadjuvant therapy.

For patients with a residual disease after standard neoadjuvant treatment (chemotherapy plus anti-HER2 agents), nodal involvement and estrogen receptor negativity have been associated with shorter event-free survival [37]. The presence of high TIL ($\geq$25%) in the residual disease was associated with worse event-free survival in a retrospective study, questioning whether in this context the use of immune checkpoint blockade might have a role in rescuing the activity of potentially dysfunctional immune cells [34]. Interestingly, the expression of Immunoglobulin (Ig)-G in the residual disease was associated with longer event-free survival [13], signifying that the presence of a well-organized adaptive immunity, including B (that produce Ig) and T lymphocytes, assures a lasting control of the disease. Hence, this highlights the need to identify the subsets of immune cells that constitute the immune infiltrate (i.e., Th, CTL, B lymphocytes, macrophages, etc.), in addition to scoring them only on HE slides.

Further, the presence of a residual disease might represent an opportunity to screen patients for anti PD-(L)1-based combinations of immune checkpoint blockade through the evaluation of the expression of PD-L1, and of other inhibitory immune checkpoint molecules, such as: Lymphocyte activation gene 3 (LAG3), T cell immunoglobulin and mucin domain 3 (TIM3) which are heterogeneously expressed in early-stage HER2-positive breast cancer [38,39] and which tightly regulate the immune response through inhibitory, non-redundant pathways.

Patients at high risk of relapse for clinicopathological factors, but with baseline high TIL and a residual disease after neoadjuvant therapy (Figure 1, panel B, left side) could be eligible to receive a rescue treatment with immune checkpoint blockade, after assessment of various immune biomarkers on the surgical specimen.

Concerning those patients with baseline intermediate TIL and a residual disease after neoadjuvant therapy (Figure 1, panel B, right side) they could all be evaluated for TIL and other immune biomarkers on the surgical specimen in order to characterize their eligibility for an immune checkpoint blockade, as an add-on treatment strategy besides standard treatments.

Whether this strategy should be given sequentially or in concomitance with standard treatments in patients with a residual disease might need to be addressed by dedicated studies.

a.   Additional multiple immune biomarkers

Beside TIL, PD-L1, LAG3 and TIM3, evaluation of other markers in the residual disease, such as CD73 and IDO, might be important, particularly in patients previously treated with PD-(L)1 blockade (i.e., administered as an upfront strategy) [40,41] (Figure 1, panel B).

So far, PD-L1 expression by IHC is performed as a biomarker for patient selection in trials of anti-PD-1/PD-L1-based immune checkpoint blockade. This also applies to LAG3 expression, which was shown to be associated with an improved benefit from PD-1 plus anti-LAG3 combinations [42]. Evaluation of the expression of multiple immune checkpoint molecules (starting from those for which drug compounds have been developed) might be achieved with the use of multiplex-IHC, a technique that allows the identification of several markers in one tissue-stain, or with the use of in situ hybridization techniques allowing the localization of the expression of genes, at both mRNA and protein levels within a histological section of a single tissue or tissue microarrays [43]. Cut-off values for positivity (usually set at >1% of positive cells, as for PD-L1 assessment) and standardization of the techniques need to be confirmed and validated.

Indeed, apart from PD-(L)1, it is not known which of these molecules is the most promising in breast cancer, considering that they can be heterogeneously expressed in tumors with intermediate or high TIL [38]. Thus, an entire panel of immune checkpoint molecules and other markers should be analyzed, also considering that they regulate non-redundant inhibitory pathways. Remarkably, by flow cytometry PD-1 and CTLA-4 are usually always expressed in inflamed breast tumors, whereas LAG3 and TIM3 are rarely highly expressed at the protein level in untreated early-stage breast tumors [38]. Ideally, the identification of different markers might represent a guide indicating which inhibitory pathway should be worthwhile as a target for immune checkpoint blockade in each patient.

6. Research Priorities in the Immunotherapy Field

To support the implementation of immune blockade strategies, some aspects need to be further investigated:

(1)   The ideal cut-off for TIL in the different settings (i.e., adjuvant, neoadjuvant, at baseline and in the residual disease), considering the wide variety of thresholds used in the literature.

(2)   The ideal cut-off (if any) for PD-L1 in early settings when considering the lesson learnt from neoadjuvant trials in triple negative breast cancer, revealing that the benefit from immune checkpoint blockade is remarkable regardless of PD-L1 status.

(3)   Concerning PD-L1 assessment: should it be done on immune cells only (as previously performed in advanced HER2-positive breast cancer) or in both immune and tumor cells (as it is through the combined positive score in early-stage triple negative breast cancer)?

(4)   The need to explore strategies that are alternatives to standard treatments (anti-HER2 agents and chemotherapy) with the aim of enhancing the immune response in hot (high TIL) tumors and convert cold (low TIL) into hot tumors in the early setting.

(5)   The potential use of immune checkpoint blockade in chemotherapy de-escalating strategies (i.e., in already inflamed, high TIL tumors) in the early setting.

(6)   The potential use of immune checkpoint blockade in escalation treatment strategies for early-stage HER2-positive low TIL breast tumors.

(7)   The difference between the hormone receptor-positive (less immunogenic) and hormone receptor-negative (more immunogenic) subgroups in HER2-positive breast cancer with regards to sensitivity to immune checkpoint blockade.

(8)   Identification of reliable novel immune (and not) biomarkers for patient selection.

Future studies will hopefully help address these research priorities.

7. Conclusions

The immune revolution challenges researchers in various ways, and the selection of patients that most likely derive lasting benefits from novel treatments represents one of the most important aspects. Diverse biomarkers have been proposed, and, among them, TIL represent the most standardized and cheaply assessed immune-related biomarker so far employed in breast cancer. However, future approaches will benefit from a more in depth characterization of the tumor microenvironment, including evaluation of the composition of TIL, of their functional profiles, of the expression of immune checkpoint molecules and from answers to open research questions as summarized above.

With this commentary, we provide an overview of the current knowledge in the field and propose an opportunity for exploitation of immune checkpoint blockade to further improve the outcome of patients with HER2-positive breast cancer.

Author Contributions: Conceptualization, C.S.; methodology, C.S., D.F., M.V.D.; validation, C.S., D.F., M.V.D.; writing—original draft preparation, C.S.; writing—review and editing, C.S., D.F., M.V.D.; supervision, M.V.D.; funding acquisition, M.V.D. All authors have read and agreed to the published version of the manuscript.

Funding: This work was not supported by any funding source. Maria Vittoria Dieci receives fundings from Celgene, Genomic Health, Eli Lilly and Novartis outside the submitted work.

Institutional Review Board Statement: Not applicable.

Informed Consent Statement: Not applicable.

Data Availability Statement: Not applicable.

Conflicts of Interest: The authors declare no conflict of interest. The institution of Debora Fumagalli receives funding from AstraZeneca, Novartis, Roche/Genentech, Pfizer, Tesaro for the conduct of clinical trials.

References

1. Sharma, P.; Allison, J.P. The future of immune checkpoint therapy. *Science* **2015**, *348*, 56–61. [CrossRef] [PubMed]
2. Lambertini, M.; Pondé, N.F.; Solinas, C.; de Azambuja, E. Adjuvant Trastuzumab: A 10-year Overview of Its Benefit. *Expert Rev. Anticancer Ther.* **2017**, *17*, 61–74. [CrossRef] [PubMed]
3. Piccart, M.J.; Hilbers, F.S.; Bliss, J.M.; Caballero, C.; Frank, E.S.; Renault, P.; Kaoudjt, R.N.; Schumacher, E.; Spears, P.A.; Regan, M.M.; et al. Road map to safe and well designed de-escalation trials of systemic adjuvant therapy for solid tumors. *J. Clin. Oncol.* **2020**, *34*, 4120–4129. [CrossRef] [PubMed]
4. Slamon, D.; Clark, G.; Wong, S.; Levin, W.; Ullrich, A.; McGuire, W. Human breast cancer: Correlation of relapse and survival with amplification of the HER-2/neu oncogene. *Science* **1987**, *235*, 177–182. [CrossRef]
5. Griguolo, G.; Pascual, T.; Dieci, M.V.; Guarneri, V.; Prat, A. Interaction of Host Immunity With HER2-targeted Treatment and Tumor Heterogeneity in HER2-positive Breast Cancer. *J. Immunother. Cancer* **2019**, *7*, 90. [CrossRef]
6. Cancer Genome Atlas Network. Comprehensive Molecular Portraits of Human Breast Tumours. *Nature* **2012**, *490*, 61–70. [CrossRef]
7. Prat, A.; Carey, L.A.; Adamo, B.; Vidal, M.; Tabernero, J.; Cortés, J.; Parker, J.S.; Perou, C.M.; Baselga, J. Molecular Features and Survival Outcomes of the Intrinsic Subtypes Within HER2-positive Breast Cancer. *J. Natl. Cancer Inst.* **2014**, *106*, dju152. [CrossRef]
8. Cejalvo, J.M.; Pascual, T.; Fernández-Martínez, A.; Brasó-Maristany, F.; Gomis, R.R.; Perou, C.M.; Muñoz, M.; Prat, A. Clinical Implications of the Non-Luminal Intrinsic Subtypes in Hormone Receptor-Positive Breast Cancer. *Cancer Treat. Rev.* **2018**, *67*, 63–70. [CrossRef]
9. Cejalvo, J.M.; Pascual, T.; Fernández-Martínez, A.; Adamo, B.; Chic, N.; Vidal, M.; Rodelo, L.; Munoz, M.; Prat, A. Distribution of the PAM50 breast cancer subtypes within each pathology-based group: A combined analysis of 15,339 patients across 29 studies. *Ann. Oncol.* **2017**, *28* (Suppl. 5), v603. [CrossRef]
10. Prat, A.; Pascual, T.; De Angelis, C.; Gutierrez, C.; Llombart-Cussac, A.; Wang, T.; Cortés, J.; Rexer, B.; Paré, L.; Forero, A.; et al. HER2-Enriched Subtype and ERBB2 Expression in HER2-Positive Breast Cancer Treated With Dual HER2 Blockade. *J. Natl. Cancer Inst.* **2020**, *112*, 46–54. [CrossRef] [PubMed]

11. Carey, L.A.; Berry, D.A.; Cirrincione, C.T.; Barry, W.T.; Pitcher, B.N.; Harris, L.N.; Ollila, D.W.; Krop, I.E.; Henry, N.L.; Weckstein, D.J.; et al. Molecular Heterogeneity and Response to Neoadjuvant Human Epidermal Growth Factor Receptor 2 Targeting in CALGB 40601, a Randomized Phase III Trial of Paclitaxel Plus Trastuzumab With or Without Lapatinib. *J. Clin. Oncol.* **2016**, *34*, 542–549. [CrossRef]

12. Cortazar, P.; Zhang, L.; Untch, M.; Mehta, K.; Costantino, J.P.; Wolmark, N.; Bonnefoi, H.; Cameron, D.; Gianni, L.; Valagussa, P.; et al. Pathological Complete Response and Long-Term Clinical Benefit in Breast Cancer: The CTNeoBC Pooled Analysis. *Lancet* **2014**, *384*, 164–172. [CrossRef]

13. Fernandez-Martinez, A.; Tanioka, M.; Fan, C.; Parker, J.S.; Hoadley, K.A.; Krop, I.; Partridge, A.; Carey, L.; Perou, C.M. Predictive and prognostic value of b-cell gene-expression signatures and b-cell receptor (BCR) repertoire in HER2+ breast cancer: A correlative analysis of the CALGB 40601 clinical trial (ALLIANCE). *Ann. Oncol.* **2019**, *30* (Suppl. 5), v55–v98. [CrossRef]

14. Denkert, C.; von Minckwitz, G.; Darb-Esfahani, S.; Lederer, B.; Heppner, B.I.; Weber, K.E.; Budczies, J.; Huober, J.; Klauschen, F.; Furlanetto, J.; et al. Tumour-infiltrating Lymphocytes and Prognosis in Different Subtypes of Breast Cancer: A Pooled Analysis of 3771 Patients Treated With Neoadjuvant Therapy. *Lancet Oncol.* **2018**, *19*, 40–50. [CrossRef]

15. Solinas, C.; Ceppi, M.; Lambertini, M.; Scartozzi, M.; Buisseret, L.; Garaud, S.; Fumagalli, D.; de Azambuja, E.; Salgado, R.; Sotiriou, C.; et al. Tumor-infiltrating Lymphocytes in Patients With HER2-positive Breast Cancer Treated with Neoadjuvant Chemotherapy Plus Trastuzumab, Lapatinib or Their Combination: A Meta-Analysis of Randomized Controlled Trials. *Cancer Treat. Rev.* **2017**, *57*, 8–15. [CrossRef] [PubMed]

16. Hendry, S.; Salgado, R.; Gevaert, T.; Russell, P.A.; John, T.; Thapa, B.; Christie, M.; van de Vijver, K.; Estrada, M.V.; Gonzalez-Ericsson, P.I.; et al. Assessing Tumor-infiltrating Lymphocytes in Solid Tumors: A Practical Review for Pathologists and Proposal for a Standardized Method From the International Immunooncology Biomarkers Working Group: Part 1: Assessing the Host Immune Response, TILs in Invasive Breast Carcinoma and Ductal Carcinoma In Situ, Metastatic Tumor Deposits and Areas for Further Research. *Adv. Anat. Pathol.* **2017**, *24*, 235–251. [CrossRef] [PubMed]

17. Salgado, R.; Denkert, C.; Campbell, C.; Savas, P.; Nuciforo, P.; Aura, C.; de Azambuja, E.; Eidtmann, H.; Ellis, C.E.; Baselga, J.; et al. Tumor-Infiltrating Lymphocytes and Associations with Pathological Complete Response and Event-Free Survival in HER2-Positive Early-Stage Breast Cancer Treated with Lapatinib and Trastuzumab: A Secondary Analysis of the NeoALTTO Trial. *JAMA Oncol.* **2015**, *1*, 448–454. [CrossRef]

18. Loi, S.; Michiels, S.; Salgado, R.; Sirtaine, N.; Jose, V.; Fumagalli, D.; Kellokumpu-Lehtinen, P.L.; Bono, P.; Kataja, V.; Desmedt, C.; et al. Tumor Infiltrating Lymphocytes Are Prognostic in Triple Negative Breast Cancer and Predictive for Trastuzumab Benefit in Early Breast Cancer: Results From the FinHER Trial. *Ann. Oncol.* **2014**, *25*, 1544–1550. [CrossRef]

19. Buisseret, L.; Garaud, S.; de Wind, A.; Van den Eynden, G.; Boisson, A.; Solinas, C.; Gu-Trantien, C.; Naveaux, C.; Lodewyckx, J.N.; Duvillier, H.; et al. Tumor-infiltrating lymphocyte composition, organization and PD-1/ PD-L1 expression are linked in breast cancer. *Oncoimmunology* **2016**, *6*, e1257452. [CrossRef] [PubMed]

20. Garaud, S.; Buisseret, L.; Solinas, C.; Gu-Trantien, C.; de Wind, A.; Van den Eynden, G.; Naveaux, C.; Lodewyckx, J.N.; Boisson, A.; Duvillier, H.; et al. Tumor infiltrating B-cells signal functional humoral immune responses in breast cancer. *JCI Insight* **2019**, *5*, e129641. [CrossRef]

21. Dieci, M.V.; Conte, P.; Bisagni, G.; Brandes, A.A.; Frassoldati, A.; Cavanna, L.; Musolino, A.; Giotta, F.; Rimanti, A.; Garrone, O.; et al. Association of tumor-infiltrating lymphocytes with distant disease-free survival in the ShortHER randomized adjuvant trial for patients with early HER2+ breast cancer. *Ann. Oncol.* **2019**, *30*, 418–423. [CrossRef]

22. Kim, R.S.; Song, N.; Gavin, P.G.; Salgado, R.; Bandos, H.; Kos, Z.; Floris, G.; Van den Eynden, G.G.G.M.; Badve, S.; Demaria, S.; et al. Stromal Tumor-infiltrating Lymphocytes in NRG Oncology/NSABP B-31 Adjuvant Trial for Early-Stage HER2-Positive Breast Cancer. *J. Natl. Cancer Inst.* **2019**, *111*, 867–871. [CrossRef] [PubMed]

23. Vanmeerbeek, I.; Sprooten, J.; De Ruysscher, D.; Tejpar, S.; Vandenberghe, P.; Fucikova, J.; Spisek, R.; Zitvogel, L.; Kroemer, G.; Galluzzi, L.; et al. Trial watch: Chemotherapy-induced immunogenic cell death in immuno-oncology. *Oncoimmunology* **2020**, *9*, 1703449. [CrossRef] [PubMed]

24. Schmid, P.; Cortes, J.; Pusztai, L.; McArthur, H.; Kümmel, S.; Bergh, J.; Denkert, C.; Park, Y.H.; Hui, R.; Harbeck, N.; et al. KEYNOTE-522 Investigators. Pembrolizumab for Early Triple-Negative Breast Cancer. *N. Engl. J. Med.* **2020**, *382*, 810–821. [CrossRef] [PubMed]

25. Schmid, P.; Adams, S.; Rugo, H.S.; Schneeweiss, A.; Barrios, C.H.; Iwata, H.; Diéras, V.; Hegg, R.; Im, S.A.; Shaw Wright, G.; et al. IMpassion130 Trial Investigators. Atezolizumab and Nab-Paclitaxel in advanced triple negative breast cancer. *N. Engl. J. Med.* **2018**, *379*, 2108–2121. [CrossRef]

26. Emens, L.A.; Esteva, F.J.; Beresford, M.; Saura, C.; De Laurentiis, M.; Kim, S.; Im, S.; Wang, Y.; Mani, A.; Shah, J.; et al. Overall survival (OS) in KATE2, a phase 2 study of Programmed Death Ligand 1 (PD-L1) inhibitor atezolizumab (atezo)+trastuzumab emtansine (T-DM1) vs placebo (pbo)+T-DM1 in previously treated HER2+ advanced breast cancer (bc). *Ann. Oncol.* **2019**, *30* (Suppl. 5), v104–v142. [CrossRef]

27. Loi, S.; Giobbie-Hurder, A.; Gombos, A.; Bachelot, T.; Hui, R.; Curigliano, G.; Campone, M.; Biganzoli, L.; Bonnefoi, H.; Jerusalem, G.; et al. International Breast Cancer Study Group and the Breast International Group.Pembrolizumab Plus Trastuzumab in Trastuzumab-Resistant, Advanced, HER2-positive Breast Cancer (PANACEA): A Single-Arm, Multicentre, Phase 1b-2 Trial. *Lancet Oncol.* **2019**, *20*, 371–382. [CrossRef]

28. Luen, S.J.; Salgado, R.; Fox, S.; Savas, P.; EngWong, J.; Clark, E.; Kiermaier, A.; Swain, S.M.; Baselga, J.; Michiels, S.; et al. Tumour-infiltrating lymphocytes in advanced HER2-positive breast cancer treated with pertuzumab or placebo in addition to trastuzumab and docetaxel: A retrospective analysis of the CLEOPATRA study. *Lancet Oncol.* **2017**, *18*, 52–62. [CrossRef]

29. Dieci, M.V.; Tsvetkova, V.; Orvieto, E.; Piacentini, F.; Ficarra, G.; Griguolo, G.; Miglietta, F.; Giarratano, T.; Omarini, C.; Bonaguro, S.; et al. Immune characterization of breast cancer metastases: Prognostic implications. *Breast Cancer Res.* **2018**, *20*, 62. [CrossRef] [PubMed]

30. Liu, J.; Blake, S.J.; Yong, M.C.; Harjunpää, H.; Ngiow, S.F.; Takeda, K.; Young, A.; O'Donnell, J.S.; Allen, S.; Smyth, M.J.; et al. Improved Efficacy of Neoadjuvant Compared to Adjuvant Immunotherapy to Eradicate Metastatic Disease. *Cancer Discov.* **2016**, *6*, 1382–1399. [CrossRef]

31. Harbeck, N. Emerging strategies in neoadjuvant treatment of patients with HER2-positive early breast cancer. *Breast* **2019**, *48*, S97–S102. [CrossRef]

32. Montemurro, F.; Nuzzolese, I.; Ponzone, R. Neoadjuvant or adjuvant chemotherapy in early breast cancer? *Expert Opin. Pharmacother.* **2020**, *21*, 1071–1082. [CrossRef] [PubMed]

33. NCCN Guidelines Breast Cancer 2020. Available online: https://www2.tri-kobe.org/nccn/guideline/breast/english/breast.pdf (accessed on 1 March 2021).

34. Hamy, A.S.; Pierga, J.Y.; Sabaila, A.; Laas, E.; Bonsang-Kitzis, H.; Laurent, C.; Vincent-Salomon, A.; Cottu, P.; Lerebours, F.; Rouzier, R.; et al. Stromal lymphocyte infiltration after neoadjuvant chemotherapy is associated with aggressive residual disease and lower disease-free survival in HER2-positive breast cancer. *Ann. Oncol.* **2017**, *28*, 2233–2240. [CrossRef]

35. Solinas, C.; Aiello, M.; Migliori, E.; Willard-Gallo, K.; Emens, L.A. Breast cancer vaccines: Heeding the lessons from the past to guide a path forward. *Cancer Treat. Rev.* **2020**, *84*, 101947. [CrossRef] [PubMed]

36. Met, Ö.; Jensen, K.M.; Chamberlain, C.A.; Donia, M.; Svane, I.M. Principles of adoprive T cell therapy in cancer. *Semin. Immunopathol.* **2019**, *41*, 49–58. [CrossRef]

37. von Minckwitz, G.; Huang, C.S.; Mano, M.S.; Loibl, S.; Mamounas, E.P.; Untch, M.; Wolmark, N.; Rastogi, P.; Schneeweiss, A.; Redondo, A.; et al. KATHERINE Investigators. Trastuzumab Emtansine for Residual Invasive HER2-Positive Breast Cancer. *N. Engl. J. Med.* **2019**, *380*, 617–628. [CrossRef]

38. Solinas, C.; Garaud, S.; De Silva, P.; Boisson, A.; Van den Eynden, G.; de Wind, A.; Risso, P.; Rodrigues Vitória, J.; Richard, F.; Migliori, E.; et al. Immune Checkpoint Molecules on Tumor-Infiltrating Lymphocytes and Their Association With Tertiary Lymphoid Structures in Human Breast Cancer. *Front. Immunol.* **2017**, *8*, 1412. [CrossRef] [PubMed]

39. Müller, P.; Kreuzaler, M.; Khan, T.; Thommen, D.S.; Martin, K.; Glatz, K.; Savic, S.; Harbeck, N.; Nitz, U.; Gluz, O.; et al. Trastuzumab emtansine (T-DM1) renders HER2+ breast cancer highly susceptible to CTLA-4/PD-1 blockade. *Sci. Transl. Med.* **2015**, *7*, 315ra188. [CrossRef]

40. Soleimani, A.; Taghizadeh, E.; Shahsavari, S.; Amini, Y.; Rashidpour, H.; Azadian, E.; Jafari, A.; Parizadeh, M.R.; Mashayekhi, K.; Soukhtanloo, M.; et al. CD73; a key ectonucleotidase in the development of breast cancer: Recent advances and perspectives. *J. Cell Physiol.* **2019**. [CrossRef]

41. Wang, Y.; Yang, B.H.; Li, H.; Cao, S.; Ren, X.B.; Yu, J.P. IDO+ DCs and signalling pathways. *Curr. Cancer Drug Targets* **2013**, *13*, 278–288. [CrossRef]

42. Solinas, C.; Migliori, E.; De Silva, P.; Willard-Gallo, K. LAG3: The biological processes that motivate targeting this immune checkpoint molecule in human cancer. *Cancers* **2019**, *11*, 1213. [CrossRef] [PubMed]

43. Jeffery, R.; Hunt, T.; Poulsom, R. In Situ Hybridization Combined With Immunohistochemistry to Localize Gene Expression. *Breast Cancer Res. Protoc.* **2006**, *120*, 323–346.

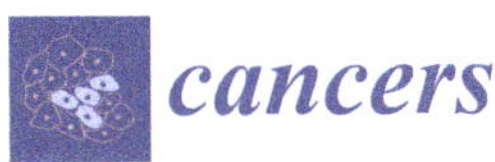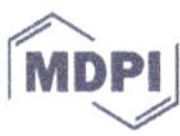

Perspective

The Influence of Chimeric Antigen Receptor Structural Domains on Clinical Outcomes and Associated Toxicities

Ashleigh S. Davey [1,2,]*, Matthew E. Call [1,2] and Melissa J. Call [1,2,]*

1 Structural Biology Division, The Walter and Eliza Hall Institute of Medical Research, Parkville 5052, Australia; mecall@wehi.edu.au
2 Department of Medical Biology, The University of Melbourne, Parkville 3052, Australia
* Correspondence: davey.a@wehi.edu.au (A.S.D.); mjcall@wehi.edu.au (M.J.C.)

Simple Summary: The development and refinement chimeric antigen receptor (CAR)-T cell immunotherapy has significantly improved the prognosis of patients with B cell malignancies. Severe treatment related toxicities however remain a significant challenge for the field. This perspective reviews 17 clinical trials of the most widely used anti-CD19 (FMC63) CAR-T cell therapies, with the aim of dissecting the contribution of the structural and costimulatory domains of the CAR to clinical outcomes and toxicities. The CD28 structural hinge and transmembrane CAR domains are highlighted as strongly associated with both clinical efficacy and severe toxicity. This perspective supports further investigation into the structural CAR domains for improved CAR design and safer CAR-T cell therapies.

Abstract: Chimeric antigen receptor (CAR)-T cell therapy has transformed the treatment of B cell malignancies, improving patient survival and long-term remission. Nonetheless, over 50% of patients experience severe treatment-related toxicities including cytokine release syndrome (CRS) and neurotoxicity. Differences in severity of toxic side-effects among anti-CD19 CARs suggest that the choice of costimulatory domain makes a significant contribution to toxicity, but comparisons are complicated by additional differences in the hinge and transmembrane (TM) domains of the most commonly used CARs in the clinic, segments that have long been considered to perform purely structural roles. In this perspective, we examine clinical and preclinical data for anti-CD19 CARs with identical antigen-binding (FMC63) and signalling (CD3ζ) domains to unravel the contributions of different hinge-TM and costimulatory domains. Analysis of clinical trials highlights an association of the CD28 hinge-TM with higher incidence of CRS and neurotoxicity than the corresponding sequences from CD8, regardless of whether the CD28 or the 4-1BB costimulatory domain is used. The few preclinical studies that have systematically varied these domains similarly support a strong and independent role for the CD28 hinge-TM sequence in high cytokine production. These observations highlight the value that a comprehensive and systematic interrogation of each of these structural domains could provide toward developing fundamental principles for rational design of safer CAR-T cell therapies.

Keywords: CAR-T cell therapy; CD19; clinical trials; CRS; toxicity

Citation: Davey, A.S.; Call, M.E.; Call, M.J. The Influence of Chimeric Antigen Receptor Structural Domains on Clinical Outcomes and Associated Toxicities. *Cancers* **2021**, *13*, 38. https://dx.doi.org/10.3390/cancers13010038

Received: 30 November 2020
Accepted: 22 December 2020
Published: 25 December 2020

Publisher's Note: MDPI stays neutral with regard to jurisdictional claims in published maps and institutional affiliations.

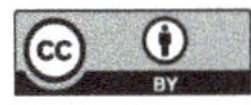

1. Introduction

Recent decades have seen the development of groundbreaking new treatments for cancer. The emergence of adoptive cellular therapies, including chimeric antigen receptor (CAR)-T cells, represents an advance that has dramatically improved upon classical cytotoxic chemotherapies and led to significant improvements in patient outcomes for advanced and refractory B cell malignancies. CAR-T cell therapy utilises engineered receptors (CARs) to redirect a patient's cytotoxic T cells to a targeted cancer antigen of choice. This therapy is a multi-step process involving leukapheresis of a patient's blood, the genetic modification of their T cells to express a tumour-antigen-specific CAR, followed by ex vivo expansion and re-infusion of the CAR-T cells back to the patient where they selectively seek out and kill target tumour cells. Following high remission rates in clinical trials, two CD19 CAR-T cell products were approved by the FDA in late 2017 for the treatment of refractory non-Hodgkin lymphoma (NHL) and for patients with relapsed or refractory B cell acute lymphoblastic leukemia (B-ALL) up to the age of 25 [1]. There are now over 200 CAR-T cell clinical trials underway for a range of cancer antigens (clinicaltrials.gov). However, safety concerns and general applicability to many tumour types are issues that still need to be resolved. A great deal of research is now underway to modulate specific properties of CAR-T cells with the aim of improving their safety and efficacy for a wider range of cancers. In this perspective, we examine the influence of CAR domain structure on the clinical outcomes and toxicities observed in the most extensively studied CAR-T cell therapies, the anti-CD19 CAR-T cells using the antibody single-chain variable fragment (scFv) FMC63. While differences in efficacy and safety profiles between the two FDA-approved anti-CD19 therapies may reasonably be ascribed primarily to their use of different costimulatory signalling domains in the CAR constructs, we highlight clinical and preclinical observations suggesting that the hinge and transmembrane (TM) domains, long considered to be functionally inert structural features, make surprisingly strong contributions to CAR-T cell toxicity. Understanding the mechanisms underlying these effects will be a key step in improving rational CAR design.

1.1. Components of the Chimeric Antigen Receptor (CAR)

Naïve T cells require dual signalling interactions for activation, first between the multi-chain T cell receptor (TCR) complex and peptides presented by an interacting cell's MHC proteins (signal 1), and additionally from costimulatory receptor:ligand interactions (signal 2). The first generation of CARs generated by Esshar and colleagues utilised the antigen specificity of an scFv fused to the entire CD3ζ protein to mimic signal 1 in T cell activation [2]. The resulting CAR was expressed well at the cell surface and was successful in redirecting T cells to target tumour antigens. However, CAR-T cell persistence was poor, and cells showed signs of exhaustion prior to tumour clearance [3–6]. This prompted the development of second-generation CARs which also contain an scFv antigen recognition domain and intracellular CD3ζ signalling tail, but additionally incorporated a flexible hinge domain for improved antigen reach and a costimulatory domain to provide signal 2 required for strong and durable T cell activation [7]. The intracellular costimulatory and signalling domains are connected to the extracellular scFv and hinge via a TM domain, which is often an extension of the costimulatory or hinge sequence. Most CAR constructs exist as dimers on the cell surface, stabilized by disulfide bonds between hinge domains and inter-monomer TM interactions [8]. Inclusion of the additional domains provided second-generation CAR-T cells with the requisite signals for activation and significantly improved persistence and clinical outcomes in treated patients [9–11]. Further iterations of CARs continue to be developed, including those with two costimulatory domains (third-generation CARs) as well as CARs with inducible expression of a transgene product such as cytokines (fourth-generation CARs/TRuCs) [12–14].

1.2. Limitations of CAR-T Cell Therapy

Since the development and initial success of second-generation CAR-T cell therapies in the clinic, many groups have now shifted focus to manipulating specific domains of the CAR with the aim of improving target cell recognition and therapeutic efficacy, and limiting CAR-associated toxicities. A significant leap in the field came with the introduction of a costimulatory domain into the CAR which significantly improved the persistence and efficacy of clinical CAR-T cell products [7]. The choice of which specific costimulatory domain is more clinically effective though is not yet unanimous. Extensive work is underway to further improve upon these current second-generation CAR-T cell constructs by altering specific CAR domains including the hinge, TM and costimulatory domains, particularly for the treatment of more difficult immunosuppressive solid tumours [8,15–22].

Clinical trials of CAR-T cell therapies all report similar treatment-related toxicities, including cytokine release syndrome (CRS) and neurotoxicity. CRS is triggered by the rapid systemic release of inflammatory cytokines including IFNγ, IL-6 and IL-1 into the blood by activated CAR-T cells and endogenous myeloid cells [23–25]. The symptoms of CRS in response to CAR-T cell therapy range from mild flu-like symptoms to severe symptoms such as hypotension, organ toxicity and acute respiratory distress, which can collectively be life threatening and often result in patients spending extended periods of time in the intensive care unit (ICU) [26]. The second major toxicity reported following CD19-targeted CAR-T cell therapy is neurotoxicity. Similar to CRS, neurotoxicity symptoms also range in severity and type, including headaches, delirium, dysphasia, ataxia, dysmetria, decrease in level of consciousness, seizures and acute cerebral edema [27–29]. The incidence of neurotoxicity among CAR-T cell-treated patients is quite variable, with some neurological events occurring in combination with CRS symptoms and others at different times or in the absence of CRS, suggesting that at least in some cases the mechanism of CAR-T cell induced neurotoxicity is different to that of CRS [30,31]. Comprehensive and timely management plans are also in place for the treatment of neurological toxicities, often involving the administration of systemic corticosteroids including dexamethasone, which has the unfortunate consequence of interfering with CAR-T cell function [32]. While both CRS and neurotoxicity symptoms can be treated in the clinic, many patients require expensive ICU administration and support, thus prevention of such severe toxicities with CAR-T cell treatment is ideal for further progression of this promising therapeutic.

It has generally been presumed that the costimulatory domains are mostly responsible for the severe toxicities observed with CAR-T cell therapies due to the increased potency and persistence observed in second-generation CARs compared to first-generation CARs [3–6]. Considering many of the costimulatory domains used clinically extend from the intracellular domain though the TM to the extracellular hinge and scFv, it is difficult to discern the contribution of the TM and hinge structural domains individually to clinical efficacy and toxicity development. We therefore examined clinical trials of the most extensively published anti-CD19 FMC63 scFv CARs, all of which contain a CD3ζ signalling tail, to understand whether CAR-related toxicities are defined by the costimulatory domain alone or whether structural features such as the hinge and TM domains of the CAR also play a role.

2. Clinical Trials of Anti-CD19 CAR-T Cell Therapy

CD19 is a cell-surface glycoprotein uniformly expressed during all stages of B cell differentiation and is present in more than 95% of B cell malignancies [33]. Under normal physiological conditions, CD19 acts as a co-receptor in complex with the B cell receptor and other surface markers to modulate downstream signalling pathways that induce B cell proliferation and activation [34]. Due to its homogenous and high expression in many B cell malignancies and the fact that bystander B cell depletion can be managed clinically, CD19 has become an attractive target for the initial testing and translation of CAR-T cell immunotherapy, evident by over half of all CAR-T cell clinical trials targeting the CD19 antigen (clinicaltrials.gov). To dissect the clinical implications of individual hinge, TM and costimulatory domains, we collected and summarised data from anti-CD19 CAR-T cell clinical trials in which the CAR construct contained the same FMC63 scFv [35] and CD3ζ signalling tail (Table 1). Clinical trials were included if they used a second-generation CAR containing these domains and provided details of clinical response rate, CRS and neurotoxicity.

Table 1. Summary of FMC63 (CD19) CAR T cells in clinical trials with published clinical outcomes.

NCT ID	Tumour Type	No. of Patients	CAR Name	CAR Domain Structure					Gene Transfer Method	CAR-T Cell Dose	Ref
				ScFv	Hinge	TMD	Costim	Signal			
NCT02842138	FL	7	CD19-BBz(86)	FMC63	CD8α	CD8α	41BB	CD3ζ	lentivirus	3×10^8–3.7×10^8	[15]
NCT02842138	DLBCL	13	CD19-BBz(86)	FMC63	CD8α	CD8α	41BB	CD3ζ	lentivirus	6×10^6–3.2×10^8	[15]
NCT02030834	DLBCL, FL	28	CTL-019	FMC63	CD8α	CD8α	41BB	CD3ζ	lentivirus	3.1×10^6–8.9×10^6/kg	[39]
NCT02445248	DLBCL	111	CTL-019	FMC63	CD8α	CD8α	41BB	CD3ζ	lentivirus	1×10^7–6×10^8	[40]
NCT01626495 NCT01029366	B-ALL, T-ALL	30	CTL-019	FMC63	CD8α	CD8α	41BB	CD3ζ	lentivirus	1×10^7–1×10^8/kg	[30,41]
NCT02435849	B-ALL	75	CTL-019	FMC63	CD8α	CD8α	41BB	CD3ζ	lentivirus	3.1×10^6/kg	[42]
NCT02631044	DLBCL	268	JCAR017	FMC63	CD8α	CD8α	41BB	CD3ζ	lentivirus	5×10^7–1.5×10^8	[43]
NCT01860937	B-ALL	25	19-28z	FMC63	CD28	CD28	CD28	CD3ζ	gamma retrovirus	1×10^6–3×10^6/kg	[44]
NCT01044069	B-ALL	53	19-28z	FMC63	CD28	CD28	CD28	CD3ζ	gamma retrovirus	1×10^6–3×10^6/kg	[23,45]
NCT00466531	CLL	16	19-28z	FMC63	CD28	CD28	CD28	CD3ζ	gamma retrovirus	2.6×10^6–3.2×10^7	[46]
NCT01840566	DLBCL, FL, MZL, MCL	15	19-28z	FMC63	CD28	CD28	CD28	CD3ζ	gamma retrovirus	5×10^6–1×10^7/kg	[47]
NCT02601313	MCL	68	KTE-X19	FMC63	CD28	CD28	CD28	CD3ζ	gamma retrovirus	2×10^6/kg	[48]
NCT02348216	DLBCL, PMBCL, TFL	101	KTE-C19	FMC63	CD28	CD28	CD28	CD3ζ	gamma retrovirus	2×10^6/kg	[49]
NCT00924326	DLBCL	17	CAR-19	FMC63	CD28	CD28	CD28	CD3ζ	gamma retrovirus	1×10^6–2×10^6/kg	[50]
NCT01593696	B-ALL	21	FMC63-28z	FMC63	CD28	CD28	CD28	CD3ζ	gamma retrovirus	3×10^4–3×10^6/kg	[51]
NCT02963038	B-ALL	10	SENL-B19	FMC63	CD28	CD28	41BB	CD3ζ	lentivirus	3×10^5–1.6×10^6/kg	[36]
NCT01865617	LBCL, FL, MCL	32	-	FMC63	IgG4	CD28	41BB	CD3ζ	lentivirus	2×10^5–2×10^7/kg	[37,38]

B-ALL, B cell acute lymphoblastic leukemia; CLL, chronic lymphocytic leukemia; DLBCL, diffuse large B cell lymphoma; FL, follicular lymphoma; MCL, mantle cell lymphoma; MZL, marginal zone lymphoma; PMBCL, primary mediastinal large B cell lymphoma.

The majority of FMC63 CAR-T cell clinical trials have been conducted on patients with B-ALL and NHLs including diffuse large B cell lymphoma (DLBCL), follicular lymphoma (FL), mantle cell lymphoma (MCL) and marginal zone lymphoma (MZL), due to their generally high and stable expression of CD19 (Table 1). These CD19 CARs generally adopt one of two multi-domain structures: 1. FMC63 scFv, CD8α hinge and TM, 41BB costimulatory domain and CD3ζ signalling tail (8-8-41BB CAR; Figure 1a), or 2. FMC63 scFv, CD28 hinge, TM and costimulatory domain, and CD3ζ signalling tail (28-28-28 CAR; Figure 1b). There is also one published clinical trial utilising a CAR with a CD28 hinge and TM but a 41BB costimulatory domain (28-28-41BB; Figure 1c) [36], and another with an IgG4 hinge, CD28 TM and 41BB costimulatory domain (IgG4-28-41BB; Figure 1d) [37,38]. In the clinical trials reviewed here, all CD28 costimulatory domain-containing CAR-T cells were transduced using gamma retrovirus, while all 41BB-containing CAR-T cells were transduced using lentivirus (Table 1). The dosage of CAR-T cells within and between clinical trials ranges significantly from 3×10^4 cells to 3.7×10^8 cells per kg (Table 1). By directly comparing the clinical trials containing each of these four iterations of the FMC63 CAR, trends towards particular structural domains that influence specific outcomes such as response rate and toxicity may be exposed.

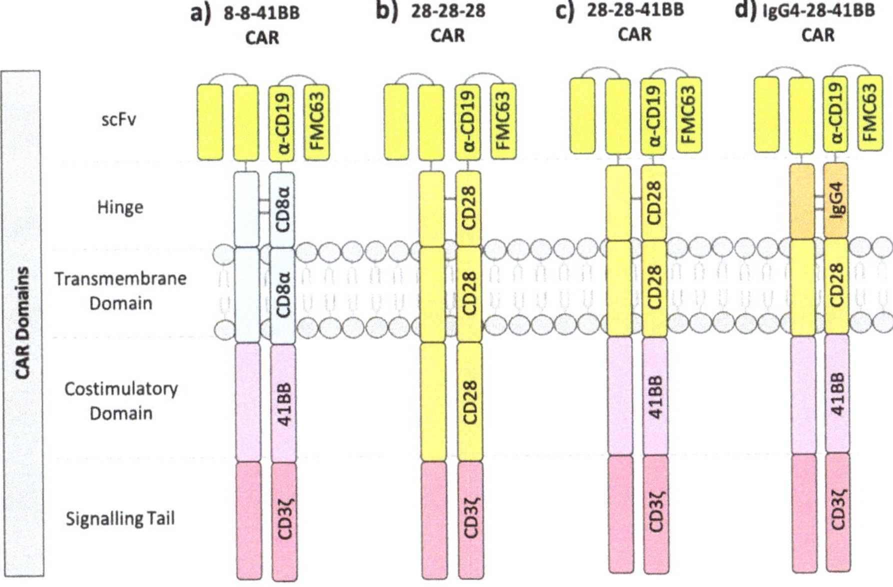

Figure 1. Structural domains of our main FMC63 anti-CD19 CARs. The structural design of the (**a**) 8-8-41BB CARs, (**b**) 28-28-28 CARs, (**c**) 28-28-41BB CARs and (**d**) IgG4-28-41BB CARs reviewed here. The individual scFv, hinge, transmembrane domain, costimulatory domain and signalling tails are labelled. Horizontal lines between hinge domains indicate disulfide bonds.

2.1. The Effect of CAR Domains on Clinical Response

Multiple factors have been reported to impact CD19 CAR-T cell therapy clinical outcome in patients, including whether a patient has received conditioning lymphodepletion therapy prior to CAR-T cell infusion, whether CAR-T cells were cultured with IL-2 prior to infusion and the extent of CAR-T cell persistence in patients [52,53]. For the studies shown in Table 1, we saw no obvious effect of age, conditioning lymphodepletion treatment or CAR-T cell dosage on patient complete response rate (Table 2). Not surprisingly, although the tumour target antigen was identical in all FMC63 CAR-T cell treatments, patient complete response rate does appear to vary depending on tumour type, with B-ALL patients gaining the highest response rates, followed by FL, DLBCL and lastly MCL (Table 2). Considering the limited number of FMC63 anti-CD19 CAR-T cell clinical trials with published results, all clinical trials in Table 1, including those with MCL patients, were included for response and toxicity CAR comparisons. The complete response (CR) rate among patients treated with the various CD19 CAR-T cell therapies was calculated as the number of patients who achieved a CR at any stage post CAR-T cell infusion as a percentage of the total number of patients treated with the CAR-T cell therapy in a single clinical trial (Figure 2). Details of the individual trial patient numbers and other reported patient responses for each clinical trial are detailed in Table S1.

Table 2. Effect of prognostic factors on complete response rate.

Prognostic Factor	No. of Patients	No. of Clinical Trials	Response Rate Mean % [95% CI]	*p*-Value
Age:				
$\leq$65	483	12	50.7% [39.1–62.3]	0.7743
>65	180	5	52.6% [24.0–81.1]	
Lymphodepletion:				
Yes	835	12	57.1% [46.9–67.4]	0.4737
No	13	3	42.9% [0–100]	
CAR-T cells infused:				
$\leq 1 \times 10^7$/kg	442	12	58.5% [47.0–70.0]	0.2043
$>1 \times 10^7$/kg	35	5	43.4% [5.8–81.0]	
Cancer type:				
B-ALL	184	5	72.3% [60.6–84.1]	
DLBCL	490	9	41.4% [32.6–50.2]	
FL	49	5	52.5% [30.2–74.7]	
MCL	73	3	22.2% [0–100]	

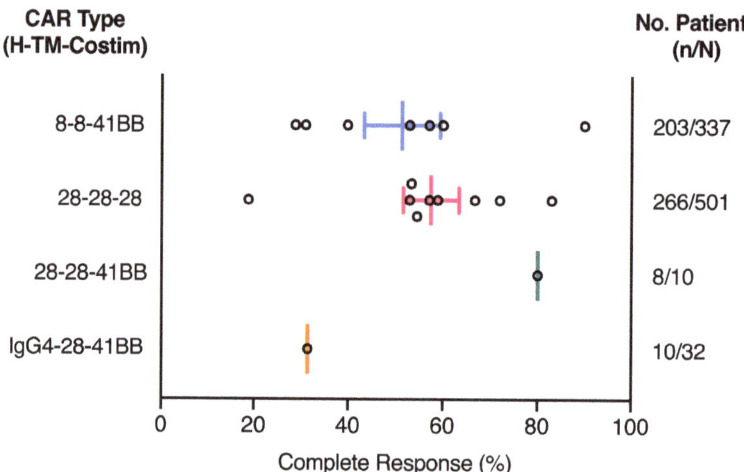

Figure 2. Effect of CAR composition on complete response in patients treated with CD19 CAR-T cell therapy. CAR type separated based on hinge (H), transmembrane (TM) and costimulatory (Costim) domain composition. All CAR constructs use the FMC63 anti-CD19 scFv and the CD3ζ-chain activation domain. Each circle represents an individual clinical trial listed in Table 1. Complete response (CR) rate calculated from the number of patients who reached a CR at any stage post CAR-T cell infusion (n) as a percentage of all patients treated with the CAR-T cell therapy (N) (Table S1). Middle line represents the mean CR and error bars represent the SEM.

Overall, 28-28-28 CARs and 8-8-41BB CARs have very similar CR rates (Figure 2). Interestingly, in a single study where B-ALL patients were treated with a 41BB CAR that used the CD28 hinge-TM domain instead of CD8α (28-28-41BB CAR), a higher CR rate was observed in comparison to the average for studies using 28-28-28 and 8-8-41BB CARs (Figure 2). Although this is only a single clinical trial of 10 patients, it highlights the 41BB costimulatory domain may be associated with improved clinical response [36]. Furthermore, comparison of this CAR with one in which only the hinge was altered, using IgG4 instead of CD28 (IgG4-28-41BB CAR), a much lower CR rate was observed [37,38]. While the IgG4-28-41BB CAR clinical trial includes a number of participants with the poorest responding MCL tumour type, it highlights the possibility that inclusion of the CD28 hinge-TM structural domains in clinical CAR constructs may also be correlated with higher complete response rate in patients. Further preclinical comparisons and clinical studies are required to investigate the full impact of the individual hinge-TM and costimulatory domain substitutions in isolation and their correlation with response rates.

2.2. CRS Toxicity Correlates with CAR Domain Design

There is currently no clear consensus on a CRS grading system for CAR-T cell therapies among institutions worldwide, making CRS severity analysis between CAR-T cell products and trials exceedingly difficult. This is largely due to the fact that the timing and definition of CRS symptoms observed following cellular therapies such as CAR-T cells differs significantly to previously described CRS responses to antibody and drug therapies [54–56]. CRS following CAR-T cell treatment was initially graded using the National Cancer Institute Common Terminology Criteria for Adverse Events (CTCAE) grading scale for adverse event reporting [57,58]. However, this scale was developed before cell therapy-induced CRS was well understood. CTCAE was more consistent with an acute cytokine storm typically observed within minutes to hours of antibody or drug treatment but did not take into consideration the more likely delayed onset of CRS symptoms up to a few days post CAR-T cell infusion [57–59]. This grading system was modified by Lee and colleagues in 2014 to more accurately define mild, moderate, severe, and life-threatening CRS symptoms regardless of the inciting agent [60]. This guideline also included treatment recommendations for each of the CRS grades described and has been consequently used by many clinical trials conducted after this date. An alternative CRS grading system was developed and used for CTL-019 CAR T cell trials from the University of Pennsylvania (Penn Grading Scale), which had a similar grading structure to the 2014 Lee et al. scale but did not use absolute cut-off values for vital signs such as % oxygen requirement to define CRS grade, as such values can vary in severity depending on the individual patient [41]. The Penn Grading System was also designed in a way that allowed for CRS symptoms to be reproducibly graded among different institutions, CAR-T cell target antigens and disease settings. While we do not provide a detailed comparison of the various CRS grading methods here, it is clear that a consensus on an accurate CRS grading program and prompt management plan for CAR-T cell induced CRS symptoms that is used worldwide in all clinical trials would be more beneficial for inter-trial analysis [61].

Despite the above limitations, we felt that the CRS grading systems used in many of the FMC63 CAR-T cell clinical trials were similar enough to yield informative comparisons among the different CAR structural designs (Table 3). To assess the effect of domain structure on CRS development, patient CRS grade was collected for each clinical trial presented in Table 1 and taken as a percentage of total patients within each clinical trial (Table S2). The percentage CRS development for each grade and clinical trial was subsequently plotted by CAR domain configuration to examine correlations between CRS diagnosis and CAR domain structure. Overall, the incidence of CRS in patients treated with CAR-T cell therapy is high, with 60–80% of patients developing some level of identifiable symptoms. While the mean percentage of patients in the highest category of CRS (grade 3+) does not differ between CAR-T cell treatment products, a clear correlation between CRS development and CAR domain configuration is observed for grade 1–2 CRS (Figure 3). The 28-28-28

CAR-T cell treatment resulted in a higher proportion of patients developing CRS compared to 8-8-41BB CAR-T cell treatment (Figure 3). It is difficult to discern the contribution of the CD28 costimulatory domain to this increased CRS toxicity, as 28-28-28 and 28-28-41BB CAR-T cell-treated patients show similar levels of grade 1–2 CRS development. However, the 28-28-41BB CAR-T cell therapy does emerge with a higher incidence of more severe grade 3+ CRS in comparison (Figure 3). Interestingly, the use of CD28 hinge and TM domains in a 41BB CAR (28-28-41BB) was associated with an increased proportion of patients developing CRS, rising to a level similar to that observed in the 28-28-28 CAR (Figure 3) [36]. While this is only a single clinical trial, it suggests that CRS severity is at least in part attributable to the CD28 hinge and TM domains independently of which costimulatory domain is used. The same degree of increase in CRS was not observed in the trial using an IgG4-CD28 hinge-TM domain configuration (IgG4-28-41BB), further underscoring that the identity and/or combination of hinge-TM structural domains can exert significant influence on manifestation of CRS toxicity even when the scFv, costimulatory and activation domains are the same (Figure 3) [37,38]. Additional research and clinical trials that make direct comparisons among CAR configurations will be required to identify the relative contributions of each individual CAR domain in developing CRS.

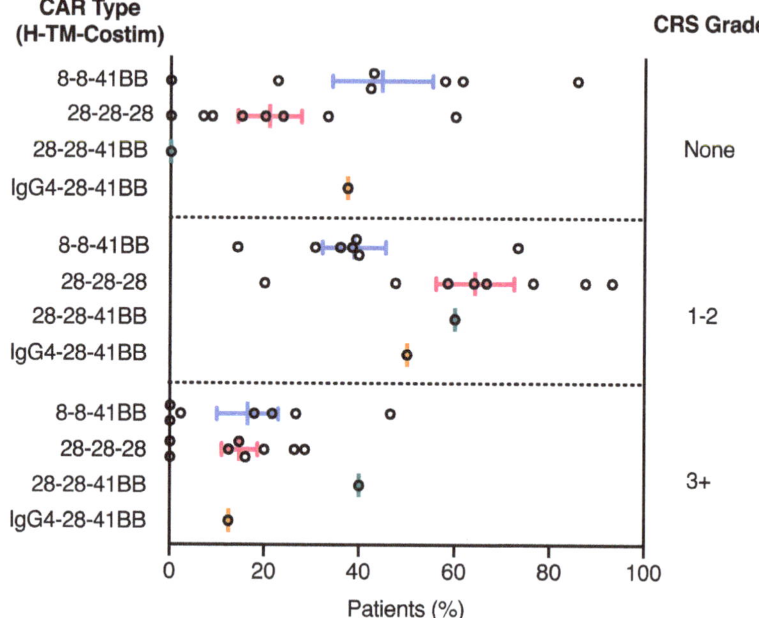

Figure 3. CAR domain structure influences CRS severity in patients treated with CD19 CAR-T cell therapies. Both CAR type, based on hinge (H), transmembrane (TM) and costimulatory (Costim) domain composition, and CRS grade, separated into none, grade 1–2 and grade 3+, are represented on the left and right *y* axis, respectively. Each circle represents the percentage of patients in a single clinical trial listed in Table 1 that developed the corresponding grade of CRS (none, grade 1–2 and grade 3+). Middle line represents the mean percentage of patients with the corresponding grade of CRS and error bars represent the SEM (Table S2).

Table 3. CRS grading systems used in published FMC63 (CD19) CAR-T cell clinical trials.

NCT ID	CAR Name	CAR Domain Structure					No. of Patients	CRS Grading System	Neurotoxicity Grading System
		ScFv	Hinge	TM	Costim	Signal			
NCT02842138	CD19-BBz(86)	FMC63	CD8α	CD8α	41BB	CD3ζ	7	CTCAE v4.03 [57]	CTCAE v4.03 [57]
NCT02842138	CD19-BBz(86)	FMC63	CD8α	CD8α	41BB	CD3ζ	13	CTCAE v4.03 [57]	CTCAE v4.03 [57]
NCT02030834	CTL-019	FMC63	CD8α	CD8α	41BB	CD3ζ	28	Penn grading system [41]	CTCAE v3.0 [58]
NCT02445248	CTL-019	FMC63	CD8α	CD8α	41BB	CD3ζ	111	Penn grading system [41]	CTCAE v4.03 [57]
NCT01626495 NCT01029366	CTL-019	FMC63	CD8α	CD8α	41BB	CD3ζ	30	Penn grading system [41]	CTCAE v3.0 [58]
NCT02435849	CTL-019	FMC63	CD8α	CD8α	41BB	CD3ζ	75	MedDRA and CTCAE v4.03 [57]	MedDRA and CTCAE v4.03 [57]
NCT02631044	JCAR017	FMC63	CD8α	CD8α	41BB	CD3ζ	268	Lee et al. 2014 [60]	CTCAE v4.03 [57]
NCT01860937	19-28z	FMC63	CD28	CD28	CD28	CD3ζ	25	CTCAE v4.0	CTCAE v4.0
NCT01044069	19-28z	FMC63	CD28	CD28	CD28	CD3ζ	53	Lee et al. 2014 [60]	CTCAE v4.03 [57]
NCT00466531	19-28z	FMC63	CD28	CD28	CD28	CD3ζ	16	CTCAE v3.0 (<2009) [58] CTCAE v4.0 (>2009)	CTCAE v3.0 (<2009) [58] CTCAE v4.0 (>2009)
NCT01840566	19-28z	FMC63	CD28	CD28	CD28	CD3ζ	15	ASBMT	CTCAE v4.03 [57]
NCT02601313	KTE-X19	FMC63	CD28	CD28	CD28	CD3ζ	68	Lee et al. 2014 [60]	CTCAE v4.03 [57]
NCT02348216	KTE-C19	FMC63	CD28	CD28	CD28	CD3ζ	101	Lee et al. 2014 [60]	CTCAE v4.03 [57]
NCT00924326	CAR-19	FMC63	CD28	CD28	CD28	CD3ζ	17	CTCAE v3.0 [58]	CTCAE v3.0 [58]
NCT01593696	FMC63-28z	FMC63	CD28	CD28	CD28	CD3ζ	21	CTCAE v4.02	CTCAE v4.02
NCT02963038	SENL-B19	FMC63	CD28	CD28	41BB	CD3ζ	10	CTCAE v4.0	CTCAE v4.0
NCT01865617	-	FMC63	IgG4	CD28	41BB	CD3ζ	32	CTCAE v4.03 [57]	CTCAE v4.03 [57]

ASBMT, American Society for Blood and Marrow Transplantation Consensus Criteria; CTCAE, National Cancer Institute Common Terminology Criteria for Adverse Event; MedDRA, Medical Dictionary for Regulatory Authorities.

2.3. Relationship between CAR Domain Structure and Neurotoxicity Development

Neurotoxicity has been reported to occur both concurrently and independently of CRS toxicity in anti-CD19 CAR-T cell clinical trials. In general, neurotoxicity events that occur concurrently with CRS are of a shorter duration and severity (grade 1–2), while delayed neurotoxicity occurring post-CRS can arise up to 3-4 weeks after CAR-T cell therapy and is more commonly associated with grade 3+ neurotoxicity [37,38,51,62]. Neurotoxicity severity has been reported to fluctuate rapidly once diagnosed, demonstrating the requirement for close patient monitoring and precise management plans to prevent rare fatal events. Similar to CRS toxicity, there are multiple grading scales that can be used to assess the level of neurotoxicity in patients receiving CAR-T cell therapy. The most common grading protocol used in the clinical trials reviewed here is the National Cancer Institute Common Terminology Criteria for Adverse Events (CTCAE), with CTCAE v3.0 used prior to 2009 [58] and CTCAE v4.0 after 2009 [57] (Table 3). The CTCAE neurotoxicity grading systems have limitations due to the unique characteristics and timing of neurotoxicity symptoms following CAR-T cell treatment compared to antibody and drug treatments. Consequently, a unique condition titled CAR-T cell-related encephalopathy syndrome (CRES) was introduced by the multi-institutional CAR-T cell therapy associated toxicity (CARTOX) working group. The CRES grading system encompasses a 10-point patient questionnaire to capture cognitive and attentive dysfunction combined with clinical tests to assess intracranial pressure and severity of seizures [32]. More recently, the American Society for Transplantation and Cellular Therapy (ASTCT; previously ASBMT) coined the term immune effector cell-associated neurotoxicity syndrome (ICANS) for CAR-T cell related neurotoxicity, using a modified version of the CARTOX screening grading system to also take into account patient consciousness, motor symptoms and cerebral edema symptoms [63]. A retrospective study using these three methods (CTCAE v4.03, CRES and ASTCT) to grade neurotoxicity events post CAR-T cell treatment in the JULIET trial uncovered the overdiagnosis of neurotoxicity using the CTCAE v4.03 grading system (45% of patients) in comparison to both CRES and ASTCT grading systems (both 17.1% of patients). Many of the patients only diagnosed with neurotoxicity using the CTCAE v4.03 and not CRES or ASTCT grading systems had mild symptoms such as headaches which were thought to be non-specific to the CAR-T cell treatment [64]. Clearly there is a disparity in the published grading systems for neurotoxicities seen after CAR-T cell therapy. A refined grading system proposed by 49 CAR-T cell experts and supported by the ASTCT was published in 2018 in the hope that future CAR-T cell clinical trials can use a consensus grading system for more accurate toxicity reporting and inter-trial analysis [63]. Use of such a universal grading system would enable better comparison of clinical trial products and outcomes.

Neurotoxicity symptoms were reported and graded in 16 of the 17 clinical trials listed in Table 1 (Table 3). To assess the effect of domain structure on neurotoxicity development, the percentage of patients that developed each grade of neurotoxicity was calculated for each clinical trial presented in Table 1 (Table S3). The percentage neurotoxicity development for each grade and clinical trial was subsequently plotted by CAR domain configuration to examine correlations between neurotoxicity diagnosis and CAR domain structure. Overall a clear increase in severe (grade 3+) neurotoxicity was observed in patients treated with the 28-28-28 CAR compared to the 8-8-41BB CAR (Figure 4). While the 8-8-41BB CAR showed on average the lowest level of severe grade 3+ neurotoxicity, use of the CD28 hinge-TM or IgG4 hinge and CD28 TM in a 41BB CAR (28-28-41BB and IgG4-28-41BB, respectively) was associated with increased incidence of grade 3+ neurotoxicity that was more in line with the 28-28-28 trials (Figure 4) [36,38]. As for CRS, these observations suggest that use of part or all of the CD28 structural domains is associated with higher toxicity. While the most relevant direct comparisons required to confirm these associations have not been made in any single large clinical trial, as outlined below, there is significant preclinical data that offer strong support for the independent contributions of hinge and TM domains to CAR function and toxicity.

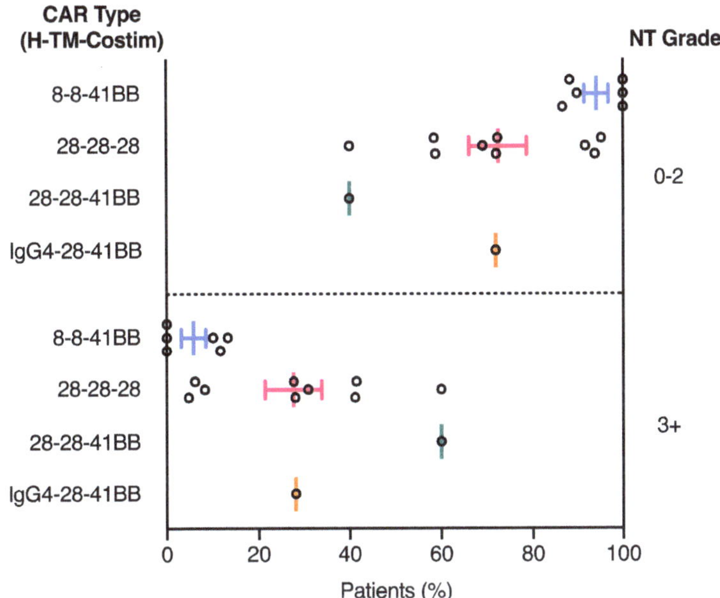

Figure 4. Grade of neurotoxicity development in patients treated with CD19 CAR T cell therapies is related to CAR domain structure composition. CAR domain structure is separated based on hinge (H), transmembrane (TM) and costimulatory (Costim) domain composition on the left *y* axis, while neurotoxicity grade is separated into grade 0–2 or grade 3+ on the right *y* axis. Each circle represents the percentage of patients in a single clinical trial listed in Table 1 that developed the corresponding grade of neurotoxicity (grade 0–2 and grade 3+). Middle line represents the mean percentage of patients with the corresponding grade of neurotoxicity and error bars represent the SEM (Table S3).

3. Preclinical Evidence of CAR Domain Design Influencing CAR-Related Toxicities

CRS symptoms are caused by a significant elevation of blood cytokine levels as a result of excessive cytokine secretion by both CAR-T cells and other immune cells. Consequently, CAR T cells which exhibit reduced cytokine secretion to levels that induce less CRS toxicity but still promote effective T cell proliferation and cytotoxicity are required. Optimisation of CAR domain configuration towards this end is a crucial goal, but unravelling the contributions of different domains is complicated by comparisons in which hinge, TM and costimulatory domains are all varied at the same time. A small number of carefully controlled preclinical studies have recently begun to address this problem systematically.

In one recent study focused on modifications to the hinge-TM domains alone, Ying and colleagues [15] generated CTL-019 variant CARs (FMC63 scFv with CD8α hinge and TM domains, 4-1BB costimulatory domain and CD3ζ tail) with small extensions to the CD8α hinge and TM domains. One of the longer hinge-TM constructs (named CD19-41BBz(86) in their study) showed a significant reduction in IFNγ, TNFα, IL-2 and IL-4 production in vitro when co-cultured with human CD19 target cells. Treatment of B cell lymphoma patients in a small phase I clinical trial with the CD19-41BBz(86) CAR-T cell therapy yielded good response rates, low circulating cytokines and little to no development of CRS or neurotoxicity symptoms post-treatment [15]. This study demonstrates that even small changes to the hinge-TM domains of a CAR can significantly impact cytokine production and CRS development. The mechanism by which this extension of only a few amino acids on each end of the hinge-TM yields such significant effects is unknown.

Another study by Alabanza and colleagues [65] directly compared FMC63 anti-CD19 CARs containing the same CD28 costimulatory domains and CD3ζ tail with either CD28 or CD8 hinge-TM regions (named FMC63-28Z and FMC63-CD828Z in their study, respectively). Both CARs showed similar cell-surface expression and induced degranulation upon target cell recognition, however secretion of IFNγ and TNFα was significantly lower in FMC63-CD828Z CAR-T cells compared to FMC63-28Z CAR-T cells. The same hinge-TM substitutions in fully human anti-CD19 (HuCD19) and human VEGFR2 (hVEGFR2) CD28 costimulatory domain-containing CARs also demonstrated reduced cytokine secretion associated with the CD8 hinge-TM region compared to the CD28 hinge-TM region [8,66]. In a separate study examining independent variations of structural and costimulatory domains, Majzner and colleagues [20] showed that both the CD28 hinge-TM and CD28 costimulatory domains contribute to the high cytokine production associated with the FMC63-CD28z configuration compared to the FMC63-CD8-41BBz configuration. Importantly, the CD28 hinge-TM domains conferred improved cytotoxic potency against low-antigen target cells, regardless of the identity of the costimulatory domain, and was associated with both higher potency and increased cytokine production even in first-generation CAR constructs containing no costimulatory domains [20]. Emerging data suggest that such effects of the CD28 hinge-TM domains are attributed to its high propensity to form heterodimers with endogenous CD28 through specific TM sequences within the membrane, thus hijacking native CD28 receptor signalling in addition to CAR-mediated signalling [17,67]. These preclinical observations support the suggestion from our review of clinical trial outcomes that the higher incidence of intermediate CRS and high-grade neurotoxicity observed in trials using FMC63 CARs with CD28-derived hinge-TM and costimulatory sequences may be more closely associated with the structural domains than the costimulatory domain.

4. Conclusions

Here we examined FMC63 anti-CD19 CAR-T cell clinical trials in an attempt to unravel the impact of the hinge, TM and costimulatory domains of the CAR protein on patient clinical outcome and toxicities. CD28 hinge-TM containing CARs were associated with a slightly higher average clinical response rate but were also associated with more severe toxicity compared to CD8 hinge-TM containing CARs. While the number of patients and clinical trials contributing to this observation are limited, several recent preclinical studies highlighted above support this association, with CD8 hinge-TM CAR-T cells consistently shown to produce lower levels of cytokines than otherwise identical CD28 hinge-TM CAR-T cells. These studies contribute to an increasing recognition within the field that the hinge-TM structural domains are not functionally inert, and work to unravel the contribution of the hinge and TM domains independently is ongoing. It remains unclear whether one or both of these structural domains contributes directly to these effects, and the mechanisms underlying these functional outcomes are still not well understood. We suggest that a broad systematic interrogation of hinge and TM domain effects on CAR structure, stability, expression levels, signalling outputs and interactions with other cell-surface signalling molecules will yield fundamental new insights into how we may rationally design safer CAR-T cell therapies that do not compromise clinical efficacy.

Supplementary Materials: The following are available online at https://www.mdpi.com/2072-669 4/13/1/38/s1, Table S1: Number and best clinical response of patients in each anti-CD19 CAR-T cell clinical trial, Table S2: Number and grade of patients diagnosed with CRS in each anti-CD19 CAR-T cell clinical trial, Table S3: Number and grade of patients diagnosed with neurotoxicity in each anti-CD19 CAR-T cell clinical trial.

Author Contributions: Conceptualization, A.S.D. and M.J.C.; writing-original draft preparation, A.S.D.; Writing-review and editing, A.S.D., M.E.C. and M.J.C. All authors have read and agreed to the published version of the manuscript.

Funding: We acknowledge NHMRC project grant 1158249 for funding and article processing charges.

Conflicts of Interest: M.E.C. and M.J.C. are inventors on a patent application related to CAR structural modifications.

References

1. June, C.H.; Sadelain, M. Chimeric antigen receptor therapy. *N. Engl. J. Med.* **2018**, *379*, 64–73. [CrossRef] [PubMed]
2. Eshhar, Z.; Waks, T.; Gross, G.; Schindler, D.G. Specific activation and targeting of cytotoxic lymphocytes through chimeric single chains consisting of antibody-binding domains and the gamma or zeta subunits of the immunoglobulin and T-cell receptors. *Proc. Natl. Acad. Sci. USA* **1993**, *90*, 720–724. [CrossRef] [PubMed]
3. Jensen, M.C.; Popplewell, L.; Cooper, L.J.; DiGiusto, D.; Kalos, M.; Ostberg, J.R.; Forman, S.J. Antitransgene rejection responses contribute to attenuated persistence of adoptively transferred CD20/CD19-specific chimeric antigen receptor redirected T cells in humans. *Biol. Blood Marrow Transpl.* **2010**, *16*, 1245–1256. [CrossRef] [PubMed]
4. Till, B.G.; Jensen, M.C.; Wang, J.; Chen, E.Y.; Wood, B.L.; Greisman, H.A.; Qian, X.; James, S.E.; Raubitschek, A.; Forman, S.J.; et al. Adoptive immunotherapy for indolent non-Hodgkin lymphoma and mantle cell lymphoma using genetically modified autologous CD20-specific T cells. *Blood* **2008**, *112*, 2261–2271. [CrossRef] [PubMed]
5. Kershaw, M.H.; Westwood, J.A.; Parker, L.L.; Wang, G.; Eshhar, Z.; Mavroukakis, S.A.; White, D.E.; Wunderlich, J.R.; Canevari, S.; Rogers-Freezer, L.; et al. A phase I study on adoptive immunotherapy using gene-modified T cells for ovarian cancer. *Clin. Cancer Res.* **2006**, *12*, 6106–6115. [CrossRef] [PubMed]
6. Park, J.R.; Digiusto, D.L.; Slovak, M.; Wright, C.; Naranjo, A.; Wagner, J.; Meechoovet, H.B.; Bautista, C.; Chang, W.C.; Ostberg, J.R.; et al. Adoptive transfer of chimeric antigen receptor re-directed cytolytic T lymphocyte clones in patients with neuroblastoma. *Mol. Ther.* **2007**, *15*, 825–833. [CrossRef] [PubMed]
7. Moritz, D.; Groner, B. A spacer region between the single chain antibody- and the CD3 zeta-chain domain of chimeric T cell receptor components is required for efficient ligand binding and signaling activity. *Gene Ther.* **1995**, *2*, 539–546.
8. Fujiwara, K.; Tsunei, A.; Kusabuka, H.; Ogaki, E.; Tachibana, M.; Okada, N. Hinge and transmembrane domains of chimeric antigen receptor regulate receptor expression and signaling threshold. *Cells* **2020**, *9*, 1182. [CrossRef]
9. Maher, J.; Brentjens, R.J.; Gunset, G.; Riviere, I.; Sadelain, M. Human T-lymphocyte cytotoxicity and proliferation directed by a single chimeric TCRzeta /CD28 receptor. *Nat. Biotechnol.* **2002**, *20*, 70–75. [CrossRef]
10. Kalos, M.; Levine, B.L.; Porter, D.L.; Katz, S.; Grupp, S.A.; Bagg, A.; June, C.H. T cells with chimeric antigen receptors have potent antitumor effects and can establish memory in patients with advanced leukemia. *Sci. Transl. Med.* **2011**, *3*, 95ra73. [CrossRef]
11. Savoldo, B.; Ramos, C.A.; Liu, E.; Mims, M.P.; Keating, M.J.; Carrum, G.; Kamble, R.T.; Bollard, C.M.; Gee, A.P.; Mei, Z.; et al. CD28 costimulation improves expansion and persistence of chimeric antigen receptor-modified T cells in lymphoma patients. *J. Clin. Investig.* **2011**, *121*, 1822–1826. [CrossRef] [PubMed]
12. Chmielewski, M.; Kopecky, C.; Hombach, A.A.; Abken, H. IL-12 release by engineered T cells expressing chimeric antigen receptors can effectively Muster an antigen-independent macrophage response on tumor cells that have shut down tumor antigen expression. *Cancer Res.* **2011**, *71*, 5697–5706. [CrossRef] [PubMed]
13. Koneru, M.; Purdon, T.J.; Spriggs, D.; Koneru, S.; Brentjens, R.J. IL-12 secreting tumor-targeted chimeric antigen receptor T cells eradicate ovarian tumors in vivo. *Oncoimmunology* **2015**, *4*, e994446. [CrossRef] [PubMed]
14. Hu, B.; Ren, J.; Luo, Y.; Keith, B.; Young, R.M.; Scholler, J.; Zhao, Y.; June, C.H. Augmentation of antitumor immunity by human and mouse CAR T cells secreting IL-18. *Cell Rep.* **2017**, *20*, 3025–3033. [CrossRef]
15. Ying, Z.; Huang, X.F.; Xiang, X.; Liu, Y.; Kang, X.; Song, Y.; Guo, X.; Liu, H.; Ding, N.; Zhang, T.; et al. A safe and potent anti-CD19 CAR T cell therapy. *Nat. Med.* **2019**, *25*, 947–953. [CrossRef]
16. Hudecek, M.; Lupo-Stanghellini, M.T.; Kosasih, P.L.; Sommermeyer, D.; Jensen, M.C.; Rader, C.; Riddell, S.R. Receptor affinity and extracellular domain modifications affect tumor recognition by ROR1-specific chimeric antigen receptor T cells. *Clin. Cancer Res.* **2013**, *19*, 3153–3164. [CrossRef]
17. Leddon, S.A.; Fettis, M.M.; Abramo, K.; Kelly, R.; Oleksyn, D.; Miller, J. The CD28 Transmembrane Domain Contains an Essential Dimerization Motif. *Front. Immunol.* **2020**, *11*, 1519. [CrossRef]
18. Finney, H.M.; Lawson, A.D.; Bebbington, C.R.; Weir, A.N. Chimeric receptors providing both primary and costimulatory signaling in T cells from a single gene product. *J. Immunol.* **1998**, *161*, 2791–2797.
19. Feucht, J.; Sun, J.; Eyquem, J.; Ho, Y.J.; Zhao, Z.; Leibold, J.; Dobrin, A.; Cabriolu, A.; Hamieh, M.; Sadelain, M. Calibration of CAR activation potential directs alternative T cell fates and therapeutic potency. *Nat. Med.* **2019**, *25*, 82–88. [CrossRef]
20. Majzner, R.G.; Rietberg, S.P.; Sotillo, E.; Dong, R.; Vachharajani, V.T.; Labanieh, L.; Myklebust, J.H.; Kadapakkam, M.; Weber, E.W.; Tousley, A.M.; et al. Tuning the antigen density requirement for CAR T cell activity. *Cancer Discov.* **2020**, *10*. [CrossRef]
21. Pegram, H.J.; Lee, J.C.; Hayman, E.G.; Imperato, G.H.; Tedder, T.F.; Sadelain, M.; Brentjens, R.J. Tumor-targeted T cells modified to secrete IL-12 eradicate systemic tumors without need for prior conditioning. *Blood* **2012**, *119*, 4133–4141. [CrossRef] [PubMed]
22. Tan, A.H.J.; Vinanica, N.; Campana, D. Chimeric antigen receptor-T cells with cytokine neutralizing capacity. *Blood Adv.* **2020**, *4*, 1419–1431. [CrossRef] [PubMed]
23. Davila, M.L.; Riviere, I.; Wang, X.; Bartido, S.; Park, J.; Curran, K.; Chung, S.S.; Stefanski, J.; Borquez-Ojeda, O.; Olszewska, M.; et al. Efficacy and toxicity management of 19-28z CAR T cell therapy in B cell acute lymphoblastic leukemia. *Sci. Transl. Med.* **2014**, *6*, 224ra225. [CrossRef] [PubMed]

24. Norelli, M.; Camisa, B.; Barbiera, G.; Falcone, L.; Purevdorj, A.; Genua, M.; Sanvito, F.; Ponzoni, M.; Doglioni, C.; Cristofori, P.; et al. Monocyte-derived IL-1 and IL-6 are differentially required for cytokine-release syndrome and neurotoxicity due to CAR T cells. *Nat. Med.* **2018**, *24*, 739–748. [CrossRef]

25. Giavridis, T.; van der Stegen, S.J.C.; Eyquem, J.; Hamieh, M.; Piersigilli, A.; Sadelain, M. CAR T cell-induced cytokine release syndrome is mediated by macrophages and abated by IL-1 blockade. *Nat. Med.* **2018**, *24*, 731–738. [CrossRef] [PubMed]

26. Fitzgerald, J.C.; Weiss, S.L.; Maude, S.L.; Barrett, D.M.; Lacey, S.F.; Melenhorst, J.J.; Shaw, P.; Berg, R.A.; June, C.H.; Porter, D.L.; et al. Cytokine release syndrome after chimeric antigen receptor T Cell therapy for acute lymphoblastic leukemia. *Crit. Care Med.* **2017**, *45*, e124–e131. [CrossRef]

27. Gust, J.; Hay, K.A.; Hanafi, L.A.; Li, D.; Myerson, D.; Gonzalez-Cuyar, L.F.; Yeung, C.; Liles, W.C.; Wurfel, M.; Lopez, J.A.; et al. Endothelial activation and blood-brain barrier disruption in neurotoxicity after adoptive immunotherapy with CD19 CAR-T Cells. *Cancer Discov.* **2017**, *7*, 1404–1419. [CrossRef]

28. Prudent, V.; Breitbart, W.S. Chimeric antigen receptor T-cell neuropsychiatric toxicity in acute lymphoblastic leukemia. *Palliat. Support. Care* **2017**, *15*, 499–503. [CrossRef]

29. Belin, C.; Devic, P.; Ayrignac, X.; Dos Santos, A.; Paix, A.; Sirven-Villaros, L.; Simard, C.; Lamure, S.; Gastinne, T.; Ursu, R.; et al. Description of neurotoxicity in a series of patients treated with CAR T-cell therapy. *Sci. Rep.* **2020**, *10*, 18997. [CrossRef]

30. Maude, S.L.; Frey, N.; Shaw, P.A.; Aplenc, R.; Barrett, D.M.; Bunin, N.J.; Chew, A.; Gonzalez, V.E.; Zheng, Z.; Lacey, S.F.; et al. Chimeric antigen receptor T cells for sustained remissions in leukemia. *N. Engl. J. Med.* **2014**, *371*, 1507–1517. [CrossRef]

31. Parker, K.R.; Migliorini, D.; Perkey, E.; Yost, K.E.; Bhaduri, A.; Bagga, P.; Haris, M.; Wilson, N.E.; Liu, F.; Gabunia, K.; et al. Single-cell analyses identify brain mural cells expressing CD19 as potential off-tumor targets for CAR-T immunotherapies. *Cell* **2020**, *183*, 126–142. [CrossRef] [PubMed]

32. Neelapu, S.S.; Tummala, S.; Kebriaei, P.; Wierda, W.; Gutierrez, C.; Locke, F.L.; Komanduri, K.V.; Lin, Y.; Jain, N.; Daver, N.; et al. Chimeric antigen receptor T-cell therapy-assessment and management of toxicities. *Nat. Rev. Clin. Oncol.* **2018**, *15*, 47–62. [CrossRef] [PubMed]

33. Nadler, L.M.; Anderson, K.C.; Marti, G.; Bates, M.; Park, E.; Daley, J.F.; Schlossman, S.F. B4, a human B lymphocyte-associated antigen expressed on normal, mitogen-activated, and malignant B lymphocytes. *J. Immunol.* **1983**, *131*, 244–250. [PubMed]

34. Wang, K.; Wei, G.; Liu, D. CD19: A biomarker for B cell development, lymphoma diagnosis and therapy. *Exp. Hematol. Oncol.* **2012**, *1*, 36. [CrossRef]

35. Nicholson, I.C.; Lenton, K.A.; Little, D.J.; Decorso, T.; Lee, F.T.; Scott, A.M.; Zola, H.; Hohmann, A.W. Construction and characterisation of a functional CD19 specific single chain Fv fragment for immunotherapy of B lineage leukaemia and lymphoma. *Mol. Immunol.* **1997**, *34*, 1157–1165. [CrossRef]

36. Ma, F.; Ho, J.Y.; Du, H.; Xuan, F.; Wu, X.; Wang, Q.; Wang, L.; Liu, Y.; Ba, M.; Wang, Y.; et al. Evidence of long-lasting anti-CD19 activity of engrafted CD19 chimeric antigen receptor-modified T cells in a phase i study targeting pediatrics with acute lymphoblastic leukemia. *Hematol. Oncol.* **2019**, *37*, 601–608. [CrossRef]

37. Turtle, C.J.; Hanafi, L.A.; Berger, C.; Hudecek, M.; Pender, B.; Robinson, E.; Hawkins, R.; Chaney, C.; Cherian, S.; Chen, X.; et al. Immunotherapy of non-Hodgkin's lymphoma with a defined ratio of CD8+ and CD4+ CD19-specific chimeric antigen receptor-modified T cells. *Sci. Transl. Med.* **2016**, *8*, 355ra116. [CrossRef]

38. Turtle, C.J.; Hanafi, L.A.; Berger, C.; Gooley, T.A.; Cherian, S.; Hudecek, M.; Sommermeyer, D.; Melville, K.; Pender, B.; Budiarto, T.M.; et al. CD19 CAR-T cells of defined CD4+:CD8+ composition in adult B cell ALL patients. *J. Clin. Investig.* **2016**, *126*, 2123–2138. [CrossRef]

39. Schuster, S.J.; Svoboda, J.; Chong, E.A.; Nasta, S.D.; Mato, A.R.; Anak, O.; Brogdon, J.L.; Pruteanu-Malinici, I.; Bhoj, V.; Landsburg, D.; et al. Chimeric antigen receptor T cells in refractory B-cell lymphomas. *N. Engl. J. Med.* **2017**, *377*, 2545–2554. [CrossRef]

40. Schuster, S.J.; Bishop, M.R.; Tam, C.S.; Waller, E.K.; Borchmann, P.; McGuirk, J.P.; Jager, U.; Jaglowski, S.; Andreadis, C.; Westin, J.R.; et al. Tisagenlecleucel in adult relapsed or refractory diffuse large B-cell lymphoma. *N. Engl. J. Med.* **2019**, *380*, 45–56. [CrossRef]

41. Porter, D.L.; Hwang, W.T.; Frey, N.V.; Lacey, S.F.; Shaw, P.A.; Loren, A.W.; Bagg, A.; Marcucci, K.T.; Shen, A.; Gonzalez, V.; et al. Chimeric antigen receptor T cells persist and induce sustained remissions in relapsed refractory chronic lymphocytic leukemia. *Sci. Transl. Med.* **2015**, *7*, 303ra139. [CrossRef] [PubMed]

42. Maude, S.L.; Laetsch, T.W.; Buechner, J.; Rives, S.; Boyer, M.; Bittencourt, H.; Bader, P.; Verneris, M.R.; Stefanski, H.E.; Myers, G.D.; et al. Tisagenlecleucel in children and young adults with B-cell lymphoblastic leukemia. *N. Engl. J. Med.* **2018**, *378*, 439–448. [CrossRef] [PubMed]

43. Abramson, J.S.; Palomba, M.L.; Gordon, L.I.; Lunning, M.A.; Wang, M.L.; Arnason, J.E.; Mehta, A.; Purev, E.; Maloney, D.G.; Andreadis, C.; et al. Pivotal safety and efficacy results from transcend NHL 001, a multicenter phase 1 study of lisocabtagene maraleucel (liso-cel) in relapsed/refractory (R/R) large B bell lymphomas. *Blood* **2019**, *134*, 241. [CrossRef]

44. Curran, K.J.; Margossian, S.P.; Kernan, N.A.; Silverman, L.B.; Williams, D.A.; Shukla, N.; Kobos, R.; Forlenza, C.J.; Steinherz, P.; Prockop, S.; et al. Toxicity and response after CD19-specific CAR T-cell therapy in pediatric/young adult relapsed/refractory B-ALL. *Blood* **2019**, *134*, 2361–2368. [CrossRef] [PubMed]

45. Park, J.H.; Riviere, I.; Gonen, M.; Wang, X.; Senechal, B.; Curran, K.J.; Sauter, C.; Wang, Y.; Santomasso, B.; Mead, E.; et al. Long-term follow-up of CD19 CAR therapy in acute lymphoblastic leukemia. *N. Engl. J. Med.* **2018**, *378*, 449–459. [CrossRef] [PubMed]

46. Hollyman, D.; Stefanski, J.; Przybylowski, M.; Bartido, S.; Borquez-Ojeda, O.; Taylor, C.; Yeh, R.; Capacio, V.; Olszewska, M.; Hosey, J.; et al. Manufacturing validation of biologically functional T cells targeted to CD19 antigen for autologous adoptive cell therapy. *J. Immunother.* **2009**, *32*, 169–180. [CrossRef] [PubMed]

47. Sauter, C.S.; Senechal, B.; Riviere, I.; Ni, A.; Bernal, Y.; Wang, X.; Purdon, T.; Hall, M.; Singh, A.N.; Szenes, V.Z.; et al. CD19 CAR T cells following autologous transplantation in poor-risk relapsed and refractory B-cell non-Hodgkin lymphoma. *Blood* **2019**, *134*, 626–635. [CrossRef]

48. Wang, M.; Munoz, J.; Goy, A.; Locke, F.L.; Jacobson, C.A.; Hill, B.T.; Timmerman, J.M.; Holmes, H.; Jaglowski, S.; Flinn, I.W.; et al. KTE-X19 CAR T-cell therapy in relapsed or refractory mantle-cell lymphoma. *N. Engl. J. Med.* **2020**, *382*, 1331–1342. [CrossRef]

49. Neelapu, S.S.; Locke, F.L.; Bartlett, N.L.; Lekakis, L.J.; Miklos, D.B.; Jacobson, C.A.; Braunschweig, I.; Oluwole, O.O.; Siddiqi, T.; Lin, Y.; et al. Axicabtagene ciloleucel CAR T-cell therapy in refractory large B-cell lymphoma. *N. Engl. J. Med.* **2017**, *377*, 2531–2544. [CrossRef]

50. Kochenderfer, J.N.; Somerville, R.P.T.; Lu, T.; Shi, V.; Bot, A.; Rossi, J.; Xue, A.; Goff, S.L.; Yang, J.C.; Sherry, R.M.; et al. Lymphoma remissions caused by anti-CD19 chimeric antigen receptor T cells are associated with high serum interleukin-15 levels. *J. Clin. Oncol.* **2017**, *35*, 1803–1813. [CrossRef]

51. Lee, D.W.; Kochenderfer, J.N.; Stetler-Stevenson, M.; Cui, Y.K.; Delbrook, C.; Feldman, S.A.; Fry, T.J.; Orentas, R.; Sabatino, M.; Shah, N.N.; et al. T cells expressing CD19 chimeric antigen receptors for acute lymphoblastic leukaemia in children and young adults: A phase 1 dose-escalation trial. *Lancet* **2015**, *385*, 517–528. [CrossRef]

52. Zhang, T.; Cao, L.; Xie, J.; Shi, N.; Zhang, Z.; Luo, Z.; Yue, D.; Zhang, Z.; Wang, L.; Han, W.; et al. Efficiency of CD19 chimeric antigen receptor-modified T cells for treatment of B cell malignancies in phase I clinical trials: A meta-analysis. *Oncotarget* **2015**, *6*, 33961–33971. [CrossRef]

53. Drokow, E.K.; Ahmed, H.A.W.; Amponsem-Boateng, C.; Akpabla, G.S.; Song, J.; Shi, M.; Sun, K. Survival outcomes and efficacy of autologous CD19 chimeric antigen receptor-T cell therapy in the patient with diagnosed hematological malignancies: A systematic review and meta-analysis. *Clin. Risk Manag.* **2019**, *15*, 637–646. [CrossRef] [PubMed]

54. Suntharalingam, G.; Perry, M.R.; Ward, S.; Brett, S.J.; Castello-Cortes, A.; Brunner, M.D.; Panoskaltsis, N. Cytokine storm in a phase 1 trial of the anti-CD28 monoclonal antibody TGN1412. *N. Engl. J. Med.* **2006**, *355*, 1018–1028. [CrossRef] [PubMed]

55. Wing, M.G.; Moreau, T.; Greenwood, J.; Smith, R.M.; Hale, G.; Isaacs, J.; Waldmann, H.; Lachmann, P.J.; Compston, A. Mechanism of first-dose cytokine-release syndrome by CAMPATH 1-H: Involvement of CD16 (FcgammaRIII) and CD11a/CD18 (LFA-1) on NK cells. *J. Clin. Investig.* **1996**, *98*, 2819–2826. [CrossRef] [PubMed]

56. Teachey, D.T.; Rheingold, S.R.; Maude, S.L.; Zugmaier, G.; Barrett, D.M.; Seif, A.E.; Nichols, K.E.; Suppa, E.K.; Kalos, M.; Berg, R.A.; et al. Cytokine release syndrome after blinatumomab treatment related to abnormal macrophage activation and ameliorated with cytokine-directed therapy. *Blood* **2013**, *121*, 5154–5157. [CrossRef] [PubMed]

57. Services, U.D.o.H.a.H. Common Terminology Criteria for Adverse Events (CTCAE). V4.03. Available online: https://evs.nci.nih.gov/ftp1/CTCAE/CTCAE_4.03/CTCAE_4.03_2010-06-14_QuickReference_5x7.pdf (accessed on 12 November 2020).

58. Services, U.D.o.H.a.H. Common Terminology Criteria for Adverse Events (CTCAE). V3.0. Available online: https://ctep.cancer.gov/protocolDevelopment/electronic_applications/docs/ctcaev3.pdf (accessed on 12 November 2020).

59. Winkler, U.; Jensen, M.; Manzke, O.; Schulz, H.; Diehl, V.; Engert, A. Cytokine-release syndrome in patients with B-cell chronic lymphocytic leukemia and high lymphocyte counts after treatment with an anti-CD20 monoclonal antibody (rituximab, IDEC-C2B8). *Blood* **1999**, *94*, 2217–2224. [CrossRef] [PubMed]

60. Lee, D.W.; Gardner, R.; Porter, D.L.; Louis, C.U.; Ahmed, N.; Jensen, M.; Grupp, S.A.; Mackall, C.L. Current concepts in the diagnosis and management of cytokine release syndrome. *Blood* **2014**, *124*, 188–195. [CrossRef]

61. Porter, D.; Frey, N.; Wood, P.A.; Weng, Y.; Grupp, S.A. Grading of cytokine release syndrome associated with the CAR T cell therapy tisagenlecleucel. *J. Hematol. Oncol.* **2018**, *11*, 35. [CrossRef]

62. Teachey, D.T.; Lacey, S.F.; Shaw, P.A.; Melenhorst, J.J.; Maude, S.L.; Frey, N.; Pequignot, E.; Gonzalez, V.E.; Chen, F.; Finklestein, J.; et al. Identification of predictive biomarkers for cytokine release syndrome after chimeric antigen receptor T-cell therapy for acute lymphoblastic leukemia. *Cancer Discov.* **2016**, *6*, 664–679. [CrossRef]

63. Lee, D.W.; Santomasso, B.D.; Locke, F.L.; Ghobadi, A.; Turtle, C.J.; Brudno, J.N.; Maus, M.V.; Park, J.H.; Mead, E.; Pavletic, S.; et al. ASTCT consensus grading for cytokine release syndrome and neurologic toxicity associated with immune effector cells. *Biol. Blood Marrow Transpl.* **2019**, *25*, 625–638. [CrossRef] [PubMed]

64. Maziarz, R.T.; Schuster, S.J.; Romanov, V.V.; Rusch, E.S.; Li, J.; Signorovitch, J.E.; Maloney, D.G.; Locke, F.L. Grading of neurological toxicity in patients treated with tisagenlecleucel in the JULIET trial. *Blood Adv.* **2020**, *4*, 1440–1447. [CrossRef] [PubMed]

65. Alabanza, L.; Pegues, M.; Geldres, C.; Shi, V.; Wiltzius, J.J.W.; Sievers, S.A.; Yang, S.; Kochenderfer, J.N. Function of novel anti-CD19 chimeric antigen receptors with human variable regions is affected by hinge and transmembrane domains. *Mol. Ther.* **2017**, *25*, 2452–2465. [CrossRef] [PubMed]

66. Brudno, J.N.; Lam, N.; Vanasse, D.; Shen, Y.W.; Rose, J.J.; Rossi, J.; Xue, A.; Bot, A.; Scholler, N.; Mikkilineni, L.; et al. Safety and feasibility of anti-CD19 CAR T cells with fully human binding domains in patients with B-cell lymphoma. *Nat. Med.* **2020**, *26*, 270–280. [CrossRef] [PubMed]

67. Muller, Y.D.; Nguyen, D.P.; Ferreira, L.M.R.; Ho, P.; Raffin, C.; Valencia, R.B.; Congrave-Wilson, Z.; Roth, T.; Eyquem, J.; Van Gool, F.; et al. The CD28-transmembrane domain mediates chimeric antigen receptor heterodimerization with CD28. *bioRxiv* **2020**. [CrossRef]

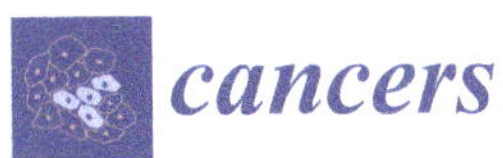 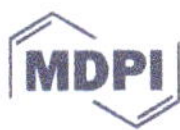

Editorial

Challenges and Opportunities for Effective Cancer Immunotherapies

Clare Y. Slaney [1,2,*] and Michael H. Kershaw [1,2,*]

1   Cancer Immunology Program, Peter MacCallum Cancer Center, Melbourne, Victoria 3000, Australia
2   Sir Peter MacCallum Department of Oncology, University of Melbourne, Parkville, Victoria 3000, Australia
*   Correspondence: clare.slaney@petermac.org (C.Y.S.); michael.kershaw@petermac.org (M.H.K.)

Received: 19 October 2020; Accepted: 24 October 2020; Published: 28 October 2020

Keywords: immunotherapy; PD-1; microenvironment; CAR T cells; immune checkpoint inhibitors

Using immunotherapy to treat cancers can be traced back to the 1890s, where a New York physician William Coley used heat-killed bacteria to treat cancer patients, which became known as "Coley's toxin". Of the almost 900 cancer patients he treated, some tumours regressed and some patients were free from recurrence for a number of years [1]. However, the toxin component was inconsistent, patients' reactions were unpredictable and the anti-cancer mechanism was not known. With the advancement of radiation therapy and chemotherapy in the 20th century, Coley's toxin was not used anymore.

In the past ten years, we have witnessed many revolutionary immunotherapies being approved to use in the clinic for treating cancer patients. These immunotherapies include the first cancer vaccine, Sipuleucel-T for advanced prostate cancer; checkpoint inhibitors such as ipilimumab, pembrolizumab and nivolumab for the treatment of advanced melanoma and other solid cancers; oncolytic virus T-Vec for melanoma; a bispecific cancer-directed T-cell engager, blinatumomab, for the treatment of acute lymphoblastic leukemia, and chimeric antigen receptor (CAR) T cells for treating certain lymphoma and leukemias [2,3]. Together, these immunotherapies have had a remarkable impact on clinical outcomes.

This year, although the majority of the world is locked down in response to the coronavirus disease (COVID-19) pandemic, a number of cancer immunotherapies were approved by the US Food and Drug Administration (FDA). The newly approved treatments include atezolizumab for advanced melanoma, brexucabtagene autoleucel (Tecartus) for mantle cell lymphoma, which is the third FDA-approved CAR T-cell therapy, pembrolizumab as the first line of treatment for colorectal cancer and pembrolizumab for cutaneous squamous cell carcinoma.

Although more and more treatment options are becoming available, challenges still remain. Immune checkpoint inhibitors (ICIs) work for certain cancer types such as melanoma, but not all cancer types respond. Even in melanoma, half of the patients do not achieve a significant beneficial response, and a substantial number of responding patients experience cancer relapse after the initial response [4]. Unfortunately, these ICI therapeutics are also often associated with a high rate of toxicity, with severe toxicities occurring in approximately 20–50% of patients [5]. Other immunotherapies can have similar problems. Certain cancers such as pancreatic cancer have proven to be difficult to treat using all the current available immunotherapies [6].

Building on the success of ICIs, numerous immunotherapies have been tested to be used in combination with other immunotherapies or with some already existing treatments. For example, anti-PD1 has been tested in combination with CAR T-cell therapy [7], oncolytic virus treatment [8,9], cyclin-dependent kinase inhibitors [10]. Given the potency of the treatment components as monotherapies, it is not surprising that a number of these combinations led to synergistic efficacy. With an abundance of combination immunotherapy trials ongoing, more and more factors that influence the therapeutic success have been revealed and synergistic design of different combination therapies may provide optimal benefit to the patients with different types of cancers.

Although yet to demonstrate efficacy in solid tumours, enormous efforts have been made in CAR T-cell research. These include the discovery of new tumour antigen targets [11], more options for combination therapy [7,12], creating T-cell products with a more desirable phenotype [13], improved manufacturing protocols [14], and novel methods for enhancing in vivo expansion of the CAR T cells [15–17]. Although most of the current immunotherapies have focused on T cells, other cellular therapies such as those utilising NK cell cytotoxicity [18,19], dendritic cells [20] and macrophages [21] are also under investigation.

Another extensively explored area lies in the understanding of immunosuppression of the tumour microenvironment (TME) [22]. The TME consists of tumour cells, immune cells, stroma, extracellular matrix and some soluble factors. This complex environment plays a fundamental role in tumour progression, shapes the tumour immune response and eventually determines the efficacy of immunotherapies [23–25]. A number of strategies have been developed in the past few years to shift the TME to favour anti-tumour immunity, and clinical studies have validated several biomarkers of the TME predicting tumour responsiveness to immunotherapies [26,27].

Much knowledge has accumulated in the past ten years, and the cancer immunotherapy field is moving forward at a fast pace. Many current obstacles will likely be overcome through improved knowledge, more advances in treatment technologies [28] and the identification of new cancer targets. In addition, new combination treatments incorporating immunotherapies, and the identification of predictive biomarkers for cancer immunotherapies, may lead to further effective treatments utilizing the immune system for a wide range of cancers.

Funding: The authors are supported by grants from the National Health and Medical Research Council and the National Breast Cancer Foundation (NBCF) of Australia.

Acknowledgments: We are grateful for all the contributing authors for their contribution to this Special Issue and the support from the *Cancers* editorial staff.

Conflicts of Interest: The authors declare no potential conflicts of interest.

References

1. Coley, W.B. The Treatment of Malignant Tumors by Repeated Inoculations of Erysipelas. With a report of ten original cases; 1893. Available online: https://pubmed.ncbi.nlm.nih.gov/1984929/ (accessed on 19 October 2020).
2. Slaney, C.Y.; Wang, P.; Darcy, P.K.; Kershaw, M.H. CARs versus BiTEs: A Comparison between T Cell-Redirection Strategies for Cancer Treatment. *Cancer Discov.* **2018**, *8*, 924–934. [CrossRef] [PubMed]
3. Kershaw, M.H.; Westwood, J.A.; Darcy, P.K. Gene-engineered T cells for cancer therapy. *Nat. Rev. Cancer* **2013**, *13*, 525–541. [CrossRef] [PubMed]
4. Testori, A.A.E.; Chiellino, S.; van Akkooi, A.C.J. Adjuvant Therapy for Melanoma: Past, Current, and Future Developments. *Cancers* **2020**, *12*, 1994. [CrossRef]
5. Johnson, D.B.; Reynolds, K.L.; Sullivan, R.J.; Balko, J.M.; Patrinely, J.R.; Cappelli, L.C.; Naidoo, J.; Moslehi, J.J. Immune checkpoint inhibitor toxicities: Systems-based approaches to improve patient care and research. *Lancet Oncol.* **2020**, *21*, e398–e404. [CrossRef] [PubMed]
6. Ali, A.I.; Oliver, A.J.; Samiei, T.; Chan, J.D.; Kershaw, M.H.; Slaney, C.Y. Genetic Redirection of T Cells for the Treatment of Pancreatic Cancer. *Front. Oncol.* **2019**, *9*, 56. [CrossRef] [PubMed]
7. John, L.B.; Devaud, C.; Duong, C.P.; Yong, C.S.; Beavis, P.A.; Haynes, N.M.; Chow, M.T.; Smyth, M.J.; Kershaw, M.H.; Darcy, P.K. Anti-PD-1 antibody therapy potently enhances the eradication of established tumors by gene-modified T cells. *Clin. Cancer Res.* **2013**, *19*, 5636–5646. [CrossRef] [PubMed]
8. Ribas, A.; Dummer, R.; Puzanov, I.; VanderWalde, A.; Andtbacka, R.H.I.; Michielin, O.; Olszanski, A.J.; Malvehy, J.; Cebon, J.; Fernandez, E.; et al. Oncolytic Virotherapy Promotes Intratumoral T Cell Infiltration and Improves Anti-PD-1 Immunotherapy. *Cell* **2018**, *174*, 1031–1032. [CrossRef] [PubMed]

9. Long, G.V.; Dummer, R.; Ribas, A.; Puzanov, I.; VanderWalde, A.; Andtbacka, R.H.I.; Michielin, O.; Olszanski, A.J.; Malvehy, J.; Cebon, J.S.; et al. Efficacy analysis of MASTERKEY-265 phase 1b study of talimogene laherparepvec (T-VEC) and pembrolizumab (pembro) for unresectable stage IIIB-IV melanoma. *J. Clin. Oncol.* **2016**, *34*, 9568. [CrossRef]

10. Hossain, D.M.S.; Javaid, S.; Cai, M.; Zhang, C.; Sawant, A.; Hinton, M.; Sathe, M.; Grein, J.; Blumenschein, W.; Pinheiro, E.M.; et al. Dinaciclib induces immunogenic cell death and enhances anti-PD1-mediated tumor suppression. *J. Clin. Invest.* **2018**, *128*, 644–654. [CrossRef]

11. Apavaloaei, A.; Hardy, M.P.; Thibault, P.; Perreault, C. The Origin and Immune Recognition of Tumor-Specific Antigens. *Cancers* **2020**, *12*, 2607. [CrossRef]

12. Mardiana, S.; John, L.B.; Henderson, M.A.; Slaney, C.Y.; von Scheidt, B.; Giuffrida, L.; Davenport, A.J.; Trapani, J.A.; Neeson, P.J.; Loi, S.; et al. A multifunctional role for adjuvant anti-4-1BB therapy in augmenting anti-tumor response by chimeric antigen receptor T cells. *Cancer Res.* **2017**. [CrossRef]

13. Cieri, N.; Camisa, B.; Cocchiarella, F.; Forcato, M.; Oliveira, G.; Provasi, E.; Bondanza, A.; Bordignon, C.; Peccatori, J.; Ciceri, F.; et al. IL-7 and IL-15 instruct the generation of human memory stem T cells from naive precursors. *Blood* **2013**, *121*, 573–584. [CrossRef]

14. Wang, X.; Popplewell, L.L.; Wagner, J.R.; Naranjo, A.; Blanchard, M.S.; Mott, M.R.; Norris, A.P.; Wong, C.W.; Urak, R.Z.; Chang, W.C.; et al. Phase 1 studies of central memory-derived CD19 CAR T-cell therapy following autologous HSCT in patients with B-cell NHL. *Blood* **2016**, *127*, 2980–2990. [CrossRef]

15. Chan, J.D.; von Scheidt, B.; Zeng, B.; Oliver, A.J.; Davey, A.S.; Ali, A.I.; Thomas, R.; Trapani, J.A.; Darcy, P.K.; Kershaw, M.H.; et al. Enhancing chimeric antigen receptor T-cell immunotherapy against cancer using a nanoemulsion-based vaccine targeting cross-presenting dendritic cells. *Clin. Transl. Immunol.* **2020**, *9*, e1157. [CrossRef]

16. Von Scheidt, B.; Wang, M.; Oliver, A.J.; Chan, J.D.; Jana, M.K.; Ali, A.I.; Clow, F.; Fraser, J.D.; Quinn, K.M.; Darcy, P.K.; et al. Enterotoxins can support CAR T cells against solid tumors. *Proc. Natl. Acad. Sci. USA* **2019**, *116*, 25229–25235. [CrossRef]

17. Slaney, C.Y.; von Scheidt, B.; Davenport, A.J.; Beavis, P.; Westwood, J.A.; Mardiana, S.; Tscharke, D.; Ellis, S.; Prince, H.M.; Trapani, J.A.; et al. Dual-specific chimeric antigen receptor T cells and an indirect vaccine eradicate a variety of large solid tumors in an immunocompetent, self-antigen setting. *Clin. Cancer Res.* **2017**. [CrossRef]

18. Xie, G.; Dong, H.; Liang, Y.; Ham, J.D.; Rizwan, R.; Chen, J. CAR-NK cells: A promising cellular immunotherapy for cancer. *EBioMedicine* **2020**, *59*, 102975. [CrossRef] [PubMed]

19. Ponath, V.; Frech, M.; Bittermann, M.; Al Khayer, R.; Neubauer, A.; Brendel, C.; Pogge von Strandmann, E. The Oncoprotein SKI Acts as A Suppressor of NK Cell-Mediated Immunosurveillance in PDAC. *Cancers* **2020**, *12*, 2857. [CrossRef]

20. Bol, K.F.; Schreibelt, G.; Rabold, K.; Wculek, S.K.; Schwarze, J.K.; Dzionek, A.; Teijeira, A.; Kandalaft, L.E.; Romero, P.; Coukos, G.; et al. The clinical application of cancer immunotherapy based on naturally circulating dendritic cells. *J. Immunother Cancer* **2019**, *7*, 109. [CrossRef]

21. Klichinsky, M.; Ruella, M.; Shestova, O.; Lu, X.M.; Best, A.; Zeeman, M.; Schmierer, M.; Gabrusiewicz, K.; Anderson, N.R.; Petty, N.E.; et al. Human chimeric antigen receptor macrophages for cancer immunotherapy. *Nat. Biotechnol.* **2020**, *38*, 947–953. [CrossRef]

22. Beavis, P.A.; Slaney, C.Y.; Kershaw, M.H.; Neeson, P.J.; Darcy, P.K. Enhancing the efficacy of adoptive cellular therapy by targeting tumor-induced immunosuppression. *Immunotherapy* **2015**, *7*, 499–512. [CrossRef]

23. Oliver, A.J.; Darcy, P.K.; Kershaw, M.H.; Slaney, C.Y. Tissue-specific tumour microenvironments are an emerging determinant of immunotherapy responses. *J. Thorac. Dis.* **2020**, *12*, 4504–4509. [CrossRef] [PubMed]

24. Oliver, A.J.; Davey, A.S.; Keam, S.P.; Mardiana, S.; Chan, J.D.; von Scheidt, B.; Beavis, P.A.; House, I.G.; Van Audernaerde, J.R.; Darcy, P.K.; et al. Tissue-specific tumor microenvironments influence responses to immunotherapies. *Clin. Transl. Immunol.* **2019**, *8*, e1094. [CrossRef] [PubMed]

25. Hass, R. Role of MSC in the Tumor Microenvironment. *Cancers* **2020**, *12*, 2107. [CrossRef]

26. Murciano-Goroff, Y.R.; Warner, A.B.; Wolchok, J.D. The future of cancer immunotherapy: Microenvironment-targeting combinations. *Cell Res.* **2020**, *30*, 507–519. [CrossRef] [PubMed]

27. Oliver, A.J.; Lau, P.K.H.; Unsworth, A.S.; Loi, S.; Darcy, P.K.; Kershaw, M.H.; Slaney, C.Y. Tissue-Dependent Tumor Microenvironments and Their Impact on Immunotherapy Responses. *Front. Immunol.* **2018**, *9*, 70. [CrossRef] [PubMed]
28. Maruoka, Y.; Furusawa, A.; Okada, R.; Inagaki, F.; Wakiyama, H.; Kato, T.; Nagaya, T.; Choyke, P.L.; Kobayashi, H. Interleukin-15 after Near-Infrared Photoimmunotherapy (NIR-PIT) Enhances T Cell Response against Syngeneic Mouse Tumors. *Cancers* **2020**, *12*, 2575. [CrossRef] [PubMed]

Publisher's Note: MDPI stays neutral with regard to jurisdictional claims in published maps and institutional affiliations.

MDPI

St. Alban-Anlage 66

4052 Basel

Switzerland

Tel. +41 61 683 77 34

Fax +41 61 302 89 18

www.mdpi.com

Cancers Editorial Office

E-mail: cancers@mdpi.com

www.mdpi.com/journal/cancers

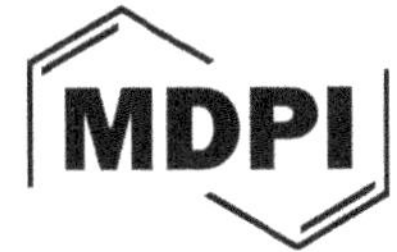